T5998/10M

KU-201-392

15 JUN 19

Clinical Pharmacology

BORDERS HEALTH SCIENCES
LIBRARY

'Patients may recover in spite of drugs or because of them.'

J. H. GADDUM, 1959

'But know also, man has an inborn craving for medicine . . . the desire to take medicine is one feature which distinguishes man the animal, from his fellow creatures. It is really one of the most serious difficulties with which we have to contend . . . the doctor's visit is not thought to be complete without a prescription.'

WILLIAM OSLER, 1894

'Morals do not forbid making experiments on one's neighbour or on one's self . . . among the experiments that may be tried on man, those that can only harm are forbidden, those that are innocent are permissible, and those that may do good are obligatory.'

CLAUDE BERNARD, 1865

'I do not want two diseases — one nature-made, one doctor-made.'

NAPOLEON BONAPARTE, 1820

'The ingenuity of man has ever been fond of exerting itself to varied forms and combinations of medicines.'

WILLIAM WITHERING, 1785

'All things are poisons and there is nothing that is harmless, the dose alone decides that something is no poison.'

PARACELSUS, 1493–1541

'First do no harm.'
'It is a good remedy sometimes to use nothing.'

HIPPOCRATES, 460–355 B.C.

Clinical Pharmacology

D. R. Laurence
MD, FRCP
Professor Emeritus of Pharmacology and Therapeutics, School of Medicine, University College London, London, UK

P. N. Bennett
MD, FRCP
Consultant Physician, Royal United Hospital, Bath and Senior Lecturer in Clinical Pharmacology, University of Bath, Bath, UK

SIXTH EDITION

With some illustrations by Peter Kneebone

CHURCHILL LIVINGSTONE
EDINBURGH LONDON AND NEW YORK 1987

CHURCHILL LIVINGSTONE
Medical Division of Longman Group UK Limited

Distributed in the United States of America by Churchill Livingstone Inc., 1560 Broadway, New York, N.Y. 10036, and by associated companies, branches and representatives throughout the world.

© D. R. Laurence 1960, 1962, 1966, 1973
© D. R. Laurence and P. N. Bennett 1980, 1987

All rights reserved. No part of this publication may be reproduced, stored in a retrieval system, or transmitted in any form or by any means, electronic, mechanical, photocopying, recording or otherwise, without the prior permission of the publishers (Churchill Livingstone, Robert Stevenson House, 1–3 Baxter's Place, Leith Walk, Edinburgh EH1 3AF).

First Edition 1960
Second Edition 1962
Third Edition 1966
Fourth Edition 1973
Fifth Edition 1980
Sixth Edition 1987

Previous editions translated into Italian, Chinese Spanish and Serbo-Croat.

ISBN 0-443-03417-6

British Library Cataloguing in Publication Data

Laurence, D. R.
Clinical pharmacology. — 6th ed.
1. Drugs 2. Pharmacology
I. Title II. Bennett, P. N.
615'.1 RM300

Library of Congress Cataloging in Publication Data

Laurence, D. R. (Desmond Roger)
Clinical pharmacology
Bibliography: p.
Includes index.
1. Pharmacology. 2. Chemotherapy. I. Bennett, P. N. II. Title. [DNLM: 1. Pharmacology, Clinical. QV 38 L379c]
RM300.L349 1987 615.7 86-29871

Produced by Longman Singapore Publishers (Pte) Ltd.
Printed in Singapore

Preface

*'For your own satisfaction and for mine, please read this preface.'**

This book is about the scientific basis and practice of drug therapy. It is particularly intended for **medical students** in their clinical years, but it contains many more facts and details than a student either needs or should attempt to learn.

The general aspects of the *how* and *why* of drugs are for students. The practical details are to help them when they begin to prescribe on their own responsibility after graduating, and the book is offered as a guide to this.

Thus **students** should read selectively, and we hope it will not be too difficult for them to do so. We would particularly suggest that students should read Chapters 1 to 10 and those parts of other chapters covering general background, principles or mechanisms of action. Unfortunately we have been unable to contrive everywhere clearly to separate these sections from the more detailed facts required for such guidance in practical prescribing as we have attempted.

In addition we hope that the book may be of use to some **more experienced doctors** in reminding them of general progress and practice in fields with which, perhaps, they are no longer primarily concerned, but which have not lost interest or all importance for them.

Justification. We believe that doctors who understand something of how drugs get into the body, of how they produce their effects, of their fate and of how evidence of therapeutic effect is assessed, will choose drugs more skilfully and use them more successfully than those who do not. They will less often expose patients to the risks of useless therapy and they will also avoid more of the hazards of adverse effects due to interaction with the patient, the disease and with other drugs. They will be less likely to mistake the ill-effects of drugs for natural disease and more likely to recognise antagonism or synergism when it unexpectedly arises either from prescribed or from self-medication.

This book represents an attempt to provide pharmacological knowledge that is both interesting† *and useful to the physician.*

Most books of moderate size either confine themselves to discussing the pharmacology of drugs without giving enough information for them to be selected and used effectively, or else they confine themselves to practical therapeutics and ignore the pharmacological background. It is too much to expect the now heavily burdened student to consult and integrate two works, one not always clearly related to clinical practice and the other often as arbitrary and as empirical as a cookery book. *This book is offered as a reasonably brief solution to the problem of combining practical clinical utility with some account of the principles of pharmacology on which clinical practice rests.*

It might be thought that the existence of big multi-author books in which each chapter is

* St. Francis of Sales: preface to *Introduction to the Devout Life* (1609).

† An author and critic (Philip Larkin: 1922–85) has told that he judged fiction by the criteria, 'Could I read it? If I could read it, did I believe it? If I believed it, did I care about it? And if I cared about it, what was the quality of my caring, and did it last?' It would be presumptuous of authors of a textbook to aspire to satisfy the criteria for good fiction, so we will only say that we have been mindful of these in writing this book. DRL, PNB.

written by a specialist would make futile a smaller book such as this, for in the available space it is not possible to give a lot of detail. But we believe it is useful to have a book of a size that is manageable other than as a work of reference—that can be compassed by individuals coming to the subject either for the first time or to refresh their general knowledge — and that may help them to use the larger discursive sources more profitably.

How much practical technical detail to include has been difficult to decide. In general, more such detail is provided for therapeutic practices that are complex or potentially dangerous as well as urgent, where there may be no time for consultation with colleagues or search in libraries (e.g. cardiac dysrhythmias) and less, or even none, on therapy that is generally conducted only by specialists or that can wait on such consultation, e.g. anticancer drugs; i.v. oxytocin.

Use of the book. Students are, or should be, concerned to *understand*, to develop a rational, critical attitude to drug therapy and they should therefore chiefly concern themselves with how drugs act and interact in disease and with how evidence of therapeutic effect is obtained and evaluated. They should not allow this to be impeded by attempts to memorise lists of alternative drugs and minor differences between them, or arbitrary practical details, such as dosage or solution strength, which should never be required of them in examinations; the only way to fix these in the mind is by actual prescribing.

The decision to try to include sufficient practical details to enable some drugs to be correctly used has inevitably made substantial parts of the book tedious. In addition, it has been thought necessary to mention numerous drugs of doubtful merit, and what have been aptly called "me-tooers", in order to enable drugs to be recognised and a choice to be made from amongst the huge number of drugs and formulations of drugs thrust at the clinician by a vigorous pharmaceutical industry.

We hope that students will readily see which sections of the book they can, and indeed should, neglect in their general reading, and that are for use when the responsibility of choice and administration becomes theirs.

Repetition. Readers may notice occasional repetition; this is often deliberate.

The 'authority' of a textbook. If a book is to be a useful guide to treatment it must offer clear conclusions and advice. If it is to be of reasonable size alternative acceptable courses of action will often have to be omitted. What is recommended should be based on sound evidence where this exists, and on an assessment of the opinions of the experienced where it does not. Exceptions to all advice will occur,* and part of the clinician's skill lies in knowing when to depart from an accepted course. Nor can a textbook take account of all possible modifying factors, e.g. personality, intercurrent disease, metabolic differences.

The status of a textbook as a practical guide has been expressed in a legal judgement where an accusation of negligent treatment made against a doctor was supported by showing that he had not followed the orthodox treatment as stated in various textbooks. The Judge said that textbook writers were writing of a subject in general and not of a particular patient. A doctor was entitled to use his common sense, his experience, and his judgement as far as they fitted into a particular case. 'It would be a sorry day for the medical profession if it were to be said that no doctor ought to depart one tittle from that which he saw written in a textbook.'† Statements in textbooks were no substitute for the judgement of the physician in charge of the case. 'His Lordship could not follow slavishly the views expressed in textbooks . . .'.† Indeed sensible authors would be troubled at the thought that they were credited with less than the usual human fallibility.

The **guide to further reading** at the end of each chapter is comprised of references to original papers and editorials (with references) from a

* Control of therapeutic claims is properly exercised by government regulary authority but limitation of doctors' freedom to prescribe what they have reason to believe best for the patients should be resisted on principle (although cost is increasingly regarded as overriding principle). The solution to bad doctoring is education, not the imposition of limitations on conscientious doctors. But if doctors will prescribe carelessly then society will take away their freedom.

† Lancet 1960; 1:593.

small number of English language journals that are likely to be available in even the most modest hospital library. This is done to enable anyone, anywhere, to gain access to the original literature and to informed opinion and also to provide interest and sometimes amusement. We do not attempt to document all the statements we make, which would be impossible without greatly enlarging this, already too long, book.

The titles of articles are included in the particular hope that students will run their eye over the list and find something that attracts them sufficiently to cause them to want to read original work. There is no substitute for contact with original minds or the excitement of following these minds through their efforts at discovery.

The general references at the end of the book are to specialist books and journals that cover the whole field.

Reasons for using non-proprietary drug names instead of the sometimes more familiar proprietary names are given in Chapter 6. The index includes an inevitably incomplete range of proprietary names.

It is assumed that the reader will possess a formulary and so the text has not been encumbered with exhaustive lists of preparations although it is hoped that enough have been mentioned to cover much routine prescribing, and many drugs have been included solely for identification.

London and Bath, 1987 D. R. L.
P. N. B.

Acknowledgements

It is not possible for two individuals to cover the whole field of drug therapy from their own knowledge and experience, and we are deeply grateful to all those who have with such good grace given us their time and energy to supply valuable facts and opinions, they principally include:

Dr E. S. K. Assem
Dr M. R. Bending
Dr N. B. Bennett
Prof Sir James Black
Dr F. R. Bompart
Prof R. J. Flower
Dr S. C. Glover
Prof Sir Abraham Goldberg
Dr Sheila Gore
Prof D. H. Jenkinson
Dr P. J. Maddison
Prof Sir William Paton
Dr Rosalind Pitt-Rivers
Prof B. N. C. Prichard
Dr J. P. D. Reckless
Dr G. M. Stern
Dr C. Ward
Dr M. E. Wilson
Dr B. Woodward
Prof O. M. Wrong

Much of any merit this book may have is due to the generosity of those named above as well as others too numerous to mention who have put their knowledge and practical experience of the use of drugs at our disposal. Responsibility for any errors rests with us.

In addition, permission to quote directly from the writings of some authorities has been generously granted and we thank the authors and their publishers who have given it.

Peter Kneebone's illustrations speak for themselves.

ERRATA

Page 233 Column 1 Line 20
for fetal read fatal

Page 320 Column 1 Line 23 to read
methadone withdrawal is less unpleasant than

Page 379 Column 2 Line 15
for 1.5 h read 6 – 50 h

Page 467 Column 1 Line 1
for cholinesterases read anticholinesterases

Page 553 Column 2 Line 1
for of the oesophagus read ulceration of the oesophagus

Page 650 Column 1 Line 26
for of read or

Page 691 Column 1 Line 9
for for read of

Page 704 Column 2 Line 10
for less than in 1000 read less than 1 in 1000

Page 714 Column 1 Line 31
for 50 h read 6 – 50 h

Contents

1

Topics in drug therapy and clinical pharmacology

Poisons in small doses are the best medicines; and useful medicines in too large doses are poisonous (William Withering, 1789).

The use of drugs to increase human happiness by elimination or suppression of diseases and symptoms and to improve the quality of life in other ways is a serious matter and involves not only technical but psychosocial considerations. We therefore begin this book with a series of essays on what we think are important topics.

1. Introduction

*Before treating any patient with drugs**, *doctors should have made up their minds on eight points:*

1. Whether they should interfere with the patient at all and if so —

2. What alteration in the patient's condition they hope to achieve.

3. That the drug they intend to use is best capable of bringing this about.

4. How they will know when it has been brought about.

5. That they can administer the drug in such a way that the right concentration will be attained in the right place at the right time and for the right duration.

6. What other effects the drug may have and whether these may be harmful.

7. How they will decide to stop the drug.

8. Whether the likelihood of benefit, and its importance, outweighs the likelihood of damage, and its importance, i.e. to consider *benefit versus risk*, or *efficacy in relation to safety*.

It is obvious that drug therapy involves a great deal more than matching the name of the drug to the name of a disease; it requires knowledge, judgement, skill and wisdom, but above all a *sense of responsibility*. A book can provide knowledge and can contribute to the formation of judgement, but it can do little to impart skill and wisdom, which are the products of experience and innate and acquired capacities.

* A World Health Organization Scientific Group has defined a drug as 'any substance or product that is used or intended to be used to modify or explore physiological systems or pathological states for the benefit of the recipient'. WHO Tech Rep Ser 1966; no. 341:7.

A *drug* is a single chemical substance that forms the active ingredient of a *medicine*, which latter may contain many other substances to deliver the drug in a stable form, acceptable and convenient to the patient. The terms will be used more or less interchangeably in this book. To use the word 'drug' intending only a harmful, dangerous or addictive substance is to abuse a respectable and useful word.

Everybody knows that drugs can do good.

Medically this good may sometimes seem trivial, as in the avoidance of a sleepless night in a noisy hotel or of social embarrassment from a profusely running nose due to seasonal pollen allergy (hay-fever). Such benefits, however, are not necessarily trivial to the recipient, concerned to be at his best in urgent matters, whether of business, of pleasure or of passion.

Or the good may be literally life-saving, as in serious acute infections (pneumonia, septicaemia) or in the prevention of life-destroying disability from severe asthma, from epilepsy or from blindness due to glaucoma.

Everybody knows that drugs can do harm.

This harm may be relatively trivial, as in hangover from a hypnotic or sleepiness from an H_1-receptor antihistamine used for hay-fever (though these effects may be a cause of serious road accidents).

The harm may also be life-destroying, as in the rare sudden death following an injection of penicillin, rightly regarded as one of the safest of antibiotics, or the slower death or disability that occasionally attends the use of drugs that are effective in asthma and rheumatoid arthritis (adrenocortical steroids, penicillamine).

There are risks in taking medicines just as there are risks in food and transport. There are also risks in not taking medicines when they are needed, just as there are risks in not taking food or in not using transport when they are needed.

Efficacy and safety do not lie solely in the chemical nature of the drug. Doctors must choose which drugs to use and must apply them correctly in relation not only to properties of the drug, but also to those of the patient and his disease (which is why prescribing cannot be delegated). Then patients must use the prescribed medicine correctly.

Drugs are used in three principal ways:

1. **Curative**, as **primary** therapy (as in bacterial and parasitic infections) or as **auxiliary** therapy (as with anaesthetics, and ergometrine and oxytocin in obstetrics).

2. **Suppressive** of diseases or symptoms, used continuously or intermittently to maintain health without attaining cure, as in hypertension, diabetes, epilepsy, asthma or to control symptoms such as pain and cough, whilst awaiting recovery from the causative disease.

3. **Preventive** (prophylactic), as when a non-immune person enters a malarial area, or contraception.

2. Benefits and risks: iatrogenic disease

Benefits of drugs are manifest to doctor and patient and also, it might be thought, obvious to even the most unimaginative healthy people who find themselves dismayed by some aspects of modern technology.

Modern technological medicine has been criticised with some justice for waiting for disease to occur and then trying to cure it rather than seeking to prevent it from occurring in the first place. It has also been criticised for failure, as judged by population health statistics. It is pointed out, for example, that improved living conditions rather than medical treatment have played the major role in the enormous decline in the death rate from infectious diseases over the past 100 years. It is true that the biggest changes in some important areas of health result from social and economic development rather than from the application of technical medicine; that 'prevention is better than cure' is a familiar saying because it is true.

But people still frequently fall sick and will continue to do so, although the pattern of disease in the community changes, infectious disease in the young giving place to degenerative disease in the old. We must look at population statistics; but we must also, in a humane society, look to the individual sufferer.

It is good to prevent tuberculosis; but those who are unfortunate enough to contract the disease will be grateful for drugs.

It is good to prevent cancer, and ways of doing so for some cancers, e.g. stopping smoking, are known, though seldom adopted; but those who fall sick will be grateful for drugs, surgery and radiation, whether these cure or whether they only ease the passage through the last phase of life.

It is better to prevent some heart disease, by moderate and sensible living, including moderation in eating, though such measures are all too little adopted; but those who fall sick will be grateful for drugs.

It would be better, if we only knew how, to prevent rheumatoid arthritis, epilepsy, pernicious anaemia, many cancers and diabetes, but we do not know how and sufferers are grateful for drugs. In any case we all have eventually to die of something, and the likelihood that the mode of death for most of us, even after practising all the excesses of advice on how to live a healthy life, will be free from pain, anxiety, cough, diarrhoea, paralysis, etc. (the list is endless) seems so small that it can be disregarded. Drugs already provide immeasurable solace in these situations, but better drugs are needed and their development should be encouraged.

Doctors know the sick are thankful for drugs just as a dedicated pedestrian struck down by a passing car is thankful for a motor ambulance to take him to hospital.

Benefits of drugs in individual diseases are discussed throughout this book and will not be further expanded here. But a general discussion of risk is appropriate.

Whenever a drug is given a risk is taken; the risk is made up of the properties of the drug, of the prescriber, of the patient and of the environment; it is often so small that second thoughts are hardly necessary, but sometimes it is substantial. The doctor must weigh up the likelihood of gain for the patient against the likelihood of loss. There is often insufficient data for a rational decision to be reached, but a decision must still be made and this is one of the greatest difficulties of clinical practice. Its effect on the attitudes of doctors is often not appreciated by those who have never been in this situation. The patients' protection lies in the doctors' knowledge of the drug and of the disease, and experience of both, together with knowledge of the patient. For instance, in typhoid fever the risk of inducing aplastic anaemia due to chloramphenicol is far less than the risk of the patient dying from untreated disease. In less dangerous infections the decision is less easy, and should chloramphenicol be used without mishap in, say, bronchitis, it may leave the patient so sensitised that a second or third course may prove fatal. It is impossible to be sure of the magnitude of such a risk in any individual case.

In some diseases in which drugs will ultimately be needed they may not benefit the patient in the early stages. For example, victims of early Parkinsonism or hypertension may be but little inconvenienced by the disease, and the premature use of drugs, whilst perhaps reducing Parkinsonian symptoms and blood pressure, can exact such a price in side-effects (including fatigue, which may be unrecognised as a side-effect and which is common with β-adrenoceptor blockers) that the patient prefers his untreated state; what patients will tolerate depends on their personality, their attitude to disease, their occupation, mode of life and relationship with the doctor.

The most shameful act in therapeutics, apart from killing the patient, is to cause disease in a patient who is but little disabled or who is suffering from a self-limiting disorder. Such **iatrogenic* disease**, induced by misguided treatment, is far from rare.

If the doctor is temperamentally an extremist, he will do less harm by therapeutic nihilism than by optimistically overwhelming his patients with well-intentioned polypharmacy. The latter course is the easier to follow because it gives more immediate satisfaction to the patient, his family and indeed to the doctor himself. All are able to feel cosily that it is clear that the doctor is doing all he can, which usually means a great deal more than is wise. Habitual prescribing in response to any complaint from a patient, and in particular habitual polypharmacy is sure to blur the process of rational thought that should precede the use of any drug, and both doctor and patient will be the worse for this.

If in doubt whether or not to give a drug to a person who will get better without it, don't.

In 1917, Sollmann felt able to write 'Pharmacology comprises some broad conceptions and generalisations, and some detailed conclusions, of such great and practical importance that every student and practitioner should be absolutely familiar with them. It comprises also a large mass

* *Iatrogenic* means 'physician-caused', i.e. disease consequent on following medical advice or intervention.

of minute details, which would constitute too great a tax on human memory, but which cannot safely be neglected.'*†

If the last sentence was true when it was written, it is many times more true now. The selection of useful drugs from the multitude, not only offered to, but thrust upon the doctor by skilful and sometimes misleading advertising, is a matter of great importance. The doctor's aim must be not merely to give the patient what will do good, but to give *only* what will do good, or at least more good than harm.

There are three major grades or risk: unacceptable, acceptable and negligible. In the presence of serious disease and with sufficient information on both the disease and the drug, then decisions in the first two categories, though they may be painful, present relatively obvious problems. But where the disease risk is remote (e.g. mild hypertension) or where drugs are to be used to increase comfort or to suppress symptoms that are, in fact, bearable, or for convenience rather than need, then the issues of risk acceptance are less obvious.

Risks should not be considered without reference to benefits any more than benefits should be considered without reference to risks.

'Risks are among the facts of life. In whatever we do and in whatever we refrain from doing, we are accepting risk. Some risks are obvious, some are unsuspected and some we conceal from ourselves. But risks are universally accepted, whether willingly or unwillingly, whether consciously or not.'‡

There are two broad *categories of risk*:

First are those that we accept by *deliberate choice*, even if we do not exactly know their magnitude, or we know but wish they were smaller, or, especially where the risk is remote though the consequences may be grave, we do not even think about the matter. Such risks include transport and sports, both of which are subject to potent physical laws such as gravity and momentum, and surgery to rectify disorder that could either be tolerated or treated in other ways, e.g. hernia, much cosmetic surgery.

Second are those risks that are *imposed* on us in the sense that they cannot be significantly altered by individual action. Risks such as those of food additives (preservatives, colouring), air pollution and some environmental radioactivity are imposed by man. But there are also risks imposed by nature such as skin cancer due to excess ultraviolet radiation in sunny climes, as well as some radioactivity.

The motives for accepting risk are various and numerous and include the general attitude of individuals to life, to work and to pleasure. There are those who enthusiastically engage in or support boxing or mountaineering or hang-gliding and there are those who feel that these risks are unacceptable and, not content with themselves abstaining from such recreations, campaign to have them stopped or controlled.

It seems an obvious truth that unnecessary risks should be avoided, but there is disagreement on what risks are truly unnecessary and, on looking closely at the matter, it is plain that many people habitually take risks in their daily life that it would be a misuse of words to describe as necessary. This is not a problem that will be resolved either simply or by further study, for there are genuine differences of opinion on absolute evaluation of risk and differences between individuals on the evaluation of risk in relation to benefit to themselves, i.e. people do what pleases themselves, and pleasure is not a rationally analysable phenomenon. However, the same people plainly resent the proposition that they should accept the inescapable risks of properly prescribed medicines.

It is also the case that some risks, though known to exist, are, in practice, ignored other than by conforming to ordinary prudent conduct, e.g. the employment of competent electricians and gas fitters in the home, looking before crossing the road, not accepting a lift in a friend's car if he is

* Sollman T A. Manual of pharmacology. Philadelphia: Saunders, 1917.

† This *information explosion* of recent decades will one day be brought under control when prescribers can, from their desk-top computer terminals, feed into a computer facts about their patient (age, sex, weight, principal and secondary diagnoses, etc.) and receive on their terminals suggestions for which drugs should be considered with proposed doses and precautions; information for the patient can also be printed. The limitations on such a service are financial and logistic; the technology exists now. In the meantime, prescribers *must* ensure that they are aware of the basic information contained in manufacturers' data sheets and standard Formularies.

‡ Pochin E E. Br Med Bull 1975; 31:184.

drunk. In the case of public transport, the acceptance of monopoly is not generally felt to pose serious safety issues since the risks are so remote in even a relatively inefficient organisation. In the case of air travel there are about two fatal accidents per million flights worldwide. Individual airline fatality rates range from 0 to 20, with most lines less than two*. There can be few passengers who seek out the figures for individual airlines and take them into account before making a booking. The reason for this is that the risks of flying by any reasonably reputable airline are so small as to be ignored by ordinary people, i.e. *the risks are negligible in the sense that they do not influence behaviour*. Also, it only needs one or two big plane crashes to alter the safety ranking of the airlines.

In general it has been suggested that, in medical cases, concern ceases when risks fall below about 1 in 100 000 so that then the procedure becomes regarded as 'safe'. In such cases, when disaster occurs, it can be difficult indeed for individuals to accept that they 'deliberately' took a risk; they feel 'it should not have happened to me' and in their distress they may seek to lay blame on others where there is no fault or negligence, only misfortune.

The benefits of chemicals used to colour food verge on or even attain negligibility; yet our society, on somewhat weak evidence, considers the risks are also negligible since it permits their use. A widely used colour in foods and medicines, tartrazine, is known to cause an allergy (asthma) in man. It is unnecessary, but it continues to be used.

The benefits of oral contraceptives and of penicillin are undoubted and the risks are equally undoubted and have been measured, and their use continues and expands because the perceived benefits outweigh the risks.

In no countries are the risks of heroin dependence acceptable, but in all countries the risks of tobacco are acceptable or, at least, accepted. Deaths from uncontrolled tobacco dependence far exceed those of therapeutic agents and road transport; the same applies to alcohol.

The risks of drugs have become a major topic of public and medical concern over the last twenty years, and this concern, often amounting to alarm, has accelerated since the thalidomide disaster of 1960–61 (p. 84), which provided an exceptionally dramatic demonstration of the worst that drugs can do.

There is general agreement that drugs prescribed for disease are themselves the cause of a serious amount of disease (adverse reactions), of death, of permanent disability, of recoverable illness and of minor inconvenience. Adverse reactions are considered in Chapter 9.

3. The public view of drugs and prescribers

Until recently, when discussing drugs in medicine it was not generally thought necessary to take serious account of the public view and indeed the public view was one of innocent acceptance; it did not significantly affect the practice of doctors and their relations with patients. But this has changed; increasingly doctors are criticised not only by individual patients, but by associations of patients formed for that purpose, amongst others; the mass media have found that drugs provide an unfailing topic for sensational entertainment, and that drugs and doctors separately and together provide the media people with occasions when 'It becomes more than a moral duty to speak one's mind. It becomes a pleasure.'†

Doctors can no longer behave as though all their prescribing decisions are a matter for themselves alone, with little or no involvement of the patient. Hence the following discussion.

The current public view of modern medicines, ably informed by the mass media, is a compound of vague expectation of 'miracle' cures with outrage when anything goes wrong. Successes soon become a routine taken for granted without thankfulness; failures, the drug accidents, are remembered (memory being assisted by repeated television programmes) and resented perpetually. But this state of affairs is a normal manifestation of human nature, and doctors who rail against it are wasting their time. The public is fickle, demanding, prone to make snap judgements and

* Consumers' Association (UK) 1986.

† O Wilde (1854–1900). *The Importance of Being Earnest*: Act II.

to righteous indignation. It is quite unrealistic to expect the public to have balanced, well-thought-out views on any complex topic: there are far too many of these anyway. It is also unrealistic to expect the public to trust the medical profession to the extent of leaving to it all drug matters. Just as 'War is much too serious a thing to be left to the military'*, so drugs are much too serious a thing to be left to the medical profession and to the pharmaceutical industry.

It has long been a source of wonder to doctors that a public that, if the mass media are to be believed, seems to fear and hate drugs, consists of individuals who when met in the clinic seem to have an insatiable appetite for drugs; 'Surely there is something you can give me, doctor?'

It is endlessly reiterated that the public does not understand that virtually all drug use carries risk and that it cannot be otherwise. If the public does not understand this, it is not for want of telling and suggests that the mass media are not as influential as they like to think; but such apparently invincible ignorance, if it exists, must have a deeper cause than mere deafness. When a drug is suspected of causing harm, then any good it may have done is discounted in the public mind by rage against doctors, drug developers, regulatory authorities and rage against technology and science itself.

The reasons for this are many and complex.

Industrially developed societies have been encouraged to believe that technology based on science would solve most, if not all their problems, including the problems of attaining happiness. Expectations have been raised and now, in the last quarter of the twentieth century with the manifest achievement of technology all around us, the naive belief that happiness can be a part of the technological package is increasingly seen to be false.

The public, fickle as always, turns on science and technology in disappointed resentment. The oft-repeated warnings of the medical profession that drugs unavoidably carry risks despite skilful development and use are treated as though they have never been. A drug accident occurs and scapegoats must be found whether or not someone is at fault.

The public wants benefits without risks and without having to alter its unhealthy ways of living; a deeply irrational position. But it is easy to understand that a person who has taken into his body a chemical with intent to relieve suffering, whether or not it is self-induced, or to prevent disease (or pregnancy), can feel a profound resentment when harm follows. Patients do not understand what has happened, all they know is that a doctor has prescribed a product of a profitable multinational industry; all they did was to swallow the tablets and now they are injured. They are not interested in being told that they voluntarily took a risk, even in the event that this was explained and that they truly understood it; and they are not interested in being told that the doctor took a risk on their behalf, for it is the patient and not the doctor who is hurt. They are also not interested in being told (should this happen to be the case) that as no one is at fault they must regard this misfortune as an accident and simply accept it. If it is added that it is likely that the injury is a consequence of the patients' own genetic make-up, then insult is added to the injury. Whether or not this attitude is reasonable is irrelevant; that is how people feel, and they will not easily change.

In addition, patients are increasingly aware that there is justified criticism of the standards of medical prescribing, indeed doctors are in the forefront of this; as well as justified criticism of promotional practices of the profitably rich, aggressive, international pharmaceutical industry.

The present situation, a mix of resentment, mistrust and misunderstanding, must at least not be allowed to get worse. There are obvious areas where some remedial action is possible.

1. Improvement of *prescribing* by doctors, including better communication with patients, i.e. doctors must learn to feel that introduction of foreign chemicals into their patients' bodies is a serious matter, which the vast majority do not feel at present.

2. Introduction of *no-fault compensation schemes* for *serious* drug injury (some countries already have these; see p. 13).

3. Free public discussion of the issues between the medical profession, industrial drug developers,

* Attributed both to C-M de Talleyrand (1754–1838) and to Georges Clemenceau (1841–1929), French statesmen.

politicians and other 'opinion-formers' in society, and patients (the public). Doctors should not hesitate to take part in such exchanges if they have any talent for exposition and can remain calm (this is essential) under provocation.

4. Restraint in promotion by the pharmaceutical industry including self-control by both industry and doctors in their necessarily close relationship. The medical and scientific departments of pharmaceutical companies generally do not have control over the marketing department and over advertising; they should.

If restraint is not forthcoming then both doctor and industry can expect more control to be exercised over them by politicians responding to public demand. If doctors do not want their prescribing to be controlled they should prescribe better.

4. Criticisms of modern drugs

Some critics have attracted public attention for their view that modern drugs, indeed modern medicine in general, does more harm than good; others, whilst admitting some benefits from drugs, insist that this is medically marginal. These opinions rest on the undisputed fact that favourable trends in many diseases preceded the introduction of modern drugs and were due to economic and environmental changes (sanitation, nutrition, housing, etc.). They also rest on the claim that drugs have not changed expectation of life or mortality (as measured by national mortality statistics) and that drugs can cause illness (adverse reactions).

If something is to be measured then the correct standards must be chosen. Overall mortality figures are an extremely crude and often an irrelevant measure of the effects of drugs whose major benefits are so often on *quality* of life rather than on its *quantity*.

Two examples of inappropriate measurements will suffice:

1. In the case of infections it is not disputed that environmental changes have had a greater beneficial effect on health than the subsequently introduced antibiotics. But this does not mean that environmental improvements alone are sufficient in the fight against infections. When comparisons of illnesses in the pre- and post-antibiotic era are made, like is not compared with like. Environmental changes achieved their results when mortality from infections was high and antibiotics were not available; antibiotics were introduced later against a background of low mortality as well as of environmental change; decades separate the two parts of the comparison, and observers, diagnostic criteria and data recording changed during this long period.* It is evident that determining the value of antibiotics is not simply a matter of looking at mortality rates.

2. About 1% of the population (UK) has *diabetes mellitus* and about 1% of death certificates mention diabetes. This is no surprise because all must die and insulin is no cure† for this lifelong disease. A standard medical textbook of 1907 stated that juvenile-onset 'diabetes is in all cases a grave disease, and the subjects are regarded by all assurance companies as uninsurable lives: life seems to hang by a thread, a thread often cut by a very trifling accident.' The modern young diabetic is accepted by most, if not all, life insurance companies with no or only modest financial penalty (premium of a person 5–10 years older). Before insulin replacement therapy was available few survived beyond 3 years‡ after diagnosis; they died for lack of insulin. The assertion that because its mention on death certificates (whether as a prime or as a contributory cause) has not changed then treatment is worthless is unjustified. The relevant criteria for juvenile onset diabetes are *change in the age* at which the subjects die and the *quality of life* between diagnosis and death, and both of these have changed enormously.

Critics naturally also point to the areas where drug benefits are controversial or absent, and there are plenty of these; but they simply tell us that medical and biological sciences, like all sciences, have a lot of unsolved problems before them. They tell nothing about what can be

* Lever A F. Lancet 1977; 1:352.

† A *cure eliminates* a disease and may be withdrawn when this is achieved.

‡ Even if given the best treatment. 'Opium alone stands the test of experience as a remedy capable of limiting the progress of the disease', wrote the great Sir William Osler, successively Professor of Medicine in Pennsylvania, McGill, Johns Hopkins and Oxford University, in 1918, only three years before the discovery of insulin.

achieved with the tools we now have. Similarly, inappropriate medical use of drugs and their social abuse are regrettable and tell us of human inadequacies, but do not diminish the successes of scientific medicine.

In addition to the critics' assertions that modern drugs are a failure, that therapeutic claims are false, and that adverse effects are too frequent (indeed they are) and are commonly concealed or ignored, it is also asserted that there is a conspiracy between the medical profession and the pharmaceutical industry to exploit the community for mutual benefit. Both industry and profession would be well advised to review their close association with a more critical eye than heretofore, and doctors should think less of their bellies ('there is no such thing as a free lunch') and their pockets and more of the fact that their first duty lies, and *must be seen to lie*, with their patients.

Finally, critics attack the low standard of prescribing (this is largely acknowledged by doctors), and a prime objective of this book is to enable doctors to prescribe better. But no book can inculcate the sense of responsibility that all prescribers should have as with their pens they flood their patients' bodies with foreign chemicals.

However, it is heartening to know that there is not a polarization of views, with assailants of drugs all outside the medical profession and champions solely within. Awareness and criticism of shortcomings of drugs and drug use is a day-to-day constituent of medical literature and meetings and there are innumerable patients with serious disease, e.g. epilepsy, glaucoma and those who have benefited from surgical anaesthesia, who know their lives and happiness are or have been transformed by drugs and who are fittingly thankful.

Doubtless doctors are as liable to be arrogant, complacent and ignorant as are all human beings, including their critics, but heat without light is generated by the angry recrimination about drugs that is so customary today.

5. Traditional and complementary (alternative) medicine

Because practitioners of complementary and traditional medicine are severely critical of modern drugs, because they use drugs according to their own special beliefs, and because they are currently attracting more attention than previously, it is appropriate to discuss drug use in complementary or alternative medical systems here.

The public disappointment that scientific medicine can neither guarantee happiness nor wholly eliminate the disabilities of degenerative diseases in long-lived populations, as well as the fact that drugs used in modern medicine can cause serious harm, naturally leads to a revival of interest in alternatives that promise efficacy with safety. These range from revival of traditional medicine to adoption of the more modern cults*, e.g. homoeopathy, which are described as *alternative, fringe* or *complementary*† medicine.‡

* A cult is a practice that follows a dogma, tenet or principle based on theories or beliefs of its promulgator to the exclusion of demonstrable scientific experience (definition of the American Medical Association).

† The term *complementary* seems to make a less ambitious claim then *alternative* medicine, and is increasingly preferred.

‡ The profusion of medical cults tells its own story. Scientific medicine changes in accord with evidence obtained by scientific enquiry applied with such intellectual rigour as is humanly possible. But this is not the case with cults, the claims for which are characterized by absence of rigorous intellectual evaluation. Medical cults and practices listed in a publication of the World Health Organization (Bannerman R H et al, eds. Traditional medicine and health care coverage. Geneva, 1983) include: homoeopathy, anthroposophical medicine, applied kinesiology, kirlian photography, reflexology, osteopathy, chiropractic, impact therapy, rolfing, breathing, cymatics, psionics, radiesthesia, radionics, orgone therapy, pyramid therapy, naturopathy, dianetics, interferential therapy, aromatherapy, flower therapy, biochemics, orthomolecular medicine, bioenergetics, enlightenment intensive, etc. The list speaks for itself, and leaves the question why, if each cult has the efficacy claimed by its exponents, orthodox medicine and indeed the other cults are not swept away. Some practitioners use orthodox medicine and, where it fails, turn to cult practices. Where such complementary practices give comfort they are not to be despised, but their role and validity should be clearly defined. 'Some of the practitioners of alternative medicine are constantly trying to obtain official recognition. The need for careful scrutiny and appraisal of all medical methods and therapies, and for quality control of drugs is likewise increasing. European health and research institutes are particularly well placed to apply modern science and technology to traditional methods of practice and therapy in order to evaluate herbal medicaments in particular. Health authorities would also wish to satisfy themselves regarding the cost-effectiveness of traditional health care in relation to official health care.' (ibid)

In other words no community can afford to take these cults at their own valuation; they must be tested, and tested with at least the rigour required to justify a therapeutic claim for a new drug. It is sometimes urged in extenuation that traditional and cult practices do not harm, unlike synthetic drugs. But even if that were true, investment of scarce resources in delivering what may be ineffective, though sometimes pleasing,

These terms are apt because when any practice, whatever its source, is shown to be effective by testing according to rational (scientific) criteria it becomes generally accepted and so ceases to be an alternative, fringe or complementary practice. Willingness to follow where the evidence leads is a distinctive feature of scientific medicine.

Note. A scientific approach does *not* mean a patient must be treated as a mere biochemical machine. It does *not* mean the exclusion of spiritual, psychological and social dimensions of human beings. But it *does* mean treating these in a rational manner.

Traditional or indigenous medicinal therapeutics has developed since before history in all societies. It comprises a mass of practices varying from the worthless to highly effective remedies, e.g. digitalis (England), quinine (South America), reserpine (India), atropine (various countries), etc. It is the task of science to find the gems and to discard the dross*, and at the same time to leave intact socially valuable supportive aspects of traditional medicine. *Complementary* medicine caters, in general, for people whom scientific medicine cannot or does not help: it does not compete with the successful mainstream of scientific medicine, but offers comfort especially to two classes of patient, (a) those with a bad prognosis or severe organic functional disability, and (b) those in whom the complaint has a major psychological component.

Features common to *complementary medicine* cults are absence of scientific thinking, naive acceptance of hypotheses, uncritical acceptance of causation (e.g. reliance on anecdote and assumption that if recovery follows treatment it is due to the treatment, the *post hoc ergo propter hoc*† fallacy) and close attention to the patient's personal feelings. Lack of understanding of how therapeutic effects may be measured is also a prominent feature. Exponents often state that comparative controlled trials of their medicines versus orthodox medicines are impracticable because the more rigid double-blind randomised controlled designs are inappropriate and in particular do not allow for the individual approach characteristic of alternative medicine. But modern therapeutic trial designs can cope with this. A few generally unsatisfactory trials comparing homoeopathic with orthodox medicines have been done‡ and perhaps this is a good omen, but a lot more study is needed if either advocates or critics are to change their attitudes.

One difficulty of doing definitive trials (which are tedious and expensive) is that so weak is the evidence for the medical cults, with regard to both empirical evidence of efficacy and theoretical basis, that those competent to do valid studies, and having a duty to use resources wisely, are liable to put the scientific evaluation of complementary medicine low on their list of priorities, at least until the alternative practitioners understand the scientific approach and are willing to accept its application. But there remain extremists who contend that they understand scientific method and reject it as invalid for what they do and believe, i.e. their beliefs are not, in principle, refutable; this is the position taken up by magic and religion where subordination of reason to faith is a virtue.

This book is not an appropriate place to attempt a broad discussion of complementary medicine. But it is useful to list some common beliefs of the practitioners and then to consider homoeopathy, for this particularly relies on drugs used in an unorthodox or unscientific way.

The following beliefs are commonly met and seem to be characteristic of complementary medicine:

experiences (e.g. dance therapy, exaltation of flowers, and the surely inexpensive urine therapy) to populations means that these resources are not available for other desirable social objectives, e.g. housing, art subsidies, medicine.

Finally, a cult called simply 'Healing', is claimed to be 'helpful for all conditions. Healing reaches the parts other therapies cannot reach . . . Healing has the greatest cost-effectiveness of all therapies. It requires no apparatus, only the fees of the healer . . . health administrators should pay more attention to promoting Healing than any other therapy.' (ibid) We do not apologise for this diversion to consider medical cults and practices, for the world cannot afford unreason, and the antidote to unreason is reason and the rigorous pursuit of knowledge.

* Traditional medicine is being fostered particularly in countries where scientific medicine is not accessible to large populations for economic reasons, and destruction of traditional medicine would leave unhappy and sick people with nothing. For this reason governments are supporting traditional medicine and at the same time initiating scientific clinical evaluations of the numerous plants and other items employed, many of which contain biologically active substances. The World Health Organization encourages these programmes.

† Latin: after this, therefore on account of this.

‡ Editorial. Lancet 1983; 1:108.

1. That synthetic modern drugs are toxic, but products obtained in nature are not; the former statement is true, but the latter is false; there is a profusion of toxic substances in nature — animal, vegetable and mineral — e.g. venoms, toxins, digitalis, laetrile, arsenic*.

2. That traditional (pre-scientific) medicines have special virtue; this belief seems to be based on a vague nostalgia for a past 'golden age' which never existed and on the grounds that natural products are used.

3. That scientific medicine will only accept evidence that remedies are effective where the mechanism is also understood. This is so plainly untrue that it is difficult to understand how the belief has gained currency; empirical evidence ('suck it and see') of efficacy has always been sufficient to justify use, e.g. penicillin, morphine, which were in use long before their mechanisms of action were understood. But knowledge of mechanisms is plainly desirable because it contributes to safer and more effective use and also allows the prospect of deliberate development of improvements.

4. Linked to 3 is the false belief that scientific medicine recognizes no form of evaluation other than the strict randomized controlled trial of single medicines, and that complementary medicine cannot be scientifically evaluated because patients receive different treatment according to their individuality.†

5. That scientific medicine rests on acceptance of rigid and unalterable dogmas; it is plainly hard for practitioners of complementary medicine to understand that in scientific medicine any belief can be and is modified or abandoned when evidence is produced that justifies this; science-based medicine is flexible (though some of the practitioners may not be) and that is the reason for its successes, which are generally not denied by practitioners of complementary medicine; scientific medicine follows, sometimes stumbling, where the evidence leads. Thus, when the claims of alternative cults have been subject to tests as intellectually rigorous as those nowadays required to justify the making of therapeutic claims, any practice that passes will become generally accepted regardless of its source.

6. That if a patient gets better when treated in accordance with certain beliefs, this provides evidence for the truth of these beliefs.

7. That because orthodox medicine and particularly the drugs it uses can cause substantial harm (iatrogenic disease) this is evidence for the therapeutic validity of alternative approaches, and for the (unwarranted) assumption that complementary medicine is not also a source of iatrogenic disease.

8. Alternative medicine charges that orthodox medicine seriously neglects the patient as a whole integrated human being (body, mind, spirit) and treats him too much as a machine. Orthodox practitioners may well feel uneasily that there has been and still is truth in this, that some doctors have been seduced by the enormous successes of medical science and technology and have become liable to look too narrowly at their patients and too easily to rely on a prescription where a much broader response is required.

The management of the patient as a whole being (holistic medicine) should be the hall-mark of good medicine, however and whenever practised; but the humane application of technology does present enormous challenges, e.g. intensive therapy units, radiotherapy, cancer chemotherapy. The management of the patient as a whole being of body, mind and spirit is a strong point of alternative medicine. Homoeopathic management,

* *Herbal teas* containing pyrrolidizine alkaloids (*Senecio, Crotalaria, Heliotropium*) cause serious hepatic veno-occlusive disease. *Comfrey* (*Symphitum*) is similar but also causes hepatocellular tumours and haemangiomas. *Sassafras* (carminative, antirheumatic) is hepatotoxic. *Mistletoe* (*Viscum*) contains cytotoxic alkaloids. *Ginseng* contains oestrogenic substances which have caused gynaecomastia: long-term users may show 'ginseng abuse syndrome' comprising CNS excitation: arterial hypotension can occur. *Liquorice* (*Glycyrrhiza*) has mineralcorticoid action: see carbenoxolone. An amateur 'health food enthusiast' made himself a tea from 'an unfamiliar (to him) plant' in his garden: unfortunately this was the familiar foxglove (*Digitalis purpurea*): happily he recovered. Other toxic natural remedies include lily of the valley (*Convallaria*) and horse chestnut (*Aesculus*). 'The medical herbalist is at fault for clinging to outworn historical authority and for not assessing his drugs in terms of today's knowledge, and the orthodox physician is at fault for a cynical scepticism with regard to any healing discipline other than his own.' (Penn R G. 1983. Adv Dr React Bull; no. 102).

† This view seems to assert that benefit, e.g. in arthritis, is measurable or not measurable according to the system of medical practice that has delivered it. There is neither intellectual nor factual basis for such belief.

for example, involves 'what might be called a short psychoanalysis, using relatively stereotyped questions'*; it attaches importance to patients' cravings and interests, their responses to hot and cold, motion, rest, moistness, dryness; 'for it is only when hidden feelings and fears are brought to the surface that the homoeopath can select a remedy that will stimulate the defence mechanism and bring about a cure'†. It is evident that such an approach is likely to give particular satisfaction in psychological and psychosomatic conditions for which orthodox doctors in a hurry have been all too ready to think that a prescription meets all the patients' needs.‡ Much of the recent increased interest in complementary medicine stems from the inadequacies of overbusy and, let us admit it, sometimes bored orthodox doctors compared with the attentiveness of practitioners of alternative medicine, as well as from the disappointment caused by inevitable failure to meet patients' over-optimistic expectations.

The following will suffice to give the flavour of one complementary medicine cult and the kind of criticism that it has to contend with. *Homoeopathy*§ is a system of medicine founded by Samuel Hahnemann (German physician: 1755–1843) and expounded by him in the *Organon of the rational art of healing*.‖ Hahnemann described his position: 'After I had discovered the weakness and errors of my teachers and books I sank into a state of sorrowful indignation, which had nearly disgusted me with the study of medicine. I was on the point of concluding that the whole art was vain and incapable of improvement. I gave myself up to solitary reflection, and resolved not to terminate my train of thought until I had arrived at a definite conclusion on the subject.¶ By understandable revulsion at the medicine of his time, by experimentation on himself (a large dose of quinine made him feel as though he had a malarial attack) and by search of records he 'discovered' a 'law' that is central to homoeopathy (and from which the name is derived)**: '*Similar symptoms in the remedy remove similar symptoms in the disease.*' 'Now as experience shows incontestably in regard to every remedy and every disease, that all remedies without exception cure swiftly, thoroughly and enduringly, the illnesses whose symptoms are of the like order with their own, we are justified in asserting that the healing power of medicines depends on the resemblance of their symptoms to the symptoms of disease: or in other words, every medicine which, among the symptoms which it can cause in a healthy body, reproduces most of those present in a given disease, is capable of curing that disease in the swiftest, most thorough, and most enduring fashion.' 'The eternal, universal law of Nature, that every disease is destroyed and cured through the similar artificial disease which the appropriate remedy has the tendency to excite, rests on the following proposition: that only one disease can exist in the body at any one time.'

In addition to the above, he 'discovered' that the effect of drugs is potentiated by dilution (provided the dilution is shaken correctly) even to the extent that an effective dose may not contain a single molecule of the drug. It has been pointed out** that the 'thirtieth potency' (1 in 10^{60}), recommended by Hahnemann, provided a solution in which there would be one molecule of drug in a volume of a sphere of literally astronomical circumference. That a dose in which no drug is present (including such preparations of sodium chloride) can be therapeutically effective is explained by the belief that there is a spiritual energy diffused throughout the medicine by the particular way in which the dilutions are shaken (succussion) during preparation or that the active molecules leave behind some sort of 'imprint' on solvent or excipient.††

* Hickman A D. Br Med J 1963; 1:523.

† Vithoulkas G. World Health Forum (WHO Geneva) 1983; 4:99. But yet homoeopathic medicines are sold directly to the public from self-selection stands, i.e. in circumstances where such exploration and counselling cannot be provided.

‡ A randomised controlled trial in irritable bowel syndrome of routine medical treatment versus the same management plus individual psychotherapy has shown that the psychotherapy was beneficial in both short- and long-term progress. Svendlund J et al. *Lancet* 1983; 2:589

§ Greek: *homos*: same: *patheia*: suffering.

‖ 1810: trans. Wheeler C E. London: Dent. 1913.

¶ Hahnemann S. Aesculapius in the balance. Leipsic. 1805.

** Clark A J. General Pharmacology, Heffter's Handbuch, Berlin: Springer. 1937.

†† Homoeopathic practitioners repeatedly express their irritation that critics give so much attention to dilution. They should not be surprised considering the enormous implications of their claim.

Thus, writes a critic 'We are asked to put aside the whole edifice of evidence concerning the physical nature of materials and the normal concentration-response relationships of biologically active substances in order to accommodate homoeopathic potency.'* But no hard evidence that tests the hypothesis is supplied to justify this, and we are invited, for instance, to accept that sodium chloride merely diluted is no remedy, but that 'it raises itself to the most wonderful power through a well-prepared dynamisation process' and stimulates the defensive powers of the body against the disease. The dogmas of homoeopathy have incurred ridicule, which is resented by its practitioners who insist that they are misunderstood and who tartly observe that critics have generally not made a serious study of homoeopathy, and that patients treated according to homoeopathic principles commonly recover, which is certainly true, but true of all forms of medicine including other cults. Pharmacologists generally feel that in the absence of conclusive evidence from empirical therapeutic trials conducted according to modern standards, there is no point in discussing the hypotheses of homoeopathy until some evidence that satisfies the ordinary criteria of scientific method is produced. But it is always necessary to bear in mind that useful discoveries may be made in pursuing unsubstantiated hypotheses, and empirical studies can be made without accepting any particular theory.

Conclusion

There is a single fundamental issue between orthodox scientific medicine and traditional and complementary medicine (though it is often obscured by detailed debates on individual practices); the issue of *what constitutes acceptable evidence* (i.e. the nature, quality, and interpretation of evidence) that can justify general adoption of modes of treatment and acceptance of hypotheses.

6. Responsibility for drug-caused injury

This topic raises important issues affecting medical practice and development of needed new drugs, as well as of law and of social justice.

All civilised legal systems provide for compensation to be paid to a person injured as a result of using a product that is defective due to *negligence* (failure to exercise reasonable care).† But there is a growing opinion that special compensation for personal injury, beyond what any available social security system provides, should be automatic and not dependent on fault and proof of fault of the producer, i.e. *'liability irrespective of fault'*, *'no-fault liability'* or *'strict liability'*‡. After all, victims need assistance regardless of the cause of disability and whether or not the producer, and, in the case of drugs, the prescriber, deserves punishment.

Many countries are now revising their laws on liability for personal injury and 'drugs represent the class of product in respect of which there has been the greatest pressure for surer compensation in cases of injury'.§

Principal causes of public anxiety include the accidents with thalidomide, practolol and clioquinol (see index) and the increased incidence of serious thromboembolism in healthy women taking combined oestrogen/progestogen oral contraceptives. From numerous public statements, it is evident that non-medical lawyers and politicians as well as the general public, understandably shocked and resentful at these and other events, have difficulty in appreciating the very special problems posed by the use of new and old drugs, e.g. as to reasonable expectation of safety, determination of cause, and the question of fault. Bad

* Cuthbert A W. Pharmaceut J; 15 May 1982: 547.

† A plaintiff seeking to obtain compensation from a defendant (via the law of negligence) must prove *three* things: 1, that the defendant owed a duty of care to the plaintiff; 2, that the defendant failed to exercise reasonable care; and 3, that the plaintiff has suffered actual injury as a result.

‡ The following distinction is made in some discussions of product liability:
(a) *strict* liability: compensation is provided by the producer/manufacturer.
(b) *no fault* liability or scheme: compensation is provided by a central fund.

§ Royal Commission on Civil Liability and Compensation for Personal Injury. 1978. London: HMSO. Cmnd. 7054. Although the Commission considered compensation for death and personal injury suffered by any person through manufacture, supply or use of products (i.e. all goods whether natural or manufactured), and included drugs and even human blood and organs, it made no mention of tobacco and alcohol.

laws, though made with the best intentions, could radically change medical practice for the worse (for the patient) and also inhibit socially desirable development of needed new drugs. It is therefore important that the medical profession try to increase general understanding of the issues raised by the public demand for special compensation for personal injury due to drugs.*

Issues that are central to the debate include:

1. *Capacity to cause harm is inherent in drugs* in a way that sets them apart from other manufactured products; harm often occurs in the absence of fault.

2. *Safety*, i.e. the degree of safety that a person is entitled to expect, must often be a matter of opinion.

3. *Causation*, i.e. proof that the drug in fact caused the injury, is often impossible, particularly where it increases the incidence of a disease that occurs naturally.

Women taking combined oestrogen/progestogen oral contraceptives have an increased liability to heart attacks and strokes (especially if they smoke) but in no one case can it be said that the contraceptive was certainly the cause. Should only some victims be compensated (how will they be chosen)? Should all get some compensation? If so, why should not compensation be paid to women who have heart attacks or strokes when not using a contraceptive? If all such diseased women are to be compensated, should not men too be compensated? If heart attacks and strokes are to be specially compensated, should not other diseases be equally compensated? etc. Jaundice due to drugs, which is indistinguishable from virus hepatitis, provides another example. Should compensation be reduced in smokers and drinkers where there is evidence that these pleasure-drugs increase liability to adverse reactions to therapeutic drugs?

4. *The concept of defect*, i.e. whether the drug or the prescriber or indeed the patient can be said to be 'defective' so as to attract liability, is a highly complex matter and indeed is a curious concept as applied to medicine.

A person who takes medication is already suffering from some form of defect (illness). He is in a situation that is complex, and one where attempts to identify specific causal relationships and to provide extra compensation for those adverse events that are due to drugs, though sometimes easy, will often present difficulties that are unresolvable. It may simply not be possible, when patients perceive an adverse change in their condition, to ascribe it confidently to drugs they have taken, to a change in the illness itself, or to one of the many possible interactions between patients' constitutions (e.g. allergy), their illness, and what enters their systems, whether this be food or medicine, or substances such as tobacco or alcohol. There is a real danger of a proliferation of claims whose justice cannot be logically ascertained, and of the public being encouraged to expect compensation for injuries where causation cannot be established.

5. *A solution.* Despite all the above there is a class of drug injury that can be identified as particularly disturbing to the public mind, its sense of justice, and as being deserving of compassion. This is the *rare serious injury* that is *totally disproportionate* to the significance normally attached to the treatment, and that was *not taken into account* (because it was so rare) when deciding to use the drug, so that it was treated as a negligible risk (p. 5), e.g. fatal blood dyscrasia from indomethacin used for dysmenorrhoea (a licenced indication) in a woman with three dependent children. But in advocating this we must remember to spare a thought for the family of a similar person who has died of natural disease and who are not offered any special compensation.

Nowhere has a scheme that meets all the major difficulties yet been implemented. This is not because there has been too little thought, it is because the subject is so difficult.

The following is offered as an outline of some of the main features of a workable scheme.

1. *New unlicenced drugs undergoing early trial in small numbers of subjects* (healthy or patient volunteers): the producer should be strictly liable for all adverse effects.

2. *New unlicenced drugs undergoing extensive trials* in patients who may reasonably expect benefit: the producer should be strictly liable for any serious effect.

* This discussion is about drugs that have been properly manufactured and meet proper standards of purity, stability etc. as laid down by regulatory bodies or pharmacopoeias. A *manufacturing defect* would be dealt with in a way no different from manufacturing errors in other products.

3. *New drugs after licensing by an official regulatory body*: liability for serious injury should now be shared with the community, which is expecting to benefit from new drugs.

4. *Standard drugs in day to day therapeutics*:

(a) there should be *no-fault scheme*, operated by or with the assent of government, that has authority, through tribunals, *quickly* to decide cases and to make awards. This body would have authority to reimburse itself from others — manufacturer, supplier, prescriber — wherever that was appropriate. An award must not have to wait on the determination of prolonged, vexatious and expensive court proceedings.

(b) *Patients would be compensated* where:
  (i) causation is proved on 'balance of probability'*
  (ii) the injury was serious
  (iii) the event was rare and remote and not reasonably taken into account in making the decision to treat.

7. Hazards of life on drugs and chronic pharmacology

The proportion of the population taking drugs continuously for large portions of their lives increases as tolerable suppressive and prophylactic remedies for chronic or recurrent conditions are developed, e.g. for hypertension, diabetes, mental diseases, epilepsies, gout, collagen diseases, thrombosis, allergies and various infections. In some cases the treatment introduces significant hazard into patients' lives and the cure can be worse than the disease if it is not skilfully managed.

1. *Chronic pharmacology: the consequences of prolonged administration of drugs and their withdrawal*. In general the dangers of a drug are not markedly increased if therapy lasts years rather than months, except perhaps for renal damage (analgesic mixtures) and carcinogenesis.

Interference with self-regulating systems: receptors; tolerance; and rebound of drug effect. When self-regulating physiological systems, (controlled by negative feedback systems, e.g. endocrine, cardiovascular) are subject to interference, their control mechanisms respond to minimize the effects of the interference and to restore the previous steady state or rhythm: this is *homeostasis*. The previous state may be a normal function, e.g. ovulation, or an abnormal function, e.g. high blood pressure. If the body successfully restores the previous steady state or rhythm then the subject has become *tolerant* to the drug. But if the homeostatic response is ineffective then the drug effect persists.

In the case of hormonal contraceptives, persistence of effect on ovulation is desired but persistence of other effects, e.g. on blood coagulation and metabolism, is not desired.

In the case of arterial hypertension, tolerance to a single drug commonly occurs, e.g. reduction of peripheral resistance by a vasodilator is compensated by an increase in blood volume that restores the blood pressure; this is why a diuretic is commonly used together with a vasodilator in therapy of the condition.

The endocrine system serves fluctuating body needs. Glands are therefore capable of either increasing or decreasing their output by means of negative feedback systems. An administered hormone or hormone analogue activates the receptors of the feedback system and high doses will cause suppression of natural production of the hormone. On withdrawal of the administered hormone the control mechanism takes time, months in the case of the hypothalamus/pituitary/adrenal cortex, to recover completely and sudden withdrawal of administered corticosteroid can result in an acute deficiency state that may be life-endangering.

The number (density) of receptors on cells (for hormones, autacoids and drugs), the number occupied (affinity), and the fit of the molecule (sensitivity) can change in response to the concentration of the specific binding molecule or ligand (Latin: ligare, to bind), whether this be agonist or antagonist (blocker), always tending to restore cell function to its normal or usual state. Prolonged high concentrations of agonist (whether administered as a drug or overproduced in the body by a tumour) cause a reduction in the number of

* This is the criterion for civil law, rather than 'beyond reasonable doubt', which is the criterion of criminal law.

receptors available for activation (*down-regulation*; and changes in receptor affinity and sensitivity), and the prolonged blocking of receptors by inert antagonists leads to an increase in the number of receptors (*up-regulation*). At least some of this may be achieved by receptors moving inside the cell and out again (*internalisation* and *externalisation*).

Down-regulation and accompanying receptor changes may explain the tolerant or refractory state seen in severe asthmatics who no longer respond to β-adrenoceptor agonists.

The occasional exacerbation of ischaemic cardiac disease on sudden withdrawal of a β-adrenoceptor blocker may be explained by up regulation during its administration, so that on withdrawal an above-normal number of receptors suddenly becomes accessible to the normal chemo-transmitter (noradrenaline). Up regulation with rebound sympathomimetic effects may be innocuous to a moderately healthy cardiovascular system, but the increased oxygen demand of these effects can have serious consequences where ischaemic disease is present and increased oxygen need cannot be met (angina pectoris, dysrhythmia, infarction). Unmasking of a disease process that has worsened during prolonged suppressive use of the drug may also contribute to such exacerbations.

The rebound phenomenon is plainly a potential hazard and the use of a β-adrenoceptor blocker in the presence of ischaemic heart disease would be safer if rebound could be eliminated. Now, some β-adrenoceptor blockers are not pure blockers (antagonists); they also have some agonist (sympathomimetic) activity, i.e. they are *partial agonists*; it seems possible that the presence of some agonist action along with the principal blocking effect might prevent the generation of additional adrenoceptors (up-regulation), and indeed there is some evidence that rebound is less or absent with partial agonist β-adrenoceptor blockers, e.g. pindolol. In general, rebound or withdrawal effects are the opposite of the main actions of the drug withdrawn.

Rebound withdrawal phenomena occur erratically. In general, they are more likely with drugs having a short half-life (abrupt drop in plasma concentration) and pure agonist or antagonist action. They are less likely to occur with drugs having a long half-life and (probably) with those having a mixed agonist/antagonist (partial agonist) action on receptors.

Clinically important consequences of abrupt withdrawal of drugs are known to occur with the following:

Cardiovascular system: antihypertensives (especially clonidine), β-adrenoceptor blockers, (warfarin provides an example of a catching-up phenomenon, p. 57, rather than of rebound).

Nervous system: all *depressants* (hypnotics, sedatives, alcohol, opioid), antiepileptics, antiparkinsonian agents. *Tricyclic antidepressants*.

Endocrine system: adrenal steroids.

Immune inflammation: adrenal steroids.

2. *Resurgence or rebound of chronic disease, the effects of which have been wholly or partly suppressed* is an obvious possible consequence of abrupt withdrawal of effective therapy. It may be worse than before because the disease process itself has worsened (autoimmune disease, ischaemic heart disease), or because there is a true rebound phenomenon (epilepsy).

This sketchy account should suffice to explain that tolerance and rebound are phenomena that are to be expected. In many cases the exact mechanisms remain obscure but clinicians have no reason to be amazed when they occur, and in the case of rebound they may particularly wish to use gradual withdrawal wherever drugs have been used to modify complex self-adjusting systems, and to suppress (without cure) chronic diseases.

3. *Metabolic changes* over a long period may induce disease, e.g. thiazide diuretics (diabetes mellitus), adrenocortical hormones (osteoporosis, etc.), phenytoin (osteomalacia). Drugs may also enhance metabolism of the primary drug and other drugs (enzyme induction).

4. *Specific cell injury or cell functional disorder* occur with individual drugs or drug classes, e.g. tardive dyskinesia (dopamine receptor blockers), retinal damage (chloroquine, phenothiazines), retroperitoneal fibrosis (methysergide). Cancer may occur, e.g. with oestrogens (endometrium) and with immunosuppressive (anticancer) drugs.

Conclusions. The objective of the above (primitive) account of some possible consequences of prolonged drug administration is to remind the user that drugs do not only induce their known listed primary actions, but they (a) evoke compensatory responses in the complex inter-related physiological systems that they perturb and that these systems need time to recover on withdrawal of the drug (gradual withdrawal can give this time; it is sometimes mandatory and never harmful); (b) drugs induce metabolic changes that may be trivial in the short term, but serious if they persist for a long time; and (c) drugs may produce localised effects in specially susceptible tissues and induce serious cell damage or malfunction. That such changes will occur with prolonged drug use is to be expected, and, with a moderate knowledge of physiology, pathology and pharmacology combined with an awareness that the unexpected is to be expected ('There are more things in heaven and earth, Horatio, than are dreamt of in your philosophy'*) patients requiring long-term therapy may be managed safely, or at least with minimum risk of harm, and enabled to live happy lives.

In addition to the above, prolonged drug therapy also exposes patients to:

5. *Dangers of intercurrent illness* — these are particularly notable with anticoagulants, adrenal steroids and immunosuppressives.

6. *Dangers of interactions with other drugs or diet* — monoamine oxidase inhibitor antidepressants (pethidine, sympathomimetics, cheese, etc.); antihypertensives (sympathomimetics, including appetite suppressants, tricyclic antidepressants), digitalis (diuretics), hypnotics and tranquillisers (alcohol), and interactions due to enzyme induction and inhibition (see *interactions*).

The patient's protection lies in the physician who should:

1. Judge the risks of permanent drug therapy against the likely benefit and act accordingly.

2. Understand the pharmacology of the drug to be used and of other drugs that may be taken if the patient has another illness or accident.

3. Ensure that patients understand what is required of them so that they will not, through ignorance, carelessness or mishap increase the inevitable minimum of risk.

8 Warnings to patients

Just as engineers say that the only safe aeroplane is the one that stays on the ground in still air on a disused airfield or in a locked hangar, so the only safe drug is one that stays in its original package. If drugs are not safe then plainly patients are entitled to be warned of their hazards.

It is self-evident to a patient that when a doctor proposes a treatment it is because he thinks it will do good. It is not equally self-evident to the patient that there is a possibility of harm and it certainly would be wrong that the onus to enquire about risk should be put on the patient; the doctor manifestly has a general duty to offer relevant information. Patients may opt to leave to the doctor the decision to use or not to use the treatment, making use of the doctor's training, knowledge of the treatment and knowledge of the patient, as it is their right to choose to do. Alternatively, patients may wish to hear a detailed explanation and decide for themselves, as is equally their right. In any case the doctor has some duty to warn.

Warnings to patients may be divided into two classes:

1. Warnings that will affect the patient's decision to accept or reject the treatment.

2. Warnings that will affect the safety of the treatment once it has begun, e.g. risk of stopping treatment, occurrence of drug toxicity.

There is no arbitrary legal or ethical obligation on doctors to warn all patients of all possible adverse consequences of treatment. It is their duty to adapt the information they give so that the best interest of each patient is served. In one court case a judge declared that there was no obligation on doctors to go over with their patients anything more than the inherent implication of the particular treatment proposed. If there was a real risk inherent in a procedure of some misfortune occurring, then doctors should certainly warn patients of the possibility that the misfortune might arise, however well the treatment was performed. Doctors should take into account the personality of the patient, the likelihood of any misfortune arising, and what warning was necessary for each particular patient's welfare.†

It is part of the professionalism of doctors to tell what is appropriate, in their patient's interest. But

* W Shakespeare (1564–1616) Hamlet: I.V.166.

† Legal correspondent. Br Med J 1980; 280:575.

this must be deliberate. If things go wrong they must be prepared to defend what they did, or, more important in the case of warnings, what they did not do, as being in their patient's best interest.

There has been public concern that doctors deliberately and arrogantly withhold information from patients. If public pressure that doctors should really try to tell all, or even most, were really to become so strong and persistent that the profession felt obliged to acquiesce, there can be no doubt the practice of medicine, for not only the doctor but also the patient, would change in a way neither party, and particularly the patient, would like. The plain impossibility of meeting the requirement verbally must result in extensive lists being printed (for all forms of treatment, including surgery). Some think this would frighten patients, and maybe it would, but it would confuse more.

A distinguished lawyer* has pointed out that even in research, where a high level of information on risks is required for the potential subject to make an understanding decision whether to participate, *total* disclosure is not mandatory. He points out that the object of offering and preserving potential subjects' choice is served by disclosure of general data they will want to know, but without requiring them to undertake a medical education. If venepuncture is proposed, for instance, warning should be given of risk of temporary soreness at the site of withdrawal, bruising and treatable infection, together with information that no medical procedure, including the proposed procedure, is free of risk . . . The medical risks of taking a common blood sample have been recorded to include haematoma, dermatitis, cellulitis, abscess, osteomyelitis, septicaemia, endocarditis, thrombophlebitis, pulmonary embolism and death. Disclosing these acknowledged possible but unlikely complications of the procedure might appear to distort rather than to preserve choice. Stating them in abstract, rather than evaluatively indicating their remote possibility, may deny rather than offer informed choice. Clearly, however, the greater the potential injury and the greater the risk of incurring it, the greater must be the level of disclosure. The intending investigator must therefore take care to accommodate the individual characteristics of each potential subject. This applies also, in principle, to treatment.

In conclusion. Doctors have a duty to warn and inform patients who undergo medical treatment or participate in research:

1. So that they can make an informed decision whether to accept treatment.
2. To render continuing treatment safer.
3. To allow medical research to be conducted to the highest ethical standard.

The profession is open to criticism in all these areas. Our principal fault is not so much arrogance or indifference as that we have not stood back and thought clearly about the principles governing our practice in giving warnings to patients and research subjects, and we have not given enough attention to ensure that patients have printed information that they need available for study when they may be in a mood and position to use it profitably (see *Information to patients*).

9. Why drug therapy carries unavoidable risk

A risk-free drug would be one for which:

1. The physician knew exactly what action was required and used the drug correctly.
2. The drug did that and nothing else, either by true biological selectivity or by selective targeted delivery.
3. Exactly the right amount of action, not too little, not too much, was easily achieved.

These criteria may be completely fulfilled, e.g. in a streptococcal infection sensitive to penicillin in a patient whose genetic constitution does not render him liable to develop an allergy to penicillin.

The criteria are partially fulfilled in insulin-deficient diabetes, in which pure human insulin may be given to replace the patient's deficiency. But the natural controls of insulin secretion in response to need (food, exercise) are lacking and even sophisticated technology cannot yet exactly mimic the normal physiological responses. Medical interference with any delicate homeostatic system responsive to rapidly changing physiological needs is inevitably crude and will bring potentially

* Dickens B M. In: Howard-Jones N, Bankowski Z, eds. Medical experimentation and the protection of human rights. Geneva: CIOMS. 1979.

serious problems for the patient. The criteria are still farther from realization in, for example, hyperlipidaemias and schizophrenia.

Some reasons why the above criteria are commonly not met:

1. Drugs are not sufficiently selective. As the concentration rises, a drug that is highly selective at low concentrations will begin to affect other target sites (receptors, enzymes); a disease process (cancer) is so close to normal cellular mechanisms that totally selective cell kill is impossible (though cure of some cancers is attainable at an acceptable price in toxicity).

2. Some effects, e.g. anticoagulation, that are desirable in one part of the body (deep veins) may lead to harm (bleeding) in another part; they cannot be localized in long-term use. Anti-inflammatory effect on a disease process may be beneficial, but the effect is not confined to disease and necessary protective responses may be reduced.

3. Similar physiological mechanisms (adrenergic, cholinergic systems) mediate a wide range of physiological functions. Selectivity in the normal functioning of the body is controlled by selective activation of the various parts of the systems and the strictly local release of chemotransmitters. Systemic administration of drugs causes general activation or deactivation of mechanisms such as does not occur naturally.

4. Prolonged modification of cellular mechanisms can lead to permanent change in structure and function, e.g. carcinogenicity.

5. Insufficient knowledge of disease processes (atherosclerosis) and of drug action (hypolipidaemics) can lead to interventions that, though undertaken with the best intentions, are harmful, i.e. an abnormal finding being treated without knowing whether the finding is a primary cause or a secondary manifestation of disease, e.g. the unexplained 47% higher (non-cardiac) mortality in clofibrate-treated patients in a trial of primary prevention of ischaemic heart disease, largely from diseases of liver and gut.*

6. Patients are genetically heterogeneous to an enormous degree and may have an unpredictable immunological response to drugs.

7. Dosage adjustment according to need is unavoidably imprecise (diabetes mellitus, depression).

8. Ignorant and casual prescribing.

Reduction of drug risk can be achieved by:

1. Better knowledge of disease (research); about 40% of useful medical advances derive from basic research that was not funded with the practical outcome in view.

2. Topical or local application of drugs to the target organ, where this is accessible.

3. Targeting of drugs inside the body:

(a) utilizing natural biochemical selectivity where it exists (molecular design).

(b) developing target-selective carriers, e.g. antibodies, that will carry active agents in an inactive form to the target site where they will be released, e.g. tumour-specific antibodies carrying anticancer drugs; macromolecules, e.g. dextrans; lectins are also being explored as carriers of drugs to cells for which they have selective affinity; cells, e.g. erythrocytes, platelets, neutrophils, fibroblasts, may also be used as carriers of drugs; artificial agents, e.g. liposomes (drugs are entrapped in a system of concentric closed phospholipid membranes), which enter cells by endocytosis, have also been developed.

4. Delivery systems that adjust drug release according to need, e.g. 'artificial pancreas'.

5. Informed, careful and responsible prescribing.

10. Reasons for taking a drug history from patients

1. Drugs are a cause of disease.

2. Withdrawal of drugs can cause disease (e.g. adrenal steroid, antiepileptic).

3. Drugs can conceal disease (e.g. adrenal steroid).

4. Drugs can interact causing positive adverse effect or negative adverse effect (therapeutic failure).

5. Drugs can give diagnostic clues (e.g. ampicillin in infectious mononucleosis, a diagnostic side-effect, not a diagnostic test).

6. Drugs can cause false results in clinical chemistry tests (e.g. plasma cortisol, urinary catecholamine, urinary glucose).

* Committee of principal investigators (WHO). Lancet 1984; 2:600.

7. Drug history can assist choice of drugs in the future.
8. Drugs can leave residual effects after administration has ceased (e.g. chloroquine, digoxin, adrenal steroid).

11. The therapeutic situation

'It is evident that patients are not treated in a vacuum and that they respond to a variety of subtle forces around them in addition to the specific therapeutic agent under investigation'*.

When a patient is given a drug his responses are the resultant of numerous factors:

1. The pharmacodynamic effect of the drug and interactions with any other drugs the patient may be taking.
2. The pharmacokinetics of the drug and its modification in the individual due to genetic causes, disease, other drugs.
3. The physiological state of the end-organ, whether, for instance, it is over- or underactive.
4. The act of medication, including the route of administration and the presence or absence of the doctor.
5. The doctor's mood, personality, attitudes and beliefs.
6. The patient's ditto.
7. What the doctor has told the patient.
8. The patient's past experience of doctors.
9. The patient's estimate of what he has received and of what ought to happen as a result.
10. The social environment, e.g. whether alone or in company.

Obviously some of the above overlap — the patient's beliefs, for example, being determined by what the doctor tells him as well as by information from other sources.

The relative importance of these factors varies according to the circumstances — an unconscious patient with meningococcal meningitis may be assumed to respond to penicillin only in so far as it affects the invading bacteria, and regardless of whether he and the doctor dislike each other. But a patient sleepless with anxiety because he cannot cope with his family responsibilities may be affected as much by the interaction of his own personality with that of the doctor as by the diazepam prescribed by the latter, and the same applies to appetite suppressants in food addicts.

The physician may consciously use all of the factors listed above in his therapeutic practice. But it is still not enough that a patient gets better, it is essential to know *why* he does so. This is because potent drugs should only be given if their pharmacodynamic effects are needed. If other factors are the effective agents, then any drug given will be a placebo and placebos should be harmless. The double-blind technique in therapeutic trials used with placebo (or dummy) medication represents an attempt to discriminate true pharmacodynamic effects from the other aspects of the therapeutic situation.

* Sherman L J. Am J Psychiatry 1959; 116:208.

12. Placebos†

All treatments have a psychological component, whether to please (true placebo effect) or, occasionally, to vex (negative placebo effect).

Placebos are used for two purposes:

1. *As a control* in scientific evaluation of drugs (see *therapeutic trials*).
2. *To benefit or please a patient* not by any pharmacological actions, but by psychological means.

A placebo is a vehicle for cure by suggestion, and is surprisingly often successful, if only temporarily. All treatments carry placebo effects — physiotherapy, psychotherapy, surgery — but it is most easily investigated with drugs, for the active and the inert can often be made to appear identical so that comparisons can be made.

The deliberate use of drugs as placebos is a confession of failure by the doctor. Failures however are sometimes inevitable and an absolute condemnation of the use of placebos on all occasions would be unrealistic for, 'to decline to humour an elderly "chronic" brought up on the bottle is hardly within the bounds of possibility'‡.

Placebos are usually given to patients with mild psychological disorders who attribute their symptoms to physical disease. There is no doubt that alleviation can sometimes be achieved but it is often only temporary, and may make any subse-

† Latin: *placebo*, I will please.
‡ Editorial. The humble humbug. Lancet 1954; 2:321.

quent attempt to face reality more difficult. The principal objection to deliberate use of placebo therapy is that the patient, not unreasonably, interprets the advice to take medicine as meaning that the doctor admits a physical basis for the symptoms; so that when, later, an attempt is made to attribute a psychological cause this will not be accepted. Placebos may also be used in patients with chronic incurable diseases when they need a prop to sustain their courage. Apart from this latter compassionate use, placebos should only be prescribed after a serious attempt to avoid using them has failed, and then only briefly; the placebo should consist of a substance innocuous and cheap, unless the patient pays for it himself, when high cost greatly potentiates its effect. Having admitted the legitimacy of their use, however rarely, it is necessary to advise a choice of substances.

'Those who have qualms of conscience about prescribing pharmacologically useless medicines tend to use semi-placebos, such as vitamins, in the vague hope that these may do some good. This is wrong, for thereby the prescriber deceives himself as well as the patient. If deception there must be, says Leslie*, let it be wholehearted, unflinching, and efficient. A placebo medicine should be red, yellow or brown; for blue and green are colours popularly associated with poisons or with external applications. The taste should be bitter but not unpleasant. Capsules should be coloured, and tablets either very small (on the *multum in parvo*† principle) or impressively large; they should not look like everyday tablets such as aspirin'‡. There is some evidence that anxiety symptoms respond particularly to green and depressive symptoms to yellow tablets and in one study on pain the efficacy of placebos declined from red to blue to green to yellow; in another, students were more sedated by blue than by pink capsules and there was a dose response in that two inert capsules were more effective than one.

In addition to the psychological suggestion inevitable in any act of medication, deliberate verbal suggestion has been shown to raise the threshold for pain and indeed to reverse potent pharmacodynamic effects at least temporarily. Such psychological effects are operative in any enthusiastically pursued therapeutic regimen.

It is of great importance that everyone who administers drugs should be aware that his attitude to the treatment may greatly influence the result. Undue scepticism may prevent a drug from achieving its effect and enthusiasm or confidence may potentiate the pharmacological actions of drugs.

An individual who reports changes of physical and mental state after taking a pharmacologically inert substance is a **placebo-reactor**. Such suggestible people are likely to respond favourably to *any* treatment. They have deceived doctors into making false therapeutic claims and have provided the basis for many therapeutic reputations. Negative reactors, who develop adverse effects when given a placebo, exist, but, fortunately, are fewer.

Some 35% of the physically ill and 40% or more of the mentally ill respond to placebos. Placebo reaction is an inconstant attribute — a person may respond at one time in one situation and not at another time under different conditions. However, there is some consistency in the type of person who specially tends to react to placebos. In one study on medical students, psychological tests revealed that those who reacted to a placebo tended to be extraverted, sociable, less dominant, less self-confident, more appreciative of their teaching, more aware of their autonomic functions and more neurotic than their colleagues who did not react to a placebo under the particular conditions of the experiment.

Tonics are placebos. They may be defined as substances with which it is hoped to strengthen those so weakened by disease, misery, overindulgence in play or work, or by physical or mental inadequacy, that they cannot face the stresses of life. The essential feature of this weakness is the absence of any definite recognisable defect for which there is a known remedy. There can be very few doctors who believe that there is any pharmacological basis for tonics. Benefits are attributable to placebo-effects and it is to be hoped that explanation and reassurance will eventually take the place of 'bottles of medicine'. Many people still expect a tonic from their doctor following an

* Am J Med 1954; 16:854.
† Latin: much in a little.
‡ Editorial Lancet 1954; 2:321.

illness and they are sceptical and shocked if told that the benefits that they feel are not the the result of pharmacological action.

If either the doctor or the patient believes in tonics to such a degree that one must be prescribed, a mineral and vitamin supplement such as those promoted specially for the aged will suffice. There are innumerable proprietary tonics, some of which contain highly active drugs including CNS stimulants; these should be avoided. The indiscriminate use of vitamins as tonics is widely advocated by pharmaceutical firms and practised by the gullible. Vitamins A and D can cause serious toxic effects.

There is every reason for doctors to cultivate techniques for the psychological potentiation of drugs, for their aim is to help patients, but it is essential that they should be aware of what they are doing and not deceive themselves about the physical power of their remedies. Some doctors can be accurately described as having placebo personalities.

13. Prescribing and drug consumption

Choice of drugs. There are national differences in prescribing that are the result of differing therapeutic approach between doctors in different countries, e.g. in hypertension, diabetes and mental disorders.

Cost and range. Pharmaceutical Services have comprised about 8–10% of the UK National Health Service expenditure over the past 25 years.

A National Health Service offers opportunities to get information on prescribing habits and costs not previously available because general practitioner prescriptions are all sent to a pricing office that arranges to pay the supplying pharmacist. It has been found that prescription frequency and cost per prescription is lower for older than for younger doctors. There is no reason to think that the patients of older doctors are worse off as a result. Perhaps age confers a relative immunity both from that occupational disease of the profession, *furor therapeuticus*, and from the belief that what is new and expensive is therefore best.

Despite enormous individual variation it seems to be approximately true that most doctors do about 75% of their prescribing from about 100 *preparations* (not different drugs), but the maximum number of preparations used by an individual doctor can be as high as 500.*

Antibiotics head the list of *prescribed* drugs, followed by diuretics, analgesics, tranquillisers, antacids plus other gastrointestinal medicines, adrenal steroid topical preparations, bronchodilators and cough medicines.

Total consumption (self-prescribed plus doctor-prescribed) of drugs comprises analgesics, cough and cold medicines and vitamins and tonics (50%) with antibiotics a close fourth, followed by drugs for skin diseases, cardiovascular diseases, hormones, tranquillisers and sedatives, antirheumatic drugs and antacids.

Amount. Consumption of drugs has become a normal part of daily life in modern society. The following supporting data are only a small proportion of what could be quoted.

In the UK on average the 57 million population (patients) consult their doctors three times a year and receive a prescription averaging 1.6 items at two of these consultations. Nearly as many prescription items again are issued without direct contact between doctor and patient.

In a study of prescriptions issued by general practitioners to a sample population of about 40 000 in the UK† in one year it was found that 54% of men and 66% of women had at least one drug dispensed. Psychotropic drugs (affecting behaviour) were prescribed to 10% of men and 21% of women. Of women aged 45–59 years, 33% received a psychotropic drug and 11% were given an antidepressant. One psychotropic drug, diazepam (Valium), generally prescribed as a sedative against anxiety and insomnia, was given to 6% of the population.

In an Australian town‡ with 15 700 inhabitants a study of drug use was conducted (in 10% of the households plus 10% of people living in insti-

* The World Health Organization publishes an updated series of reports on *The use of essential drugs*, which gives guidance for establishing national programmes for supply of drugs; the pharmaceutical industry dislikes the concept that some drugs may be classed as *essential* and therefore others, presumably, as *inessential*. But the WHO programme has attracted much interest and approval. See WHO Tech Rep Ser 1977; 615: 1979; 641: 1983; 685: 1985; 722.

† Skegg D C G et al. Br Med J 1977; 1:1561.

‡ Quoted in Wade D N. Clin Pharmacol Ther 1976; 19:651.

tutions, hotels, etc.). In the two weeks immediately preceding enquiry:

only 11% of people reported neither illness nor drug usage,

66% of people had taken some medication; more than half of these had taken more than one drug, and

6% had taken four or more drugs,

almost 60% of the medication taken was self-prescribed,

slightly less than 40% was prescribed by a doctor, 2% was prescribed by a pharmacist.

In another study in Melbourne (Australia) it was found that 30% of the population regularly took drugs.

A survey in nine Western European countries* disclosed that the proportion of all people using a tranquilliser or sedative drug was 17% in Belgium and France, 14% in the UK and 10% in Spain. The proportion of women was twice that of men and use increased with age.

In Eastern Quebec (Canada), medication, at the time of an enquiry, was being taken by 37% of females and 27% of males, and regular medication was being taken by 65% of women aged over 60 years.

In Denmark it is calculated that every person is prescribed a dose of a tranquilliser every second or third day and an analgesic every eighth day per annum.

In a study in the UK†, in the two weeks prior to enquiry of adults aged over 55 years, 32% had taken self-prescribed, 52% had taken doctor-prescribed medicines, and 44% had taken some of each. Amongst adults, aspirin and other analgesics, and amongst children, skin ointments and antiseptics, were the most frequently used medicines; the majority of these were not prescribed by a doctor. One-fifth of the medicines prescribed by doctors had actions on the nervous system. It was also found that 40% of adults took some medicine every day in the two weeks before enquiry. 75% of these daily medicines were obtained on repeat prescriptions and 25% of regular medicine takers were using medicines prescribed a year or more ago. *'So, for a sizeable proportion of people, medicine taking has become a habit often encouraged, or at least supported by their doctors.'*†

Consumption of both self- and doctor-prescribed drugs has increased rapidly over the past 10 years in Australia, the USA and the UK.

The author of the Australian study already quoted writes, 'By any standards Australians are near the top of the world "Hit Parade" of drug takers'. It seems that 60% of Australians average two or more doses of analgesics per day. In the UK it is estimated that one night's sleep in 10 is drug assisted.

In the UK, prescribing by family doctors grows at 5% per annum (in real terms, i.e. allowing for inflation). It is one of the fastest-growing sectors of the health and personal social services budget.

It is evident that people have an increasing desire for medicines and that this is well catered for by manufacturers and doctors. The question arises whether this desire is solely the result of a true medical need, i.e. whether the drugs are curing or preventing disease. We do not think it is. We agree with the Australian author who suggests that drug consumption in our societies is unnecessarily high and that it causes a significant burden of drug-induced disease, that current levels of drug use are probably symptomatic of underlying stresses and pressures in urban societies together with a cultural background that accepts the social use of drugs and encourages unduly high expectations in relation to heath, with a low threshold of what constitutes illness.

A curious by-way of medicine has been revealed in investigations of patients who are having **repeat prescriptions** from their doctors.

About two-thirds of general practice prescriptions are for repeat medication (half issued by the doctor at a consultation and half via the receptionist),

95% of patients' requests are acceded to without further discussion,

25% of patients who receive repeat prescriptions have had 40 or more repeats,

55% of patients aged over 75 years are on repeat medication.

* Balter M B et al N Engl J Med 1974; 290:769.

† Dunnell K, Cartwright A. Medicine takers prescribers and hoarders. London: Routledge & Kegan Paul, 1972. A classic study.

In a survey* of over 50 000 patients of 20 general practitioners it was revealed that:

2.8% of patients had been receiving a daily dose of a psychotropic drug (e.g. tranquilliser, sedative) for at least one year.

The average time since starting this was 5.2 years.

80% of these long-term consumers were aged over 40 years.

75% of them were women.

The numbers of these patients had increased by 80% in 10 years.

Of 31 patients taking a psychotropic drug in 1957, 24 were still doing so 10 years later.

An analysis of patients who received the same preparation for above 6 months, and often for years — 'long-repeat patients' — concluded that the patients are unhappy and their unhappiness manifests itself as unpleasant bodily sensations. The doctor can find no definite disease but he goes on trying and makes multiple diagnoses, often psychiatric. However, since no satisfactory diagnosis is established, no rational therapy can be provided. The patient continues to complain and the doctor continues to try unsuccessfully. Eventually doctor and patient take refuge uneasily in 'long-repeat prescriptions'. Of course, many patients taking the same drug for years are doing so for the best reasons, i.e. firm diagnosis for which effective therapy is available, e.g. epilepsy, diabetes, hypertension; but many do not.

Summary. Repeat prescriptions can be classified† thus:

1. For the *specific pharmacological effect* of the drug.
2. As a way of *maintaining a relationship* (by both doctor and patient); the prescription provides contact, but it can be kept impersonal; anxious phobic patients use this relationship to escape the pain of trying to eliminate their phobia, and the doctor may collude with them in this.
3. As *a gift* — a symbol of a wish to do something when the prescriber cannot think of anything better.
4. To fulfil *socially motivated patient demands*, e.g. weight reduction.
5. As a way of *getting rid of the patient*.

The list speaks for itself.

14 Economics: cost-benefit, cost-effectiveness, quality of life

The appetite of citizens for health care based on their real needs, on their wants and on their unrealistic expectations exceeds the capacity of even the richest societies to deliver. Health care resources are therefore rationed in one way or another, whether according to national social policies or to individual wealth. The debate on supply is not about whether there should be rationing, but about what form rationing should take.

Drugs comprise a significant element in the cost of health services (about 10% of expenditure in the UK National Health Service) — major items ranging from enormous use of cheap non-proprietary (generic) drugs (penicillin, diazepam) to limited use of high-cost patented agents (some anticancer drugs). In the UK a family doctor prescribes drugs to an annual value of well above his earnings, i.e. collectively family doctors dispose of enormous resources and are visibly the objects of assiduous courtship by a hospitable pharmaceutical industry. Traditionally the doctor thinks only of his individual patients' needs. But the individual patient also wants a good general service, which cannot be provided if resources are squandered in any one area, e.g. overprescribing.

Increasing attention therefore, is now being given to economics in health care, including drug use. *Economics is the science of the distribution of resources*. There are three economic concepts that have particular importance to the thinking of every doctor who takes out his pen to prescribe, i.e. to distribute resources.

1. *Opportunity cost* means that which has to be sacrificed in order to carry out a certain course of action, i.e. costs are benefits foregone elsewhere — if money is spent on presribing that money is not available for another purpose; wasteful prescribing can be seen as an affront to those who are in serious need, e.g. institutionalised mentally

* Balint M et al. Treatment or diagnosis: a study of repeat prescriptions in general practice Lippincott: Tavistock, 1970.
† Harris C M. Br Med J 1980; 281:57.

retarded citizens who everywhere would benefit from increased resources.

2. *Cost-effectiveness analysis* is concerned with how to attain a given objective at least cost, e.g. prevention of postsurgical venous thromboembolism by heparin, warfarin, aspirin, external pneumatic compression; analysis includes cost of materials, of adverse effects, of any tests, of nursing and doctor time, etc.

3. *Cost-benefit analysis* is concerned with issues of whether (and to what extent) to pursue objectives and policies, it is thus a broader activity than cost-effectiveness analysis and has to concern itself with the quality as well as the quantity (duration) of life.

Some doctors in richer societies, unfamiliar with these concepts and feeling uneasily or resentfully that material values (prices) cannot or should not be placed on life and its quality, refuse to agree that economics can have a role in the practice of medicine, declaring that a doctor must do his best for each individual patient regardless of cost. We all wish this could be so, but it cannot be, and there are two replies to those who take up that position:

1. There is no society in the world where all can have medical care regardless of cost and

2. By their daily intuitive decision-taking doctors are directing resources to selected individuals and therefore necessarily depriving others of the opportunity to use these same resources for what may be their greater need.

The economists' objective is to ensure that needs are defined and that available resources are deployed according to priorities set by society, which has an interest in fairness between its members. The question is whether resources are to be distributed in accordance with unregulated power struggle between professionals and associations of patients and public pressure groups, all, no doubt, warmhearted towards deserving cases of one kind or another, but none able to see the whole scene. Or whether there is to be a planned evaluation that allows division of the resources on the basis of some visible attempt at fairness.

Resources spent, or wasted, on say, drugs or physiotherapy, are not available for other worthy purposes, such as the upgrading of institutions or the treatment of disease, whether or not it is self-induced (alcohol, tobacco, motor-cycles), or for heart transplants or rheumatism or diabetes mellitus.

But the enemies of cost-benefit appraisal have a valid point when they challenge the economists to show that *quality* of life can be measured. This challenge is now being met.

Everyone is familiar with the measurement of the benefit of treatment in saving or extending life, i.e. life expectancy: the measure is the *quantity* of life (in years). But it is evident that life may be extended and yet have a low *quality*, even to the point that it is not worth having. It is therefore useful to have a unit of health measurement that combines the *quantity* of life with its *quality* to allow individual and social decisions to be made on a sounder basis than mere intuition.

To meet this need there has been developed the *quality-adjusted-life-year* (QALY); estimations of years of life expectancy are modified according to estimations of quality of life.

*Quality of life has four dimensions**:

1. physical mobility
2. freedom from pain and distress
3. capacity for self-care
4. ability to engage in normal social interactions

The approach to measure it has been developed into a questionnaire, *measure of perceived (by the subject) health*†. This explores *the six areas that best reflect problems with health*: sleep, physical mobility, energy, pain, emotional reactions, and social isolation; and also investigates *the seven areas of daily life most often affected by health or its diminution*: paid employment, looking after the house, social life, home life, sex life, hobbies and interests, and holidays.

Already studies in which quality-of-life measures are included have been done in drug therapy of peptic ulcer‡ and rheumatism§, and the assessments are being refined to provide improved

* Williams A. In Smith G T, ed. Measuring the social benefits of medicine. London: Office of Health Economics, 1983.
† McEwen J. In Smith G T, ed. Measuring the social benefits of medicine. London: Office of Health Economics, 1983.
‡ Culyer A J et al. Soc Sci Med 1981; 15c:3.
§ Proceedings of the conference on outcome measures in rheumatological clinical trials. J Rheumatol 1982; 9:753.

assessment of the benefits and risks to the individual and to society of medicines.

15. Whether patients take prescribed medicines: patient compliance*

It might seem reasonable to assume that a patient given a prescription will obtain the medicine and actually consume it. The assumption would be wrong, for example approximately 7% of prescriptions issued in an English mining community† were never presented for dispensing. Where patients have to pay the full cost of a prescription this can have a simple economic explanation. But in this case the prescription charge in the National Health Service was modest and it was men aged 25–34 years who were least likely to present the prescription, whereas in the same community those of children and the old were nearly always presented. The reason suggested was that these relatively young men had to go to the doctor for a sickness certificate to claim National Insurance pay when unable to work, and that they considered the medical content of the consultation as irrelevant and rejected the offered medication. In other communities the rate of non-presentation of prescriptions has been estimated as 1–5%.

Further, having obtained the medicine, some 30–70% of patients do not accurately follow the prescriber's instructions or do not take it at all.

There are two major aspects of *patient compliance*:

1. *non-comprehension* of instructions, so that the patient *cannot* comply:
   (a) due to inadequacy of the doctor
   (b) due to inadequacy of the patient.
2. *comprehension* of instructions, but failure to carry them out.

The *major factors* established‡ as associated with non-compliance can be summarised:

Disease: psychiatric diagnosis
Regimen: complexity (more than two administrations per day), long duration
Source of medicine: time-wasting or inconvenient clinics
Doctor/patient relation: inadequate supervision; patient dissatisfaction with doctor, including the feeling he or she does not know the doctor well
Patient: inappropriate health beliefs, family instability
Adverse effects

Many investigations are somewhat contradictory of each other but other factors affecting compliance of mature and mentally normal people include a variety of psychosocial factors (including the patients' personality, social isolation, etc.), what patients think they have to gain (i.e. understanding of the seriousness of their condition) and whether the gain is immediate and obvious (e.g. peptic ulcer relapse) or remote (e.g. hyperlipidaemia) and whether they feel ill (e.g. acute infection) or well (e.g. moderate hypertension), the number of medicines to be taken concurrently, whether the instructions fit the daily routine, and the possession of stores of medicines previously used but now obsolete (these should be removed).

Level of intelligence and education are not, it seems, important factors in compliance.

The wide range of factors to be taken into account in special cases is illustrated by the use of a single dose of radioactive iodine to treat hyperthyroidism in patients likely to be non-compliant with continuous antithyroid medication (carbimazole). Since patients will inevitably become hypothyroid years hence due to the radioactive iodine, and will then have to take thyroxine daily for the rest of their lives, the problem of compliance is merely postponed, it is not eliminated.

The patient's relationship with the doctor, including the amount of supervision provided, is important. It has been found that if patients feel satisfied with the consultation, feel that they know and are known by the doctor, and the interviews are conducted in a friendly rather than in a business-like fashion, then he or she (there is no sex

* The term *compliance* has been objected to as having overtones of obsolete, arrogant attitudes, implying 'obedience' to doctors' 'orders'. But this seems oversensitive and the suggested alternative, *adherence*, does not have quite the right meaning. We retain *compliance* and point out that it applies also to doctors who do not follow prescribing instructions in official Data Sheets, etc. (Doctor compliance must, of course, precede *patient compliance* (see below).

† Waters W H R et al. Br Med J 1976; 1:1062.

‡ After Haynes R B Compliance with Therapeutic Regimens, *In* Sacket, Haynes, eds. Baltimore: Johns Hopkins University Press. 1976.

difference here) is more likely to comply with prescribing instructions. Unfortunately, in more that half of doctor-patient consultations patients do not overtly state their expectations, so that patient satisfaction will be highly dependent on the intuition, willingness to take time and even on the mood of the doctor, as well as on the interaction of the doctor's personality with that of the patient. Everyone knows that some patients dislike some or all doctors; it is also the case that some doctors dislike some, let us hope not all, patients; no doubt this should not be so, but it is.

Simple failure of comprehension and memory are also obviously important in complying with instructions and these are not helped by a general absence, in most patients, of even the most elementary concept of how the body works and of disease; 'Thus approximately 50% of a lay population will not be able to point to the general area of the kidneys, heart, stomach or lungs when presented with outline drawings of the body'. This is demonstrated from time to time on television shows and much laughter is generated by the grotesque concepts of anatomy revealed.

'Patients often have active misconceptions. Only about 10% of patients with peptic ulcer have a reasonably clear idea that acid is secreted by the stomach. Many think that it comes from the teeth when food is chewed, or from the brain when food is swallowed.'

'Another (misconception) is that medication can be discontinued as soon as the patient starts to feel better, a situation commonly seen when antibiotics have been prescribed.'* In one study of sore throat in children treated at home, penicillin by mouth was prescribed for 10 days. By the third day over half the children were no longer receiving the drug and by the sixth day nearly three-quarters had ceased to take it. It has been estimated that one-third of prescribed antibiotics are never taken.

Patients also are often diffident about asking nurses and doctors for explanations or repetitions when they are not clear or have forgotten. This is particularly important at first consultations when the patient may be told his diagnosis for the first time and it applies even where the patient shows no overt anxiety.

Patients should not be blamed for non-compliance where the prescriber has failed to give adequate instructions. Clear and repeated instructions using short words and supplemented by written matter (especially for the old) can greatly improve compliance, as can engaging the patient as an understanding participant in the management of his disease, e.g. high blood pressure, rather than as a simple recipient who is subject only to exhortation to do as he is told with threats of displeasure or disaster if he does not.

Studies of what patients remember of what the doctor has told them give results that will occasion no surprise. About one-third of patients have been found unable to recount instructions immediately on leaving the doctor's consulting room; brevity, clarity and repetition by the doctor improve patient recall. Proper labelling of the container supplied to the patient or special packaging (calendar packs for oral contraceptives) naturally also helps, as may pamphlets of standard written advice on management of chronic diseases, e.g. diabetes, hypertension.

It is unlikely that any patient will reliably take more than three drugs without special supervision.

What every patient needs to know†:

1. The *name* of the medicine.
2. The *objective*
   (a) to treat the *disease*
   (b) to relieve *symptoms*

i.e. how important the medicine is, whether the patient can judge its efficacy and *when* benefit can be expected to occur.

3. How and when to *take* the medicine.
4. Whether it matters if a dose is *missed* and what, if anything, to do about it.
5. How *long* the medicine is likely to be needed.
6. How to recognize *side-effects* and any action that should be taken, including effects on car driving.
7. Any *interaction* with alcohol or other medicines.

Note: It is plain that all this cannot be told to the patient briefly with any hope that it will be remembered; directions on the container, special packaging and other written matter will be useful

* Ley P. Prescribers Journal 1977; 17:15.

† After Drug and Ther Bull 1981; 19:73.

in addition to verbal instructions from doctor and pharmacist.

A remarkable instance of non-compliance with hoarding was that of a 71-year-old man who attempted suicide and was found to have in his home 46 bottles containing 10 685 tablets. Analysis of his prescriptions showed that over a period of 17 months he had been expected to take 27 tablets of several different kinds daily* (see *opportunity cost*).

Obviously small children, the old and mentally incapacitated patients cannot comply with instructions and family aid must be obtained. But evidence suggests that any psychiatric diagnosis (except perhaps an obsessional state) is likely to be associated with low compliance. Anecdotes circulate concerning the effect of psychotropic drugs on the vegetation in the grounds of psychiatric hospitals and one of the adverse effect of discarded drugs on the aerodynamic capacities of seagulls visiting a hospital in the UK.

Evaluation of compliance. Merely asking patients whether they have taken the drug as directed is not likely to provide reliable evidence.† The figures for non-compliance are based on studies that include interview, counting tablets that remain when the patient attends the doctor, blood or urine testing for the drug or a marker included in the tablet (e.g. riboflavin, phenol red) and measuring pharmacodynamic effect.

Of course undiscovered non-compliance can invalidate therapeutic trials.

In one study on compliance‡ 674 children with acute otitis media prescribed an oral antibiotic and a nasal decongestant for 10 days were studied. The first major non-compliance was the failure of 374 patients to return for review. Of the 300 who did return, the following was found:

86% of parents thought their child's illness moderate or severe

7% of children received the full course.

Treatment had stopped by the fourth day in over one third, especially in children of poorly educated or unmarried mothers

28% of children refused or vomited the medicine

3% had spilled the medicine or broken the bottle

20 had side-effects

Some pharmacists dispensed less than the full 10-days course (expecting parents to retun for the remainder)

Some labels were illegible or legible but incorrect

70% of parents used teaspoons with capacities varying from 2.5 to 9 ml

Doctors gave poorly memorable information, did not provide medicine for immediate use to cover the period until the prescription could be dispensed, and they prescribed in fractions of a spoonful (see *doctor compliance* below).

Successful drug therapy evidently comprises a great deal more than choosing the right drug.

16. Errors of prescribing: doctor compliance

It would be inappropriate to discuss the failings of patients to take prescribed drugs without reference to the errors of doctors in prescribing and other staff in administering drugs in hospital. Compliance is not a concept for patients alone; doctors have a *duty* to comply, i.e. not to be ignorant, to tell patients what they need to know, to warn (p. 16), and quite simply to recognize the importance of what they are doing; if doctors wrote cheques as badly as they commonly write prescriptions, they would soon be in trouble.

In one study in a university hospital,§ where standards might be expected to be high, of 7526 prescriptions written for 840 patients, there was an error of drug use (dose, frequency, route) in 3% of prescriptions and an error of prescription writing (in relation to standard hospital instructions) in 30%. In 79% of patients there was at least one error in prescription writing. Many errors were trivial, but many could have resulted in overdose, serious interaction or undertreatment.

In other hospital studies error rates in drug administration of 15% to 25% have been found, rates rising rapidly where four or more drugs are being given concurrently, as is so often the case; studies on hospital in-patients show that each

* Smith S E et al. Lancet 1974; 1:937.

† The way the patient is questioned may be all-important, e.g. 'were you able to take the tablets?' may get a truthful reply where, ' Did you take the tablets?' may not, because the latter question may be understood by the patient as implying personal criticism. (Pearson R M. Br. Med J 1982; 285:757.)

‡ Mattar M E et al. J Pediatr 1975; 87:137.

§ Tesh D E et al. Br J Clin Pharmacol 1975; 3:1057.

receives about six drugs, and up to 20 during a stay is not rare. Error rates can be reduced by well-planned hospital and ward practice.

It has been found that merely providing information (on antibiotics) did not influence prescribing, but gently asking physicians to justify their prescriptions caused a marked fall in prescribing.

17. Self-medication* and medicines in the home

To feel unwell is common, though the frequency varies with social and cultural circumstances, and it is both natural and desirable that people should care for themselves as far as is practicable, which includes medicating themselves.

People commonly experience symptoms or complaints and commonly want to take remedial action. In one study of adults randomly selected from a large population, nine out of ten had one or more complaints in the two weeks before interview; in another of premenopausal women a symptom occurred as often as one day in three; in both studies a medicine was taken for more than half these occurrences.

About one in 30–40 symptoms is taken to a doctor. Self-medication is not a substitute for visiting the doctor (though this has been commonly supposed and frequently asserted) and purchasers of these 'home medicines' visit their doctors as often as the rest of the population. It seems that the public is sensible enough to realize that doctors have little to contribute to many minor ills and, taking into account the natural reluctance to visit a doctor that sensible people feel, as well as the inconvenience, it is easily understandable that patients prefer 'do it yourself' (DIY), i.e. self-medication. The commonest symptoms experienced are 'undue' tiredness, pain (headache, backache), indigestion, 'nerves' and depression, and cough; medication is taken in anything from 40% to 70% of incidents.

The medicines most commonly purchased from pharmacies are analgesics, antacids, laxatives,† antitussives and expectorants. About 20% of purchases are for long-term use. Experience of adverse effects is low (8%) and knowledge of them is also low (8–20%). When purchasers are asked their reason for choosing a medicine they give first the user's own assessment of need closely followed by advice from pharmacist and doctor; promotion via the mass media is thought least influential (though advertisers might well claim that their skills are so subtle as to account for users thinking they are making their own judgement when they are not).

Half the purchasers of home medicines are aged above 65 years; some studies have found a marked preponderance (×4) of women purchasers; women experience more symptoms than men, but they may also more often be making purchases for others — spouses, old parents or children.

Self-medication is appropriate for:

1. short-term relief of symptoms, where
2. accurate diagnosis is unnecessary and for
3. the relief of mild cases of some chronic or recurrent diseases, e.g. eczema, with
4. drugs that have a large margin of safety.

In general modern drugs will only be deemed suitable for self-medication by direct sale to the public after prolonged and safe use as prescription-only medicines.

It is desirable that there be home prescribing or self-medication wherever medicines may be made available without unacceptable risk. The decision as to what risk is unacceptable should be made by level-headed members of the public in consultation with doctors. The fact that some accidents will happen and some abuses will occur is not a reason for refusing to consider enlarging the range of home remedies. Whether aspirin would, if it were now discovered, be considered suitable for general sale is certainly debatable; but despite the deaths and illness aspirin causes no-one now seriously advocates restricting it to a doctor's prescription only. It was undoubtedly right initially to restrict oral contraceptives to doctor's prescription, but now that so much is known about them many reasonable people experienced in the area consider that prescription could safely be widened to other health workers, though not

* See Anderson J A D. Self medication. Lancaster: MTP Press. 1979.

† Extensive use of laxatives indicates that patients/the public do *not* know best, and need advice.

at present to direct supply to the public for self-prescription.

But antibiotics should remain available only on a doctor's prescription, for indiscriminate use promotes the spread of drug-resistant bacteria so that infections become untreatable or treatable only with the less safe drugs. In addition some particularly serious bacterial infections, e.g. of the heart valves, are partially suppressed by casual use or wrong choice of antibiotic, so that accurate diagnosis is prevented or delayed until fatal damage has been done by the smouldering infection.

In the UK, a survey* has shown that 99% of a sample of homes contained one or more medicines. The average number of items was 10.3 (3 doctor-prescribed, 7.3 non-prescribed); nearly all had some kind of analgesic and skin cream; one-fifth had sedatives, tranquillisers or sleeping tablets and two-fifths had one or more items that the informant could not identify. In only two of 686 homes were any medicines locked up; medicines were most commonly kept in the kitchen.

From time to time there are campaigns† to collect all unwanted drugs from homes in an area. Usually the public are asked to deliver the drugs to their local pharmacies. In one UK city of 600 000 population, 500 000 'solid dose units' (tablets, capsules, etc.) were handed in. In another of about one million population about one million solid dose units were recovered. Liquid preparations were not accurately measured but over 450 litres were returned. The organisers of the second study thought the amounts would have been larger if there had been better organisation. It should be remembered that these are preparations that are unwanted in the sense that the owners no longer feel any need to keep them; they are not the whole medicine store of the households.

GUIDE TO FURTHER READING

1 Editorial. The real world of drug prescribing. Lancet 1979; 2:781.
2 Editorial. The right to prescribe. Lancet 1976; 2:352.
3 Grant G B et al. Development of a limited formulary for general practice. Lancet 1985; 1:1030.
4 Michel J-M. Why do people like medicines? A perspective from Africa. Lancet 1985; 1:210.
5 D'Arcy P F. Essential medicines in the third world. Br Med J 1984; 289:982.
6 Andrews G. On the promotion of non-drug treatment. Br Med J 1984; 289:994.
7 Melmon K L et al. The undereducated physician's therapeutic decisions. N Engl J Med 1983; 308:1473.
8 Gosney M et al. Prescription of contraindicated and interacting drugs in elderly patients admitted to hospital. Lancet 1984; 2:564.
9 Myers E D et al. Information, compliance and side-effects: a study of patients on antidepressant medication. Br J Clin Pharmacol 1984; 17:21.
10 Schaffner W et al. Improving antibiotic prescribing in office practice. A controlled trial of three educational methods. JAMA 1983; 250:1728.
11 Fox W. Compliance of patients and physicians: experience and lessons from tuberculosis. Br Med J 1983; 287: 33, 101.
12 Drury V W M. Patient information leaflets. Br Med J 1984; 288:427.
13 Skegg D C G et al. Use of medicines in general practice. Br Med J, 1977; 1:1561.
14 Steel K et al. Iatrogenic illness on a general medical service at a university hospital. N Engl J Med 1981; 304:638.
15 Laporte J-R et al. Drug utilisation studies: a tool for determining the effectiveness of drug use. Br J Clin Pharmacol 1983; 16:301.
16 Diamond A L et al. Product liability in respect of drugs. Br Med J 1985; 290:365.
17 Roberts C J et al. How much can the National Health Service afford to spend to save a life or avoid a severe disability. Lancet 1985; 1:89.
18 Freireich E J. Can we afford to treat leukaemia? N Engl J Med 1980; 302:1084.
19 Shapiro M et al. Benefit-cost analysis of antimicrobial prophylaxis in abdominal and vaginal hysterectomy. JAMA 1983; 249:1290.
20 Mooney G H et al. What is economics? Br Med J 1982 285:949, 1024.
21 Drummond M G et al. Assessing the costs and benefits of treatment alternatives. Br Med J 1982; 285: 1561, 1638.
22 Reilly D et al. Is homoeopathy a placebo response? Controlled trial of homoeopathic potency, with pollen in hay fever as a model. Lancet 1986; 2:881, and subsequent correspondence, p. 1106.
23 Smith T. Alternative medicine. Br Med J 1983; 987:307.
24 Editorial. Alternative medicine is no alternative. Lancet 1983; 2:773.
25 Skrabanek P. Acupuncture and the age of unreason. Lancet 1984; 1:1169.
26 Lieter J. Current controversy on alternative medicine. N Engl J Med 1983; 309:1524.
27 Gillon R. Justice and allocation of medical resources. Br Med J 1985; 291:266.
28 Editorial. The trial of homoeopathy. Lancet 1983; 1:108.

* Dunnel, K., Cartwright, A. (1972) Medicine takers prescribers and hoarders. London: Routledge Kegan Paul.
† DUMP: Disposal of Unwanted Medicines and Poisons

2

Clinical pharmacology

It is only over the past 70 years or so in Britain and 90 years on parts of the European mainland and North America that the manifest need to make a special study of the biological effects of the rapidly increasing number of potential drugs made by organic chemists has led substantial numbers of research workers to devote themselves to pharmacology. So important has this work become that departments of pharmacology have long ago ceased to be subdivisions of physiology, and pharmacology has become an independent discipline with its own attitudes and techniques.

This has been followed by what has aptly been called the 'drug explosion' of the past 40 years*. The eruption into therapeutics of thousands of new drugs, as well as a general 'information explosion' in medicine, has called into being workers specialising in **scientific study of drugs in man** or **clinical pharmacology**. The subject is increasingly recognised as both a health care and an academic speciality, indeed no medical school can be considered complete without a department or sub-department of Clinical Pharmacology.

The clinical pharmacologist's work is to provide facts and opinions that are useful for optimising the treatment of patients, and therapeutic success with drugs is becoming more and more dependent on the user having a technical knowledge of both pharmacodynamics and pharmacokinetics; a humane and caring doctor cannot dispense with technical skill.

Clinical pharmacology comprises two major parts:

* Modell W. Clin Pharmacol Ther 1961; 2:1.

1. **Pharmacology:**
   (a) *pharmacodynamics*: investigation of *how* drugs, alone and in combination, affect the body (young, old, well, sick);
   (b) *pharmacokinetics*: absorption, distribution, metabolism, excretion or how the body, well or sick, affects drugs.
2. **Therapeutic evaluation**: *whether* a drug is of value and *how* it may best be used:
   (a) *formal therapeutic trials*
   (b) *surveillance studies* for both efficacy and adverse effects.

In addition clinical pharmacologists engage in various other activities related to these two main areas, e.g. prescribing systems, cost-benefit analysis, official drug regulation, etc.

Work in these categories has long been done well by clinical scientists and physicians, but has largely resulted from the chance availability of a drug having particular interest for them; it has not been systematic. The magnitude of the need for clinical pharmacology, as shown by the disagreements on when and how to use many drugs (tranquillisers; adrenal steroids) and their safety in relation to their benefits (drugs in pregnancy; antidepressants) now demands the full-time attention of clinical workers, whether or not they care to call themselves clinical pharmacologists. All that is needed in addition to training in medicine and pharmacology is 'enthusiasm, stemming from the knowledge that through the study of drugs, medicine can be changed even more in the next fifty years than it has been in the past fifty' (H F Dowling).

In 1934 the advent of clinical pharmacology was foreshadowed by Sir Thomas Lewis*, one of the founders of modern clinical science, when he wrote of the early investigations of quinidine 'these problems were attacked simultaneously, and almost exclusively by *clinicians, many of whom, while studying the therapeutic effects, became at the same time their own pharmacologists*. Thus from the first the work was co-ordinated and the various problems were quickly solved.'

If it is desired to single out a pioneer clinical pharmacologist it would surely be Harry Gold (1899–1972) of Cornell University, USA, whose influential studies in the 1930s showed us how to be clinical pharmacologists. In 1952 he wrote a seminal article, '*The proper study of mankind is man*'†, which deserves re-reading. He writes, 'a special kind of investigator is required, one whose training has equipped him not only with the principles and technics of laboratory pharmacology but also with knowledge of clinical medicine . . .'

Clinical scientists of all kinds do not differ fundamentally from other biologists, they are set apart only to the extent that there are special difficulties and limitations, ethical and practical, in seeking knowledge from man. Many clinical problems can best be tackled by using animals to fill in the inevitable gaps resulting from the exigencies of clinical practice. 'Clinical science has the long established right to wander unimpeded into any branch of medical science in search of information directly relevant to the problems of human disease. These excursions into animal physiology, pharmacology, and into all branches of general pathology, are not only legitimate, they are also quite necessary', for 'the worker in the allied science is rarely so aware of the precise need of clinical science as is the worker in this field'.

'It is essential that those who in studying human patients perceive opportunities for putting questions to the test of animal experimentation should themselves engage in such work; that correlation should not be left to the chance meeting and union of clinical and laboratory studies.' Again, writing on his classic investigations into atrial fibrillation, Lewis made the point that the clinical scientist, trying to elucidate a human problem, should not hesitate to pass from one field to another — 'the observations began with man; animal experimentation was called in aid; it led to further investigations in man . . .'*.

Pharmacology is the same science whether it is animal or man that is investigated. The need for it grows rapidly as not only scientists but now the whole community can see its promise of release from distress and death over yet wider fields. The concomitant dangers of drugs (fetal deformities, adverse reactions, dependence) only add to the need for the effective and ethical application of science to drug invention, evaluation, and use.

* Lewis T. Clinical science. London: Shaw, 1934.
† Gold H. Am J Med 1952; 12:619.
The quotation is from *An Essay on Man* by Alexander Pope (1688–1744); the whole passage is relevant to modern clinical pharmacology and drug therapy.

Know then thyself, presume not God to scan,
The proper study of mankind is man,
Placed on this isthmus of a middle state,
A being darkly wise, and rudely great:
With too much knowledge for the sceptic side,
With too much weakness for the stoic's pride,
He hangs between; in doubt to act or rest;
In doubt to deem himself a god or beast;
In doubt his mind or body to prefer;
Born but to die, and reas'ning but to err;
Alike in ignorance, his reason such,
Whether he thinks too little or too much;
Chaos of thought and passion, all confused;
Still by himself abused, or disabused;
Created half to rise, and half to fall;
Great lord of all things, yet a prey to all;
Sole judge of truth, in endless error hurled;
The Glory, jest and riddle of the world!

GUIDE TO FURTHER READING

1 Modell W. The drug explosion. Clin Pharmacol Ther 1961; 2:1.
2 Gold H. 'The proper study of mankind is man.' Am J Med 1952; 12:619.
3 Laurence D R. Clinical pharmacology. Lancet 1964; 1:1173.
4 Lasagna L. The role of a division of clinical pharmacology in a university environment. Postgrad Med 1961; 29:525.
5 Gaddum J H. Clinical Pharmacology. Proc Roy Soc Med 1954; 47:195.
6 Modell W et al. Special subcommittee report. Commission on Drug Safety, USA. On position and status of the clinical pharmacologist in drug research. Clin Pharmacol Ther 1964; 5:226.
7 Lewis T. Clinical science. Shaw: London, 1934.
8 Dollery C T. Clinical pharmacology. Lancet, 1966; 1:359.
9 Prichard B N C et al. Clinical pharmacology: function, organization, and training. Lancet 1971; 2:653.
10 World Health Organization. Clinical pharmacology, scope, organization, training. WHO Tech Rep Ser 1970; 446.
11 Davies D M. Clinical pharmacology in a district general hospital. Lancet 1976; 1:1063.
12 Smith A et al. Clinical pharmacology clinics in general practice. Br Med J 1977; 2:169.
13 Conference. Geographic determinants in clinical pharmacology. Clin Pharmacol Ther 1976; 19: 605–724.
14 Crooks J. Drug epidemiology and clinical pharmacology. Their contribution to patient care. Br J Clin Pharmacol 1983; 16:351.
15 Atkinson A J et al. University and pharmaceutical industry co-operation: the need to plan for the future. Clin Pharmacol Ther 1984; 35:431
16 Fraser H S Clinical pharmacology in developing countries. Br J Clin Pharmacol 1981; 11:457.
17 Alvan G et al. Problem-oriented drug information: a clinical pharmacological service. Lancet 1983; 2:1410.
18 Shirkey H C. Clinical pharmacology in pediatrics. Clin Pharmacol Ther 1972; 13:827.
19 Vesell E S. Clinical pharmacology: a personal perspective. Clin Pharmacol Ther 1985; 38:603.
20 Hassar M et al. Free-living volunteers' motivations and attitudes toward pharmacologic studies in man. Clin Pharmacol Ther 1977; 21:515.
21 Anglo-American Workshop on Clinical Pharmacology. Present status and future directions of clinical pharmacology. Clin Pharmacol Ther 1986; 39: 435–480.

3

Discovery and development of drugs

More and more doctors are playing a role in evaluation of new drugs, and those that are not are faced with the problems of whether to prescribe them, or they meet patients taking them. It is, therefore, not only of some interest, but it is desirable that all doctors should have a general knowledge of the process of drug discovery in an industry that actively seeks to influence what they do, that delivers enormous benefits, but which is also subject to rising criticism of its role in medicine and society. When making criticisms it should be borne in mind that the pharmaceutical industry is also heavily regulated by governments acting on behalf of society and that the official regulators play a decisive role in deciding what shall and what shall not be made available for general prescribing and the therapeutic claims that a manufacturer may make.

It will be obvious from the account that follows that drug development is an extremely arduous, highly technical and enormously expensive operation. Successful developments (<1% of compounds that go into test eventually become licenced medicines) must carry the cost of the failures (>99%).* It is also obvious that such programmes are likely to be carried to completion only when the organisations and the individuals within them are motivated overall by the challenge to succeed, to serve society and to make money (no doubt these motives are present to varying degrees in the various sections — business, administrative, scientific, manufacturing — that go to make up a research-based company). Indeed, these three incentives operate generally in society, including doctors and journalists.

There are innumerable complex and potentially useful, as well as harmful, substances found in nature, made by animals, plants, bacteria and fungi. Some are themselves useful medicines, others can be used as a starting point by the synthetic chemist, but most new drugs are now synthetic chemicals.

Until the end of the 19th century the discovery of drugs was entirely a matter of chance and serendipity. Paul Ehrlich (1854–1915) put an end to this by developing the idea and the scientific basis for selective toxicity.

The whole business of drug development rests on biological *selectivity* and *prediction* of this in man.

Pharmacology in drug development

Most new drugs are developed in industrial rather than in academic laboratories. These two kinds of laboratory are complementary, having important, though different, approaches, the 'organised opportunism' of the industrial and the 'knowledge for its own sake' of the academic laboratory. The academic workers are often fired with interest to use the discoveries of the industrial scientists as tools to explore fundamental mechanisms and indeed industrial discoveries make a major contribution to basic pharmacology as their mechanism

* One substantial research-based company (Janssen) made, over 32 years (1953–85), approximately 70 000 new molecules of which, in 1985, 50 were in use as human and 14 as veterinary medicines; 5 as antimycotics for plants; and one for wood protection. The company's biological screening system was capable of making 'go or no-go' decisions at a rate of 25 new molecules per working day, i.e. up to 5000 per year (Dr Paul Janssen, personal communication, 1985).

Medicinal drugs produced by this company include, diphenoxylate, loperamide, domperidone, ketanserin, haloperidol, dextromoramide, cinnarizine, miconazole, and mebendazole.

of action is probed and defined, e.g. aspirin, cimetidine. The rational development of new drugs by industry is easier when the fundamental biochemical nature of normal and diseased processes, more widely, though not exclusively, studied in academic laboratories, is understood; for example, the development of histamine receptor blockers depended on knowledge that histamine was released in the body and was a mediator in urticaria, hay fever and normal gastric acid secretion; the efficacy of allopurinol in gout could be predicted from knowledge of the path of synthesis of uric acid in the body. A cure for human cancer is more likely to be found if details of the biochemistry of malignant and normal cells are known than it is by empirically testing tens of thousands of chemicals selected at random or because they are related to existing relatively unselective and inefficient anticancer drugs. Drugs are tested in animals in which cancer has been artificially induced or which have been bred to have a high incidence of the disease, as well as in tissue culture (though cells in tissue culture develop new characteristics).

'The most frequent purpose of research in the drug industry can be stated simply; it is to discover profitable drugs. For a drug to be profitable it should be both useful and safe, properties that are evaluated eventually by the clinician. The task of the pharmacologist is to predict these properties from animal experiments, within the limitations imposed by availability of facilities and staff. This must be done in such a way that the possibility of missing a useful drug is minimised; in other words, the 'screening' programme must be efficient'.*†

The greatest difficulties for the laboratory pharmacologist lie in designing his animal experiments to yield the maximum information from a relatively few animals and to be relevant to human physiology and disease. It is, for example, particularly difficult to design animal experiments to test drugs for their possible efficacy in human mental disorders, but relatively easy to test them for anticoagulant effects because animal and human blood clots by similar mechanisms and because measurement of clotting is easy.

At long last it is now possible to claim that drugs may actually be *designed* and *purpose made* reasonably frequently. There are *four principal approaches* to drug discovery:

1. *Synthesis of analogues or antagonists of natural hormone, autacoid or transmitter substances, or of molecules that modify understood biochemical processes* may create real novelty in therapeutics, e.g. histamine H_2-receptor blocking drugs, dopamine agonists and antagonists, calcium channel blockers, and prostaglandins. The successes of this approach provide strong arguments for society to support research in the basic medical sciences, for to know how the body works normally and how it goes wrong (disease) allows rationally planned interference for the health and happiness of mankind (the fact that well-meant attempts can go badly wrong provides an argument for more and better science, not for giving up and stopping research).

2. *Modification of the structures of a known drug* is obviously likely to produce more agents with similar properties or only minor differences, and this is much complained of ('me-too' or 'me-again' drugs). *But* molecular design is now so sophisticated that it is possible to take a molecule and eliminate one or more actions and enhance another to produce novel results, e.g. sulphonamides (antimicrobials), sulphonylureas (antidiabetics), thiazides (diuretics), acetazolamide (carbonic anhydrase inhibition for glaucoma), which are all derived from the first sulphonamides synthesised in the early 1930s.

3. *Random screening.* When completely novel chemicals are made and unfamiliar substances isolated from natural sources there is a case for screening them in a battery of animal tests designed to detect 'interesting' effects. Such screening is now highly sophisticated.

4. *Discovery of new uses for drugs already in general use* as a result of intelligent observation and serendipity, e.g. β-adrenoceptor block for hypertension, aspirin for antithrombotic effect.

The process of new drug development‡ may

* Vane J R. In: Laurence D R, Bacharach AL, eds. *Evaluation of Drug Activities*. London: Academic Press, 1963.

† It has been remarked that drug developers seek to make 'forgeries' to 'deceive' the body, and there is truth in this.

‡ Based on regulatory guidelines in the UK, but they are broadly similar worldwide.

be summarized as follows:

A. **Idea** or *hypothesis*

B. **Synthesis** of substances

C. **Studies in animals*** of:

1. *Pharmacology*

a. The action relevant to the proposed therapeutic use.

b. Other actions: classified according to the principal physiological systems.

c. Interaction with other drugs as far as is relevant to the proposed use, i.e. drugs that are likely to be given concurrently (this can be delayed to a late stage).

d. Pharmacokinetics: it is clearly not possible to design satisfactory toxicology studies without knowledge of pharamacokinetics in the species to be used.

2. *Toxicology*

a. *Single dose studies* (acute toxicity).

b. *Repeated dose studies*: (subacute, intermediate and chronic or long-term toxicology).

c. *General*

(i) at least two mammalian species are used (only one being a rodent).

(ii) at least two different routes of administration, one being the route proposed for use in man.

(iii) signs of toxicity should be revealed and the mode of death and organs injured (target organs) determined, i.e. it is not sufficient to state that, 'at *x* times the proposed human dose no injury occurred'.

d. Duration of repeated-dose studies:

Intended duration of use in man	*Duration of studies in animals*
Single dose (or several doses on one day)	14 days
up to 10 days	28 days
up to 30 days	90 days
beyond 30 days	180 days

e. *Repeated dose* animal studies are generally divided into two: *short-term* (2–4 weeks), which provide information for designing the *long-term* studies.

(i) Three doses are used: the lowest approximating to the proposed therapeutic dose in man, the highest to produce recognizable toxicity, and one in between.

(ii) If the drug is a pro-drug (i.e. it is inert and requires to be metabolised into active form) then this conversion must be demonstrated to occur in each animal species used.

(iii) Dosing must (obviously) be done on seven days a week. But this has not, in the past, been obvious to some companies who have conveniently assumed that the human five-day working week will be also recognized by the animals as providing continuous exposure.

(iv) Monitoring of animals should include: food consumption, body weight, behaviour and condition, haematology, biochemistry and urinalysis (for organ function); plus other monitoring as appropriate to the particular drug or its use, e.g. eye.

(v) All animals that die during the test should be autoposied (cannibalism must be prevented as it destroys potentially valuable evidence).

(vi) On completion of the test the animals are killed ('sacrificed') and extensive histological studies are done. The list (UK) of tissues to be examined contains 30 items.

(vii) There are exceptions to most or all of the above, e.g. the therapeutic effect (hypoglycaemia) may make high-dose studies impracticable; target organ toxicity also may not be attainable.

3. *Special toxicology*

a. *Mutagenicity*. A bacterial mutagenicity test demonstrates the induction of point mutations (base-pair changes and frame-shift mutations). This is always required. It is not sufficient to apply the drug to bacteria *in vitro* since metabolites that will be formed in animals or man are absent. Tests involving animals (e.g. intraperitoneal injection of bacteria) are required.

b. *Definitive carcinogenicity tests* are not required prior to the early studies in man unless there is serious reason to be suspicious of the drug, e.g. the mutagenicity test is unsatisfactory; the structure, including likely metabolites in man, gives rise to suspicion; or the histopathology in repeated-dose animal studies is suspicious.

Full scale (most of the animals' life) carcinogenicity tests will generally only be required if the drug is to be given to man for above one year.

Carcinogenicity (oncogenicity) studies comprise:

* Mouse, rat, hamster, guinea pig, rabbit, cat, dog, monkey. Not all are used for any one drug.

(i) two animal species having known low incidence of spontaneous tumours.

(ii) metabolic data for the drug are required

(iii) 3 dose levels: *high* — chosen to produce minimum toxic effect; *low* — 2–3 times therapeutic (pharmacologically effective) dose in the animal; *intermediate* — geometric mean of high and low doses.

(iv) *Duration*: rat: 24 months administration (plus six months for the evaluation); mouse, hamster: 18 months, i.e. most of animal's life. (The animals become extremely valuable as the test progresses for if they are wiped out by epidemic infection or muddled up, the safety programme may be set back by years.)

(v) At conclusion of the test: the (UK) guidelines list 30 tissues to be examined histologically, but remark that the list is not comprehensive and intelligent account should be taken of any special circumstances.

(vi) *Definition*. 'A neoplasm (tumour) is regarded as a population of abnormal cells with uncontrolled and usually increased proliferative activity and other less well defined morphological and functional features. With the exception of virus-induced neoplasms they are independent of the continued presence of the inciting agent(s).' 'A malignant neoplasm is one which invades surrounding tissues and/or metastasises.'

(vii) *Interpretation of the results*. 'The strongest evidence that a compound is a carcinogenic hazard for man is epidemiological. Although most known human carcinogens are found to be carcinogenic for experimental animals, there is no evidence that all substances which are carcinogenic for animals are also carcinogenic for man.'

'Extrapolation to man is a difficult, sometimes arbitrary procedure. . .'

'The likelihood of a carcinogenic risk in man is increased if there is a high yield of malignant tumours involving a specific tissue when the test animal is given the test substance, by the route to be used in man, at a dosage equal to or lower than that which induces minimal toxicity. In other circumstances, the agent may be regarded as a weak carcinogen and the risk may more easily be reconciled with benefits associated with the therapeutic use of the compound.'

(viii) Short-term reliably predictive carcinogenicity tests are much needed not only because they would be cheaper but because they could easily be done before a compound is given to man, however, 'available techniques involving short-term testing of chemicals for mutagenicity/transformation are not at present capable of replacing formal carcinogenicity testing in animals as a means of evaluating a drug's carcinogenic potential. Short-term studies giving positive results will always indicate the need for formal carcinogenicity studies; those giving negative results do no preclude the need for formal studies where these are indicated.'

It may be asked why any novel compound should be given to man before full-scale formal carcinogenicity studies are completed. The answers are that animal tests are uncertain predictors (above), that such a requirement would make socially desirable drug development expensive to a seriously damaging degree, or might even cause novel ventures to cease. This would be caused by delay and the cost of the greatly increased number of tests that would have to be done on compounds that are eventually abandoned for other reasons. This may seem right or wrong, but it is how things are at present.

c. *Reproduction* studies are conducted to detect:

— damage to male and female gametes
— effects on intra-uterine homeostasis
— embryogenesis
— toxic effect on the fetus
— effects on maternal metabolism damaging to the fetus
— effects on uterine growth and development
— effects on parturition
— effects on post-natal development, suckling of the young and maternal lactation
— late effects on the progeny, e.g. behaviour, fertility.
— second generation effects

Some of the above investigations use a minimum of two animal species (embryotoxicity) and some (fertility, perinatal) one species.

Three dose levels are ordinarily used.

Pharmacokinetic studies should be done in pregnant animals and drug concentrations should be measured in both mother and fetus.

Autopsy and histological examination is conducted. This is a *major* laboratory exercise.

*Ethics of using animals in drug development**

No one will read the above scheme with satisfaction and some will read it with disgust. Many tests in drug development are done on anaesthetised animals and many on isolated organs of animals killed 'humanely'. But there is at present no substitute for the whole animal with intact integrated physiological systems and capable of forming the often biologically active metabolites of drugs. It cannot be seriously doubted that, especially in toxicology testing, a lot of suffering is caused.

All this would be totally unjustified if results useful to man could not be obtained. In many known respects animals are similar to man, but in many respects they are not.

It would be hypocritical for a society that tolerates first the mutilation (e.g. castration) and later, after short confined lives, the killing of animals for food — let alone chasing them about the field to their death (or escape) or driving them towards lines of gunmen for recreation — to shrink from employing them for maintaining health and life in other ways. At present, in order to begin to decide whether a chemical is a medicine or merely a chemical, either animal experiments (involving whole animals or animal tissues) must be done, or substances of almost totally unknown biological effect must be given to man. Failing either of these, drug therapy must cease to advance. We prefer, though we regret, the first course.

As knowledge of basic mechanisms advances, *in vitro* biochemical preparations and tissue cultures may one day allow prediction of what effect a drug will have in intact man, and whole animals will not be necessary. This time is a long way off for cells in tissue culture develop characteristics, e.g. new receptors, that they did not have when subject to the control mechanisms of the body. However, we welcome research designed to reduce the need to use animals.

* An admirable discussion of the issues will be found in Paton W. Man and mouse. London: Oxford, 1984.

Animals are also used to test cosmetics, food additives, such as preservatives which are necessary to allow food to be supplied in big cities, as well as colouring, which is unnecessary, and chemicals used in industry, etc. Plainly these activities all pose ethical problems.

General discussion

It is frequently pointed out that regulatory guidelines are not rigid requirements to be universally applied. But whatever the intention, they do tend to be treated as minimum requirements if only because research directors fear to risk holding up their expensive co-ordinated programmes with disagreements that result in their having to go back to the laboratory, with consequent delay and financial loss.

Knowledge of the *mode of action* of a potential new drug obviously greatly enhances prediction from animal studies of what will happen in man. Whenever practicable such knowledge should be obtained; sometimes this is quite easy, but sometimes it is impossible. Many drugs have been introduced safely without such knowledge, the later acquisition of which has not always made an important difference to their use (e.g. antibiotics, hormones for replacement). The mode of action of drugs in many areas remains obscure (e.g. psychiatry), and any requirement that it be defined before exploratory clinical use could delay valuable therapeutic advance.

But in many areas, a lot that is relevant to prediction can be discovered, and so should be required before clinical trial (e.g. antihypertensives, anticoagulants, β-adrenoceptor blocking drugs). In the development of new drugs, there can be no general invariable rule. But failure to take this matter seriously can lead to disaster, e.g. a drug may lower the plasma lipids, but if this is at a late stage of synthesis, it may be at the cost of accumulation of precursors that may themselves be damaging. On the other hand, to refuse to allow clinical investigation of a potential antiepileptic, antipsychotic, anaesthetic or antibiotic where the developer had found himself unable to define the detailed mode of action would be perverse.

The pharmacological studies are integrated with those of the toxicologist to build up a picture of the undesired as well as of the desired drug effects. Some information on toxicity will generally have been got during the initial pharmacological testing, and this is extended by the toxicologist's special investigations.

Initial pharmacological testing comprises examination of the effects of graded single doses, but chronic studies with regular dosage for days or weeks are sometimes needed, for there are drugs that, as well as acutely altering some bodily functions, also change others more slowly (e.g. some tranquillisers and drugs for hypertension; oral contraceptives), and many drugs are now given to man for years.

Generally, in *pharmacological testing* the investigators know what they are looking for and choose the experiments to gain their objectives.

But in *toxicological testing* the investigators have less clear ideas of what they are looking for; they are screening for risk and certain major routines must be done. Toxicity testing is liable to become mindless routine to meet regulatory requirements to a greater extent than are the pharmacological studies.

All drugs are poisons and the task of the toxicologist is to find out how a compound acts as a poison to animals, often using very high doses, and to give an opinion on the significance of his data in relation to risks likely to be run by human beings receiving the drug at much lower doses. This will remain a nearly impossible task until biochemical explanations of all effects can be provided. The toxicologist is in an unenviable position. When a useful drug is safely introduced he is considered to have done no more than his duty. When an accident occurs he is invited to explain how this failure of prediction came about. When he predicts that a chemical is unsafe in a major way for man, his prediction is never tested.

Acute toxicity tests are performed to determine the adverse effects of increasing single doses and how death is caused. They are also used to establish what is unsuitably called the *therapeutic index* or ratio. This concept was devised by Ehrlich as: maximum tolerated dose ÷ minimum curative dose, to give some indication of the safety of antimicrobial drugs. In clinical practice the index is never calculated, for the data are not available in a suitable form, especially for drugs used over long periods. However, the concept embodies a sensible way of thinking about drugs, i.e. safety in relation to efficacy.

In a drug development laboratory practical use can be made of a modification of this concept provided it is recognised that, as with all animal data, it cannot be arbitrarily transferred to man. The *therapeutic index for animals* is nowadays calculated as: plasma concentration causing adverse effect ÷ plasma concentration causing therapeutic effect. The objective is to get some notion of benefit: risk ratio.

But it is more important to discover *how* the compound acts as a poison and this may need microscopical and biochemical studies with repeated or chronic administration.

Short-term (subacute) and long-term (chronic) toxicity tests are performed to determine the effects of exposing animals to a range of doses (usually three) of the drug over periods between one week and the lifetime of the animals, generally rats and dogs, and whether the effects are reversible or irreversible. Except for testing for oncogenesis, little is generally gained by exceeding six months' daily administration by the route that will be used in man. Duration of the tests and their exact nature will differ widely according to whether a drug may be given once or a few times (e.g. general anaesthetic) or continuously for years (e.g. antiepileptic).

Species differences between animals, and between animals and man, are a source of problems of interpretation. Perhaps the most famous species difference is the lethal bleeding from the intestine of guinea pigs following penicillin administration (due to an effect on the gut bacteria on which obligatory vegetarian species rely to break down cellulose) and its almost negligible toxicity to non-herbivores, including man.

Fortunately such differences of the effect of a drug on the body (pharmacodynamics) are less common than are differences in the effect of the body on a drug (pharmacokinetics), but gross differences in rate or path of metabolism may make nonsense of chronic toxicity studies undertaken to predict toxicity to man, as may unanticipated environmental influences, e.g. drug metabolising enzyme induction due to insecticide used routinely in an animal house for pest control.

It is clear that many common unwanted effects that limit the use of a drug in man cannot be predicted from animals, e.g. malaise and many cardiovascular and central nervous system symptoms. Nor, at present, can allergic reactions, e.g. some blood disorders and urticaria.

Special toxicology. There are three additional areas in which a drug accident might occur on a substantial scale. All are concerned with the interaction of the drug with genetic material or its expression in cell division (reproduction, mutagenesis, oncogenesis).

In all three areas there is particular concern because the effect may be delayed and hard to recognise at an early stage and may be the same as natural disease so that it is particularly difficult reliably to identify its cause.

1. *Reproduction, including fertility and teratogenesis* (teratos = monster: genesis = production). An accident in this area has already happened with thalidomide. The thalidomide disaster was dramatic, i.e. there was an epidemic of rare, gross and consistent abnormality with the result that it was soon realised that something new was happening, a cause was sought and comparatively easily found.

But lesser, though serious, abnormalities, especially if diverse in kind, could occur on a much larger scale before it was recognised that anything new or unusual was happening.

Increasingly, national registers of birth defects are being kept so that changes in incidence of abnormalities may be detected at an early stage. But these depend on easy recognition of the abnormality at or near birth and on reliable information on drug consumption of the mother. A drug or other environmental factor, e.g. virus, could cause a drop in intelligence without this being noticed by any existing monitoring system.

For detection to be at all easy, positive suspicion must be aroused as in the case of thalidomide (dramatic abnormality); or of smoking (always suspect) by mothers during pregnancy; investigations suggest that smoking mothers have more still births and smaller babies, perhaps of slower development and lower intelligence. Another drug could be having effects of this kind in the community and remain unsuspected for a long time; indeed, unless its use was extremely common in women of reproductive capacity, an effect might well never be detected.

Extensive testing of new drugs in pregnant animals has been mandatory since the thalidomide disaster. At first, administration of the drug in early pregnancy in two animal species was thought sufficient. But now animal tests are much more extensive. How far such tests, especially when giving positive results only at high dose, provide genuine prediction and so protection for humanity remains uncertain. But as a consequence of thalidomide no new drug now reaches the market without such testing.

This problem of predicting from animal experiments what new substances will cause fetal damage in man, when there is not even a reliable list of existing drugs that have the effect in man to provide a guide to devising animal tests, will be neither easily nor soon solved. Two illustrations suffice — it has been found that salicylates are teratogenic in rats and that this effect is enhanced if the pregnant animals are immobilised. There is no reason to believe salicylates to be seriously teratogenic in man at present, though aspirin is not clear of suspicion. Some adrenal steroids are highly teratogenic in rabbits, but do not appear to be so in man.

2. *Mutagenesis*. Drugs may cause abnormalities of genetic material (genes, chromosomes) of cells so that a permanent change in the hereditary constitution (mutation) occurs.

When a mutation occurs in reproductive cells (spermatozoa, ova) then a hereditary defect occurs. This defect may appear in the first generation progeny of the individual, or it may be of a recessive kind that will only become evident if two individuals affected by the chemical mutagen mate. Thus the effect of a mutagenic drug might not appear for months or even years. The longer the interval the more difficult attribution of the true cause is likely to be.

Where a mutation occurs in somatic (non-reproductive) cells, then these tissues, e.g. bone marrow cells, may develop abnormal characteristics and become malignant (cancer); in the case of the bone marrow this is leukaemia. In this area of risk too, it can be difficult to establish a causal association with the drug, which may have been taken and then stopped a long time previously; there is some hope of doing so where an effect is dramatic in frequency or in kind, but where there is merely a moderate increase in the incidence of a common condition then there is little prospect of detecting it and finding the cause.

Epidemiological rather than experimental laboratory techniques are required to determine what *is* happening in man rather than what *might* be happening. Medical record-linkage schemes are being developed so that it will become possible, for example, to examine the drug history of all patients having a particular disease; also prescription monitoring so that the medical history of those taking a particular drug can be studied.

It is known that in appropriate experimental situations anti-cancer drugs, nitrite ion (used as a food preservative), caffeine (coffee) and ionising radiation can be mutagenic, as also may be habitual tobacco smoking.

What is not known is how much hazard, if any, these pose to man in the actual conditions of ordinary life. At present no systematic monitoring of populations for mutations is taking place, except insofar as birth defect and cancer registries may be recording effects of mutation.

3. *Oncogenesis*. Malignant and benign tumours occur spontaneously and can also be induced by drugs and other chemicals, sometimes as a result of mutation. The possibility of malignant tumours being caused by drugs (carcinogenesis) is a major concern.

The topic is extremely complex and controversial. There are two important stages in carcinogenesis — initiation and promotion. Thus two substances may be necessary to cause cancer, an initiator and a promoter. But virtually any irritant substance seems to be carcinogenic in animals under the right experimental conditions. Glass, platinum foil, plastics (credit cards), American dimes* and strong glucose solutions have been found to be carcinogenic in animals.

Cytotoxic anticancer drugs are carcinogenic. They are usually also teratogenic and mutagenic; there is reason to believe that at least some cancers are the result of genetic mutations in the somatic cells causing a hereditary change from normal organ cell type, e.g. liver, blood, to cancer cells.

Carcinogens may act directly on cells or secondarily through changes in the hormone balance of the body. Some cancers (e.g. prostate, breast) are hormone-dependent and male and female sex hormones are used in treatment, e.g. oestrogen for prostate cancer, where the price of local comfort and longer life for the male patient may be the appearance of breasts of female size.

Since appearance of cancer may be delayed until long after the drug has ceased to be used, epidemiological methods monitoring populations will be required to detect the unexpected in man, i.e. cancer caused by a drug that is not under special suspicion.

Where a drug is under suspicion then case-control studies (see index) become practicable.

It might be thought reasonable that a drug should be banned if it comes under the slightest suspicion of oncogenicity or mutagenicity. But slight suspicions are easy to arouse and hard to verify. Possibly definitive investigations are so enormously time-consuming and expensive that, when suspicion is only slight, it becomes impossible to assert that 'where safety is concerned expense is no object'. Precipitate action on only slight suspicion (especially that aroused by limited laboratory experiments in animals) is likely to do more harm than good in disrupting medical practice without corresponding benefit to patients. When a useful drug is under consideration to be banned then it is necessary to consider the alternatives that replace it and whether there is adequate knowledge of them; commonly there is not. This may at first sight seem a callous attitude but a blind 'safety at all costs' approach, in these as in many other areas of life, may in fact incur costs in deprivation of benefits, costs that are excessive even in these important and emotionally charged areas.

If it should occur that a new drug is found to be mutagenic or carcinogenic in man and that it had not been tested for these properties in animals before being introduced to man, there can be little

* Moore G E et al. JAMA 1977; 238:397. The authors advised the government to consider banning money as unsafe.

doubt that there will be a public outcry. Parallels will be drawn with thalidomide. The pharmaceutical company and the national regulatory authority will be accused of negligence and incompetence.

It will be asserted that the possibility of a disaster was known (as it was), that laboratory tests for these properties existed (as they did) and that to fail to use them was plainly negligent (which is by no means necessarily the case). The predictive value of these tests is uncertain and so the results are liable to be controversial. But at least new drugs in suspect areas should not give *worse* results in animals than any similar drugs already in use.

The moment the predictive value for man of any safety test is reasonably certain it will be made mandatory and indeed the pharmaceutical industry will be only too ready to use it, however costly it may be.

It is in the public interest, that public fear does not push drug developers into doing, and regulatory bodies into demanding massive, mindless, routine testing programmes of dubious significance. On the other hand, public and professional pressure for research into development of reliable predictive tests can only do good.

Until the science is more developed it should probably remain the case that oncogenicity testing is sometimes demanded and sometimes not, and that a simple mutagenicity test is always required.

D. Drug quality

It is easy for an investigator or prescriber, interested in pharmacology, toxicology and therapeutics, to forget the fundamental importance of chemical and pharmaceutical aspects. An impure, unstable drug is useless. A pure drug that remains a pure drug after 5 years of storage in hot, damp climates is vital to therapeutics. The record of manufacturers in providing this is impressive.

Applications for licences to regulatory bodies must contain information on, for example, structural and molecular formula and the evidence for this, synthetic route and how this is monitored for quality, impurities and analytical methods to detect these, the tests to be applied to each batch manufactured, conditions of storage that may affect stability (humidity, temperature, acidity, alkalinity, light), the composition of the dosage form (which may be complex), its properties, disintegration, dissolution (pharmaceutical bioavailability) and so on.

Conclusion on pre-clinical testing

The dominant feature of the problem of finding new drugs to alleviate or cure disease is that of predicting from experiments with chemicals on animals what effect these chemicals will have in man, often in situations that cannot be mimicked in the animal laboratory.

As drugs are developed and promoted for long-term use in more and relatively trivial conditions, e.g. minor anxiety or slight high blood pressure, and affluent societies become less and less willing to tolerate small physical or mental discomforts, demanding relief without even minor inconvenience, drug therapy will continue to increase and the problem of demonstrating not only the efficacy, but also the safety of drugs, will grow. Only profound knowledge of biochemical mechanisms will eliminate risk in the introduction of new drugs, and this is a long way off. In the meantime failures of prediction will continue to occur. Another disaster as horrible as thalidomide may happen although, with growth of adequate systems for monitoring possible adverse reactions, it should be on a smaller scale; even so the recent history of drug withdrawals gives little ground for confidence.

Limited resources of scientific manpower and money will not be used to the best advantage if the public shock over thalidomide and subsequent events is allowed to express itself in governmental regulations requiring a plethora of expensive tests (and toxicity testing is very expensive) of dubious meaning for anything other than the animal concerned, for this would prevent industrial laboratories from devoting resources to investigation of fundamental mechanisms of drug action, in the knowledge of which alone lies health with safety.

The path of industrial drug developers is a stony, even if sometimes a highly profitable, one.

They risk huge sums of money*, but clinicians, sympathetic though they should be, must ruthlessly resist any development that they believe will add to the risks of clinical trial. Whilst clinicians must not demand too much, equally they must not allow commercial pressures, including the often substantial sums of money offered to investigators, to affect their judgement of what is best for healthy volunteers or for the sick.

This account of drug development, largely stressing the difficulties and the imponderables, may be put into perspective (before we proceed to evaluation in man) by the following figures on the general safety of drugs in relation to *accidents* and to *smoking* (per annum) in recent times in the UK (pop. 57 million).

Deaths due to:	
therapeutic use of drugs (named on death certificate)	40–50
accidents in the home	6000
motor vehicle accidents	7000
malignant pulmonary neoplasms	28 000

When the pre-clinical testing has been completed to the satisfaction of the developer, of any national regulatory requirements, and of the clinical investigator who will carry the programme forward, the time has come to administer the drug to man and so to launch the experimental programme that will decide whether the drug is only a drug or whether it is also a medicine. This is the subject of the next chapter.

GUIDE TO FURTHER READING

1 Brodie B B. Difficulties in extrapolating data on metabolism of drugs from animal to man. Clin Pharmacol Ther 1972; 3:374

2 Tishler M. Drug discovery — background and foreground. Clin Pharmacol Ther 1973; 14:479.

3 O'Donnell M. The demands of public opinion. Proc Roy Soc Med 1974; 67:1300.

4 Melmon K L. The clinical pharmacologist and scientifically unsound regulations for drug development. Clin Pharmacol Ther 1976; 20:125.

5 Gross F. The present dilemma of drug research. Clin Pharmacol Ther 1976; 19:1.

6 Schrogie J J et al. Evaluation of the prison inmate as a subject in drug assessment. Clin Pharmacol Ther 1977; 21:1.

7 Lasagna L. Will all new drugs become orphans? Clin Pharmacol Ther 1982; 31:285.

8 Gross F. Drug research: dead end or new horizon? Br Med J 1982; 285:1444.

9 Smith R. Doctors and the drug industry in Sweden. Br Med J 1985; 290:448.

10 Goldberg A et al. Pharmaceutical medicine. Lancet 1985; 1:447.

11 Editorial. Doctors and the drug industry. Br Med J 1983; 286:579.

12 Weatherall M. An end to the search for new drugs? Nature 1982; 296:387.

13 Sheck L et al. Success rates in the United States drug development system. Clin Pharmacol Ther 1984; 36:574.

* But they are seldom willing to invest these sums if they do not see a profitable market if they succeed. Thus research for diseases specially prevalent in developing (poor) countries and rare diseases (e.g. hepatolenticular degeneration) in any country, is commercially unattractive because, even if a drug is successfully developed, either the countries that need it are too poor to buy it or patients are too few to provide a profit. Thus these are *'orphan' diseases*. An *'orphan' drug* is a drug that, though known to be effective, is not worth making available because it is not patentable or there are too few patients, or a drug having interesting actions but that has not yet found a use, e.g. dopamine and levodopa were orphan drugs, but are so no longer.

4

Evaluation of drugs in man: therapeutic trials

When studies in animals predict that a new chemical may be a useful (i.e. effective and safe) medicine then the time has come to put it to the test in man.

We devote substantial space to clinical evaluation of drugs for the reasons given at the start of Chapter 3 and because the topic provides an exercise in logical thinking that can only benefit all who have to choose therapy for patients.

When the new agent offers a possibility of doing something that has not been done before or of doing something familiar in a different way, it can be seen to be worth testing. But where it is a new member of a familiar class of drug, potential advantage may be harder to see. Yet these 'me-too' drugs are often worth testing. Prediction from animal studies of modest but useful clinical advantage is uncertain and therefore if the new drug seems reasonably effective and safe in animals it is also reasonable to test it in man. The point has been put cogently: 'it is possible to waste too much time in animal studies before testing a drug in man'*: though satisfactory both qualitatively and quantitatively in animals, it may be useless in man solely because its duration of action is too short or too long, so that 'the practice of studying the physiologic disposition of a drug in man only after it is clearly the drug of choice in animals not only may prove short-sighted and time consuming, but also may result in relegating the best drug for man to the shelf for evermore.'*

Rational introduction of a new drug to man

This proceeds in a commonsense manner that is conventionally divided into *four phases*.

These phases are divisions of convenience in what is a continuous expanding process beginning with a single subject closely observed in the laboratory and proceeding to tens of subjects (healthy subjects and volunteer patients) through hundreds of patients, to thousands before the drug is agreed to be a medicine by a national regulatory authority and is licenced for general prescribing. The process may be abandoned at any stage. The phases may be defined as follows:

* Brodie B B. Clin Pharmacol Ther 1962; 3:374.

Phase 1

Clinical pharmacology (20–50 subjects)
- Healthy volunteers (*or patients*), according to class of drug and its safety
- Pharmacokinetics (absorption, distribution, metabolism, excretion).
- Pharmacodynamics (biological effects) where practicable; tolerance; safety; efficacy.

Phase 2

Clinical investigation (50–300)
- Patients
- Pharmacokinetics; pharmacodynamics, dose-ranging in expanding carefully controlled studies for efficacy and safety.

Phase 3

Formal therapeutic trials (randomised controlled trials; 250–1000+)
- Efficacy on a substantial scale; safety; comparison with other drugs.

Phase 4

Post-licencing (marketing) studies (2000–10 000+)
- Surveillance for safety and efficacy: further formal therapeutic trials, including comparisons with other drugs.

As in the case of pre-clinical testing, regulatory authorities issue *guidelines* as to the scope and amount of data likely to satisfy them. They do not demand studies in healthy volunteers (it is obviously impossible to *demand* that healthy people volunteer to take drugs), but developers know that the passage of their drug into patients will be eased if such studies are available and provide some assurance of safety. Developers are willing to pay substantial sums for healthy volunteer studies, and contract companies have been formed to meet this need. The commercialisation of such research raises ethical problems.

Regulatory guidelines for studies in man ordinarily include:

a. Studies of *bioavailability* and (when other manufacturers have similar products) of *bioequivalence* (equal bioavailability between products used for the same purpose is plainly important).

b. *Clinical trials* (reported in detail) that substantiate the safety and efficacy of the drug under conditions of use, e.g. a drug for long-term use in a common condition will require a total of at least 100 patients (preferably more) treated continuously for about one year as well as hundreds more treated for shorter periods. At least three independent trials are likely to be required.

c. If the drug will be used in the *elderly* then elderly people should be studied if there are reasons for thinking they may react to or handle the drug differently.

d. *Fixed-dose combination* products may improve patient compliance for long-term therapy but will also require other explicit justification, e.g. potentiation of therapeutic effect, less toxicity for each ingredient, and all must be needed for every claimed therapeutic indication: inclusion of one component to counteract an adverse effect of another component will sometimes be justified if that adverse effect is common: inclusion of a component to prevent abuse by producing an unpleasant effect is undesirable.

e. *Interaction studies* with other drugs likely to be taken simultaneously (plainly all possible combinations cannot be evaluated; an intelligent choice, based on knowledge of pharmacodynamics and pharmacokinetics, is made).

f. The application for a licence for general use (Product Licence) should include a draft *Data (information) Sheet** for prescribers and sometimes for patients. This should include information on the form of the product (tablet, capsule, delayed release, liquid form, etc), its uses, dosage (adults, children, elderly where appropriate), contra-indications (strong recommendation), warnings and precautions (less strong), side-effects/adverse reactions, overdose and how to treat it, etc.

Experimental therapeutics

As the number of potential drugs produced increases, the problem of who to test them on

* Medicines need instruction manuals just as do domestic appliances.

grows. Clearly there are two main groups, healthy volunteers, volunteers patients (and, very rarely, non-volunteers patients); it is relevant that some drug actions can be demonstrated on normals (anticoagulant, anaesthetic, antihypertensive) whereas others cannot (antiparkinsonian, antimicrobial) so that to try the latter on healthy volunteers to obtain pharmacokinetic and safety data is to treat man formally as an experimental animal, risking toxicity, however remotely, to obtain information of no benefit to the subject; this is increasingly often done; it poses ethical problems.

There are two main types of human investigation in the context of this book, *non-therapeutic* (pharmacological) and *therapeutic*, and they often overlap.

In the *non-therapeutic* experiment the individual is the chief subject of a special pharmacodynamic or pharmacokinetic investigation, often using complex physiological and biochemical techniques, and although the data obtained may be useful in advancing drug therapy, they may not have any direct use in therapy of the patient from whom they were obtained and indeed much of this work is done in healthy volunteers.

In the *therapeutic investigation* the measurements made on individuals are often simpler; studies involve patients treated in a carefully planned experiment or else the observation (surveillance) of routine therapy conducted by clinicians.

Only the therapeutic investigations (experimental and observational) will be discussed further because doctors may reasonably feel they can dispense with the details of how changes in, say, various vascular beds are detected, until such time as they may take a specialised interest in the subject. But they cannot afford to ignore the principles of therapeutic evaluation, for such studies provide the basis of choice of drugs for individual patients, and enable prediction of the outcome of treatment with less uncertainty. It is useful to know a good therapeutic study from a bad, for the latter are common, and both good and bad are thrust at doctors by vested interests in the hope that they will accept their verdict. More difficult, some bad studies, previously easily detectable, are now replete with the jargon of the formal therapeutic trial; the terms random allocation, double-blind, statistically significant, and probability, are draped around what on close inspection is seen to be, scientifically, a fraud. Some critics of anti-scientific mind have condemned valid techniques (e.g. double-blind) rather than workers who have misused them and others have pointed out that the randomised controlled therapeutic trial is not the only path to truth, omitting to notice that nobody who knows about the subject has actually made the claim they dispute.

Throughout this book, lists of alternative drugs are given without any serious attempt to discriminate between them. The reason for this is that useful discrimination is impossible because it is not easy to find people prepared to carry out detailed comparative trials on closely similar drugs; therefore, non-experimental surveillance techniques that evaluate drugs under conditions of ordinary use are an increasingly important development.

Therapeutic investigations employ two classes of outcome in which the effect measured is —

1. *The therapeutic effect itself*, e.g. sleep, eradication of infection, and
2. *A factor related to the therapeutic effect* (with varying degrees of certainty), e.g. blood lipids or glucose, or blood pressure; in these diseases true therapeutic effect, i.e. healthy life free from complications, can only be measured by studying large numbers of patients over years. Such long-term studies are indeed necessary, but are impracticable on organisational and financial grounds prior to releasing all new drugs for general prescription. It is in such areas as these that techniques of large-scale surveillance for efficacy, as well as for safety, under conditions of ordinary use, are needed to supplement the necessarily smaller and shorter formal therapeutic trials.

Thus *therapeutic evaluation* is conducted in two principal ways:

1. *Formal therapeutic trials* (experimental cohort studies)
2. *Surveillance programmes*, e.g. case-control studies, and observational cohort studies (large-scale monitoring for efficacy and/or adverse reactions).

When a new drug is being developed, the first therapeutic trials are devised to find out the best the drug can do under conditions ideal for showing efficacy, e.g. uncomplicated disease of mild-to-moderate severity in patients taking no other drugs, with carefully supervised administration by specialist doctors. Interest lies particularly in patients who complete a full course of treatment. If the drug is ineffective in these circumstances there is no point in proceeding with an expensive development programme. Such studies are sometimes called, a little inappropriately, 'explanatory' trials.

If the drug is found useful in these trials, then it becomes desirable next to find out whether it can be successful and safe in the rough and tumble of routine medical practice, in patients of all ages, at all stages of disease, with complications, taking other drugs and relatively unsupervised. Interest continues in all patients from the moment they are entered into the trial and it is maintained if they fail to complete, or even to start, the treatment, for what is wanted is to know the outcome in all patients deemed suitable for therapy, not only in those who successfully complete it. The reasons some drop out may be related to aspects of the treatment. Such trials are therefore analysed on *intention to treat* rather than on completion of treatment; the investigator is not allowed to risk introducing bias by exercising his own judgement as to who should or should not be excluded from the analysis.* In these real life, or naturalistic, conditions the drug may not perform so well, e.g. minor adverse effects may now cause patient non-compliance, which had been avoided by supervision and enthusiasm in the early trials. These naturalistic studies are sometimes called 'pragmatic' trials.

Formal therapeutic trials are expensive and are hard to administer. Surveillance studies are less precise but compensate for this by their convenience and/or large size and closeness to the realities of ordinary medical practice.

Formal therapeutic trials are unlikely to reveal:

a. *adverse effects that are uncommon or occur only after prolonged use*, e.g. oral contraceptives and vascular disease; renal damage due to analgesics.

b. *effects in special population groups*, e.g. pregnancy, renal or hepatic disease, since these are generally excluded, reasonably, from formal therapeutic trials.

c. *unexpected therapeutic effects*, i.e. potential new uses.

d. *drug interactions*.

Thus, *drug evaluation comprises formal therapeutic trials followed by surveillance studies* (p. 61).

Discussion of experimental therapeutics and of formal therapeutic trials and surveillance programmes follows.

Pickering has written, '. . . therapeutics is the branch of medicine that, by its very nature, should be experimental. For if we take a patient afflicted with a malady and we alter his conditions of life . . . we are performing an experiment. And if we are scientifically minded we should record the results. Before concluding that the change for better or for worse in the patient is due to the specific treatment employed, we must ascertain . . . whether the result was merely due to the natural history of the disease . . . or whether it was due to some other factor which was necessarily associated with the therapeutic measure in question. And if, as a result of these procedures we learn that the therapeutic measure employed produces a significant, though not very pronounced improvement, we would experiment with the method, altering dosage or other detail to see if it can be improved. This would seem the procedure to be expected of men with six years of scientific training behind them.

'But it has not been followed. Had it been done we should have gained a fairly precise knowledge of the place of individual methods of therapy in disease, and our efficiency as doctors would have been enormously enhanced'.†

There are some who dislike or reject the notion of deliberate experimentation on the sick, feeling that a scientific approach implies an unsympathetic or even a malevolent disposition. They forget that in the past positively harmful treatments have been widely used for many years (bleeding for pneumonia, for example) because of the lack of recognition of the need, as well as lack

* Analysis excluding patients who have failed to complete may be presented provided the full 'intention to treat' analysis is also displayed.

† Pickering G W. Proc Roy Soc Med. 1949, 42:229.

of knowledge of the techniques, of scientific evaluation of therapy. It has been pointed out that where the worth of a treatment, new or old, is in doubt, there may be a greater obligation to test it critically than to go on prescribing it supported only by habit or wishful thinking.*

The choice before the doctor is not whether he should experiment on his patients, but whether he should do so in a planned or in a haphazard fashion; whether he should try to organise his experience so that it is of value to himself and to others or to follow the notoriously unreliable 'clinical impression'. The latter is the less ethical course.

Doctors who think they can assess the value of a treatment by using it on patients in an uncontrolled fashion have the whole history of therapeutics against them. It is given to only a few to test a treatment that dramatically alters disease and whose efficacy is obvious with casual use, and even then details of its application will generally need carefully planned studies, e.g. adrenal steroids in rheumatoid arthritis and asthma, where wrong use may be more dangerous than no use.

Modern scientific techniques uncover the most effective treatments whilst exposing the smallest numbers to the less effective or positively harmful; they save lives, time and money. They are not unethical for they are only properly used when the relative merits of treatments are genuinely unknown.

Some patients find it hard to put their confidence in a doctor who, openly admitting uncertainty, is using two treatments concurrently in order to achieve a true measure of their relative values. They need the emotional security that is provided by doctors who behave as though they know, indeed, who sometimes themselves believe they know, even though patients may rightly suspect that there are others of equal authority who take an opposite view.

Though the 'statistical therapeutic comparision' or 'formal therapeutic trial' or 'randomised controlled trial,' discussed below, is a powerful tool for advancing therapy, it does not suit every occasion. Sometimes, as in malaria or diabetes, there are clinical or laboratory tests that will rapidly tell whether a treatment is effective, though they may not provide evidence of a marginal difference between effective drugs, and in tuberculous meningitis a single recovery was considered adequate evidence of therapeutic efficacy.

* Green F H K. Lancet 1954; 2:1085.

The need for statistics

In order to decide whether patients treated in one way are benefitted more than those treated in another, there is no possibility of avoiding the use of numbers. The mere statement by a clinician that patients do better with this or that treatment is due to his having formed an opinion that more patients are helped by the treatment he advocates than by other treatments. The opinion is based on numbers, but having omitted to record exactly how many patients have been treated by different methods and having omitted to ensure that the only variable factor affecting the patient was the treatment in question, only a 'clinical impression', instead of facts, can be stated. This is a pity, for progress is delayed when convinced opinions are offered in placed of convincing facts. The former, though not necessarily wrong, are unreliable, despite the great assurance with which they are often advanced. This is not to dismiss the anecdotal clinical survey or the case-report, for they tell what *can* happen, which is useful. Also, formal therapeutic trials are commonly done because someone has formed an impression that is thought to deserve testing.

Above 100 years ago Francis Galton saw this clearly. 'In our general impressions far too great weight is attached to what is marvellous. . . . Experience warns us against it, and the scientific man takes care to base his conclusions upon actual numbers. The human mind is . . . a most imperfect apparatus for the elaboration of general ideas. . . . General impressions are never to be trusted. Unfortunately when they are of long standing they become fixed rules of life, and assume a prescriptive right not to be questioned. Consequently, those who are not accustomed to original enquiry entertain a hatred and a horror of statistics. They cannot endure the idea of submitting their sacred impressions to cold-blooded verification. But it is the triumph of scientific men to rise superior to such superstitions,to devise tests by which the value of beliefs may be ascertained, and to feel sufficiently masters of themselves to discard contemptuously whatever may be found untrue . . . the frequent incorrectness of notions derived from general impressions may be assumed. . . .'*

Therapeutic trial design: the randomised controlled trial: general aspects

The aims of a therapeutic trial, not all of which can be attempted on any one occasion, are to decide the folllowing:

1. whether a treatment is of value,
2. how great its value is (compared with other remedies, if such exist),
3. in what types of patients it is of value,
4. what is the best method of applying the treatment, how often, and in what dosage if it is a drug,
5. what are the disadvantages and dangers of the treatment.

Bradford Hill† defines the therapeutic trial as 'a carefully, and ethically, designed experiment with the aim of answering some *precisely framed question*. In its most rigorous form it demands *equivalent groups* of patients *concurrently treated* in different ways. These groups are constructed by the *random allocation* of patients to one or other treatment. . . . In principle the method is applicable with any disease and any treatment. It may also be applied on any scale; it does not necessarily demand large numbers of patients'. This is the classic *randomised controlled trial*.

Three important points in the above definition may be stressed. *Equivalent groups of patients*: if the treatment groups differ significantly in age, sex, race, duration of disease, severity of disease or in any other possibly relevant factor, it will not be possible to attribute differences in outcome to the treatment under investigation, unless there is some way of eliminating the bias that has entered. The best way of getting equivalent groups is by alloting patients to them by *random allocation*.‡

The function of randomisation is to eliminate systematic biases, known (personal judgements of clinicians or patients) or unknown, that could affect assignment to treatment.

To allot patients alternately or otherwise systematically is not satisfactory as investigators almost inevitably know into what treatment group a patient will go whilst engaged in deciding whether the patient should enter the trial, and may be unconsciously influenced by this if they have strong feelings about either the patient or the value of the respective treatments. With random allocations in sealed envelopes the treatment groups into which the patients go is only discovered after it has been decided to enter them into the trial. It is plainly 'embarrassing to have recourse to opening a sealed envelope — and still more to tossing a coin', if a decision has to be made in front of the patient, and randomization can be achieved by a simple mental trick.§

Treatments must be carried out *concurrently* (at the same time) and *concomitantly* (at the same place) partly for the reasons given above and partly because diseases may vary in severity with time and place, and virulence of an organism may change, especially in epidemics; the weather and industrial atmospheric pollution may influence respiratory and cardiac diseases; or a hospital may even get a reputation, for good or ill, so that more or less severe cases may be sent to it, and doctors and nurses change in number and quality; diagnostic criteria and skill also vary with time and place. Thus controls from the past (*historical controls*) are nearly always unacceptable.

Before commencing any therapeutic trial it is essential *to formulate exactly the question that is to*

* Galton F. Generic images. Proceedings of the Royal Institution 1879.

† Bradford Hill A. Principles of medical statistics. London. Hodderand Stoughton, 1977.

‡ It is not necessary to have equal numbers in each group, especially if the natural history of the disease is well known, when a 2:1 ratio can be used instead of the usual 1:1. Random number series can be adapted to provide unequal groups or allocation may be devised to change during the trial so that more patients are progressively allocated to the most successful treatment — 'play the winner' allocation.

§ Such as by adding the day of the month to the last two digits of the patient's case number or year of birth and giving treatment A to odd and B to even numbers. But sceptical statisticians do not trust doctors to refrain from doing this prematurely and demand allocation to be totally independent of the investigator. They may be wise. Doll W R S. In: Laurence D R, ed. Quantitative methods in human pharmacology and therapeutics, London: Pergamon, 1959.

be answered. For example: 'Is drug X capable of relieving the pain of osteoarthrosis more or less completely, with greater or fewer side-effects and for a shorter or longer time than is drug Y?' The question should be as simple as possible, for to try to discover too much can be a cause of failure, and it should be kept in mind throughout the whole process of designing the trial. Neglect to set down at the start exactly what is the objective of the study invites failure.

Ethics of research in man and particularly of the randomised controlled trial

Modern medicine is accused of callous application of science to human problems. Official regulatory bodies rightly require scientific evaluation of drugs. Drug developers need to satisfy the regulators and they also seek to persuade an increasingly sophisticated medical profession to prescribe their products. For these reasons scientific drug evaluation as described here is likely to increase in volume and more and more doctors will be personally involved.

Therefore we provide discussion of the ethics of medical research in man.

Ethics of human experimentation are of grave concern to all who use drugs, especially new drugs, and some aspects have already been mentioned.

Human experiments are of two main kinds, (1) **therapeutic**: those that may actually have a therapeutic effect or provide information that can be used to help subjects, and (2) **non-therapeutic**: those that provide information that cannot be of direct use to them (e.g. healthy volunteers always and patients sometimes). In practice, experiments often do not fall clearly into one or other group and attempts to lay down codes of behaviour based on the assumption that they do have so far failed to achieve their object of allowing medicine to advance whilst certainly preventing abuse.

The issue of *consent* bulks large in discussions of the ethics of human experimentation and is a principal concern of the ethical review committees that are now the norm in medical research.

Some dislike the word 'experiment' in relation to man, thinking that its mere use implies a degree of impropriety in what is done. It is better, however, that all should recognise the true meaning of the word, 'to ascertain or establish by trial',* that the benefits of modern medicine derive wholly from experimentation and that some risk, however slight, is inseparable from medical advance. The duty of all doctors lies in ensuring that in their desire to help patients in general they should never allow themselves to put the individual who has sought their aid at any disadvantage, for '*the scientist or physician has no right to choose martyrs for society*'.†

Physicians deal with individuals and have sometimes argued against the statistical therapeutic trial that it does not tell what will happen to any one individual who consults them. This is obviously true, but the knowledge gained from such studies that, with a treatment, *x*% recover, *y*% improve and *z*% are unchanged, with details of unwanted effects, provides a better basis for the choice of therapy for individuals than the often divergent clinical impressions of doctors.

It is, of course, only proper to perform a therapeutic trial when the doctors genuinely do not know which treatment is best, and if they are prepared to withdraw individual patients or to stop the whole trial if at any time they become convinced that it is in the patients' interest to do so.

If it is not known whether one treatment is better than another, then nothing is lost by allotting patients at random to those treatments under test, and it is in everybody's interest that good treatments should be adopted and bad treatments abandoned as soon as possible. It is, of course, more difficult to justify testing a new treatment when existing treatments are fairly good than when they are bad, and this difficulty is likely to grow. With a new drug the situation is generally clear — its efficacy is unknown — but when a drug has been licenced and used for years without proper scientific evaluation, so that unsupported claims surround it, then the difficulties of getting true scientific evaluation are multiplied, for 'long years of habitual prescribing based on early and authoritative impressions and optimism confers on a drug qualities of survival which have a high

* Oxford English Dictionary.

† Kety S. Quoted by Beecher H K. JAMA 1959; 169:461.

degree of immunity against the disqualifying actions of scientific experiment in man'.* Ill-performed scientific tests have the same effect.

Doctors must consider the ethical implications of their acts, the casual use of drugs as much as the planned evaluation, and none can fail to profit by reading some of the references at the end of this chapter.

The randomised controlled trial, particularly, has been subject to ethical criticism. Objections have always, often justly, been raised to the conduct of individual randomised controlled trials, but of recent years these have been extended to the principles on which such trials are based. It is worth considering these criticisms, for the conduct of clinical science puts a grave responsibility on the investigator.

Ethical objections that have been raised to the randomised controlled trial may be summarised as follows:

a. the interest of the individual is always subordinated to the interest of society, or 'group' ethics supersede 'individual' ethics, and this is unethical.

b. the null hypothesis (i.e. the postulate that there is no difference between the treatments under test) is virtually never valid.

c. a physician's opinion is what matters, it provides a valid basis for treating the individual and a physician must have an opinion; he is not allowed to 'retreat to a position of scientific ignorance'; if he is wrong, his errors will be corrected 'when confronted with the results of other clinicians.'

d. the double-blind technique is an unethical deception.

e. the use of dummy or placebo controls is an unethical deception.

f. random allocation is unethical as it overrides the physician's judgement, see (b) and (c) above.

g. patients in one group will get inferior treatment.

h. as the point of statistical significance is approached the clinician will find his opinion on relative efficacy being influenced and he can no longer ethically continue; he may not seek to escape this by using the double-blind technique.

These views have been put forward by critics of modern science and its method, including lawyers, who urge that the randomised controlled trial can only be legally conducted when there is a formal 'contract for experimentation' in which it is made explicit that the patient agrees to receive a treatment that the doctor judges to be inferior, and that, when mortality is the criterion of efficacy, he might die for that reason.

Such extreme views are the result of ignorance of medical practice, of unawareness of the uncertainty of medical knowledge, of the value of opinions of physicians, and also of defects in logical thinking. Nevertheless, they highlight very real ethical issues. A badly conceived, designed and conducted trial may indeed qualify for the harshest criticisms and it is the task of clinical investigators to ensure that their conduct is above reproach, and seen to be so.

The ethical position of the critics is itself dubious. Their doctrines expose people to receiving inferior treatment through ignorance and, by preventing the degree of certainty about a treatment needed to convince others, delay the worldwide use of effective treatments. It is impossible to define clearly 'group' ethics and 'individual' ethics; groups are made up of individuals; it is in the interest of both that knowledge be gained; but gaining knowledge always has a cost; therefore, we explore improvements in trial design and use ethics review committees to minimise unintended exploitation of individuals and groups.

The *interaction of ethical and scientific issues* has been well summarised in a Report†:

'An analysis of the ethical problems of therapeutic trials might begin with a question long familiar to moral philosophy: what is the nature and degree of certitude required for an ethical decision? More precisely, *is there any ethically relevant difference between the use of statistical methods and the use of other ways of knowing, such as experience, common sense, guessing, etc? When decisions are to be made in uncertainty, is it more or less ethical to choose and abide by statistical methods of defining 'certitude' than*

* Gold H. In: Laurence D R, ed. Quantitative methods in human pharmacology and therapeutics, London: Pergamon, 1959.

† Eur J Clin Pharmacol 1980; 18:129.

to be guided by one's hunch or striking experience? These questions are raised by the assertion that it is ethically imperative to conclude a clinical trial when a 'trend' appears. . . . . . the choice of statistical methods can constitute in many circumstances an acceptable ethical approach to the problem of decision in uncertainty.

'As physician-investigators seek knowledge about safety and efficacy of medicines, which is a social good, the dignity of individuals must not be overridden. The ethical principles of research, namely, informed and voluntary participation of subjects, and assessment of risks and benefits and protection of subjects by ethical review boards, must be rigorously applied, for indeed there are serious ethical considerations. But in well-designed therapeutic trials these ethical principles of responsibility to the individual are preserved.

'Sometimes, therapeutic trials may be necessary in special categories of patients, e.g. those who are critically ill, children, the mentally retarded, or the mentally disturbed. These special groups are rightly the subject of special discussion. In general, the principles mentioned above also apply to these special groups, although details may differ, most particularly with regard to procedures for obtaining consent, whether it be from the patient or a surrogate.

'Different research methods should be used in accordance with different research problems, always favouring those methods which pose the least risk to subjects. In addition, experimental design and statistical methods must provide for ascertaining and implementing the needs and wishes of individual subjects. When it becomes clear that continued inclusion in a therapeutic trial may be to the disadvantage of patients, the ethical researcher will withdraw the patients or even terminate the whole study. The therapeutic trial is both ethically required for the social good of more effective medical care and is capable of being designed in ways which respect the wellbeing and rights of individual participants.'

We briefly discuss *a few of the principal ethical issues*, some of which receive further discussion in this chapter:

1. *Ethics of starting a randomised controlled trial and number of patients*

There must be a genuine problem that deserves a clear answer and for which the randomised controlled trial is an appropriate instrument. A physician who is quite sure that he knows the best treatment cannot ethically participate in a trial. A physician who has an opinion but who is aware of the fallibility of clinical impressions may feel free to participate.

Forecasting the number of patients (see below) needed to obtain an answer to the question is a major scientific issue with great ethical implications. Here scientific skill and medical knowledge together must be integrated to ensure that a trial does not expose patients to inferior treatment unnecessarily. Equally, a trial that is so small that there is not hope for a useful result is unethical because it fruitlessly exposes patients to risk. Bad clinical science is always unethical.

2. *Research Ethics Review Committees*

It is now generally conceded that so great are the ethical problems that the decisions as to what is or is not ethical cannot be left to the investigators alone; it is necessary that they convince their equals (peers), including lay (non-medical) people that their proposals are ethical. Since bad science is unethical because it exposes subjects to inconvenience, expense or risk, with little or no gain, ethics committees also consider, at least to some extent, the scientific quality of the studies they review.

3. *Consent: 'informed' or understanding consent*

Consent is central to the whole conduct of clinical research; if it is not 'informed', i.e. the subject or parent does not understand the essentials of what is involved, then consent is meaningless and must be invalid. It is sometimes said 'there is no such thing as informed consent', but this is less than fair, though to purist theory, out of touch with the real world, it may seem so. Informed consent is an ideal to which we should aspire even if we seldom attain it. Plainly, research ethics committees have a major role in considering the quality of consent, and this is why there should always be *local* ethics committees, which understand their own people and know the investigators, to consider each study. This does not diminish the ethical role of a body such as the World Health Organization, which rightly reviews the ethics of the research it sponsors, but such review does not replace local review.

4. *Ethics of stopping a trial* (see also p. 57).
Once one treatment has shown itself to be better than another then the trial must not be prolonged. In planning the trial these two points must be carefully considered:

a. What is the degree of certainty required?
b. How may that point be recognised so that the trial may be stopped when it is reached and prolongation will unnecessarily expose patients to an inferior treatment?

Here again the achievement of an ethical position is based on the use of appropriate scientific design.

5. *New treatments*
The best time to achieve a scientific evaluation is when a treatment is new and no one has formed firm opinions of its value.

6. *Old, standard or traditional treatments*
It can be difficult to arrange evaluation because their general acceptance on poor evidence has resulted in beliefs that may be strongly held and habits that are hard to break. But yet the ethical course is to undertake scientific evaluation so that the ineffective and/or less safe treatments can be abandoned.

7. *Withholding treatment: placebo or dummy treatment*
The use of a *placebo* or *dummy treatment* poses ethical problems but is often preferable to the continued use of treatments of unproven efficacy or safety. It is not inherently unethical. Investigators who propose to use a placebo or otherwise withold effective treatment should specifically justify their intention. Frequently, consent can be obtained to the use of a placebo without impairing the scientific validity of the procedure if the patient is invited to agree that an inert preparation will (or may) be used (and why it will be used) at some time during the course of treatment, but without specifying exactly when. The way in which the proposal is put to patients will vary with circumstances: the Ethics Committee should satisfy itself that it will be done in such a way as to create genuine understanding in the patient. Generally, patients easily understand the concept of distinguishing between the imagined effects of treatment and those due to a direct action on the body.

In conclusion — On ethics

*The objective must be that no patient should be worse off than he might have been in the hands of a reasonable and competent physician.** When placebos or suspected inert treatments (that may be part of a local tradition) are used as scientific controls, it must be done in such a way that a patient who deteriorates will be detected and transferred to active treatment within the trial or else withdrawn from the trial.

The ethical quality of trials can be enhanced by skilled and ingenious scientific techniques; ethics and science cannot be considered as independent items.

'In developing new medicines, ethical, scientific and economic aspects are interdependent. Expensive resources (time, money, scientific manpower) must not be wasted; the smallest possible number of patients or healthy volunteers should be exposed to substances which prove to be ineffective or to have untoward effects.

'Much harm can follow flawed or premature judgements about the efficacy or safety of a new treatment. When uncertainty exists about either new or old [treatments], it is scientifically and ethically imperative to resolve doubts efficiently by controlled trials. Admittedly, uncontrolled clinical observation has identified drugs that have dramatic effects in well-defined diseases (malaria, septicaemia, reduction of blood pressure and blood sugar). But such major advances in treatment are rare; most therapeutic advance occurs in modest steps, and here clinical opinions have all too often been in error and sometimes only discovered to be so after decades.

'Numerous examples attest to strong beliefs being held widely and for long periods both for and against the same treatment, and forms of treatment which were considered as effective on grounds of clinical impression, have turned out to be ineffective or even harmful.

'By contrast, scientifically designed trials of drugs, e.g. in tuberculosis, have allowed precise evaluations of benefits and risks and provided the physician with reliable data for the choice of drug

* Glaser E M. In: Witts L J, ed. Medical Surveys and Clinical Trials London. Oxford University Press, 1964.

and drug combinations, including safer and cheaper intermittent therapy.

'The decision to mount a formal trial depends on there being genuine doubt as to whether there is a true difference between two treatments; or where there is no existing treatment, whether the treatment proposed has any efficacy. The theoretical basis for the study is to test the null hypothesis, i.e. that the regimens to be compared are equally effective. Where it is genuinely reasonable to propose the null hypothesis then a study is ethical, and indeed necessary.'*

Hypothesis of no difference; statistical significance; confidence intervals

When it is suspected that treatment A may be superior to treatment B and it is wished to find out the truth it is convenient, and only seemingly eccentric, to set about it by testing the hypothesis that the treatments are equally effective, or ineffective, as the case may be — the 'no difference' hypothesis (*null hypothesis*). Thus, when two groups of patients have been treated (between-patient comparison) or each patient has had a course of each drug (within-patient comparison) and it has been found that improvement has occurred more often with one treatment than with the other, it is necessary to decide how likely it is that this difference is due to a real superiority of one treatment over the other. *A statistical significance test will tell how often a difference of the observed size would occur due to chance (random influences) if there is, in reality, no difference between the treatments*. If the result of the test is that the observed difference is unlikely if there is truly no difference between treatments, we may choose to believe, or at least to act as though there is a real superiority of one treatment and to adopt it in preference to the other in our practice.

A difference may be statistically significant but clinically unimportant.

Equally, a trial result may show no difference between treatments, yet there is a chance that there may, in reality, be a difference. In a properly designed trial it is possible to calculate the probability that if the real difference is of certain magnitude it may have been missed in a trial of the size performed.

In clinical practice most agree that if the statistical significance test shows that, the no-difference hypothesis being true, a difference as large as that observed would only occur five times if the experiment were repeated 100 times, then this is acceptable as sufficient evidence that the null hypothesis is unlikely to be true (but not impossible), i.e. that there is a real difference between the treatments. This level of probability is generally expressed in therapeutic trials as, the difference was 'statistically significant' 'significant at the 5% level' or 'P† = 0.05'. *'Statistical significance'* simply means, unlikely in the event of no genuine treatment difference.

If the analysis reveals that, the no-difference hypothesis being true, the observed difference, or greater, would only occur *once* if the experiment were repeated 100 times, the results are generally said to be 'statistically highly significant', 'significant at the 1% level' or '$P = 0.01$'.

The statistical tests do not prove that a difference is due to one treatment being better than another or not better than another, as the case may be, they merely provide probabilities. A clinician who would act on the results of an experiment that provided a 'statistically significant' result ($P = 0.05$) when there were good theoretical reasons for expecting that result, might refuse to accept a theoretically improbable conclusion or one that went against his 'experience' unless the difference was 'statistically highly significant' ($P = 0.01$) and this would be reasonable. It is as important not to allow oneself to be bludgeoned by statistics as it is important not to disregard strong evidence. *Statistics may be defined as 'a body of methods for making wise decisions in the face of uncertainty'*‡. Used properly, it is a tool of great value for promoting efficient therapy.

Many investigators and many medical editors think that a significant statistical test is all that is needed (editors tend to publish trials having

* Eur J Clin Pharmacol 1980; 18:129.

† P = percentage divided by 100 (chance proportion).

‡ Wallis W A et al. Statistics, a new approach. London: Methuen, 1957.

positive tests and to reject those having negative tests because no-difference studies seem to them boring). But both parties are wrong. There is also need to know the *precision* or *power* of the statistical test, whether the particular trial shows a difference or no difference, i.e. what assurance can we have that the test represents truth or reality (as opposed to the chance or probability of the particular result). We need to have an estimate of the likelihood of occurrence of the *two kinds of error of therapeutic experiments* —

Type I error, i.e. finding a difference between treatments when in reality they do not differ, and

Type II error, i.e. finding no difference between treatments when in reality they do differ to an extent doctors would want to know about — the *target* difference.

It is up to the clinician to decide the target difference and what probability level (for either type of error) he will accept if he is to use the result as a guide to action; this the statistical significance test alone cannot tell him (see *trial size*, below).

For example, a trial result reported as *not statistically significant* means only that the result is *compatible* with there being no real difference between the treatments under comparison; it does not mean that there *is* no real difference, and this fact is all the more important when the trial is small and the statistical test is therefore of low power. The *power* of a therapeutic trial is the probability of a statistically significant finding in favour of the better treatment when the difference between treatments equals or exceeds the realistic target difference in which doctors are interested.

Not statistically significant has a very different interpretation if the patients in the trial number 50 or 500. Large numbers of patients give high precision and allow a high chance of achieving statistical significance when treatments differ by the target amount. Small numbers of patients inevitably give low precision (or power) and there is little assurance of achieving statistical significance when the actual treatment difference is modest yet useful (i.e. is on target).

A finding of *not statistically significant* can only be interpreted as meaning there is no clinically useful difference if the *confidence interval* of the result is also stated in the report and is narrow. Therapeutic trials involve the measurement of a quantity, e.g. amount of pain or swelling, blood pressure, incidence of heart attacks, and the 95% *confidence interval* of the mean indicates:

a. the lowest and the highest true values with which the data collected are compatible (at the 5% significance level) and

b. the range within which it is possible to be (95%) certain that the real or true value lies.

'Confidence intervals reveal the precision of an estimate. A wide confidence interval points to a lack of information, whether the difference is statistically significant or not, and is a warning'* against placing much weight on, or confidence in, the results of small studies. 'Confidence intervals are extremely helpful in interpretation, particularly of small studies, as they show *the degree of uncertainty related to a result* — such as the difference between two means — whether or not it was statistically significant. Their use in conjunction with non-significant results may be especially enlightening'.*

Thus, a treatment difference that is not statistically significant and that has a wide confidence interval is compatible with the null hypothesis being true and there being no real difference between the treatments *or* a substantially adverse effect *or* a substantially beneficial effect, which is hardly very useful to know. This situation occurs with small trials and can be avoided only by proper foresight, with calculation of the minimum number of subjects needed to detect at high probability a useful effect (which has been defined by the clinician in advance) or lack of it. Trials of inadequate power cannot achieve the investigator's objective and therefore are not worth undertaking, indeed worthless studies are unethical in that they inconvenience patients or put them at risk and waste professional time and resources without any possibility of gain.

Plainly trials should be devised to have adequate *power*, e.g. an at least 80% chance of detecting the defined useful target effect within narrow confidence limits, at 5% statistical significance ($P = 0.05$). It is not worth starting a trial that has less than a 50% chance of achieving the set objective, because the power of the trial is too low; but such small trials are frequently done and published

* Altman D et al. Br Med J 1983; 286:1489.

without any statement of power or confidence interval, which would reveal their inadequacy. What is required in trial reports are statements such as the following:

a. the observed difference between the treatment groups is not *statistically significant* ($P > 0.05$) but this result is compatible (95% confidence interval) with there being a real difference between the treatments with a range as wide as + 30% to − 20% (i.e. almost as large in the opposite direction), which wide range means the trial is useless as a guide to action; not only is the range wide, but it spans zero.

b. the observed difference between the treatment groups is *statistically significant* ($P < 0.05$), but this result is compatible with there being a real difference with a range of 2–35% (same direction). With such a wide range the trial may be thought inadequate, e.g. the target (useful) difference may have been set at 20%.

But where the range is narrow, 30–38%, it is above the target difference (20%) and so is clinically important as well as statistically significant) then the trial will be thought to give reliable information that may (provided it is independently confirmed) provide a basis for action.

If all reports were presented with such information on *both* statistical significance *and* confidence intervals the literature would be less burdened by valueless and potentially misleading trials because journal editors would refuse to publish those that were condemned as valueless by their authors' own calculations.

The size of a therapeutic trial; number of subjects; fixed-sample and sequential designs

Before starting a therapeutic trial it is necessary to decide when it should stop.

The number of patients required for a therapeutic trial depends on what difference the investigator regards as clinically important and, in reality, worth detecting. If the investigator can state this (as he will have to eventually when he comments on the importance of his results) it is possible to calculate the number of patients needed to have a high probability of detecting the target (worthwhile) difference if the actual difference between treatments measures up to the realistic expectation. This is the concept of *power* of a therapeutic trial that is discussed above. Obviously it is better to make this calculation before embarking on a trial rather than to make it after its completion and risk finding that the power is so low that the trial is worthless. Overambition to detect small differences is liable to lead to impossibly large trials; compromise is often necessary having regard to the number of patients likely to be available (commonly overestimated by investigators), management problems, and a realistic assessment of what difference is really of clinical importance (target difference).

A clinician contemplating a **fixed-sample** therapeutic trial wants to know how many patients should be treated in order to decide whether one treatment is better than another, and he turns to a statistician to help him. An estimate can only be provided if he will tell the statistician what magnitude of difference he is interested in detecting* *and* the risks he will tolerate of errors of Types I and II, i.e. of accepting a difference where it does not exist and of missing a difference that does exist. The result of this calculation is commonly a shock to the clinician who may have, a little vaguely, and full of therapeutic enthusiasm, begun by saying that he wants to detect 'any' difference, however small, and to be 'quite certain' that it is real. What, to the doctor, may seem quite modest requirements may only be realisable with an impossibly large number of patients.

Two examples will suffice.

A trial that offers a better than even chance of detecting a difference of 2:3, i.e. 2 deaths (or other event) in one treatment group against 3 deaths in the other, which can well be a clinically important difference, will require numbers of patients that provide for about 100 deaths (or other event) in the trial. But such a probability (better than even chance) may be thought insufficient, and to become reasonably sure that a difference of this magnitude (2:3) will be detected, a trial involving about 200 deaths will be needed. If the death rate is 20% (as in tetanus in some

* The *target difference*. Differences fall into three grades: (1) that the doctor will ignore, (2) that will make the doctor wonder what to do (more research needed), and (3) that will make the doctor act, i.e. change prescribing practice.

parts of the world), then the trial should be planned to include about 1000 patients — a daunting prospect, though it has been done.*

A trial that would detect (with statistical significance at 5% level, see above) a treatment that raised a cure rate from 75% to 85% would require 500 patients for 80% power. Obviously larger differences require fewer patients, and smaller differences require more patients (these figures make it clear why surveillance techniques of therapeutic evaluation are attracting increasing interest). A well-conducted trial giving a modest probability that is soon confirmed by other workers is preferable to a mammoth undertaking the aim of which is near certainty and which either breaks down from boredom and other human weakness, or else provides its result after the drug being tested has become obsolete.

The obvious course would seem to be to make a start and perform a statistical significance test every week/month and to stop as soon as a significant result was obtained but, unfortunately, it is not permissible to use two treatments concurrently and to perform an orthodox significance test at convenient intervals to 'see how things are going', or with the intention of stopping the trial as soon as 'the results are significant'. This is because chance must be the only factor operating in addition to the treatments to be tested, and such a practice introduces the workers' own preconceptions or wishes as a factor in determining when the trial should end. Differences between treated groups fluctuate as the trial proceeds and at one moment a 'significant' difference will occur due to chance if the trial goes on long enough. It is essential that this moment should not be watched for and grasped by the investigators — to pick it out will lead to a greater number of false positive results and so to false therapeutic claims.

It is therefore necessary, after deciding in consultation with a statistician what difference it is realistic to seek and with what precision, having regard to the time, energy and number of patients available, to agree on the number of patients to be treated, to treat them and then to test the results.† Then there is less likelihood of hitting on a falsely 'significant' difference. This is a **fixed-sample trial** and at the end there may be disappointment if, when the results are examined, they just miss the agreed acceptable level of statistical significance. Here, having presented their results, clinicians are entitled to express their opinion on their meaning, and the size of the confidence interval will be of great assistance (see above). It is here too that the results of independent workers are helpful; *confirmation by others is an essential process in therapeutic advance* as in all science. It is *not* legitimate, having just failed (say, $P = 0.06$) to reach the agreed level (say, $P = 0.05$) to take in a few more patients in the hope that they will bring P down to 0.05 or less,† for this is deliberately not allowing chance and the treatment to be the sole factors involved in the outcome, as they should be. At least this is the theory, but 'only an investigator with superhuman will power or completely chaotic records could supervise a clinical trial for months or years without ever looking to see which way the results were drifting' and being influenced by them in deciding when to stop the trial. Strictly this is not in accordance with statistical principles, but it will doubtless continue to be done. It has been suggested that 'the simplest solution is to continue as at present, where most published P-values need to be mentally doubled. The only completely ethical and valid alternative is for every clinical trial to have a professional statistician, using weekly computerised analyses to administer a sequential design.†

The **sequential design** was developed in response to the evident need for a design that allows *continuous* assessment and stops the study *either* as soon as a statistically significant result is reached *or* when such a result becomes unlikely. The essential feature has to be that the trial is terminated at a *pre*-determined point and not when the investigator, looking at the results to date, thinks it appropriate; (few investigators would be able to resist picking out the moment when the difference was statistically significant, which inevitably would mean a high rate of false-positive results). The technique of sequential analysis allows continuous monitoring but it has

* Vakil B J et al. Clin Pharmacol Ther. 1968; 9:465. A sequential trial that required 796 patients with tetanus.

† Peto R et al. Br J Cancer 1976; 34:585; 35:1.

disadvantages, e.g. a single unequivocal end-point is needed (and many trials, e.g. in rheumatism, require multiple assessments). A compromise between simple fixed-sample and truly sequential designs has been attained; it allows a formal analysis to be conducted at several *pre-determined* intervals and a decision made to stop or to continue. Such interim analyses reduce the statistical significance of the trial, but not to a serious degree if they are done, say, less than four times in a big trial.* Such modified sequential designs recognise the realities of medical practice and provide a reasonable trade-off between statistical and medical needs. It is virtually a necessity to have expert statistical advice when undertaking such trials. Indeed, common prudence dictates that anyone contemplating a therapeutic comparison of any kind should consult a statistician during the planning and not after the trial is over, for the function of statisticians is to help the clinician obtain a reliable result with minimum waste. They cannot convert a bad trial into a good one after it has finished and they tend to be annoyed if asked to do so, particularly after an editor has rejected the investigators' report.

If an experiment is ill-designed or ill-conducted it cannot be salvaged by statistics. Significance tests can be legitmately applied only to an experiment in which the sole variable that differs systematically between groups is the treatment to be tested. Bias in selection, allocation, observation and assessment of patients renders significance tests invalid. The application of such tests to data collected from old case records is more misleading than useful and is scientifically invalid.

The sensitivity of therapeutic trials

This, sadly, is not as great as clinicians would like: 'The practical conclusion is that clinical trials can easily monitor death rate ratios between two treatments which are 1:3 or better, but that detection of anything less extreme than 2:3 is very difficult. These summary ratios are very important, and should be written on the shirt-cuffs of all trial organisers, as attempting to study a difference which could not plausibly be as extreme as 2:3 by a clinical trial is a common mistake.'†

* But it is usual to make interim analyses at a higher (more extreme) level so that the overall risk of Type I error adopted in the trial design is not increased.

It is plain that a single trial will seldom give a conclusive answer to a therapeutic question. Confirmatory trials by other people in other centres play a major role in reaching reasonable certainty in therapeutics.

But where numerous trials have been done and the outcomes vary, it is tempting to collect them all together and **pool** the results using appropriate statistical methods (it is *not* acceptable to do a simple addition of groups). This can be enlightening, but the trials selected must be of good quality and the final result treated with caution.

Double-blind and single-blind techniques

The fact that both doctors and patients are subject to bias due to their beliefs and feelings has led to the invention of the double-blind technique. This is a '*control device to prevent bias from influencing results*. On the one hand it rules out the effects of hopes and anxieties of the patient by giving both the drug under investigation and a placebo (dummy) of identical appearance in such a way that the subject (the first "blind" man) does not know which he is receiving. On the other hand, it also rules out the influence of preconceived hopes of, and unconscious communication by, the investigator or observer by keeping him (the second "blind" man) ignorant of whether he is prescribing a placebo or an active drug. At the same time, the technique provides another control, a means of comparison with the magnitude of placebo effects.

'The device is both philosophically and practically sound. In addition, perhaps because of the widespread attention it has attracted, or the magic quality it appears to have, the double-blind technique has been assumed to be a complete method of drug evaluation in itself. Indeed, it is often called the double-blind test. Many seem to believe that all that is necessary for a good clinical study is to use it, and, since it is relatively easy to apply, many are exploiting it in just this way. A number of papers emphasise in the very title that this type

† Peto M et al. Br J Cancer 1976; 34:585.

of control was used, not only as if the use of a control were worthy of special mention, but also as if to warn the reader in advance that a special type of insurance has been taken out to guarantee that the results about to be recounted were beyond reproach.'*

The double-blind technique should be used if possible whenever evaluation depends on other than strictly objective measurements. There are occasions when it might at first sight seem that criteria of clinical improvement are objective when in fact they are not, for example the range of voluntary joint movement in rheumatoid arthritis has been shown to be greatly influenced by psychological factors, and a moment's thought shows why, for the amount of pain a patient will put up with is influenced by his mental state. Assessment of progress of chest radiographs in pulmonary tuberculosis is also liable to bias, due to enthusiasm or lack of it, and in the classic Medical Research Council chemotherapy trials† it was arranged that the radiologist commenting on the serial films should do so in ignorance of what treatment the patient was having.

Sometimes the double-blind technique is not possible because, for example, side-effects of an active drug reveal which patients are taking it or tablets look or taste different, but it never carries a disadvantage, 'only protection against spurious data'. It is not, of course, used with drugs fresh from the animal laboratory, whose dose and effects in man are unknown, although the subject may legitimately be kept in ignorance (single-blind) of the time of administration. Single-blind technique has little use in therapeutics research as it is equally important that the observer also be blind.

Ophthalmologists are understandably disinclined to refer to the double-blind technique; they call it double-masked.

Placebo or dummy medication as a control device in therapeutic trials

The foregoing quotation refers to occasions when a dummy or placebo treatment would be used, but this is not invariably necessary or indeed ethical, for it is not permissible to deprive patients of seriously effective therapy. In drug trials in, say, epilepsy or tuberculosis, the control groups comprise patients receiving the best available therapy.

The inert placebo or dummy is useful to:

1. Distinguish the pharmacodynamic effects of a drug from the psychological effects of the act of medication and circumstances surrounding it, e.g. increased interest by the doctor, more frequent visits, etc.
2. Distinguish drug effects from fluctuations in disease that occur with time and other external factors, e.g. in ulcerative colitis, rheumatoid arthritis (untreated controls also achieve this).
3. Avoid false negative conclusions. For example, a therapeutic trial of a new analgesic should consist of comparison of the new drug with a dummy as well as with a proved active analgesic. If all three treatments give the same result, a likely explanation is that the method used (including trial size) is incapable of distinguishing between an active and an inactive drug and so should be modified; whereas if only the new drug and the dummy are used and give identical results, there are two possible explanations, first that the method used is insensitive and second that the new drug has only placebo-effect, i.e. is pharmacologically inactive at the dose used.

It was found, for instance, in one trial in which angina pectoris was being treated and the progress of the disease determined by recording the frequency of attacks of pain, that 60% of patients improved over, on average, the first 11 weeks, regardless of whether they were receiving an active drug, a dummy (using double-blind technique) or no treatment at all. This meant that this particular method was less sensitive over this period and improvement genuinely due to a drug was masked, at least partially, until after the eleventh week. This early improvement regardless of drug therapy could partly be attributed to the establishment of a good psychological relationship between patient and physician.‡

* Modell W. JAMA 1958; 167:2190.

† Medical Research Council Br Med J 1955; 1:435.

‡ Cole S L et al. JAMA 1958; 68:275.

Controls: within-patient or between-patient (parallel group) studies

Sometimes in chronic stable disease that cannot be cured but can be alleviated it is possible to give each of the treatments under test, including placebo, to each patient, thus conveniently using them as their own controls (a cross-over study) for example in parkinsonism or hypertension. When this is done it is important to ensure in a small series that each drug both precedes and follows each other drug the same number of times, to avoid the risk of systematic bias due to changes with time and 'carry-over' effect, i.e. interaction of the drug given first with that given second. If in an analgesic trial a less effective drug always follows a more effective, the weaker drug may be dismissed as ineffective because the patient's standard has become influenced by the high degree of relief provided by the more effective drug. The less effective drug must precede as well as follow both the more effective drug and the dummy (if any) if error is to be avoided. In addition, persistence of a drug or metabolites and enzyme induction may influence the response to a subsequent drug.* For these reasons between-patient studies are preferred, but they require more subjects.

In acute self-limiting diseases it is plainly impossible to given more than one treatment to one patient and the controls must be other patients, i.e. between-patient or parallel groups.

Naturally there is a temptation simply to give a new treatment to all patients and to compare the results with the past, i.e. historical controls. Unfortunately this is almost always† unacceptable, even with a disease such as leukaemia, for standards of diagnosis and treatment change with time, severity of disease (infections) fluctuates. The provision that controls must be concurrent and concomitant (p. 50) stands.

Some mortal sins of clinical assessment‡

a. *Enthusiasm and scepticism* — 'a marvellous/useless drug, this.'

b. *Change of assessor* — 'do the measurements for me Jim/Miss Jones/darling.'

c. *Change of time* — 'don't worry about the assessment. Go ahead with lunch/X-rays/physiotherapy/your bath.'

d. *Squeezing* — 'you're much better, aren't you, Miss B?' 'Any indigestion yet, Miss B?'

e. *Pride*. 'I'm honest. No need for placebo in my trials'.

f. *Impurity* — 'We're short of cases: she'll have to do.' 'A few aspirins won't make much difference.'

g. *Imbalance* — 'Sex/severity/treatment order, doesn't matter.'

h. *Error* — 'Not quite significant. Let's try sequential analysis'.

Surveillance studies

There are *two important epidemiological approaches* that are applied to the study of drugs, especially to the detection of uncommon adverse reactions. They are not experimental (as is the randomised trial where entry and allocation of treatment are strictly controlled). They are *observational* in that the groups to be compared have been assembled from subjects who already are, or who are not (the controls), taking the treatment in the ordinary way of medical care.

The observational cohort§ study

Patients receiving the drug are collected and followed up to determine the outcomes (therapeutic and adverse). This is forward-looking (prospective) research. Prescription event monitoring (p. 63) is an example, and there is an increasing tendency to recognise that many new drugs should be monitored in this way when prescribing becomes general. Major difficulties include selection of an appropriate control group, the need for large numbers of subjects and for prolonged surveillance. This sort of study is scientifically inferior to the experimental cohort study (randomised controlled trial) and is cumber-

* 'Carry-over' can be minimised by inserting 'washout' periods between active treatments, but these are not always ethically acceptable.

† Criteria for cautiously but usefully employing historical controls are suggested by Bailar J C et al. Studies without internal controls. N Engl J Med 1984; 311:156.

‡ Hart F D et al. Measurement in rheumatoid arthritis. Lancet 1972; 2:28.

§ Used here for a group of people having a common attribute, e.g. they have all taken the same drug.

some for research on drugs. Happily, clever epidemiologists have devised an alternative, the case-control study.

The case-control study

This reverses the direction of scientific logic from forward-looking (prospective) to backward-looking (retrospective)* investigation. The investigator assembles a group of patients who have the condition it is desired to investigate, e.g. women who have had an episode of thromboembolism. A control group of women who have not had an episode of thromboembolism is then assembled, e.g. similar age, parity and smoking habits, for example from hospital admissions for other reasons, or primary care records, and a complete drug history is taken from each group, i.e. the two groups are 'followed up' backwards to determine the proportion in each group that has taken the suspect agent, in this case the oral contraceptive pill.

To solve the question of thromboembolism and the combined oestrogen-progestogen contraceptive pill by means of an observational cohort study requires enormous numbers of subjects† (the adverse effect is, happily, uncommon) followed over years. An investigation into cancer and the contraceptive pill would require follow-up for 10–15 years. This approach is evidently cumbersome and expensive, and cannot satisfy the urgent need for an answer once a suspicion is raised.

A case-control study can be done quickly; it has the advantage that it begins with a much smaller (compared with the cohort) number of cases (hundreds or less) of disease, but it has the disadvantage that it follows up subjects backwards and there is always suspicion of the intrusion of unknown and so unavoidable biases in selection of both patients and controls. Here again, independent repetition of the studies, if the results are the same, greatly enhances confidence in the outcome.

* For this reason Feinstein has named these *trohoc* (*cohort* spelled backwards) studies.

† The Royal College of General Practitioners (UK) recruited 23 000 women takers of the pill and 23 000 controls in 1968 and issued a report in 1973. It found an approximate doubled incidence of venous thrombosis in combined-pill takers (the dose of oestrogen has been reduced since this study).

A major disadvantage of the case-control study is that it requires a definite hypothesis or suspicion of causality. A cohort study on the other hand does not; subjects can be followed 'to see what happens' (event recording).

Case-control studies do not prove causation.† They reveal associations and it is up to investigators and critical readers to decide what is the most plausible explanation of the associations revealed.

Feinstein has pointed out that the validity of case-control studies can be increased if the standards of entry and evaluation are raised to those applied to experimental studies in the same field (randomised controlled trials). He concludes that 'Epidemiologic research has become increasingly important because it offers a substitute for the unattainable scientific "gold standard" of a randomised experimental trial . . . An insistence on high scientific quality can help epidemiologic studies achieve the standards and rigor of research in other branches of modern science.'‡

Doctors should be familiar with the case-control study and Table 4.1 illustrates its conduct and value. It speaks for itself and shows particularly the importance of confirmatory studies to strengthen assurance.

Readers can decide for themselves how convincing are these studies taken singly and together; for those who have a low threshold of suspicion we list the references in the table so that they can examine the choice of controls (particularly), on which all depends. In determining causation other knowledge of hormonal effects on coagulation is taken into account.

General discussion

Observational cohort studies in which large numbers of patients under routine care are monitored to obtain information of the dosage, route, adverse effects, efficacy, etc. of drugs

† Experimental cohort studies (randomised controlled trials) are on firmer ground with regard to causation. In the experimental cohort study there should be only *one* systematic difference between the groups (i.e. the treatment being studied). In case-control studies the groups may differ systematically in several ways.

‡ Feinstein A et al. N Engl J Med (1982); 307:1611.

Table 4.1 Case-control studies of oral contraception and thromboembolic diseases*

Event	Country, date	*Thromboembolic events* Total number of patients	Contraceptive users	*Controls*: Number of contraceptive users
Deaths	UK, 1968[1]	26	16	4
Hospital admissions	UK, 1969[2]	84	42	12
	USA, 1969[3]	129	53	19
	Sweden, 1971[4]	84	55	12
Primary care consultation	UK, 1967[5]	20 (deep vein)	5	2
		72 (superficial vein)	11	4

* Data summarised from: Bradford Hill A. Meeting on pharmacological models to assess toxicity and side-effects of fertility regulating agents. Geneva. 1973.

1. Br Med J 1968; 2:193.
2. Br Med J 1969; 2:651.
3. Am J Epidemiol 1969; 90:365.
4. Acta Med Scand 1971; 190:455.
5. J R Coll Gen Pract 1967; 13:267.

provide advantages in that the physician is practising the way he thinks best, is not confined to a rigid pre-planned scheme and his discretion about using alternative drugs can often be unfettered. Such techniques are likely to be useful not only for monitoring new drugs, but for comparing minor variants of, e.g. hypnotics and analgesics, for which it is already difficult to find skilled workers who are willing to devote time to formal comparative studies.

a. *In hospitals* the system is organised to that ward routine is not disturbed (the most developed example is the Boston [USA] Collaborative Drug Surveillance Program). Such systems, which may operate internationally, employ pharmacists or nurses to collect data on standardised self-coding forms from consecutively admitted patients (using the clinical records and interviews with clinical staff and patients). The range of data collected can be as wide or as narrow as circumstances and resources permit. Generally there will be included patients' characteristics (age, sex, weight, consumption of tobacco, alcohol), previous drugs and details of present therapy, reasons for its discontinuation, adverse or beneficial events during stay in hospital (whether or not they are thought to be caused by drugs), etc. After the patient has left hospital the final editing of the data sheets 'is done by a computer program that checks the data for completeness, plausibility and internal consistency. Recently acquired data are added to the master files periodically, and routine analyses are performed to evaluate suspected and unsuspected drug effects'.†.

b. *Outside hospitals*, surveillance programmes present obvious additional difficulties including expense. Techniques include *prescription event monitoring*, i.e. surveillance of prescriptions where these are eventually handled in a central office (as in the UK National Health Service where they are sent to a pricing office) and questionnaires sent to doctors using the drugs that are being monitored asking for report of *all events* that have happened to the patient (good and ill), not merely events that the doctor thinks may be drug caused. This potentially important field of surveillance is relatively undeveloped as yet. Increasingly it is recognised that many, if not all, new medicines should be subject to such safety monitoring when they are released for general prescribing.

† Miller R R et al. Drug effects in hospitalized patients: experiences of the Boston Collaborative Drug Surveillance Program 1966–1975. New York: Wiley, 1976.

Reliability of published therapeutic trials

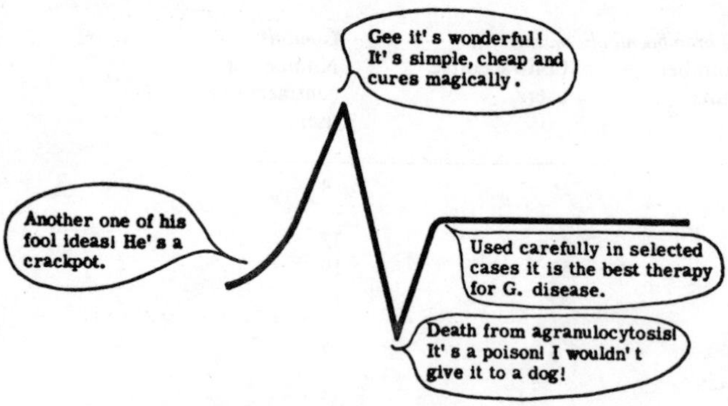

Fig. 4.1 Oscillations in the development of a drug.*

From time to time people experienced in therapeutic evaluation study published therapeutic trials and report their conclusions.

In one study it was concluded that about 66% of published papers are acceptable and 33% unacceptable according to what are now generally agreed criteria.

In another study 50% of papers were found to have statistical errors of which half were serious, and in 8% of papers a claim was made that was unsupportable on re-examination of the data.

In conclusion

This account of some aspects of therapeutic evaluation may be sufficient to show with what care studies must be designed. The possibilities of error are legion. Throughout this book there are references to examples of well-designed studies that show how the same principles are adapted to suit widely different circumstances. The reader is recommended to consult them both for instruction and entertainment and to pursue the subject further in the list of references at the end of this Chapter.

It is increasingly appreciated that rigorous randomised controlled trials of classic design constitute only a part, though a vital part, of drug evaluation. The conclusion, in such a trial, that treatment A is better than treatment B, for disease C, may distract attention from the fact that the disease may have multiple aetiology and that 'therapeutics' often involves a lot more than prescribing a drug or other regimen. For example, bronchospasm due to an antigen–antibody reaction may be completely relieved by orthodox drug therapy, whereas bronchospasm precipitated by domestic unhappiness, whether or no there is a true allergic basis, may get only trivial relief from drugs. The therapy of anxiety is another florid example. It is as vital that the advocates of the individual approach should not discount the value of the randomised controlled trial, which has done so much for the improvement and rationalisation of therapeutics, as it is that the practitioners who wisely base their choice of treatment on the results of therapeutic experiments, wherever possible, should realise that the treatment preferred in such a study may sometimes be inappropriate for an individual patient.

It has been pointed out† that the more an illness resembles an accident (e.g. most infections), the more effective will be so-called scientific treatments and the more applicable will be the randomised controlled trial in evaluating treatment; but where illness can be due, wholly or partly, to lack of integration between individual and environment (e.g. anxiety, depression, asthma, eczema, hay fever, ulcerative colitis) the more treatments has to be related to the individuals' life history, to enable them to achieve the integration that they could not achieve alone, and then drugs may take second place or may not be needed at all.

This book is not a book of 'therapeutics' but of clinical pharmacology and drug therapy, which may constitute a negligible part of the therapy of some patients and the determining factor in the outcome for others. The fact that general aspects of therapy will be seldom referred to here does not imply that they are thought to lack importance.

* By courtesy of Dr. Robert H. Williams and the Editor of JAMA.

† Balint M Lancet 1961; 1:40.

GUIDE TO FURTHER READING

On Ethics

1 Hill A B Medical ethics and controlled trials. Br Med J 1963; 2:1043, and subsequent correspondence.
2 Beecher H K. Some fallacies and errors in the application of the principle of consent in human experimentation. Clin. Pharmacol. Ther 1962; 3:141.
3 Beecher H K. Experimentation in man. JAMA 1959; 169:461.
4 Religious statements on human experimentation, Roman Catholic, Protestant, Jewish. World Medical Journal 1960; 7:80, and after
5 Editorial. Secret randomized clinical trials. Lancet 1982; 2:78.
6 Cancer Research Campaign Working Party in Breast Conservation. Informed consent: ethical, legal, and medical implications for doctors and patients who participate in randomized clinical trials. Br Med J 1983; 286:1117.
7 Schafer A. The ethics of the randomized controlled clinical trial. N Engl J Med 1982; 307:719.
8 CIOMS/WHO. Proposed international guidelines for biomedical research involving human subjects. p 49 Geneva: WHO, 1982.
9 Altman D G. Statistics and ethics in medical research: misuse of statistics is unethical. Br Med J 1980; 281:1182.

On Therapeutic Evaluation

1 Pickering G W The place of the experimental method in medicine. Proc Roy Soc Med 1949; 42:229.
2 Hill A B. Principles of medical statistics. London: Hodder & Stoughton, 1984. A classic book.
3 Wolf S. et al. Effects of placebo administration and occurrence of toxic reactions. JAMA 1954; 155:339.
4 Beecher H K. Analgesic power and the question of 'acute tolerance' to narcotics in man. J Pharmacol Exp Ther 1953; 108:158.
5 Modell W et al. Factors influencing clinical evaluation of drugs with special reference to the double-blind technique. JAMA 1958; 167:2190.
6 Gore S M et al. Misuse of statistical methods: critical assessment of articles in B.M.J. from Jan to Mar 1976. Br Med J 1977; 1:85.
7 Peto R et al. Design and analysis of randomized clinical trials requiring prolonged observation in each patient. Br J Cancer 1976; 34:585; 35:1.
8 Modell W. Anyone for a symposium? Clin Pharmacol Ther 1960; 1:689.
9 Beecher H K. Surgery as placebo. JAMA 1961; 176:1102.
10 Joyce C R B et al. The objective efficacy of prayer. J Chron Dis 1965; 18:367.
11 Feinstein A R. Hard science, soft data, and the challenges of choosing clinical variables. Clin Pharmacol Ther 1977; 22:485. One of a long series of important articles on clinical biostatistics.
12 Wade O L et al. Significant or important. Br J Clin Pharmacol 1977; 4:411.
13 Gore S M. Statistics in question: a series of articles. Assessing clinical trials (1980/81) Br Med J; 282: 1605, 1687, 1780, 1861, 1958, 2036, 2114. 283: 40, 122, 211, 296, 369, 426, 486, 548, 600, 660, 711, 775, 840, 901, 966. These articles have been published as a book, Statistics in practice, with Altman D G. London: British Medical Association 1982.
14 Mainland D. Statistical ritual in clinical journals: is there a cure? Br Med J 1984; 288:841, 920.
15 Altman D G et al. Statistical guidelines for contributors to medical journals. Br Med J 1983; 286:1489.
16 Pocock S J. Current issues in the design and interpretation of clinical trials. Br Med J 1985; 290:39.
17 Strom B L et al. Postmarketing studies of drug efficacy: when must they be randomized? Clin Pharmacol Ther 1983; 34:1.
18 Bland J M et al. Is the clinical trial evidence about new drugs statistically adequate? Br J Clin Pharmacol 1985; 19:155.
19 Castle W M et al. Problems of postmarketing surveillance. Br J Clin Pharmacol 1983; 16:581.
20 DerSimonian R. et al. Reporting on methods in clinical trials. N Engl J Med 1982; 306:1332.
21 Guyatt G. Determining optimal therapy — randomized trials in individual patients N Engl J Med 1986; 314:889.
22 Sacks H S et al. Meta-analyses of randomized controlled trials [pooling]. N Engl J Med 1987; 316:450.
23 Editorial. The controlled trial: consensus? Lancet 1987; 1:547.

5

Official regulation of drugs: disasters and follies

Medicines are part of our way of life from birth, when we enter the world with the aid of drugs, to death where drugs assist (most of) us to depart with minimal distress and perhaps even with a remnant of dignity. In between these events we regulate our fertility, often, with drugs. We tend to take such usages for granted.*

But during the intervals remaining, an average family experiences illness on one day in four and between the ages of 20 and 45 years a lower-middle-class man experiences approximately one life-endangering illness, 20 disabling (temporarily) illnesses, 200 non-disabling illnesses and 1000 symptomatic episodes,† and medicines play a major role in these.

But neither patients nor doctors are in a position to decide for themselves across the range of medicines that they use, which ones are pure and stable and effective and safe. They need some assurance that the medicines they are offered fulfil these requirements and are also supported with information that permits optimal use. Only governments can provide such assurance, insofar as it can be provided.

Official or statutory regulation of medicines provides a perfect example of *the role of governments*:

a. To enable citizens to undertake jointly tasks that they cannot undertake individually, and
b. to protect individual citizens from the actions of others.

The objective of official regulations is to ensure a supply of effective and safe medicines whether by selection from amongst those used in traditional systems or by modern invention. Unsafe or ineffective medicines should be identified and eliminated, whilst bearing in mind that an unduly purist approach based on the assumption that what is not demonstrable by modern techniques of drug evaluation is not knowledge, may both result in wrong judgements and unnecessarily deprive the community of comforts that are harmless but which provide psychological support. In respect of these latter it is the function of official drug regulation to ensure that any such placebo medicines are known for what they are and that unjustified therapeutic claims are not made.

Official (statutory) drug regulation is therefore concerned with:

1. **quality**, i.e. purity, stability (shelf-life)
2. **safety**
3. **efficacy**
4. **supply**, i.e. whether the drug is to be unrestrictedly available to the public or confined to

* Doris: I'd be bored.
Sweeney: You'd be bored. Birth, and copulation, and death. That's all the facts when you come to brass tacks.

T S Eliot (Poet: 1888–1965): Sweeney Agonistes

† Quoted In: Anderson J A D, ed. Self medication. Lancaster: MTP Press, 1979.

sales through pharmacies or to doctors' prescriptions.

A basic requirement of any control system is that no medicine may be sold or supplied without prior licencing or registration by government. If there is no licencing system there is no control.

Plainly, manufacturers and developers need to be told what kinds of data and in what amount are likely to persuade the regulatory authority to grant a licence. Therefore the authority issues 'guidelines', generally stating that these will be interpreted and applied 'flexibly'. But, almost inevitably, flexible guidelines tend to become minimal requirements in the day-to-day operation of a legislative act by government servants.

A summary of guidelines for *pre-clinical tests* begins on p. 37, and for *clinical tests* on p. 46.

Some history

The beginning of substantial government intervention in the field of medicines paralleled the proliferation of synthetic drugs in the early 20th century when the traditional and familiar pharmacopoeia expanded slowly and then, in mid-century, with enormous rapidity; intervention was initially confined to safety aspects and was developed piecemeal as issues arose, until the thalidomide disaster of 1961 caused governments all over the world to rationalise, formalise and extend their control of medicines in single, though often complicated, laws.

Governmental controls developed approximately as follows. **Safety** came first, with restrictions on supply of 'dangerous drugs' especially drugs of addiction, and it is significant that there was actually a UK Act of Parliament entitled The Dangerous Drugs Act.

Then followed controls on **quality** in manufacture which were stimulated by the introduction of preparations of substances occurring naturally in the body, e.g. insulin (1922) on accurate dose of which the life of large numbers of diabetics depends. Inefficient or incompetent manufacture (impurity, inefficacy, instability) will cause deaths, and since consumers are not able to determine for themselves whether the preparation offered is reliable, they require protection against defective products. Therefore government control is essential in the public interest.

Efficacy at first received less attention. In the first half of this century drug therapy was relatively uncritical, though in the UK a law was passed forbidding advertising to the public of 'cures' for veneral disease, tuberculosis and epilepsy. Drug therapy was based on the assertions derived from the impressions of physicians. In mid-century, methods of formal therapeutic evaluation, though foreshadowed by isolated individuals in the previous 200 years, became established, and scientific comparisons of the efficacy of new and old medicines became commonplace.

But governments did not act to extend control of medicines to include efficacy as well as safety; there was no public pressure for them to do so. The most effective pressure that persuades politicians that they should act radically and quickly is a public scandal where failure to respond will make them so unpopular that they fail to achieve re-election.

The first comparatively comprehensive drug regulatory law prior to thalidomide was passed in the USA in 1938, following the death of about 107 people due to the use of diethylene glycol (a constituent of antifreezes) as a solvent for a liquid formulation of sulphanilamide for treating common infections. The sulphonamides, introduced in 1935, were the first major therapeutic advance against common bacterial infections.

In early 1937, in the USA, tablets and capsules of sulphanilamide were marketed by a number of firms including the S. E. Massengill Company of Tennessee. In June 1937 the firm's salesmen reported a demand for the drug in liquid form (easier for children to take, etc).

Since sulphanilamide is relatively insoluble in the usual vehicles, a number of other solvents used in industry were tried. Diethylene glycol was effective and an 'elixir' was made of drug, solvent, flavouring and water.

No tests in animals were made to determine the toxicity either of the ingredients separately or of the finished product, or to determine whether the mixture was stable, i.e. whether the drug decomposed in the solvent when stored. The company's laboratory merely checked the mixture for appearance, flavour and fragrance. No special trials were conducted in man; 1100 litres of the mixture were made and marketed. This procedure was compatible with the then existing law in the USA.

In October 1937, news of deaths in Oklahoma was telephoned to the US Food & Drug Administration (FDA) by a physician. Eight children with sore throats and one adult with gonorrhoea had died after taking the 'elixir'. When the Massengill Company heard of the deaths it sent out 1100 telegrams to its customers and salesmen asking for recovery of all 'elixir' that had been sold. Since these requests seemed unlikely to impress receivers with the true urgency of the situation, the investigating FDA inspectors insisted, on October 19, that a more cogent telegram be sent:

'Imperative you take up immediately all elixir sulphanilamide you dispensed. Product may be dangerous to life. Return our expense.'

Large amounts were sent back, but it was essential that *all* be recovered. Almost all the 239 FDA inspectors and chemists were assigned to this task. Warnings were broadcast by radio and newspaper. Individual prescriptions were identified and pursued, though the pursuit was hampered by prescriptions such as, 'Betty Jane, 9 months old' and 'Mrs Jackson' (no address). But some elixir had been sold directly to the public and the purchasers were unknown.

Massengill Company travelling salesmen were pursued from hotel to hotel and interviewed. One salesman was uncooperative, but changed his mind when jailed. Most doctors and pharmacists cooperated. But one doctor who had admitted dispensing to five patients refused their names though claiming they were all alive. Enquiry revealed he had supplied seven patients and four were dead.

'One of the fatal prescriptions was traced through neighbourhood gossip describing the symptoms of the fatal illness of a Negro employee of a lumber mill. The inspector recognised the symptoms as characteristic of 'elixir' poisoning and through the mill superintendent found the victim's sister. She remembered the doctor had given her brother some red medicine about October 2 or 3. She said that in accordance with their custom, all medicines, glasses, spoons, etc. had been placed on the grave, which was about $1\frac{1}{2}$ miles back in the fields. Accompanied by the Negroes, the inspector walked to the wooded knoll with its single mound of fresh earth on which lay several bottles, dishes and spoons. One 4 ounce bottle contained about one ounce [28 ml] of the "elixir". It bore the weatherbeaten but legible prescription label of the doctor.'*

Typical effects occurred 24–48 hours after taking the elixir, with nausea, vomiting, malaise, severe abdominal pain, sometimes diarrhoea, and anuria, the patient became unconscious and either died after 2–7 days or recovered over 7–21 days. Autopsy disclosed renal and hepatic damage.

As soon as its help was asked by physicians (October 11, 1937) the American Medical Association asked the Massengill Company the composition of the 'elixir' since this was not declared on the label. The Company provided the information, though requesting that it should be treated as confidental. On October 20 the Company telegraphed the American Medical Association, 'Please wire . . . suggestion for antidote and treatment . . .' and the Association replied, 'Antidote for Elixir Sulfanilamide-Massengill not known . . .'

About 107 people died. The only basis for action under the Food and Drugs Act was that the word 'elixir' traditionally implied an alcoholic solution, whereas this contained diethylene glycol.

On October 23, Dr. Massengill issued a press statement: 'My chemists and I deeply regret the fatal results, but *there was no error in manufacture of the product*. We have been supplying legitimate professional demand and *not once could have foreseen the unlooked-for results*. I do not feel that there was any responsibility on our part. The chemical sulfanilamide had been approved for use and had been used in large quantities in other forms, and now its many bad effects are developing.'

The bad effects were in fact due to the diethylene glycol solvent and evidence of possible harm

* Quoted from Report of the Secretary of Agriculture submitted in response to resolutions in the House of Representatives and Senate (USA): JAMA 1937; 109: 1985, the principal source of this story.

was available prior to marketing this 'elixir'. Effects similar to those in man are easily shown in animals.

In November, Dr. Massengill stated (in a letter to the American Medical Association) *'I have broken no law.'* In fact a federal court later found that he had broken the law in relation to 'adulteration and misbranding' of an 'elixir' and he was fined $150 on each of 112 counts, making a total of $16 800.

But 'Federal officials were miserably handicapped by the weak law'*.

The USA Congress now acted quickly and passed a bill providing that no new drug or any modifications of old drugs should be placed on the market until the entire formula had been submitted to the Food and Drug Administration of the US Department of Agriculture and the firm licensed to market the drug. Claims made on labels, advertisements, etc. were also brought under supervision of the Federal Trade Commission*. These requirements remain the basis of effective drug control systems.

All this took place 9 years after a pharmacologist speaking before the Section of Pharmacology and Therapeutics of the American Medical Association (1929) said: 'Many drug firms make the mistake of believing that their chemists can furnish trustworthy pharmacologic opinion. Indeed, some eminent chemists, impatient with careful pharmacologic technic have ventured to estimate for themselves the clinical possibilities of their own synthetics . . . *There is no short cut from chemical laboratory to clinic, except one that passes too close to the morgue.*'†

Other specialists in 1938 listed the technical requirements for developing a drug and commented, 'many more lives will be sacrificed if such standards are not put into effect. Any essential compromise with these requirements will inevitably exact a toll of deaths or injuries among the public. The life and safety of the individual should not be subordinated to the competitive system of drug exploitation.'†

Other countries did not learn the lesson provided by the USA and it took the thalidomide disaster of 1960–61 to make governments all over the world initiate comprehensive control over all aspects of drug introduction, prescribing and supply. Those governments that already had some control system extended it.

But no regulatory system can guarantee complete safety. Therefore it is interesting to consider whether the thalidomide disaster might have been prevented in Europe by a control system such as was then in force in the USA.

Thalidomide was developed in West Germany and introduced thence into other countries.

The USA and the UK have similar attitudes to technical medicine. The former had a comprehensive regulatory body (FDA) in 1960 and the latter did not. It might be thought that this would provide a field test of the usefulness of official drug regulation. But it did not.

Thalidomide was marketed in the UK, according to accepted practice at the time, without official review or hindrance but it was delayed in the USA by the routine administrative machinery. During this delay period it was discovered and published in the UK that thalidomide could cause peripheral neuritis in man. Naturally this led to further cautious delay in the USA and during this further period the harmful effect on the fetus was revealed in other countries (see p. 84).

It is hard to be sure, but it seems likely that if thalidomide had been first developed in the USA the drug would have been marketed there. There will continue to be speculation, informed by hindsight, whether the substantial freedom of the USA from thalidomide (there was some in clinical trial) was the result of scientific insight or of bureaucratic delay giving time for the adverse effects to be identified elsewhere.

Mere delay protects, provided others are using the drugs concerned. But it can also deprive populations of valuable drugs.

A modern drug regulatory authority

A modern drug regulatory authority requires the following:

1. **Pre-clinical tests**
   a. Tests carried out in animals to allow some prediction of potential efficacy and safety

* JAMA 1938; 111:583.

† JAMA 1938; 111:919

in man (see p. 37 for an outline of the tests).

b. Chemical and pharmaceutical quality (purity, stability, formulation, etc.)

2. **Regulatory review.** At this stage the authority may review the data and decide formally whether clinical tests may begin or it may accept notification of the developer's intention in the form of a certified summary (to which it may object if it chooses).

3. **Clinical (human) tests.** Phases 1, 2, 3 to determine whether the drug deserves to be licensed or registered for general prescription (the drug being supplied for these trials by the developers without payment, for it is not yet a medicine; see p. 46 for an outline of the tests).

4. **Regulatory review.** The authority formally reviews both pre-clinical and clinical data and decides whether the drug can be granted a licence for general prescribing (Product Licence), i.e. it is deemed to be a medicine and it can be marketed with therapeutic claims. The regulatory authority decides what therapeutic claims can be made and also must be satisfied of the adequacy of the information to be provided to prescribers (Data Sheet) and also, where appropriate, any Patient Information Leaflet (which is particularly important with preparations for long-term use such as oral contraceptives).

When a novel drug is granted a Product Licence it is recognised as a medicine by independent critics and there is rejoicing amongst those who have spent many years developing it. But the testing is not over, the most stringent test of all is about to begin. It will be used in all sorts of people of all ages and sizes and having all sort of other conditions. Its use can no longer be so closely supervised as hitherto. Doctors will prescribe it and patients will use it correctly and incorrectly. It will have effects that have not been anticipated. It will be taken in overdose. It has to find its place in therapeutics.

5. **Post-licencing/marketing surveillance** (p. 46) has thus become an essential stage of drug evaluation. It is neither easy nor cheap to accomplish.

The important objective is to obtain information on large numbers of patients, 10 000–20 000, in observational cohort studies, e.g. prescription event monitoring (p. 63) and case-control studies where appropriate; spontaneous reporting of suspected adverse reactions is also encouraged, e.g. by marking the drug with a special symbol, ▼ in formularies (in the UK).

Further randomised controlled trials (experimental cohort studies) especially comparing the new drug with those already available will continue, for a long time in the case of really novel advances.

6. **Duration of a Product Licence** should always be limited (5 years in UK). This reminds producers to keep up an interest in their products since they may be asked to justify renewal of their licence at regular intervals. Of course, in the light of experience, it is always open to the regulatory authority to challenge the licence-holder at any time and to ask for more data on safety (usually) or efficacy. Producers who do not keep the dossier on their products up-to-date may, and often have, found themselves in difficulty when the safety of a product is suddenly questioned. Lack of data is one of the most certain ways of ensuring adverse decisions by regulatory authorities, particularly when there is mass-media pressure.

General discussion

It may be wondered why post-licencing/marketing surveillance should be necessary. Commonsense would seem to dictate that safety and efficacy of a drug should be fully defined before it is granted a Product Licence (marketed). Pre-licencing trials with very close supervision are commonly limited to hundreds of patients and this is unavoidable, chiefly because this close supervision is impracticable on a large scale for a very long time.

Closely supervised pre-marketing trials (particularly when no exciting result is anticipated but merely a possibility of modest advance) constitute a tremendous burden on both investigators and patients. Interest of the doctor flags, willingness of patients to accept the inconvenience of close supervision declines, precise records become imprecise, patients drop out. Even if mammoth controlled trials are done, and they have been done and are very expensive, there is no assurance of a useful result.

An 8-year study of treatment of diabetes*,

* JAMA 1975; 231:583.

which started in 1961, cost US $7.7 million and did not answer the problems of long-term management of maturity-onset diabetes.

Current multicentre and international studies of drug treatment of mild high blood pressure will take years to complete and already the cost is running into the equivalent of millions of US dollars.

Both the above examples concern drugs already marketed and shown effective in controlling the blood sugar and the blood pressure respectively. But it still has to be conclusively proved that close control of blood sugar and of *mild* high blood pressure is actually accompanied by fewer major complications and longer life, though this seems likely in both cases. The end result of long-term treatment over many years can only be discovered by following treated patients over many years. It is vital that correct answers be obtained (for social and economic reasons).

Definitive therapeutic studies in such diseases require large-scale production of drugs and their use in many thousands of patients over years. In medical and social terms it seems irrelevant whether the drug is 'marketed' or not; in any case it must be paid for by somebody, and, in fact, always ultimately by the public.

Medicines must be allowed to be sold (they are supplied free for clinical trials) at a reasonably early stage if research-based industry is to continue to operate. Of course there will be no question of granting a licence to sell until there is evidence that the majority of patients will benefit. But the rarer risks cannot be accurately determined until as many as 100 000 or even more patients have used the drug and their experience been recorded. Such experience may take years. The only way in which this experience can be financed is by selling the drug. Selling the drug need not mean its use is not being closely supervised. It is supervision and evaluation that is important to patients rather than whether it is supplied 'free' or for money. But a flow of money is essential to industry to support manufacture, distribution and research into further new drugs.

It is for these reasons that post-licencing schemes are increasingly regarded as essential to complete the definitive evaluation of drugs under conditions of ordinary use on a large scale, these programmes being preferable to attempts to enlarge and prolong formal therapeutic trials.

The regulatory organisation has the power to control the claims and to ensure that necessary information is provided to prescribers and patients so they will not be misled. But allowing sale and general prescribing no longer means the end of the period of formal evaluation.

It is now recognised that full evaluation of medicines commonly takes extensive use over many years* and techniques are being adapted to this fact and devised to reduce the period to a minimum.

Oral contraceptives, antidiabetic agents and hormone replacement therapy for post-menopausal women are examples where benefit: risk evaluation proceeds over decades. Major tranquillisers are still controversial after more than 20 years of widespread use.

It is evident that when a drug increases the incidence of a disease that occurs spontaneously and commonly, no monitoring system, however efficient, can identify the first drug-induced cases for what they are. For example, the use of oestrogen alone, or 'unopposed' by a progestogen as in oral contraceptives, to relieve unpleasant menopausal symptoms and subsequent continuous and indefinite use as hormone replacement therapy (HRT) has recently been shown probably to cause endometrial cancer, and the incidence increases as therapy is more prolonged (some investigators disagree, stating that these studies are biased).

Such a consequence can only reliably be discovered and confirmed by epidemiological methods (p. 61) and this means large-scale use in women, and certainty grows as more women develop cancer. If this is not acceptable practice then therapy of this kind cannot be introduced at all for the foreseeable future.

* For these reasons the UK and many other countries having a research-based industry do not require that a drug or medicine (formulation) be shown to be better than others as a condition for marketing. But Norway approaches this by requiring that medical 'need' be shown as a condition for marketing. Norway has available about 1900 formulations (chemical entities plus dose forms) and the UK has about 6000.

Professional medical caution over the possible hazard of HRT has been condemned by some vocal women as an example of the indifference of a male-dominated profession to the suffering of women, and even as a sexist desire (conscious or unconscious) in men to make women suffer. The fact that women doctors expressed equal concern merely shows, it is implied, how successfully men dominate the profession.

The benefit of oestrogens used briefly for menopausal symptoms are not controversial. The benefits used as long-term replacement therapy are controversial. That long-term continuous use reduces post-menopausal osteoporosis is now reasonably sure, but that it also increases the incidence of cancer seems probable. It is not merely important to know that this cancer risk is there, but it is essential to know, if at all possible, the magnitude of the effect, because only then can a sensible decision be taken on acceptance or non-acceptance of risk.

It seems that the increased risk is less than that of heavy smoking.

In the light of such knowledge the options are to:

1. abandon the use of oestrogens for this purpose altogether,

2. use oestrogens in short courses at the lowest effective dose to relieve particularly troublesome symptoms.

3. accept the risk wherever women feel more comfortable taking oestrogen and to prescribe the hormone indefinitely; the woman herself will decide this, for only she can tell how important are such subjective issues as feelings of well being, possibly postponed facial wrinkling, etc.

4. follow the most recent evidence, which suggests that oestrogen combined with progestogen carries little or no risk of cancer.

In such a situation the function of a drug regulatory body is to ensure that the public and the medical profession are properly informed and to offer advice, prepared in consultation with experts in the field, so that those who do not have the skill, the time or the wish to study the evidence and form their own opinion can yet feel that the best opinion is available to them. It is our opinion that the course suggested in (4) above is the wisest when there is no overt clinical need, but the patient seeks therapy. We are aware that to some women a wrinkled face is worse than death, and we would not wish to prevent them making their own choice and taking a risk whether or not it can be precisely quantified.

Though efficacy of a new drug for the intended uses must be shown, safety is the chief concern behind official drug regulation, as is shown by the name of the UK drug regulatory organisation, the Committee on *Safety* of Medicines (a body of independent people which makes recommendations that are implemented [or not] by the Licensing Authority [i.e. government]).

There is an understandable tendency to feel that a substance developed with the objective of relieving suffering should itself be incapable of causing suffering, and that if suffering ensues some persons must be at fault and that they can be discovered and punished. But this feeling is not based on reason, and hazard is as inseparable from introducing chemicals (drugs) into the body as it is from surgery. Everybody knows, indeed it is self-evident, that surgery and anaesthesia carry risks and most people readily accept them. But the act of prescribing is so brief and seems so trivial that it is hard for many to accept that the result can have widespread and even catastrophic effects. It is from irrational feelings that all drug-induced disease is or should be avoidable that there arise public pressures and outcry when things go wrong due to the inevitable inadequacies of drug science.

Those responsible to the public or who might be blamed for an accident, naturally find it hard to resist this pressure. They attempt to meet the essentially unreasonable demand for virtually total safety by increasing the requirements for testing, even where there is no good reason to believe that increased testing gives increased assurance of safety.

For example, before thalidomide (1961) it was not a routine practice to test new drugs on pregnant animals. After thalidomide it became the routine to test all new drugs during early pregnancy in animals, at which stage the major organ forming processes take place. Now testing has expanded to cover risk at all stages of the reproductive process (p. 38). Thus it is hoped to avoid future accident. In fact, little is known of the predictive value of such tests. But there is no doubt whatever as to their cost in money and scientific resources.

Increasingly drugs are tested for carcinogenicity and mutagenicity.

And so it goes on, the labour and cost of drug testing prior to administration to man steadily increases. This could be justified if there were good assurance that the increase really gave extensive protection to man. But there are grounds for believing that such tests have a limited and uncertain value except where precise mechanisms have been determined.

We are not saying that tests in animals are of no use. They are essential within their limitations. We would regard the administration to man of chemicals on which there was no information on their effects in animals in these special areas as quite unacceptable.

We consider that the pursuit, by public demand and by the natural desire of drug scientists and official regulatory bodies, of virtually absolute safety, or 'safety at any cost', even when lip service is sometimes paid to the inevitability of hazard, is now reaching a point where it may, paradoxically, act against the public interest. It may stop the development of new drugs for serious and untreatable (especially for rare) disease by rendering research programmes prohibitively costly, and by causing the withdrawal of drugs before their risks have been quantified and calmly reviewed in relation to the risks of disease and of daily life in general.

Already an oral contraceptive must undergo research and safety testing for about 8 years (carcinogenicity tests in beagles for 7 years were until recently thought necessary) before trial in woman (or man), and there is then no substantial certainly that it will not then fail the necessarily large and rigorous human testing programme.

Whether drugs are developed by private or state enterprise, considerations of investment of the now enormous resources demanded are liable to turn those responsible to seek other outlets for their skills and for their investment.

We consider that there is a solution.

Put bluntly it is based on the fact that if we want to know for certain if a drug is effective in human disease, it must be put to the test in human disease. If we want to know for certain whether a drug damages human beings (at therapeutic doses) we must put it to the test in human beings. It is only after a human has been damaged that we can know for certain that the drug damages humans.

This means that drugs should undergo a reasonable (in current scientific terms) testing programme in animals. They should then enter a limited period (that will be defined for each drug) of closely supervised testing in man to define provisionally efficacy and safety.

If the drug is judged to pass these tests successfully then it should be made generally available for prescription, but under special defined conditions of post-licencing surveillance (according to whether it is an anaesthetic, an ointment for eczema, an inhalation for asthma, etc.) that will ensure that patients receiving it are individually monitored for unexpected events or for changes in incidence of coincident disease for a period that will often be years. For example, if an adverse effect occurs in 1 in 10 000 (0.01%) patients treated, then to determine this reliably (95% probability) it will be necessary to study 30 000 treated patients and often the same number of controls.

Such a programme will allow the public to be provided with the new drugs it needs with a minimum of risk. Always it must be remembered that though there are risks in taking drugs, there are also risks is not taking drugs, and there are risks in not developing new drugs.

Decision taking and subjective aspects of official drug regulation*

Official regulators and their advisers decide not only what new medicines shall be made available to medical practice but also what existing medicines shall remain available. For example, in one period of 20 months in the UK, six recently introduced medicines were withdrawn (five nonster-

* One of us (DRL) has been an adviser in drug regulation since 1964.

oidal anti-inflammatory drugs [NSAIDs] and one antidepressant) due to regulatory action of one kind or another. In addition, one long-established NSAID (oxyphenbutazone) was withdrawn and another (phenylbutazone) had its licence restricted to ankylosing spondylitis and availability was restricted to hospitals (i.e. primary care doctors were no longer considered fit to prescribe it). Whilst the objectives of regulators are plain enough, i.e. to do what is best for the sick without exposing themselves to censure, the above record cannot be thought satisfactory. Doctors, and particularly rheumatologists, have forcefully expressed doubts whether regulation is operating optimally. In fact drug regulation is not a matter for medicine, pharmacy and science alone. There is substantial indirect input from consumer groups and politicians, from the injured, the supposedly injured, and the mass media, as well as from vocal health groups and cults, which are disturbed at what they see as unconsidered and excessive use of hazardous synthetic chemicals. Their input is erratic, but collectively it is influential. It pressures regulators to act defensively. Thus drug regulation is a complex activity subject to many influences. Its practice has a major influence on medicine and doctors would be wise to take a closer interest than they usually do.

Statutory regulation has risks as well as benefits. Wrong or hasty decisions may often affect only individual drugs, but wrong policies may have widespread adverse effects on socially desirable drug development and use.

It has been pointed out that in medicine, 'The trend of greater risks for greater gain is likely to continue.'* The fact that society wants the benefits of medical advance but pays only lip-service to the proposition that risks are inescapable puts a heavy mental burden on drug regulators. Regulators are in the business of taking risks on behalf of society, and, through their political masters, are answerable to society.

The principal theme of regulation is, inevitably, *risk avoidance*. Those who engage in statutory regulation are to some extent prisoners of its post-thalidomide origin and of the enormous labour of the operation. Drug developers, whilst they accept the principle of official regulation, resent its rigidities and what they see as excessive requirements, believing many of them to be harmful, but they also need to know where they stand and so they encourage, whether consciously or not, the development of the very regulations they so often deplore. This applies particularly to arbitrary safety requirements, when a research director cannot afford to be told that an expensive programme is deemed insufficient for reasons that are simply a matter of opinion or that a clinical trial that was terminated after ten months should have lasted one year, and it must be done again.

It is difficult to stand back and view the general scene. But anyone who does this is likely to agree that we are operating a system that is based on unproved predictive assumptions. This was unavoidable in the immediate aftermath of thalidomide when, understandably, the pressures to get something started quickly were irresistible. But there has been no scientific monitoring of the performance of regulation (not an easy task) with provision for change in the light of the results.† Twenty-five years after thalidomide the operation remains essentially unchanged. A perceptive comment on one drug withdrawal was, 'The present system is too slow at detecting risk as well as unduly apt to slam the brakes on hard once it is detected.'‡

In taking decisions, it has been pointed out,§ there are *three kinds of uncertainty*:

of the *facts*
of the *public reaction to the facts*
of the *future consequences of decisions*.

Regulators are influenced not only to *avoid risk* but to *avoid regret* later and this latter consideration has a profound effect whether or not the decision taker is conscious of it.

Therefore there are two important subjective human factors, *uncertainty* and *regret avoidance* and it is easy to agree that, 'Balancing the benefits

* Royal Commission of Civil Liability and Compensation for Personal Injury London: HMSO, Cmnd 7054–I, 1978.

† A start has been made. Lunde I, Dukes M N G. On regulating regulation. Eur J Clin Pharmacol 1981; 19:1.
‡ *Times*, 24 August 1982.
§ Lord Ashby. Proc Roy Soc Med 1976; 69:721.

against the risks belongs not in the domain of science but to society. The judgement is a value judgement — a social rather than a scientific decision.' (B. Commoner, 1977) All this tends to promote defensive regulation.

The kind of risk-taking that is in the interest of society requires high-quality data at the licencing stage plus a sound plan of post-licencing (marketing) investigation. If this latter is not done, any adverse events or scandal will almost unavoidably result in the condemnation of the drug. No regulatory body can face the prospect of being in the position of ignoring bad data until good data can be obtained and then later finding that the good data confirm the condemnation already demanded by the mass media. For this reason alone we must give priority to raising the standard of data at all stages of drug development and ensuring that its collection continues after a product licence has been granted. This is in the interest of the pharmaceutical industry. In a crisis, a company that has not good data can expect no help from the regulatory body; indeed it can only expect a negative decision.

Collective decision-making by advisory groups (as in UK) of people of different disciplines who comparatively seldom meet, who are in uncertainty as described above and who are subject to considerable pressure of regret avoidance must tend to defensive policies and to discourage innovatory thinking.

The practical situation is that there is always an insufficiency of knowledge on which to make rational and reliable judgements and there is no prospect of this situation changing. We all know this, but we behave much of the time as though it were not so.

Advisory committees are formed of a mix of those involved in drug development and use and sometimes include consumer or lay representation.* They know, intellectually, that drugs cannot be wholly safe and that they are called upon to take reasonable risks on behalf of society.

They also know from experience that society as a whole (or as represented by politicians and the mass media), though it may 'know' that 'there is no such thing as a safe drug' will not behave as if it really understood this when an unpredicted risk eventuates; blame will be allocated and a scapegoat will be sought, and protestations by developers and regulators are vain because data are always inadequate and, with hindsight, there is always something more that could have been done.

It is self-evident that it is much harder to detect and quantitate a *good* that is *not* done, than it is to detect and quantitate a *harm* that *is* done. Therefore, although it is part of the decision-taker's job to facilitate the doing of good, the avoidance of harm looms larger. The risk of a decision that results in harm being done and detected dominates the mind in a way that the risk of possible failure to do good, even if it is detected, cannot do. Attempts to convict regulators of failing to do good (e.g. the delay in introducing valuable new drugs in the USA due to regulatory procrastination, the 'drug lag') do not induce the same feelings of horror in regulators that are induced by the prospect of finding they have approved a drug that has, or may have, caused serious injury and that the victims are about to appear on television.†

This is not to ridicule the regulators and their advisers. They are doing their best, and commonly make good and sensible decisions that receive no congratulations. But we do not often think of the human aspects of their work.

The future

Specialists in the study of risk management do not agree that current approaches to drug regulation can be effective, and think that as long as they continue to be used the future is bleak.

One of them‡ illustrates attitudes to the prob-

* In the UK, the Committee on Safety of Medicines and the Medicines Commission. These are QUANGOS (*q*uasi-*a*utonomous *n*on-*g*overnment *o*rganizations; their membership, appointed by government to give independent advice, is sarcastically said to consist of 'the good and the great').

† The very last thing a drug regulator wishes to be able to say is, 'I awoke one morning and found myself famous': (Lord Byron (1788–1824) on the publication of his poem Childe Harold's Pilgrimage).

‡ William C. Clark of the International Institute for Applied Systems Analysis (Austria) to whom we are grateful for permission to quote: Clark W C. In: Schwing R C, Albers W A, eds. Societal risk assessment. New York: Plenum Press, 1980.

lems of coping with the unknown (as drug regulators have to do) by adapting the ancient myth of *the Lady or the Tiger*:

There are two doors; behind one is a hungry tiger (risk) and behind the other is a beautiful lady (benefit).

Three young men are placed in turn before the doors and invited to open one and take the consequences, i.e. to make a benefit/risk assessment.

'The *first man* refused to take the chance', he would not face risk; 'he lived safe and died chaste'; he had retreated from reality; he wanted the simple risk-free life that never was; for him there will be no new drugs; there are such people in our society.

'The *second man* hired risk-assessment consultants. He collected all the available data on lady and tiger populations. He brought in sophisticated technology to listen for growling and to detect the faintest whiff of perfume. He completed check-lists. He developed a utility function and assessed his risk averseness. Finally, sensing that in a few more years he would be in no condition to enjoy the lady anyway, he opened the optimal door . . . and was eaten by a low probability tiger'. This man indulged in the fantasy that besets current drug regulators; that the unknown can be overcome by multiplying technical tests.

'The *third man* took a course in tiger taming. He opened a door at random and was eaten by the lady.'* This is the traditional empirical approach but it is increasingly acknowledged to have become inadequate for the growing complex problems it has to address. There is a lesson here for some mindless large-scale programmes of post-licencing (marketing) surveillance.

'We are, sadly but simply, hooked on a risk control policy which gives us little but which we can no longer do without.'* This is shown by the behaviour of regulators and the public with each new drug accident (or presumed drug accident). On each occasion they re-fight the old battles. They seem wedded to belief in 'Prospective, knowledge-presuming notions of rationality in which optimal or best-possible decisions and rules are derived from existing available information and are implemented by virtue of their assumed rationality. Subsequent performance is assumed to be optimal if these rules are rigorously enforced. Success is deemed to be within our grasp if we persist in this course.'* This quote is a little difficult to follow at first reading, but it is worth trying again and reflecting on it.

We are faced with 'risk assessors' sincere knowledge-seeking efforts to identify potential dangers' and to construct a rigid or near-rigid framework for detecting dangers. The regulator in fact agrees he always has too little knowlege but he behaves as though the unknown is a 'wrinkle to be ironed out of a fabric.'* In this he is wrong and the history of risk management shows the inadequacy of the approach. Our ignorance will always remain greater than our knowledge.

It is pointed out that the practical mainstay of man and beast in daily life may be a better model, i.e. the acceptance of the inevitability of incomplete knowledge as central, to be lived with and accommodated rather than overcome. 'The fundamental question is not how to calculate, control, or even reduce risk' which is what we currently attempt, 'it is how to increase our risk-taking abilities'*; to develop rational coping systems, i.e. institutions that can continuously respond to and learn from the inevitable surprises awaiting us, and our future may depend on our ability to design such institutions for 'adaptive risk management'*.

For drug regulation this means continuous evaluation of the efficacy of regulations, the kinds of risks detected and the kinds that go undetected (we are just beginning to do this), so that armed with such knowledge we can decide what are the tasks that post-licencing surveillance schemes can fulfil and the kinds of situations best solved by intensive pre-licencing studies. 'Only when we begin to blend the results of such studies in the careful design of integrated risk management strategies will we be able to move much beyond the present unsatisfactory state of management by polemic.'*

We should seriously try to understand that salvation does not lie in lists of requirements

* William C Clark: ibid: the carnivorous lady variation is due to Anna Maria Krebl.

modified intermittently and almost always upwards, and indeed it is not to be found in a traditional scientific approach. Risk-management, which is what we are talking about, belongs, it is suggested, in the realm of 'trans-science' and not science. Trans-science treats questions that transcend science, i.e. 'questions that can be asked *of* science and yet which cannot be answered *by* science', e.g. How safe is safe enough? Plainly scientists have a role but it is a role different from that in which questions can be unambiguously answered by science. We see what is meant by this when we read that Congress of the USA 'has failed repeatedly to meet FDA's [Food and Drug Administration] own requests for an unambiguous legislative mandate specifying what balance of risks and benefits *does* constitute the public good, how this is to be democratically determined and achieved.'* The FDA will have known that Congress could not answer, yet Congress repeatedly intervenes in the functioning of the FDA, interventions that have been described as resembling 'nothing so much as Keystone Cops† Scenarios.'

'The most important lesson of both experience and analysis is that societies' abilities to cope with the unknown depend on the flexibility of their institutions and individuals, and on their capability to experiment freely with alternative forms of adaptation to the risks which threaten them'.

'Neither the witch hunting hysterics nor the mindlessly rigid regulations characterizing so much of our present chapter in the history of risk management say much for our ability to learn from the past.'*

Appendix 1
A personal view of drugs and drug regulation

The following controversial account, titled *the seven pillars of foolishness*,‡ synthesises the complexities of drug regulation, development and the interest of patients through the eyes of one person of unique experience. We are grateful to Dr Graham Dukes for allowing us to republish it here.§ Dr Dukes has experience of the practice of medicine, of the pharmaceutical industry, of official drug regulation (Netherlands), of the World Health Organization and of an academic Chair of Drug Policy Science (Groningen University, Netherlands).

Has it ever struck you that, for some of us who live in the world of drug therapy, a medicine so very easily becomes more important — certainly more central and more tangible — than the hundreds of thousands of people who take it? It has a name, protected by law and patent, whilst its users are but a grey, anonymous, heterogeneous mass. It is fathered by proud men in white coats, who conceived its origins upon laboratory blackboards. It is born in a retort. It is developed and nurtured like any infant to adulthood. It curtsies before the scientific world as might the most select of society *debutantes*, and then, somewhat incongruously, it is often promoted into fame in the medical marketplace in a manner of which a rock star might be envious. The mere patient has no say over the drug; he is ordered to take it by his physician, and if he does as he is bid the doctors pat him on the head and condescendingly call him compliant. If all goes well from the drug's point of view it has its long day of acclaim, bringing its industrial godfathers fame and fortune. If at any time its name and reputation are besmirched, grave advocates will be at hand to defend it. It may be a long time before the glory fades and other medicines take their place before the footlights. And even then, the old drug may be an unconscionable time a-dying.

I do not see any real alternative at present to this process; this is the way that technological society in the west chooses to advance and the way good business apparently must be done. If, in the interests of progress, mankind has to live with image-builders and the ever more subtle machinery of hidden persuasion, applied to a range of goods ranging from video-recorders and benzodiazepines to politicians, then there is not very much mankind can currently do about it. But some-

* Ibid.
† Early Hollywood silent slapstick comedy films.
‡ Wisdom has built herself a house, she has erected her seven pillars.' The Bible: Proverbs; 9:1.

§ Also to Elsevier Science Publishers B V. The text has appeared as the introductory essay In: Side-effects of Drugs. Annual 8. Amsterdam: Elsevier, 1984.

where limits must surely be set. One such limit must apply when one defines what can reasonably be regarded as progress, in the name of which this whole process is maintained. Not every new molecule which acquires a sales licence can claim to represent a step ahead; many a new drug is merely a step aside, some are quite distinctly a step backwards. How much sales talk can one tolerate for such fruits of pseudo-innovation? It has very often been argued that when a new drug appears in the medical marketplace it is still too early to decide whether or not it represents a useful advance in therapy, and that many a new drug should be given a chance to prove itself in this respect over a period of years before the world passes judgment. So it may be, but did you ever see a drug introduced to physicians like that? 'Dear Doctor', the introductory letter might run, 'we do not really know whether our new product is any better, or safer, or more convenient to use than those which you already have, but we surely hope so. We would also like to earn back some of the money which we have spent on developing it, so that we can go on trying. Will you kindly give it a chance?' Oddly, if medical society had not grown so used to hyperbole, such an honest approach might prove to have some appeal to the prescriber. But nothing of this: the physician is beaten about the ears with the name of the new nostrum, with its supposed advantages, and with pictures which imply what words must not promise; all this goes on until he is so conditioned (compliant, perhaps) that he begins to prescribe it. If the truth be exactly as its founder fathers may have believed at the start, namely that the drug has nothing new to offer, this will in due time become evident; but that will happen only very slowly, for it will be a matter, not merely of confirming or rejecting a calm hypothesis, but of gradually eroding the inflated image of the drug which Madison Avenue advertising has built around it. And if the truth of the matter be that the drug is in fact risky the slowness with which that truth emerges in the face of many triumphal fanfares can mean unnecessary suffering.

Lest anyone think that this is another diatribe against the drug industry and its promotional techniques, let me at once take some people to task. Where a flicker of a risk seems to be emerging it is not merely the marketing managers who will at first be loath to admit it. What about the regulators in their ministerial offices? They have only just licensed the drug. If it is indeed problematical, what will parliament be saying about their licensing policies and their technical competence? Then there is the doctor. He has prescribed it and his first few patients appear happy. Is he very anxious to hear that he has been reckless or uncritical? Are his patients willing to have the new remedy, with the hope which it might bring, taken away from them? All these things can delay the admission, even where convincing evidence comes forward, that a hypothesis of risk is anything more than a hypothesis. Once a drug has got onto the market, the dice are heavily loaded in favor of its remaining there, with the reputation originally accorded to it, for a long time.

It has been said often enough but I have to say it again: drug risks are inevitable. Much drug therapy as it exists today is still a lamentably crude means of influencing the workings of a machine as complex as the human body. It may one day be possible to make fine adjustments to physiological balances, and indeed there are a few instruments, such as the hormonal releasers, which render it possible to do so already; all too often however the only drugs available are pharmacotherapeutic blunderbusses which present a known or unknown degree of risk. That being so, one has to be extraordinarily careful about handling them socially and administratively in ways which may raise the measure of risk still further. Loading the dice in the way I have already described increases the risks; so for example does the use of fancy algorithms to test every shred of evidence of a drug's noxiousness before one is prepared to take it seriously. But the risks are raised to a wholly irresponsible degree if one puts the interests of the drug in the middle of the picture and those of the patient at the periphery. Yet that happens, and in some areas it is getting worse rather than better.

People still point to thalidomide as a monumental disaster, *the* monumental disaster, fortunately now a quarter of a century behind us; then they add blissfully that things like that do not happen nowadays. Unhappily they do. Not in exactly the same horrifying way, but in a multitude of others. During the last two years there has been a new epidemic of misery, and one cannot continue to pretend that all is well. The most unhappy aspect of it all has been that things have been made worse than they need have been; much of the misery could have been prevented entirely, much more cut short quickly, had society been awake, and honest, and interested.

Let me recall seven stories. They are seven aspects of the recent history of antirheumatic drug treatment, and since they have been well documented in these volumes* and elsewhere I shall not repeat every detail; but I shall attempt to put all seven stories into some perspective. For they stand like seven pillars of foolishness, some taller than others, yet all monuments to human error, greed, vanity, self-interest, gullibility or short-sightedness. Thanks to such things, most of these stories are worse then they need have been.

Benoxaprofen

Benoxaprofen was (or is) an antirheumatic drug which was submitted to various drug regulatory agencies for licencing from about 1979 onwards. It was structurally related to many well-known antirheumatic drugs and most of its effects appeared very similar. There was, however, some qualitative shift as regards the relative importance of the two modes of action often described for these drugs; as compared with its predecessors, benoxaprofen seemed to have a little less effect on prostaglandin synthetase and a little more on leukocyte migration. The hypothesis was raised that this might result in a reduced incidence of those adverse effects — notably gastric bleeding — which seem to be linked to prostaglandin synthetase inhibition. The early clinical studies indeed suggested some practical benefit, but this is quite usual with most antirheumatic drugs of this type — the real gastric problems usually emerge later.

When the real problems emerged with benoxaprofen they were however more serious than with other drugs of its type. Not only was it causing the usual pattern of gastric irritation, but it was also apparently killing old people from hepatic disorders and it was inducing photosensitivity on a massive scale; it was also causing onycholysis† in a frequency of anything up to fifteen percent. The brief and destructive career of benoxaprofen ended with its withdrawal in the summer of 1982 from the very few markets in which it had been accepted by regulatory agencies.

No party emerges very creditably from this story. The world's regulatory authorities found themselves from the start in disarray, handing down decisions on the original new drug application which ranged from complete rejection to open-armed acceptance. The company which marketed the drug, a highly respected and usually very sober organization, launched it with reckless, hysterical, preposterous advertising; whatever one may think of the words in which it was couched, visually it clearly conveyed the impression that one was dealing with a breakthrough of world-shattering importance. As a result, the drug was prescribed on a massive scale and when the troubles came they came in battalions. It seems probable that at least seventy elderly patients died‡ and a great many more people suffered. Yet even then the foolishness was not over. Some regulatory agencies, conveniently forgetting the emphatic recommendation of the World Health Organization that drugs likely to be used in the elderly should be investigated in the elderly at an early stage, sought in retrospect to whitewash their acceptance of the drug despite the almost total lack of such geriatric trials. Company lawyers continued to deny cause and effect, no doubt in the hope of fending off liability proceedings. Even after the drug had been quietly abandoned, a vigorous defence of it was still being put up by gentlemen whose own adverse reaction monitoring systems had failed to detect the harm which was being done; in such cases, no doubt, one's own reputation weighs more heavily than anything else.

Benoxaprofen was a compound which seemed

* In: Dukes M N G, ed. Side-effects of drugs. Annual volumes. Amsterdam: Elsevier.

† Separation of the nail from the nail bed.

‡ Whether these drug-*related* deaths were all drug-*caused* remains a matter of disagreement.

to bear promise of better things to come, and it is sad that it has gone; but the patients who were killed by benoxaprofen, many of them unnecessarily, are dead as well; no amount of whitewash and denial will bring them back to us.

Zomepirac

Like the benoxaprofen drama, that involving zomepirac was limited largely to one country — in this instance the United States. Zomepirac is basically a traditional antiinflammatory analgesic agent. It is extremely closely related to tolmetin which has been sold in some countries for many years as an antirheumatic drug. Tolmetin is a perfectly usable compound, though a little too prone to cause anaphylactoid reactions, and had zomepirac been presented as its twin sister it would no doubt have been used in the same way and treated with the same respect. But the image builders took over; zomepirac was selectively investigated as an analgesic; with its other properties relegated to the small print it took its bow in the advertising columns as heaven's own gift to pain sufferers. This time, the advertising men appear to have had not only the doctors but even the stock market and the regulators in their pockets; when zomepirac turned out to induce anaphylaxis on a scale commensurate with the scale of its promotion, astonishment and dismay were expressed on all sides. The drug was withdrawn in March 1983, and the accusations as to who was responsible for it all are still flying; but at least eight people are dead, and to judge from scattered news items rather more. Given a little more caution by everyone involved — need any of them have died at all?

Osmosin

Osmosin was laid to rest by its founder fathers in January 1984; its victims had been laid to rest the previous year. Developed at a time when the patents on indometacin* were running out, Osmosin provided it with an elegant but costly kinetic face-lift. Its osmotic tablets released the drug slowly through a semipermeable membrane as they travelled down the gastrointestinal tract, thereby prolonging the duration of activity and perhaps promising to reduce gastric irritation. Even at the time when it was developed, there were murmurings to the effect that in this way gastric problems might merely be shifted to a lower level. As things turned out, this is apparently what happened; the Osmosin tablets seem either to have adhered to the intestinal mucosa, became lodged in diverticula or peppered the gut with potassium which, astonishingly, was used as an excipient. When perforations resulted, the anti-inflammatory effect may well have masked the consequences until it was too late; certainly people who had tolerated plain indometacin well for a long time died when they were needlessly switched to Osmosin. In the drug's own obituary, the company claimed that extensive studies had failed to demonstrate any special risk; so they may have done, but that presumably only reflects the inadequacy of the studies. There is a splendid company there in Rahway which had done fine things for medicine and will do fine things again; it should not have its monuments in the churchyards.

* Indometacin = indomethacin

Two butazones

The double story of phenylbutazone and oxyphenbutazone is quite a different one. These drugs have been with us for a generation. They arrived at a time when in the field of antirheumatic treatment there was little to choose from, and they found their place. They caused their problems, but the nature of these became known very early; the 1960 edition of Meyler's *Side Effects of Drugs* recorded a series of cases of agranulocytosis as well as a range of other complications and their incidence. Twenty years later, the 'butazones' as they were loosely called, were almost hidden among the throng of newer nonsteroidal antirheumatic agents which now jostled one another in the market place. Nevertheless they had retained something of their early reputation for the treatment of ankylosing spondylitis, though it is not clear whether they really deserved it. Things might have gone on as they were for another generation, with both products falling gently into obscurity, had not, in the summer of 1983, an internal memorandum from Messrs Ciba-Geigy dropped into the hands of Dr Sidney Wolfe of America's Public Citizen action group. The memorandum estimated that there had been 1182 deaths due to these drugs worldwide and it not unreasonably raised the question within the company whether it was not time to stop promoting them. Public Citizen called for an immediate ban on both drugs as an 'imminent hazard to public health'. Dr Ole Hansson of Sweden, who appears to be deeply convinced that Ciba-Geigy is incorrigibly wicked in its ways, took up the cry in the Scandinavian newspapers; on December 14th Norway banned both products and throughout the world regulatory agencies sat down to consider whether or not they should follow suit; some seemed very likely at least to make gestures of concern.

From what I have already said it will be clear that my main concern is with patients dying or suffering needless injury; but in the way in which society is now suddenly reacting to Dr Wolfe and Dr Hansson there is something very wrong as well. Most of the evidence of the harm which these drugs can do was available two decades ago, largely quantified. If it is true that, because of the arrival of somewhat safer products, one should reevaluate and perhaps discard these old stalwarts, then that could have happened any time from 1970 onwards, certainly by 1975, on the basis of a careful comparison of the benefit-to-risk ratio of all the compounds available. Alas, regulatory agencies do not usually do these things; they are too busy approving new drugs to take a hard look at old ones; when they do so, it all too often happens because people like Dr Wolfe and Dr Hansson have raised the hue and cry. I have a shrewd suspicion that aspirin has killed a multiple of those who are said to be victims of the butazones, and that several other drugs are rather worse than these two; but I have to suspend judgement because I do not have the comparative data available. Unhappily, neither does anyone else; the medical world too has been much too busy testing new antirheumatic drugs to learn much more about the comparative merits of those it already has. Is there not something amiss with our priorities?

Pyrithioxine

Pyrithioxine hydrochloride is what my friend Dr Leo Offerhaus calls a chameleon. It is a vitamin B6 derivative and reputed to be an anabolic for the brain, very good for confusion, behavioural disorders in children and senile dementia. Even for these purposes it is sold under thirty of the most musical names with which a drug was ever blessed, including Cerebrotrofina, Musa, Gladius, Scintidin, Tonomentis and Life. Small wonder that when it suddenly surfaced in France, chameleon-like, as an antirheumatic agent physicians had no idea what it was and compliantly prescribed it. When it began to cause rashes and stomatitis did one in a thousand physicians know of its structural link — the dithio group — to penicillamine, with which some of these rheumatic patients must have been treated earlier? Had they known, they might have prescribed it more critically. Some elderly rheumatic patients were indeed already receiving the same compound under another connotation for their ailing medical state. But do you know what the physician who asked about the chemical nature of this new antirheumatic drug was told? He was solemnly informed that it was 3, 3′-dithiodimethylenebis (5-hydroxy-6-methyl-4-pyridylmethanol) dihydrochloride monohydrate. Mercy be with us — will doctors never insist on having generic names and some intelligible indication of what they are really dealing with before they write a prescription?

Oxametacin

Space is at a premium, and I must be brief. Oxametacin, by all accounts, is a miracle, for the clinical papers which I have seen conclude that it is the equivalent of indometacin without its side effects. I am nevertheless also assured that it has been discussed around certain regulatory tables and gave rise there to some amusement. Privately, all I can conclude is that the published material is not all of a standard which I would like to see, that the drug is metabolized in part as indometacin and that the patients without side-effects did not receive an effective dose. If better work proves the contrary, I shall be delighted to be corrected; so far, I am forced to believe that this is not the way to help rheumatic patients to avoid adverse reactions. This gem, should you require it, is to be found in the pharmacies of Italy; you will be hard put to it to find it in most other places.

Seven stories and many morals

The chain of stories could continue; the particular nastinesses or oddities associated with indoprofen, ibufenac, aclofenac, mefenamic acid, acemetacin, fenclofenac and glafenine are much in the same vein. For the present purpose, these seven tales must suffice. Not all of them had a tragic ending, but all of them illustrate some of the absurdities in the way in which the community has behaved and continues to behave when it deals with drug safety. Even from the purely scientific and epidemiological point of view it is difficult enough to come by reliable information on adverse reactions, and to spot it sufficiently early to prevent much injury being caused. Yet, even as the facts begin to emerge, any attempt to interpret and objectify them may be bedevilled by the machinations of people who have their own interests to defend and their own axes to grind. It is entirely proper that the truth about side effects and benefit-risk ratios should emerge from a weighing of a mass of conflicting evidence, but the process is immeasurably complicated and delayed where costly reputations and much money are at stake. Doctors, companies, regulatory agencies, politicians, consumers and nowadays even stockbrokers (yes, *stockbrokers*!) all throw up their own particular smokescreens when suspicions of major adverse reactions are discussed; all that one can do, and must do, is to set aside most of the commentary and interpretation that is cast around on such a vexed issue, go back to the patients who are at the centre of the problem and verify the facts. For let me say it once again; it is only the patient who matters. For him or her a serious side effect is of course not a side effect at all; it is a very central effect indeed, perhaps one of life and death.

These problems can arise in every field of drug therapy, but it is today tragically easy to identify them in the field of antirheumatic treatment. For two decades most nations have in good faith accepted the argument that every nonsteroidal antiinflammatory drug which shows promise must be given a chance, since it may contribute something to therapeutic progress. As a result, the financially profitable field of antirheumatic drug therapy has in many countries become a fairground, the noise in which is utterly confusing to pharmacologists, physicians and patients alike. No one particular segment of the community is really to blame; society has created a situation in which everyone is under pressure to behave in a particular way; if I had a good new antirheumatic drug to sell I too would be obliged to sell it with trumpets and bells, however distasteful I might find it, since otherwise no-one would notice. It is clear that too much injury is being caused by drugs in this field; the proportion of drugs which come, kill and go is too high, and amid all the clamour it is now impossible for the doctor to decide which risks are worth taking in his patient's interest.

Should one not, to begin with, look very carefully at the comparative merits of all the antirheumatic drugs currently known, sponsoring impartial research where necessary to find the data needed to prune the market and update the textbooks? If no-one else will do it, the drug regulatory agencies of the world, which are very slowly closing their ranks, might share out the task, if possible in collaboration with the pharmaceutical industry. It has to be done. As recently as January 1984 one could find statements in the medical literature to the effect that aspirin, after three generations, was still the drug of choice in rheumatoid arthritis. That may not always be true, but the fact that in 1984 it can still be said with some authority and backed by substantial evidence surely makes one wonder whether society has been using its resources optimally to find better and safer antirheumatic medicines. The fact alone that the number of nonsteroidal antiinflammatory drugs licensed for sale in various European countries varies sevenfold reflects the uncertainly as to how the situation should now be handled.

Again, I think the medical profession should be taking a hard look at the way in which new antirheumatic drugs are currently sold to it, and the consequences which that has for everyone. More restrained promotion could be more informative and a great deal less wasteful. If only a fraction of the money currently being spent, at the community's expense, on breathless four-colour advertisements and double teams of detailmen were to be diverted into basic research in the better industrial laboratories society might be on the way to developing the truly new and truly safer antirheumatic drugs which patients need. Whether one believes that industry can regulate itself into a more balanced situation, or whether one expects governments to impose a solution will depend on one's own private philosophies, but I know it must happen if there are not going to be a series of other pillars of foolishness lining our way through the 'eighties'. Accidents will still happen, patients will still be injured and killed by the unforeseen and unforeseeable, but people will hopefully no longer die merely because society has been as hesitant to admit the risks as is currently the case.

There is an unhappy turn of phrase currently going around medical meetings which refers to patients as 'the people out there . . .' Perhaps that is merely symptomatic of the wrongheadedness which besets the world of drug experts. The patients are indeed out there, and the drugs are in here with us, being coddled in the warmth. It may be the destiny of the clinical pharmacologists to bring drug policies and policy makers back where they belong, at the bedside and in the consulting room, with the patient — every patient — at the heart of things, whilst the chemists, the stockbrokers, the image makers and the detailmen wait, cap in hand, at the door for judgement to be pronounced.

Appendix 2:
A tale to remember: the thalidomide disaster

Thalidomide has provided a terrible lesson to the world in regard to drug development, testing, naming, prescribing and consumption. It deserves to be remembered as follows:

Until 1961 the public took a largely romantic interest in the development and introduction of new drugs and its attention was only turned to the subject when it learned from the press, generally incorrectly, and several times a year, that a major advance or 'breakthrough' had taken place. In 1961 a major breakthrough did occur — man discovered that drug introduction was more hazardous than he had previously believed. The thalidomide disaster aroused public opinion, forced governments to supervise drug introduction and therapeutic claims and all concerned with this process got a salutary shock. Our attitude to casual use of drugs can never be and should never be the same since thalidomide, and therefore the story is given in some detail here.

In 1960–1961 in West Germany an outbreak of phocomelia occurred. Phocomelia means 'seal extremities'; it is a congenital deformity in which the long bones of the limbs are defective and substantially normal or rudimentary hands and feet arise on, or nearly on, the trunk, like the flippers of a seal; other abnormalities may occur simultaneously. Phocomelia is ordinarily exceedingly rare.

Most West German clinics had no cases during the 10 years up to 1959. In 1959, in 10 clinics, 17 were seen; in 1960, 126; in 1961, 477. The European outbreak seemed confined to West Germany (though a similar but smaller occurrence was simultaneously noted in Australia), and this, with the steady increase, made a virus infection, such as rubella, seem unlikely as a cause. Radio-active fall-out was considered and so were X-ray exposure of the mother, hormones, foods, food preservatives and contraceptives. One doctor, investigating his patients retrospectively with a questionnaire, found that 20% reported taking Contergan in early pregnancy. He questioned the patients again and 50% then admitted taking it; *many said they had thought the drug too obviously innocent to be worth mentioning initially.**

In November 1961, the suggestion that a drug, unnamed, was the cause of the outbreak was publicly made by the same doctor at a paediatric meeting, following a report on 34 cases of phocomelia. 'That night a physician came up to him and said, "Will you tell me confidentially, is the drug Contergan? I ask because we have such a child and my wife took Contergan."' Several letters followed, asking the same question, and it soon became widely known that thalidomide (Contergan, Distaval, Kevadon, Talimol, Softenon) was prob-

* Illustrating the problems of retrospective research, e.g. case-control studies; enquiries of patients are unreliable.

ably the cause. It was withdrawn from the West German market in November 1961 and from the British market in December 1961. By that time reports had also come from other countries.

A *case-control study* showed that of 46 cases of phocomelia 41 mothers had taken thalidomide and of 300 mothers with normal babies none had taken thalidomide, between the fourth and ninth week of pregnancy.

Soon more reports were forthcoming and despite the fact that such retrospective studies do not provide conclusive evidence of cause and effect, judgement could no longer be suspended on such an important matter, for the drug was not a vital one. Prospective observational cohort studies were quickly made in ante-natal clinics where women had yet to give birth — though few, they provided evidence incriminating thalidomide. The worst had happened, a trival new drug was the cause of the most grisly disaster in the short history of modern scientific drug therapy. Many thalidomide babies died, but many live on with deformed limbs,* eyes, ears, heart and alimentary and urinary tracts.

The West German Health Ministry estimated that thalidomide caused about 10 000 birth deformities in babies, 5000 of whom survived and 1600 of whom would eventually need artificial limbs. In Britain there were probably at least 600 live births of malformed children of whom about 400 survived. The world total was probably about 10 000.

Thalidomide had been marketed in West Germany in 1956 as Contergan, and in Britain in 1958 as Distaval, as a sedative and hypnotic. Its chief merit seemed to be that overdose did not cause coma, probably because, with suitable particle size, elimination balanced absorption; given orally to animals a lethal dose could not be reached. Suicides were disappointed by thalidomide. Liquid formulations introduced later did not have this advantage and serious overdose could occur.

Thalidomide seemed a safe and pleasant hypnotic, and no doubt some patients found it preferable to others, but in the context of all drug therapy any advantages were trival, and there were reasonable alternatives.

Despite the absence of any other notable properties, thalidomide, skilfully promoted and credulously prescribed and taken by the public — it was also sold without prescription — achieved huge popularity, it 'became West Germany's baby-sitter'. It was a routine hypnotic in hospitals and was even recommended to help children adapt themselves to a convalescent home atmosphere and was sold mixed with other drugs for symptomatic relief of pain, cough and fever (Grippex, Polygripan, Peracon Expectorans, Valgis, Tensival, Valgraine, Asmaval, etc.). This may help explain the difficulties of patients and of doctors in determining who had had thalidomide and who had not, and the statement, probably true, that some women, knowing the danger of thalidomide from press publicity, but not the confusion that reigns amongst drug names, continued to use their supplies of the drug alone or in a mixture, for none of these prominently featured the non-proprietary name on the label. When a drug is in disfavour the advantages of its non-proprietary name become suddenly obvious to those who normally promote the use of proprietary names, and so more publicity of its teratogenic effect was under the name, thalidomide, than under the numerous proprietary names.

In 1960–1961 it had become evident that prolonged use of thalidomide could cause hypothyroidism and peripheral neuritis. The latter effect was the principal reason why approval for marketing in the USA, as Kevadon, had been delayed by the US Food and Drug Administration. Approval had still not been given when the fetal effects were discovered and so general distribution was avoided. Nonetheless some 'thalidomide babies' were born in the USA following indiscriminate pre-marketing clinical trials by 1270 doctors who gave the drug to 20 771 patients, of whom at least 207 were pregnant. Other countries in which cases of thalidomide phocomelia occurred include Australia, Belgium, Brazil, Canada, East Germany, Egypt, Israel, Lebanon, Peru, Spain, Sweden and Switzerland, although the drug was not marketed in all these.

When a drug becomes popular it crosses frontiers. It is interesting to speculate why modest

* For pictures of thalidomide deformities, see Br Med J 1962; 2:646, 647, and JAMA 1962; 180:1106.

apparent improvements can give a drug a therapeutic reputation such that people will go to great trouble to get it. Responsibility may perhaps be divided amongst manufacturers who over-promote, doctors who write testimonials on inadequate evidence, encouraging over-promotion, the mass-media which so ably both satisfy and stimulate the public appetite for 'wonder drugs' and the stupid vanity of some patients that makes them feel it a desired distinction to be able to boast of being under treatment with the latest drug, particularly if it is one which is not available to their associates.

Perhaps the fact that the incidence of phocomelia was greater amongst children of professional classes reflects the urge of doctors to ensure that their own families, as well as those of their perhaps most demanding or critical patients, should get the very newest and therefore, it is optimistically assumed, the best, drugs.

So rapidly did the news of the thalidomide disaster spread that some mothers who had taken it knew of the risk weeks before their babies were born. Of course, not all who took thalidomide during the crucial period (37th to 54th days from the first day of the last menstruation) had abnormal babies, perhaps no more than 20%, there is no reliable figure.

In 1977 in the UK there were still heard demands for an official public enquiry into the thalidomide disaster.

The present position is that after a long struggle the victims of thalidomide have received a substantial sum of money from the company that marketed thalidomide. It is unlikely that a court of law would have awarded more in the event of the producer being found guilty of negligence, an outcome that remains uncertain.

In the UK, the medical/scientific lessons provided by the episode have been learned in that an official advisory regulatory body (Committee on Safety of Medicines) has been set up and no new drug is marketed until a body of independent experts has agreed that testing is adequate to support the therapeutic claims which are also controlled under law.

The only remaining issue would seem to be whether the company is liable *in law* for the consequences of thalidomide. This has not been tested in the courts since the firm concerned paid out, having admitted 'moral' but not 'legal' liability. The law on 'product liability' ('strict' liability, 'no fault' liability) is under review in many countries and there seems little point in embarking on what could be an enormous and expensive legal exercise under laws that are about to be changed, partly, indeed, as a result of the thalidomide disaster.

GUIDE TO FURTHER READING

1 Lasagna L. Drug discovery and introduction: regulation and over-regulation. Clin Pharmacol Ther 1976; 20:507.
2 Workshop Report. Clinical trials of drugs. Clin Pharmacol Ther 1975; 18:629–662. Topics include clinical trials as seen by investigators, industry and regulatory authority, paediatric trials and new uses for old drugs.
3 Freis E D. The drug lag. JAMA 1976; 235:473.
4 Melmon K L. The clinical pharmacologist and scientifically unsound regulations for drug development. Clin Pharmacol Ther 1976; 20:125.
5 Bokke O M et al. Drug discontinuations in the UK and USA, 1964–1983. Clin Pharmacol Ther 1984; 35:559.
6 Alloza J L et al. A comparison of drug product information in four national compendia. Clin Pharmacol Ther 1983; 33:269.
7 Editorial. Crying wolf on drug safety. Br Med J 1982; 284:219.
8 Herxheimer A. Immortality for old drugs. Lancet 1984; 2:1460, and subsequent correspondence.
9 Smith T. Image and reality: drugs for the future. Br Med J 1982; 285:761.
10 Masson A et al. Matching prescription drugs and consumers: the benefits of direct advertising. N Engl J Med 1985; 313:513. A controversial view: see subsequent correspondence.
11 Richards T. Drugs in developing countries: inching towards rational policies. Br Med J 1986; 292:1347.

On Thalidomide

1 Woollam D H M. Thalidomide disaster considered as an experiment in mammalian teratology. Br Med J 1962; 2:236.
2 Taussig H. A study of the German outbreak of phocomelia. JAMA 1962; 180:1106.
3 Mellin G W et al. The saga of thalidomide. N Engl J Med 1962; 267:1184, 1238.
4 Smithells R W et al. The incidence of limb and ear defects since the withdrawal of thalidomide. Lancet 1963; 1:1095.
5 Editorial. Thalidomide's long shadow. Br Med J 1976; 4:1155.
6 Editorial. Thalidomide: 20 years on. Lancet 1981; 2:510.

6

Classification of drugs, names of drugs

In any science, however undeveloped, there are two basic requirements, *classification* and *nomenclature (names)*.

1. **Classification**. It is evident from the way this book is organised that there is no homogeneous system for classifying drugs that suits all purposes. Drugs are commonly categorised according to the convenience of who is discussing them — clinicians, pharmacologists or medicinal chemists.

Drugs may be classified by:

a. *Therapeutic use*, e.g. antimicrobial, antidiabetic, antihypertensive, analgesic, tranquilliser.

b. *Mode or site of action*,
   (i) *molecular interaction*, e.g. receptor blockers, enzyme inhibitors
   (ii) *cellular site*, e.g. loop diuretic, catecholamine uptake inhibitor (imipramine)
   (iii) *physiological system*, e.g. vasodilator, hypolipidaemic, anticoagulant.

c. *Molecular structure*, e.g. barbiturate, glycoside, alkaloid, steroid.

2. **Names**. Any drug may have names in all three of the following classes:

a. the *full chemical* name
b. a *non-proprietary** (official or approved) name used in pharmacopoeias and chosen by official bodies.
c. a *proprietary* name or names that are the commercial property of a pharmaceutical company/ies.

Example:

a. 3-(10, 11-dihydro-5H-dibenz [*b, f*]-azepin-5-yl)-N, N-dimethylpropylamine
b. imipramine
c. Tofranil, Praminil, Berkomine (UK): Prodepress, Surplix, Deprinol, etc. (various countries).

In this book proprietary names are distinguished by a capital letter.

The principal features of the names are:

a. *Full chemical name* describes the compound for chemists. It is obviously unsuitable for prescribing.

b. *Non-proprietary name*. 'Three principles remain supreme and unchallenged in importance: the need for distinction in sound and spelling, especially when the name is handwritten; the need for freedom from confusion with existing names, both non-proprietary and proprietary, and the desirability of indicating relationships between similar substances,'† e.g. diazepam, nitrazepam, flurazepam are all benzodiazepines.

c. *Proprietary name* is a trade mark applied to a particular formulation(s) of a particular substance by a particular manufacturer. It is designed to distinguish as far as possible between related substances for obvious commercial reasons. Thus the three drugs in (b) above are named Valium, Mogadon and Dalmane.

* This is not the same as a 'generic' name. 'Sulphonamide', 'barbiturate' are generic names, i.e. refer to a class or genus of compounds. But 'generic' is often misused to mean 'non-proprietary'. Unfortunately this misuse has become standard practice.

† Trigg R B. 1978; Pharmaceutical Journal 220:181.

The principal reasons for advocating the habitual use of non-proprietary names in prescribing are:

1. *Clarity*: because it gives information of the class of drug, e.g. nortriptyline and amitriptyline are plainly related, but their proprietary names are Allegron and Lentizol.

There have been cases of prescribers, when one drug had failed, unwittingly changing to another drug of the same group or even to the same drug, thinking that such different names must mean different drugs. Multiple names for the same drug are commonly totally uninformative, see example on previous page (imipramine). Such occurrences are a criticism of the prescriber, but they are also a criticism of the system that allows such confusion.

2. *Economy*: drugs sold under non-proprietary names are usually, but not always, cheaper than those sold under proprietary names.

3. *Convenience*: the pharmacist can supply whatever he stocks whereas if a proprietary name is used he is usually obliged to supply that preparation alone. He may have to send for the preparation named although he has an equivalent in stock. But hospitals commonly allow substitution so that drugs can be bought in bulk. Mixtures of drugs are sometimes given non-proprietary names, e.g. co-trimoxazole for Bactrim and Septrin, but most are not, no doubt largely because the details of the mixture are liable to be changed by the manufacturer, whether for medical or for commercial reasons, so that the official specification would be liable quickly to become incorrect. No prescriber can be expected to write out the ingredients, so proprietary names are used in many cases, there being no alternative.

International travellers with chronic illnesses will be grateful for international non-proprietary names* (proprietary names often differ from country to country: the reasons are linguistic as well as commercial).

The principle non-commercial reason for advocating the use of proprietary names in prescribing is consistency of the product, so that problems of quality, especially bioavailability, are reduced. There is substance in this argument, though it is sometimes exaggerated.

It is reasonable to use proprietary names when dosage, and therefore pharmaceutical bioavailability, are critical so that small variations in the amount of drug available for absorption can have big effects on the patient, for example, drugs with low therapeutic ratio, e.g. digoxin, hormone replacement therapy, adrenocortical steroids (all uses), antiepileptics, cardiac antidysrhythmics, warfarin. Also, with the introduction of complex formulations (e.g. sustained release) it is important clearly to identify these, and use of proprietary names has a role.

The pharmaceutical industry regards freedom to market under brand names and to advertise or, as it calls the latter, to 'effectively (bring) to the notice of the medical profession',† as two of the essentials of the 'process of discovery in a vigorous competitive environment'.†

Industry resents criticism of these activities for, rightly knowing itself to have contributed immensely to the relief of human suffering, it believes that it knows what is best for the community, particularly as much criticism has undoubtedly been made from frankly political motives. As a result the resonable protests by doctors who simply want to practice rational medicine undistracted by a hubbub of names and claims are unregarded.

The present situation is that industry spends a lot of money promoting its many names for the same article; and the community, as represented by the UK Department of Health, spends a small sum trying to persuade doctors to forget the brand names and to use non-proprietary names.‡ The ordinary doctor who prescribes for his ordinary patients is the target of both sides.

Whatever the theoretical pros and cons, one thing is plain, that until non-proprietary names approach in brevity and euphony those coined by the drug firms, the fight for their general use is a losing one. If one of the chief purposes of a drug name is that it should be used by doctors when prescribing, then provision of such non-proprietary

* Selected by the World Health Organization.

† Annual Report, 1963–1964. Association of British Pharmaceutical Industries.

‡ In 1984 Some UK general practitioners were concerned about increased workloads, saying that generic names take longer to write and have to be looked up; easily believable by anyone who has spent his life among doctors.

names as ceftazidime for Fortum, or even benzathine penicillin for Penidural defeats this purpose.

The search for proprietary names is a 'major problem' for pharmaceutical firms, increasing, as they are, their output of new preparations. One well-known firm *averages* 30 new preparations a year, another warning of the urgent necessity for the doctor to cultivate eclecticism, which he can do only on a foundation of knowledge of drugs and of criteria for their clinical assessment. The bleak outlook for practising doctors is shown by the following.

One firm (in the USA) has 'commissioned an IBM machine to produce a dictionary of forty-two thousand nonsense words of an appropriate scientific look and sound'. An official said 'Thinking up names has been driving us cuckoo around here . . . proper chemical names are hopeless for trade purposes, of course . . . We manufacture what are known as ethical drugs, sold on prescription. Doctors are the market we shoot for. A good trade name carries a lot of weight with doctors . . . they're more apt to write a prescription for a drug whose name is short, and easy to spell and pronounce, but has an impressive medical ring. . . . We believe there are enough brand new words in this dictionary to keep us going for years. . . . We don't yet know what proportion of names is unpronounceable . . . how many are obscene, either in English or in other languages, and how many are objectionable on grounds of good taste: "Godamycin" would be a mild example.' The names which 'look and sound medically seductive' are being picked out. 'Words that survive scrutiny will go into a stock-pile and await the inexorable proliferation of new drugs.'*

Perhaps the doctors have themselves to blame for this prospect which is made more appalling by the news that 'no other industry has a faster rate of innovation and product obsolescence.'†

About names of drugs, the medical profession is irritated by the pharmaceutical industry and the pharmaceutical industry is irritated by the medical profession. From time to time the issue is raised yet again in the medical press. In 1977 the *British Medical Journal (BMJ)* responded.‡

'Our reluctance to consider printing the proprietary names of drugs in *BMJ* articles has stimulated further correspondence . . . There is a good case for including the name of the specific preparation used in reports of side effects and in trials of new drugs, since a proprietary or non-proprietary "equivalent" may differ in the preservatives used or in bioavailability. The real problems arise with teaching and review articles in the Medical Practice section, which may mention a score or so of commonly used drugs on a single page. While we recognise the irritation that may be caused our readers by our description of all these drugs simply by their approved or generic names, there is no satisfactory alternative. We tried to provide a glossary of the manufacturers' names a few years ago, but it proved dauntingly difficult. What do we do, for example, when an article refers to prednisolone? MIMS (The Monthly Index of Medical Specialities) lists Codelcortone, Codelsol, Cordex, Cordex Forte, Delta-Cortef, Deltacortril, Deltastab, Di-Adreson, Precortisyl, Prednesol, and Sintisone, and a further group of various methylprednisolone preparations. Similar lists need to be made for compounds such as phenobarbitone, and indeed any widely prescribed drug that is no longer covered by patent. New proprietaries are introduced each month, others are withdrawn; but pharmaceutical firms are rightly indignant if their latest product is omitted from such lists. About one-quarter of *BMJ* readers live outside Britain, and drugs used in all parts of the world (such as ampicillin or propranolol) may have different proprietary names in each continent.

'In practical terms, most doctors have a *British National Formulary* on their desks, which includes a reasonably comprehensive glossary of proprietary drugs with their approved names. A similar list is published by the British Pharmacopoeia Commission. *The range of drugs prescribed by any individual is remarkably narrow, and once the decision is taken to "think generic" surely the effort required is small.*'§

* *New Yorker*, 14 July 1956.

† Annual Report, 1963–64. Association of British Pharmaceutical Industries.

‡ Editorial Br Med J 1977; 4:980, see also subsequent correspondence.

§ Our italics; DRL, PNB.

Confusing names

The need for both clear thought and clear handwriting is shown by the frequency with which medicines of totally different class have closely similar names, both proprietary and non-proprietary, e.g. Asilone/Ilosone, atropine/Intropin, chlorpromazine/chlorproramide, cotrimoxazole/clotrimazole, Daonil/De-Nol/Danazol, etc. Serious injury has occurred due to confusion of names and the dispensing of the wrong drug.

GUIDE TO FURTHER READING

1 Miller L C. Doctors drugs and names JAMA 1961; 177:27.
2 Dowling H F. The pharmaceutical industry and the doctor. N Engl J Med 1961; 264:75.
3 Editorial. Industry and profession. Lancet 1961; 2:411, and subsequent correspondence.
4 Taussig H B. The evils of camouflage as illustrated by thalidomide. N Engl J Med 1963; 180:92, and Editorial, p. 108.
5 Editorial. Brand names. Br Med J 1968; 1:781.
6 Webb V J. Non-proprietary names. Br Med J 1968; 1:484.
7 Huskisson E C Trade names of proper names? — a problem for the prescriber. Br Med J 1973; 4:225.
8 Turner P. Brand names for drugs. Lancet 1976; 2:797.
9 Vere D. Brand names for drugs. Lancet 1976; 2:911.

7

J. W. Black, FRS*

How drugs act

All living things can be seen struggling to achieve 'self' or identity. Assertions of 'self' by living things are often expressed by chemicals that are repellant or poisonous to other forms of life. Man's experience of these poisonous effects of plants and animals, paradoxically, has often led to the development of new remedies for treating his own diseases.

William Withering†, who defined the use of digitalis (foxglove leaves) in heart disorders, wrote in 1787, 'Poisons in small doses are the best medicines; and useful medicines in too large doses are poisonous', i.e. **drugs are useful poisons**.

Bacteria, the simplest of free-living organisms, produce some of the most lethal poisons known to man. For example, botulinum and tetanus toxins are several million times more toxic than strychnine. However, the really interesting thing is that bacterial toxins can damage and kill in many different ways. For example, botulinum toxin produces respiratory paralysis, tetanus toxin produces muscular spasm and convulsions, diphtheria toxin damages the heart and the toxins of staphylococci rupture red blood corpuscles. Much has been learned about the way drugs act from studying these toxins. Happily, bacteria and fungi often produce substances that are toxic to other microorganisms but not to man and these, the antibiotics, have been a therapeutic gold-mine. Not all of the thousands of known antibiotics are useful to man, but finding out how they interfere with living processes has told us a lot about the way biological machines work.

Bacteria and fungi are not the only source of poisons; jelly-fish, starfish, sting rays, spiders, scorpions and snakes are all venomous animals, i.e. they produce poisons. The human species has had to contend with all of these and much more besides. Poisonous plants must have been a bane of his early life and even today the injudicious and the ignorant are doomed by plant poisons. Just like bacterial toxins, plant poisons can produce an enormous variety of effects in man. Early man didn't know about bacteria but he soon knew his onions, his tea and his coffee as well as his deadly nightshades and poison ivy. He must have learned very early that certain plants could not only harm him but give him useful poisons. There is no doubt that folk medicine was not all hocus-pocus. The virtues of the opium poppy, the deadly nightshade, the purple foxglove and ergot from fungus-infected rye, employed in old herbal remedies are now used in modern medicine as their purified active ingredients — morphine, atropine, digitoxin and ergotamine.

For centuries, it was known that eating ergot, the name for the reproductive bodies of a fungus infecting rye grains, interfered with pregnancy and it was used for inducing labour. Ergot could also constrict the small arteries and when eaten for any considerable time as bread made from infected rye, could produce gangrene of the limbs. The disease became known as St Anthony's Fire,

* This account of how drugs work was written for a non-specialist readership, but it will not be despised by readers of this book because, not only is its author an experienced pharmacologist, but he has been leading scientist in the teams that conceived and carried through the research programmes which resulted in the introduction into routine therapeutics of both β-adrenoceptor and of histamine H_2-receptor blocking drugs, the basis of the action of which are here so clearly described. We are grateful to be allowed to reproduce this updated account from Laurence D R, Black J W. The medicine you take: Benefits and risks of modern drugs. London: Fontana, 1978. DRL. PNB.

† William Withering, MD, FRS (1741–1799), physician.

because the long journey to the Saint's shrine at Padua (Italy) was often associated with relief, no doubt because victims escaped from the supply of infected grain. It took man till the 17th century to learn to avoid making bread from infected rye but by the end of the 19th century he was still fumbling to exploit its value as a medicinal herb in obstetrics.

The young Henry Dale*, fresh from his training by the great physiologists of the day at Cambridge, brought modern pharmacological science to ergot with extraordinary success, at the beginning of this century.

First (1906) he found that an extract of ergot had sympatholytic actions, that is, the ergot extract could annul the blood pressure-raising effect of adrenaline (epinephrine). In fact, it reversed the effects so that adrenaline now caused a fall in blood pressure. Adrenaline, as every journalist knows, is produced in the body in response to stress and changes the activity of every organ in the way most suitable to meet the emergency. The heart is stimulated to beat faster and the bowel is inhibited into quiescence; the pupils are stimulated to dilate but the bladder is inhibited; the blood vessels to the skin are stimulated into contraction so that blood can be shunted towards the muscles in arms and legs where the blood vessels are inhibited and dilated; the subject is made ready for urgent action, for fight or flight. Dale found that his ergot extract was a particular selective antagonist to adrenaline; the excitatory actions were reduced but the inhibitory actions were untouched. Paul Ehrlich† had introduced the idea of *selective toxicity* ('magic bullet') twenty years earlier to explain how his arsenicals would poison parasites without destroying the host i.e. chemotherapy. But here was selective action or toxicity between the tissues of a single animal and this, as we will see, is the heart of modern pharmacology.

Dale went on to look at the chemical nature of his ergot extract, and ergotoxine was the name given to the 'pure' substance found in it. Ergotoxine is now known to be a mixture of three different but closely related derivatives of lysergic acid. Another simple derivative of this substance, lysergic acid diethylamide, is better known as LSD 25, famous for its ability to disturb consciousness and produce hallucinations. But the sympatholytic actions, mentioned above, were found not to be the basis of ergot's stimulant action on the uterus in obstetrics; Dale had to wait nearly 30 years to see the agent responsible for this effect, another related derivative of lysergic acid, ergometrine (ergonovine), to be isolated from ergot.

Although Dale didn't find ergometrine in his ergot extract he did find two other substances which led to a revolution in pharmacology. Unlike the ergot alkaloids, which are complex chemicals, these 'new' substances, histamine and acetylcholine, were very simple. Dale showed that *histamine* acted on tissues and organs throughout the body to produce a picture almost identical with anaphylactic shock although it took nearly 30 years to prove that it was actually responsible for this dangerous condition.

Anaphylactic shock occurs when a foreign protein is given to a sensitised person. We become sensitised to a protein when, our normal first-line mechanisms for keeping foreign substances outside our system having failed the second line of defence, the manufacture of new proteins, antibodies, operates. These antibodies are 'designed' to recognise and combine with the foreign protein and they are fixed to the outer surface of tissue cells that make and store histamine. Anaphylaxis occurs when a second invasion of the foreign protein is detected and bound by the antibody; this binding of antigen to antibody makes the defending cell release its stored histamine. The histamine, in turn, opens up millions of pores in the blood capillary walls to flood the area invaded by the foreign protein with plasma and blood cells to dilute, neutralize and ingest the foreign molecules.

Histamine has many other actions on tissues that seem to be designed to repel invaders, but as in every war, there are innocent victims; in this

* Sir Henry H. Dale (1875–1968): his revolutionary studies in physiology and pharmacology were carried out in industrial laboratories (Burroughs Wellcome Ltd.) and in the laboratories of the Medical Research Council (UK): his collaboration with the medicinal chemist George Barger (1878–1939) was vital to his success.

† Paul Ehrlich (1854–1915) developed the concept of 'aiming with chemicals', i.e. selective toxicity, i.e. chemotherapy, and realised it in practice in Frankfurt, Germany.

case there is also stimulation of secretion in eyes and nose, contraction of the muscles in the bronchi narrowing the airways (asthma) and dilatation of blood vessels, leading to low blood pressure and shock; the whole reaction can be unpleasant, dangerous or even lethal*.

Dale's work not only led to this understanding of the pathology of anaphylaxis but, many years later, it also led to the development of drugs that would block the actions of histamine on tissues in much the same way as he had shown that ergotoxine blocked some of the actions of adrenaline. The *antihistamines*, as they were called, were also able to block only some of the actions of histamine. These discrepancies in the spectrum of activity of the antihistamine and anti-adrenaline compounds led to the development, in the last 20 years, of a further series of antagonists (see later) so that now all the actions of adrenaline and histamine can be annulled if necessary.

Finally, Dale found a new substance, which he identified as *acetylcholine*, in one of his ergot extracts. Again, he discovered some fascinating differences: he found that acetylcholine had two distinct types of action. One type could be paralyzed by atropine and the other type by nicotine. Just as there was delay with ergometrine, many years had to elapse before acetylcholine was also shown to occur in mammalian tissues and his demonstration of the selective blocking actions of atropine and nicotine played a major part in understanding the physiological function of acetylcholine.

Indeed, Dale had a central role in establishing what we now refer to as the Chemical Theory of Nervous Transmission. When impulses travel along the nerve fibres that pass between brain and muscles, they release, at the end of the nerve, the contents of millions of tiny vesicles, each of them having contained a few thousand molecules of acetylcholine. These molecules of acetylcholine convey 'information' from nerve ending to muscle fibre and initiate its contraction. Drugs having actions like nicotine, including the arrow poison curare, can annul this action of acetylcholine and produce muscular paralysis. However, when acetylcholine is released at nerve endings in certain organs such as the heart and blood vessels, atropine but not curare is able to block this action.

How does it come about that drugs can pick and choose in this way? How is it that substances foreign to the body can produce such selective actions? Can we learn the rules so that we could produce new selective actions at will? To see the outline of an answer to these questions, we must look at the inner workings of ourselves and related mammals more closely, and this involves considering technicalities of **molecules, enzymes and receptors**.

Living things are chemical machines that get their energy by burning up (metabolizing) sugars. Sugars are difficult to store in tissues and they are converted into fats, which constitute the main fuel store. However, very large molecules (proteins) are used in the structure of tissues from cell walls to skin and bone, the contraction of muscles and the secretions of glands, the transport of oxygen and vitamins in blood, the protection by antibodies, in the manufacture (synthesis) of every piece and component of cells and in the controlled release of energy from sugars and fats. Proteins are made by joining a large number of small molecules, amino acids, into long chains called polypeptides and there are usually several polypeptide subunits in each protein. Although there are only 20 primary amino acids, they are arranged in a precise order in each particular protein (determined by other proteins, of course, the genes). The fixed order of the sequence of amino acids in proteins allows these few amino acids to be the basis of everything from viruses to man. A little mental arithmetic informs us that 20 amino acids can be arranged in 2400 000 000 000 000 different ways and, when we know that each protein may contain several thousand amino acids we can begin, just begin, to appreciate the complex beauty of living things. However, the real beauty of the proteins lies not so much in their strict sequence of amino acids as in their predetermined three-dimensional structure, that is, the way the chain of amino acids arranges itself in space like a skein of wool and the way the polypeptide subunits dovetail into each other. The arrangement is precise but flexible, for the

* Anaphylactic shock can result from non-protein drugs that have combined with a protein in the body to form an antigen; penicillin does this and kills about 20 people a year in the UK as a result.

subunits can adjust their position in a limited way, backwards and forwards.

The three-dimensional arrangement and the relative movement of subunits provide the basis of the catalytic function of proteins. Protein catalysts are called **enzymes** and catalysis is the facilitation of chemical reactions; but an essential feature of a catalyst is that it is not itself structurally altered when it facilitates the marriage of two other molecules; like the priest (catalyst) after completing one marriage ceremony, he is free to do it again and again! Imagine two species of molecules mixed in a solution which, though they are capable of joining together to form a new third species of molecules, are disinclined to do so. Like all molecules they are dashing about at high speed in a totally random way. When they bump into each other the energy of motion making them tend to spin away again, like colliding billiard balls, is greater than the energy needed to join them together so that not many new molecules are formed. Now add some enzyme that is suitably adapted to catalyse this reaction, i.e. on the surface of the enzyme there is a region, usually a narrow cleft, called the active site, which is adapted in a reciprocal or inverse way to the two 'unwilling' molecules. If one of the molecules gets into the cleft the fit is so precise and snug that it is 'disinclined' to leave. If the other molecule also gets into its (adjacent) site then for a brief moment their vigorous motion is stilled and chemical union can occur. If, now, a third molecule is added to the mixture which also has affinity for the active site, that is it can fit into one of the sites, but which is incapable of forming a chemical union with the other molecule, then the catalytic function of the enzyme will be blocked. This third molecule is called a *competitive inhibitor* of the enzyme.

Many useful drugs act as enzyme inhibitors. Gout is due to excessive formation of uric acid in the body so that solid crystals of sodium urate form in the tissues, particularly in the joints, causing extremely severe pain. Uric acid is formed from the precursor substances hypoxanthine and xanthine at the final stages of purine metabolism. The combination of both these bases with oxygen (oxidation) to form uric acid is catalyzed by the enzyme xanthine oxidase. Inhibition of this enzyme will thus slow down the synthesis of uric acid. **Allopurinol** (Zyloric) is chemically almost identical to hypoxanthine, a carbon and a nitrogen atom are simply transposed in one of the structural rings. But that is enough. Allopurinol has affinity for the active site of xanthine oxidase but since the enzyme fails to combine it with oxygen (oxidation) the enzyme becomes and stays blocked and is prevented from making uric acid. Allopurinol thus successfully prevents attacks of gout. However, the unoxidised precursors, xanthine and hypoxanthine, now accumulate in the tissues and blood. Fortunately in this case the accumulation of precursors does not matter because they are readily eliminated by the kidneys into the urine. Occasionally these substances are present in such large amounts that they crystallise out to form a urinary stone, but drinking extra water and making the urine alkaline with sodium bicarbonate is usually sufficient to keep them soluble and easily eliminated.

As well as causing molecules to marry, enzymes can also cause them to break apart or divorce. Acetylcholine is an ester that can be rapidly broken down to acetic acid and choline by the catalytic enzyme cholinesterase. As described above, the acetylcholine is released at the junction between nerve terminals and muscle fibres. As soon as the acetylcholine has stimulated the muscle, the cholinesterase, located on the outside of the muscle fibre, rapidly destroys the transmitter. If the enzyme is inhibited, the effects of nerve impulses become greatly exaggerated and the muscles are thrown into irregular twitching and spasm; if the enzyme is completely inhibited, the muscles become effectively paralysed by the build-up of acetylcholine. The so-called nerve gases (war gases) are capable of forming irreversible chemical bonds with this enzyme and other cholinesterase inhibitors, e.g. malathion, are used as insect poisons. However there are also reversible inhibitors of the enzyme, such as *neostigmine*, that are valuable for treating myasthenia gravis. In this disease the patient suffers from muscle weakness, which is often severe. The muscles behave as though there was not enough acetycholine being produced. When the cholinesterase is inhibited muscle power returns dramatically because the acetylcholine now stays around longer and gives prolonged stimulation to the muscles.

The introduction of treatment by cholinesterase inhibition is described elsewhere.

Occasionally, drugs can be used to play tricks on enzymes. The enzyme is offered a drug that closely resembles the molecules which it normally unites or divides (substrates), but which, unlike the unalterable competitive antagonists, is still capable of being handled by the enzyme. The enzyme can be persuaded to make counterfeit molecules! For example the transmitter at sympathetic nerve endings, that is the visceral (involuntary) nerves that adjust our systems for fight, fright or flight, is not adrenaline as Dale thought at the time but an immediate precursor, noradrenaline (norepinephrine). The enzymes that synthesize noradrenaline from DOPA, an earlier amino acid precursor, can also act on administered methylDOPA to produce methylnoradrenaline, which has been described as a 'false transmitter' because it is less effective than the normal transmitter. **Methyldopa** (Aldomet) is used successfully to lower high blood pressure, and this effect may be due to the reduction in the effectiveness of the sympathetic nerves that normally constrict blood vessels or to a similar action in the brain.

Most enzymes are not found free in cell fluid but are firmly fixed to cell membranes. There may be several ranks of enzymes so arranged that the products of one reaction immediately become the substrate for the next. Cell membranes are highly specialised structures, made of a mosaic of proteins and fats (lipoproteins), and the movement of molecules and ions across the membrane is strictly regulated. Impedence to the **flow of ions** gives cell membranes a static charge like an electrified perimeter fence, which can be switched on and off as pores in the membrane are opened or closed. This is the mechanism by which cells are sensitive to changes in their environment, the basis of their excitability. Each beat of heart muscle is preceded by a regulated switching off of the cell membrane voltages and the synchronized voltage changes can be detected on the surface of the body with an electrocardiograph. Some drugs used to treat irregular heart beat, the antidysrhythmics, act on the cell membranes, particularly of the heart, to alter the flux of ionic currents across cell membranes. **Lignocaine** (Xylocaine) alters the pores through which the sodium ions flow into the heart cells just before each contraction and so can control the speed with which the wave of excitability passes across the heart; it is effective in controlling some disordered rhythms of the heart.

All membranes restrict the movement of other molecules into and out of cells and there are special arrangements to restrict the penetration of substances between other places, such as from the blood into the brain and across the placenta into the fetus. To compensate for this, cell membranes are supplied with special chemical pumps, or **active transport** processes, to move particularly valuable substances either way across the membranes. Regulated penetration is particularly important in the kidneys. In the kidneys, blood plasma, that is the fluid non-cellular part of the blood, is first filtered indiscriminately, like filter coffee, into long tubes. The cells lining these tubes have highly-developed systems of transport processes located on their membranes and they actively pick out and return to the blood the molecules they 'want' such as glucose and amino acids and leave behind the 'useless' end-products of protein metabolism such as urea and uric acid. The tubular cells also actively secrete substances, particularly organic acids, including some drugs such as penicillin, directly into the tubular fluid from the blood. Here, where there are specialised chemical processes at work, is another site of drug action.

Penicillin is an organic acid and is eliminated at high speed mainly because it is secreted out of the body by the tubular cells of the kidney. In the early days of penicillin development, when it was extremely expensive to make, this represented a waste of valuable drug. Even today when penicillin is quite cheap to make, rapid elimination by the kidneys can make it difficult to keep the blood levels high enough to treat serious diseases such as bacterial infection of the heart (endocarditis) or to treat gonorrhoea, when the need is to make a simple massive dose of drug last as long as possible. The answer was found in drugs such as probenecid (Benemid). **Probenecid** is also an organic acid and competes for the same secretory process as used by penicillin so that the elimination of penicillin is impeded by competition and usefully higher blood levels of drug are attained.

The cell membrane is also the point at which one cell receives chemical messages from other cells. We have already seen how noradrenaline and acetylcholine act as chemotransmitters — released from nerve endings to the reponding cells, e.g. muscles, which are caused to contract. Histamine has been seen to link invading foreign proteins with blood vessels and other tissues. However we now know that there are many, probably thousands, of chemical regulators in the body. The chemical structure of some of these is known and where they are distributed to all cells in the body by the blood rather than released strictly localized to the site of action, they are classed as hormones. The sex hormones, oestradiol and androsterone, are examples, so are the thyroid hormones (iodothyronines) and insulin. Others are less clearly established, but the existence of numerous chemical regulators to orchestrate the activities of the millions of cells in our bodies is no longer doubted. How does any one cell know what is going on if it is being bombarded by large numbers of different regulators?

Receptors provide the answer. Each chemical regulator has built into its conformation and chemical properties some specific piece of biological information. For that information to be received by a cell the information has to be decoded in the same kind of way that a radio receiver decodes radio waves that it is tuned to receive and no others. A receptor has some similarity to the active site on an enzyme, that is a macromolecular site which shows chemical complementarity in its spatial arrangement and distribution of ionic charges, to the corresponding hormone. However, whereas at an enzyme the substrate is chemically altered and the enzyme remains unchanged, at a receptor the hormone is not altered but the interaction changes the receptor. Changes in the conformation and charge distribution at a receptor then trigger off some predetermined change in cellular activity.

Receptors, like enzymes, are also common sites for drugs to act. After all both of these sites are designed to be the basis for selective chemical effects in physiology and, if drugs happen to contain enough of the recognizable information they will be able to deceive the body's own selective machinery. Just as enzyme inhibitors, allopurinol for example, are often closely related chemically to the normal substrate, so receptor antagonists are often closely related chemically to the natural hormone. Knowledge about the physiological function of a specified hormone/receptor system can be used to guess what the properties of a new interfering substance (antagonist) might be. There are many examples of this kind of speculation but here is an example which led to the development of **propranolol** (Inderal), which is valuable in heart disease and high blood pressure.

Man can live for a few months without food and for a few days without water but even a few minutes without air and oxygen destroys him. Survival depends on how much food, water and oxygen is stored in the body, and not much oxygen can be held in blood, the main oxygen store. To hoard a day's supply of oxygen, about 1710 litres of blood, or more than 20 times the body weight, would be needed; the normal blood volume is about 5.5 litres.

When the oxygen supply fails, the heart is an early casualty. Oxygen is supplied to the heart muscle by arteries through which blood flows mainly during the brief pause between beats, and this delivery is so vital that the heart has its own special blood supply, the coronary arteries. Without oxygen the heart muscle first fails to beat, then dies; the coronary arteries are the heart's own life line.

The heart responds to an increase in bodily activity, be it during exercise or excitement, by beating faster and by pumping more powerfully. The increased force and rate of beating is due to noradrenaline being released at special (sympathetic) nerve endings on the heart muscle fibres. To do this extra work the heart must have more oxygen, and so the coronary arteries must respond by delivering blood faster. Healthy arteries do this, like water taps, by widening the bore. However, diseased arteries have swellings in their inner linings which narrow the bore so that blood flow cannot increase to meet the demand; if the pipe is furred up, opening the tap wider no longer increases flow. The first sign of trouble that the patient experiences occurs when the coronary arteries fail to deliver enough blood and oxygen to match the needs of the heart when it is working harder, as during exercise. At the critical point in oxygen delivery when demand exceeds supply, there is pain, which may be severe — angina pectoris. The muscle may recover when the exercise is stopped by the pain so that the heart work is reduced to a level which the coronary arteries can sustain, but the patient's activity is now limited. However part of the muscle may become damaged beyond repair. This is a myocardial infarct and the cause of 'heart attacks'. After a substantial infarct adequate pumping can still be maintained by the undamaged areas of the muscle provided that enough noradrenaline is secreted at the nerve endings in the heart. The irony of a heart infarct is that the level of stimulation by noradrenaline that is needed to maintain adequate pumping also increases the likelihood that abnormal stimulation of the heart occurs at the boundary between normal and damaged muscle. This abnormal stimulation can wreck coordinated beating of the heart — the wall of the heart becomes a twitching mass of unsynchronized contractions and it suddenly ceases to be an effective pump. This is called fibrillation and usually means sudden death, though prompt application of an electric shock from a 'defibrillator' machine may restore normal rhythm.

Traditionally, angina pectoris has been treated with nitrates and infarction with rest and analgesics. A patient taking nitrates felt warm and flushed in the face and everyone assumed that a similar dilatation of blood vessels occurred in the heart so that more blood could be delivered. A big search went on for drugs that would be better dilators of coronary blood vessels, more selective and longer-lasting, and the search was fairly successful. The newer drugs increased coronary blood flow all right but they often failed to prevent or relieve angina pectoris! Probably there was nothing mysterious about this: diseased arteries cannot dilate as well as healthy ones and the drug actions on blood vessels that tend to increase oxygen supply to the heart also, by inducing nervous reflex changes, act indirectly on heart muscle to increase oxygen demand. If we cannot effectively increase oxygen supply by drugs, why not try to reduce the heart's demand for oxygen? This is what happens anyway when a man with angina pectoris stops for a rest or the patient with an infarct is immobilised in bed. The trouble is that stimulation of the heart by noradrenaline, which mainly determines the heart's demand for oxygen, is only partly controlled by physical exercise — excitement, fear, pain and even lack of physical fitness also promote stimulation of the heart. Physical rest is not enough. Hence the suggestion; why not look for drugs that would prevent noradrenaline acting on the heart as a way of controlling the heart's demand for oxygen.

The noradrenaline receptors are the special chemical sites on heart muscle cells that first recognise and combine with noradrenaline and then trigger the changes in cellular enzymes that make the heart beat faster and more strongly. Propranolol has been found to be a drug that is recognised and bound by the heart's noradrenaline receptors but which not only fails itself to trigger the usual changes in enzyme activity but also, by occupying the receptor, prevents noradrenaline from doing so. This property of propranolol might have been enough to make it useful but it was found to have an additional property which was crucial. The noradrenaline receptors in blood vessels appear to be different from those in the heart. Those in the blood vessels are now classified as mostly alpha-adrenoceptors and propranolol appears to be a selective antagonist of the **beta-adrenoceptors** found in heart muscle. This means the propranolol interferes with the changes in the heart that occur during exercise or emotion without significantly interfering with the nervous control of the blood vessels. During exercise, the noradrenaline-secreting nerves that supply blood vessels shunt the blood away from skin and abdominal organs and increase the supply to the muscles; this action is not altered by propranolol because beta-adrenoceptors are not significantly involved.

When patients with coronary artery disease are treated with propranolol they are able to do more work without pain and they get short-term relief. However, there is also evidence that long-term blockade of beta-adrenoceptors increases life-expectancy. An unexpected bonus has been the clinical finding that propranolol is an effective treatment for high blood pressure. If this action, as seems likely, is also due to propranolol's capacity to moderate heart work and output during exercise, new light may be thrown on the origin of this widespread disease.

Here is a drug, then, which not only brings relief to sick people but is also invaluable in helping us to understand the function of noradrenaline and related hormones in health and disease. This is one of the most important points about drugs today. They do more than bring relief; they are now also important tools in medical research, helping us to understand the nature of disease.

Histamine gives another example of this double use of new drugs. The beta-adrenoceptor blockers were discovered after it was found that the early antagonists, the alpha-adrenoceptor blockers, were unable to prevent the heart responding to adrenaline. New histamine blockers were discovered after it was found that the old antihistamines were unable to prevent the glands in the stomach, the gastric glands, responding to histamine. Gastric glands secrete hydrochloric acid which, contrary to popular belief, is probably less concerned with digestion than with protecting us by sterilising the upper gut; the incidence of tuberculosis, for example, is higher in people who are unable to secrete acid. Every time we eat, this acid secretion in the stomach is switched on. Some people secrete too much acid either because the stimulus is too strong or perhaps because there is a fault in the mechanism which switches the secretion off once digestion is complete. Either way, excess secretion of acid is associated with ulceration in the stomach and/or duodenum. These ulcers (peptic ulcers) can either make life miserable through pain and indigestion or they may lead to the serious, even lethal, complications of severe bleeding or perforation, when the stomach contents leak into the peritoneal space and produce peritonitis. Surgery can excise the glands, removing the ability to secrete acid, or cut the nerves, removing the stimulus to secrete. But these are major operations and more than 1 in 200 patients die as a result.

The nerves which the surgeon cuts secrete acetylcholine at their terminals so that atropine, which is a competitive antagonist to acetylcholine, should be able to achieve the same effect as surgery. **Atropine** and related drugs have been used to treat peptic ulcers for many years but the results have been disappointing to patient and doctor alike. Doses of atropine that would be needed to reduce acid secretion also block other acetylcholine receptors causing blurred vision, a distressingly dry mouth and trouble in emptying the bladder. Atropine also blocks receptors serving the nerves going to the muscle in the wall of the stomach so that the emptying of the stomach contents is delayed and prolonged and this might do as much harm as the reduced acid would do good. Atropine just isn't selective enough, not nearly as selective as surgery.

Besides acetylcholine, two other substances are found in the stomach that are powerful stimulants of gastric secretion — histamine and gastrin. **Gastrin**, a polypeptide released by food from another part of the gut, is the main gastric hormone for controlling gastric secretion. Gastrin reaches its receptors on cells in the gastric mucosa indirectly via the blood. Gastrin stimulates the secretion of digestive enzymes as well as acid. Histamine is made from a single amino acid (histidine) and is concentrated in the region of the acid-secreting cells. Histamine only stimulates acid secretion. Some investigators believe that gastrin stimulates acid secretion indirectly by releasing histamine locally from its storage sites.

Just as noradrenaline acts on two different kinds of receptors so too does histamine. The **histamine receptors** are identified as H_1- and H_2-types. The antihistamines which we take for hay fever block the H_1-receptors. A few years ago new antagonists were found which could block the H_2-receptors. One of these H_2-receptor antagonists, called **cimetidine** (Tagamet), is now being used clinically. Although cimetidine is a competitive antagonist of histamine, the effects of gastrin are also suppressed. This could be good news for people with peptic ulcers because gastric acid secretion can now be reduced in a very selective way. More patients can now get the benefit of rapid healing of their ulcers than they could with the previous treatment with drugs that blocked the effects of acetylcholine. They also have the chance of avoiding the serious implications of abdominal surgery. In 1985, after about 10 years extensive clinical use, no serious unpredicted effects of cimetidine have so far been discovered.

Medical scientists have also got a new tool for

probing the function of histamine. It is possible to think of histamine having a protective function in inflammation and tissue repair, even gastric acid secretion can be seen as part of a protective system. But the puzzling area is the presence of histamine in the brain. Histamine is manufactured in the brain and its function is unknown. However, now that we can classify histamine receptors by using drugs like cimetidine some progress is likely which may or may not lead to the development of new medicines.

More and more, we are understanding how drugs make use of the body's own control machinery — receptors, hormones, transport processes, binding sites and so on — to produce selective actions. This understanding gives us a good chance, in the future, of producing many more entirely new drugs which will increase the number of people who can benefit from modern medicine.

However, no matter how skilled we become at making more selective and effective drugs, we will never escape from the problem of **drug toxicity**. This is an axiom, not an argument. Interaction between a drug and its elective site of action is determined by its goodness-of-fit for the active site plus the likelihood that random molecular motion will bring a molecule into contact with that site. The likelihood of such a molecular encounter is mainly determined by the concentration of molecules. Where a molecular species has high affinity for a site, a low concentration of molecules will achieve interaction. But as the concentration is increased, effective interaction may begin to take place at lower affinity sites and new actions, perhaps unwanted and even damaging ones, can then occur; the drug becomes less selective. This will be true whether the molecule is a natural or a foreign substance. A polypeptide hormone secreted by the pituitary gland regulates the water content of the body by controlling its reabsorption in the kidney; if, however large unphysiological doses are given into a vein, a new action, constriction of the blood vessels, appears; even the blood vessels to the heart, the coronary arteries, constrict and a large enough dose can kill an animal by stopping the heart. The latter action was discovered first and the hormone was called vasopressin; the former action was discovered later and so it is now called the antidiuretic hormone. All kinds of hormones and chemical regulators in the human body, such as insulin, histamine, vitamin D, can be lethal when used as drugs and given in overdose.

Except for suicides, the answer to overdose toxicity lies in careful prescribing, the prescriber should give as little of a drug as is necessary to produce the desired effect and carefully monitor his patients.

8

General pharmacology

We earnestly commend this chapter to our readers. In it are discussed the general topics of how drugs act and interact, how they enter the body, what happens to them inside the body, how they are eliminated from it, and other topics of importance such as the effects of genetics, age and disease on drug action. These topics are important to all who use drugs, for although all considerations will not be in the front of the conscious mind of the prescriber, an understanding of these matters will enhance rational decision taking and handling of drugs and will minimise unpleasant surprises for the doctor, and for the patient. Knowledge of the requirements for achieving success and the possible explanations for failure and for adverse events will enable the doctor to maximise the benefits and minimise the risks of drug therapy.

Pharmacology, the study of the effects chemical agents on living processes, comprises two broad divisions, which are:

1. **Pharmacodynamics** — the biological and therapeutic effects of drugs.
2. **Pharmacokinetics** — the absorption, distribution, metabolism and excretion of drugs.

The distinction can be put crudely thus — *pharmacodynamics is what drugs do to the body: pharmacokinetics is what the body does to the drugs*. It is self-evident that knowledge of pharmacodynamics is essential to the choice of drug therapy. But the well-chosen drug may fail (or be poisonous) because too little or too much is present at the site of action for too short or too long a time. Drug therapy can fail for pharmacokinetic as well as for pharmacodynamic reasons. Those who try to practise drug therapy by remembering an apparently arbitrary list of actions or indications cannot provide the standard of care that patients now have a right to expect.

Technical incompetence in the modern doctor is inexcusable and technical competence and a humane approach are not incompatibles as is sometimes suggested.

PHARMACODYNAMICS

Understanding mechanisms of drug action is not only an objective of the pharmacologist who seeks to develop better drugs, it also permits a more intelligent use of medicines. Consider the treatment of hypertension or asthma for example — using combinations of drugs with the *same mode of action* will provide additive therapeutic effect but also additive adverse effects. Selection of combinations of drugs having *different modes of action* will also provide additive therapeutic efficacy and reduce the risk of additive adverse effects.

Qualitative aspects of drug action

It is appropriate to begin by considering *what* drugs do and *how* they do it, that is, the *nature* of drug action.

Body functions are mediated through control systems that involve receptors, enzymes, carrier molecules and specialised macromolecules such as DNA. Most drugs act by altering the body's control systems. Some do so non-specifically, for example general anaesthetic agents and ethanol, and such substances tend to interfere with several systems, thereby causing unwanted effects. The majority of medicinal drugs act through binding to some specialised constituent of the cell to alter its function and that of the system to which it contributes. These drugs tend to be biologically selective, having an action on particular cells, and structurally specific in that small modifications to their structure may profoundly alter their effect.

An overview of the **mechanisms of drug action** may appear thus:

1. **The cell membrane,**

a. Action on specific receptors*, e.g. agonists and antagonists on adrenoceptors, antihistamine drugs on histamine receptors, anticholinergic drugs on acetylcholine receptors.

b. Interference with selective passage of ions across membranes, e.g. antidysrhythmia and antiepilepsy drugs.

c. Inhibition of membrane bound enzymes and pumps, e.g. membrane-bound ATPase by cardiac glycoside; tricyclic antidepressants block the pump by which amines are actively taken up from the exterior to the interior of nerve cells.

d. Interaction with cell membranes, e.g. general and local anaesthetics appear to act on the lipid, protein or water constituents of nerve cell membranes.

2. **Metabolic processes within the cell**

a. Enzyme inhibition, e.g. monoamine oxidase by phenelzine, cholinesterase by pyridostigmine, xanthine oxidase by allopurinol.

b. Inhibition of transport processes that carry substances across cells, e.g. blockade of anion transport in the renal tubule cell by probenecid can be used to delay excretion of penicillin, which is eliminated by this mechanism.

c. Incorporation into larger molecules, e.g. 5-fluorouracil, an anticancer drug, is incorporated into messenger-RNA in place of uracil.

3. **Outside the cell**

a. Successful antimicrobial agents alter metabolic processes unique to the microorganism (e.g penicillin interferes with formation of the bacterial cell wall) or show enormous quantitative differences in affecting a process common to both humans and microbes (e.g. inhibition of folic acid synthesis by trimethoprim).

b. Direct chemical interaction, e.g. chelating agents, antacids.

c. Osmotic purgatives (e.g. magnesium sulphate) and diuretics (e.g. mannitol) are active because neither they nor the water in which they are dissolved are absorbed by the cells lining the gut or kidney tubules, respectively.

The more important mechanisms will now be considered further.

Receptors

The concept that some drugs exert their effects by combining with specialised recognition sites on cells dates from the early years of this century. Based on the observation that curare antagonised the muscle contraction produced by nicotine but

* A *receptor* mediates a biological effect (e.g. adrenoceptor); a *binding site* (e.g. plasma albumin) does not.

could not prevent the contraction caused by electrical stimulation of muscle, Langley* reasoned that nicotine and curare must act by combining with some component of the muscle cell other than the contractile substance. This unknown constituent was a 'receptive substance' or receptor. For many years thereafter, pharmacologists regarded receptors only as conceptual entities necessary for developing and discussing hypotheses of drug action. In 1964, de Jongh† wrote: 'To the modern pharmacologist the receptor is like a beautiful but remote lady. He has written her many a letter and quite often she has answered the letters. From these letters the pharmacologist has built himself an image of this fair lady. He cannot, however, truly claim to have seen her, although one day he may do so.' His words were prophetic. The discovery that snake venom α-toxins (which can be radio-labelled) bind selectively to acetylcholine receptors of the kind found in skeletal muscle opened the way for quantification of the distribution of the acetylcholine receptor at the synapse. Indeed in this tissue the receptor molecules can clearly be seen on electron micrographs. It has also become evident that the classical lock-and-key concept gives too restricted a picture of the interaction between drug and receptor. New light on this has come from the use of the radioligand binding technique‡ in which the number and binding properties of receptors in or on whole cells or, more often, membrane preparations is studied by counting the amount of radio-labelled drug that becomes bound. Such studies have shown that the receptor numbers do not remain constant but change according to circumstances. When tissues are continously exposed to an agonist, the number of receptors decreases (*down regulation*) and this may be a cause of tachyphylaxis (loss of efficacy with frequently repeated doses), e.g. in asthmatics who use sympathomimetic bronchodilator drugs excessively. Prolonged contact with an antagonist leads to formation of new receptors (*up regulation*). Indeed, one explanation for the worsening of angina pectoris or cardiac ventricular dysrhythmia in some patients from whom a β-adrenoceptor blocker has been withdrawn abruptly is that normal concentrations of circulating catecholamines now have access to an increased (*up regulated*) population of β-adrenoceptors.

Most receptors are protein molecules. When the agonist binds to the receptor, the proteins undergo an alteration in conformation which induces changes in systems within the cell that in turn bring about the drug response. For example, activation of β-adrenoceptors by a catecholamine (the first messenger) increases the activity of adenylate cyclase, which raises the rate of formation of cyclic AMP (the second messenger), a modulator of the activity of several enzyme systems that cause the cell to act. Other drug-receptor effects are mediated through control of membrane ion channels closely associated with the receptor, e.g. nicotinic acetylcholine receptors, or through modulation of intracellular calcium, e.g. some acetylcholine muscarinic effects.

Agonists. Drugs that activate receptors do so because they resemble the natural transmitter or hormone, but their value in disease states may rest on their greater capacity to resist degradation and so to act for longer than the natural substance they mimic; bronchodilation produced by salbutamol, for example, lasts longer than that induced by adrenaline.

Antagonists. Antagonists (blockers) for receptors are sufficiently similar to the natural agonist to be 'recognised' by the receptor and to occupy without activating it, therapy preventing the natural agonist from exerting its effects. Drugs that have no activating effect on the receptor are termed *pure antagonists.*

Partial agonists. Some drugs, in addition to blocking access of the natural agonist to the receptor, are capable of a degree of activation, i.e. they have both antagonist and agonist action. Their effects can vary with circumstances, e.g. nalorphine in moderate doses antagonises opioid-induced respiratory depression, but in large doses increases it. For this reason, nalorphine became obsolete as soon as naloxone (a pure antagonist)

*Langley J N. J Physiol (Lond) 1905;33:374.

† de Jongh D K. In: Ariens E J, ed. Molecular Pharmacology, Vol 1. New York: Academic Press. 1964.

‡ The extraordinary discrimination of this technique is shown by the calculation that the total β-adrenoceptor protein in a large cow amounts to 1 mg. Maguire M E et al. In: Greengard P, Robison G A, eds. Adv Cycl Nucleotide Res 1977; 8: 1–83

was introduced. Such substances, e.g. pentazocine, are said to show *partial agonist activity* (PAA). The beta-adrenoceptor antagonists pindolol and oxprenolol have partial agonist activity (in their case it is often called *intrinsic sympathomimetic activity*; (ISA), while propranolol is devoid of agonist activity, i.e. it is a pure antagonist. The difference is readily apparent clinically in that a patient will have a lower resting heart rate on propranolol than on pindolol when with both drugs the blockade of the β-adrenoceptor, i.e. protection against fluctuating concentrations of catecholamines, as shown by the absence of tachycardia in response to exercise, is equally effective. It is possible that this difference is of practical therapeutic importance (p. 498).

Receptor binding. If the forces that bind drug to receptor are weak (hydrogen bonds, van der Waals bonds, electrostatic bonds), the binding will be reversible; if the forces involved are strong (co-valent bonds), then binding will be effectively irreversible. An antagonist that binds *reversibly* to a receptor can by definition be displaced from the receptor by mass action*. If the concentration of agonist increases sufficiently (competition; see also Chapter 7) the response is then restored. This phenomenon is commonly seen in clinical practice — the patient who is taking a β-adrenoceptor blocker and whose low resting heart rate can be increased by exercise is showing that he can raise his sympathetic drive to release enough noradrenaline (agonist) to diminish the prevailing degree of receptor blockade. Increasing the dose of β-adrenoceptor blocker will limit or abolish exercise-induced tachycardia, showing that the degree of blockade is enhanced as more drug becomes available to compete with the endogenous transmitter. Since agonist and antagonist compete to occupy the receptor according to the law of Mass Action, this type of drug action is termed *competitive antagonism* (see p. 502 for an example of the application of this theory to the treatment of overdose of β-adrenoceptor blocker). When receptor-mediated responses are studied either in isolated tissues or in intact man, a graph of the logarithm of the dose given plotted against the response obtained commonly gives an S-shaped (sigmoid) curve, the central part of which is a straight line. If the measurements are repeated in the presence of an antagonist, and the curve obtained is parallel to the first one but displaced to the right, then antagonism is said to be competitive.

Drugs that bind *irreversibly* to receptors include phenoxybenzamine (to the α-adrenoceptor). Since such a drug cannot be displaced from the receptor, increasing the concentration of agonist does not fully restore the response and antagonism of this type is said to be unsurmountable. The log-dose-response curve for the agonist in the absence of and in the presence of a non-competitive antagonist are not parallel. Some toxins act in this way, for example α-bungarotoxin, a constituent of some snake venoms, binds irreversibly to the acetylcholine receptor and is used as a tool to study it. Restoration of the response after irreversible binding requires elmination of the drug from the body and synthesis of new receptors and for this reason the effect may persist long after drug administration has ceased (hit and run drug).

Enzymes

Interaction between drug and enzyme is in many respects similar to that between drug and receptor (p. 96). Drugs may alter enzyme activity because they resemble a natural substrate and hence compete with it for the enzyme. For example, captopril is effective in hypertension because it is structurally similar to that part of angiotensin I which is attacked by angiotensin-converting enzyme; by occupying the active site of the enzyme and so inhibiting its action, captopril prevents formation of the pressor substance angiotensin II. Likewise, drugs or other foreign substances may compete for the same enzyme. Carbidopa competes with levodopa for dopa decarboxylase and the resulting reduction in metabolism of levodopa in the blood (but not in the brain, to which carbidopa does not penetrate) is the basis for the use of this combination in Parkinson's disease. Ethanol prevents metabolism of methanol to its toxic metabolite, formic acid, by competing for occupancy of the enzyme alcohol dehydrogenase; this is the rationale for using ethanol in methanol poisoning (p. 184). The

* The Law of Mass Action states that the rate of a chemical reaction is proportional to the concentration (mass) of reacting substances.

above are examples of competitive inhibition of enzyme activity, i.e. inhibition that is *reversible*. Inhibition of enzyme activity may also be *irreversible*, as in the case of organophosphorous insecticides, which combine covalently with the active site of acetylcholinesterase; recovery of cholinesterase activity depends on the formation of new enzyme. Covalent binding of aspirin to cyclo-oxygenase inhibits the enzyme in platelets for their entire lifespan because platelets have no system for synthesising new protein and this is why low doses of aspirin are sufficient for antiplatelet action (p. 579).

An action on the same receptor or enzyme is not the only mechanism by which one drug may oppose the effect of another. Extreme bradycardia following overdose of a β-adrenoceptor blocker can be relieved by atropine, which accelerates the heart by blockade of the parasympathetic branch of the autonomic nervous system, the cholinergic tone of which (vagal tone) operates continuously to slow it. Bronchoconstriction produced by histamine released from mast cells in anaphylactic shock can be counteracted by adrenaline, which relaxes bronchial smooth muscle (β_2-adrenoceptor effect). In both cases, a pharmacological effect is overcome by a second drug, which acts via a different physiological mechanism, i.e. there is *physiological* antagonism.

Selectivity of drug action

The pharmacologist who produces a new drug and the doctor who gives it to a patient share the desire that it should possess a selective action so that management of the patient is not complicated by additional unwanted (adverse) effects.

That drugs were selective to varying degrees in their effects had been obvious from their first use, but it was not until the end of the 19th century that Paul Ehrlich began to develop new selective drugs systematically in the laboratory (see *chemotherapy*).

There are in general two approaches to obtaining selectivity of drug action:

1. By modification of drug structure.

Many drugs are designed to have a structural similarity to some natural constituent of the body, e.g. a neurotransmitter, a hormone, a substrate for an enzyme, and achieve selectivity of action by replacing or competing with the natural constituent in the biological system of which it is a part. Enormous scientific effort and expertise goes into the synthesis and testing of analogues of natural substances in order to create drugs that ideally are capable of obtaining a specified effect and that alone. The approach is the basis of modern drug design and it has led to the production of adrenoceptor antagonists, histamine receptor antagonists and many other important medicines. But there are biological constraints to selectivity. Anticancer drugs that may act against rapidly dividing cells also damage other tissues with a high cell replication rate, such as bone marrow and gut epithelium. β_1-adrenoceptors predominate in the myocardium and the β_2-receptors in bronchial smooth muscle. However, the fact that some β_1-receptors can be identified in the bronchi and some β_2-receptors are found in the heart places a limit on the degree to which β_1 or β_2-adrenoceptor agonists or antagonists can be expected to act selectively on the heart or on the bronchi.

2. By selective delivery of the drug to the desired site of action alone.

When the circumstances lend themselves to it, the objective of target tissue selectivity can sometimes be achieved by special drug delivery systems, for example by intrabronchial administration of β_2-adrenoceptor agonists or corticosteroids (inhaled pressurised metered aerosol for asthma), by corticosteroid retention enema for ulcerative colitis, or by pilocarpine ocular inserts for glaucoma. Selective targeting of drugs to sites of disease in the body offers considerable scope for therapy as technology develops, e.g. attaching drugs to antibodies selective for cancer cells.

Quantitative aspects of drug action

That a drug has a desired *qualitative* action is obviously all-important, but it is not enough by itself. There are also *quantitative* aspects, i.e. the right *amount* of action is required, and with some drugs the dose has to be very precisely adjusted to deliver this, neither too little nor too much, to escape both inefficacy and toxicity, e.g. digoxin, lithium, and gentamicin. While the general correlation between dose and response may evoke no surprise, certain characteristics of the relation are fundamental to the way drugs are used. These are:

1. The extent to which the desired response alters as the dose is changed

Change in response with alteration of dose is defined by the shape of the dose-response curve, which conventionally has dose plotted on the horizontal and response on the vertical axis. A steep and prolonged rising curve thus indicates that a small change in dose produces a large change in drug effect over a wide dose range. This is the case with the loop diuretics; frusemide, for example, causes progressively greater diuresis as the dose is increased from 20 mg to 500 mg per day. By contrast, the dose-response curve for the thiazide diuretics soon reaches a plateau; the clinically useful dose range for bendrofluazide, for example, is between 2.5 and 10 mg and increasing the dose beyond this produces no added diuretic effect. Toxicity is commonest with drugs that have steep dose-response curves for both the wanted and unwanted effects.

2. Potency

The terms *potency* and *efficacy* (below) are often used confusingly. It is pertinent to make a clear distinction between them, particularly in relation to claims made for usefulness in therapeutics. *Potency* is the amount (weight) of drug in relation to its effect, e.g. if weight-for-weight drug A has a greater effect than drug B, then drug A is more potent than drug B, but the maximum therapeutic effect obtainable may be similar with both drugs. Differences in potency are usually without clinical importance — the diuretic effect of bumetanide 1 mg is equivalent to frusemide 50 mg, thus bumetanide is more potent than frusemide but both drugs achieve about the same maximum effect. The difference in weight of drug that has to be administered is of no significance unless it is very great.

3. Efficacy or therapeutic efficacy

Efficacy is the capacity of a drug to produce an effect and refers to the maximum such effect, e.g. if drug A can produce a therapeutic effect that cannot be obtained with drug B, however much of drug B is given, then drug A has the higher therapeutic efficacy. Differences in therapeutic efficacy are of great clinical importance. The diuretics again provide an example; amiloride (low efficacy) can at best cause no more than 5% of the filtered sodium load to be excreted and there is no point in increasing the dose beyond that which achieves this for no greater diuretic effect can be attained; bendrofluazide (moderate efficacy) can cause no more than 10% of the filtered sodium load to be excreted no matter how much drug is administered; frusemide (high efficacy) can cause 25% and more of filtered sodium to be excreted and the effect continues over a wide range of doses (hence it is called a high efficacy diuretic).

4. The therapeutic index

When the dose of a drug is increased progressively, the response in the patient usually rises to a maximum beyond which further increases in dose do not elicit a greater effect but induce only unwanted effects. This is because *a drug does not have a single dose-response curve, but a different curve for each action*, so that new and unwanted actions are recruited if dose is increased after the maximum therapeutic effect has been achieved. Thus a sympathomimetic bronchodilator exhibits one dose-response relation for decreasing airways resistance and another for increase in heart rate. Clearly the usefulness of any drug is intimately related to the extent to which such dose-response relations overlap. Ehrlich introduced the concept of the *therapeutic index* as the maximum tolerated dose divided by the minimum curative dose but since there are no single such doses that apply to all individuals, the index is never calculated in this way. The index can be calculated for animals by using the ratio LD_{50}/ED_{50}, i.e. the dose that is lethal in 50% of animals (LD_{50}) divided by the dose that has the desired effect in 50% of animals (ED_{50}). Similarly, a dose that has some unwanted effect in 50% of humans (e.g. a specified increase in heart rate say, in the case of an adrenoceptor agonist bronchodilator) can be related to that which is effective in 50% (e.g. a specified decrease in airways resistance) although in practice such information is not available for many drugs. Nevertheless the therapeutic index does embody a concept that is fundamental in comparing the usefulness of one drug with another, namely, **safety** in relation to **efficacy**.

5. Acquired and natural tolerance

Tolerance is said to have developed when it becomes necessary to increase the dose of a drug to obtain an effect previously obtained with a smaller dose. *Acquired tolerance* is familiar especially with opioids and is due to reduced efficacy at receptor sites. It can also be due to increased metabolism as a result of enzyme induction. There is commonly cross-tolerance between drugs of similar structure and sometimes between those of dissimilar structure. There is also *natural tolerance*, which is not induced by the drug but is due to inherent genetic factors (see pharmacogenetics).

6. Biological assay and standardisation

Biological assay, of which the therapeutic trial can be considered a special form, is the process by which the activity of a substance (identified or unidentified) is measured on living material, e.g. contraction of bronchial, uterine or vascular muscle. It is only used when chemical or physical methods are not practicable, as in the case of a mixture of active substances or of an incompletely purified preparation or where no chemical method has been developed. The activity of a preparation is expressed relative to that of a standard preparation of the same substance.

Biological standardisation is a specialised form of bioassay. It involves matching of material of unknown potency with an international or national standard with the objective of providing a reliable preparation for use in therapeutics and research. The results are expressed as *units* of a substance rather than its weight.

PHARMACOKINETICS

The action of a drug that is desired is a *qualitative* choice, but having made the qualitative choice, considerations of *quantity* inevitably arise; it is possible to have too much or too little of a good thing. To obtain the right effect at the right intensity, at the right time, for the right duration, with minimum risk of unpleasantness or harm, is what pharmacokinetics is about.

Dosage regimens of long-established drugs were devised by trial and error. Doctors learned by experience the dose, the frequency of dosing, and the route of administration that was most likely to give a beneficial effect and least likely to be toxic. Apart from being laborious and putting patients at risk, this empirical approach left a number of questions unanswered. It did not explain, for example, why digoxin is effective in a once-daily dose, whereas aspirin may need to be given four times daily; why a dose of morphine is more effective if it is given intramuscularly than if the same amount is taken by mouth. The answers to these questions lie in understanding how drugs cross membranes to enter the body, how they are distributed round it in the blood and other body fluids, how they are bound to plasma proteins and tissues (which act as stores) and how they are eliminated from the body. Because these processes can now be understood in mathematical terms, they can be quantified and the information may be used to develop dosing regimens that are not dependent on the slow process of trial and error.

Pharmacokinetics* is concerned with the *rate* at which drug molecules cross cell membranes to enter the body, to distribute within it and to leave the body, as well as with the chemical changes (metabolism) to which they are subject within it.

The subject will be discussed under the following headings:

The time course of drug concentration and effects

The order of reaction — whether processes are first or zero order.

Plasma half-life and steady state concentration.

Plasma concentration and pharmacological effect.

* Greek: *Pharmakon* drug, *Kinein* to move

The individual processes
Absorption
Distribution
Metabolism
Elimination

The time course of drug concentration and effects

A number of important topics are fundamental to the understanding of this process.

The order of reaction

1. **First Order Processes**. Drugs taken into the body are subject to the processes of absorption, distribution, metabolism and excretion. In the majority of instances, the rates at which these processes occur are proportional to the concentration of the drug. In other words, transfer of drug across a cell membrane or formation of a metabolite is *high at high concentrations* and falls in proportion to be *low at low concentrations*. This is because the processes follow the Law of Mass Action, which states that the rate of reaction is directly proportional to the active masses of reacting substances. In order words, at high concentrations, there are more opportunities for crowded molecules to interact with each other or to cross cell membranes than at low, uncrowded concentrations. Processes for which rate is proportional to concentration are called *first order**. In doses used clinically, most drugs are subject to first order processes of absorption, distribution, metabolism and elimination and the knowledge that a drug exhibits first order kinetics is useful — for example it can be predicted that a 50% or 100% increase in dose will lead to an increase in steady-state plasma concentration by the same percentage. The converse will also be true: since rate and concentration are in proportion, when dosing is discontinued, the rate of elimination from plasma falls as the plasma concentration falls and the time for *any* plasma concentration to fall by 50% ($t_{\frac{1}{2}}$, the plasma half-life, see p. 109) will always be the same; thus it is possible to quote a single figure for the $t_{\frac{1}{2}}$ of the drug.

* Some further explanation: if the rate (R) of elimination of a drug is directly proportional to its concentration (C), i.e. $R \propto (C)^1$, then the elimination is said to show *first order* kinetics.
When, however, the rate of elimination of a drug remains constant, regardless of changes in concentration, i.e. $R \propto (C)^0$, then it is said to show *zero order* kinetics.
It may be noted for completeness that if the elimination rate were to be proportional to the square of the concentration, i.e. $R \propto (C)^2$, *second order* kinetics would be said to apply. Second order kinetics would also apply if the rate of elimination depended on both the concentration of the drug and also that of a second substance, A, present in limited amount: the rate of elimination would then be given by $R \propto (C)\,(C_A)$.
Thus the 'order' of a reaction is the sum of the powers of the concentration terms appearing in the equation that relates rate to concentration.

Zero Order Processes. As the amount of drug in the body rises, those processes that have limited capacity become saturated, that is, the rate of the process reaches a maximum at which it stays constant (e.g. due to limited amount of enzyme) despite an increase in the dose of drug. Clearly, these are circumstances in which the rate of reaction is *not* proportional to dose and processes that exhibit this type of kinetics are described as *rate-limited* or as *zero order* or as showing *saturation kinetics*. In practice, enzyme-mediated metabolic reactions are the most likely to show rate-limitation because the amount of enzyme present is finite and can become saturated. Passive diffusion does not become saturated. There are some important consequences of zero-order kinetics.

Alcohol (ethanol) is a drug whose kinetics have considerable implications for society as well as for the individual, as follows.

Alcohol is subject to first-order kinetics with a $t_{\frac{1}{2}}$ of about one hour at plasma concentrations below 10 mg/100 ml (attained after drinking about two-thirds of a *unit*, see p. 412). Above this concentration the enzyme process that converts the alcohol into acetaldehyde (alcohol dehydrogenase) approaches and then reaches saturation at which point alcohol metabolism cannot proceed any faster. Thus as the subject continues to drink, *the blood alcohol concentration rises disproportionately for the rate of metabolism remains the same* (at about 10 ml or 8 g/h for a 70 kg man), and alcohol shows zero-order kinetics.

Consider a man of average size whose life is unhappy to a degree where he drinks about half a bottle of whisky (alcohol content 120 g or 150 ml) over a short period, absorbs it, and goes very drunk to bed at midnight with a blood alcohol concentration of about 250 mg/100 ml.

If alcohol metabolism were subject to *first-order* kinetics, with a $t_{\frac{1}{2}}$ of one hour throughout the whole range of social consumption, the subject would halve his blood alcohol concentration each hour and when he drove his car to work at 8:00 the next morning, it is easy to calculate that he would have a negligible blood alcohol concentration (less than 1 mg/100 ml), though no doubt, a severe hangover, which might reduce his driving skill.

But alcohol is subject, at these high levels, to *zero-order* kinetics and so, metabolising about 8 g (10 ml) of alcohol per hour, after 8 h the subject will have eliminated 64 g (80 ml), leaving 56 g (70 ml) in his body, giving a blood concentration of about 120 mg/100 ml. The legal limit for car driving in the UK is a generous 80 mg/100 ml and at 120 mg/100 ml a serious accident is likely. The subject will be convicted of drunk driving on his way to work despite his indignant protests that the blood or breath alcohol determination must be faulty since he has not touched a drop since midnight. He will, deservedly, be banned from the road, and will thus have leisure to reflect on the difference between *first-order* and *zero-order* kinetics.

This is an example thought up for this occasion, although no doubt something close to it happens in real life often enough, but an example important in therapeutics is provided by phenytoin. At low doses the elimination of phenytoin proceeds as a first-order process, i.e. as dose is increased there is a *proportional* increase in the steady-state plasma concentration because elimination increases to match the increase in dose. But gradually, the elimination process approaches saturation and attains a maximum rate beyond which it cannot increase; the process thus becomes constant and zero order. Further increases in dose cannot be matched by increase in the rate of elimination and so the plasma concentration rises steeply and *disproportionately*, with danger of toxicity. No doubt many drugs could achieve saturation kinetics if a high enough dose were taken. The distinction between first-order and zero-order kinetics becomes a clinically important issue when the change from one to the other occurs *within the therapeutic scale of dosing*. This is the case with phenytoin and also with salicylate at high therapeutic doses. Clearly saturation kinetics may also explain delay in recovery from drug overdose.

When a drug is subject to first-order kinetics, and by definition the rate of elimination is proportional to plasma concentration, then the $t_{\frac{1}{2}}$ is a constant characteristic, i.e. a single value can be quoted throughout the plasma concentration range, and this is convenient. If the rate of a process, e.g. removal from the plasma by metabolism, is not directly proportional to plasma concentration, then the $t_{\frac{1}{2}}$ cannot be constant. Consequently, when a drug exhibits zero-order elimination kinetics no single value for its $t_{\frac{1}{2}}$ can be quoted for, in fact, $t_{\frac{1}{2}}$ decreases as plasma concentration falls. Certain simple and valuable calculations are dependent on knowing the $t_{\frac{1}{2}}$: estimation of time to eliminate a drug; construction of dosing schedules; prediction of the time to achieve steady state plasma concentration. These become too complicated to be of much practical use when elimination kinetics approach zero order.

Plasma half-life and steady-state concentration

This section examines the manner in which the concentration of a drug in the plasma rises when a patient begins dosing and falls after dosing ceases. These processes follow certain simple rules that also give the prescriber a knowledge of the amount of change in plasma concentration in response to alteration of dose. This knowledge provides a means for accurate control of drug effect. Consider first the time course of a drug in the blood after an i.v. bolus injection (a single dose injected in a period of some seconds as distinct from a continuous infusion); as is expected, plasma concentration will quickly reach a peak from which there will be a sharp drop as the drug distributes in the body (*distribution phase*) and which will then be followed by a steady decline (*elimination phase*) and, if the elimination processes are first order, the time taken for *any* concentration point to fall to half its value is always the same. In other words, the half life ($t_{\frac{1}{2}}$), which is the time taken for the plasma concentration to fall by half, is a constant*. Either the *blood* $t_{\frac{1}{2}}$ or the *plasma* $t_{\frac{1}{2}}$ may be quoted, depending simply on whether the drug is measured in blood or plasma and since the latter is more common the term *plasma* $t_{\frac{1}{2}}$ is preferred in this text. **The $t_{\frac{1}{2}}$ is the single most useful characteristic of a drug in pharmacokinetic terms**. It can be used to predict the following:

1. *Decline in plasma concentration after dosing ceases*

Consider a drug with a $t_{\frac{1}{2}}$ of 6 h, which after a constant intravenous infusion is present in plasma at a steady concentration of 100 mg/l.

If the infusion is discontinued, the plasma concentration will decline as follows:

Hours	*No. of $t_{\frac{1}{2}}$s*	*Plasma concentration (mg/l)*
0	–	100
6	1	50
12	2	25
18	3	12.5
24	4	6.25
30	5	3.125

Thus, the extent of decline in plasma concentration can be predicted at various times after the last dose, including the time in which elimination from plasma is virtually complete.

2. *Increase in plasma concentration after dosing begins*

When a drug is given by constant intravenous infusion or repeatedly by other routes, the amount of drug in the body and with it the plasma concentration rise until a state is reached at which the rate of administration of drug to the body is exactly equal to the rate of elimination. This is referred to as the **steady state** and when it is attained the amount of drug in the body is constant and it follows that the plasma concentration is at a **plateau**. The importance is, or course, that once steady state has been reached on any particular dosing schedule then, provided the desired effect is being attained, adherence to this schedule will ensure a constant amount of drug action and the patient will experience neither toxicity nor decline of effect. Thus, having taken the decision to start a patient on a drug, the doctor next needs to know the *time it will take to reach steady state*. The $t_{\frac{1}{2}}$ provides this, for the relation is the *inverse* of that between $t_{\frac{1}{2}}$ and decline in plasma concentration after dosing ceases.

The rise in plasma concentration to steady state of a drug having a $t_{\frac{1}{2}}$ of 6 h and administered at 6-hourly intervals is as follows:

Hours	*No. of $t_{\frac{1}{2}}$s*	*% of ultimate steady state*
0	0	0
6	1	50
12	2	75
18	3	87.5
24	4	93.75
30	5	96.875

(Note: each step rises by half the difference between current concentration and ultimate [100%] concentration).

The significant fact is that **the time to reach steady state is a function only of $t_{\frac{1}{2}}$** and on regular dosing it can be predicted that after five half-lives, for all practical purposes, the amount of drug in the body will be constant and the plasma concentration will be at a plateau.

Clearly if a drug is given by repeated oral administration rather than by constant i.v. infusion, the plasma concentration will fluctuate between peaks and troughs, but in time all the peaks will be equal height and all the troughs will be of equal depth; this is also called a steady-state concentration, since the mean concentration is constant.†

Change from steady state. The same principle holds for change from any steady state plasma

* Some further explanation: the constant relationship arises because the graph relating logarithm of plasma concentration to time is a straight line. An approach for analysing pharmacokinetic data follows: it is more convenient to think of the body in a simpler form than the complex collection of tissues and fluids which we know it to be — indeed, the simplest model of the body is a single homogenous unit or compartment into which drug is placed and is very evenly distributed, and from which elimination occurs as a first-order process. This oversimple concept of the body has yet proved useful. In such a system, the mathematical prediction is that drug concentration declines exponentially with time and the relationship between the logarithm of drug concentration and time is a straight line — just what is observed in practice, ie the drug appears to behave as though the body were a single compartment. More elaborate models of two and three compartments can be made but need not be discussed here.

† The peaks and troughs can be of practical importance with drugs of low therapeutic index, e.g. aminoglycoside antibiotics, and it is necessary to measure both to monitor therapy (p. 223).

concentration to a new steady state brought about by either

a. alteration in the rate of drug administration or

b. alteration in the rate of drug elimination and provided the kinetics remain first order. Thus, if elimination is increased by enzyme induction or is decreased by development of renal impairment, plasma concentration will *fall* or *rise* to a new steady state, and will take five times the new $t_{\frac{1}{2}}$ to get within 97% of the new steady state.

An illustration. On a constant daily dose of digoxin ($t_{\frac{1}{2}}$, 1.5 d), a patient can be expected to have a plasma concentration 97% of steady state within 7.5 d (5 × $t_{\frac{1}{2}}$). A blood sample to check that the plasma concentration is in the therapeutic range would be reasonable at this stage but an estimate, say, at 3 days could be misleading because it would represent only 75% of the ultimate steady state. This relation is particularly important when the patient's renal function is impaired, as $t_{\frac{1}{2}}$ is then increased, digoxin being largely excreted by the kidney. If, in such a patient, $t_{\frac{1}{2}}$ of digoxin is extended to 3 days, then an estimation of plasma concentration at 6 days, even if it gives a result within the therapeutic range, would represent only 75% of the ultimate steady state and the patient may be at risk of toxicity from continued dosing. Likewise, in the patient whose blood concentration is at steady state, a 50% increase or 75% decrease in *daily dose* of digoxin will eventually give a new steady state that will be 50% greater or 75% less than the original. The time to get to within 97% of the *new* steady state blood concentration is still 5 × $t_{\frac{1}{2}}$, i.e. 7.5 days, in the patient with normal renal function, 15 days in the patient whose renal function is impaired.

The relation between $t_{\frac{1}{2}}$ and time to reach steady-state blood concentration applies to all drugs, as much to dobutamine ($t_{\frac{1}{2}}$, 2 min), when it is useful to know that an alteration of infusion rate will reach a plateau within 8–10 min, as to amiodarone ($t_{\frac{1}{2}}$, 700 h), when a constant dose will give a steady blood concentration only after 21 weeks.

Plasma $t_{\frac{1}{2}}$ values are given in the text when they are known and seem particularly relevant. **A few $t_{\frac{1}{2}}$ values are listed below** so that they can be pondered upon in relation to clinical practice.

Drug	$t_{\frac{1}{2}}$
dobutamine	2 min
aspirin	15 min
benzylpenicillin	30 min
ampicillin	1.25 h
paracetamol	2 h
propranolol	3 h
tolbutamide	6 h
atenolol	7 h
oxazepam	10 h
imipramine	15 h
diazepam	30 h
digoxin	36 h
chlorpropamide	36 h
warfarin	44 h
phenobarbitone	85 h
chloroquine	72 h (single)
	150 h (repeated)
digitoxin	150 h
amiodarone	700 h

(Drugs that induce their own hepatic metabolism show shorter $t_{\frac{1}{2}}$ with chronic therapy)

The **biological effect** $t_{\frac{1}{2}}$ is the time in which the biological effect of a drug declines by one half. The biological effect $t_{\frac{1}{2}}$ is more difficult to establish than the plasma $t_{\frac{1}{2}}$ and is not usually quoted. However, certain comments are appropriate.

1. For most drugs over a certain range, the *logarithm of plasma concentration* has a straight-line relation with *effect*; but *logarithm of plasma concentration* is also linearly related to *time*. It would be usual therefore, on cessation of dosing, to expect a straight line relation between decline in *effect* and passage of *time*.

2. Sometimes the biological effect $t_{\frac{1}{2}}$ can be provided with reasonable accuracy, e.g. with drugs that act competitively with receptors (α-and β-adrenoceptor agonists and antagonists).

3. Sometimes the biological effect $t_{\frac{1}{2}}$ cannot be provided, e.g. with antibiotics when the number of infecting organisms and their sensitivity determines the outcome.

The use of plasma and biological $t_{\frac{1}{2}}$ values. The issues that concern the practising doctor are not primarily those of changing drug plasma concentration but relate inevitably to drug action, that is, to the time of onset and offset of effect in relation to dosing and to the useful duration of individual doses. Accurate data on drug action are more difficult to obtain and therefore scarcer than information about plasma concentration. Thus the plasma $t_{\frac{1}{2}}$ is often taken as a general guide to the time course of drug action but its limitations in this respect must be recognised, for implications as to the relation between drug plasma concentration and effect immediately arise. These are discussed in the next section.

*Plasma concentration and pharmacological effect**

Experience shows that patients may vary greatly in the amount of drug required to achieve the same response, in other words response to drug can be represented as a normal distribution curve. The dose of warfarin that maintains a therapeutic concentration may vary as much as five-fold between individuals, and there are many other examples. This is hardly surprising considering known variation in drug metabolism, disposition and tissue responsiveness discussed in this chapter and it raises the issue of how optimal drug effect can be achieved quickly in each patient, i.e. can drug therapy be 'individualised'? A logical approach is to assume that effect is related to drug concentration at the receptor site in the tissues and that in turn the plasma concentration is likely to be related to, though not necessarily the same as, tissue concentration. Indeed, for many drugs, correlation between plasma concentration and clinical effect is better than that between dose and effect. Yet monitoring therapy by measuring drug in plasma is of practical use only in selected instances and the reasons for this are now discussed:

1. *Plasma concentration is obviously not worth measuring* if dose can be titrated against a quickly and easily measured effect such as blood pressure (antihypertensives), weight (diuretics), prothrombin time (oral anticoagulants) or blood sugar (hypoglycaemics).

2. *Plasma concentration may have no correlation with effect.* This is the case with drugs that act irreversibly and these have been named *hit and run drugs* because their effect persists long after the drug has left the plasma. Such drugs destroy or inactivate target tissue (enzyme, receptor) and restoration of effect occurs only after days or weeks, when resynthesis takes place, e.g. monoamine oxidase inhibitors, reserpine, some anticholinesterases and anticancer drugs.

3. *Plasma concentration may correlate poorly with effect*

a. Many drugs produce metabolites that are pharmacologically active but may not be identified by the assay procedure, e.g. benzodiazepines, several β-adrenoceptor antagonists.

b. Conversely, a non-specific assay may measure a pharmacologically inactive metabolite.

Correlation between plasma concentration and effect is inevitably weakened in both (a) and (b) above.

c. Total drug in plasma (free+bound) is usually monitored rather than free unbound drug because to measure free drug alone is technically more difficult. The best correlation is likely to be achieved by measurement of free (active) drug in plasma water as opposed to total drug in plasma. This was shown with propranolol, the total concentration of which correlated poorly with reduction of exercise tachycardia whereas the unbound fraction correlated well*. Many basic drugs, e.g. lignocaine, disopyramide, bind to acute-phase proteins (e.g. α_1-acid glycoprotein), which are present in greatly elevated concentration in inflammatory states. The consequent rise in total drug concentration is due to increase in *bound* (inactive) but not in the *free* (active) concentration and correlation with effect will be lost if only total drug is measured.

d. A further cause of poor correlation is introduced if the effect of a drug declines as dose is increased beyond an optimum point. Nortriptyline is most effective in a range 50–150 ng/ml of plasma. The lack of benefit below 50 ng/ml is expected, and presumably represents concentrations too low to inhibit the amine pump; loss of effect at concentrations in excess of 150 ng/ml is unexpected, and may be due to the α-adrenoceptor blocking effect of nortriptyline, which

* Concentration of drugs in biological fluids (and in gas, e.g. alcohol) is currently expressed in a dangerously confusing variety of notations (e.g. μg/ml, mmol/l). Standardisation is desirable and the convention is likely to become molar unit per litre, i.e. SI (Système International) units.

* McDevitt D G et al. Clin Pharmacol Ther 1976; 20: 152.

becomes important only at higher concentration. The phenomenon arises because drugs may have more than one action (and dose-response curve) depending on the dose used (see Therapeutic Index, p. 106). An intermediate range in which the desired action is obtained is called a *therapeutic window*. A similar phenomenon occurs with clonidine, which has a maximum antihypertensive effect at a plasma concentration of about 1.5 ng/ml. At or below this concentration clonidine reduces blood pressure by activating α-adrenoceptors in the brain; above this concentration, clonidine exerts a peripheral α-adrenoceptor agonist effect, which causes blood pressure to *rise*.

4. *Plasma concentration may correlate well with effect*. When this is the case, and when the effect is inconvenient to measure, dosage may best be monitored according to the plasma drug concentration (in relation to a previously defined optimum range).

Plasma concentration monitoring has proved useful in the following situations:

a. when the desired effect is suppression of infrequent sporadic events such as epileptic seizures or episodes of cardiac dysrhythmia.

b. when there is no quick and reliable assessment of effect, e.g. mood changes in a depressed patient, and where social environment plays a role as great or even greater than that of the drug.

c. when lack of therapeutic effect and toxicity may be difficult to distinguish. Digoxin illustrates this case best, for the drug is both a treatment for, and sometimes the cause of supra-ventricular dysrhythmia; a plasma digoxin measurement will help to distinguish whether a dysrhythmia is due to too much or too little digoxin.

d. to reduce the risk of adverse drug effects, e.g. otic or renal damage with aminoglycoside antibiotics or lithium, when therapeutic doses are close to toxic doses (low therapeutic index).

e. to diagnose and treat drug overdose.

f. to check patient compliance on a drug regimen, e.g. when there is failure of therapeutic effect at a dose that is expected to be effective.

g. when metabolic or elimination mechanisms are impaired.

h. to define dosage schedules of new drugs.

Timing of blood samples for plasma concentration monitoring

The *interpretation* of drug concentration measurements must take into account the time at which a blood sample is taken in relation to dosing and the following should be considered:

1. Whether dosing with the drug being monitored is at *steady state* conditions, i.e. whether 5 $t_{\frac{1}{2}}$ periods have elapsed since dosing commenced or since the last change in dose. In the case of drugs that alter their own rates of metabolism by enzyme induction (e.g. carbamazepine, phenobarbitone, phenytoin) it is best to allow 2–4 weeks to elapse between change in dose and plasma concentration measurement. Plasma concentration measurements undertaken when the patient is not at steady state are likely to be misleading.

2. Whether *peak* or *trough* concentration is measured. As a general rule, when a drug has a short $t_{\frac{1}{2}}$ it is desirable to know both; monitoring peak (usually 15 min after i.v. dose) and trough (just before the next dose) concentrations of gentamicin ($t_{\frac{1}{2}}$, 2.5 h) helps to obtain efficacy without incurring toxicity. With a long $t_{\frac{1}{2}}$ drug, it is usually best to sample just before a dose is due or at least to avoid the time of the absorption peak; for example, the concentration of digoxin ($t_{\frac{1}{2}}$, 36 h) should be measured 6–9 h after the last oral dose.

Concentration ranges that are useful for monitoring therapy are given in this book with descriptions of individual drugs.

Individual pharmacokinetic processes

This section considers the processes whereby drugs are absorbed into, distributed around, metabolised by and excreted from the body. Common to all these is the necessity for drugs to pass across cell membranes, a discussion of which now follows.

Drug passage across cell membranes

Our bodies are labyrinths of fluid-filled spaces. Some, such as the lumina of the kidney tubules or intestine, are connected to the outside world; the blood, lymph and cerebrospinal fluid (CSF) are enclosed. These spaces are lined by sheets of cells and the extent to which a drug can cross epithelia or endothelia is fundamental to its clinical use. It is the major factor that determines whether a drug can be taken orally for systemic effect or whether within the glomerular filtrate it will be reabsorbed or excreted in the urine.

Cell membranes are essentially bilayers of lipid molecules, though with 'islands' of protein, and they preserve and regulate the internal environment. Lipid-soluble substances diffuse readily into cells and therefore throughout body tissues. Adjacent epithelial or endothelial cells are joined by so-called tight junctions, some of which are believed to contain water-filled channels through which water-soluble substances of small molecular size may filter.

The jejunum and proximal renal tubule contain many such channels and are called *leaky* epithelia, whereas the tight junctions in the stomach and urinary bladder do not have these channels and water cannot pass; they are termed *tight* epithelia. Protein molecules within the lipid bilayer allow specific substances to enter or leave the cell preferentially (carrier proteins).

The passage of drugs across membranes is determined by the natural processes of diffusion, filtration and active transport.

Diffusion is the most important means by which a drug enters the tissues and is distributed through them. It refers simply to the natural tendency of any substance to move from an area of high concentration to one of low concentration. In the context of an individual cell, the drug moves passively at a rate proportional to the concentration difference across the cell membrane, i.e. it shows first-order kinetics; cellular energy is not required, which means that the process does not become saturated and is not inhibited by other substances. Diffusion across the lipid component of cell membranes is effectively limited to substances that are lipid soluble.

Filtration. Aqueous channels in the tight junctions between adjacent epithelial cells allow the passage of some water-soluble substances. Neutral or uncharged (i.e. non-polar) molecules pass most readily since the pores are believed to be electrically charged. Within the alimentary tract, pores are largest and most numerous in jejunal epithelium and filtration allows for rapid equilibration of concentrations and so of osmotic pressures across the mucosa. Ions such as sodium enter the body through the aqueous channels and pore size probably limits passage to substances of low molecular weight, e.g. methanol (32) or glycerol (92). Filtration seems to play at most a minor role in drug transfer within the body except for glomerular filtration, which is an important mechanism of drug excretion.

Active transport mechanisms enable some drugs to move into or out of cells against a concentration gradient. These processes expend cellular energy and are more rapid than transfer by diffusion. Competition for the carrier molecule involved may occur between substances of similar molecular structure. The mechanisms show a high degree of specificity for particular compounds because they have developed from biological needs for the uptake of essential nutrients or elimination of metabolic products. Thus, drugs that are subject to them are those that bear some structural resemblance to natural constituents of the body. Examples of the use of active transport systems by drugs are the absorption of 5-fluorouracil (a pyrimidine analogue used in cancer) and iron by the gut, the crossing of the blood-brain barrier by levodopa and the secretion of many organic acids and bases by renal tubular and biliary duct cells.

Passive facilitated diffusion is the mechanism by which vitamin B_{12} is absorbed from the gut and possibly the means by which catecholamines enter nerve cells. Cellular energy is not expended but since a carrier is involved, the system is saturable and specific for certain substrates.

The dominating effect of lipid solubility on drug transfer across membranes is clear. Drugs exhibit greater or lesser degrees of lipid solubility according to environmental pH and the structural properties of the molecule. Broadly speaking, water solubility is favoured by the possession of alcoholic (–OH), amide (–CO.NH_2) or carboxylic (–COOH) groups, and the formation of glucuronide and sulphate conjugates. Presence of a benzene ring, a hydrocarbon chain, a steroid nucleus or halogen (–Br, –Cl, –F) groups favours lipid solubility.

It is convenient and useful to classify drugs in a physicochemical sense into:

1. Those that are *charged or uncharged* according to environmental pH (electrolytes).

2. Those that are *incapable of assuming a charge* whatever the environmental pH (uncharged, non-polar substances).

3. Those that are *permanently charged* whatever the environmental pH (charged, polar substances).

1. **Drugs that are charged or uncharged according to environmental pH** Many drugs are weak electrolytes, i.e. their structural groups ionise to a greater or lesser extent, according to environmental pH. Usually most molecules are present partly in the ionised and partly in the un-ionised state. The degree of ionisation influences lipid solubility (and hence diffusibility) and so affects absorption, distribution and elimination.

Ionisable groups in a drug molecule tend either to lose a hydrogen ion (acidic groups) or to add on a hydrogen ion (basic groups). The extent to which a molecule has this tendency to ionise is given by the dissociation (or ionisation) constant (Ka). This is usually expressed as the pKa, i.e. the negative logarithm of the Ka (just as pH is the negative logarithm of the hydrogen ion concentration). It is convenient to remember that when the pH of a solution is the same as the pKa of a drug within it, then the drug is 50% ionised and 50% un-ionised.

If the pH is *decreased* from the pKa value by one unit, an acid becomes 91% un-ionised and a base becomes 91% ionised; if the pH decreases from the pKa value by two units, an acid becomes 99% un-ionised and a base becomes 99% ionised. Correspondingly, if the pH is *increased* from the pKa value by one unit, an acid becomes 91% ionised and a base becomes 91% un-ionised and so on. Thus, aspirin, which is a moderately strong acid (pKa 3.5), is 99% *un-ionised* at pH 1.5 (gastric lumen) and 99% *ionised* at pH 5.5 (urine); the base pethidine (pKa 8.6) is 99% ionised at pH 6.6 (urine). *See* pH variation and drug kinetics *below*.

In summary:

acidic groups become less ionised in an acid environment and *basic groups become less ionised in a basic* (*alkaline*) *environment and vice versa*.

This in turn influences diffusibility since:

un-ionised drug is lipid soluble and diffusible.

ionised drug is lipid insoluble non-diffusible.

The above is a useful general rule for drugs that have one main ionisable group. However, a pair of drugs that have ionisable groups of similar pKa will not automatically have the same lipid solubility, and therefore diffusibility, for *lipid solubility is a property of the whole molecule*, not only of ionisation. For example, the pKa of the ionising group responsible for much of the pharmacological activity of propranolol is 9.41, and that of metoprolol is 9.68 — little different. However, in a chemical test system to study how the drug molecules will partition between an aqueous and a lipid solvent, propranolol will enter a lipid phase at least 20 times more readily than metoprolol, which contains another ionising group. The greater lipid solubility of propranolol is also expressed clinically, since it crosses the blood–brain barrier much more readily than metoprolol and has a greater likelihood of causing central nervous side effects.

pH variation and drug kinetics. Studies of the partitioning of a drug across a lipid membrane according to differences in pH have been developed as the **pH partition hypothesis**. There is a wide range of pH in the gut (pH 1.5 in the stomach; 6.8 in the upper and 7.6 in the lower intestine). But the pH inside the body is maintained within a limited range, pH 7.4 ± 0.04 so that only drugs that are substantially un-ionised at this pH will be lipid soluble, diffuse across tissue boundaries and so be widely distributed, e.g. into the CNS. Urine pH varies between the extremes of 4.6 and 8.2; thus the amount of drug reabsorbed from the renal tubular lumen by passive diffusion can be very much affected by the prevailing urine pH.

Consider how the disposition of an acidic drug, aspirin (pKa 3.5), is affected by these differences in pH. Aspirin, entering the acidic environment of the stomach, where it is unionised and so lipid soluble and diffusible, ought to be readily absorbed. In practice, because of constant gastric emptying, relatively little of a swallowed dose enters the body this way. On the other hand, such aspirin as does enter the gastric epithelial cells (pH 7.4) will ionise when it encounters the higher pH and will localise there — this *ion trapping* may be one mechanism whereby aspirin is concentrated in, and so harms, the gastric mucosa.

In the more alkaline environment of the small intestine, although aspirin is ionised and less lipid soluble, the vastly greater absorbing surface is capable of taking up most of a dose. Once inside the body, because it is almost completely ionised at body pH, the drug remains predominantly in extracellular fluid. Passing via the glomerulus into the renal tubular fluid, the elimination of aspirin is promoted if the urine pH is high, for this renders aspirin ionised and lipid insoluble so that the drug does not re-enter tubular cells. This principle is put to use in the alkalisation of urine in the treatment of salicylate overdose.

The converse occurs with basic drugs, e.g. pethidine.

2. **Drugs that are incapable of assuming a charge** include digoxin, chloramphenicol and cyclandelate. Having no ionisable groups, they are unaffected by environmental pH, are lipid soluble and so diffuse readily across tissue boundaries. These drugs are also referred to as non-polar.

3. **Drugs that are permanently charged** carry groups whose ionisation is so strong that they remain charged at all values of the body pH. Such compounds are termed polar, for their groups are either negatively charged (acidic, e.g. heparin) or positively charged (basic, e.g. propantheline, tubocurarine, suxamethonium) and all have very limited capacity to cross cell membranes. This is a disadvantage in the case of heparin, which is not absorbed by the gut and must be given parenterally. Conversely, heparin is a useful anticoagulant in pregnancy because it does not cross the placenta (which warfarin does and is liable to cause haemorrhage as well as being teratogenic).

Brain and cerebrospinal fluid (CSF). The capillaries of the cerebral circulation differ from those in most other parts of the body in that they lack the fenestrations between endothelial cells through which substances in the blood normally gain access to the extracellular fluid. Indeed there are tight junctions between adjacent capillary endothelial cells which, together with their basement membrane and a thin covering from the processes of astrocytes, separate the blood from the brain tissue. This *barrier* places certain constraints on the passage of substances from the blood to the brain and CSF. Compounds that are lipid insoluble do not cross it readily. For the *same* concentration in the *plasma* the brain concentration will be *lower* with the *water-soluble* (lipid insoluble) *atenolol* than with the *lipid-soluble propranolol*, and CNS side-effects are more prominent with the latter. Penicillins and methotrexate are water-soluble and gain little access to the brain and CSF. Infection breaks down the usual behaviour of the barrier; in acute bacterial meningitis, penicillins will penetrate readily but, as recovery occurs and normal function is restored, antibiotic is excluded with risk of relapse, since the CSF concentration falls prematurely. Systemic methotrexate therapy may have no effect on leukaemic deposits in the CNS. Conversely, lipid-soluble substances enter brain tissue with ease; diazepam given intravenously is effective within one minute for status epilepticus; the level of general anaesthesia can be controlled closely by altering the concentration of inhaled anaesthetic gas.

Some substances cross the blood–brain barrier by active transport. Levodopa and methyldopa make use of such processes and penicillin is removed from the CSF by active transport (as in the renal tubule), which can be inhibited by probenecid.

About one-tenth of CSF is changed every hour, so there is also a washout effect, which reduces the concentration of drugs in the CSF.

Since CSF protein concentration is low in relation to plasma, total CSF concentrations of drugs that are substantially bound to protein are lower than in plasma, although the free concentration may be similar.

Placenta. Chorionic villi, consisting of a layer of trophoblastic cells that enclose fetal capillaries, are bathed in maternal blood. The large surface area and blood flow (500 ml/min) are essential for gas exchange, uptake of nutrients and elimination of waste products. The fetal and maternal blood streams are therefore separated by a barrier that has the general characteristics of lipid membranes elsewhere in the body, allowing the ready passage of lipid-soluble substances but excluding water-soluble compounds, especially those with molecular weight exceeding 600.* This exclusion is of particular importance with short-term use, e.g. neuromuscular block, but with long-term use all compounds will eventually enter the fetus to some

* Most drugs have a molecular weight of less than 600, e.g. diazepam 284, morphine 285, but some have more, erythromycin 733, digoxin 780, gallamine 891 (which is relevant to Caesarian section).

extent. However, the mature placenta is much more than a passive membrane for there are active processes that transport amino acids, sugars and vitamins into the fetal circulation, and uric acid and creatinine into the mother's blood. Furthermore, the placenta contains monoamine oxidase, cholinesterase and a microsomal enzyme system like that in the liver, which can metabolise drugs and can respond to enzyme-inducing drugs taken by the mother. The physicochemical and metabolic properties of the placental barrier should be taken into account as well as the duration of use in assessing the risk of fetal exposure to drugs in the maternal circulation.

Absorption

Commonsense considerations of anatomy, physiology, pathology, pharmacology, therapeutics and convenience determine the route by which a drug is administered. Usually these are:

Enteral, by
- mouth (swallowed) or by buccal (sublingual) absorption
- rectum

Parenteral, by
- intravenous injection or infusion
- intramuscular injection
- subcutaneous injection or infusion
- inhalation
- topical application

Other routes, intrathecal, intradermal, intranasal, intrapleural, etc. are used when appropriate.

Irrespective of the route chosen, *three factors are important* in determining the rate at which a drug is absorbed from its site of administration, namely:

a. dosage form (tablet, suppository, aerosol);
b. solubility in the tissue in which it is placed;
c. blood flow through the tissue.

Drug absorption from the gastrointestinal tract

Issues relevant to the absorption of drugs from the gastrointestinal tract will first be considered as this is the commonest route by which drugs are given.

The *small intestine* is the principal site for absorption of nutrients; it is also where most orally administered drugs enter the body. This part of the gut has two important attributes, an enormous surface area (estimated to be that of a tennis court, singles size), and an epithelium through which fluid readily passes in response to osmotic differences caused by the presence of food in the gut. It follows that drug access to the small-intestinal mucosa is important and disturbed alimentary motility can reduce absorption, i.e. if gastric emptying is slowed by food, or intestinal transit is accelerated by gut infection. The degree to which a drug is lipid soluble and ionised at intestinal pH also influences its absorption from the gut. The pH in the fluid immediately adjacent to the enterocytes (biophase) is thought to be about 5, which is less than that of the general intestinal contents. Some drugs (levodopa, methyldopa) are actively transported into the blood, but this seems to confer no special advantage. The stomach does not play a major role in absorbing drugs, even those that are acidic and thus unionised and lipid soluble at gastric pH, because its area is much smaller than that of the small intestine and gastric emptying is speedy ($t_{\frac{1}{2}}$, 30 min). The colon is certainly capable of absorbing drugs and many sustained-release formulations probably depend on absorption at this site. Absorption of ionisable drugs from the buccal mucosa is influenced by the prevailing pH, which is 6.2–7.2. Lipid-soluble drugs are rapidly effective by this route because blood flow through the mucosa is abundant and entry is directly into the systemic circulation, avoiding the process of first-pass inactivation in the liver (see below).

Enterohepatic circulation. This phenomenon is well illustrated by the conservation of bile salts, which normally circulate between liver and intestine about eight times a day. A number of drugs form conjugates with glucuronic acid in the liver and are excreted in the bile. Being polar, these glucuronides are not reabsorbed. However, intestinal enzymes and bacteria in the gut lumen may hydrolyse the conjugate to release the parent drug, which is then reabsorbed and reconjugated in the liver. Enterohepatic recycling appears to help maintain the effect of sulindac, pentaerythritol tetranitrate and ethinyloestradiol. Indeed, in the case of oral contraceptives, recycling may expose the drug to a possible interaction. Broad-spectrum antibiotics in high dose by mouth may cause diarrhoea so that ethinyloestradiol conjugate escapes recycling and the plasma concentration falls. Use of antibiotics, possibly at a sensitive stage in the menstrual cycle, has been proposed as a cause of oral contraceptive failure.

Systemic availability. When a drug is injected intravenously it gains access to the systemic circulation and thence to the tissues and receptors, i.e. 100% is available to exert its therapeutic effect. If the same quantity of the drug is swallowed, it does not follow that the entire amount will reach first the portal blood and then the systemic blood, i.e. its availability for therapeutic effect may be less than 100%. The anticipated response to a drug may not be achieved unless biological availability is taken into account. In a strict sense, considerations of reduced availability apply whenever any drug intended for systemic effect is given by any route other than the intravenous, but in practice the issue concerns enteral administration. This may be thought of in three main ways:

1. **Pharmaceutical factors.** The amount of drug that is released from a dose form is highly dependent on its formulation. With tablets, for example, particle size (surface area exposed to solution), diluting substances, tablet size and pressure used in the tabletting machine can affect the disintegration and dissolution and so the biological availability of the drug. The term *bioavailability* is conventionally attached to this category. Manufacturers are expected to produce a formulation with an unvarying bioavailability so that the same amount of drug is released with the same speed from whatever brand the patient may be taking. Substantial differences in bioavailability of digoxin tablets from one source occurred when the technique and machinery for making the tablets were changed; also tablets from different sources have been shown to have different bioavailability and therefore they are therepeutically unequivalent. Differences in bioavailability can be demonstrated if differing blood concentration-time profiles are obtained when several formulations of the same amount of drug are given to a single individual one after another. But in manufacturing practice measurement of the time a tablet takes to break up in water (*disintegration time*) and the time for the particles to dissolve (*dissolution time*) are used to check consistency of different batches. Physicians tend to ignore pharmaceutical formulation as a factor in variable or unexpected responses, probably because they do not understand it and feel entitled to rely on others to provide reliable preparations. Good pharmaceutical companies reasonably point out that, having a reputation to lose, much trouble is taken to make their preparations consistently reliable. This is a matter of great importance when dosage requires to be precise (anticoagulants, antidiabetics, adrenal steroids). A particularly florid example (phenytoin) is described under *interactions*. The following account by Lauder Brunton in 1897 is also relevant: 'A very unfortunate case occurred some time ago in a doctor who had prescribed aconitine to a patient and gradually increased the dose. *He thought he was quite certain that he knew what he was doing.* The druggist's supply of aconitine ran out, and he procured some new aconitine from a different maker. This turned out to be many times stronger than the other and the patient unfortunately became very ill. *The doctor said, "It cannot be the medicine"*, and to show that this was true, he drank off a dose himself with the result that he died.* So you must remember the difference in the different preparations of aconitine.'

2. **Biological factors** related to the gut. These include destruction of drug by gastric acid, e.g. benzylpencillin, and impaired absorption due to intestinal hurry, which is important for all drugs that are slowly absorbed. Drugs may also bind to food constituents, e.g. tetracyclines to calcium and to iron, or to other drugs, e.g. acidic drugs to cholestyramine, and the resulting complex is not absorbed.

3. **Pre-systemic (first-pass) elimination.** Despite the fact that they pass readily through the gut mucosal cell membrane, some drugs appear in low concentration in the *systemic* circulation. The reason lies in the considerable extent to which such drugs are metabolised in a single passage through the gut wall and liver, and an important feature of the oral route is that all drug that is

* The doctor died of cardiac dysrhythmia and/or cerebral depression. Aconitine is a plant alkaloid and has no place in medicine.

absorbed cannot escape these elimination processes. As little as 10–20% of the parent drug may reach the systemic circulation unchanged. This is also called the **hepatic first-pass effect**. By contrast, if the same dose is given intravenously, 100% is systemically available and the patient is exposed to higher concentrations with greater effect. Once a drug is in the systemic circulation, irrespective of which route is used, about 20% is subject to the hepatic metabolic processes in each circulation because that is the proportion of cardiac output that supplies the liver. Most drugs that are subject to the first-pass effect are extensively cleared by the liver, but it does not automatically follow that a drug with high hepatic clearance has a short plasma $t_{\frac{1}{2}}$. If a drug is highly bound in tissues, i.e. has a large distribution volume (see p. 122), then only a small proportion of the total drug in the body is present in the plasma and exposed to the elimination process. For example, though nortriptyline is subject to extensive hepatic clearance, less than 1% of the drug is present in plasma, the distribution volume is 1000 l/70 kg and $t_{\frac{1}{2}}$ is 50 h.

Drugs for which pre-systemic elimination is significant include:

analgesics	*adrenoceptor blockers*	*others*
morphine	propranolol	chlorpromazine
pentazocine	metoprolol	nortriptyline
pethidine	oxprenolol	isosorbide dinitrate
propoxyphene	labetalol	chlormethiazole

If the reader cares to list the *enteral* and *parenteral* doses of the above drugs that achieve comparable effects, the difference introduced by pre-systemic elimination will be apparent. Note that if a drug produces active metabolites, differences in dose may not be as great as those anticipated on the basis of differences in plasma concentration of the parent drug after intravenous and oral administration.

Drugs exhibit the hepatic first-pass phenomenon because of the rapidity with which they are metabolised. Indeed, the rate at which drug is delivered to the liver, i.e. blood flow, is the main determinant of metabolism. Many other drugs are completely metabolised by the liver but at a slower rate and consequently loss in the first pass through the liver is unimportant. The parenteral dose of these drugs does not need to be reduced to allow for pre-systemic elimination.

Drugs for which pre-systemic elimination is not significant, include: chloramphenicol, clindamycin, diazepam, phenytoin, quinine, theophylline, and warfarin.

In severe hepatic cirrhosis with both impaired liver cell function and well-developed channels shunting blood into the systemic circulation without passing through the liver, first-pass elimination is reduced and systemic availability is increased. The result of these changes is an increased likelihood of exaggerated response to normal doses of drugs having high hepatic clearance and, on occasion, frank toxicity.

It is convenient now to consider *the advantages and disadvantages of the different routes by which drugs may be given.*

Enteral administration

1. **By swallowing**

a. *For systemic effect:*

Advantages: convenience and acceptability, but whether given before or after food is of importance for some drugs. An antibiotic should in general be given on an empty stomach to prevent interference with absorption by food; an oral hypoglycaemic gives best control of blood sugar if taken just before or with food; potential gastric irritants, e.g. non-steroidal anti-inflammatory drugs should be taken after food.

Disadvantages: absorption may be delayed, reduced or even enhanced after food*, or slow or irregular after drugs that inhibit motility (anticholinergics); some drugs are not absorbed (gentamicin); some drugs are destroyed in the gut (insulin, oxytocin, some pencillins); tablets taken with too small a quantity of liquid and in the supine position, may lodge in the oesophagus with delayed absorption and even ulceration, especially in the feeble elderly and those with enlargement of the left atrium (impinging on the oesophagus); sustained-release potassium chloride, emepronium and doxycycline tablets may cause ulceration. Ideally solid-dose forms should be taken standing up and washed down with 150 ml (tea cup) of

* Welling P G. Clin Pharmacokinet 1984; 9(5):404.

water; even sitting (higher intraabdominal pressure) is less efficient. At least patients should be told to sit and take 3 or 4 mouthfuls of water (a mouthful ≡ 35 ml) or a cupful. Some patients do not even know they should take water.

b. *For effect in the gut*:

Advantages: drug is introduced at the site of action (neomycin, anthelmintics), and with non-absorbed drugs the local concentration can be higher than would be safe in the blood.

Disadvantages: drug distribution may be uneven, and in some diseases of the gut the whole thickness of the gut wall is affected (severe bacillary dysentery, typhoid) and effective blood concentrations (as well as intraluminal concentrations) may be needed.

2. **Buccal for systemic effect**

Advantages: oral mucosa has an abundant blood supply that enters the systemic circulation directly, so that a quick effect can be obtained (glyceryl trinitrate, nifedipine and ergotamine can be given thus); the possibility of degradation by gastric acid, delayed effect by slow gastric emptying or first-pass metabolism in the liver is avoided; the effect can be terminated by spitting out the tablet (or swallowing it in the case of glyceryl trinitrate for which the first-pass metabolism is sufficient to eliminate it).

Disadvantages: inconvenient for frequent regular use; irritation of the mucous membrane; excessive salivation promotes swallowing so losing the advantages of this route.

3. **Rectal administration**

a. *For systemic effect* (suppositories or solutions). Although the rectal mucosa is not a naturally important absorption site, it has a rich blood and lymph supply. The suggestion has been made that drugs which are subjected to hepatic first-pass elimination might escape this if given by rectum. This is true only for drugs absorbed from the lower rectum via the inferior haemorrhoidal veins, which drain to the systemic circulation. Substances that cross the upper rectal mucosa will be carried by the superior haemorrhoidal vein to the hepatic portal circulation. The route a drug takes depends on how it distributes within the rectum and this is somewhat unpredictable. In general, dose requirements are either the same or slightly greater than those needed for oral use.

Advantages: a drug irritant to the stomach can be given by suppository (aminophylline, indomethacin); suitable in vomiting, motion sickness, migraine or when a patient cannot swallow, and when cooperation is lacking (sedation in children).

Disadvantages: psychological, the patient may be embarrassed or may like the route too much; rectal inflammation may occur with repeated use; absorption can be unreliable, especially if the rectum is full of faeces.

b. *For local effect*, e.g. proctitis, colitis; an obvious use. A survey in the UK showed that a substantial proportion of patients did not remove the wrapper before inserting the suppository. A 2nd century AD Greek physician named Soranus described soothing intrarectal instillations to treat diarrhoea.

Some definitions of enteral dose-forms

Tablet: a solid dose-form in which the drug is compressed or moulded with pharmacologically inert substances (excipients); variants include sustained-release and coated tablets.

Capsule: the drug is provided in a gelatin shell or container.

Mixture: a liquid formulation of a drug for oral administration.

Suppository: a solid dose-form shaped for insertion into rectum (or vagina); it may be designed to dissolve or it may melt at body temperature (in which case there is a storage problem in countries where the environmental temperature may exceed 37°); the vehicle in which the the drug is carried may be fat, glycerol with gelatin, or macrogols (polycondensation products of ethylene oxide) with gelatin.

Syrup: the drug is provided in a concentrated sugar (fructose or other) solution.

Linctus: a viscous liquid formulation.

Parenteral administration

1. **Intravascular administration**

An intravenous bolus (i.e. rapid injection) passes round the circulation, being progressively diluted each time; it is delivered principally to the organs with high blood flow (brain, liver, heart, lung, kidneys).

Advantages: gives immediate, effective and highly predictable blood concentration; allows rapid modification of dose; immediate cessation of administration is possible if unwanted effects occur; is suitable for administration of drugs that are not absorbed from the gut or are too irritant (anticancer agents) to be given by other routes; drugs that are rapidly destroyed ($t_{\frac{1}{2}}$ a few min) can be infused continuously (oxytocin) to provide a steady state.

Disadvantages: hazard if drug is given too quickly, as blood concentration may rise at such a rate that normal mechanisms of distribution and elimination are outpaced. The heart and brain are particularly liable to give a dramatic response and some drugs will act within one circulation time. The arm-to-tongue circulation time is 13 ± 3 sec and with most drugs an injection given over 4 or 5 circulation times seems sufficient to avoid excessive plasma concentrations. Local venous thrombosis is liable to occur with prolonged infusion due to irritant formulations (e.g. diazepam) or microparticulate components of infusion fluids. Infection of the intravenous catheter is also a risk during prolonged infusions and the site and giving set should be changed every few days.

2. **Intramuscular injection**

Blood flow is greater in the muscles of the upper arm than in the gluteal mass and thigh, and also increases with physical exercise. Usually these influences are unimportant, but one football-playing patient who was given an intramuscular injection of a depot (sustained-release) phenothiazine had to be substituted towards the end of the game when he developed an extrapyramidal disorder, presumably due to excessive absorption of the drug.

Advantages: reliable and more rapid absorption than subcutaneous injection (soluble preparations are absorbed within 10 to 30 min); irritant drugs can be given; depot preparations (pencillins, neuroleptics, medroxyprogesterone) can be used.

Disadvantages: not acceptable for self-administration; liable to be painful; tissue binding or precipitation from solution may delay the appearance of drug in the systemic circulation (phenytoin, diazepam); delayed absorption in peripheral circulatory failure; risk of infection (abcess).

3. **Subcutaneous injection**

Advantages: reliable action; acceptable for self-administration; some depot preparations (hormone implants) can be used but most require an i.m. injection.

Disadvantages: less convenient than oral administration; irritant drugs cause pain, poor absorption in peripheral circulatory failure. Repeated injections can cause lipoatrophy, resulting in erratic absorption (see insulin).

4. **Inhalation**

a. as *a gas* (e.g. volatile anaesthetics)

b. as *an aerosol* (e.g. β_2-adrenoceptor agonist bronchodilators). Aerosols are particles dispersed in a gas, the particles being small enough to remain in suspension for a long time instead of sedimenting rapidly under the influence of gravity (i.e. colloidal); the particles may be liquid (fog) or solid (smoke).

c. as a *powder* (e.g. sodium cromoglycate). Particle size and air flow velocity are important. Most particles above 5 μm in diameter impact in areas of the upper respiratory tract; particles of about 2 μm reach the terminal bronchioles; a large proportion of particles less than 1 μm will be exhaled. Air flow velocity diminishes considerably as the bronchi progressively divide, promoting drug deposition peripherally.

Advantages: drugs as gases can be rapidly taken up or eliminated giving the close control that marked the use of this route in general anaesthesia from its earliest days. Aerosols provide high local concentration for effect on bronchi (salbutamol, beclomethasone), minimising systemic effects; self-administration is practicable.

Disadvantages: needs special apparatus (some patients find pressurised aerosols difficult to use to best effect); a drug must be non-irritant if the patient is conscious; for local effect, bronchi should not be obstructed (mucus plugs in asthma).

5. **Topical** (local) application (to skin, eye, anal canal and rectum, vagina, etc.)

Advantage: provides high local concentration without systemic effect (usually*).

Disadvantage: absorption can occur, especially when there is tissue destruction so that systemic effects result (adrenal steroids and neomycin to the skin: atropine to the eye).

Transdermal delivery systems (TDS) release drug through a rate-controlling membrane into the skin and so into the systemic circulation. Fluctuations in plasma concentration associated with other routes of administration are largely avoided, as is first-pass elimination in the liver. Glyceryl trinitrate may be given this way, in the form of a sticking plaster attached to the skin. Hyoscine administered via a TDS to sailors was effective at preventing motion sickness in continuous heavy seas with no significant ocular side effects and a tolerable degree of dry mouth.† But TDS may have an unexpected outcome, for not only may the sticking plaster drop off unnoticed, it may find its way onto another person. A hypertensive father rose one morning and noticed that his clonidine plaster was missing from his upper arm. He could not find it and applied a new plaster. His nine-month-old child, who had been taken into the paternal bed during the night because he needed comforting, spent an irritable and hypoactive day, refused food but drank and passed more fluid than usual. The missing clonidine patch was discovered on his back when he was being prepared for his bath. No doubt this was accidental, but children also enjoy stick-on decoration and the possibility of poisoning from misused, discarded or new drug plasters means that these should be kept and disposed of as carefully as oral formulations.‡

* A cautionary tale. A 70-year-old man reported left breast enlargement and underwent mastectomy; pathological examination revealing benign gynaecomastia. Ten months later the right breast was noted to be enlarged. Tests of endocrine function were normal but the patient himself was struck by the fact that his wife had been using a vaginal cream (containing 0.01% dienestrol) initially for atrophic vaginitis but latterly the cream had been used to facilitate sexual intercourse which took place two to three times a week. On the assumption that penile absorption of oestrogen was responsible for the disorder, exposure to the cream was terminated. The gynaecomastia in the remaining breast then resolved. Di Raimondo CV et al. N Engl J Med 1980; 302:1089.

† van Marion W F et al. Clin Pharmacol Ther 1985; 38:301.

‡ Reed M T et al. N Engl J Med 1986; 314:1120.

Distribution

If a drug is required to act throughout the body or to reach an organ inaccessible to topical administration, it must be got into the blood and into other body compartments. Most drugs distribute widely — some dissolved in plasma water, some bound to plasma proteins, some to tissues. Distribution is often uneven for drugs may bind selectively to plasma or tissue proteins or be localised within particular organs. Clearly, the site of localisation of a drug is likely to influence its action, e.g. whether it crosses the blood–brain barrier to enter the brain, and the *extent* and *strength* (tenacity) of protein or tissue binding will affect the time it spends in the body and thereby its duration of action. Drug distribution, its quantification and its clinical implications are now discussed.

Distribution volume. The distribution volume of a drug is the volume in which it appears to distribute (or would require) if the concentration throughout the body were equal to that in plasma, i.e. as if the body were a single compartment. An explanation follows.

The pattern of distribution from plasma to other body fluids and tissues is a characteristic of each and every drug that enters the circulation and it varies enormously between drugs. Precise information on the concentration attained by a drug in various tissues and fluids requires biopsy samples and for understandable reasons this is usually not available for humans§, although it often is practised in animals. What can be sampled readily in humans is *plasma*, the drug concentration in which, taking account of the dose given, is a measure of whether a drug tends to remain in the circulation or to distribute from the plasma into the tissues. If a drug remains mostly in the plasma, its distribution volume will be about that of plasma, i.e. small; if it is present mainly in the tissues, its distribution volume will include most of the body, i.e. it will be large. Such information is clinically useful. Consider drug overdose. Removing a drug by haemodialysis is likely to be a beneficial exercise only if a major proportion of

§ Fingernail clippings excepted; chloroquine can be detected in these for up to one year after stopping the drug. Ofori-Adjei D, Ericsson O. Lancet 1985; 2:331.

the total body load is in the plasma. That aspirin/salicylate is such a drug is indicated by the knowledge that it has a small distribution volume, but haemodialysis is obviously an inappropriate treatment for overdose with pethidine, which has a very large distribution volume, since most of this drug is outside the blood and is localised in the tissues. Drug interactions provide another example for, as is explained below (Protein Binding), the knowledge that a drug is present mainly in the tissues predicts for example that adverse reaction due to displacement from plasma proteins is unlikely. But these are qualitative considerations and if knowledge of distribution volume is to be of practical and scientific value it must be *quantified*.

The principle for establishing the distribution volume is essentially that of using a dye to find the volume of a simple container filled with liquid. The weight of dye that is added divided by the concentration of dye once mixing is complete gives the distribution volume of the dye, which is the volume of the container. Similarly, the distribution volume of a drug in the body is found (a) after a single intravenous bolus dose by dividing the amount of drug given by the concentration achieved in plasma* or (b) at steady-state dosing conditions, by dividing the amount of drug calculated then to be in the body† by the plasma concentration, which by definition is constant.

The result of this calculation, the **distribution volume**, in fact only rarely corresponds with a physiological body space such as extracellular water or total body water, for it is a measure of volume a drug would **apparently** occupy knowing the dose given and the plasma concentration achieved and assuming the entire volume is at that concentration. For this reason, it is often referred to as the **apparent** distribution volume. Indeed, for some drugs that bind extensively to tissues, the apparent distribution volume, which is based on the resulting low plasma concentration, is many times total body volume.

Thus the distribution volume may be defined as *the volume of fluid in which the drug appears to distribute with a concentration equal to that in plasma*.

The following list illustrates a range of apparent distribution volumes. The names of those substances that distribute within (and have been used to measure) physiological spaces are in italics.

* Using the intravenous route ensures that all the drug enters the systemic circulation, i.e. that bioavailability is 100%. But clearly a problem arises in that the plasma concentration is not constant but falls after the bolus has been injected. To get round this, use is made of the straight line relation between logarithm of plasma concentration and the time after a single intravenous dose (p. 110). The log concentration-time line extended back to zero time gives the theoretical plasma concentration at the time the drug was given. In effect, the assumption is made that drug distributes instantaneously and uniformly through a single compartment, the distribution volume. This mechanism, although seeming artificial, does usefully characterise drugs according to the extent to which they remain in or distribute out from the circulation.

† Rowland R, Tozer T N. Clinical pharmacokinetics. New York: Lea and Febiger, 1980:177.

Apparent distribution volumes of some drugs
(Figures are in litres for a 70-kg person.*)

Drug	*Vol*	
Evans blue	3	(plasma volume)
tolbutamide	7	
frusemide	7	
warfarin	8	
salicylate	10	
inulin	15	(used to measure extracellular water)
gentamicin	18	
ampicillin	27	
isoniazid	42	
antipyrine	43	(used to measure total body water)
rifampicin	65	
lignocaine	90	
diazepam	210	
propranolol	280	
metoprolol	390	
pethidine	500	
digoxin	600	
nortriptyline	1 000	
desipramine	3 000	
chloroquine	12 000	

Selective distribution within the body occurs because of special affinity between particular

* Litres per kg are commonly used, but give a less vivid image of the implication of the term 'apparent', e.g. chloroquine.

drugs and particular body constituents. Many drugs bind to proteins in the plasma; in the tissues methotrexate binds for weeks to the enzyme dihydrofolate reductase and phenothiazines and chloroquine bind to melanin-containing tissues, including the retina, which may explain the occurrence of retinopathy; highly lipid-soluble drugs are sequestered in fat and muscle (thiopentone, DDT).

Drugs may also concentrate selectively in a particular tissue because of specialised transport mechanisms, e.g. iodine in the thyroid. Administration of a radio-labelled drug to animals followed by whole-body autoradiography, can reveal such 'deep compartments', which is useful to know at an early stage of a new drug development.

Plasma protein and tissue binding. Many natural substances circulate around the body partly free in plasma water and partly bound to plasma proteins; these include cortisol, thyroxine, iron, copper and in hepatic or renal failure, by-products of metabolism. Drugs, too, circulate in the protein-bound and free states, and the significance is that the *free* fraction is pharmacologically active whereas the *protein bound* component is a reservoir of drug that is inactive because it is bound to protein. Free and bound fractions are in equilibrium and free drug removed from the plasma by metabolism and excretion is replaced by drug released from the bound fraction. Association and dissociation between drug and plasma protein is usually rapid although an exception is suramin, which is bound so avidly and released so slowly that a single dose exerts a trypanocidal effect for three months.

Albumin is the main binding protein for many natural substances and drugs. Each albumin molecule consists of a chain of 584 amino acids held in a series of loops by bridging disulphide bonds. This complex polypeptide structure has a net negative charge at blood pH and a high *capacity* but low (weak) *affinity* for many cationic (basic) drugs, i.e. a lot is bound but it is readily released. Two particular sites on the albumin molecule bind acidic drugs with high affinity (strongly) but these sites have low capacity. Saturation of binding sites on plasma proteins in general is unlikely in the doses at which most drugs are used. Other binding proteins in the blood include lipoprotein and α_1-acid glycoprotein, both of which carry basic drugs, e.g. quinidine, chlorpromazine, imipramine. The particular significance of α_1-acid glycoprotein is that it is an acute-phase reactant, i.e. one of several proteins that increase in the plasma in states of physiological stress, such as myocardial infarction, and inflammation, such as Crohn's disease. Plasma concentration monitoring of basic drugs bound to α_1-acid glycoprotein may therefore give spuriously high values if total and not free drug is assayed. Certain globulins bind hormones, including the contraceptive steroids.

Disease may modify protein binding of drugs to an extent that is clinically relevant (Table 8.1). In chronic renal failure, hypoalbuminaemia and retention of (as yet unidentified) products of metabolism that compete for binding sites on protein, are both responsible for the decrease in protein binding of drugs. Most likely to be affected are the acidic drugs that are highly protein bound. These include phenytoin and diazoxide, and care is needed in initiating and

Table 8.1 The free, unbound and therefore pharmacologically active percentage of some drugs to illustrate the range and, in some cases, the changes caused by disease.

Drug	% unbound in plasma
Warfarin	1
Chlorpromazine	2
Diazepam	2 (6% in liver disease)
Frusemide	2 (6% in nephrotic syndrome)
Tolbutamide	2
Clofibrate	4 (11% in nephrotic syndrome)
Cloxacillin	5 (20% in renal disease)
Imipramine	5
Propranolol	5
Phenytoin	9 (19% in renal disease)
Diazoxide	10 (13% in renal disease)
Quinidine	14 (42% in liver disease)
Thiopentone	16 (28% in renal disease)
Triamterene	19 (40% in renal disease)
Trimethoprim	30
Theophylline	35 (71% in liver disease)
Pethidine	36
Sulphamethizole	38 (62% in renal disease)
Chloramphenicol	49
Morphine	65
Digoxin	75 (82% in renal disease)
Ampicillin	80
Paracetamol	>95

modifying dose with this type of drug in patients with renal failure (see also Drugs and Renal Disease, p. 563).

Chronic liver disease also leads to hypoalbuminaemia and increase of endogenous substances such as bilirubin, which may compete for binding sites on protein. Drugs that are normally highly protein bound should be used with special caution and increased free concentration of diazepam, tolbutamide and phenytoin have been demonstrated in patients with this condition (see also Drugs and Liver Disease, p. 643).

Drugs may *interact* at plasma protein binding sites. Increased free concentrations of phenytoin are found when sodium valproate is added to therapy. Both drugs occupy the same binding site on the albumin molecule but sodium valproate has greater affinity and displaces bound phenytoin. Similarly, warfarin is displaced from protein-binding sites by phenylbutazone and azapropazone, leading to transient increased anticoagulant effect. In general, however, the importance of drug interactions purely due to displacement from protein binding sites has been overstated. A moment's thought about drug distribution is relevant. The effects of displacement from the binding protein depend on the following:

1. the amount of displaced drug that is added to the free fraction
2. the volume into which that amount of drug is displaced (see distribution volume, p. 122) and
3. the disposition of drug receptors.

Clearly, drugs that are *both* extensively protein bound and have a small distribution volume (e.g. warfarin, 99% bound, distribution volume 8 l/70 kg) are most probable candidates to create adverse effects due to displacement from plasma proteins. Drugs that have a large distribution volume are unlikely to exhibit adverse effects from this type of drug interaction, even if they are extensively bound. In the case of nortriptyline the fraction of the drug that is in the plasma is 94% bound, but the distribution volume of 1000 l indicates that most of the drug is present in tissues and alteration in the fraction-free in plasma is unlikely to be important. Furthermore, drug that enters the free fraction is immediately available for metabolism and excretion, which attenuates the biological effects so that they are brief. Indeed, in displacement interactions that are clinically important, additional mechanisms may operate. For example, sodium valproate displaces phenyloin from its protein binding site but also impairs its metabolism.

Plasma protein binding has obvious implications for *monitoring drug therapy* according to plasma concentration. Total drug in plasma is easiest to measure but may give wildly misleading results for drugs that bind to α_1-acid glycoprotein. The free fraction rather than the total is more likely to correlate with therapeutic effect. It is probable that as the technology of drug measurement becomes more sophisticated, regular monitoring of the free fraction will become feasible as a routine.

A glance at the table of distribution volumes (p. 123) shows that a number of drugs distribute much more readily to **tissues** than to plasma. These include many basic, lipid-soluble drugs such as diazepam, propranolol and desipramine. Less is known about tissue, e.g. muscle, binding than about plasma protein binding because solid tissue samples can be obtained only by invasive biopsy. Extensive binding to tissues delays elimination from the body, even of drugs that are rapidly cleared from the plasma. Amitriptyline, for example, has a distribution volume of 1000 l and despite a high plasma clearance (700 l/min) the $t_{\frac{1}{2}}$ is 24 h.

Selective binding of drug to certain tissues may lead to toxicity, as is shown by the strong affinity of chloroquine for the retina. Displacement from tissue binding sites may be a mechanism for drug interaction. When quinidine is given to patients who are receiving digoxin, the plasma concentration of digoxin may double. Studies in healthy volunteers have shown that the distribution volume of digoxin falls when quinidine is given, and that quinidine displaces digoxin from binding sites in tissue. As with interaction due to displacement from plasma proteins, however, an additional mechanism contributes to the overall effect in that quinidine also impairs renal excretion of digoxin.

Metabolism

Drugs are treated by the body as foreign

substances and become subject to its various mechanisms for ridding itself of chemical intruders. Some highly water-soluble drugs can be eliminated unchanged by the kidney but others must first undergo structural modification, usually by enzyme action. **Metabolism** is a general term for chemical transformations that occur within the body and its processes change drugs in two major ways:

1. by reducing lipid solubility and
2. by reducing biological activity.

1. **Reducing lipid solubility**

Metabolic reactions tend to make a drug molecule progressively more water soluble and so favour its elimination in the urine. The detail of how this is achieved is described later in this section but its significance deserves comment here. Consider the situation if there were no drug metabolising enzymes. 'For simplicity let us assume that a drug is evenly distributed throughout body water. If the compound has a low lipid solubility, about five hours would elapse before half the substance is lost from the body; if the drug is also secreted by the (renal) tubules, this time will be shortened to as little as one hour. However, if the drug is lipid-soluble, the excretion rate will be drastically reduced by back diffusion into the plasma from the tubular segment where the urine in concentrated. About thirty days would elapse before half the drug leaves the body. This extended duration might be an advantage with an antibacterial agent but would be of doubtful value with an anaesthetic agent. If a drug . . . is also reversibly localised in tissues its half-life would be about 100 years — considerably longer than those of the physician and patient combined!'*

Drug metabolising enzymes usually differ from those of intermediary metabolism and (probably) developed during evolution to enable the body to dispose of lipid soluble substances such as hydrocarbons, sterols and alkaloids, that are ingested with food.† 'Of course, it is not conceivable that nature should have prepared, in advance, a specific microsomal enzyme for the oxidation of every existing or yet-to-be synthesised foreign substance; this would require an endless number of enzymes'*.

2. **Altered biological activity**

The end result of metabolism usually is the abolition of biological activity but various steps in between may have the following consequences:

a. *Conversion of a pharmacologically active to an inactive substance* (most drugs).

b. *Conversion of a pharmacologically active to another active substance.*

active drug	*active metabolite*
amitriptyline	nortriptyline
codeine	morphine
chloroquine	hydroxychloroquine
diazepam	oxazepam
phenylbutazone	oxyphenbutazone
spironolactone	canrenone

c. *Conversion of a pharmacologically inactive to an active substance*, i.e. a *pro-drug*

inactive substance	*active metabolite(s)*
azathioprine	mercaptopurine
benorylate	salicylic acid and paracetamol
cyclophosphamide	4-ketocyclophosphamide
enalapril	enalaprilat
sulindac	sulindac sulphide
talampicillin	ampicillin
cholecalciferol	1α-hydroxycholecalciferol (alfacalcidol)

A number of tissues, including the kidney, gut mucosa, lung and skin metabolise drugs but the liver is by far the most important. Many hepatic enzymes are present in the smooth endoplasmic reticulum, a system of intracellular membranes that is responsible for a host of metabolic reactions including drug biotransformation. When cells are homogenised, the endoplasmic reticulum rolls up into small dense bodies that can be isolated by centrifugation and these (partial artefacts) are called microsomes. Other drug metabolising enzymes are found in the mitochondria and in the cell sap or cytosol. *It is useful to think of drug metabolism in two broad phases, as follows:*

* Brodie BB. In: Binns TB, ed. Absorption and distribution of drugs. London: Livingstone, 1964.

† Fish lose lipid-soluble substances through the gills. They do not need such effective metabolising enzymes and they have not got them.

Phase 1 metabolism brings about a change in the drug molecule by oxidation, reduction or hydrolysis and often introduces a chemically active site into it. The new metabolite may retain its biological activity but have different pharmacokinetics, e.g. diazepam ($t_{\frac{1}{2}}$, 30 h) and desmethyldiazepam ($t_{\frac{1}{2}}$, 65 h). The most important single group of reactions are the oxidations, in particular those undertaken by the so-called mixed-function oxidases, which are present in microsomes. The final components of this system are the cytochrome P_{450} isoenzymes, which are capable of oxidising a number of aromatic or aliphatic compounds, hence the term 'mixed-function'. This system appears to be a defence mechanism that has evolved to oxidise compounds that are foreign to the body. Significantly, the cells of the gut wall and liver, which are the first to experience ingested foreign substances, are particularly rich in cytochrome P_{450} enzymes. *Examples of reactions that take place in the smooth endoplasmic reticulum are*:

— addition of an -OH group, e.g. tolbutamide to hydroxytolbutamide (inactive)
— removal of a $-CH_3$ group, e.g. imipramine to desipramine (active)
— removal of a $-C_2H_5$ group, e.g. lignocaine to an active metabolite
— removal of a $-NH_2$ group, e.g. amphetamine to phenylacetone.
— hydrolysis, e.g. pethidine (meperidine) to meperidinic acid (active).

Other metabolic reactions take place elsewhere in the cell. Xanthine oxidase (inhibited by allopurinol in the treatment of gout) is present in the cytosol, as are the enzymes that metabolise ethanol. Monoamine oxidase is present in mitochondria. Plasma contains histaminase.

Phase II metabolism involves union of the drug with one of several polar (water soluble) endogenous molecules that are products of intermediary metabolism, to form a water-soluble conjugate that is readily eliminated by the kidney or, if the molecular weight exceeds 300, in the bile. The drug must possess a chemically active site to which the conjugating molecule can attach and this is often a hydroxyl group introduced in Phase I metabolism. Conjugation with a more polar molecule is also a mechanism by which natural substances are eliminated, e.g. bilirubin as glucuronide, oestrogens as sulphates. Phase II metabolism almost invariably terminates biological activity.

Examples are:

— *glucuronide conjugation*; glucuronic acid, derived from glucose, is the most important conjugating agent in man because it is so highly water soluble. Morphine, paracetamol, salicylates and numerous other drugs are excreted as glucuronides. Neonates are deficient in the capacity to form glucuronides, which is why they experienced lethal toxicity with chloramphenicol (the 'grey syndrome'). Congenital deficiency of the ability to form bilirubin glucuronide is the basis of familial unconjugated hyperbilirubinaemia (Gilbert's syndrome).
— *sulphate conjugation*: the body needs enzymes or systems that make sulphates, e.g. for the formation of heparin or chondroitin sulphate. The same mechanisms are called into use to metabolise paracetamol, isoprenaline, oral contraceptive steroids and other drugs. The pool of sulphate available to conjugate is limited and after overdose of paracetamol, for example, the pathway to form glucuronide compensates.
— *acetylation*: acetylcoenzyme A reacts with the amino ($-NH_2$) group of a number of drugs to form a polar acetyl conjugate. Some individuals are genetically unable to produce more than a limited amount of the enzyme responsible for this reaction, N-acetyltransferase, and they are termed slow acetylators. Their reduced ability to acetylate is reflected in toxicity to normal doses of isoniazid (peripheral neuropathy), hydralazine (systemic lupus erythematosus), phenelzine, dapsone and sulphapyridine.
— *glutathione conjugation*: Phase I oxidation of some drugs gives rise to the formation of epoxides which are short-lived and highly reactive metabolites. Epoxides are important because they can bind irreversibly through covalent bonds to cell constituents — indeed, this is one of the principal ways in which drugs are toxic to body tissues. Glutathione is a tripeptide that combines with epoxides, rendering them inactive. The presence of glutathione in the liver

is part of an important defence mechanism against hepatic damage by halothane and in overdose, paracetamol.

Enzyme induction. The capacity of the body to metabolise drugs can be altered by medicinal drugs themselves and by other substances; clearly this phenomenon has implications for drug therapy. The term *enzyme induction* refers to an absolute increase in enzyme amount and activity as a consequence of exposure to particular chemicals. It is accompanied by hypertrophy of liver cell endoplasmic reticulum, which contains most drug-metabolising enzymes.

Inducing substances do not all show an obvious similarity of structure but in general share some important properties; they tend to be lipid-soluble, they are substrates, though sometimes only minor ones (e.g. DDT), for the enzymes they induce; they generally have long plasma half-lives.

Stimulation of our own metabolism can be seen as a mechanism that allows us to adapt to the foreign substances we meet in our environment in large or in small amounts, e.g. drugs, tobacco smoke, hydrocarbon pollutants, insecticides. Any individual's enzymes are in a greater or lesser state of induction, depending on the degree of exposure to these agents.

For example, a first alcoholic drink taken after a period of abstinence from alcohol may have quite a significant effect on behaviour but the same drink taken at the end of two weeks' regular imbibing may pass almost unnoticed because the individual's liver enzymes are in a higher state of induction, so that alcohol is metabolised more rapidly and has less effect. The time for onset and offset of induction depends on enzyme half-life, but significant induction generally occurs within a few days and it passes off over 2–3 weeks following withdrawal of the inducer.

More than 200 substances have been shown to induce enzymes in animals but the list of *proven enzyme inducers in man* is much more restricted. It includes:

barbecued meats	griseofulvin
Brussels sprouts	meprobamate
barbiturates	methaqualone
carmabazepine	phenylbutazone
DDT (dicophane; and other insecticides)	phenytoin
	progesterone
ethanol	rifampicin
tobacco smoke	glutethimide

Rifampicin appears to have a differential inducing effect in that some metabolic reactions are accelerated to a greater extent than are others. As a rule, however, most of the inducers to which man is exposed during drug therapy exert the same general effect of increasing the rate of drug metabolic reactions.

Enzyme induction is relevant to drug therapy for the following reasons:

1. *Clinically important drug interactions* may be caused, as the following examples illustrate.

a. Pregnancy can result in users of the oral contraceptive pill if potent inducers such as antiepilepsy drugs or rifampicin are taken concurrently. In this circumstance an oral contraceptive of high estrogen content may be used (or an alternative contraceptive method); if breakthrough bleeding occurs, the oestrogen content is not high enough. The metabolism of progestogens is also increased by enzyme induction.

b. Antiepilepsy drugs also increase the breakdown of dietary and endogenously formed vitamin D, producing an inactive metabolite — in effect a vitamin D deficiency state, which can result in osteomalacia. The accompanying hypocalcaemia can increase the tendency to fits and a convulsion may lead to fracture of demineralised bones.

c. Anticoagulant control with warfarin is dependent on a steady state of elimination by metabolism. Enzyme induction can lead to reduction of plasma warfarin, loss of anticoagulant control and danger of thrombosis. Conversely, if a patient's anticoagulant control is stable on warfarin plus an inducing agent, there is a danger of haemorrhage if the inducing agent is discontinued because warfarin will be eliminated at a slower rate.

2. *Tolerance to drug therapy* may result and provide an explanation for sub-optimal treatment, e.g. with an antiepilepsy drug.

3. *Drug toxicity* may be more likely. Ethanol drinkers are probably more likely to develop liver toxicity after paracetamol overdose; increased production of an hepatotoxic metabolite may explain this.

4. *Variability in response to drugs* is

increased. Enzyme induction caused by heavy drinking or heavy smoking may be an unrecognised cause for failure of an individual to achieve the expected response to a normal dose of a drug.

5. *Enzyme induction offers scope for therapy*. Phenobarbitone given for 7–14 days before labour reduces severe neonatal hyperbilirubinaemia by stimulating fetal hepatic glucuronyl transferase (the enzyme that conjugates bilirubin with glucuronic acid). The water-soluble glucuronide is more readily excreted than bilirubin itself. It may be worth using phenobarbitone when bilirubinaemia is to be anticipated, e.g. in Rhesus haemolytic disease (in which it may reduce the need for repeated exchange transfusions).

Patients with familial unconjugated hyperbilirubinaemia (Gilbert's syndrome) and a degree of icterus that is socially embarrassing have been helped by deliberate enzyme induction.

Enzyme inhibition. Consequences of inhibiting drug metabolism as a general rule are even more profound than those of enzyme induction. Reduced effect due to enzyme induction may be mitigated if accelerated metabolism gives rise to pharmacologically active products. For example, effects of reducing plasma concentration of propranolol by enzyme induction are likely to be offset by increased production of its main metabolite, 4-hydroxypropranolol, which is pharmacologically active. But inhibition of propranolol metabolism by cimetidine raises plasma propranolol concentration and causes excessive effect (bradycardia).

Effects of enzyme inhibition by drugs also tend to be more selective than those of enzyme induction. Consequently, **enzyme inhibition offers more scope for therapy as the following list indicates:**

Drug	*Enzyme inhibited*	*Treatment of*
phenelzine	MAO A, B	depression
selegiline	MAO B	Parkinson's disease
captopril	angiotensin converting enzyme	hypertension, cardiac failure
benserazide	DOPA decarboxylase	Parkinson's disease
disulfiram	aldehyde dehydrogenase	alcoholism
allopurinol	xanthine oxidase	gout
acetazolamide	carbonic anhydrase	glaucoma

Enzyme inhibition by drugs is also the basis of a number of important drug interactions as the following examples show:

Drug	*Inhibits metabolism of*
allopurinol	azathioprine
chloramphenicol	phenytoin chlorpropamide tolbutamide
cimetidine	propranolol
isoniazid	phenytoin
metronidazole	ethanol
MAOIs	6-mercaptopurine, some sympathomimetics, e.g. phenylpropanolamine, amphetamine
sodium valproate	phenytoin phenobarbitone primidone

Other examples appear under Drug Interactions (p. 144). Sodium valproate, as an inhibitor of drug metabolism, is an exception among the anticonvulsants, which are generally enzyme inducers. Phenytoin toxicity may result if sodium valproate is taken concurrently because metabolism is inhibited, but also because sodium valproate displaces phenytoin from its protein binding site.

Elimination

Clearance is a useful way of expressing removal of drug from blood or plasma. The term has the same meaning as the familiar *renal creatinine clearance*, which is a measure of removal of endogenous creatinine from the plasma and is used to monitor renal function. The units of clearance are volume and time (ml/min, l/h, etc). Just as creatinine clearance is found by dividing the rate of appearance of creatinine in the urine by its plasma concentration, so *total body clearance of a drug* is calculated by dividing the amount that enters the systemic circulation* by the area under its blood or plasma concentration time curve.

Clearance values can provide useful information about the biological fate of a drug. *Renal clearance* of a drug that is elminated only by filtration by the kidney obviously cannot exceed the glomerular filtration rate (127 ml/min in the adult male). If a drug is found to have a renal clearance in excess of this, then it must in addition be actively secreted by the kidney tubules. This is true for benzylpenicillin (renal clearance 480 ml/min), which is secreted by the renal anion transport mechanism and also for cationic substances like paraquat (clearance above 200 ml/min). Renal clearance of a drug is readily determined — the amount of a dose recovered in the urine in a specified time is divided by the area under the plasma concentration time curve in that time.

Most drugs are eliminated either by the kidneys or by the liver. Hence the *total body clearance* is the sum of the *hepatic* and *renal* clearances, and the hepatic clearance is found simply by subtracting value for renal clearance from that for total clearance.

Knowing the hepatic clearance of a drug can be useful. Certain drugs are cleared so rapidly by the liver that the clearance value is almost equal to the figure for liver blood flow, e.g. lignocaine, dextropropoxyphene. Indeed, for such drugs, liver blood flow is the main determinant of clearance and if blood flow falls (cardiac failure, haemorrhage) clearance also falls and plasma concentration rises. Poor hepatic clearance may thus explain an adverse reaction in a patient with cardiac failure who receives a standard dose of lignocaine after myocardial infarction.

Some drugs, however, despite being totally metabolished by the liver, have an inherently slow rate of elimination and low hepatic clearance values, e.g. diazepam, warfarin, tolbutamide. It follows that changes in liver blood flow will not affect the rate of elimination and plasma concentration of such drugs.

* The dose given by intravenous injection or infusion is preferred, for the entire amount is known to enter the systemic circulation; if the drug is given by mouth, poor absorption from the gut and presystemic elimination (see p. 118) must be taken into account to find the amount that reaches the systemic circulation.

Renal elimination. *The mechanisms that affect drugs and their metabolites as they are excreted by the kidney are*:

1. **Glomerular filtration.** The rate at which a drug enters the glomerular filtrate depends on its concentration in plasma water, its molecular weight and its charge. Substances that have a molecular weight >50 000 are excluded from the glomerular filtrate while those of molecular weight <10 000 (the vast majority of, if not all, drugs)† pass easily across the glomerulus. Binding to plasma proteins slows the filtration rate because drug bound to plasma proteins (molecular weight >70 000) is not filtered.

2. **Renal tubular excretion.** An important part of the excretory function of the kidney is the ability of cells of the proximal renal tubule actively to transfer charged (acidic or basic) molecules from the plasma to the tubular urine. There are two such systems, one for *acids*, e.g. penicillin, frusemide, and one for *bases*, e.g. amiloride, amphetamine.

3. **Renal tubular reabsorption**. The glomerular filtrate contains drug at the same concentration that it is free in the plasma, but the fluid is concentrated progressively as it flows down the nephron so that a gradient develops, drug in the tubular fluid becoming more concentrated than in the blood perfusing the nephron. Since the tubular epithelium has the properties of a lipid membrane, the extent to which a drug diffuses back into the blood will depend on its lipid solubility, i.e. on its pKa and on the pH of tubular urine. If urine becomes more alkaline, acidic drugs ionise, become less lipid soluble and their reabsorption diminishes, but basic drugs become unionised (and therefore more lipid soluble) and their reabsorption increases. Manipulation of urine pH is given useful expression when bicarbonate is used to treat overdose with aspirin. If the urine becomes more acid the ionisation process and effects are reversed.

Faecal elimination. When a drug intended for systemic effect is taken by mouth, a proportion may be excreted in the faeces without ever having been absorbed. Sometimes the objective of

† Almost all drugs have a molecular weight of less than 1000.

therapy is that drug be not absorbed from the gut, e.g. neomycin. Drug in the blood may diffuse passively into the gut lumen, depending on its pKa and the pH difference between blood and gut contents.

The most important mechanism by which drugs are actively transported into the gut is by:

Biliary excretion. There is one transport system for acids and one for bases, similar to those in the proximal renal tubule, and in addition, there is a system that transports unionised molecules, e.g. digoxin, into the bile. Small molecules tend to be reabsorbed by the bile canaliculi and in general only compounds that have a molecular weight > 300 are excreted in bile.

Drug that reaches the intestine in the bile may be reabsorbed and re-excreted, so establishing an *enterohepatic cycle*, which prolongs life of the drug in the blood, e.g. oral contraceptives.

Pulmonary elimination. The lungs are the main route of elimination (and of uptake) of volatile anaesthetics. Apart from this case, the lungs play only a trivial role in drug elimination. The route however, acquires notable medico-legal significance when ethanol concentration is measured in the air expired by drivers (breathalyser).

Breast milk. Most drugs that are present in a mother's plasma appear to some extent in her milk. The amounts are so small that loss of drug in milk is of no significance as a mechanism of elimination, but sometimes there are consequences for the suckling infant.

Unbound drug in plasma and milk can be expected to partition according to pH, pKa and lipid solubility. The pH of milk is more acidic than that of plasma and basic drugs ionise and accumulate in milk (ion trapping, p. 115). Milk also contains more fat than plasma, which favours retention of lipid-soluble drugs. The amount of drug bound to milk proteins is generally about half that bound to plasma proteins. The effects on an infant depend on the amount of drug ingested, on the inherent properties of a drug, e.g. toxicity in small dose, and on the functioning of the infant's metabolic and excretory systems. These mechanisms are notably immature in the neonate.

Drug taking can be timed to reduce risk — a drug with a short milk half-life taken immediately after feeding may be present in negligible amounts by the time the next feed is due. It may not be assumed, however, that the concentration-time profile in plasma is the same as that in milk, for the appearance of some drugs in milk is delayed, e.g. aminophylline.

Data on the extent of drug transfer from plasma to breast milk and other potential risks are summarised in Table 8.2.

Table 8.2 Drugs and breast milk

Drug	Comment/effect on Infant
1. *Drugs that are contraindicated during breast-feeding*	
Anticancer drugs	possible immune suppression reported with methotrexate and cyclophosphamide plus general hazard of late effects
Bromocriptine	suppresses lactation
Chloramphenicol	(genetic) bone marrow depression
Ergot alkaloids	hazard when used in repeated doses for migraine; single dose post-partum is safe
Clemastine	drowsiness, irritability, refusal to feed
Gold salts	rash, hepatitis, nephritis
Phenindione	haemorrhage
2. *Drugs that should be avoided or used with caution*	
Alcohol	high dose may affect infant
Aminophylline	irritability
Amiodarone	significant amounts in milk
Aminoglycosides	avoid; low therapeutic ratio and
Antibiotics	prolonged $t_{\frac{1}{2}}$ in neonates
Aspirin	avoid high, repeated dose but occasional use appears safe
Atropine	anticholinergic effects in some intolerant infants
Benzodiazepines	sedation with repeated doses
β-adrenoceptor blockers	monitor infant but most are probably safe, except sotalol
Calciferol	hypercalcaemia in high dose
Carbimazole	hypothyroidism, but propylthiouracil may be used
Chlorpromazine	drowsiness
Clindamycin	bloody stools
Corticosteroids	adrenal suppression in high (prednisolone >10 mg/day) but not in replacement doses
Diuretics	some may suppress lactation before it is well established
Iodine, iodides	iodine is concentrated in milk: avoid povidone-iodine in vaginal preparations and iodides in cough mixtures

Drug	Comment/effect on Infant
Isoniazid	convulsions, neuropathy, hepatic injury; if used, observe infant carefully and give pyridoxine to mother and child
Laxatives	avoid anthraquinones (cascara, senna, danthron) and phenolphthalein
Lithium	avoid, but if used, careful observation of infant and monitoring of maternal plasma concentration are essential
Meprobamate	high milk concentration: sedation
Metronidazole	discontinue breast feeding for 12–24 h after a single dose; avoid breast-feeding if repeated doses used
Nalidixic acid	haemolysis in glucose-6-phosphate dehydrogenase (G-6-PD) deficient infant
Nitrofurantoin	haemolysis in G-6-PD deficient infants
Opioid analgesics	appear safe in therapeutic doses but withdrawal symptoms may occur in infants of addicted mothers
Penicillins	safe except for allergy
Phenobarbitone	drowsiness if maternal plasma concentration is high
Radiopharmaceuticals	discontinue breast-feeding with ^{125}I and ^{131}I, which may persist for 2 weeks in milk; temporary cessation may be adequate with shorter $t_{\frac{1}{2}}$ isotopes
Reserpine	galactorrhoea, and nasal stuffiness and respiratory problems may occur
Sex hormones	oestrogens, progestogens and androgens suppress lactation in high doses; androgens may induce masculinisation in female or precocious development in male infants; cyproterone may have an anti-androgenic effect; oestrogen/progestogen oral contraceptives appear in milk in amounts too small to be harmful but may suppress lactation if it is not well established
Sulphonamides	risk of kernicterus in jaundiced and haemolysis in G-6-PD deficient infants; sulphafurazole and sulphamethoxazole (also co-trimoxazole) and sulphasalazine appear to be safe but avoid sulphamethoxypyridazine, which has a long $t_{\frac{1}{2}}$

It has been necessary to put a limit to the antibiotic content of cow's milk for sale (antibiotics are injected directly into the udder to treat bacterial mastitis as well as i.m.) because cases of drug allergy have occurred in man, particularly from penicillin in milk. Also, penicillin in milk has been found to interfere with production of the more desirable types of cheese, e.g. Stilton. Veterinary antibiotic preparations should contain a suitable marker substance to increase ease of detection of contamination by a range of antibiotics. If a cow or a woman eats garlic, onions or other strongly flavoured substances, her milk may be flavoured; the possibility of encouraging infants with flavoured breast milk remains unexploited.

Drug dosage

Drug dosage can be of five main kinds:

1. **Fixed dose.** The effect that is desired can be obtained at well below the toxic dose (many mydriatics, diuretics, analgesics, oral contraceptives, antimicrobials) and enough drug can be given to render individual variation clinically insignificant.

2. **Variable dose with crude adjustments.** Here fine adjustments make comparatively insignificant differences and the therapeutic end-point may be hard to measure (depression, anxiety), may change only slowly (thyrotoxicosis, epilepsy), or may vary because of pathophysiological factors (analgesics, adrenal steroids for suppressing disease).

3. **Variable dose with fine adjustments.** Here a vital function (blood pressure, blood sugar) that often changes rapidly in response to dose changes and can easily be measured repeatedly, provides the end-point. Adjustment of dose must be accurate. Adrenocortical replacement therapy falls into this group, whereas adrenocortical pharmacotherapy falls into (2), above.

4. **Maximum tolerated dose** is used when the ideal therapeutic effect cannot be achieved because of the occurrence of unwanted effects (anticancer drugs; some antimicrobials). The usual way of finding this is to increase the dose until unwanted effects begin to appear and then to reduce it slightly.

5. **Minimum tolerated dose.** This concept is not so common as (4), above, but it applies to long-term adrenocortical steroid therapy against inflammatory or immunological conditions, e.g. in asthma, rheumatoid arthritis, when the dose that provides symptomatic relief may be so high that

serious adverse effects are inevitable if it is continued indefinitely. The patient must be persuaded to accept incomplete relief on the grounds of safety. This can be difficult to achieve.

Dosing schedules, whatever their type, are simply schemes aimed at achieving a desired effect whilst avoiding toxicity. Such regimens can be arrived at by trial and error, but applying simple pharmacokinetic principles can add precision and logic to a dosing schedule.

The discussion that follows applies where drug effect relates closely to plasma concentration, which in turn relates closely to the amount of drug in the body.

The objectives of a dosing regimen where continuing effect is required are:

a. to define an *initial* dose that attains the desired effect rapidly without causing toxicity.

Often the dose that is capable of *initiating* drug effect is the same as that which *maintains* it. However on repeated dosing it takes five $t_{\frac{1}{2}}$ periods to rise to steady-state concentration in the plasma and this lapse of time may be undesirable. The effect may be achieved earlier by giving an initial dose that is larger than the maintenance dose; the initial dose is then usually called the *priming* or *loading* dose.

The **priming dose** is that which will achieve a therapeutic effect in an individual whose body does not already contain the drug. It is found by experiment when a drug is introduced into clinical use. Sometimes a standard dose will suffice for most adults but for drugs with a narrow therapeutic ratio, e.g. anticancer drugs, the initial or priming dose may be scaled according to body weight. Knowing the distribution volume may also be useful, for this volume multiplied by the desired plasma concentration gives the required dose. Gentamicin, for example, has a distribution volume of 18 l/70 kg and in order to achieve a plasma concentration of 8 mg/l, a dose of 8 × 18 = 144 mg would be given.

b. to define a dose which, given at intervals, maintains the effect; the **maintenance dose**.

This raises the issue as to how much drug should be given, and how frequently. Intuitively, the solution might be to give half the initial dose at intervals equal to the plasma half-life, for this by definition is the time in which the plasma concentration declines by half. Whether or not this approach is satisfactory or practicable, however, depends very much on the half-life itself, as is illustrated by the following cases:

1. **The half-life is 6–12 h.** In this instance, replacing half the initial dose at intervals equal to the $t_{\frac{1}{2}}$ can indeed be a satifactory solution because dosing every 6–12 h is acceptable.

2. **The half-life is greater than 24 h.** With once-daily dosing (which is desirable for compliance) giving half the initial dose every half-life means that more drug is entering the body than is leaving it each day, and the drug begins to accumulate towards toxic amounts. The solution is to replace only that amount of drug that leaves the body in 24 h. This quantity can be calculated* once the initial dose, plasma half-life and dose interval have been established in man.

3. **The half-life is less than 3 h.** Dosing at intervals equal to the $t_{\frac{1}{2}}$ would be so frequent as to be unacceptable. To take an extreme case, maintaining the plasma concentration of dobutamine ($t_{\frac{1}{2}}$, 2 min) by repeated administration would demand an unrealistic frequency of dosing. The answer, of course, is to use *continuous intravenous infusion* because steady state plasma concentration will be reached in 10 min (5 × $t_{\frac{1}{2}}$) and thus a priming dose would not be neccessary. Alternatively, for a drug with a rather longer $t_{\frac{1}{2}}$, a priming dose may be given as an intravenous bolus followed by a constant intravenous infusion, to maintain the effect as in the case of lignocaine

* This is in fact straightforward for people who are not paralysed by the proposal they should make a simple calculation. Assume that a initial dose (D_i) has been given and achieves the desired effect. Some time later, say *t* hours, there is a certain amount of drug left in the body, D_t. The maintenance dose (D_m) must be the difference between the initial dose and the amount of drug that is present in the body *t* hours after the time the initial dose was given. Thus $D_m = D_i - D_t$. D_t is given by the expression $D_t = D_i.e^{-kt}$. Hence, $D_m = D_i.(1 - e^{-kt})$.

Here k is the elimination constant of the drug and equals $0.693/t_{\frac{1}{2}}$ and if dosing is once daily, *t*, the dose interval, is 24 h. The value of D_m can be found by using a pocket calculator with a natural logarithm (base e) function and the only information needed is the initial dose, the half-life and the dose interval. The reader may care to calculate the maintenance dose of digoxin for a patient who requires an initial (priming) dose of 1.5 mg and in whom the half-life of the drug is 36 h. See Rowland M, Tozer T N. Clinical Pharmacokinetics. Philadelphia: Lea and Febiger, 1980:179. (Answer: 0.56 mg.)

($t_{\frac{1}{2}}$, 90 min). The rate of the infusion is calculated to equal the rate of removal of lignocaine from plasma, as described above.

Intermittent administration of drug with short $t_{\frac{1}{2}}$ is nevertheless reasonable provided large fluctuations in plasma concentration are acceptable, ie that the drug has a wide therapeutic range. The pencillins are a good example; benzylpencillin has a $t_{\frac{1}{2}}$ of 30 min but is effective in a 6-hourly regimen because the drug is so non-toxic that it is possible safety to give a dose that achieves a plasma concentration many times in excess of the minimum inhibitory concentration (MIC) for sensitive organisms. Thus, the plasma concentration remains above the MIC for much of the dose interval despite the elapse of twelve half-lives between doses. But few drugs are so non-toxic as to be used thus. Alternative techniques are described below.

Prolongation of drug action

The most obvious way to prolong a drug action is to give a larger dose (above).

Pharmacological prolongation of the action of local anaesthetics is achieved by their combination with adrenaline, which reduces blood flow and so the distribution of drug away from the injection site. In some instances drug action may be usefully extended by slowing the rate of *metabolism*, as when a dopa decarboxylase inhibitor, e.g. carbidopa, is combined with levodopa (as Sinemet) for parkinsonism. *Delayed excretion* is seldom practicable, the only important example being the use of probenecid to block renal tubular excretion of penicillin, e.g. when the latter is used in single dose to treat gonorrhoea.

The objective of an *even* as well as a *prolonged* effect is more often achieved by altering the molecular structure (e.g. benzodiazepines) or the pharmaceutical formulation in which a drug is presented. Much effort has gone into the development of *depot (injectable) or sustained-release (oral)* preparations. Clearly there is no point in a sustained-release formulation of a drug that has a long $t_{\frac{1}{2}}$. One drug manufacturer is said to have taunted his competitors by preparing a sustained-release placebo.*

Oral preparations designed to give slow continuous sustained release of drugs in the intestine are now popular. The possible advantages are obvious. Frequency of medication is reduced but, clearly, it must be at least once a day, which is convenient for the patient and can improve compliance for that reason. Most long-term medication for the elderly can now be given as a single morning dose, which is much less likely to be forgotten than three or four doses of the same or different drugs in a day. In addition sustained-release preparations may avoid local bowel toxicity due to high local concentration (e.g. ulceration of the small intestine with KCl tablets) and may also avoid the toxic peak plasma concentrations that can occur when dissolution and absorption of the formulation are rapid. Oral sustained-release preparations call for careful evaluation as there is great variability in the functions of the stomach and intestine; release rates demonstrated *in vitro* may not be reflected in release or absorption in everyday use.

Techniques for prolonging release† include various tablet coatings that dissolve at different rates — chelates, resins, plastic matrices and a formulation from which drug egress is controlled osmotically (Oros). Drugs that irritate the stomach are sometimes given special 'enteric' coatings (varnish, hardened gelatin) to delay disintegration of the tablet until it has reached the intestine. Some of these enteric-coated tablets probably pass intact into the toilet.

Long-acting, or depot, *injectable* preparations are more reliable because the environment in which they are deposited is more constant than can ever be the case in the alimentary tract and medication can be given at longer intervals, even weeks e.g benzathine penicillin, some neuroleptics, some contraceptives. The usual aim with these formulations is to render the drug relatively insoluble so that it dissolves slowly at the site of injection. In general such preparations are chemical variants, e.g. microcrystals, or the original drug in oil, wax, gelatin or synthetic media. They include phenothiazine tranquillisers, the various insulins and penicillins, and preparations

* Dragstedt C. JAMA 1958, 168:1652.

† Self-poisoning with sustained-release formulations has caused death because observation of the patient was withdrawn too soon.

of vasopressin. Solid tablets of hormones are sometimes implanted subcutaneously. The advantages of infrequent administration and patient compliance in a variety of situations are obvious. Some risk of prolonged adverse effects is inescapable, though implants can be removed.

For the eye a plastic device is available to place under the lid where it delivers pilocarpine for a week (Ocusert). Since users must be unaware of its presence (or they would not use it), there is risk of its falling out unnoticed with potentially serious consequences to a glaucomatous eye.

Reduction of absorption time

This can be achieved by making a soluble salt of the drug which is then rapidly removed from the site of administration. In the case of s.c. or i.m. injections the same objective may be obtained with *hyaluronidase*. This enzyme depolymerises hyaluronic acid, a constituent of connective tissue that prevents the spread of foreign substances, e.g. bacteria, drugs. By combining an injection with hyaluronidase a drug spreads rapidly over a wide area and so is absorbed more quickly, e.g. ergometrine i.m. in the hands of nurses who are not trained to give i.v. injections.

When an i.v. injection of an irritant drug has accidentally leaked into perivenous tissue and there is pain, or risk of damage to another structure (e.g. thiopentone in the antecubital fossa may damage the median nerve), hyaluronidase and saline may be injected locally to dilute the irritant and hasten its absorption.

Dose, weight and surface area

When a fixed dose is inappropriate, it may be desirable to adjust the dose to the patient. It is usual then to calculate dose according to *weight*. There is, however, evidence that *surface area*, which is directly related to metabolic rate, may be more appropriate. Drugs whose dosage needs calculating (in adults or children), are probably best related to surface area, although the same result is obtained by taking the body weight to the power of 0.7. Fig. 8.1 relates body weight to percentage of adult dose on this basis, and its use is recommended where a calculation has to be made and only the adult dose is known (p 141).

For infants there is no reliable formula and if the proper dose of a drug is not known it must be ascertained, because the risk of intolerance is substantial (see p. 140).

Fixed-ratio drug combinations

This section refers to *combinations of drugs in a single pharmaceutical formulation*. It does not refer to concomitant drug therapy, e.g. in infections, hypertension and in cancer, when several drugs are given separately to obtain increased therapeutic effect or range, or to treat more than one disease.

Combinations should not be prescribed unless there is good reason to consider that the patient needs *all* the drugs in the preparation and that the doses are appropriate and will not need to be adjusted separately.

Advantages of fixed-dose drug combinations

1. *Convenience with improved patient compliance*. This case is particularly appropriate when two drugs are used at constant dose on a long-term basis for an asymptomatic condition as in mild or moderate hypertension, e.g. thiazide plus a β-adrenoceptor blocker. The fewer tablets the patients have to take, the more reliably will they use them, especially the elderly who as a group tend to receive more drugs because they tend to have multiple pathology.

2. *Enhanced effect*. Single drug treatment of tuberculosis leads to the emergence of resistant mycobacteria; this effect is prevented or delayed by using two or more drugs simultaneously. Combining isoniazid with rifampicin (Rifinah, Rimactazid) ensures that single drug treatment cannot occur; treatment has to be two drugs or no drug at all. Oral contraception (with an oestrogen and progestogen combination) is given for the same reason. It is astonishingly reliable.

3. *Minimisation of unwanted effects*. Decarboxylase inhibition prevents the extracerebral decarboxylation of levodopoa to dopamine, which will not enter the brain. Combining levodopa with benserazide (Madopar) or with carbidopa (Sinemet) slows its metabolism in the body so that smaller amounts of levodopa can be used; this reduces side effects, which would normally limit treatment with the necessarily

higher doses of levodopa alone. Giving a potassium-retaining diuretic in combination with a thiazide prevents potassium depletion (more effectively than by attempting to replace potassium).

Disadvantages of fixed-dose drug combinations

1. *Dosage of one drug cannot be altered without altering that of others.* A drug with a wide range of dose that must be adjusted to suit the patients' reponse (calcium channel blocker) is best not combined with a drug for the same disease with a narrow dose range (thiazide). Adrenocortical steroids should *never* be combined in one tablet with other drugs.

2. *Impractability of providing individualised multi-drug preparations* because of the amount of labour and the complex pharmaceutical technology required.

3. *Time course of drug action* often demands different intervals between administration.

4. *Irregularity of administration*, e.g. in response to symptom, pain, cough, may be desirable for some drugs but not for others.

5. *Confusion of therapeutic aims*: use of combinations of iron with folic acid and cyanocobalamin are hazardous if they delay diagnosis of pernicious anaemia. The fact that iron plus a little folic acid is properly used in pregnancy for routine anaemia prophylaxis simply confirms that combinations must be rationally thought out and adjusted to meet particular needs.

6. *Identification of the drug causing an adverse effect* is more difficult when a combination is used.

Conclusions. A great many marketed combinations are open to criticism, some are positively desirable and some have the sanction of time alone. Occasionally, an advantage can be justified in theory but may be insignificant in practice. Some combinations are marketed to fulfil a commercial purpose rather than a medical need. But rational combinations are acceptable. Too often, critics of irrational combinations attack all fixed-dose formulations; in doing this, it is the critics who are irrational (and ignorant).

Before prescribing a combination, the doctor should pause to consider whether any of the ingredients is unnecessary; if it is, the combination should not be prescribed. It can never be justifiable to give patients drugs they do not need in order to provide them with one that they do need. The fact that doctors sometimes prescribe combinations in ignorance of the exact ingredients, which are commonly not indicated by the name, and are then surprised to find the patient is taking an undesired drug provides a sad criticism of the medical profession, as does the fact that some of the available combinations are prescribed at all.

Iron formulations with vitamins, caffeine, etc. provide examples of objectionable combinations. Prescription of hormones requires particular attention to detail of the amount, the timing and the duration of dose; in some countries hormones combined with other classes of drugs are marketed and these provide some of the most offensive products that discredit the producer, the regulatory authority and, above all, the doctor who prescribes these horrors.

INDIVIDUAL OR BIOLOGICAL VARIATION

That individuals respond differently to drugs, both from time to time and from other individuals is a matter of everyday experience. Doctors need to accomodate for individual variation for it may explain both adverse response to a drug and failure of therapy; the skills of using drugs require that variation in response be recognised and taken into accout when prescribing. Sometimes there are obvious physical characteristics such as the patient's age, race or disease that warn the prescriber to adjust drug dose, but there are no convenient external features that signify, for example, pseudocholinesterase deficiency, which causes prolonged paralysis after suxamethonium, or slow acetylators, who may not tolerate hydralazine. An understanding of the reasons for individual variation in response to drugs is therefore relevant to all prescribers. Considerations of both pharmacodynamics and pharmacokinetics are entailed and the issues will be discussed under the following headings: *inherited influences* and *environmental and host influences*.

Variability due to inherited influences

Consider how individuals in a population might be expected to respond to a fixed dose of a drug – some would show less than the usual response, most would show the usual response and some would show more than the usual response. This type of variation is described as *continuous* and in a graph the result would appear as a normal or Gaussian distribution curve, similar to the type of curve that describes the distribution of height, weight or metabolic rate in a population. The curve is the result of a multitude of factors, some *genetic* (multiple genes), some environmental, that contribute collectively to the response of the individual to the drug; they can include race, sex, diet, weight, environmental and body temperature, circadian rhythm, mental state and expectation, absorption, distribution, metabolism, excetion and receptor density, but no single factor has a predominating effect. Less commonly, variation is *discontinuous* when differences in response (a) reveal a distinct sub-group of the general population who, for example, are resistant to normal doses of coumarin anticoagulants or (b) separate the general population into two discrete groups, for example, fast and slow acetylators of isoniazid and other drugs. Discontinuous variation occurs when a *single* genetic factor dominates response to a drug, as does possession of the gene for the N-acetylase enzyme that metabolises isonizid.

Pharmacogenetics* is that branch of pharmacology that is concerned with drug responses that are governed by heredity. Inherited factors causing different responses to drugs are commonly biochemical because genes govern the production of enzymes. Less often the factors are anatomical as is the occurrence of glaucoma due to mydriatics in patients with a shallow anterior eye chamber.

* Some terminology: An individual's *genotype* refers to his or her genetic constitution and the *phenotype* to the observable characteristics, such as hair colour. At any one position (*locus*) on a chromosome a gene may have a number of different forms, which are termed *alleles*. The range of genetic characteristics that is exhibited by individuals in a population is determined by the play of a number of alleles – this is called *genetic polymorphism*.

Inherited abnormal responses to drugs mediated by single genes may be classified as follows:

A. **Heritable conditions causing decreased drug responses**

1. *Resistance to coumarin anticoagulants*. Those who exhibit this rare inherited or familial abnormality possess a variant of the enzyme that converts vitamin K to its reduced and active form, which the coumarins normally inhibit; patients require 20 times or more of the usual dose of these drugs to obtain an adequate clinical response. A similar condition also occurs in rats and has practical importance as warfarin, a coumarin, is used as a rat poison (rats with the gene have been dubbed 'super rats' by the mass media.)

2. *Resistance to suxamethonium*. This rare condition is characterised by increased cholinesterase activity and failure of normal doses of suxamethonium to cause muscular relaxation (cf. cholinesterase deficiency, below).

3. *Resistance to vitamin D*. Individuals who exhibit this condition develop rickets that responds only to huge doses of vitamin D.

4. *Resistance to mydriatics*. Response to sympathomimetics is related to iris colour in that light eyes (commoner in whites) dilate more than dark eyes (commoner in blacks). Furthermore, atropine causes less pupillary dilation in blacks than in whites.

B. **Heritable conditions causing increased or toxic drug responses**

1. *Pseudocholinesterase deficiency*. The neuromuscular blocking action of suxamethonium is terminated by plasma pseudocholinesterase ('true' cholinesterase, acetylcholinesterase, hydrolyses acetylcholine released by nerve endings, whereas various tissues and plasma contain other non-specific, hence 'pseudo', esterases). Certain individuals form so little plasma pseudocholinesterase that metabolism of suxamethonium is seriously impaired. The deficiency classically comes to light when a patient fails to breathe spontaneously after a surgical operation and artificial ventilation may have to be undertaken for some hours. Plasma pseudocholinesterase activity is controlled by several allelic genes at the same locus, which give

rise to various phenotypes with varying amounts of pseudocholinesterase in the plasma. Relatives of an affected individual, for this as for other inherited abnormalities carrying avoidable risk, should be sought out and checked to assess their own risk, *and told of the result*. Pseudocholinesterase deficiency is rare in the UK, the prevalence being about 1 in 2500 (0.04%).

2. *Hereditary methaemoglobinaemias*. Due to deficiency of methaemoglobin reductase methaemoglobin, which cannot carry oxygen, forms more readily with certain drugs, e.g. nitrates, sulphonamides, causing cyanosis.

3. *Poor oxidation*. Certain individuals have a limited capacity to oxidise drugs. Poor oxidisers, who comprise 2–9% of most populations, are probably homozygous for an autosomal recessive gene that controls the metabolism of several drugs. Therefore when standard doses of any of the following are used, poor oxidisers are at high risk of side effects — debrisoquine (hypotension), phenytoin, nortriptyline. Poor oxidisers of tolbutamide have also been identified but these individuals metabolise debrisoquine at normal rates, indicating that they have a different genetic defect.

The poor oxidiser state was first revealed in rather dramatic circumstances in the laboratory of Professor R L Smith*, who writes:

Recollections of a poor metaboliser of debrisoquine. 'In the early 1970s we embarked upon a research programme directed towards elucidating the basis for the variable dose requirements of patients receiving the two antihypertensive drugs, debrisoquine and bethanidine. As part of this study I took 40 mg of debrisoquine sulphate; within two hours my blood pressure crashed to 70/50 mm Hg and I was unable to stand for four hours due to incapacitating postural hypotension. Significant hypotensive effects persisted and it was two days until the blood pressure returned to normal. Analysis of my urine revealed that, unlike the other subjects studied, who showed little if any cardiovascular response to the same dose of debrisoquine, nearly all the dose was excreted as unchanged drug whereas other subjects converted it to the 4-hydroxy metabolite. Studies several years earlier had shown me to be a deficient metaboliser of amphetamine and a related drug, p-methoxyamphetamine and because of these experiences, I had already been dubbed an "odd metaboliser". However the drama of the clinical response to a single dose of debrisoquine catalysed a search for its explanation and culminated in the uncovering of the first example of a genetic polymorphism of drug oxidation.'

* Professor of Biochemical Pharmacology, St Mary's Hospital Medical School, London.

4. *Glucose-6-phosphate dehydrogenase (G-6-PD) deficiency*. G-6-PD activity is important to the integrity of the red blood cell through a chain of reactions: the enzyme is an important source of reduced nicotinamide-adenine dinucleotide phosphate (NADPH), which maintains erythrocyte glutathione in its reduced form. Reduced glutathione in turn is necessary to keep haemoglobin in the reduced (ferrous) rather than in its ferric form (methaemoglobin), which is useless for oxygen carriage. Build-up of methaemoglobin in erythrocytes impairs the function of sulphydryl groups, especially those associated with the cell membrane, and leads to haemolysis if red cells are exposed to certain oxidant substances, including drugs. G-6-PD deficiency is common in African, Mediterranean and South East Asian races and in their descendants. Affected individuals may suffer acute haemolysis if they ingest nitrates, naphthalenes, anilines and the following drugs:

Antimalarials:	4- and 8-aminoquinoline antimalarials, e.g. chloroquine, primaquine; quinine
Antimicrobials:	sulphonamides, nitrofurantoin, nalidixic acid, chloramphenicol, PAS
Others:	quinidine, probenecid

Some individuals experience haemolysis after eating the broad bean, *vicia fava* — hence the term *favism*. Curiously, this genetic defect may confer a biological advantage — G-6-PD-deficient individuals appear to resist carriage of falciparum malaria, presumably because their red cells do not survive well in the circulation.

5. *Malignant hyperthermia*. After exposure to general anaesthetic agents, individuals develop muscular rigidity, fever and lactic acidosis. A family history helps to identify potential sufferers from this rare and serious condition (p. 457).

6. *Acetylator phenotypes*. Acetylation is an important route of metabolism for many drugs

that possess an $-NH_2$ group. Population studies have shown that individuals are either rapid or slow acetylators but the proportion of each varies greatly between races as follows:

Ethnic group	*Rapid acetylators* (%)
Inuit (Canadian Eskimos)	95
Japanese	88
Thais	72
Latin Americans	70
Black Americans	52
White Americans	48
Britons	38
Swedes	32
Egyptians	18

Acetylator status is relatively simple to establish. After a standard test dose of sulphadimidine by mouth, the percentage recovered in urine as acetylsulphadimidine is 65–90% in fast acetylators and 40–55% in slow acetylators. The importance of acetylator status to therapy is illustrated by the following drugs:

Isoniazid. Slow acetylators on standard doses are at risk of peripheral neuropathy because isoniazid interferes with pyridoxine metabolism; in practice it is simpler routinely to add pyridoxine to the anti-tuberculosis regimen than to establish every patient's acetylator status. Tuberculosis responds well in fast and slow acetylators when isoniazid is taken daily but on a once-weekly regimen fast acetylators relapse more readily because they then have time to reduce the amount of drug below effective concentrations.

Hydralazine. Fast acetylators require a higher dose to control hypertension but if more than 200 mg per day is taken, slow acetylators are likely to have antinuclear antibodies in their plasma and some of these patients develop systemic lupus erythematosus.

Procainamide. On a standard regimen, plasma concentration is higher, and dysrhythmia control is better in slow acetylators but more of these patients develop antinuclear antibodies and systemic lupus erythematosus.

Phenelzine. Both antidepressant and toxic effects are greater in slow acetylators.

Sulphasalazine (salicylazosulphapyridine). Nausea, headache, abdominal discomfort and red cell haemolysis occur more frequently in slow acetylators, presumably because of the sulphapyridine component of this drug (used for ulcerative colitis).

Dapsone. Evidence is conflicting but slow acetylators may experience more red cell haemolysis and rapid acetylators may need higher doses to control dermatitis herpetiformis and leprosy.

7. *Porphyria* (p. 160).

8. *Glaucoma* (a) with adrenal steroids develops in about 5% of the US population. (b) with shallow anterior chamber of the eye: when the pupil is dilated with a mydriatic, the iris blocks the outflow of aqueous humour and angle-closure glaucoma results.

C. **Innocent heritable conditions recognised by the use of chemicals**

1. Ability to taste phenylthiourea.
2. Characteristic-smelling urine after eating asparagus (methylmercaptan is formed).
3. Red urine after eating beetroot: this has led to erroneous diagnosis of haemoglobinuria.
4. Ability to smell cyanide (this would not be innocent in a factory using or making cyanide).

It is likely that many clinically important single gene differences (*idiosyncracies*) in response to drugs remain to be discovered. Once a genetic difference, e.g. metabolic reaction, is understood, it will be possible to predict what will happen when drugs of particular molecular structures are administered. But whether patients should be screened routinely for such differences in drug response is a matter of economics and logistics.

Bacterial resistance to drugs is genetically determined and is of great clinical importance.

Insect resistance to insecticides is also genetically determined; the use of insecticide selects out the naturally tolerant insects that breed and fill the biological vacuum made available by the death of the rest.

Variability due to environmental and host influences

A multitude of factors related to both the individual and his or her environment contribute to differences in drug response. In general, their precise role is less well documented than is the case with genetic factors but their range and complexity is illustrated by the folllowing list of likely candidates: age, sex, pregnancy, lactation, exercise, sunlight, disease, infection, occupational exposures, drugs, circadian and seasonal variations, diet, stress, fever, malnutrition, alcohol intake, tobacco or marijuana smoking and the functioning of the cardiovascular, gastrointestinal, hepatic, immunological and renal systems*. Some are now discussed further.

Age

a. **The neonate and infant**

The young human being differs greatly from the adult, not merely in size but also in the proportions and constituents of the body and the functioning of its physiological systems. These differences are reflected in the way the body handles and responds to drugs in this age group and they are relevant to prescribing for them.

Absorption of drugs from the gastrointestinal tract is slower because gastric emptying is slower and may be irregular and intestinal transit time is longer; the increased contact time of drug with the mucosa favours its absorption. Gastric acidity is low and acidic drugs may be less well absorbed than in the adult (see pH variation and drug kinetics, p. 115). Rectal absorption is efficient with an appropriate formulation and this route may be preferred with an uncooperative infant. Intravenous drug administration is preferred in the seriously ill newborn because its relatively low proportion of skeletal muscle and fat render unsuitable the intramuscular or subcutaneous routes. Drugs or chemicals that come in contact with the skin are readily absorbed as the skin is well hydrated and the stratum corneum is thin; adverse reactions may result, e.g. with hexachlorophane used in dusting powders and emulsions to prevent infection.

Distribution of drugs is influenced by the lower proportion of fat and the higher proportion of water in the neonate. Calculation of the neonatal dose as a weight-related fraction of the adult dose will therefore overestimate the actual tissue concentration. The blood–brain barrier is more permeable and drug binding to plasma proteins is less than in the adult.

Metabolism. Although the enzyme systems that inactivate drugs are present at birth, the rate of metabolism is reduced, especially in the first two weeks of life, both in respect of Phase 1 (oxidation, reduction, etc.) and Phase 2 (synthetic) reactions. Inability to conjugate and thus inactivate chloramphenicol causes the grey syndrome in neonates.

Elimination by the kidney is reduced in the neonate, whose glomerular filtration rate at birth is relatively low compared with the adult; gentamicin, digoxin and indomethacin have long $t_{\frac{1}{2}}$ periods in the neonate because they depend on glomerular filtration. Tubular function is also immature and penicillins and sulphonamides, which are secreted by the tubules, are cleared more slowly than in the adult.

b. **The elderly**

The incidence of adverse drug reactions rises with age in the adult, especially after 65 years. The disproportionally large number of drugs that the elderly are required to take, poor compliance with dosing regimens and the presence of disease, all contribute to this outcome. In addition, however, medication in this age group carries a risk because the dosing regimens must be modified to suit the characteristics of the elderly body, as is now discussed.

Absorption of drugs may be slightly slower because gastrointestinal blood flow and motility are reduced but the effect is rarely important.

Distribution is influenced by the following changes: body weight is reduced so that standard doses provide a greater amount of drug per kg; body water is less and water-soluble drugs tend to be present in higher blood concentration (and distribution volume decreased); body fat increases, which tends to lower the blood concentration of lipid-soluble drugs (and increase distribution volume); plasma albumin concentration is reduced, giving scope for increased free drug.

Metabolism of some drugs is reduced and hepatic enzyme induction appears to be lessened. Liver blood flow diminishes and drugs that are normally extensively eliminated in first-pass

* Vessell E S. Clin Pharmacol Ther 1982; 31(1): 1.

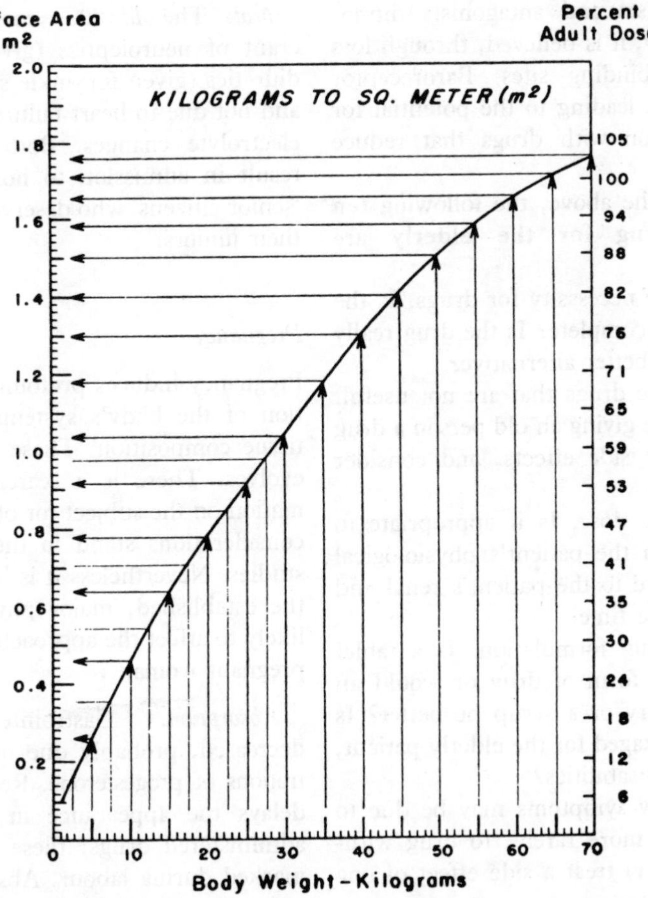

Fig. 8.1 Chart for estimation of dose from body weight and surface area. The figures on the right show what per cent of the adult dose should be given. (By courtesy of the authors and publishers; Talbot N B, Richie R H, Crawford J D Metabolic Homeostasis: a syllabus for those concerned with the care of patients. Cambridge; Mass Harvard University Press. 1959.)

through the liver (p. 118) appear in higher concentration in the plasma (greater systemic availability) and persist in it for longer.

Elimination. Renal blood flow, glomerular filtration and tubular secretion decrease with ageing, a decline that is not signalled by raised serum creatinine concentration because production of this metabolite is diminished by virtue of the relatively low muscle mass in the age group. Indeed, in the elderly, serum creatinine may be within the concentration range for normal young adults even when the creatinine clearance is 50 ml/min (127 ml/min in adult male). Particular risk of adverse effects arises with renally eliminated drugs that have a small therapeutic ratio, e.g. aminoglycoside antibiotics, digoxin, procainamide and chlorpropamide. Even drugs that are normally eliminated by metabolism may pose a problem through the accumulation of water-soluble metabolites, which retain pharmacological activity, e.g. hydroxylated metabolites of propranolol and tricyclic antidepressants.

Drug response may alter with ageing, to produce either a greater or lesser effect than is anticipated in younger adults. Drugs that act on the central nervous system appear to produce an exaggerated response in relation to that expected from the plasma concentration and sedatives and hypnotics may have a pronounced hangover effect. These drugs are also more likely to depress respiration because vital capacity and maximum breathing capacity are lessened in the elderly. Response to β-adrenoceptor agonists and antagonists diminishes in old age partly, it is believed, through loss of specific receptor-binding sites. Baroreceptor sensitivity is reduced, leading to the potential for orthostatic hypotension with drugs that reduce blood pressure.

Having regard to the above, the following **ten rules for prescribing for the elderly** are recommended*:

1. Think about the necesssity for drugs. Is the diagnosis correct and complete? Is the drug really necessary? Is there a better alternative?

2. Do not prescribe drugs that are not useful. Think carefully before giving an old person a drug that may have major side effects, and consider alternatives.

3. Think about the dose. Is it appropriate to possible alterations in the patient's physiological state? Is it appropriate to the patient's renal and hepatic function at the time?

4. Think about drug formulation. Is a tablet the most appropriate form of drug or would an injection, a suppository or a syrup be better? Is the drug suitably packaged for the elderly patient, bearing in mind his disabilities?

5. Assume any new symptoms may be due to drug side effects or, more rarely, to drug withdrawal. Rarely (if ever) treat a side effect of one drug with another.

6. Take a careful drug history. Bear in mind the possibility of interaction with substances the patient may be taking without your knowledge, such as herbal or other non-prescribed remedies, old drugs taken from the medicine cabinet or drugs obtained from friends.

7. Use fixed combinations of drugs only when they are logical and well studied and they either aid compliance or improve tolerance or efficacy. Few fixed combinations meet this standard.

8. When adding a new drug to the therapeutic regimen, see whether another can be withdrawn.

9. Attempt to check whether the patient's compliance is adequate, e.g. by counting remaining tablets. Has the patient (or his relatives) been properly instructed?

10. Remember that stopping a drug is as important as starting it.

* In Caird F I, ed. Drugs for the elderly. Copenhagen: WHO (Europe), 1985.

Note. The *old* (80+ years) are particularly intolerant of neuroleptics (given for confusion) and diuretics (given for ankle swelling that is postural and not due to heart failure), which cause adverse electrolyte changes. Both classes of drug may result in admission to hospital of semicomatose 'senior citizens' who deserve better treatment from their juniors.

Pregnancy

Pregnancy induces profound changes in the function of the body's systems and in its fluid and tissue composition. These alter as the pregnancy evolves. There is a scarcity of definitive information on the subject for obvious ethical and legal considerations stand in the way of experimental studies. Nevertheless it is helpful to consider how the established, major physiological changes are likely to affect the approach to drug dosing for the pregnant woman.

Absorption. Gastrointestinal motility is decreased, probably due to high plasma concentrations of progesterone. Reduced gastric emptying delays the appearance in the plasma of orally administered drugs; these changes are especially marked during labour. Absorption from an intramuscular site is likely to be efficient as tissue perfusion is increased due to vasodilatation.

Distribution. Cardiac output increases by about 30% during pregnancy, reaching its maximum between 30 and 34 weeks. Changes in its distribution also take place; renal blood flow increases by 50% but flow to the liver does not appear to alter. The mother gains fluid throughout pregnancy and at term the increase in total body water (including the fetus, placenta and amniotic fluid) amounts to 8 litres, with 80% in the extracellular space. Blood volume expands by about one-third. These changes account for the decreased haemoglobin concentration in pregnancy and drugs given in standard doses would be expected to achieve lower concentrations than in the non-pregnant state; this has been found to be the case with a number of antibiotics. Body fat increases by 4–5 kg and provides a reservoir for fat-soluble drugs. Plasma albumin declines by up to 10 g/l in the first half of pregnancy and the free fraction of drug in the plasma can be expected to increase; any consequences of this change are most likely to occur with heavily protein-bound drugs (anticoagulants, antiepilepsy drugs).

Elimination. Creatinine clearance increases by about 50% in pregnancy and drugs that are mainly eliminated by the kidney are also more rapidly cleared (ampicillin, lithium, digoxin).

In summary, drug disposition is altered in a number of ways by the physiological changes of pregnancy. Drug dosage may need to be adjusted as pregnancy evolves and then readjusted in the puerperium; when drug dosage is normally controlled by plasma concentration monitoring, measurements may need to be undertaken more frequently. (*See also* Placenta, p. 116, and Drugs and the Embryo/Fetus, p. 171.)

Disease

Disease can modify drug kinetics and response in a number of ways, some of which are listed below:

Absorption

a. Surgery that involves resection and reconstruction of the gut may lead to malabsorption — after partial gastrectomy, of iron, folic acid and fat soluble vitamins, and after ileal resection, of vitamin B_{12}, for example.

b. Delayed gastric emptying and intestinal stasis during an attack of migraine interferes with absorption of drugs from the gastrointestinal tract.

c. Coeliac disease appears to have variable effects on drug absorption, which may be increased (trimethoprim, sodium fusidate) or decreased (pivampicillin).

d. Severe low output cardiac failure or shock (with peripheral vasoconstriction) delays absorption from subcutaneous or intramuscular sites; reduced hepatic blood flow prolongs the presence in the plasma of drugs that are so rapidly extracted by the liver that removal depends on the rate of presentation to it, e.g. lignocaine.

Distribution. Hypoalbuminaemia, from any cause (burns, malnutrition, sepsis) allows more free drug to be present in plasma, with the risk of enhanced or adverse responses especially to those that are highly protein bound, e.g. phenytoin, clofibrate. When renal function is poor there is decreased binding of several drugs, e.g. phenytoin, salicylate, diazoxide, thiopentone; in addition to low plasma albumin concentration, accumulated (and as yet unidentified) products of body metabolism may displace bound drug.

Inflammation is associated with increase in the concentration of the acute-phase protein, α_1-acid glycoprotein, which binds a number of basic drugs (lignocaine, disopyramide), monitoring of which may thus give misleadingly high results.

Metabolism. Acute inflammatory disease of the liver (viral, alcoholic) and cirrhosis affect both the functioning of the hepatocytes and blood flow through the liver. The magnitude of effect and the duration of action of drugs that normally undergo hepatic metabolism are inevitably affected (increased) by these changes. There is less hepatic extraction of drugs that would normally be substantially removed from the plasma in the first pass through the liver, e.g. propranolol, labetalol, chlormethiazole. Since such drugs have higher *systemic availability* after oral dosing to patients with liver disease, the amount of drug given by that route should be less than normal. Many other drugs exhibit prolonged $t_{\frac{1}{2}}$ and reduced clearance in patients with chronic liver disease, e.g. diazepam, tolbutamide, rifampicin, phenobarbitone. (See Drugs and the Liver, p. 641.)

Elimination. Disease of the kidney (p. 559) has profound effects on the pharmacokinetics and actions of drugs that are eliminated by that organ.

Diet

a. The presence of food in the stomach, especially if it is fatty, delays gastric emptying. Plasma concentration of some antimicrobials, e.g. cloxacillin, may be much reduced if they are taken on a full stomach, but food enhances the absorption of some drugs (e.g. hydrochlorothiazide) by increasing splanchnic blood flow, which may also reduce the opportunity for hepatic first-pass metabolism. More specifically, calcium (e.g. in milk) interferes with absorption of tetracyclines (by chelation). Hepatic microsomal enzymes may be induced by many dietary factors including alcohol, charcoal grilled (broiled) beef and Brussels sprouts; a high protein–low carbohydrate diet appears to stimulate drug metabolism, while a low protein–high carbohydrate intake has the opposite effect.

b. Protein malnutrition causes changes that influence pharmacokinetics, e.g. loss of body weight, reduced hepatic metabolising capacity, hypoproteinaemia.

Pollutants

Many insecticides, e.g. DDT, are enzyme inducers, as are the hydrocarbons in cigarette smoke.

Circadian rhythms

Circadian* rhythms occur in many physiological functions relevant to drug action, e.g. hepatic metabolic activity, CNS sensitivity to depressants, urinary excretion, adrenocortical function, blood pressure and volume. Knowledge is still limited and there has been little recognition in prescribing except with adrenal steroid replacement (larger doses in the morning) and antihypertensives with long $t_{\frac{1}{2}}$ (low morning blood volume with morning hypotension). There appear to be well marked circadian rhythms in the anticoagulant effect of heparin infused at a constant rate†. In childhood acute lymphoblastic leukaemia, a maintenance treatment regimen administered in the morning was associated with a risk of relapse 4.6-times greater than that of the same treatment given in the evening‡.

Drugs

See Drug Interactions (below).

DRUG INTERACTIONS

Drug interactions may be *desired* or *undesired*, *beneficial* or *harmful*. They are deliberately sought when drugs are given together, e.g. in tuberculosis or hypertension, when the benefits to the patient may be increased by using two additive therapeutic actions of drugs having different, and so not additive, adverse effects; they are deliberately sought in the management of morphine overdose with naloxone. On the other hand 'every time a physician adds to the number of drugs a patient is taking he may devise a novel combination that has a special risk.'§

Although dramatic and unintended interactions attract most attention and are the principal subject of this section they should not distract attention from the many therapeutically useful interactions that are the basis of rational polypharmacy. These useful interactions are referred to throughout the book whenever it is relevant to do so and can be classified similarly.

It is salutary to be reminded that 'when a patient receiving one kind of tablet is given another in addition, he sometimes hesitates thinking that the second may 'interfere' with the first. A similar, though more sophisticated, notion should induce some thoughtful hesitation among the prescribers.'‖

Doctors provide generous opportunity for the occurrence of interactions.

In a hospital study, more than 40% of patients receiving drugs were taking six or more. The incidence of unwanted effects (not all of them were drug interactions, of course) in this group was about seven times that amongst patients taking less than six drugs.¶

Clinical importance of drug interactions. That one drug can be shown measurably to alter the disposition or effect of another drug does not mean that the interaction is necessarily of clinical importance (though it may be, and often is, statistically significant).

Clinically important drug interactions are most likely with drugs that have a *steep dose-response curve* and a *small therapeutic ratio* so that relatively small quantitative changes at the target site (receptor, enzyme, etc.) will lead to substantial changes in effect (therapeutic or adverse). Drugs falling into this class, which are in fact the chief

* *circa* about, *diem* day
† Decousus H A et al. Br Med J 1985; 290: 341.
‡ Rivard G E et al. Lancet 1985; 2: 1264.
§ Dollery C T. Pro Roy Soc Med 1965; 58:943.
‖ Editorial. Lancet 1962; 2: 818.
¶ Wade O L. Br Med Bull 1970; 26: 240.

sources of serious interactions, include *oral anticoagulants, cardiac glycosides and antidysrhythmics, sympathomimetics, antihypertensives, anticancer drugs, antiepileptics and oral hypoglycaemics*. The chance of two drugs that may interact being used together is obviously much greater if both are used to treat the same disease, e.g. digoxin and quinidine for cardiac dysrhythmia.

Some knowledge of the *pharmacological basis* of how one drug may change the action of another will be useful in obtaining those interactions that are wanted, as well as recognising and preventing those that are not, for the numbers of drugs and of facts are too great for it to be possible to remember them all.

Drug interactions are of two principal kinds:

1. **Pharmacodynamic interaction: both drugs act on the target site of clinical effect**, exerting synergism, potentiation or antagonism. The drugs may act on the same or different receptors or processes, mediating similar biological consequences. Examples: alcohol + benziodiazepine (to produce sedation): morphine + naloxone (to reverse opioid overdose): bethanidine + imipramine (loss of antihypertensive effect): rifampicin + isoniazid (effective antituberculosis combination), etc.

2. **Pharmacokinetic interactions: the drugs interact remotely from the target site** to alter plasma (and other tissue) concentrations so that the amount of the drug at the target site of clinical effect is altered, e.g. enzyme induction (rifampicin/warfarin), competition for plasma protein binding sites (sodium valproate/phenytoin).

Interaction may result in *antagonism* or *synergism*.

Antagonism occurs when the action of one drug opposes the action of another. It may be that the two drugs simply have opposite pharmacological effects (histamine and adrenaline on the bronchi), i.e. *physiological or non-competitive antagonism*; or, it may be that they compete reversibly for the same drug receptor (morphine/naloxone), i.e. *competitive antagonism*.

Synergism.* The probability that pharmacologists will, in the foreseeable future, agree on the terminology to describe drug synergism is remote. Therefore, the following will suffice: synergism is of two sorts:

1. **Summation** or **addition** occurs when the effects of two drugs having the same action are additive, i.e. 2+2=4 (bethanidine plus a thiazide diuretic have an additive antihypertensive effect).

2. **Potentiation** (to make more powerful) occurs when one drug increases the action of another, i.e. 2 + 2 = 5. Sometimes the two drugs both have the action concerned (trimethoprim/sulphonamide) and sometimes one drug lacks the action concerned (MAOI/amphetamine).

Drugs can interact at any stage from when they are mixed with other drugs or with substances used in pharmaceutical formulation, in i.v. infusion or syringe, to their final excretion either unchanged or as metabolites.

Interactions are exceedingly varied in kind, and in the following categorisation there has been some sacrifice of scientific precision in favour of simplicity, e.g. class 3(b) below.

Drug interactions occur —

1. *Outside the body*: formulation or mixing by giver.
2. *At site of entry*: before or at point of absorption.
3. *Inside the body*: after absorption.
   a. *at transit and storage sites*: non-specific binding sites.
   b. *at site of action or nearby*: specific receptors, enzymes, parasites, etc.
   c. *by interference with biotransformations*: metabolism.
   d. *at exit*: excretion.

The examples that follow are all potentially important in therapy, and the topic has, for convenience, been extended to include stability in solution and interaction with food and with natural substances in the body. Interactions are also mentioned throughout the book.

Interactions outside the body

A. *Pharmaceutical interaction.* The preparation becomes offensive or the ingredients separate. This is rare since doctors nowadays wisely confine their prescribing to preparations whose detailed

* Greek: *syn* together, *ergos* work

constitution has been devised by pharmacists; the subject will not be considered further.

B. *Chemical interaction* is rare for the same reason. A case in which the interaction was between drug and pharmaceutical diluent has occurred. In 1968 in several Australian cities there was an outbreak of neurological disorder in epileptics.* Initially, posterior fossa tumour was often suspected, but the clinical picture was compatible with drug intoxication. The only drug being taken by all the patients (in Brisbane there were 51) was phenytoin, and they got better when phenytoin dosage was reduced. It was at first difficult to understand why patients, most of whom had not altered their dosage, should suddenly develop toxic effects. In most of the cases who could be investigated, the blood level of phenytoin was found to be above the therapeutic range.

The affected patients were all taking the same brand of phenytoin. It was possible, therefore, that the currently used capsules might have accidentally been filled with too much phenytoin or that the previously used capsules might have contained too little phenytoin. Samples were investigated and both were found to have the correct total amount of drug. Enquiries revealed that some months before the first cases appeared the manufacturer had changed the diluting substance from a calcium compound to lactose. Patients were therefore treated alternately with the two types of capsule each containing the same total phenytoin, but different diluents. Substantially higher blood levels occurred with the lactose diluent. Probably the phenytoin was interacting with the calcium diluent to form an insoluble complex so that absorption was reduced.

Some patients suffered, but there were others who became better controlled, showing that they previously had been treated inadequately.

Examples. Thiopentone and suxamethonium interact chemically and should not be put in the same syringe.

Protamine zinc insulin contains excess of protamine, which interacts with soluble insulin if this is drawn up in the same syringe.

* Tyrer J H et al. Br Med J 1969; 4:271.

Intravenous fluids offer special scope for interactions (incompatibilities) when drugs are added to the reservoir. A principal factor causing interaction is change of pH. The concentration of drug in a mixture is also relevant to its stability, e.g. the more concentrated a solution of ampicillin, the greater its stability.

Drugs are commonly weak organic acids or bases. They are often insoluble and to make them soluble it is necessary to prepare salts. Plainly, the mixing of solutions of salts can result in precipitation or instability.

General advice

1. Do not add drugs to blood, amino acid solutions or to fat emulsions.
2. In the absence of special knowledge, a drug should be added only to simple solutions (dextrose, sodium chloride or a mixture of these). Sodium chloride (0.9%) is acid (pH 4.5–7) due to dissolved CO_2. Dextrose (5%) is acid (pH 3.5–6.5) due to some breakdown to acid products resulting from heat sterilising and storage. The solutions have very little buffering capacity and pH readily changes with added drugs.
3. Interaction may occur without visible change in the solution, though if the infusion is to be brief, absence of visible change during the course of the infusion gives grounds for optimism that acceptable activity is retained.
4. All mixtures should be made immediately before use; do not make up a supply for the whole weekend on Friday night.
5. Single drug additions to simple solutions are likely to be safe; two or more are likely to interact, e.g. heparin and benzylpenicillin.
6. The pharmacy or manufacturers' package inserts should be consulted wherever possible, for what you are using is not simply a drug, it is a preparation containing drug, stabiliser, preservative, etc., any of which may be a source of interaction.
7. The examples given here apply to mixing a drug in the infusion reservoir. Where the drug is injected over a few minutes into the giving set near the patient and flushed in, there is little time for interaction to occur.

Some examples

a. Retention of major (about 90%) activity of antibiotics:*

benzylpenicillin: 16 h in sodium chloride (0.9%) and in dextrose (5%).

ampicillin: 8 h in sodium chloride: 4 h in dextrose.

gentamicin: 24 h in sodium chloride and in dextrose.

erythromycin varies according to salt.

cephalosporins: 24 h in sodium chloride and in dextrose.

It is plain that the most recent information from the manufacturer should be sought when it is desired to add antimicrobial drugs to the reservoir of an i.v. infusion.

b. Heparin is stable in sodium chloride (0.9%) for up to 24 h but loses activity rapidly if put into the reservoir of infusions containing dextrose, antibiotics, hydrocortisone or sympathomimetics.

c. Noradrenaline (4 mg in 1 litre, ie 4 μg/ml) in dextrose or dextrose saline retains its potency (above 80%) for about 5 h; in blood or sodium chloride (0.9%) it is rapidly oxidised and this may be reduced by adding ascorbic acid (10 mg/litre).

d. Other sympathomimetics, also aminophylline, compound vitamin preparations and vitamin C are liable to interact with a wide range of drugs.

e. Insulin is stable in dextrose and sodium chloride solutions, though about 20% is lost by binding to reservoir and tubing.

It is convenient to mention here the local *thrombophlebitis* that is a complication of i.v. infusions. Its frequency increases with the duration of the infusion, the acidity of the fluid (due to manufacturing requirements most i.v. infusion fluids are acid) and the amount of obstruction and damage to the vein caused by the catheter or needle. Protection lies in giving brief infusions into large veins, and in changing the site daily, if possible (a counsel of perfection), where they must be prolonged.

* Formulations differ, data are incomplete, there are many variables, e.g. pH, temperature, concentration; any data given by good manufacturers about their preparations take precedence.

Interactions at site of entry, before absorption

The complex environment of the gut offers extensive opportunities for drugs to interfere with each other as well as with gut physiology.

a. *Gut motility*. Since drug absorption is influenced not only by the properties of the drug and its formulation but also by the varying physiological conditions (pH, permeability) at different levels of the gut, it is to be expected that changes in gut motility may influence rate and extent of absorption of drugs, and that the detailed consequences of such changes will vary according to the drug.

Duration of stay in the stomach before passing its contents on to the intestine is probably the single most important factor.

Drugs having anticholinergic effects (including some antidepressants, antihistamines and phenothiazine tranquillisers) reduce gastric and intestinal motility as do opioid analgesics; the time spent by drugs in the stomach is prolonged.

Metoclopramide accelerates gastric emtying so that drugs stay in the stomach for less time.

Purgatives reduce the time spent in the small intestine, though this is unlikely to be of consequence unless the patient has a daily purgative habit and even then only in the case of sustained-release formulations.

In fact, drug-induced motility changes are not a source of serious interactions, though differences that can have clinical importance have been shown with levodopa (delay in the stomach allows metabolism of drug and reduces the amount available for absorption by an active transport mechanism in the small intestine); adrenal steroids and digoxin (are poorly soluble and rapid transit may reduce the amount absorbed); paracetamol (the *rate* of absorption, though not the total, of drug absorbed is reduced by anticholinergics).

b. *pH of gut contents*. Changes in pH, e.g. due to antacids, by altering drug ionisation and so solubility in lipids, alter the rate of absorption.

When used in ordinary therapy, however, these effects of antacids are probably of little practical importance, for an oral dose has soon substantially passed into the intestine where the absorbing area is much greater than that of the stomach and pH effects are trivial in relation.

c. *Direct interaction in the gut.* Tetracyclines chelate with metals and in the presence of calcium, magnesium and aluminium-containing antacids absorption may be seriously reduced. Milk contains sufficient calcium to warrant its avoidance as a major article of diet when taking tetracyclines. Iron, even in small amounts, seriously reduces tetracycline absorption.

Cholestyramine interferes with absorption of thyroxine and some acidic drugs. Iron absorption is enhanced by ascorbic acid and reduced by carbonates, tetracyclines and desferrioxamine. Liquid paraffin reduces absorption of fat-soluble vitamins.

d. *Alterations in gut flora* by antimicrobials may potentiate oral anticoagulant (by reducing bacterial synthesis of vitamin K in the large gut), or possibly render oral contraceptives ineffective by preventing bacterial reactivation of conjugated steroid secreted in bile.

e. *Interference with absorptive mechanisms.* Monoamine oxidase inhibition in gut mucosa allows increased absorption of tyramine (from foods) and other sympathomimetics that are substrates for MAO; liver MAO is also reduced, with consequent increase in systemic biovailability.

f. Other than in the gut.
(i) See hyaluronidase.
(ii) Vasoconstrictors (adrenaline, felypressin) are added to local anaesthetics to delay absorption and usefully prolong anaesthesia.

Interactions inside the body, after absorption

A. Transit and storage sites

1. Drugs sometimes interact directly with each other in the *plasma*, e.g. protamine with heparin; desferrioxamine with iron; dimercaprol with arsenic.

2. More important in clinical practice is the result of administering a drug with a high affinity for plasma protein to a patient who is already taking another drug which is extensively *protein bound*. When this is done, there may be competition for protein binding sites; if the second drug successfully competes with and displaces the first, the fraction of the first drug that is free and available to act pharmacologically, will rise and there may be an immediate increase in effect. If the first drug is, say, more than 95% protein bound, it is only necessary to displace a very small percentage to *double* the concentration of free drug and substantially to alter its distribution.

Certain factors mitigate the displacement effect. First, consider distribution volume. If the drug is displaced into a large distribution space then any increase in free concentration will be small. Imipramine, although it is 95% protein bound, has a distribution volume of 1000 l/70 kg and displacement interactions are not a problem, but difficulties may arise with non-steroidal anti-inflammatory drugs, which tend to be highly protein bound and to occupy small distribution spaces. Second, the rise in concentration of free drug also means that more is available for metabolism and elimination; the potentiating effect of displacement is thus temporary provided both drugs continue to be taken, for the free concentration will fall until a new equilibrium is established. Unwanted effects are likely to arise when the displacing drug is taken intermittently or in varying amounts and will be most significant where precise control of the plasma concentration of one drug is required. Fluctuations in control of anticoagulant and oral hypoglycaemic therapy can be due to this.

Unfortunately, because there are numerous protein binding sites, and because drugs have different affinities for these sites, knowledge that a drug binds extensively with plasma protein is not, of itself, sufficient to allow prediction of clinically important interactions. In addition, small structural difference between members of a series may be accompanied by big differences in protein binding so that generalisation to a group of drugs from knowledge of a single member is not necessarily valid.

Some clinically important protein-binding interactions include:

clofibrate, a *chloral metabolite* (trichloracetic acid), *aspirin* (salicylate), *phenylbutazone* and analogues, and *indomethacin* all displace and so potentiate *warfarin*.

sulphonamides, dicoumarol and *salicylate* displace

and so potentiate *tolbutamide* and *methotrexate*. *sulphonamides* and *vitamin K* displace *bilirubin* and can cause kernicterus in the newborn.

3. Displacement by competition for proteins in *tissues* other than blood can also occur. Quinidine displaces digoxin from its tissue binding site(s); in addition quinidine impairs the excretion of digoxin by the kidney and there is risk of digoxin toxicity if quinidine is added to a drug regimen unless the dose of digoxin is lowered.

B. Metabolism

1. **Enzyme induction** (see also p. 128). Many drugs that are substrates for drug metabolising enzymes can induce an increase in synthesis of these enzymes with the result that the rate of metabolism of the inducing drug and of other drugs is increased. Chlorinated hydrocarbon insecticides (DDT group), alcohol, some hypnotics, antiepilepsy drugs, some antirheumatics, adrenocortical steroids, griseofulvin, and probably a wide variety of substances in the environment, including food additives, are enzyme inducers and enzyme induction can be considered a contributory factor to the normally encountered individual variation, i.e. much of the population is induced to varying degrees.

However, there are specially important situations in which a potent inducer is administered to a person who is being treated with a drug the action of which requires to be precisely controlled. Examples are:

Oral anticoagulant therapy. Metabolism of warfarin (and its dose requirements) is increased by enzyme inducers including rifampicin, carbamazepine and phenytoin; if any such drug is added to a regimen containing warfarin, anticoagulant control will be lost unless the dose of warfarin is increased.

It is a relief to know that benzodiazepine hynotics do not significantly induce drug metabolising enzymes or otherwise interfere with anticoagulant therapy, but other hypnotics do, e.g. dichlorphenazone.

Oral contraceptive therapy. Oestrogen–progestogen mixtures, especially in low dose, may be rendered ineffective by enzyme inducers. Before prescribing, for example, phenytoin or phenobarbitone for epilepsy, a doctor should check that the patient is not taking the oral contraceptive pill lest an unplanned pregnancy result (such cases have occurred and compensation has been paid to patients).

Chronic alcohol ingestion causing enzyme induction is a likely explanation of the tolerance shown by alcoholics to hydrocarbon anaesthetics and to tolbutamide.

2. **Enzyme inhibition** (see also p. 129). Drugs that interfere with metabolising processes are an important source of interaction for this action will potentiate other drugs whose intensity and duration of effect are limited by being metabolised.

Examples of clinically important interactions are:

Phenytoin metabolism in inhibited by coumarin anticoagulants, by isoniazid (important with slow inactivators only), by phenylbutazone, cimetidine, disulfiram and by sulthiame, so that phenytoin intoxication may occur.

Tolbutamide metabolism is inhibited, so that hypoglycaemia may occur, by phenylbutazone, coumarin anticoagulants, chloramphenicol and sulphonamides.

Purine analogues such as azathioprine and 6-mercaptopurine are metabolised by xanthine oxidase. Allopurinol (a xanthine oxidase inhibitor), which is used in gout to block the part played by xanthine oxidase in the synthesis of uric acid, can potentiate these toxic drugs.

Alcohol metabolism is blocked by disulfiram and, to a lesser extent, by sulphonylurea antidiabetics and metronidazole, leading to accumulation of the unpleasant intermediary, acetaldehyde.

Monoamine oxidase inhibitors (MAOI) are not completely selective for MAO and they also interfere with metabolism of opioid analgesics, especially pethidine, of barbiturates, anticholinergics and tricyclic antidepressants.

Anticholinesterases, see index.

Chloramphenicol inhibits metabolism of warfarin, tolbutamide and chlorpropamide and enhances the action of these drugs.

C. Site of action and nearby

This imprecise heading includes interactions at specific receptors. There are numerous examples of competition for specific receptors and use is made of, for example, selective anatagonists to acetylcholine (atropine-like drugs, anticholinergics), and to catecholamines (α and β-adrenoceptor blockers) in therapeutics. Strictly, interaction with the agonist when administered as a drug is sought only in cases of overdose (cholinergic drugs, including anticholinesterases, and adrenergic or sympathomimetic drugs).

Examples, some of which are more complicated than the classic simple competition for receptors but which involve competition, include:

α-adrenoceptor block against monoamine oxidase inhibitor/cheese interaction (tyramine).

Naloxone against morphine.

Anticholinesterase against curare.

Atropine against anticholinesterases.

This category includes other interactions of considerable variety. The following list shows something of the range of possibilities (see also under individual drugs):

Indirectly acting sympathomimetics, e.g. most appetite suppressants, and tricyclic antidepressants reduce the effectiveness of adrenergic neurone blocking antihypertensive drugs.

Levodopa induces hypertension in presence of a monoamine oxidase inhibitor.

Sympathomimetic amines that are substrates for monoamine oxidase (phenylephrine, orciprenaline, tyramine in foods), when taken orally after a monoamine oxidase inhibitor, are readily absorbed instead of being destroyed in the gut wall and so are greatly potentiated.

Tricyclic antidepressants potentiate catecholamines.

Aminophylline potentiates β-adrenergic effects: a cardiac risk in treating asthma.

Neomycin and *streptomycin* have neuromuscular blocking activity and synergise with curare.

Thiazide diuretics potentiate curare probably by inducing hypokalaemia.

D. At site of exit from the body

The clinically important interactions occur in the kidney by:

1. *Interference with passive diffusion.* Drugs that are soluble in lipids are reabsorbed from the glomerular filtrate by diffusing across the renal tubular cell membranes. Most drugs are weak electrolytes and the degree of solubility in lipids depends on the proportion of drug that is ionised (lipid insoluble) or un-ionised (lipid soluble). The degree of ionisation is affected by pH (see pH partition hypothesis, p. 115). The pH of the urine can be easily raised (by sodium bicarbonate) or lowered (by ascorbic acid). Thus, the amount of drug that remains in the tubule lumen and is excreted in the urine can be influenced by the physician. *pH influences on renal excretion are only of practical importance with drugs*:

a. *that are excreted largely unchanged in the urine*, and

b. *whose ionisation constant (pKa) is such that important changes in ionisation will occur over the range of pH (4.6–8.2) obtainable in urine. These are, for bases pKa 7.5–10.5 and for acids pKa 3.0–7.5.*

Alkalinisation of urine is clinically useful in aspirin and phenobarbitone poisoning. With phencyclidine, fenfluramine and amphetamine, excretion is enhanced by urinary acidification; this is not usually necessary in the treatment of poisoning, though it can be used to increase the ease of detection of the drugs in the urine of 'sportsmen' or of suspected addicts who deny taking the drugs. Reliable chemical identification allows the investigator the psychologically satisfying experience of accusing others of falsehood out of a sense of professional duty.

2. *Interference with active transport.* Organic acids are passed from the blood into the urine by active transport across the renal tubular epithelium. Penicillin is mostly excreted in this way. Probenecid, an organic acid that competes successfully with pencillin for this transport system, may be used to prolong the action of penicillin when repeated administration is impracticable, e.g. in sexually transmitted diseases, where compliance is notoriously poor. Salicylates block the uricosuric effect of probenecid.

GUIDE TO FURTHER READING

1 Langley J N. On the reaction of cells and of nerve-endings to certain poisons, chiefly as regards the reaction of striated muscle to nicotine and to curare. J Physiol (Lond) 1905; 33: 374–413
2 Dale H H. Some physiological actions of ergot. J Physiol (Lond) 1906; 34: 163–206
3 Ehrlich P. Chemotherapeutics: scientific principles, methods and results. Lancet 1913; 2: 445–451
4 Ahlquist R P. A study of the adrenotropic receptors. Am J Physiol 1948; 153–586–600
5 Lands A M et al. Differentiation of receptor systems activated by sympathomimetic amines. Nature 1967; 214: 597–598
6 Motulsky H J, Insel P A. Adrenergic receptors in man. Direct identification, physiologic regulation and clinical alterations. N Engl J Med 1982; 307: 18–29
7 Editorial. What therapeutic drugs should be monitored? Lancet 1985; 2: 309–310
8 Milne M D et al. Non-ionic diffusion and the excretion of weak acids and bases. Am J Med 1958; 24: 709
9 Editorial. Clinical aspects of the blood–brain barrier. Br Med J 1976; 3: 133
10 Editorial. Drug absorption: The solution is solution. Lancet 1979; 2: 1003–1004
11 Scott A K, Hawksworth G M. Drug absorption. Br Med J 1981; 282: 462–463
12 Editorial. Food, drugs and bioavailability. Br Med J 1984; 289: 1093–1094
13 Lindup W E, Orme M C L'E. Plasma protein binding of drugs. Br Med J 1981; 282: 212–214
14 Gibaldi M, Levy G. Effect of plasma protein and tissue binding on the biologic half-life of drugs. Clin Pharmacol Ther 1978; 24(1): 1–4
15 Dent C E et al. Osteomalacia with long-term anticonvulsant therapy in epilepsy. Br Med J 1970; 4: 69–72
16 Gelehrter T D. Enzyme induction. N Engl J Med 1976; 294: 522–526, 589–595, 646–651
17 Alvares A P et al. Intraindividual variation in drug disposition. Clin Pharmacol Ther 1979; 26(4): 407–419
18 Dormandy T L. An approach to free radicals. Lancet 1983; 2: 1010–1014
19 Committee on drugs. The transfer of drugs and other chemicals into human breast milk. Pediatrics 1983; 72(3): 375–383
20 Vessell E S. Pharmacogenetics: Multiple interactions between genes and the environment as determinants of drug response. Am J Med 1979; 66: 183–187
21 Editorial. Pharmacokinetics in the elderly. Lancet 1983; 2: 568–569

9

Unwanted effects of drugs: adverse reactions

Cur'd yesterday of my disease,
I died last night of my physician.*

Nature is neutral, i.e. it has no 'intentions' towards humans, though it is often unfavourable to them. It is mankind, in its desire to avoid suffering and death, that decides that some of the biological effects of drugs are desirable (therapeutic) and others are undesirable (adverse). In addition to this arbitrary division, which has no fundamental biological basis, unwanted effects of drugs are promoted, or even caused, by numerous non-drug factors. Because of the variety of these factors, attempts to make a simple account of the unwanted effects of drugs must be imperfect, but an attempt is made here under the following headings:

- Introductory discussion
- Terminology and definitions
- Kinds of adverse reactions
- Degrees of certainty in attributing adverse events to drugs
- Methods of collecting data on adverse reactions
- Discovery of drug-induced illness
- General data and general discussion
- Causes of adverse reactions
  - non-drug factors
  - drug factors
- Allergy in response to drugs
- Pseudo-allergic adverse drug reactions
- Miscellaneous
- Drugs and the embryo/fetus

* From *The Remedy Worse than the Disease*. Matthew Prior (1664–1721).

Introductory discussion

There is general agreement that drugs prescribed for disease are themselves the cause of a serious amount of disease (adverse reactions), ranging from mere inconvenience to permanent disability and death.

Since drugs are intended to relieve suffering, it may be felt peculiarly offensive that they can also cause disease. Therefore it is important to know how much disease they do cause and why they cause it, so that preventive measures can be taken wherever possible.

It is not enough to measure the rate of adverse reactions to drugs, their nature and their severity, though accurate data on these are obviously useful. It is necessary to take, or to try to take, into account which effects are avoidable (by skilled choice and use) and which unavoidable (inherent in drug or patient). Also, different adverse effects can matter to a different degree to different people. In addition, prescribing patterns can vary greatly from one region of a country to another and there are substantial differences between countries.

Since there can be no hope of eliminating all adverse effects of drugs it is necessary to evaluate patterns of adverse reaction against each other. One drug may frequently cause minor ill-effects but pose no threat to life, though patients do not like it and may take it irregularly, to their own detriment. Another drug may be pleasant to take, so that patients take it consistently, with benefit, but it may rarely kill someone. It is not obvious which drug is to be preferred.

Some patients, e.g. those with a history of allergy or previous reactions to drugs, are up to four times more likely to have another adverse reaction, so that the incidence does not fall evenly on the population taking a drug.

It is also useful to discover the causes of adverse reactions, where these are unknown, for such knowledge can be used to render what are at present unavoidable reactions avoidable.

Avoidable adverse effects will be reduced by more skilful prescribing and this means that doctors, amongst all the other claims on their time, must find time better to understand drugs, as well as to understand their patients and their diseases.

Estimates of the incidence and severity of adverse reactions to drugs are various, for reliable data are hard to get; but see p. 156.

Terminology

Many **unwanted effects** of drugs are medically trivial, and in order to avoid inflating the figures of drug-induced disease, it is convenient to retain the term **side effects** for minor effects of Type A class, below. The term **adverse reaction** should be confined to *harmful or seriously unpleasant effects occurring at doses intended for therapeutic (prophylactic or diagnostic) effect and which call for reduction of dose or withdrawl of the drug and/or forecast hazard from future administration*; it is effects of this order that are of importance in evaluating drug-induced disease in the community.

Other terms used:

Intolerance means a low threshold to the normal pharmacological action of a drug. Individuals vary greatly in their susceptibility to drugs, those at one extreme of the normal distribution curve being intolerant of the drugs, those at the other, tolerant.

Idiosyncrasy (see *pharmacogenetics*) implies an inherent qualitative abnormal reaction to a drug, usually due to genetic abnormality, e.g. porphyria.

Adverse reactions are of two principal kinds:

Unwanted effects that will occur in everyone if enough of the drug is given because they are due to excess of normal predictable, dose-related, pharmacological effects. They are common, and skilled management reduces their incidence, e.g. postural hypotension, hypoglycaemia, hypokalaemia, etc. This class is called *Augmented* or *Type A* reactions.

Unwanted effects that will occur only in some people. They are not part of the normal pharmacology of the drug and are due to unusual properties of the patient interacting with the drug. These effects are predictable where the mechanism is known (though predictive tests may be expensive or impracticable), otherwise they are unpredictable for the individual, although the incidence may be known. The class includes unwanted effects due to inherited abnormalities (see *pharmacogenetics*) and immunological processes (see *drug allergy* below); it is call *Bizarre* or *Type B* reactions.

Reliable *attribution of a cause-effect relationship* provides the biggest problem in this field.

Degrees of certainty

Karch and Lasagna* propose the following **degrees of certainty for attributing adverse events to drugs:**

Definite:	time sequence from taking drug is reasonable
	event corresponds to what is known of drug
	event ceases on stopping drug
	event returns on restarting drug
Probable:	time sequence reasonable
	corresponds to what is known of drug
	ceases on stopping drug
	not reasonably explained by patient's disease
Possible:	time sequence reasonable
	corresponds to what is known of drug
	could readily have been result of patient's disease or other therapy
Conditional:	time sequence reasonable
	does not correspond to what is known of drug
	could not reasonably be explained by the patient's disease

* JAMA 1975; 234:1236.

Doubtful: event not meeting the above criteria.

Methods of collecting data

The principal **methods of collecting data on adverse reactions** are:

1. **Formal therapeutic trials**. These provide reliable data only on the commoner events as they involve small numbers of patients (hundreds); they detect an incidence of up to about 1:200.

2. **Epidemiological techniques** used for post-marketing studies include:

The *observational cohort study* and the *case-control study* and are described on p. 61 of Chapter 4. These are extremely important in the detection and quantification of adverse reactions. They detect an incidence of 1:5000–1:10 000.

One form of observational cohort study is *prescription event monitoring*. Prescriptions for a drug (5000–20 000) are collected (in the UK this is made practicable by the existence of a National Health Service in which prescriptions are sent to regional offices for pricing and payment of the pharmacist). The prescriber is sent a questionnaire and asked to report all *events* that have occurred (*not* only suspected adverse reactions). By this means unsuspected effects may be detected. Prescription event monitoring can be used routinely on newly licenced drugs and it can also be implemented quickly in response to a suspicion raised, e.g. by spontaneous reports.

3. **Spontaneous reporting systems** depend on doctors' intuitions and willingness to respond. They are therefore erratic, but really have no upper limit of qualitative sensitivity and may detect the rarest events; they are plainly useless for quantification.

4. **National vital statistics**, e.g. birth defect registers and cancer registers, are insensitive unless a drug-induced event is highly unusual or very frequent. If suspicions are aroused then case-control and observational cohort studies will be initiated.

5. **New drugs**. Patients taking new drugs are increasingly subject to formal surveillance (see above) after the necessarily limited therapeutic trials have justified release for general prescribing (post-marketing/licencing surveillance), and efforts are made to stimulate spontaneous reporting. Indeed it may be made a condition of licencing that records be kept of the first few thousand patients (monitored release).

Drug-induced illness

The discovery of drug-induced illness has been usefully analysed by Jick* thus:

1. Drug *commonly* induces an otherwise *rare* illness: this effect is likely to be discovered by clinical observation in the pre-registration (pre-marketing) formal therapeutic trials and the drug will almost always be abandoned: but some patients are normally excluded from such trials, e.g. pregnant women, and detection will then occur later (e.g. thalidomide).

2. Drug *rarely* induces an otherwise *common* illness: this effect is likely to remain undiscovered.

3. Drug *rarely* induces an otherwise *rare* illness: this effect is likely to remain undiscovered before the drug is released for general prescribing: the effect should be detected by informal clinical observation or during any special post-registation surveillance and confirmed by a case-control study (see above), e.g. chloramphenicol and aplastic anaemia, practolol and oculomucocutaneous syndrome.

4. Drug *commonly* induces an otherwise *common* illness: this effect will not be discovered by informal clinical observation: it may, if great, be discovered in formal therapeutic trials and in case-control studies, but if moderate or small it may require observational cohort studies, e.g. sulphonylureas and cardiovascular mortality in diabetics.

5. Both drug and illness rates in *intermediate* range: both case-control and cohort studies may be needed.

The practicalities of detecting rare adverse reactions can be illustrated:

For reactions with no background incidence the number of patients required to give a good (95%) chance of detecting the effect is given in table (below). Assuming that three events are required before any regulatory or other action should be taken, it shows the large number of patients that must be monitored to detect even a relatively high incidence adverse effects.

* N Engl J Med 1977; 296:481

Expected incidence of adverse reaction	*Required number of patients for event*★ *1*	*2*	*3*
1 in 100	300	480	650
1 in 200	600	960	1 300
1 in 1000	3 000	4 800	6 500
1 in 2000	6 000	9 600	13 000
1 in 10000	30 000	48 000	65 000

The problem can be many orders of magnitude worse if the adverse reactions closely resemble spontaneous disease with a background incidence in the population.

Adverse reactions to drugs: general data and general discussion

1. Cause 2–3% of consultations in general practice.

2. Cause up to 3% of admissions to acute care hospital wards (and 0.3% of general hospital admissions).

3. Overall incidence in hospital in-patients 10–20%, and possible prolongation of hospital stay in 2–10% of patients in acute medical wards.

4. Predisposing factors: age over 60 years or under one month, female, previous history of adverse reaction, hepatic or renal disease.

5. Cause death in up to 0.3% hospital in-patients (or 1% if intravenous fluids are included), largely in patients already seriously ill.

6. Most commonly occur early in therapy (days 1–10).

7. Most common diseases of sufferers: cardiovascular, diabetes mellitus, respiratory (infection, chronic obstructive lung disease).

8. Most common drugs in *hospital*: digitalis, antibiotics, diuretics, potassium, analgesics, tranquillisers, insulin: *causing admission*: digitalis, aspirin, adrenocortical steroids, diuretics, antihypertensives, warfarin.

9. Mechanism: pharmacological 80%, immunological 20%.

★ By permission from: Safety requirements for the first use of new drugs and diagnostic agents in man. Geneva: CIOMS 1983.

10. Most commonly affect: gastrointestinal tract, skin, mental alertness, plasma K concentration.

11. Fatal adverse reactions to drugs (notified on death certificate) in one year (UK) included:

anticoagulants	11	chiefly bleeding
adrenal steroids	35	chiefly adrenal failure, bowel perforation
chloramphenicol	5	blood disorders
phenylbutazone	17	blood disorders
aspirin	2	gastric erosion

Deaths were also notified as due to insulin, lignocaine, penicillin, gold, phenytoin, monoamine oxidase inhibitors, imipramine and phenothiazine tranquillisers.

These figures are almost certainly underestimates, for doctors are understandably reluctant to attribute a patient's death to therapy with such certainty that they notify it as principal cause, and they attribute it to disease if it is at all reasonable to do so.

12. Study of 26 462 consecutive hospital patients in seven countries[†]: 24 (0.09%) considered to have died as a result of drugs administered: most were severely ill prior to the event that caused death (leukaemia, heart failure, cancer, etc.). The principal drugs were anticancer, digoxin and heparin: five died from i.v. fluid overload and one from excess KCl: these latter may be considered preventable by skill. Bearing in mind that the skill to avoid these can be considerable, this record is not a cause for shame.

13. Study of 10 280 surgical inpatients[‡]: two elderly women died from haemorrhage due to heparin.

14. Studies of spontaneous reporting by doctors do not provide incidence figures but suggest that in out-patients deaths are most commonly due to haematological (including thromboembolism) and anaphylactic events.

Caution. About 80% of well people not taking any drugs admit on questioning to symptoms (often several) such as are commonly experienced as lesser adverse reactions to drugs. These symptoms are intensified (or diminished) by adminis-

† Porter J. et al. JAMA 1977; 237:879.
‡ Armstrong B. et al. Am J Surg 1976; 132:643.

tration of a placebo. Thus, many symptoms may be wrongly attributed to drugs.

On the other hand people may take drugs without realising they are doing so. The quinine in tonic water was responsible in the following example of intolerance*†:

> I saw a 43-year-old man in consultation who had a 7-week history of tinnitus and hearing loss. He had consulted an otologist, who found bilateral diminution in hearing, and a neurologist, who suggested the diagnosis of bilateral angle meningioma. Because of the history of ingestion of seven to eight drinks per day he was sent for a medical evaluation prior to further work-up for neurosurgery. The history of alcohol ingestion was correct, but his diet was in general adequate. After a physical examination, which was not remarkable except for the facts already noted, casual discussion brought out the fact that the drinks were always gin and tonic. Since I had seen cinchonism in the south-west Pacific, I thought it worthwhile to change the beverage to Tom Collins‡. Within 48 hours the symptoms had disappeared. A test dose of 300 mg of quinine brought a return of the tinnitus. Later, a test dose of 150 mg produced the same effect. Three weeks after the discontinuance of the quinine, audiogram showed restoration of hearing.
>
> While I have not obtained the exact formula of quinine water, I am informed that the Schweppes brand contains about 30 mg per pint [568 ml]. The man was ingesting about 100 mg daily. It is clear that it would take an enormous consumption to produce the symptoms in the normal adult.

It is important to avoid alarmist or defeatist extremes of attitude. Many treatments are dangerous, e.g. surgery, electroshock, drugs, and it is irrational to accept the risks of surgery for peptic ulcer or hernia and refuse to accept any risk at all from drugs for conditions of comparable seriousness.

Many patients whose death is deemed to be partly or wholly caused by drugs are dangerously ill already; justified risks may be taken in the hope of helping them; ill-informed criticism in such cases can act against the interest of the sick. On the other hand there is no doubt that some of these accidents are avoidable. Avoidability is often more obvious when reviewing the conduct of treatment after death (i.e. with hindsight) than it was at the time.

Sir Anthony Carlisle,§ in the first half of the 19th century, said that *medicine is 'an art founded on conjecture and improved by murder'*. Although medicine has advanced so rapidly, there is still a ring of truth in that statement‖ to anyone who follows the introduction of new drugs and observes how, after the early enthusiasm, the reports of serious toxic effects appear.

Another cryptic remark of this therapeutic nihilist was 'Calomel is poison and digitalis kills people'. This disparaging statement is of interest because the latter is one of the essential drugs in modern therapy. One reason it is essential is that it is effective, and it can kill when used ignorantly or carelessly. William Withering in 1785 laid down rules for the use of digitalis that would serve today. Neglect of these rules resulted in needless suffering for patients with heart failure for more than a century until the therapeutic criteria were rediscovered. Any drug that is really worth using can do harm, and *it is an absolute obligation on the doctor to use only drugs about which he has troubled to inform himself*. The following report of a coroner's inquest shows the reality of this:

'. . . an inquest has been held on a woman who died from internal hæmorrhage due to dicoumarol which had been given for thrombosis in the leg veins. The doctor is reported to have said that he gave the dose recommended in the manufacturer's literature; he confessed his ignorance of the dangerous properties of dicoumarol and complained that these were not mentioned in the instructions for use.'¶

It may be hoped that such irresponsibility is rarer than the ignorance that contributes to the misuse of drugs, using them where none are

* Yohalem S B. JAMA 1953; 153:1304.

† See also, Cundall R D. Hypersensitivity to quinine in Bitter Lemon. Br Med J 1964; 1:1638.

‡ Tom Collins: iced drink of gin with soda water, lemon or lime juice, and sugar.

§ Noted for his advocacy of the use of 'the simple carpenter's saw' in surgery.

‖ In the less candid language of our times the opinion has been repeated; 'The trend of greater risks for greater gain is likely to continue'. *Royal Commission on Civil Liability and Compensation for Personal Injury*. London: HMSO, Cmnd. 7045, 1978.

¶ Editorial. Lancet 1949; 1:698.

needed, inappropriate choice where they are needed, and not only over-dosage but inadequate dosage when the doctor is uninformed and does not have clear aims.

Effective therapy depends not only on the *correct choice* of drugs but also on their *correct use*. This latter is sometimes forgotten and a drug is condemned as useless when it has been used in a dose or way which absolutely precluded a successful result; which can be regarded as a negative adverse effect.

Causes of adverse reactions

Adverse reactions to drugs are due to:

1. Non-drug factors
   - (a) intrinsic to the patient: age, sex, genetics, tendency to allergy, disease, personality and habits.
   - (b) extrinsic to the patient: the prescriber, the environment.
2. Drug factors
   - (a) intrinsic to the drug.
   - (b) choice of the drug.
   - (c) use of the drug.
   - (d) interactions between drugs.

Non-drug factors

Factors intrinsic to the patient: age, sex, genetics, allergy (tendency to), **disease, personality and habits.**

Age. The very old and the very young are liable to be intolerant of many drugs, largely because the equipment for disposing of them in the body is less efficient. The young, it has been aptly said, are not simply 'small adults'.

The **newborn**, see p. 140.

Older children may metabolise some drugs more rapidly than adults. They are more tolerant than adults of digitalis, but tolerance to atropine and morphine is probably normal, although the contrary is sometimes stated. Amphetamine sedates hyperkinetic children.

For drug dosage in children, see Fig 8.1 and text nearby.

In the aged. The practical importance of this topic is so great that it will be considered in some detail here. The elderly tend to show an increased response to standard drug dosage and an increased incidence of adverse reactions is due to a combination of factors:

1. lower body size (body water and lean mass) with consequent changes in apparent volume of distribution (some drugs),
2. lower glomerular filtration and renal tubular function,
3. lower blood flow to vital organs, kidney, etc.,
4. lower concentration and lower binding capacity of plasma proteins,
5.* lower hepatic metabolic capacity (for some drugs),
6. homeostatic mechanisms less effective (confusion induced by sedatives, falls due to drug-induced giddiness),
7. tendency to multiple diseases with consequent multiple prescribing,
8. tendency to suboptimal nutrition.

Drug therapy in the elderly should be kept to a minimum, both for number of drugs and dosage of each drug.

Glomerular filtration rate declines after the age of 50 years and is reduced by as much as 30% in the mid-sixties; renal tubular function also declines. Increased $t_{\frac{1}{2}}$ of drugs (digoxin, gentamicin) has been shown despite normal plasma creatinine concentration (creatinine production is less in the old).

There is little evidence that the ageing process slows drug absorption, which is not surprising since most drugs enter gut cells by passive diffusion. Plasma albumin concentration tends to fall in old age but for several drugs (diazepam, salicylate, benzylpenicillin) no change in binding has been found. By contrast the binding of pethidine reduces with increasing age which may partly explain relative intolerance to this drug in the elderly.

Metabolism also diminishes with age. In one study of geriatric in-patients the mean plasma half-life of antipyrine (phenazone) was increased by 45% and that of phenylbutazone by 29% above that in young controls. Prolongation × 4 of the $t_{\frac{1}{2}}$ of diazepam in the elderly has also been

* Items 1 to 5 may be summed up, 'Respect for their pharmacokinetic variability should be added to the list of our senior citizens' rights.' Fogel B S. N Engl J Med 1983; 308:1600.

observed, but with accompanying changes in the volume of distribution and clearance.* Thus increasing $t_{\frac{1}{2}}$ of metabolised drugs cannot always be ascribed to slowing metabolic rates. Standard doses of propranolol produce higher plasma concentrations in the elderly, possibly due to reduced blood flow to and reduced first-pass extraction by the liver.

All central nervous system depressants are especially liable to have greater effect than normal, and acute and chronic confusional states may occur, which is why atropine is often substituted for hyoscine in anaesthetic premedication and a benzodiazepine or chloral hydrate or derivative is preferred to a barbiturate. Phenothiazines with extrapyramidal effects are liable to lead to immobility which causes pressure sores and also to overt Parkinsonism, but phenothiazines are probably drugs of choice in severe senile restlessness, confusion and agitation. Hangover from hypnotics and giddiness from antihypertensives may cause falls with broken bones in old people whose homeostatic mechanisms are no longer what they were. There may be truth in the claim that the high clinical reputation of some geriatricians is based on their simply stopping the prescriptions of their colleagues and allowing old people to regain their natural health.

The old are relatively intolerant of digitalis and of anticoagulants.

The time of onset of an initial dose of i.v. anaesthetic in the old can be twice as long as in younger subjects due to prolonged circulation time; this has led to overdose when a second dose is given before the first has had time to act. Epidural anaesthetics may spread more extensively in the old.

Sex. There are no clinically important qualitative sex differences in adverse effects of drugs except, of course, to drugs affecting sex characteristics and fertility, but the subject is poorly documented. Women are said to be more liable to become excited by morphine than are men; in this respect they resemble cats. In a study on depression, women responded more than men to electroconvulsion therapy and less to antidepressant drugs. Women have a higher incidence of adverse reactions than do men and are poisoned by a lower intake of alcohol.

Genetics: see *pharmacogenetics*.

Allergy: see *allergy to drugs*.

Disease. Examples of the modification of drug action by disease are legion. Disease not only alters target organs, but also the organs of metabolism and elimination, i.e. both pharmacodynamics and pharmacokinetics.

Hepatic and renal insufficiency often result in defective metabolism and excretion (see special sections).

Hypoalbuminaemia reduces the binding capacity for drugs and concentrations of free (and active) drug may be excessive.

In *congestive heart failure* there is decreased hepatic and renal perfusion and sometimes cellular damage due to hypoxia is added. Patients will require lower doses of drugs that normally have a high metabolic clearance rate, e.g. lignocaine. Fluid retention may be accompanied by lower than usual plasma concentration because of the increased volume of distribution of a drug.

Thyroid disease. High and low metabolic rates have the expected effects. In hyperthyroidism drug metabolism is accelerated and in hypothyroidism it is diminished; the latter is particularly important clinically.

Respiratory disease. Patients with a malfunctioning respiratory centre (raised intracranial pressure, severe pulmonary insufficiency) are intolerant of drugs that are well known to depress respiration (opioids) but *any* sedative, e.g. benzodiazepines, may precipitate respiratory failure in such patients. The respiratory depressant effect of morphine is first manifested by slowing of the rate and normal people compensate for this by breathing more deeply, but patients with *severe emphysema* cannot do this and should therefore be treated circumspectly. Patients with raised intracranial pressure may be restless and it is important to avoid respiratory depression when using drugs to quieten them.

Other examples include:

Asthmatic attacks may be precipitated by cholinergic drugs and by β-adrenoceptor block (eye drops for glaucoma have killed).

Patients with *myocardial infarction* are especially

* *Clearance* is what is important (see p. 129) but figures of $t_{\frac{1}{2}}$ are commonly what is available to prescribers.

liable to develop cardiac dysrhythmias with digitalis or sympathomimetic amines.

In *infectious mononucleosis* and other disorders affecting lymphocytes (leukaemia, some viral infections) rashes with ampicillin are usual; this is important as the patients commonly present with a sore throat and are liable to receive the drug; the mechanism is probably allergic, the rash may not recur with subsequent administration but it cannot be assumed that any penicillin is safe.

Myasthenia gravis is made worse by quinine and myasthenics are intolerant of competitive neuromuscular blocking agents including aminoglycoside antibiotics, and resistant to depolarising agents. Patients with this disease or *dystrophia myotonica* are liable to develop respiratory failure under general anaesthesia.

Patients with *hypopituitarism* and *hypothyroidism* are intolerant of cerebral depressants and probably other drugs, due to their low metabolic rate.

In *shock*, drugs injected subcutaneously may not be absorbed owing to existing intense vasoconstriction and then, as this passes off, all doses previously given may be absorbed simultaneously with dire results, e.g. repeated doses of morphine to travelling casualties of accident or battle. In both severe *oedema* and shock, drugs should be injected i.m. or i.v., not s.c.

Schizophrenics are often tolerant of drugs affecting the central nervous system and high doses may be needed.

Hysterics sometimes show exaggerated responses, especially to sedatives, and stagger and fall about on the smallest doses.

Men with *prostatic enlargement* are liable to develop urinary retention if a vigorous diuresis is induced, and with sympathomimetic and anticholinergic drugs. *Pyloric stenosis* may be converted to an obstruction if gastric peristalsis is abolished by anticholinergic drugs.

In a variety of *malignant diseases*, particularly Hodgkin's disease, alcoholic drinks induce pain. This can give a diagnostic clue.

A patient in severe *pain* may become confused if given a hypnotic without an accompanying analgesic, for the pain keeps him awake.

Some drugs may be given in a chemical form unsuited to a particular occasion, e.g. high doses of antibiotics presented as sodium salts, and sodium-containing antacids should not be used in patients with heart failure, and *potassium* citrate to alkalinise the urine is dangerous in renal failure. Drug absorption, metabolism and excretion can be impaired by the circulatory changes of heart failure.

It is impossible to list completely the possible important alterations of drug effects caused by disease. The examples given above suffice to show that safety lies in knowledge of both drug and disease and an awareness of the possibilities.

An uncommon but particularly important example is the **hepatic porphyrias** (acute intermittent p., variegate p., hereditary coproporphyria, p. cutanea tarda) caused by genetically determined single enzyme defects.

In healthy people the rate of haem synthesis is dependent on the enzyme δ-aminolaevulinate (ALA) synthetase, which responds, by negative feed-back, to the amount of haem present, i.e. if there is insufficient haem, enzyme activity increases and vice versa. But the haem precursor, porphobilinogen, that is produced by the activity of ALA-synthetase cannot, in people with the enzyme defect of porphyria, be converted to haem, and so porphobilinogen accumulates. A vicious cycle occurs, less haem, more ALA synthetase, more porphobilinogen, the metabolism of which is blocked and a clinical attack occurs. The exact precipitating mechanism of the clinical features of an acute attack of porphyria is uncertain, but it would be rational to use any safe means of depressing the formation of ALA synthetase. Fructose (laevulose) will do this, and up to 400 g has been given i.v. per day in acute attacks with apparent benefit within 24 hours; glucose may be substituted; haematin infusion (haem arginate, Normosang) has also been found effective if given early and may prevent chronic neuropathy.

Increase in the haem-containing hepatic oxidising enzymes of the cytochrome P_{450} group causes an increased demand for haem. Therefore drugs that induce these enzymes would be expected to precipitate acute attacks of porphyria and they do so, see below.

It is of interest that those who inherited acute intermittent porphyria and variegate porphyria suffered no biological disadvantage from the

Table 9.1 Evaluation of drugs in acute porphyria.* This table is organised under the therapeutic headings given in the British National Formulary. The drugs are categorised as follows: **A** — those in the unsafe group which have been reported by three or more workers in the field to be associated with clinical exacerbations of porphyria; or, in the safe group, those considered by three or more authorities to be harmless to porphyric patients on the basis of their clinical experience. **B** — those in the unsafe group which have been reported by two or less workers in the field to be associated with clinical exacerbations of porphyria; or, in the safe group, those considered by two or fewer authorities to be harmless to porphyric patients on the basis of their clinical experience. In many instances, the clinical experience with drugs in the above two groups will have been corroborated by experimental data, of type: **C** — those which have been evaluated only in animals with experimentally produced porphyria. **D** — those which have been evaluated only in cell culture systems. No clinical experience has been reported with the drugs in the latter two groups. Finally, those drugs for which **conflicting data** are available have been listed and classified where possible as: (S) probably safe, (U) probably unsafe.

Unsafe		Thought to be safe		Contentious	
1. *GASTROINTESTINAL SYSTEM*					
Aluminium preparations	C	Atropine	A	Cimetidine	U
		Domperidone	C	Metoclopramide	U
Hyoscine butylbromide	A	Magnesium sulphate	B	Ranitidine	S
		Propantheline	B		
2. *CARDIOVASCULAR SYSTEM*					
		Adrenaline	B	Disopyramide	S
		Atropine	A	Prazosin	S
		Clofibrate	D		
		Digoxin	A		
Diuretics					
Spironolactone	C	Acetazolamide	D		
		Bumethanide	B	Frusemide	S
		Ethacrynic Acid	B		
		Triamterene	C		
				Thiazides	S
Antihypertensive Agents					
Methyldopa	A	Atenolol	B		
Clonidine	D	Diazoxide	D		
Hydralazine	B	Guanethidine	A		
Phenoxybenzamine	D	Labetalol	B		
		Propranolol	A		
		Reserpine	A		
		Tolazoline	A		
Anticoagulants					
		Heparin	B		
		Warfarin	B		
3. *RESPIRATORY SYSTEM*					
Bemegride	B				
Guaiphenesin	C				
Nikethamide	C				
Pentylenetetrazol	C				
Theophylline	B				
Antihistamines					
Clemastine	C	Chlorpheniramine	A	Diphenhydramine	S
Dimenhydrinate	B	Tripelennamine	B	Promethazine	U
Terfenadine	B				

Unsafe		Thought to be safe		Contentious	
4. *CENTRAL NERVOUS SYSTEM*					
Hypnotics, Sedatives and Anxiolytics					
Barbiturates	A	Chloral hydrate†	A	Chlormethiazole	S
Carbromal	B	Chlorpromazine	A	Clobazam	U
Carisoprodol	A	Droperidol	B	Clonazepam	U
Chlordiazepoxide	B	Lorazepam	C	Diazepam	U
Chlormezanone	B	Methylphenidate	B	Methotrimeprazine	S
Dichloralphenazone†	A	Prochlorperazine	B	Oxazepam	U
Ethchlorvynol	B	Promazine	A	Promethazine	U
Ethinamate	C	Triazolam	C		
Flunitrazepam	B	Trifluoperazine	B		
Flurazepam	A				
Glutethimide	A				
Lofepramine	A				
Meprobamate	A				
Methyprylone	A				
Nitrazepam	B				
Tranquillisers/Anti-Emetics					
Cinnarizine	C	Chlorpromazine	A	Promethazine	U
Dimenhydrinate	C	Cyclizine	B	Metoclopramide	U
Dixyrazine	C	Domperidone	C		
Hydroxyzine	C	Meclozine	A		
Isometheptene	C	Prochlorperazine	B		
		Trifluoperazine	B		
Psychoanaleptics					
Iproniazid	B	Lithium salts	B	Amitriptyline	U
		Methylphenidate	D	Imipramine	U
Phenelzine	C			Nortriptyline	S
Tranylcypromine	C				
Viloxazine	C				
Anticonvulsants					
Barbiturates	A	Bromides	A	Chlormethiazole	S
Carbamazepine	A	Magnesium sulphate	B	Clonazepam‡	U
Ethosuximide	A	Paraldehyde	B	Diazepam‡	U
Ethotoin	B			Sodium valproate‡	S
Hydantoins	A				
Methsuximide	A				
Oxazolidinediones	B				
Paramethadione	A				
Phenobarbitone	A				
Phensuximide	A				
Phenytoin	A				
Succinimides	A				
Sulthiame	B				
Troxidone	B				
Analgesics: Non-Narcotic					
Amidopyrine	C	Aspirin	A	Indomethacin	S
Antipyrine	C	Codeine	B		
		Diamorphine	B		
		Fenoprofen	C		
		Glafenine	C		
		Ibuprofen	B		
		Mefenamic Acid	B		
		Naproxen	B		
		Paracetamol	A		
Analgesics: Narcotics					
Oxycodone	C	Buprenorphine	B	Dextromoramide	S
Pentazocine	A	Diamorphine	B	Dextropropoxyphene	U

Unsafe		Thought to be safe		Contentious	
Phenacetin	C	Droperidol	A		
Tilidate	B	Methadone	A		
		Morphine	A		
		Pethidine	B		
Migraine					
Clonidine	B	Prochlorperazine	B		
Dihydroergotamine	A				
Ergotamine	A				
Isometheptene	B				
Lysuride	C				
Orphenadrine	C				
Appetite Suppressants					
Diethylpropion	C				
Methamphetamine	B				
5. *INFECTION*					
Colistin	B	Aminoglycosides	B	Cephalosporins	U
Chloramphenicol	C	Gentamicin	C	Chloroquine	S
Cycloserine	B	Hexamine	C	Isoniazid	U
Dapsone	A	Penicillins	A	Mebendazole	S
Erythromycin	B	Primaquine	B	Nitrofurantoin	U
Griseofulvin	A	Quinine	B	Pyrimethamine	
Metronidazole	C	Sodium Fusidate	B	Tetracyclines	S
Nalidixic acid	B				
Novobiocin	B				
Pyrazinamide	A				
Rifampicin	C				
Sulphonamides	A				
6. *ENDOCRINE SYSTEM*					
Hormone preparations					
Danazol	B	Corticotrophine (ACTH)	B	Androgens	U
Dydrogesterone	C	Dexamethasone	B	Corticosteroids	S
Metyrapone	D	Methyluracil	B	Cyproterone	S
		Propylthiouracil	B	Ethinyloestradiol	U
		Prednisolone	B	Oestrogens	U
		Thiouracil	B	Oral contraceptives	U
		Thyroxine	B	Progestogens	U
Antidiabetic Agents					
Sulphonylureas	A	Biguanides	C		
		Glipizide	C		
		Insulin	A		
7. *OBSTETRICS, GYNAECOLOGY AND RENAL*					
Ergometrine	A	Oxytocin	B	Oestrogens	U
Hyoscine butylbromide	A	Propantheline	B	Oral contraceptives	U
Phenoxybenzamine	B				
Lignocaine	C				
8. *MALIGNANT DISEASE — IMMUNOSUPPRESSION*					
Antineoplastic agents					
Aminoglutethimide	B	Doxorubicin	C	Cyproterone	S
Busulphan	C			Ethinyloestradiol	S
Chlorambucil	C			Melphalan	S
Cyclophosphamide	C			Vincristine	S
Mercaptopurine	B				
Methotrexate	C				

Unsafe		Thought to be safe		Contentious	
9. *NUTRITION AND BLOOD*					
Ethanol	A	Alpha tocopheryl acetate	A		
		Ascorbic Acid	A		
		B Vitamins	B		
		Folic Acid	B		
		Fructose	A		
		Glucose	A		
		Pyridoxine	A		
		Sodium Calcium edetate (EDTA)	A		
10. *MUSCULOSKELETAL AND JOINT DISEASE*					
i. *Non-steroidal anti-inflammatory agents*					
Amidopyrine	A	Alclofenac	C	Indomethacin	S
		Aspirin	A	Phenylbutazone	U
Azapropazone	C	Codeine	A		
Benoxaprofen	C	Dihydrocodeine	A		
Dichloralphenazone	A	Fenoprofen	C		
Diclofenac	A	Flurbiprofen	B		
Dipyrone	A	Ibuprofen	B		
Flufenamic acid	B	Ketoprofen	C		
Oxyphenbutazone	A	Mefenamic acid	B		
		Naproxen	B		
Piroxicam	B	Paracetamol	B		
		Sulindac	C		
ii. *Corticosteroids*					
		Dexamethasone	B	Hydrocortisone	S
		Prednisolone	C		
iii. *Specific anti-rheumatic agents*					
Gold (Sodium aurothiomalate)	C	Penicillamine	B	Chloroquine	S
iv. *Anti-gout agents*					
Piroxicam	C	Allopurinol	C	Probenecid	U
		Colchicine	B		
v. *Muscle relaxants and antispasmodics*					
Carisoprodol	A	Domperidone	C	Diazepam	U
Chlormezanone	B	Neostigmine	A	Metoclopramide	U
Chlorzoxazone	B	Propantheline	B	Pancuronium	S
Dipyrone	A	Suxamethonium	A		
Hyoscine butylbromide	A	Tubocurarine	B		
Oxanamide	C				
11. *EYE*					
Chloramphenicol	A	Acetazolamide	B	Tetracyclines	S
Hyoscine butylbromide	A	Amethocaine	C	Cocaine	S
Mercuric Oxide	B	Atropine	A		
Oxyphenbutazone	B	Dexamethasone	B		
Proxymetacaine	C	Gentamicin	A		
Sulphacetamide	C	Guanethidine	C		
		Oxybuprocaine	C		
		Prednisolone	C		
		Zinc sulphate	B		
12. *EAR, NOSE AND OROPHARNYNX*					
Oxymetazoline					

Unsafe		Thought to be safe		Contentious	
13. *SKIN*					
Crystal Violet	B				
		Resorcinol	B		
		Zinc preparations	B		
14. *VACCINES* — none proven unsafe					
15. *ANAESTHESIA*					
Alcuronium	C	Amethocaine	C	Cocaine	S
	B	Bupivacaine	C	Halothane	U
		Cyclopropane	C	Ketamine	S
Barbiturates	A	Diethylether	A	Pancuronium	S
Chloroform	B	Droperidol	C	Propanidid	U
Enflurane	C	Fentanyl	C	Proxymetacaine	S
Etidocaine	C	Minaxolone	C		
Etomidate	C	Nitrous oxide	A		
Fluroxene	B	Prilocaine	B		
Lignocaine	C	Procaine	B		
Methohexitone	C	Suxamethonium	C		
Thiopentone	C	Tetracaine	C		
		Tubocurarine	C		

* We are grateful to Prof. Sir Abraham Goldberg for permission to base this text on the comprehensive Report of the Porphyria Research Unit (Univ. of Glasgow), and to Dr M. R. Moore.

† Note that chloral is in one group and dichloralphenazone is in another; this is because of the phenazone component.

‡ Diazepam has been used safely in status epilepticus. Seizure prophylaxis: clonazepam and sodium valproate may be used, though sporadic reports of porphyrogenicity do exist.

natural environment and bred as well as the normal population until the introduction of barbiturates and sulphonamides. They are now at serious disadvantage, for many drugs can precipitate fatal acute attacks.

Apparently unexplained attacks of porphyria should be an indication for close enquiry into all possible chemical intake, e.g. surreptitious ingestion of mouthwash containing alcohol, eucalyptol, menthol, etc. caused attacks in one patient. Studies showed that the mouthwash, in particular the eucalyptol, induced hepatic ALA-synthase activity.*

Personality and habits. Not enough is known to enable any generalisations of practical utility to be made, but there is no doubt that the response to drugs acting on the central nervous system is influenced by personality.

It is a commonplace that the response to alcohol is different and characteristic for some individuals and this is probably a personality difference. Pavlov noted that dogs of 'excitatory' temperament might need eight times as much sedative as dogs of 'inhibitory' temperament. Another prominent example is the response to placebo or dummy administration. It is also known that placebo-reactors are liable to respond atypically to other drugs and that the response to a drug may vary with alterations in mental state.

Alcohol and smoking induce drug metabolising enzymes and smokers have an increased liablity to thromboembolism from oral contraceptives. *Diet* (nutrition) has already been mentioned.

* Bickers D R. et al. N Engl Med 1975; 292:1115.

Factors extrinsic to the patient

The prescriber. It is obvious that the choice of drug and the skill with which it is used will have an important bearing on the occurrence of adverse reactions. There can be no doubt that many avoidable, and so unnecessary, adverse reactions occur from low standards of skill and knowledge and lack of a sense of professional responsibility†.

The environment. Significant environmental factors causing adverse reactions to drugs include

† Examples can be found in the annual reports of the medical protection organisations.

simple pollution by drugs, for example halothane in the air of surgical operating theatres causing abortions amongst female staff, penicillin in the air of hospitals or in the milk of cows treated for mastitis, causing allergy.

Drug effects may also be modified by hepatic enzyme induction from insecticide accumulation (DDT) and from alcohol and the tobacco habit.

Antimicrobials used in feeds of animals for human consumption have given rise to concern in relation to the spread of resistant bacteria that may affect man.

Drug factors

Factors intrinsic to the drug. These include:

Side-effects, i.e. effects that are an inevitable part of the pharmacological action of the drug at therapeutic doses, but which are undesired, e.g. drowsiness from phenobarbitone when used against epilepsy, vomiting with digoxin or morphine, respiratory depression from morphine, hypokalaemia from thiazide diuretics, failure of ejaculation with adrenergic neurone blocking drugs, and so on.

Secondary effects are the indirect consequences of a primary drug action. Examples are vitamin deficiency or opportunistic infection which may occur in patients whose normal bowel flora has been altered by antibiotics; diuretic-induced hypokalaemia causing digoxin intolerance; the Herxheimer reaction (probably due to products released by killed organisms, usually spirochaetes) is another type of secondary effect.

Toxicity. Toxic effects are due to a direct action of the drug, often at high dose, and a damaging effect on tissue is implied, for example liver damage from paracetamol overdose or from a non-steroidal anti-inflammatory drug, eighth cranial nerve damage from gentamicin. All drugs, for practical purposes, are toxic in overdose and *overdose can be absolute or relative*; in the latter case an ordinary dose may be administered but may be toxic due to an underlying abnormality in the patient, for example, disease of the liver or kidney. Mutagenicity, carcinogenicity and teratogenicity (see index) can be regarded as special cases of toxicity.

Choice of drug. Inappropriate choice can obviously be a cause of adverse reactions. It is in the hands of the prescriber.

Use of the drug. The technique of use of a drug can be important. It also is in the hands of the prescriber; obviously, unskilled administration of general anaesthetics or anticancer drugs, however well chosen, is more serious than unskilled administration of correctly chosen penicillin.

Drug regulatory authorities that collect and evaluate spontaneously reported adverse reactions seldom have information to allow them to determine whether an adverse reaction should be primarily attributed to the prescriber's choice or skill and so regarded as avoidable, rather than inherent to the drug and unavoidable.

Interactions between drugs: see p. 144.

Allergy in response to drugs

Allergic reactions to drugs are the resultant of the interaction of drug or metabolite (or a non-drug element in the formulation) with patient and disease, and subsequent re-exposure.

Lack of previous exposure is not the same as lack of *history* of previous exposure. Exposure is not necessarily medical, e.g. penicillins occur in dairy products following treatment of cattle, and penicillin antibodies are commonly present in those who deny having received the drug.

Immune responses to drugs may be harmful (allergy) or harmless; the fact that antibodies are produced does not mean a patient will necessarily respond to re-exposure with clinical manifestations; most of our population have antibodies to penicillins, but, fortunately, comparatively few are allergic to them.

Whilst macromolecules (proteins, peptides, dextran polysaccharides) can act as complete antigens, most drugs are simple chemicals (mol. wt. less than 1000) and act as *incomplete antigens or haptens*, which become complete antigens in combination with a body protein.

The chief target organs of drug allergy are the skin, respiratory tract, gastrointestinal tract, the blood and the blood vessels.

Drugs may elicit allergic reactions of all principal types:

Type I reactions. *Immediate-type* (anaphylactic). The drug causes formation of tissue-sensitising antibodies that are fixed to mast cells or leucocytes; on subsequent administration the allergen (conjugate of drug or metabolite) reacts with these antibodies, activating but not damaging the cell to which they are fixed and causing release of pharmacologically active substances, e.g. histamine, leukotrienes, prostaglandins, platelet-activating factor, and causing effects such as urticaria, anaphylactic shock and asthma. Allergy develops within minutes and lasts 1–2 hours.

Type II reactions. *Autoallergy*. The drug or metabolite combines with a protein in the body so that the body no longer recognises the protein as self, treats it as a foreign protein and forms antibodies, e.g. methyldopa or penicillin-induced haemolytic anaemia.

Type III reactions. Antigen and antibody form large complexes and activate complement. Small blood vessels are damaged or blocked. Leucocytes attracted to the site of reaction engulf the immune complexes and release pharmacologically active substances (including lysosomal enzymes), starting an inflammatory process. These reactions include serum sickness, glomerulonephritis, vasculitis and pulmonary disease.

Type IV reactions. *Delayed type* (*cell-mediated*) *allergy* in which antigen-specific receptors develop on T-lymphocytes. Subsequent administration leads to a local or tissue allergic reaction, e.g. contact dermatitis.

Cross-allergy within a group of drugs is usual.

Why allergy is commoner with some drugs, e.g. penicillins, than with others and why the same drug produces different effects in different people is unknown; a genetic basis in the host is likely. In addition, patients with allergic diseases, e.g. eczema, are more likely to develop allergy to drugs.

Assem* has summarised *distinctive* (*though not invariable*) *features of allergic reactions to drugs*:

1. no correlation with known pharmacological properties of the drug,

2. no linear relation with drug dose (very small doses may cause very severe effects),

3. often include rashes, angioedema, serum sickness syndrome, anaphylaxis and asthma; characteristics of classical protein allergy,

4. require an induction period on primary exposure, but not on re-exposure,

5. disappear on cessation of administration and reappear on re-exposure to a small dose,

6. occur in a minority of patients receiving the drug,

7. desensitisation may be possible.

Principal clinical manifestations of drug allergy and their treatment (with adrenocortical steroid, histamine H_1-receptor blocker and adrenaline).

1. **Urticarial rashes and angioneurotic oedema** (Types I, III). These are probably the commonest type of drug allergy. They are usually accompanied by itching. The eyelids, lips and face are usually most affected; oedema of the larynx is rare but may be fatal if tracheostomy is not done. The itching oedematous lesions are due to the liberation of histamine, etc. in the skin. Such reactions may be generalised, but frequently are worst in and and around the area of administration of the drug. They respond to adrenaline (i.m. if urgent), ephedrine, H_1-receptor antihistamines and adrenal steroids.

2. **Non-urticarial rashes** (Types I, II, IV) occur in great variety; frequently they are weeping exudative lesions. It is often difficult to be sure when a rash is due to a drug. Apart from stopping the responsible drug, treatment is non-specific; in severe cases an adrenal steroid should be tried. Skin sensitisation to antibiotics may be very troublesome, especially amongst those who handle them. See *drugs and the skin*.

3. **Anaphylactic shock** (Type I). It occurs with penicillin, horse serum passive immunisation and a huge variety of other drugs. The combination of antigen with antibody on the cells is followed by release of histamine and other substances from basophils or mast cells, with a severe fall in blood pressure, bronchoconstriction, angioedema (including larynx) and sometimes death due to loss of fluid from the intravascular compartment. Anaphylactic shock usually occurs suddenly, in less than an hour after the drug, but within

* Assem E-S K. In: Davies D M, ed Textbook of adverse drug reactions. London: Oxford University Press, 1981.

minutes if it has been given i.v. Treatment is urgent. *First* 0.5–1.0 ml of Adrenaline Inj. (1 mg/ml: 1 in 1000) should be given i.m.* to raise the blood pressure and to dilate the bronchi; it may be repeated after 3 min according to the clinical condition. Noradrenaline would ordinarily be preferred to constrict the dilated arterioles and veins (α effect), but it lacks any useful bronchodilator action (β effect) and adrenaline is the best compromise in this emergency. The adrenaline should be accompanied by an H_1-receptor antihistamine (say, chlorpheniramine 10 mg i.v.) and hydrocortisone (100 mg i.m. or i.v.). The adrenal steroid may be of benefit by reducing vascular permeability and by suppressing further response to the antigen–antibody reaction. Benefit from an adrenal steroid is not immediate; it is unlikely to begin for 30 min and takes hours to reach its maximum. Any ward or other place where anaphylaxis may be expected should have all the drugs and tools necessary to deal with it in one convenient kit, for when they are needed there is little time to think and none to run about from place to place.

A reaction is said to be *anaphylactoid* if it clinically resembles anaphylactic shock but does not have an immunological basis, i.e. it is a *pseudo-allergic reaction* (p. 170).

4. **Pulmonary reactions: asthma** (Type I). The antigen–antibody reaction causes local liberation of substances, including histamine, which cause contraction of smooth muscle. Stimulation of the bronchial muscle may result in an asthmatic attack which can be fatal. 0.25 to 1.0 ml of Adrenaline Inj. (1 mg/ml) s.c., will usually cut short an attack; the other treatments for asthma are also effective.

Organic dusts (e.g. posterior pituitary powder taken by insufflation for diabetes insipidus, as well as dusts met occupationally) cause not only asthma, but also syndromes resembling acute and chronic lung infections.

5. **The serum-sickness syndrome** (Type III) occurs about 1 to 3 weeks after administration. Treatment is by an adrenal steroid, and as above if there is urticaria.

6. **Blood disorders:**†

a. **Thrombocytopenia** (Type II, but also pseudo-allergic; see p. 170) due to drugs is not common except with apronal (Sedormid) which is deservedly obsolete, but it has been reported occasionally after a large number of drugs, including phenylbutazone, gold, sulphonamides, quinine, quinidine, antimitotic agents, phenazone, rifampicin, tetracycline, PAS, phenobarbitone, thiourea derivatives, thiazides, oestrogens, digitoxin. Adrenal steroids may help.

b. **Granulocytopenia** (Type II, but also pseudo-allergic) sometimes leading to agranulocytosis, is a very serious, though rare, allergy which may occur with many drugs, e.g. chloramphenicol, sulphonamides including diuretic and hypoglycaemic derivatives, colchicine, gold, anticonvulsants, methyldopa, etc. Amidopyrine and derivatives are notorious in this respect and need never be used, as there are adequate substitutes. Treatment of agranulocytosis involves both stopping the drug responsible and giving a *bactericidal* drug (e.g. penicillin) to treat or prevent infection. If the blood picture does not rapidly improve following withdrawal of the drug an adrenal steroid plus an androgen (e.g. fluoxymesterone) should be given in severe granulocytopenia and in all cases of agranulocytosis, but proof of its beneficial effect is naturally hard to get.

c. **Aplastic anaemia** (Type II, but not always immunological). About 50% of cases of aplastic anaemia may be drug-induced. Chloramphenicol is the most important cause but others include sulphonamides and derivatives (diuretics, antidiabetics), phenylbutazone, hydantoin anticonvulsants, gold, perchlorate and some insecticides, e.g. dicophane (DDT). In the case of chloramphenicol, bone marrow depression is a normal pharmacological effect of the drug, although aplastic anaemia may also be due to idiosyncrasy or allergy.

* Not s.c. for the intense local vasoconstriction added to the low blood pressure will result in low tissue perfusion and so in delayed absorption. In extreme urgency 0.5 ml diluted × 10 may be given slowly i.v. It can cause ventricular fibrillation, but this may be thought to be the lesser risk.

† Where cells are being destroyed in the periphery and production is normal, transfusion is useless or nearly so, as the transfused cells will be destroyed, though in an emergency even a short cell life (platelets, erythrocytes) may tip the balance usefully. Where the bone marrow is depressed, transfusion is useful as the tranfused cells will survive normally.

Death occurs in about 50% of cases, and treatment is as for agranulocytosis, with, obviously, blood transfusion.

d. **Haemolysis** of all kinds is included here for convenience. There are three principal categories.

(i) *Dose-related pharmacological action on normal cells*, e.g. lead, benzene, phenylhydrazine, chlorates, methyl chloride (refrigerant), some snake venoms.

(ii) *Idiosyncrasy* — cells are genetically defective in the enzyme glucose-6-phosphate dehydrogenase and haemolyse readily in the presence of oxidant drugs such as 8-aminoquinoline antimalarials (primaquine, pentaquin, pamaquine), quinine, sulphonamide, sulphones, nitrofurans (nitrofurantoin, furazolidone), phenacetin, aspirin and other antipyretic analgesics, PAS, ascorbic acid, probenecid, fava beans. The defect is commonest in blacks, Sephardic Jews and Filipinos. Characteristically there is an acute haemolytic episode 2–3 days after starting the drug. The haemolysis is self-limiting, only older cells with least enzyme being affected.

(iii) *Allergy* (Type II) occurs with methyldopa, levodopa, phenacetin, PAS, penicillin, quinine, quinidine, sulphasalazine and organic antimony. It may be that in some of these cases a drug–protein–antigen/antibody interaction involves eythrocytes casually, i.e. a true 'innocent bystander' phenomenon.

Precipitation of a haemolytic crisis may also occur with the above drugs in the rare chronic haemolytic states due to unstable haemoglobins.

Treatment is to withdraw the drug, and an adrenal steroid is useful in severe cases if the mechanism is immunological. Blood transfusion may be needed.

7. **Fever** (mechanisms obscure). Treatment is to stop the drug.

8. **Syndromes resembling the collagen diseases** (Type II) are sometimes caused by drugs, e.g. hydralazine, procainamide, isoniazid, anticonvulsants, sulphonamides. Adrenal steroids are useful.

9. **Hepatitis and cholestatic jaundice** are sometimes allergic (Type II, see *drugs and the liver*). Adrenal steroids may be useful.

10. **Nephropathy** of various kinds (Types II, III) occur as does damage to other organs, e.g. myocarditis. Adrenal steroid may be useful.

Diagnosis of drug allergy is still largely on clinical criteria, history, type of reaction, response to withdrawal and systemic rechallenge (if thought safe to do so).

Simple skin testing is naturally most useful in diagnosing contact dermatitis, but it is unreliable for other allergies; also it is not necessarily safe and can cause anaphylactic shock.

Detection of drug-specific circulating antibodies only proves that an immunological response has occurred; it does not prove clinical allergy. Development of reliable *in vitro* predictive tests (e.g. employing human tissue or leucocytes) is a matter of considerable importance, not merely to avoid hazard to patients but to avoid depriving them of a drug that may be useful, for drug allergy, once it has occurred, is not necessarily permanent, e.g. less than 50% of patients giving a history of allergy to penicillin have a reaction if it is given again.

Hyposensitisation. Once a patient becomes allergic to a drug, it is better that he should never again come into contact with it. However, this can be inconvenient, for instance in allergy to antituberculosis drugs both in patients and in nurses. Such people can be hyposensitised by giving very small amounts of allergen, which are then gradually increased (usually every few hours) until a normal dose is tolerated. This may have to be done under cover of either an H_1-receptor antihistamine or of an adrenal steroid, or both, to prevent reactions during the procedure. A full kit for treating anaphylactic shock should be handy.

The ease and safety of hyposensitisation varies with different drugs; penicillin is troublesome and antituberculosis drugs generally less so.

The mechanism underlying hyposensitisation is not understood but may involve the production by the patient of blocking antibodies that compete successfully for the allergen but whose combination with it is innocuous. Sometimes allergy is to an ingredient of the preparation other than the essential drug and merely changing the preparation is sufficient. Impurities are sometimes responsible and purified forms of penicillins have been shown to induce fewer reactions than standard forms.

Prevention of allergic reactions is important since they are unpleasant and may be fatal. Patients should always be told when they are thought to be allergic to a drug, and it is essential that if a patient says he is allergic to some drug then that drug should *not* be given without careful testing. But if the drug *must* be given these are precautions, e.g. rapid (rush) hyposensitisation with prophylactic drugs as above.

Assumption that patients are all either ignorant or stupid has caused deaths: a young man was admitted to hospital for an interval appendicectomy, but had a sore throat and slight fever. The house surgeon said this would soon clear up with penicillin, but the patient at once protested, saying that he was seriously allergic to penicillin. The doctor said that in that case he would use another drug, but in fact he gave penicillin and the patient died from anaphylactic shock.*†

A doctor has also been known, when choosing an alternative drug to avoid a reaction, to prescribe inadvertently another drug from the same group, because the proprietary name gave no indication of the nature of the drug; another good reason for adopting the commonsense system of one drug, one sensible non-proprietary name.

Repeated blood counts in patients taking drugs known to cause *allergic* blood disorders, especially agranulocytosis, appear at first sight to be desirable, but as the onset is ordinarily sudden they commonly fail to give protection and may give a false sense of security.‡ In addition, spontaneous fluctuations in the number of granulocytes make the interpretation of such counts difficult, especially in children. Routine blood counts are probably not worth doing§ except with drugs having a particularly high incidence, when they can provide some protection by allowing early diagnosis (if done often enough, at least weekly). The best protection is to tell the patient to report at once any fever, enlarged glands or sore throat‖ (evidence of infection) and to stop taking the drug until he has had advice. Unfortunately, this can lead to frequent interruption of therapy in nervous patients. Although innumerable drugs are capable of causing blood disorders, antithyroid drugs, phenylbutazone, gold and prolonged courses of sulphonamides are particularly notorious. A few drugs, such as amidopyrine and phenazone, have been abandoned because of the risk of blood disorders, and courses of others, such as chloramphenicol, are kept short for this reason.

The only way completely to prevent allergic reactions to drugs is to cease to use drugs; but at least the unnecessary use of drugs for trival complaints should be avoided.

* Quoted in: Rosenheim M L. et al., eds. Sensitivity reactions to drugs. Oxford: Blackwell Scientific Publications, 1958.

† Failure to ask a patient about previous adverse reaction to penicillin before starting treatment has been judged negligent in the courts.

‡ *Not* a sense of false security.

§ Though where a drug that causes bone marrow depression as a pharmacological dose-related effect (rather than because of idiosyncrasy or allergy) blood counts are part of the essential routine monitoring of therapy, e.g. anticancer drugs.

‖ Though one patient's agranulocytosis was first manifested clinically by an acute infection of pre-existing haemorrhoids.

Pseudo-allergic reactions

These are effects that mimic allergic reactions but have no immunological basis; they are largely genetically determined and are due to release of endogenous biologically active substances, e.g. histamine or leukotrienes, by the drug, probably through a variety of mechanisms, direct and indirect, including complement activation leading to formation of polypeptides that affect mast cells as in true immunological reactions.

Pseudo-allergic effects mimicking Type I reactions (above) are called *anaphylactoid*, and they occur with aspirin and other non-steroidal anti-inflammatory drugs (indirect action as above): corticotrophin (direct histamine release): i.v. anaesthetics and a variety of other drugs i.v. — morphine, tubocurarine, dextran, radiographic contrast media — and cromoglycate (inhaled).

Type II reactions are mimicked by the haemolysis induced by drugs (antimalarials, sulphonamides and oxidizing agents) and fava beans in subjects with inherited abnormalities of erythrocyte enzymes or haemoglobin.

Type III reactions are mimicked by nitrofurantoin (pneumonitis) and penicillamine (nephropathy). Lupus erythematosus due to drugs (procainamide, isoniazid, phenytoin) may be pseudo-allergic.

Miscellaneous adverse reactions

Reaction to *intravenous injections* are fairly common — hypotension, renal pain, rigors and fever may occur, especially if the injection is very rapid. Some are due to foreign substances in the solutions and some just due to excessive speed causing a transient very high blood level in, say the brain.

Toxicity to the eye. Toxic *cataract* can be due to chloroquine (retina also affected) and related drugs, adrenal steroids (topical and systemic), phenothiazines, naphthalene, carbromal, ergot, dinitrophenol, galactose, lactose, paradichlorobenzene and alkylating agents. *Corneal opacities* occur with amiodarone, phenothiazines and chloroquine. *Retinal* injury with thioridazine (particularly, of the neuroleptics), chloroquine and indomethacin.

Drugs and the embryo/fetus

Drugs may act on the embryo/fetus:

1. *Directly* (thalidomide, anticancer drugs, antithyroid drugs): any drug affecting cell division, enzymes, protein synthesis, or DNA synthesis, is a potential teratogen, e.g. all antibiotics except penicillin.
2. *Indirectly*:
   (a) on the placenta (vitamin A, isotretinoin, 5-HT)
   (b) on the uterus (vasoconstrictors reduce blood supply and cause fetal anoxia);
   (c) on the mother's hormone balance and biochemistry;
   (d) on the father's sperm (uncertain).

Tests in animals are poor predictors for man. Proposals to do tests on pregnant women who await abortion have met with both practical and ethical problems.

Passage of drugs into the fetus. The placenta is not simply a passive 'barrier' between mother and fetus. The majority of substances essential for fetal growth (e.g. amino acids) are transferred actively *against* a concentration gradient. However, drugs administered to the mother pass across principally by passive diffusion *down* a concentration gradient. For practical purposes the placental 'barrier' may be considered equivalent to the blood–brain 'barrier'. The principal property affecting transfer is solubility in lipids (see *pharmacokinetics*), and lipid-soluble drugs pass rapidly into the fetus. Drugs that are relatively insoluble in lipids will, if present in high concentration, eventually enter the fetus. But the rate (i.e. amount of drug in unit time) is slow and single moderate doses to the mother may leave the fetus unaffected, e.g. tubocurarine given as a muscle relaxant during Caesarian section does not affect the infant, whereas used in high doses over a prolonged period to control convulsions it has resulted in a paralysed infant. Thus accurate prediction of entry into the fetus depends on knowledge of the rate of transfer and the dose and duration of administration. Since maternal erythrocytes and immune globulins have been shown to enter the fetus, it is plain that any drug may do so.

Once a drug is in the fetus its kinetics may differ from those in the mother (see *age and drug action*), and the drug and its metabolites may persist due to undeveloped metabolic and excretory processes, e.g. CNS depressants given to the mother may persist in the baby for days after birth.

Fetal therapeutics. *Syphilis* is treated *in utero* by giving penicillin to the mother.

Enzyme inducers (e.g. phenobarbitone, alcohol) are also effective in the fetus and can be given to the mother before labour to enhance the ability of the newborn to conjugate free bilirubin (by inducing the hepatic enzyme glucuronyl transferase) and so to prevent kernicterus (see *enzyme induction*).

Early pregnancy. If drugs can enter the fetus it is not surprising that they are capable of modifying development in the early stages before a placenta has developed (embryo) and when the organs are being formed (organogenesis). The most vulnerable period for major abnormality, i.e. *teratogenesis* (teratos = monster) is weeks 3–10 of intrauterine life, which corresponds to about 5–12 weeks after the first day of the last menstruation. Before that time drugs are likely to cause abortion and after it the organs are formed and abnormalities are less anatomically dramatic; thus the activity of a teratogen is most devastating soon after implantation, at a time when the woman may not know she is pregnant.

Selective interference can produce characteristic abnormalities, and this was one factor that caused thalidomide to be so readily recognised; the others were the previous rarity of phocomelia and the widespread use of the drug.

Teratogenic effects can occur at doses that do not harm the mother and they are associated with increased intra-uterine mortality, i.e. if the abnormality is gross enough, abortion occurs.

Drugs known to be teratogenic include anti-cancer drugs, warfarin, alcohol, adrenocortical steroids and isotretinoin.

Drugs probably teratogenic include antiepileptics and sex hormones in general. Tobacco smoking retards growth; it does not cause anatomical abnormalities in man as far as is known.

Innumerable drugs including aspirin, gastric antacids, co-trimoxazole, iron, neuroleptics, benzodiazepines and diuretics have come under suspicion.

Naturally the subject is a highly emotional one for prospective parents. Much depends on dose and stage of pregnancy. A definitive list of drugs is not practicable; the topic must be followed in the current literature.

Late pregnancy. Because the important organs are already formed, drugs will not cause the gross anatomical defects that can occur when they are given in early pregnancy. Administration of hormones, androgens or progestogens, can cause fetal masculinisation; iodide and antithyroid drugs in high dose can cause fetal goitre, as can lithium; tetracyclines can interfere with tooth and bone development.

Inhibitors of prostaglandin synthetase (aspirin, indomethacin) may delay onset of labour and, in the fetus, it is possible they may interfere with cardiovascular function (maintenance of a patent ductus arteriosus is dependent on prostaglandins, which relax the ductus muscle).

It is probable that drug allergy in the mother can also occur in the fetus and it is possible that the fetus may be sensitised where the mother shows no effect, e.g. neonatal thrombocytopenia from thiazide diuretics used in toxaemia of pregnancy.

Other drugs suspected of harming the fetus at some stage include anticoagulants, sulphonamides and oral antidiabetics; aminoglycoside damage to the fetal eighth nerve is rare, if it occurs.

The suggestion that congenital cataract (due to denaturation of lens protein) might be due to drugs has some support in man, and aromatic compounds can cause cataract in animals. Chloroquine and chlorpromazine are concentrated in the fetal eye. Since both can cause retinopathy it would seem wise to avoid them in pregnancy if possible.

Throughout pregnancy if an anticoagulant is needed heparin is preferred (large mol. wt. so does not readily cross placenta) and because warfarin is teratogenic.

Drugs given just **prior to labour** can cause post-natal effects: reserpine (nasal discharge, costal retraction, lethargy, feeding difficulty); chloramphenicol collapse due to failure to conjugate); vasoconstrictors (fetal distress by reducing uterine blood supply): β-adrenoceptor blockers may impair fetal response to hypoxia; sulphonamides (displacement of bilirubin from plasma protein); anticoagulants (haemorrhage).

Babies born to mothers dependent on opioids may show a physical withdrawal syndrome.

Drugs given **during labour**. Any drug that depresses respiration in the mother can cause respiratory depression in the newborn; opioid analgesics are notorious in this respect, but there can also be difficulty with any sedatives and general anaesthetics; they may also cause fetal distress by reducing uterine blood flow, and prolong labour by depressing uterine muscle.

Drugs used to relax the uterus in premature labour, e.g. β-adrenoceptor agonists (isoxsuprine) may affect the fetal circulatory adjustments (closure of ductus arteriosus) that occur at birth. Diazepam (and other depressants) in high doses may cause hypotonia in the baby and possibly interfere with suckling. There remains the possibility of later behavioural effects due to delayed development of the central nervous system due to drugs used during pregnancy; such effects have been shown in animals, including impaired ability to learn their way around mazes if the mothers received drugs during pregnancy.

Detection and causality. Whilst anatomical abnormalities are the easiest to detect, growth retardation and behavioural disorders can result from drugs. There is also a substantial spontaneous background incidence in the community (up to 2%) so that the detection of a low-grade teratogen that increases the incidence of one of the commoner abnormalities presents an intimidating task (see p. 155). Also most teratogenic effects are probably multifactorial.

Detection of teratogens will be accomplished by combinations of the techniques previously described.

In this emotionally charged area it is indeed hard for the public and especially for parents of an affected child to grasp that:

'The concept of absolute safety of drugs needs to be demolished. It has been suggested that a particular antinauseant used in pregnancy (Debendox, Bendectin)* should have been taken off the market until it could be proved to be safe. In real life it can never be shown that a drug (or anything else) has no teratogenic activity at all, in the sense of never being a contributory factor in anybody under any circumstances. This concept can neither be tested nor proved.

'Let us suppose for example, that some agent doubles the incidence of a condition that has natural incidence of 1 in 10,000 births. If the hypothesis is true, then studying 20,000 pregnant women who have taken the drug and 20,000 who have not may yield respectively two cases and one case of the abnormality. It does not take a statistician to realise that this signifies nothing, and it may need ten times as many pregnant women (almost half a million) to produce a statistically significant result. This would involve such an extensive multicentre study that hundreds of doctors and hospitals have to participate. The participants then each tend to bend the protocol to fit in with their clinical customs and in the end it is difficult to assess the validity of the data. Alternatively, a limited geographical basis may be used, with the trial going on for many years. During this time other things in the environment change, so again the results would not command our confidence. If it were to be suggested that there was something slightly teratogenic in milk, the hypothesis would be virtually untestable.

'In practice we have to make up our minds which drugs may reasonably be given to pregnant women. Do we start from a position of presumed guilt or from one of presumed innocence? If the former course is chosen then we cannot give any drugs to pregnant women because we can never prove that they are completely free of teratogenic influence. It therefore seems that we must start from a position of presumed innocence and then take all possible steps to find out if the presumption is correct.

'Finally, we must put the matter in perspective by considering the benefit/risk ratio. The problem of prescription in pregnancy cannot be considered from the point of view of only one side of the equation. Drugs are primarily designed to do good, and if a pregnant woman is ill it is in the best interests of her baby and herself that she gets better as quickly as possible. This often means giving her drugs. We can argue about the necessity of giving drugs to prevent vomiting, but there is no argument about the need for treatment of women with meningitis, septicaemia or venereal disease.

'What we must try to avoid is medication by the media or prescription by politicians. A public scare about a well-tried drug will lead to wider use of less-tried alternatives. We do not want to be forced to practise the kind of defensive medicine that is primarily designed to avoid litigation. The best decisions for patients are made by well-informed doctors.'†

General discussion. Whilst everyone will wish to avoid giving to women drugs that have been shown to cause fetal abnormalities in animals, they will also properly be reluctant at present to accept the corollary that failure to induce such abnormalities in animals means that a drug is safe.

Human toxic effects not predicted from animal experiments are often reversible, but even the

* A combination of anticholinergic (dicyclomine, later omitted), antihistamine (doxylamine) and vitamin (pyridoxine).

† By permission from Smithells R W. In: Hawkins D F, ed. Drugs and pregnancy. Edinburgh: Churchill-Livingstone, 1983.

most optimistic enthusiast for drugs must shrink from the thought that his hand wrote a prescription resulting in a deformed, surviving baby.

Clinical data are, at present, inevitably open to doubt, and any list of suspected drugs must, so slight is our knowledge, become obsolete and misleading very quickly. This topic must, therefore, be followed in the periodical press and manufacturers' up-to-date Data Sheets.

It is possible that some drugs in common use may be undetected low-grade teratogens. In one retrospective (case-control) study of the drug consumption of mothers of infants with congenital abnormalities it was found that more of these took aspirin, antacids, amphetamine, barbiturates, iron, cough medicines and sulphonamides in early pregnancy than did those in the control group (mothers of infants without congenital abnormalities). The authors acknowledge that such studies do not give proof of cause, e.g. a drug may be taken to control symptoms of a disease that causes the abnormality. But they conclude that it would be wise to avoid these drugs (prescribed or self medication) on which suspicion falls unless there is a specific indication for them, not only during known pregnancy but also in any women of childbearing age in whom conception is likely; a counsel of perfection, perhaps.

The medical profession clearly has a grave duty to refrain from all inessential prescribing of drugs with, say, less than 10–15 years' widespread use behind them, for all women of childbearing age. It is not sufficient safeguard merely to ask a woman if she is or may be pregnant (the natural reluctance to broach this subject to unmarried women may, even in our permissive society, act as a salutary check to casual prescribing), but it will also be necessary to consider the possibility of a woman who evidently is not pregnant at the time of prescribing, becoming so whilst taking the drug.

Since morning sickness of pregnancy occurs during the time when the fetus is vulnerable, it is specially important to restrict drug therapy of this symptom to a minimum; but severe vomiting with its accompanying biochemical changes may itself harm the fetus.

Thus, before a drug is condemned as a cause of fetal damage, it is necessary to consider whether the disease for which it was given, or other intercurrent disease, might perhaps be responsible.

Since the only way to be certain whether a drug causes fetal damage in man is to test it in man, it is necessary that doctors should (a) suspect a drug-induced abnormality when it occurs and (b) report it to a central organisation (Committee on Safety of Medicines) or (c) to a national register of all birth defects (such a register ideally should be kept plus a full drug history of the mother from prior to conception). Unfortunately, none of these requirements is easily satisfied. Minor congenital abnormalities are common in the absence of drug therapy and some may be virtually undetectable, e.g. reduced intelligence or learning ability. Human frailty also causes any reporting system based on voluntary co-operation to be less than perfect. For example, the UK Committee on Safety of Medicines has found that when a letter exhorting doctors to report drug reactions is sent out, there is a large, but very short-lived increase in reports.

In addition, the more cautiously a new drug is introduced, the more difficult it is going to be to detect, by epidemiological methods, a capacity to cause fetal abnormality. This is especially so if the abnormality produced is already fairly common.

The possibility of fetal abnormalities resulting from drugs taken by the father exists but has only begun to be explored in animals.

GUIDE TO FURTHER READING

1 Dukes M N G, ed. Meyler's side effects of drugs. Amsterdam-Oxford: Excerpta Medica, 1975 and subsequent annual volumes. Standard comprehensive reference work.

2 Editorial. Deaths due to drug treatment. Br Med J 1977; 2:1492.

3 Greenberg G et al. Maternal drug histories and congenital abnormalities. Br Med J 1977; 2:853.

4 Editorial. Vaginal adenocarcinomas and maternal oestrogen administration. Lancet 1974; 1:250.

5 Von Felsinger J M et al. Drug-induced mood changes in man. Personality and reactions to drugs. JAMA 1955; 157:1113.

6 Jick H. Drugs — remarkably non-toxic. N Engl J Med 1974; 291:824.

7 Hurwitz N. Predisposing factors in adverse reactions to

drugs. Br Med J 1969; 1:536. Admission to hospital due to drugs, 539.
8 Scott J L et al. A controlled double-blind study of the hematologic toxicity of chloramphenicol. N Engl J Med 1965; 272:1137.
9 Shapiro S et al. Common drugs responsible for deaths in hospital. JAMA 1971; 216:467.
10 Klotz U et al. The effects of age and liver disease on the disposition of diazepam in adult man. J Clin Invest 1975; 55:347.
11 Editorial. Drugs and the elderly. Lancet 1977; 2:693.
12 Show S M et al. Need for supervision in the elderly receiving long-term prescribed medication. Br Med J 1976; 1:505.
13 Parker C W. Drug allergy. N Engl J Med 1975; 292: 511, 732, 957.
14 Smith A P Response of aspirin-allergic patients to challenge by some analgesics in common use. Br Med J 1971; 1:494.
15 Black S. Inhibition of immediate-type hypersensitivity response by direct suggestion under hypnosis. Br Med J 1963:1:925.
16 Austen K F. Systemic anaphylaxis in the human being. N Engl J Med 1974; 291:661.
17 Bickers D R et al. Exacerbation of hereditary hepatic porphyria by surreptitious ingestion of an unusual provocative agent — a mouthwash preparation. N Engl J Med 1975; 292:1115.
18 Lamon J M et al. Prevention of acute porphyric attacks by i.v. haematin. Lancet 1978; 2:492.
19 Heinonen O P et al. Cardiovascular birth defects and antenatal exposure to female sex hormones. N Engl J Med 1977; 296:67.
20 Kygegombe D et al. Drug metabolizing enzymes in the human placenta, their induction and depression. Lancet 1973; 1:405.
21 Editorial. Noxious transplacental influences. Lancet 1974; 1:1267.
22 Ferber E. Chemical carcinogenesis. N Engl J Med 1981; 305:1379.
23 Kalter H et al. Congenital malformations. N Engl J Med 1983; 308: 424, 491.
24 Hemminki K et al. Spontaneous abortions in hospital staff engaged in sterilising instruments with chemical agents. Br Med J 1982; 285:1461.
25 Kramer M S et al. An algorithm for the operational assessment of adverse drug reactions. JAMA 1979; 242:623.
26 Inman W H W. Postmarketing surveillance of adverse drug reactions in general practice. Br Med J 1981; 282: 1131, 1216.
27 Rawlins M D. Postmarketing surveillance of adverse reaction to drugs. Br. Med J 1984; 288:879.
28 Editorial. Adverse drug reactions. Br Med J 1981; 282:1819.
29 Temple R J et al. Adverse effects of newly marketed drugs. N Engl J Med 1979; 300:1046.

10

Drug overdose, poisoning and antidotes

The principles of treatment, and miscellaneous antidotes and poisons are dealt with in this chapter. The management of poisoning due to therapeutic agents is largely dealt with in the appropriate chapter (see index).

Deliberate self-poisoning. Formerly, most of those who poisoned themselves were seriously trying to commit suicide. A curious by-product of the modern 'drug and prescribing explosion' is that this is no longer so and 'self-poisoning' flourishes, 'since few who practice it have minds set on dying' (parasuicide), and live to give another display as they often do ('repeaters').* 'To take tablets knowing that this will remain undiscovered for many hours is a very different matter from promptly entering the living room and brandishing the offending bottle before the assembled family's startled gaze.'†

* An extreme example is that of a young man who, over a period of six years, was admitted to hospital following 82 episodes of self-poisoning, 31 employing paracetamol; he had had a disturbed, unhappy upbringing and had been expelled from both the Danish Navy and the British Army. Prescott L F et al. Br Med J 1978; 2:1399

† Kessel N Br Med J 1965; 2:1265, 1336.

More than one in every thousand of the adult population of Edinburgh have been admitted to hospital each year after an act of self-poisoning. Drugs are used in more than 90% of instances, chiefly benzodiazepines, antidepressants, paracetamol and aspirin. Forty-five years ago domestic coal gas and corrosives, e.g. lysol, accounted for the majority of cases. Domestic gas is now the relatively non-toxic natural gas (methane) replacing the toxic coal gas (carbon monoxide).

The mortality rate of self-poisoning is very low, less than 1% of acute hospital admissions, and 'completed' suicides occur chiefly among the despondent elderly, whilst parasuicide flourishes amongst the young, often using drugs prescribed for another member of the family.

Accidental self-poisoning causing admission to hospital occurs predominantly amongst children under five years, usually with medicines left within reach and less often with domestic chemicals, e.g. bleach (calcium hypochlorite), detergents. The introduction of child-resistant packaging (containers requiring special manoeuvres, and strip or blister packaging of individual tablets) has been accompanied by a substantial fall in hospital admissions of small children. Unfortunately the arthritic elderly are also liable to be defeated by such packaging.

SOME ASPECTS OF ACUTE POISONING

For centuries it was supposed not only that there could be, but that there actually was, a single antidote to all poisons. This was Theriaca Andromachi, a formulation of 72 (a magical number) ingredients amongst which particular importance was attached to the flesh of a snake (viper). The antidote was devised by Andromachus, whose son was physician to the Roman Emperor, Nero* (AD 54–68).

In practice most emergency treatment of acute poisoning is symptomatic and not specific to the poison, success depending on a combination of speed and common sense as well as on the nature of the poison, the amount taken and the time that has since elapsed. Where there is a specific antidote, its use can be vital, e.g. naloxone against opioid drugs, N-acetylcysteine against paracetamol, desferrioxamine against iron.

It is essential that the immediate aim be clear, for without this, treatment will not combine maximum efficiency with minimum risk. In poisoning by a CNS depressant, for example, the aim is to keep the patient oxygenated, to sustain circulation and electrolyte balance until the poison has been eliminated, and to prevent pneumonia. It is *not* to wake the patient up at once, for this, though satisfying to the physician, may be impossible to achieve without poisoning him or her with convulsant drugs.

In the UK the centres of the National Poisons Information Service† provide information and advice over the telephone throughout the day and night.

The principles of treatment may be stated thus:

1. Identification of the poison(s)

The following may assist: the circumstances in which the subject is found, e.g. with a labelled medicine container; some clinical features, e.g. overbreathing (salicylate toxicity); chemical analysis of plasma, urine or gastric aspirate. A thin-layer chromatography system that is capable or identifying a wide range of drugs in biological fluids (Toxilab) can provide an answer within 6 hours. When poisoning is due to deliberate self-administration the history that the patient gives is often unreliable, which is hardly surprising.

2. Prevention of further absorption of the poison

A. *External*: wash with water, sodium bicarbonate, vinegar, alcohol, as appropriate.

B. *From the gut*:

(i) by *gastric lavage* (using a cuffed endotracheal tube if the patient is unconscious). Whether or not this procedure is used depends on the assessment of each case but it should be adopted if a potentially toxic dose has been ingested within the past 5 hours, or 8–12 hours with salicylates or drugs with anticholinergic activity e.g. tricyclic antidepressants, for these delay gastric emptying. It has been suggested that of patients who are subjected to this unpleasant experience, it is unnnecessary in 50%. It is however easier to decide retrospectively that gastric lavage was unnecessary because the overdose was small or the substance innocuous than to face a possible challenge of negligently failing to undertake a potentially life-saving procedure. Conscious children should rarely if ever be subjected to gastric lavage. The technique of lavage (with repeated small volumes) is important but will not be considered here. The chief danger is aspiration into the lungs. When it is thought necessary to pass a stomach tube, this may have to take second place to emergency resuscitative measures, controlled respiration or suppression of convulsions. Nothing is gained by aspirating the stomach of a corpse.

(ii) *by emesis*, in conscious patients only, especially if solids (e.g. berries), which might block a gastric tube, have been eaten. Vomiting may be induced by oral ipecacuanha* (contains emetine, a centrally active emetic). Of other options, saline solution is dangerous and has

* A remarkable man whose subjects believed him to be a god. He even believed it himself, with results that were as inevitable as they were disastrous. His conduct soon caused him to have an urgent need for a universal antidote, 'But the domestic infelicities of the Caesars are no part of our present story. The reader greedy for criminal particulars must go to the classical source, Suetonius' (Wells H G. The Outline of History. 1920, revised 1931).

† For telephone numbers see British National Formulary (BNF).

‡ *Ipecacuanha Emetic Mixture, Paediatric* (BNF) is used for adults as well as for children: dose — adults, 30 ml; child, (6–18mths), 10 ml; older children, 15 ml: followed by a drinking glass of water and repeated (once only) after 20 min if vomiting has not occurred. Some ipecacuanha preparations are as much as × 15 stronger. It is *vital* to choose the correct preparation.

induced fatal hypernatraemia. Apomorphine may depress the CNS or cause intractable vomiting and shock. Copper sulphate is dangerous.

The amount of drug recovered will obviously vary with the time since the episode and with the vigour of vomiting, but more than 30% of recovery cannot be counted on. The advantage of emesis is that it can be done on first seeing the patient, whereas gastric aspiration and lavage should be done in hospital. Ipecacuanha can cause prolonged unpleasant vomiting.

Mechanically induced vomiting, by putting the patient's *own* fingers down his or her throat is less effective.

Both emesis and lavage are *contraindicated* for corrosive poisons (increased corrosion leading to perforation), and petroleum distillates (inhalation chemical pneumonia).

(iii) *by oral adsorbents*. Activated charcoal (Medicoal, Carbomix) consists of a very fine black (carbonised) power prepared from vegetable matter (e.g. sawdust, coconut shell), it adsorbs indiscriminately and most efficiently; the adult dose is 5–10 g (with 100–200 ml water), repeated in 15–20 min up to a total of 50 g, or 5–10 times the estimated weight of ingested poison, whichever is the greater. More than 50 g total may cause vomiting. Charcoal is most beneficial for poisons that are toxic in small quantities, such as tricyclic antidepressants. Other substances adsorbed by activated charcoal include: aspirin, amphetamines, barbiturates, cocaine, carbamazepine, digoxin (cholestyramine is also effective), glutethimide, mercuric chloride, also paracetamol, phenothiazines, mercury salts, iodine, theophylline.

There is little risk in administering activated charcoal but note that:

a. it should be used *in addition to emesis*, which it in no sense replaces.

b. it should only be given after ipecacuanha has been effective, for it adsorbs that substance.

c. it may absorb other antidotes, such as methionine (for paracetamol poisoning).

Prolonged use is described as enteral dialysis (below).

3. Specific antidotes

Those agents that are readily available are listed and described later in this chapter. Use of specific antibodies to bind and so neutralise an administered toxic substance has made a first step with digoxin (see p. 532)

4. Acceleration of elimination of the poison

From the gut. Purgation, e.g. if sustained-release formulation is thought to remain after emesis.

From the blood. The techniques of diuresis with alteration of urine pH, dialysis and haemoperfusion are assumed to make a contribution to recovery when used *skilfully* in the *right* patients but they all have hazards and can themselves kill. Such techniques are appropriate in less than 5% of cases.

Diuresis with alteration of urine pH

The rationale is that most drugs are weak electrolytes and at physiological pH exist partly as ionised and partly as un-ionised molecules. Weak acids become more ionised (and less lipid soluble) in an alkaline environment, weak bases become more ionised (and less lipid soluble) in an acid environment and vice versa. Urine pH can be manipulated so that a drug is present in the tubular fluid predominantly in the ionised state. Being then lipid insoluble, it cannot diffuse back through the lipid membranes of the tubular cells, remains in the lumen and is eliminated in the urine.

Maintenance of a good urine flow helps this process and is desirable anyway, but the practice of forcing diuresis (with frusemide and i.v. fluid) in addition to alteration of urine pH is questionable on grounds of safety. In the treatment of aspirin (salicylate) overdose, simply infusing sodium bicarbonate intravenously to keep the urine alkaline is as at least as efficient as forced alkaline duiresis, and is probably safer. It is the alteration of urine pH rather than the fast urine flow that is important*.

Alteration of urine pH is a reasonable treatment technique for poisons that are:

* Prescott L F et al. Br Med J 1982; 285:1383.

a. acids of pKa 3.0–7.5 or bases of pKa 7.5–10.5.
b. distributed principally in the extracellular fluid.
c. not strongly protein bound.
d. normally eliminated in the urine

In practice, alteration of urine pH and diuresis should be considered and may be indicated for poisoning as follows:

Alkalinisation for aspirin (salicylate), phenobarbitone and phenoxyacetate herbicides (2,4-D; MCPA). The objective is to maintain a urine pH of 7.5–8.5 by intravenous infusion of sodium bicarbonate and urine pH should be checked at least hourly. Available preparations of sodium bicarbonate vary between 1.26–8.4% and the concentration given will depend on the patient's fluid needs and the urine flow that is desired. A flow of 3 ml/min is adequate and can be achieved by supplementing the sodium bicarbonate with infusion of dextrose 5% and correcting for hypokalaemia by adding potassium 10–20 mmol periodically.

In conscious cooperative subjects oral sodium bicarbonate will not only enhance elimination but also reduce absorption of any drug remaining in the gut.

Acidification for *phencyclidine* (also amphetamine and fenfluramine, but sedation alone is likely to be adequate).

The objective is to maintain a urine pH of 5.5–6.5 by giving ascorbic acid. In practice urinary acidification is rarely necessary (see also Table 10.1).

Peritoneal dialysis. Peritoneal dialysis involves instilling dialysis fluid into the peritoneal cavity. Poison in the blood enters the dialysis fluid, which is then drained and replaced. The technique is readily available because little equipment is needed but it depends on adequate peritoneal blood flow and becomes inefficient if the patient is hypotensive. Haemodialysis or haemoperfusion is substantially more effective.

Haemodialysis and haemoperfusion. Both haemodialysis and haemoperfusion involve establishing a temporary extracorporeal circulation, usually from an artery to a vein in the arm. In haemodialysis, a semipermeable membrane separates blood from dialysis fluid and the poison passes passively from the blood, where it is present in high concentration, into the fluid. The principle of haemoperfusion is that blood flows over activated charcoal or an appropriate ion-exchange resin, which adsorbs the poison. Loss of blood cells and activation of the clotting mechanism are largely overcome by coating the charcoal with an acrylic hydrogel that does not reduce adsorbing capacity, though the patient requires to be heparinised.

These techniques require for success that:

a. a substantial amount of the poison be present in the plasma water, i.e. the poison should have a relatively small apparent volume of distribution.

b. the poison should dissociate readily from any plasma protein binding sites.

c. the effects of the poison should relate to the plasma concentration.

d. the poison should readily pass through the dialysis membrane, or should be avidly adsorbed onto the charcoal or resin of the haemoperfusion column.

e. removal by haemoperfusion or dialysis should constitute a significant addition to natural methods of elimination.

Such artificial methods of removing poison from the body are invasive, demand skill and experience on the part of the operator and are expensive in manpower. Their use should therefore be confined to cases of severe, prolonged or progressive clinical intoxication when other methods have failed or when high plasma concentration indicates a dangerous degree of poisoning. Controlled trials of efficacy are, not surprisingly, lacking. Thrombocytopenia, leucopenia and loss of clotting factors may occur in the artificial circulation leading to the risk of infection or bleeding and the latter may be aggravated because heparin is given.

Indications for the use of elimination techniques based on plasma concentration* are summarised below and we are grateful to the authors and to the editor of the *British Medical Journal* for permission to publish this material.

* Vale J A, Meredith T, Buckley B. Br Med J 1984; 289:366.

Summary of selection of elimination techniques

*Salicylates**		
	>500 + metabolic acidosis >750 mg/l	Alkaline diuresis
	750–900 mg/l + renal failure >900 mg/l	Haemodialysis or haemoperfusion
Meprobamate	>100 mg/l	Haemoperfusion
Trichloroethanol derivatives (chloral hydrate, triclofos)	>50 mg/l	Haemoperfusion
*Phenobarbitone, barbitone**	>75–100 mg/l	Alkaline diuresis
	>100 mg/l	Alkaline diuresis, haemodialysis or haemoperfusion
	>150 mg/l	Haemodialysis or haemoperfusion
Other barbiturates	>50 mg/l	Haemoperfusion
Methanol, ethylene glycol	>0.5 g/l	Peritoneal dialysis or haemodialysis (Dialysis is indicated if more than 30 g has been ingested or there is metabolic acidosis, mental, visual or fundoscopic abnormality. Many antifreeze solutions now contain methanol as well as ethylene glycol)
Lithium	>5 mmol/l	Peritoneal dialysis or haemodialysis (Forced diuresis is ineffective and an infusion of sodium chloride is dangerous)
Theophylline	>60 mg/l	Haemoperfusion (Correction of hypokalaemia is most important and may obviate the need for haemoperfusion)

Enteral dialysis (*lavage*). This term is used for the practice of continuing administration of adsorbent activated charcoal, beyond the immediate need of binding a swallowed poison in the gut. The objective is to adsorb poison that diffuses into the gut from the blood and enters it in the bile (enterohepatic circulation). The full value of this practice has yet to be determined but it may accelerate elimination of aspirin (salicylate), theophylline and phenobarbitone even where they have been injected.

5. General supportive treatment is of prime importance

This cliché can be taken to mean measures directed towards maintaining circulation, respiration and electrolyte balance, and to preventing pneumonia in unconscious patients. The salient fact is that patients recover from most poisonings provided they are adequately oxygenated, hydrated and the vital organs adequately perfused, for in the majority of cases, the most efficient mechanisms of elimination are the patients' own and, given time, will remove all the poison.

Care may be summarised thus:

1. Treatment of the cause of unconsciousness, if possible.

2. Preservation of respiration and oxygenation, which may involve:

a. controlled ventilation.

b. prevention of *hypostatic pneumonia* by altering the posture of the patient regularly and by suction of airways as needed. It is better to watch for and then to treat pneumonia vigorously, than to use antimicrobials prophylactically.

c. treatment of *aspiration pneumonia* by airway clearance, early administration of methylprednisolone up to 30 mg/kg by i.v. infusion, bronchodilators and, if necessary, mechanical ventilation.

d. management of special problems created by the poisoning, e.g. respiratory centre depression (opioids), respiratory muscle spasm (strychnine, phencyclidine), respiratory muscle paralysis (anticholinesterase insecticides), adult respiratory distress syndrome (opioids, aspirin, barbiturates, paraquat), pulmonary oedema (β-adrenoceptor blockers, mexiletine, disopyramide).

3. Preservation of the circulation.

* NB: Haemodialysis or haemoperfusion are two or three times more efficient than forced diuresis or peritoneal dialysis.

a. poisoning not uncommonly causes *hypotension*, either through myocardial depression (β-adrenoceptor blockers, tricyclic antidepressants, dextropropoxyphene), peripheral vasodilatation (barbiturates) or fluid loss from hyperventilation, aspirin (salicylate) or vomiting. Measures that restore the circulation include elevation of the legs, correction of fluid deficit and infusion of colloid. If these fail, dopamine may be given, for it has both cardiac inotropic and renal vasodilating actions.

b. cardiac dysrhythmias are caused by many drugs (tricyclic antidepressants, digoxin, anticholinergics, phenothiazines, theophylline). Provided the cardiac output is maintained, it may be wiser not to treat a dysrhythmia than to risk adding to the patient's problem by giving antidysrhythmic drugs. Electrical pacing may be used.

c. resuscitation after *cardiac arrest* in poisoning should be continued for longer than is customary; fixed and widely dilated pupils may be due to the poison (tricyclic antidepressants, plants containing anticholinergic substances, e.g. deadly nightshade) or to hypothermia and not to irreversible cerebral anoxia.

4. Prevention of:

a. starvation, dehydration and electrolyte imbalance.

b. bladder distension.

c. hypothermia.

d. pressure sores.

ANTIDOTES

Readily available agents used for the listed indications appear in Table 10.1. We are grateful to Drs Meredith, Caisley and Volans and to the Editor of the *British Medical Journal* for permission to reproduce the data*.

CHELATING AGENTS

A chelating agent renders an ion (generally a metal) biologically inactive by incorporating it into an inner ring structure in the molecule (Greek, *chele* claw). It does this by means of structural binding groups (ligands). Where the stable complex is non-toxic and is excreted in the urine, this offers a way of inactivating and eliminating toxic metals.

The principal uses of chelating agents

Dimercaprol (BAL) for *arsenic mercury*, *gold*, lead, antimony, bismuth, thallium.

Sodium calcium detate (*Ca EDTA*) for *lead*, copper, manganese and radioactive plutonium, uranium, thorium, yttrium.

Penicillamine (dimethylcysteine) for *copper*, *lead*, *gold*, mercury and zinc: also in cystinuria.

Desferroxamine for *iron*, (which see).

* Meredith T et al. Br Med J 1984; 289:742.

Table 10.1 Antidotes

Drug	Indication	Mode of action	Dose
Acetylcysteine	Paracetamol ? Carbon tetrachloride	Restores depleted glutathione stores; protects against hepatic and renal failure.	150 mg/kg initial dose in 200 ml dextrose 5% i.v. over 15 min, followed by an i.v. infusion of 50 mg/kg in 500 ml of 5% dextrose over 4 h, then 100 mg/kg in one litre of dextrose 5% over 16 h. Total dose 300 mg/kg of acetlycysteine in 20 h. Most effective up to 8 h after ingestion. ? effective after 15 h.
Ammonium chloride	Phencyclidine ? Fenfluramine	Acid diuresis	4 g orally every 2 h preceded by arginine hydrochloride 10 g i.v. over 30 min.

Table 10.1 (cont'd)

Drug	Indication	Mode of action	Dose
Atropine	Organophosphorus and carbamate insecticides. Choline esters, e.g. carbachol	Competitive inhibition of muscarinic receptors.	1.2–2.4 mg i.v. repeated every 5–10 min until full atropinisation is achieved (dry mouth & pulse rate more than 70/min). Continue for 2–3 days; large quantities may be necessary.
Benztropine	Movement disorders or psychotropic effects due to: butyrophenones, e.g. haloperidol, diphenylbutylpiperidines, e.g. fluspirilene or pimozide, domperidone, metoclopramide, phenothiazines, thioxanthenes, e.g. clopenthixol.	Competitive inhibition of muscarinic receptors; blocks dopamine reuptake.	1–2 mg by i.m. or i.v. injection, repeated as necessary.
Benzylpenicillin	*Amanita phalloides*	Displaces toxin from plasma albumin and enhances urinary excretion.	250 mg/kg i.v. daily in divided doses.
Calcium gluconate	Fluorides Hydrofluoric acid	Binds or precipitates fluoride ions.	Hydrofluoric acid skin burns: apply as 2.5% gel repeatedly, but if pain does not subside, inject 10% solution under burn (0.5 ml/cm^2); 10–20 g in 25 ml water orally followed by 10 ml of 10% solution by i.v. injection.
	Hyperkalaemia Hypermagnesaemia (antacids)	Reverses neuromuscular paralysis due to raised K^+ & Mg^{2+}.	Hyperkalaemia & hypermagnesaemia: 10 ml of 10% solution by slow i.v. injection.
	Oxalates	Reverses hypocalcaemia.	Oxalate: 10 ml of 10% solution by i.v. injection.
Desferrioxamine	Iron	Chelation of ferrous ions.	(1) 2 g in 10 ml sterile water by i.m. injection. (2) Undertake gastric lavage with desferrioxamine solution (2 g in 1 litre of warm water). (3) After gastric lavage, leave 5 g (in 50 ml water) in stomach. (4) 5 mg/kg/h by slow i.v. infusion (maximum 80 mg/kg in 24 h) or 2 g by i.m. injection 12 hourly.
Dextrose	Insulin Oral hypoglaecamic agents	Increases blood sugar.	50 ml 50% by i.v. injection, repeated as necessary.
Dicobalt edate	Cyanide & cyanide derivatives, e.g. acrylonitrile	Chelates to form non-toxic cobalti- and cobalto-cyanides.	600 mg by i.v. injection over 1 min followed by a further 300 mg injection if response does not occur within 1 min. But see p. 188.

Table 10.1 (cont'd)

Drug	Indication	Mode of action	Dose
Dimercaprol	Arsenic, copper, lead, gold, mercury	Chelation of metal ions.	2.5–5 mg/kg by deep i.m. injection 4 hourly for 2 days then 2.5 mg/kg twice daily on the 3rd day and once daily thereafter.
Ethanol	Ethylene glycol Methyl alcohol (methanol)	Inhibits metabolism of methanol to formaldehyde & formic acid. Inhibits metabolism of ethylene glycol to glycoaldehyde & glycolate.	(1) 50 g orally or i.v. followed by infusion of 10–12 g/h to maintain plasma ethanol level of 1–2 g/l. For those with induced liver enzymes e.g. alcoholism or chronic epilepsy, give ethanol at rate of 12–15 g/hour. (2) If haemodialysis is used, infusion rate should be increased to 17–22 g/h because ethanol is readily dialysable, or ethanol may be added to peritoneal dialysate fluid at concentration of 1–2 g/l of diasylate.
Folinic acid	Folic acid antagonists e.g. methotrexate, trimethoprim, pyrimethamine. ?Methanol	Bypasses blocked folate metabolism. Stimulation of folate dependent one-carbon pool pathway for methanol metabolism.	(1) Methotrexate: up to 60 mg twice daily by i.v. injection followed by 15 mg six hourly by mouth for 5–7 days. (2) Trimethoprim: 3–6 mg by i.v. injection followed by 15 mg daily by mouth for 5–7 days. (3) Pyrimethamine: 6–15 mg i.v. (4) Methanol: 30 mg i.v. 6 hourly for 2 days.
Fuller's earth (aluminium silicate, bentonite)	Paraquat Diquat	Adsorption within the gut.	250 ml of 30% suspension 4-hourly for 24–48 hours. Always given with magnesium sulphate.
Glucagon	β-adrenoreceptor blocking drugs.	Bypasses blockade of β_1 β_2 receptors; stimulates cyclic AMP formation with positive inotropic effect.	50–150 μg/kg i.v. over one minute followed by infusion of 1–5 mg/h.
Heparin	Ergotamine (chronic poisoning) Aminocaproic acid Tranexamic acid	Reverses hypercoaguable state.	30 000–50 000 units daily by i.v. infusion.
Hydrocortisone	?Prevention of stricture formation due to ingestion of corrosives.	Anti-inflammatory agent.	200 mg 6-hourly by i.v. injection initially, followed by reducing doses as the clinical state permits.
	Hypercalcaemia due to alfacalcidol & vitamin D.	Decreases gut absorption & increases renal excretion of calcium.	
Magnesium sulphate	Paraquat Diquat Delayed release preparations	Osmotic purgative to assist passage of delayed release preparations through gastrointestinal tract.	100 ml of (BNF) mixture in 250 ml of water, repeated every 2 h until diarrhoea occurs.

Table 10.1 (cont'd)

Drug	Indication	Mode of action	Dose
Methionine	Paracetamol	Restores depleted glutathione stores; protects against renal & hepatic failure.	2.5 g initially, then 2.5 g 4-hourly for 3 doses (10 g over 12 h). Most effective up to 8 h after ingestion. ? Effective after 15 h.
Methylene blue	Chemicals causing methaemoglobinaemia, e.g. cetrimide, cresols, dapsone, nitrates, paradichlorobenzene, phenols, primaquine.	Promotes conversion of methaemomethaemoglobin to haemoglobin.	1–2 mg/kg (0.1 ml of 1% solution per kg) by slow i.v. infusion. In patients with glucose-6-phosphate dehydrogenase deficiency, use vitamin C 1 g i.v. slowly, or 200 mg orally three times daily as methylene blue causes haemolysis.
Naloxone	Narcotics (opioid)	Competitive inhibitor at opioid receptor sites.	0.4–2.4 mg initially i.v. repeated every 2–3 min up to 10 mg. May also be given as an infusion.
Neostigmine	Anticholinergic drugs	Anticholinesterase which causes accumulation of acetylcholine at cholinergic receptor sites	0.25 mg subcutaneously reverses peripheral but not central effects.
Pencillamine	Copper, gold, lead, mercury, zinc.	Chelation of metal ions.	250 mg–2 g orally daily.
Phenoxybenzamine	Severe hypertension due to clonidine, methylphenidate, methysergide, monoamine oxidase inhibitors, oxedrine, and phenylephrine.	Long acting alpha-adrenoceptor antagonist, causes peripheral vasodilation.	1 mg/kg diluted in 250 to 500 ml 5% dextrose and infused i.v. over 60 min.
Phentolamine	Severe hypertension due to clonidine, methylphenidate, methysergide, monoamine oxidase inhibitors, oxedrine, and phenylephrine.	Short acting α-adrenoceptor antagonist causes peripheral vasodilation.	5–60 mg i.v. (over 10–30 min), repeated as necessary.
Prenalterol	β-adrenoceptor blocking agents	Cardioselective β-adrenoceptor partial agonist.	2–15 mg by slow i.v. injection, repeated as necessary.
Propranolol	β_2-adrenoceptor stimulant drugs, e.g. salbutamol. Ephedrine Theophylline Thyroxine	Non-selective β-adrenoceptor blocking drug. Suppresses sympathetic over-activity and rate-related myocardial ischaemia. Reverses hypokalaemia due to beta adrenoceptor stimulants and theophylline.	1–2 mg i.v. over 1 min initially. Repeat every 2 min up to 5–10 mg or 40 mg orally 6–8-hourly. NB: atropine 0.6–1.2 mg i.v. should be given before propranolol injection (to avoid excess bradycardia).
Sodium bicarbonate	Alkalinisation of urine; to prevent crystallisatiaon of sulphonamides in renal tubules; to correct metabolic acidosis.	Alkalinisation and enhanced excretion of bicarbonate ions in the urine.	Dose according to urinary pH or severity of metabolic acidosis.

Table 10.1 (cont'd)

Drug	Indication	Mode of action	Dose
Sodium calcium edetate (Ca EDTA)	Lead	Chelation of lead ions.	50–75 mg/kg by i.v. infusion over 1 h for 5 days (every 2 g of EDTA should be diluted with 200 ml normal saline). NB: There is evidence that the addition of dimercaprol 5 mg/kg by deep i.m. injection 4-hourly for 24 h adds to effectiveness of EDTA regimen. Penicillamine 0.25–2 g daily by mouth may be used in place of EDTA.
Sodium chloride	Silver nitrate Bromides	Precipitates silver as silver chloride. Specifically enhances urinary excretion of bromide ions.	10 g/l orally, repeated as necessary to precipitate silver ions or to produce sodium chloride diuresis for bromide toxicity.
Sodium nitrite	Cyanide & cyanide derivatives e.g. acrylonitrile Hydrogen sulphide	Produces methaemoglobinaemia, which has special affinity for CN-, and HS-, ions to form cyanmethaemoglobin & sulphmethaemoglobin.	10 ml of 3% solution i.v. over 3 min followed, in poisoning from cyanide and cyanide derivatives, by 25 ml of 50% sodium thiosulphate over 10 min.
Sodium nitroprusside	Severe hypertension due to ergotamine & methysergide.	Peripheral vasodilator reversing vasoconstriction & severe hypertension.	50–400 μg/min by i.v. infusion. Adjust dose to patient's response. Do not continue for longer than 48 h.
Sodium thiosulphate	Cyanide & cyanide derivatives, e.g. acrylonitrile	Replenishes depleted thiosulphate stores necessary for the conversion of CN^- to thiocyanate.	25 ml of 50% sodium thiosulphate over 10 min preceded by 10 ml of 3% sodium nitrite solution i.v. over 3 min.
Sulphadimidine	*Amanita phalloides*	Displaces toxin from plasma albumin & enhances urinary excretion.	3 g initially than 1.5 g 6-hourly by slow i.v. or deep i.m. injection.
Vitamin C	Chemicals causing methaemoglobinaemia; use in patients with G6PD deficiency instead of methylene blue.	Promotes conversion of methaemoglobin to haemoglobin.	1 g slowly by i.v. injection or 200 mg orally three times daily.
Vitamin K	Coumarin & indanedione anti-coagulants.	Bypasses inhibition of vitamin K epoxide reductase enzyme.	10–20 mg by slow i.v. injection, repeated as necessary.

Individual chelating agents

Dimercaprol (BAL, British Anti-Lewisite) competes with body enzymes for toxic metal ions. It was synthesised during a systematic study of possible antagonists to arsenical vesicant war gases such as Lewisite. Arsenic and other metal ions are toxic in relatively low concentration, probably because they combine with the –SH groups of essential enzymes, thus inactivating them. Dimercaprol acts as a provider of –SH groups; it protects by combining its –SH groups with the metal ions to form relatively harmless ring chelates, which are excreted mainly in the urine. Dimercaprol is therapeutically effective because the ring compound formed with many heavy-metal ions is more stable than is the ring structure that the ions form with enzymes. It is obviously desirable that there should be an excess of dimercaprol available until all the metal has been eliminated, and as it is both oxidised in the body and excreted in the urine, repeated administration is necessary.

Use: Dimercaprol is useful and may be life-saving in poisoning with the metals listed above. It is ineffective primary therapy in lead poisoning because it does not combine with the metal sufficiently firmly, but its efficacy may be enhanced by combining it with sodium calciumedetate.

Dimercaprol, as 5% solution, is given by deep and painful i.m. injection. The dose in chronic poisoning is 2.5–5 mg/kg, 4-hourly for 2 days, then 2.5 mg/kg 12-hourly on the third day and then daily for 7 days. In severe acute poisoning, the course can be started with 5 mg/kg 4-hourly during the first 24 hours.

Adverse effects are common, particularly with the larger doses. They include nausea and vomiting, lachrymation and salivation, paraesthesiae, muscular aches and pains, urticarial rashes, tachycardia and a raised blood pressure. Gross overdosage may cause overbreathing, muscular tremors, convulsions and coma. The mechanism of toxic effects is not known, but it has been suggested that the removal of metallic groups from essential enzymes may be responsible. Ephedrine or a H_1-receptor antihistamine may reduce adverse reactions if given 30 min before an injection.

Dimercaptosuccinic acid (DMS) is structurally similar to dimercaprol.

Sodium calciumedetate (calcium disodium edathamil: the calcium chelate of the disodium salt of ethylenediaminetetraacetic acid, EDTA) is a chelate that has revolutionised the treatment of lead poisoning. The chelating agent combines more avidly with lead than with calcium. The lead chelate is formed by this exchange and is excreted in the urine, leaving behind a harmless amount of calcium. Dimercaprol combines with lead less firmly but is useful given with sodium calciumedetate in acute lead poisoning. The symptoms and signs of lead poisoning respond dramatically to this treatment.

Sodium calciumedetate 50–75 mg/kg daily is given by i.v. infusion over 1 h, daily for 5 days and repeated after a 7-day interval, as is indicated by the blood lead concentration. Dimercaprol 5 mg/kg 4-hourly may be given in addition during the first 24 h.

Ill-effects are fairly common and include hypotension, lachrymation, nasal stuffiness, sneezing, muscle pains and chills. Renal damage can occur.

Disodium edetate forms sodium calciumedetate in the body, inducing hypocalcaemia so that tetany may occur. This action can be used in hypercalcaemia, and is so effective that dangerous hypocalcaemia can result. Dicobalt edetate: see *cyanide* below.

Penicillamine (dimethylcysteine) is a metabolite of penicillin that contains -SH groups, so that it is similar to dimercaprol in action. It can be given orally or injected.

Its principal use is to prevent copper absorption from the diet in *hepatolenticular degeneration* (Wilson's disease) in which there is an inherited defect that prevents normal copper disposal so that the metal accumulates in the body. Although dimercaprol can be useful in this disease, penicillamine is more effective and can be taken orally, which is important because therapy must be life-long.

Penicillamine can halt the progress of the disease, but improvement is limited by the amount of irreversible brain damage that has already occurred. Therefore, early diagnosis of hepatolenticular degeneration is important. Where pencillamine is not tolerated, *trien* (triethylene-tetramine) can be used.

Potassium sulphide, orally, after meals, may be given as well as the chelating agent to reduce absorption of copper from the intestine by forming insoluble copper sulphide.

Pencillamine combines with cystine and prevents formation of stones in *cystinuria*; it also combines with pyridoxine and can cause pyridoxine deficiency. An effect on collagen may explain its benefit in advanced rheumatoid arthritis.

SOME POISONINGS

Cyanide poisoning. Effects of cyanide (used in industry: burning plastic upholstery) appear so rapidly that usually the patient is either dead before treatment can be started or else has taken so little that recovery is inevitable if left alone. However, speedy treatment can save an occasional life. Patients who have had a journey to hospital and have no symptoms, e.g. drowsiness, though they be very frightened, probably do not need specific treatment.* But early symptoms of cyanide poisoning are similar to anxiety (tachypnoea, excitement, etc.). Cyanide causes cellular anoxia by chelating the metallic (Fe) part of the intracellular respiratory enzyme, cytochrome P_{450} oxidase. The combination is reversible.

Specific therapy consists of measures to *chelate cyanide* in the blood by the following techniques:

1. by dicobalt edetate (Kelocyanor), which directly chelates cyanide (but which is relatively toxic if given in the absence of cyanide, so that accurate diagnosis is important; cobalt poisoning is treated by sodium calciumedetate), and
2. by forming methaemoglobin, the ferric ion of which takes up cyanide as cyanmethaemoglobin.

Dose: (1) 300 mg i.v., immediately followed by glucose (50 ml of 50% solution), the whole repeated after 1 min and in 5 min if no response (adverse effects include vomiting, chest pain and anaphylactic shock). (2) If dicobalt edetate is not available or is ineffective give sodium nitrite i.v. (10 ml of 3% solution over 3 min). Sodium thiosulphate i.v. (25 ml of 50% solution over 10 min) should then be given to convert the cyanide slowly released from the methaemoglobin to the inactive thiocyanate.

Gastric lavage with an oxidising solution to convert cyanide to inactive cyanate may be undertaken after the formation of methaemoglobin, e.g. sodium thiosulphate (5%); potassium permanganate (0.2%); hydrogen peroxide (3%).

There is evidence that oxygen, especially if at high pressure (hyperbaric), overcomes the cellular anoxia in cyanide poisoning; the mechanism is uncertain, but oxygen should be administered.

In carbon monoxide poisoning, oxygen also hastens the conversion of carboxyhaemoglobin. *Hyperbaric oxygen* is additionally useful because enough can dissolve in *plasma* to oxygenate tissues.

* Bryson D D. Lancet 1978; 1:92.

Methanol poisoning used to arise from the substitution of methanol for ethanol in illicit production of 'moonshine' but in the UK most cases result from deliberate ingestion by those who have access to it at work (paint, antifreeze solutions). As little as 10 ml may cause permanent blindness and 30 ml may kill. Confusion, ataxia, epigastric pain and vomiting are followed by metabolic acidosis and coma (see also CNS Ch 20 p. 422). Methanol is metabolised to formaldehyde and formic acid by alcohol and aldehyde dehydrogenases that are present in the retina (for the interconversion of retinol and retinene) and accumulation of these toxic metabolites may cause blindness, although this may not be the entire explanation. Acidosis appears to be the result of formate and possibly lactate production. Therapy is directed at

1. correcting acidosis by administering sodium bicarbonate intravenously.
2. eliminating methanol and formate by haemodialysis if plasma methanol exceeds 0.5 g/l or more than 30 g has been ingested.
3. inhibiting methanol metabolism by giving ethanol which has a much greater affinity for the dehydrogenase enzymes (see Table 10.1 for details, also p. 423).

Ethylene glycol is readily available as a constituent of antifreezes. In the first 12 hours after ingestion the patient appears as though intoxicated with alcohol but does not smell of it; subsequently there is increasing acidosis (due to production of lactic acid), pulmonary oedema and cardiac failure, and in 2–3 days renal pain and tubular necrosis develop because calcium oxalate crystals form in the urine.

In addition to general supportive measures against shock and respiratory distress, acidosis should be corrected with intravenous sodium bicarbonate and hypocalcaemia with calcium gluconate. As with methanol (above), ethanol should be given to inhibit the metabolism of ethylene glycol and haemodialysis used to eliminate the poison. Ethylene glycol has been used criminally to give 'body' and sweetness to white table wines.

Paraquat is a widely used herbicide. It is extremely toxic if it is ingested; a mouthful of commercial solution taken and spat out may be enough to kill. The earliest sign of ingested paraquat is redness of the fauces, which progresses to ulceration and usually involves the oesophagus as well. Subsequently renal tubular necrosis develops and later there is pulmonary oedema followed by pulmonary fibrosis; whether the patient lives of dies depends largely on the severity of the lung lesion.

Paraquat is absorbed rapidly from the upper small intestine but only slowly from the lower gut. It is not metabolised and is eliminated in the urine, which it enters by active secretion through the renal tubules in addition to glomerular filtration. Unfortunately, quite small amounts are toxic to the kidney, and when renal damage occurs, the only route of elimination of absorbed paraquat is impaired. It then accumulates in the lung as a result of a slow but selective and active uptake mechanism. Lung damage appears to be due to the formation of superoxide, a chemically reactive radical of oxygen.

A urine test for paraquat is available to confirm absorption (sodium bicarbonate plus sodium dithionite causes the urine to turn blue). Plasma concentration measurements can assist in predicting the likely outcome.

Treatment is *urgent*, including gastric lavage, adsorbent orally, e.g. fuller's earth (aluminium silicate), activated charcoal and osmotic purgation. Haemodialysis or haemoperfusion probably have a role in the first 24 hours, the rationale being that lowering the plasma concentration by these methods protects the kidney, failure of which allows the slow but relentless accumulation of paraquat in the lung.

Diquat is similar but the late pulmonary changes may not occur.

Dinitro-compounds. Dinitrophenol, abandoned as an explosive, had a short career in therapy of obesity, but it was so toxic that it shortened life more than obesity does. It was tried because it increased cellular respiration (by uncoupling oxidative phosphorylation), and increased the metabolic rate so that the surplus fat would be used up.

Related compounds, dinitro-orthocresol (DNOC) and dinitrobutylphenol (DNBP) are used as selective weed killers and insecticides, and cases of poisoning occur accidentally and when safety precautions are ignored. They can be absorbed through the skin, and the hands, face and are usually stained yellow. Symptoms and signs are mainly those associated with a very high metabolic rate. Copious sweating and thirst are early warning signs and may proceed to dehydration and vomiting, weakness, restlessness, tachycardia and deep, rapid breathing. Eventually, convulsions and coma may occur. Treatment is urgent and consists of cooling the patient and attention to fluid and electrolyte balance. It is essential to differentiate this type of poisoning from that due to cholinesterase inhibitors because if atropine is given to patients poisoned with dinitro-compound, they may stop sweating and die of hyperpyrexia.

Pentachlorophenol is similar (used as insecticide and preservative, e.g. of canvas).

Organophosphorus pesticides are anticholinesterases (see index); they also cause delayed neurotoxicity. Organic carbamates are similar.

Organochlorine pesticides (e.g. DDT) may cause convulsions in acute overdose. Treat as for status epilepticus.

Rodenticides. *Fluoracetamide and relatives* cause muscular twitching and convulsions with death from cardiorespiratory collapse. Selective antidotes have been found in the laboratory but have not been proved in man. Other rodenticides include *warfarin plus vitamin D* (see index), and *thallium* (treat with Prussian blue, i.e. potassium ferric cyanoferrate, which exchanges potassium for thallium; give 10 g by mouth twice daily); for *strychnine* give diazepam to control muscle spasm. Numerous other substances are used as rodenticides.

Kerosene (paraffin or diesel oil), petrol (gasoline) chiefly cause CNS depression and pulmonary damage from inhalation. It is vital to avoid aspiration into the lungs during attempts to remove the poison or in spontaneous vomiting; gastric aspiration should be performed only if a cuffed endotracheal tube is efficiently in place. It may be necessary to anaesthetise the subject to do this.

Fungus (mushroom) poisoning is commonest in

late summer and early autumn when wild fungi are most easily available. Some are greatly prized by epicures but the danger is that edible and non-edible varieties may be confused. The range of toxins that these plants produce is reflected in the diversity of symptoms caused. Patients should receive ipecacuanha to induce vomiting unless it has already occurred; activated charcoal may then be given to adsorb toxin in the gastrointestinal tract. Table 10.2 is based on information in the *Medical Letter on Drugs and Therapeutics* and we are grateful to the Chairman of the Editorial Board for permission to reproduce this.

Harassing agents (short-term incapacitants; anti-riot agents)

'Harassing agents may be defined as chemical agents that are capable when used in field conditions, of rapidly causing a temporary disablement that lasts for little longer than the period of exposure'.* They are sensory irritants that cause pain in the most sensitive tissues with which they come into contact, i.e. the eyes and respiratory tract. This results in reflex lachrymation (*lachry-*

* Health aspects of chemical and biological weapons. Geneva: WHO 1970.

Table 10.2 Poisonous fungi ('mushrooms')

Toxin	Contained in†	Symptoms and signs	Comment
Cyclopeptides	*Amanita phalloides* other Amanita species *Galerina* species *Cortinarius orellanus* *Lepiota* species	Nausea, vomiting, colicky pain, diarrhoea. Temporary recovery with relapse on day 2–4 followed by increasingly abnormal tests of hepatic function, renal shutdown, convulsions and coma. Symptoms of *Cortinarius orellanus* poisoning may be delayed 3–14 days.	Cyclopeptides in *Amanita phalloides* cause >90% of fatal mushroom poisoning. One mushroom can cause severe poisoning, three (50 g) are usually fatal. Gastric lavage, repeated duodenal aspiration, rehydration, charcoal haemoperfusion, thioctic acid 200–300 mg/day i.v. in two doses and penicillin in high dose are recommended.‡
Methylhydrazine ('rocket fuel' toxin)	*Gyromitra* species	Nausea, vomiting, diarrhoea, abdominal cramps. May develop abnormal tests of hepatic function, haemolysis, seizures, fever, incoordination and coma.	Methylhydrazine, formed by some who ingest this mushroom, is a component of rocket propellants. Pyridoxine, parenterally in large dose, is advocated.
Coprine (disulfiram-like toxin)	*Coprinus* species	Flushing, paresthesiae, palpitations, followed by nausea, vomiting and sweating. Rarely, visual disturbances, vertigo, confusion, hypotension, arrhythmias, respiratory problems and coma.	Mushrooms contain a compound that is metabolised after ingestion to an acetaldehyde dehydrogenase inhibitor.
Muscarine	*Inocybe* species	Combination of perspiration, salivation and lachrymation is typical. Miosis, bradycardia, hypotension, bronchoconstriction may occur.	Atropine can block the cholinergic (muscarinic) effects (but can aggravate other types of mushroom poisoning).
Ibotenic acid, muscimol, pantherin	*Amanita* species	Ataxia and disturbed vision. Patient may report visions and appear intoxicated	Psychoactive mushrooms: no specific treatment is usually required but diazepam may be helpful for agitated patients.
Psilocybin	*Psilocybe* species	Hallucinations, dilated pupils vertigo, ataxia, weakness and drowsiness. Symptoms progress over about 12 h	
Other toxins	Many genera	Gastrointestinal symptoms	Symptomatic treatment, plus general measures indicated above.

† And other species and genera
‡ Editorial. Lancet 1980; 2:351.

mators), sneezing (*sternutators*) and cough. If the agent is a gas or an aerosol of particles less than 0.5 μm in diameter, it will penetrate to the small bronchi and cause chest pain.

The pharmacological requirements for a safe and effective harassing agent (it is hardly appropriate to refer to benefit versus risk) must be stringent. As well as high potency and efficacy and rapid onset and offset of effect in open areas under any atmospheric condition, it must be safe in confined spaces where concentration may be very high and may affect an innocent, bedridden invalid should a projectile enter the window.

A favoured substance at present is CS (orthochlorobenzylidene malononitrile). This is a solid that is disseminated as a particulate aerosol by including it in a pyrotechnic mixture. The spectacle of its dissemination has been rendered familiar by television. It is not a gas, it is an aerosol or smoke. The particles aggregate and settle to the ground in minutes so that the risk of exposure out of doors being prolonged is not great.

'According to the concentration of CS to which a person is exposed, the effects vary from a slight pricking or peppery sensation in the eyes and nasal passages up to the maximum symptoms of streaming from the eyes and nose, spasm of the eyelids, profuse lachrymation and salivation, retching and sometimes vomiting, burning of the mouth and throat, cough and gripping pain in the chest'.* The onset of symptoms occurs immediately on exposure (an important factor from the point of view of the user) and they disappear dramatically; 'At one moment the exposed person is in their grip. Then he either stumbles away, or the smoke plume veers or the discharge from the grenade stops, and immediately, the symptoms begin to roll away. Within a minute or two, the pain in the chest has gone and his eyes, although still streaming, are open. Five or so minutes later, the excessive salivation and pouring tears stop and a quarter of an hour after exposure, the subject is essentially back to normal'.*

Exposed subjects absorb small amounts only, and the plasma $t_{\frac{1}{2}}$ is about 5 seconds.

* Home Office. Report of the enquiry into the medical and toxicological aspects of CS. pt II. London: HMSO. 1971: Cmnd 4775.

Investigations of the effects of CS are difficult in 'field use', but some have been done and at present there is no evidence that even the most persistent rioter will suffer any permanent effect. The hazard to the infirm or sick seems to be low, but plainly it would be prudent to assume that asthmatics or bronchitics could suffer an exacerbation from high concentrations, though bronchospasm does not occur in normal persons. Whether or not CS can cause unconsciousness is uncertain and is difficult to investigate for, 'in the highly charged circumstance of a riot, unconsciousness can occur for a variety of reasons', and deliberate use of CS in training operations has induced panic and fainting at first contact. Vomiting seems to be due to swallowing contaminated saliva. Transient looseness of the bowels may follow exposure.

Hazard from CS is probably confined to situations where the missiles are projected into enclosed spaces.

Various formulations of CS can be prescribed, e.g. *Cartridge, 1.5 inch, Anti-riot, Irritant* and *Grenade, Hand, Anti-riot, Irritant*.

CN (α-chloroacetophenone), tear gas, is generally used as a solid aerosol or smoke; solutions (Mace) are used at close quarters.

DM (adamsite) is relatively toxic; it was used in the 1914–1918 war.

CR (dibenz[b,f]oxazepine) was put into production in 1973 after testing on 150 army volunteers. In addition to the usual properties (above) it may induce a transient rise in intraocular pressure, which is dismissed by the investigators as unimportant on the grounds 'of the likely youth of those against whom CR will be used'.†

'Authority' is reticent about the properties of all these substances and no further important information is readily available.

This brief account has been included, because in addition to helping victims (wash them, calm them) even the most well-conducted and tractable students and doctors may find themselves exposed to CS smoke in our troubled world; and some may even feel it their duty to incur exposure. That an account of such substances should seem appro-

† Editorial. Lancet 1973; 2:1184.

priate for inclusion in a book on clinical pharmacology, is sad, for it is a science that exists for the purpose of increasing happiness by relief of suffering.

Drugs used for torture and interrogation

Regrettably, drugs have been and are being used for torture, sometimes disguised as 'interrogation' or 'aversion therapy'. Facts are, not surprisingly, hard to obtain, but it seems that suxamethonium, hallucinogens, thiopentone, neuroleptics, amphetamines, apomorphine and cyclophosphamide have been employed to hurt, frighten, confuse or debilitate in such ways as callous ingenuity can devise.

Drugs are also used for judical execution, e.g. i.v. thiopentone, potassium, curare.

It might be urged that it is justifiable to use drugs to protect society by discovering serious crimes such as murder. But there always must be uncertainty of the truth of evidence, obtained with drugs, that cannot be independently confirmed, and there is no such thing as a 'truth drug'* in the sense that it guarantees the truth of what the subject says; also, the employment of drugs offers inducement to inhuman behaviour. In addition, the definition of criminal activity is so easily perverted to include activities in defence of human liberty, and opinions on what is desirable social change vary so widely that this use of drugs and any doctors or others who engage in it or who misguidedly allow themselves to be persuaded that to monitor such use by others can be in the interest of victims, must surely be outlawed.

* Use of drugs ('truth serum') such as thiopentone to obtain evidence in more ordinary judicial circumstances has been, and in some countries still is, practised. Accused people convinced of their own innocence sometimes volunteer to undergo such tests. The problem of discerning truth from falsehood remains.

GUIDE TO FURTHER READING

1 Editorial. Patients who take overdoses. Br Med J 1985; 290: 1297–1298.
2 Alderson M R. National trends in self-poisoning in women. Lancet 1985; 1: 974–975.
3 Editorial. "Overdose — will the psychiatrist please see?" Lancet 1981; 1: 195–196.
4 Platt S, Kreitman N. Trends in parasuicide and unemployment among men in Edinburgh, 1968–82. Br Med J 1984; 289: 1029–1031.
5 Proudfoot A T, Park J. Changing pattern of drugs used for self-poisoning. Br Med J 1978; 1: 90–94.
6 Prescott L F. New approaches in managing drug overdose and poisoning. Br Med J 1983; 287: 274–276.
7 Editorial. Gastrointestinal clearance of drugs with activated charcoal. N. Engl J Med 1982; 307: 676–678.
8 Editorial. Benzodiazepine overdose: are specific antagonists useful? Br Med J 1985; 290: 805–806.
9 Smith T W et al. Treatment of life-threatening digitalis intoxication with digoxin-specific Fab antibody fragments. N Engl J Med 1982; 307: 1357–1362.
10 Editorial. Methanol poisoning. Lancet 1983; 1: 910–912.
11 Craft A W et al. Accidental childhood poisoning with household products. Br Med J 1984; 288:682.
12 Editorial. Solvent misuse. Br Med J 1985; 290:94–95.
13 ABC of Poisoning. (A series of articles). Br Med J 1984; 289: 39–40, 94–95, 172–174, 240–241, 304–305, 366–369, 426–428, 486–489, 546–548, 614–618, 681–686, 820–822, 907–908, 990–993, 1062–1064, 1133–1135, 1214–1217, 1291–1294, 1361–1364. These articles have been published as a book; Volans G, Hendry J, eds. ABC of Poisoning. London: British Medical Association, 1985.
14 Amnesty International. Report on Torture. Duckworth. 1973.
15 United Nations. Report of Secretary-General. Chemical and bacteriological weapons and the effects of their possible use. New York; UN, 1969.
16 World Health Organization. Health aspects of chemical and biological weapons. Geneva, 1970.
17 Editorial. Chemical and bacteriological warfare in the 1980s. Lancet 1984; 2:141.
18 Vale J A et al. Syrup of ipecacuanha: is it really useful? Br Med J 1986; 1321

11

Infection I: Chemotherapy

The term **chemotherapy** is used for the drug treatment of parasitic infections in which the parasites (viruses, bacteria, protozoa, fungi, worms) are destroyed or removed without injuring the host. The use of the term to cover all drug or synthetic drug therapy needlessly removes a distinction that is convenient to the clinician and has the sanction of long usage. By convention the term is used to include therapy of cancer.

History

Chemotherapy has been practiced empirically since ancient times. The Ancient Greeks used male fern, and the Aztecs chenopodium, as intestinal anthelmintics. The Ancient Hindus treated leprosy with chaulmoogra; there are numerous other examples. For hundreds of years moulds have been applied to wounds, but, despite the introduction of mercury as a treatment for syphilis (16th century) and the use of cinchona bark against malaria (17th century), the history of modern rational chemotherapy does not begin until the late 19th century.

It is not surprising that the differential staining of tissues and bacteria should have been the basis of early chemotherapeutic research, for it was an obvious instance of chemicals affecting the parasite and host differently and gave hope of usefully selective toxicity. Aniline dyes were used for staining, and, when it was shown that these dyes could also kill bacteria, Paul Ehrlich*, already interested in differential staining of leucocytes, tried the effect of dyes on infected experimental animals. In 1891 he cured experimental malaria in guinea pigs with methylene blue, but it was less effective than quinine. In 1904 he controlled trypanosome infections in mice with another dye, trypan red, but it was ineffective in other species.

Ehrlich thus developed the idea of chemotherapy and he invented the word. In 1906 he wrote: 'In order to use chemotherapy successfully, we must search for substances which have an affinity for the cells of the parasites and a power of killing them greater than the damage such substances cause to the organism itself, so that the destruction of the parasite will be possible without seriously hurting the organism. This means we must strike the parasites and the parasites only, if possible, and to do this *we must learn to aim, learn to aim which chemical substances*!' Or, as a modern microbiologist has put it in reverse,

* 1854–1915. The German scientist who played a major role in developing haemotology and immunology, he was also the pioneer of chemotherapy and discovered the first cure for syphilis.

formaldehyde 'admittedly will fix the patient's bacteria, but will also fix the patient'*.

By 1906 it was clear that chemotherapy was a practical proposition and not the fantasy that eminent contemporaries declared it. Inorganic arsenic had been shown to clear trypanosomes from the blood of infected horses and an organic arsenical had been used successfully on man. This inspired Ehrlich to make and test further compounds. His efforts resulted in the introduction of arsphenamine (Salvarsan) for the treatment of syphilis and it was soon followed by neoarsphenamine (Neosalvarsan), which was widely used until 1945 when penicillin superseded it.

After neoarsphenamine there was a lull. Then the antimalarials pamaquin and mepacrine were developed from dyes and, in 1935, the first sulphonamide, linked with a dye (Prontosil), was introduced as a result of systematic studies by Domagk† who noted its antistreptococcal action in mice.

The results obtained with sulphonamides in puerperal sepsis, pneumonia and meningitis were dramatic and caused a reorientation of medical thought. Up to then chemotherapy had been virtually confined to protozoa and metazoa, spirochaetes being considered as a special case; to kill pyogenic bacteria in the body had seemed impossible.

In 1928, seven years before the discovery of the sulphonamides, Fleming‡ had long been interested in wound infections. He had also discovered the antibacterial constituent of tears (lysozyme), for which research he obtained a supply by squirting lemon juice into the eyes of himself, his colleagues and students (the latter for a small payment). His discovery of penicillin was made at St. Mary's Hospital, London, when, whilst studying colony variation in staphylococci, on his return from holiday he noticed one of his culture plates contaminated with a fungus that destroyed surrounding bacterial colonies. This accidential rediscovery of the long-known ability of penicillium fungi to suppress the growth of bacterial cultures was now followed up. Fleming investigated the properties of 'mould broth filtrates', which, for brevity, he named 'penicillin'. He described penicillin as an antiseptic more powerful than phenol, which yet could safely be applied to the tissues. The name 'penicillin' has since been applied to the pure antibiotic substances.

Attempts to isolate penicillin from the crude preparations were made, but lack of appreciation of its potentialities as well as the difficulty of preparing enough for experiments caused it to be put aside as a curiosity, although Fleming used it in his laboratory as a method of differentiating bacterial cultures throughout the 1930s.

In 1939, principally as an academic exercise, Florey§ and Chain‖ undertook an investigation of *antibiotics*, i.e. substances produced by micro-organisms that are antagonistic to the growth or life of other micro-organisms.¶ They prepared penicillin, discovered its *systemic* in addition to its local chemotherapeutic power against experimental infections in mice, and confirmed its remarkable lack of toxicity.

The importance of this discovery for a nation at war was obvious to these workers, but the time, July 1940, was unpropitious, for London was being bombed and invasion was feared. It was necessary to manufacture penicillin in the Oxford University Pathology Laboratory.**

* Jawetz E. Br Med J 1963; 2:951.

† Gerhard Domagk (1895–1964). Bacteriologist and pathologist who made his discovery while working in I G Farbenindustrie (Bayer) (Germany). Awarded the 1939 Nobel Prize for Physiology or Medicine, he had to wait until 1947 to receive the medal because of Nazi German policy at the time.

‡ Alexander Fleming (1881–1955). Lesser mortals sometimes feel encouraged to know that the lucky, the great and the famous are actually human too. It may cheer some to know that Fleming 'was certainly one of the worst lecturers I have ever heard' (R. Hare, a colleague of Fleming: The birth of penicillin and the disarming of microbes. London: Allen and Unwin, 1970. Highly recommended reading).

§ Howard Walter Florey (1898–1969). Professor of Pathology at Oxford University.

‖ Ernst Boris Chain (1906–79). Biochemist. Fleming, Florey and Chain shared the 1945 Nobel prize for Medicine or Physiology.

¶ Strictly, the definition should refer to substances that are antagonistic *in dilute solution* for it is appropriate to exclude various metabolic products such as alcohol and hydrogen peroxide.

** The mood of the time is shown by the decision that by the time the invaders reached Oxford, the essential records and apparatus for making penicillin should have been deliberately destroyed; but the productive strain of *Penicillium* mould was to be secretly preserved. To this end, several of the principal workers smeared the spores of the mould into the linings of their ordinary clothes where it could remain dormant but alive for years, and any member of the team who escaped (wearing the right clothes) could use it to start the work again. (Macfarlane G. Howard Florey. Oxford. 1979.)

Fletcher, who at the time had just been appointed a research fellow in medicine at Oxford, was asked to help with the first clinical trials of penicillin in 1941. He writes:*

It was characteristic of Florey that the first thing that he did was to ask me to go over to the Dunn Laboratory (where all the penicillin work had been carried out), to meet the rest of the team. Ernst Chain — small, dark, excitable, bubbling with enthusiasm — showed me his apparatus for freeze drying the extracts of penicillin to produce a powder. Norman Heatley quietly showed me the stacks of bed pans in which he had succeeded in producing just enough penicillin to make it possible to consider starting clinical trials and his ingenious extraction columns for getting the pencillin out of the culture medium into aqueous solution.

Florey explained that although penicillin had been found to be entirely harmless to leucocytes, tissue cultures, and a wide variety of laboratory animals, he did not want to risk giving the first injection to a healthy volunteer in case of some unique adverse reaction in man. So he asked me to find a patient with some inevitably fatal disorder who might be willing to help. There were no ethical committees in those days that had to be consulted, so I looked around the wards and found a pleasant 50-year-old woman with disseminated breast cancer and who had not long to live. I explained to her that I wanted to try a new medicine that could be of value to many people, and asked if she would agree to a test injection of it. This she readily did.

Florey and Witts came with me on 17 January to witness the first injection of 100 mg (about 5000 units) of penicillin which was expected to produce a bactericidal concentration in the blood. I gave it slowly into an antecubital vein, and the patient at once said that she had a curious musty taste in her mouth but suffered no other immediate harm. A few hours later, however, she developed a rigor and her temperature rose for a few hours, but there were no other ill effects. Before clinical trials could be carried out, the pyrogen was removed by further purification and rabbits were used to ensure that no pyrogen remained.

The time had now come to find a suitable patient for the first test of the therapeutic power of penicillin in man. Every hospital then had a 'septic' ward, filled with patients with chronic discharging abscesses, sinuses, septic joints, and sometimes meningitis. Patients with staphylococcal infections would be ideal because sulphonamides had no effect on them and were inactivated by pus. In the septic ward at the Radcliffe Infirmary there was then an unfortunate policeman aged 43 who had had a sore on his lips four months previously from which had developed a combined staphylococcal and streptococcal septicaemia. He had multiple abscesses on his face and his orbits (for which one eye had been removed): he also had osteomyelitis of his right humerus with discharging sinuses, and abscesses in his lungs. He was in great pain and was desperately and pathetically ill. There was all to gain for him in a trial of penicillin and nothing to lose.

Penicillin treatment was started on 12 February 1941, with 200 mg (10,000 units) intravenously initially and then 300 mg every three hours. All the patient's urine was collected, and each morning I took it over to the Dunn Laboratory on my bicycle so that the excreted penicillin could be extracted to be used again. There I was always eagerly met by Florey and Chain and other members of the team. On the first day I was able to report that for the first time throughout his illness, the patient was beginning to feel a little better. Four days later there was a striking improvement, and after five days, the patient was vastly better, afebrile, and eating well, and there was obvious resolution of the abscesses on his face and scalp and in his right orbit. But alas, the supply of penicillin was exhausted: the poor man gradually deteriorated and died a month later. The total dose given over five days had been only 220,000 units, much too small a dose, as we know now, to have been able to overcome such extensive infection; but there was no doubt about the temporary clinical improvement, and, most importantly, there had been no sort of toxic effect during the five days of continuous administration of penicillin. This remarkable freedom from side effects, apart from allergy, has remained one of penicillin's most fortunate features.

Since 1939, large programmes of screening fungi and bacteria for antibiotic production have been conducted. The next success was the isolation of streptomycin from a soil organism and this was followed by tetracycline, erythromycin and others. Simultaneously, there have been developments in synthetic agents, especially against tuberculosis and tropical diseases, including malaria, leprosy and amoebiasis. That nothing is beneath the notice of some investigators is illustrated by the discovery of antibacterial substances in the anal gland secretion of the Argentine ant and in the faeces of blow-fly larvae.

Classification of antimicrobial† drugs

Antimicrobial agents may broadly be classified according to the type of organism against which

* Fletcher C. Brit Med J 1984; 289: 1721.

† The classic definition of *antibiotic*, see above, is increasingly ignored at least in clinical practice where it is now commonly used as synonymous with antimicrobial. It would be pedantic to object.

they are active and in this book follow the sequence:

Antibacterial drugs
Antiviral drugs
Antifungal drugs
Antiprotozoal drugs
Anthelmintic drugs

Further sub-classifications appear where relevant under each main division.

Antibacterial chemotherapeutic agents may also be classified into those that act primarily by stopping bacterial growth (bacteristatic) and those that act primarily by killing bacteria (bactericidal).

Primarily bacteristatic antimicrobials include the sulphonamides, the tetracyclines, chloramphenicol and para-aminosalicylate (for tuberculosis).

Primarily bactericidal drugs include the penicillins and cephalosporins, the aminoglycosides, isoniazid and rifampicin.

The classification is somewhat arbitrary because most bacteristatic drugs can be shown to be bactericidal at high concentrations. It does retain a certain usefulness in that *when a bacteristatic drug is used, the defence mechanisms of the body are relied on to destroy the organisms* whose multiplication has been stopped by the drug. These mechanisms are inadequate for the purpose in carriers, in infective endocarditis, in some debilitated patients and in those whose immune systems are compromised by disease or drugs. In these cases, bactericidal drugs should be used. In addition, bactericidal drugs act best against dividing organisms so that a bacteristatic drug may protect the organisms, and this can have clinical importance when combinations are used.

General principles of antimicrobial chemotherapy

The following principles, many of which apply to drug therapy in general, are a guide to good practice with antimicrobial agents.

1. *Make a diagnosis* as precisely as is possible, defining the site of infection, the organism(s) responsible and antimicrobial sensitivity. This objective will be more readily achieved if all relevant biological samples reach the laboratory before treatment is begun. It is an abuse of antimicrobials to use them simply as antipyretics. This causes diagnostic confusion, may fail to cure and can even kill the patient.

2. *Remove barriers* to cure, e.g. lack of free drainage of abcesses, obstruction in the urinary or respiratory tracts.

3. *Decide whether chemotherapy is really necessary*. As a general rule, acute infections require chemotherapy whilst chronic infections may not. Chronic abscess, empyema or osteomyelitis respond poorly, although chemotherapeutic cover is essential if surgery is undertaken in order to avoid a flare-up of infection or its dissemination due to the breaking down of tissue barriers. Even some acute infections such as gastroenteritis may be better managed symptomatically than by antimicrobials.

4. *Select the best drug*. This involves consideration of:

a. *specificity*, for ideally the antimicrobial activity of the drug should match that of the infecting organisms. Indiscriminate use of broad spectrum drugs encourages opportunistic infections. There are, however, times when, because of the absence of precise information about the responsible microbe, 'best guess' chemotherapy of reasonably broad spectrum must be given.

b. *pharmacokinetic factors*, to ensure that the chosen drug is capable of reaching the site of infection in adequate amounts, e.g. by crossing the blood–brain barrier.

c. *the patient*, who may previously have been allergic to antimicrobials or whose routes of elimination may be impaired, e.g. by renal disease.

5. Administer the drug in *optimum dose* and *frequency* and by the most *appropriate route(s)*. Inadequate dose may lead to the development of microbial resistance. In general, intermittent dosing is preferred to continuous infusion, which creates the risk of incompatibility with infusion fluids and loss of drug potency. Plasma concentration monitoring is often a guide to the adequacy of therapy.

6. Continue therapy until apparent cure has been achieved, *and then for about three days further to avoid relapse*. If an infection deserves treatment, it deserves at least five days.

There are many exceptions to this, such as typoid fever, tuberculosis and infective endocarditis, in which it is known that relapse is possible long after apparent clinical cure and so the drugs are continued for a longer time determined by experience.

7. *Test for cure.* In some infections, microbiological proof of cure is desirable because disappearance of symptoms and signs occurs before the organisms are eradicated, e.g. urinary infections. Microbiological examination must be done, of course, after withdrawal of chemotherapy.

8. *Prophylactic chemotherapy* for surgical and dental procedures should be of very limited duration. It should start *at the time of surgery* and continue for say 48 hours, to reduce the risk of producing resistant organisms.

9. *Carriers* should, in general, not be treated with antimicrobials to remove the organisms, for it is better to allow natural re-establishment of a normal flora. Attempts to treat are likely to prolong rather than to shorten this process (but see typhoid).

How antimicrobials act

There are five principal sites of action.

1. *The cell wall* gives the bacterium its characteristic shape and provides protection against the much lower osmotic pressure of the environment. The peptidoglycan component of the cell wall (which is not present in man) is very important for its integrity. Bacterial growth involves breakdown and extension of this layer. Penicillins and cephalosporins interfere with the formation of the peptidoglycan layer so that the cell absorbs water and bursts. Obviously, they can only act against growing cells.

2. *The cytoplasmic membrane* inside the cell wall is the site of most of the cell's biochemical activity. Colistin disorientates the molecules (like a detergent at an oil–water interface) so that the membrane becomes permeable and vital metabolites escape. The cytoplasmic membrane of fungi contains sterol components, which are essential to its structure. Amphotericin selectively attacks fungi by complexing with the sterol and disorganising the membrane.

3. *Inhibition of protein synthesis.* Tetracyclines, chloramphenicol, erythromycin, fusidic acid and the aminoglycosides interfere at various points with the build-up of peptide chains on the ribosomes.

4. *Nucleic acid metabolism.* Nalidixic acid, rifampicin and actinomycin interfere with RNA and DNA metabolism.

5. *Intermediary metabolism.* Sulphonamides, trimethoprim, PAS and isoniazid interfere with bacterial metabolism as described elsewhere.

Use of antimicrobial drugs

Choice of antimicrobials

From the point of view of treatment, infections fall into two main classes in which —

1. **Choice of antimicrobial follows automatically from the clinical diagnosis** because the causative organism is always the same, and is virtually always sensitive to the same drug, e.g. segmental pneumonia in a young person, which is almost always caused by *Streptococcus pneumoniae* (penicillin); acute osteomyelitis, which is likely to be due to *Staphylococcus aureus* (flucloxacillin in the UK); some haemolytic stretococcal infections, e.g. scarlet fever, erysipelas (penicillin), typhus (tetracycline), leprosy (dapsone with rifampicin).

2. **Choice of antimicrobial should be based, wherever possible, on bacterological identification and sensitivity tests because:**

a. *The infecting organism is not identified by the clinical diagnosis*, for instance, in bronchopneumonia, meningitis, urinary tract infection, although a useful guess can often be made.

b. *The infecting organism is identified by the clinical diagnosis*, but no assumption can be made as to its sensitivity to any one antimicrobial, for instance, carbuncle, tuberculosis, gonorrhoea.

In infections in either sub-division of the second group above there are a number of courses of action:

1. *When microbiological services are not available at all* it is necessary to choose an antimicrobial based on the best guess, knowing the likely pathogens in a given clinical situation. Thus, trimetho-

prim alone is a reasonable first choice for the coliform organisms, normally responsible for lower urinary tract infection; but septicaemia related to bowel or genital tract surgery and probably involving coliforms, streptococci and anaerobes calls for a broad spectrum of cover, e.g. gentamicin plus amoxycillin plus metronidazole or a cephalosporin plus metronidazole. Treatment should be changed only after adequate trial, usually three days, for over-hasty alterations cause confusion and tend to produce resistant organisms. Lack of bacteriological assistance is not an excuse for indiscriminate polypharmacy.

2. *When microbiological services are available but treatment cannot be delayed* it is obviously necessary to act if they are absent, except that all appropriate specimens (blood, pus, urine, sputum, cerebrospinal fluid) *must* be taken for examination before administering any antimicrobial, so that modification of treatment can be made later if necessary, after identification and sensitivity tests.

3. *When microbiological services are available but treatment can only be delayed until simple staining tests have been done*, the antimicrobial will be selected on the knowledge that the organism is a Gram-positive or a Gram-negative coccus or bacillus, and the clinical setting. It is necessary, therefore, to know the approximate range of antimicrobial drugs over organisms so classified. For example, a penicillin may be indicated when Gram-positive cocci are found or an aminoglycoside if Gram-negative rods are present. Full details appear in the tables at the end of this chapter and in the descriptions of individual drugs.

4. *When microbiological services are available and treatment may reasonably be delayed for up to 48 hours*, then therapy may be chosen with knowledge of both the organism and its sensitivity to drugs. This course should be followed whenever possible because it gives the best results.

5. *Initial treatment of serious infections*. In such serious infections as meningitis, Gram-negative bacillary sepsis, and endocarditis, prompt 'best guess' treatment is essential and antimicrobial drugs should not be withheld until laboratory tests are completed. Parenteral administration, preferably i.v. is usually mandatory. After the infection is under control, an oral formulation may be substituted.

Administration of antimicrobials

Oral administration is convenient, less unpleasant than parenteral administration and is commonly adequate. Food retards absorption and peak plasma concentrations are therefore lower. In general, antimicrobials should be taken between meals or at least one hour before a meal. In the case of cloxacillin the timing in relation to food can make the difference between success and failure.

Parenteral administration is often required in hospital practice. The i.v. route is preferred for serious infection and has the advantage over i.m. injection in that it is less painful, more secure when circulatory failure may hamper absorption from an injection site, and can be used when the patient has a bleeding disorder. Furthermore, some drugs are simply too irritant or too bulky to be given i.m. Intermittent i.v. injection by bolus or infusion (20–30 min) are preferred to continuous infusion, which introduces risk of incompatibility or drug instability. However, the i.m. route is cheaper, less complicated and is quite satisfactory, even in some serious infections when parenteral therapy need be only brief (pneumonia, cellulitis, osteomyelitis) before resorting to the oral route.

Combinations of antimicrobials

A critical attitude is essential towards the use of two or more antimicrobials, prescribed separately to suit the patient and the infection. *The indications for use of two or more antimicrobials concomitantly are four:*

1. *To obtain potentiation*, i.e. an effect unobtainable with either drug alone, e.g. co-trimoxazole; penicillin plus gentamicin (in enterococcal endocarditis).

2. *To delay development of drug resistance*, especially in chronic infections, e.g. tuberculosis.

3. *To broaden the spectrum of antibacterial activity* in a known mixed infection or where treatment is essential before a diagnosis has been reached; full doses of each drug are needed.

4. *To reduce severity or incidence of adverse reactions* where the organism is fully sensitive to each drug, but only if doses liable to cause adverse

reactions are used; here, lower therapeutic doses of each drug are used. This use is uncommon.

The attitude 'if one drug is good, two should be better and three should cure almost anybody of anything'* is naive and irrational.

Bactericidal drugs act most effectively on rapidly dividing organisms. Thus, a bacteristatic drug, by reducing multiplication, may protect the organism from the bactericidal drug.† When a combination must be used blind, it is best to use two bacteristatic or two bactericidal drugs. But the matter of mutual antagonism of antimicrobials is complex; drugs are not purely bacteristatic or bactericidal at all concentrations and microbiologists will advise special combinations for particular organisms.

Disadvantages of combined therapy include:

1. A false sense of security, discouraging efforts towards accurate diagnosis.

2. Broader suppression of normal flora with increased risk of opportunistic infection with resistant organisms.

3 Increased incidence and variety of adverse reactions.

Chemoprophylaxis and suppressive therapy

It is sometimes assumed that what a drug can cure it will also prevent, but this is not necessarily so.

The basis of effective true chemoprophylaxis is the use of a drug against one organism of virtually uniform susceptibility, e.g. penicillin against a group A streptococcus. But the term chemoprophylaxis is commonly extended to include prevention of *disease* as well as prevention of *infection*.

The main categories of chemoprophylaxis may be summarised as follows:

1. *True prevention of infection*: recurrent rheumatic fever‡, recurrent urinary tract infection, protection of immunocompromised patients.

2. *Suppression* of existing infection before it causes overt disease (tuberculosis, malaria, animal bites).

3. *Prevention of exacerbations* of a chronic infection (bronchitis, cystic fibrosis).

4. *Prevention of opportunistic infections* due to commensals getting into the wrong place (bacterial endocarditis after dentistry and peritonitis after bowel surgery); note that these are both high-risk situations of short duration. Prolonged administration of drugs before surgery would result in the areas concerned (mouth and bowel) being colonised by drug-resistant organisms with potentially disastrous results (see below).

5. *Epidemics* of meningococcal meningitis, dysentery, rickettsial infection and plague, as well as trypanosomiasis and syphilis and gonorrhoea. The indications for chemoprophylaxis vary and may be non-existent in some cases, e.g. sexually transmitted diseases.

6. *Contacts*: influenza A can be partially prevented by amantadine; in an epidemic of meningitis or when there is a case in the family, rifampicin is accepted as protective; very young and fragile non-immune child contacts of pertussis *might* benefit from erythromycin or amoxycillin.

In *hepatic failure*, the suppression of bowel flora to prevent coma due to absorption of toxic protein metabolites can also be considered a form of chemoprophylaxis.

Prophylaxis of bacterial infection can be achieved often by doses that are inadequate for therapy. Details of the practice of chemoprophylaxis are given in the appropriate sections.

Attempts to use drugs routinely in groups specially at risk to prevent infection by a range of organisms, e.g. pneumonia in the unconscious or in patients with heart failure and in the newborn after prolonged labour, have not only failed but have sometimes permitted infections with less susceptible organisms. Attempts routinely to prevent bacterial infection secondary to virus infections, e.g. in respiratory tract infections or measles, have not been sufficiently successful to

* Jawetz E. Ann Rev Pharmacol 1968; 8:151.

† Antagonism has been shown to occur in clinical practice when penicillin has been combined with a tetracycline or erythromycin (bacteristatic).

‡ Rheumatic fever is caused by a large number of types of group A streptococci. But immunity is type specific, so that recurrent attacks are commonly due to infection with different strains. All strains are sensitive to penicillin and so chemoprophylaxis is effective. Acute glomerulonephritis is also due to group A streptococci. But only a few types cause it, so that natural immunity is more likely to protect and, in fact, second attacks are rare. Therefore, chemoprophylaxis is not used.

outweigh the disadvantages of drug allergy and infection with drug-resistant bacteria. It is probably generally better to await complications and then to treat them vigorously, than to try to prevent them.

Chemoprophylaxis in surgery

This topic deserves fuller discussion. The principles governing use of antimicrobials in the context are:

1. Chemoprophylaxis is justified:
— when the risk of infection is high because of bacteria in the viscus that is being operated on, e.g. the large bowel,
— when infection, though rare, may have disastrous consequences, e.g. infection of diseased heart valves,
— when the patient is specially susceptible to infection, e.g. because of leukaemia, diabetes.

2. Antimicrobials should be selected with a knowledge of the likely pathogens at different sites.

3. Antimicrobials should be given i.m., i.v. or occasionally rectally at the beginning of anaesthesia and for no more than 48 hours. Specific instances are:

a. *colorectal surgery*: because there is a high risk of infection with *Escherichia coli*, clostridia and bacteroides that inhabit the gut: a cephalosporin plus metronidazole is satisfactory.

b. *gastric surgery*: colonisation of the stomach with gut organisms (above) occurs especially when acid secretion is low, e.g. in gastric malignancy, following use of histamine H_2-receptor blocker or following previous gastric surgery to reduce acid; usually a cephalosporin alone provides adequate chemoprophylaxis.

c. *gynaecological surgery*: because the vagina contains bacteroids, coliforms and lactobacilli, especially during reproductive life: metronidazole and a cephalosporin are used. Chemoprophylaxis is indicated for hysterectomy, particularly by the vaginal but also by the abdominal route, and for perineal floor repair, but probably not for other elective procedures.

d. *leg amputation*: because there is a risk of gas gangrene in an ischaemic limb (the skin is contaminated by bowel organisms from waist to knee), and the mortality is high: penicillin should be given, or metronidazole for the patient with allergy to penicillin.

e. *insertion of prostheses*: many would regard chemoprophylaxis as justified because infection almost invariably means that the artificial joint, valve or vessel must be replaced. Staphylococci are most often responsible and fluoxacillin should be used.

f. *prevention of endocarditis*: see infective endocarditis, p. 242.

Problems with antimicrobial drugs

Microbial resistance to drugs

Resistance of antimicrobials is a matter of great importance; if sensitive strains are supplanted by resistant ones, then a valuable drug may become useless. So far, new discoveries have kept pace with development of resistance, but it is sometimes necessary to use the more toxic antimicrobials, and there are no grounds for assuming that new drug development will always outrun resistance. For several years penicillinase-producing staphylococci were a grave clinical problem and killed many people.

Types of drug resistance

1. *Drug tolerant* (primary or acquired): the organism is capable of growing in the presence of the antimicrobial. This is the most usual form.

2. *Drug destroying*: the organisms inactivate the drug: examples include penicillinase- (β-lactamase-) producing staphylococci and the production of aminoglycoside-inactivating enzymes by other bacteria (see below — plasmids).

Origins of resistance in clinical practice:

1. *Selection* of primary or natural resistant strains. In the course of therapy, the naturally sensitive strains are eliminated and those naturally resistant (whether drug tolerant or drug destroying) proliferate and occupy the biological space created for them by the drug. This has happened in the case of gonococci and of penicillinase-producing staphylococci. Such natural selection by the environment is why resistant strains are much more common in hospitals where, for example,

there may even be important amounts of penicillin in the air.

2. *Spontaneous mutation* with selective multiplication of the resistant strain so that it eventually dominates as in (1) above. A high degree of resistance may occur in a single-step mutation (e.g. streptomycin) or it may develop gradually in a series of small steps over a period of days (e.g. erythromycin) or even more slowly, but in general, bacterial resistance developing by the latter mechanism is uncommon.

3. *By transmission of genes from other organisms*, the commonest and most important mechanism. The processes by which genetic material is transferred are:

a. *conjugation*: this is in effect carnal intercourse between cells and requires that bacteria, not necessarily of the same species, come into contact with each other. The genetic material is transferred in the form of *plasmids*, which are circular twin-helical strands of DNA that lie outwith the chromosomes and contain up to 100 genes capable of controlling various metabolic processes including formation of β-lactamases that inactivate penicillins and cephalosporins, and enzymes that destroy aminoglycosides. Plasmids that are encoded for multiple antibiotic resistance are called R-plasmids.

b. *transduction*: genetic transfer occurs through a bacteriophage (a virus that infects bacteria), particularly in the case of staphylococci.

Conjugation and *transduction* are the usual mechanisms and conditions suitable for gene transfer to occur in clinical practice, especially in the large bowel.

Resistance genes are often located on discrete moveable DNA elements called *transposons*, and in effect, plasmids and bacteriophage act as vectors for transposon spread. Transposons have the ability to enter and remain stable in different bacteria even though the plasmid or phage that allowed their entry is destroyed. The significance of transfer of quantities of DNA through R-plasmids or their contained transposons is that bacteria develop resistance, not necessarily to a single drug, but more commonly to a number of antibiotics. Multiple antibiotic resistance confers a considerable advantage on the bacteria in environments in which antibiotics are widely used, e.g. hospitals.

Some mechanisms of resistance to antimicrobial drugs:

1. *Inactivation by enzyme(s) produced by bacteria*. Penicillin and cephalosporins contain a β-lactam ring — they are inactivated by β-lactamase enzymes.

Chloramphenicol resistance develops in the presence of chloramphenicol acetyl transferase (plasmid mediated).

Aminoglycoside-inactivating enzymes are produced (mostly by coded plasmids).

2. *Modification of the site of antibacterial action*. Trimethoprim inhibits bacterial dihydrofolate reductase. Plasmid-mediated resistance can arise from the synthesis of a dihydrofolate reductase with much less sensitivity to the drug. It is relatively uncommon.

3. *Impaired access to the site of antibacterial action*. Antibacterial effects of tetracycline are partly due to the capacity of sensitive organisms to accumulate the drug within the cell. Plasmid-mediated antagonism of this transport process results in resistance to tetracycline.

The problem is complex, for some organisms have not yet become resistant to certain antimicrobials, whereas others readily do so. For example, clostridia and *Streptococcus pyogenes* have not yet developed penicillin resistance, whereas enterobacteria readily acquire resistance to most drugs.

Some microbiologists treat the fact that a microbe does not become resistant to a drug as a challenge to be met rather than a blessing for which to give thanks. Their laboratory efforts in this field have not, so far, led to clinical disaster.

Gonococci rapidly became sulphonamide resistant. By 1945, 10 years after the introduction of sulphonamides, the incidence of resistant strains had risen from less than 30% to over 70% but fortunately, by this time, the efficacy of penicillin had been established. By 1959, strains of gonococci, relatively penicillin-resistant (drug tolerant), were reported and penicillin dosage was being increased in some clinics. In the 1970s, penicillinase-producing (drug destroying) gonococci made their appearance. Since sulphonamides for gonorrhoea have been abandoned, the oganism has gradually regained sensitivity to sulphonamides.

Antibiotic use in humans is not the only source of resistant bacteria. Sub-therapeutic doses of broad spectrum antibiotics have for years been added to animal feeds to promote growth. Outbreak of intestinal infection in eighteen people of whom one died, was probably due to a multiply-resistant salmonella originating in calves fed on chlortetracycline*.

Limitation of resistance to antimicrobials may be achieved by:

1. avoidance of indiscriminate use by ensuring that the indication for, dose of and duration of treatment are appropriate,
2. using antimicrobial combinations in selected circumstances, e.g. tuberculosis,
3. constant monitoring of resistance patterns in a hospital or community,
4. restricting control of drug use, which involves agreement between clinicians and microbiologists, e.g by limiting the use of the newest member of a group of antimicrobials so long as the currently-used drugs are effective.

Opportunistic infection

When any antimicrobial drug is used, there is suppression of part of the normal bacterial flora of the patient, which varies according to the drug. Often, this causes no ill effects, but sometimes a drug-resistant organism, freed from competition, proliferates to an extent that can even be fatal. The principal responsible organisms are *Candida albicans*, *Proteus* spp, pseudomonads and staphylococci. The mere presence of yeasts in the sputum does not mean they are causing disease.

Antibiotic-associated colitis is an example of an opportunistic infection. Almost any antimicrobial that can alter bowel flora may initiate this condition, but the drugs most commonly associated are lincomycin, clindamycin, amoxycillin, ampicillin and cephalosporins. It takes the form either of an acute, non-specific colitis or pseudomembranous colitis that may endanger life, with diarrhoeal stools containing blood or mucus, abdominal pain, leucocytosis and dehydration. A history of antibiotic use in the previous 3 weeks, even if the drug therapy has been stopped, should alert the physician to the diagnosis, which is confirmed by proctosigmoidoscopy and the isolation of *Clostridium difficile* or its toxin from the stools, for it is this toxin that causes the colitis. It is not yet fully understood how antimicrobial therapy allows *Clostridium difficile* to flourish opportunistically in certain cases, but recognition of its causal role in antibiotic-associated colitis provides a rational basis for therapy with vancomycin 125–500 mg by mouth, 6-hourly for 5 days. Metronidazole is also effective.

A special problem of opportunistic infection arises in patients whose *immune systems* are compromised by disease or drugs. Bacterial infection causes about two-thirds of deaths in such patients, the remainder being mainly due to fungi. The requirements are:

1. that treatment be prompt and should be initiated before the results of bacteriological tests are known.
2. that drugs be given parenterally and
3. that bactericidal agents are used, usually in combination, e.g. an aminoglycoside plus a β-lactam antibiotic.

A famous example of opportunistic infection is that induced in guinea pigs by penicillin. The drug that is so remarkably non-toxic (except for allergy) in man and other species is highly noxious to guinea-pigs. Deaths do not occur in germ-free guinea pigs, and can be prevented by a mixture of non-absorbed antibiotics that are active against coliform bacteria. The pencillin, by interfering with normal gut flora, allows an enormous proliferation (10-million-fold) of coliform bacteria in the caecum, with enterocolitis and fatal bacteraemia. This condition may be analagous to the enterocolitis described above that occurs in humans during broad spectrum antibiotic treatment.†

Masking of infections. Masking of infections by chemotherapy is an important possibility. The risk cannot be entirely avoided but it can be minimised by intelligent use of antimicrobials. For example, a course of penicillin adequate to cure gonorrhoea

* Holmberg S D et al. N Engl J Med 1984; 311:617.

† Farar W E et al. Am J Pathol 1965; 47:629.

may prevent simultaneously contracted syphilis from showing primary and secondary stages, and a serological test for syphilis should be done three months after treatment for gonorrhoea. Acrosoxacin will cure gonorrhoea but not syphilis.

Adverse reactions to antimicrobials

Antimicrobials commonly cause allergic-type adverse reactions and it is prudent always to take a drug history before prescribing. When there is doubt, skin-test challenge should be considered, for it is as much a disservice to patients to deny them the use of an effective drug to which they are mistakenly believed to be sensitive, as it is to prescribe one to which they react adversely.

Other adverse reactions, e.g. organ toxicity, are given with the account of individual drugs.

Life-endangering antibiotic (antimicrobial) enterocolitis can occur with a number of agents; it is discussed above.

Drug interactions with antimicrobials

Antimicrobials may interact with each other and with other drugs. Examples are:

1. on absorption: tetracycline chelates iron and calcium and absorption from the gut of all is diminished.

2. on metabolism: rifampicin induces hepatic drug metabolising enzymes and may cause an oral conceptive to fail; metronidazole, cephamandole and latamoxef inhibit alcohol metabolism to cause a disulfiram-like reaction.

3. on elimination: probenecid competes successfully with penicillin for the renal tubular anion transport mechanism, causing pencillin to be retained.

4. on organs: gentamicin and frusemide in high dose create increased risk of ototoxicity; certain cephalosporins have increased chance of nephrotoxicity when used with loop diuretics.

Treatment failure

Treatment failure may be due to drug resistance, natural or acquired. Where the organism is sensitive to the drug used, failure is usually due either to the way the drug is used or to some factor peculiar to the patient, as follows:

1. Treatment begun too late to save patient.
2. Suboptimal use of drug,
   a. dose too small
   b. intervals between doses too long
   c. duration of course too short
   d. unsuitable route
   e. adjuvant medications not used.
3. Organisms present in altered state (dormancy, variant forms).
4. Substances antagonising effect of drug present in the patient, e.g. pus or unsuitable pH.
5. Barriers to adequate access of drug to organism,
   a. natural, e.g. poor entry into eye, cerebrospinal fluid.
   b. pathological, e.g. abscess, fibrosis.
6. Reduced host defences,
   a. disease, e.g. hypogammaglobulinaemia, leukaemia, old age, diabetes, cystic fibrosis.
   b. immunosuppression, e.g. anticancer drugs or adrenal steroids.
7. The organism isolated is not that causing the disease.

Antimicrobial drugs of choice

The following notes and Table 11.1 provide a summary of the choice of antimicrobial drugs. They are published here by permission of the Chairman of the Editorial Board of the *Medical Letter on Drugs and Therapeutics* (USA; 1986). We are very grateful to him for permission to use this material.

The table should be used in conjunction with the text. There is some repetition between text and table, but presenting the data in different ways may be helpful. There are also some differences for there is no single correct procedure for each infection. Resistance may be a problem with drugs marked* and susceptibility tests should be performed.

Table 11.1 Antimicrobial drugs of choice

Infecting organism	Drug of first choice	Alternative drugs
Gram-positive cocci		
★ *Staphylococcus aureus* or *epidermidis*		
Non-penicillinase producing	Penicillin G or V[1]	A cephalosporin[2,3]; vancomycin; imipenem; clindamycin
Penicillinase-producing	a penicillinase-resistant penicillin[4]	A cephalosporin[2,3]; vancomycin; amoxicillin-clavulanic acid; ticarcillin-clavulanic acid; imipenem; clindamycin
Methicillin-resistant[5]	Vancomycin, with or without rifampin[6] and/or gentamicin	Trimethoprim-sulfamethoxazole[6]
Streptococcus pyogenes (Group A) and Groups C and G	Penicillin G or V[1]	An erythromycin[7]; a cephalosporin[2,3]; vancomycin
Streptococcus, Group B	Penicillin G or ampicillin	A cephalosporin[2,3]; vancomycin[6]; an erythromycin[6]
Streptococcus, viridans groups[8]	Penicillin G with or without streptomycin or gentamicin[6]	A cephalosporin[2,3]; vancomycin[6]
Streptococcus bovis[8]	Penicillin G	A cephalosporin[2,3]; vancomycin[6]
Streptococcus, *enterococcus* group		
Endocarditis[8] or other severe infection	Ampicillin or penicillin G with gentamicin[6] or streptomycin	Vancomycin[6] with gentamicin[6] or streptomycin
Uncomplicated urinary tract infection[9]	Ampicillin or amoxicillin	Nitrofurantoin
Streptococcus, anaerobic (peptostreptococcus)	Penicillin G	Clindamycin; chloramphenicol[6,10]; a cephalosporin[2,3]
★ *Streptococcus pneumoniae*[11] (pneumococcus)	Penicillin G or V[1]	An erythromycin[7]; a cephalosporin[2,3]; chloramphenicol[6,10]; vancomycin[6]
Gram-negative cocci		
Branhamella (Neisseria) *catarrhalis*	Amoxicillin-clavulanic acid	Trimethoprim-sulfamethoxazole[6]; an erythromycin[6]; a tetracycline[6,12]
★ *Neisseria gonorrhoeae*[13] (gonococcus)	Amoxicillin (with probenecid) or ceftriaxone	Penicillin G; ampicillin; cefoxitin[2]; spectinomycin; trimethoprim-sulfamethoxazole; chloramphenicol
Neisseria meningitidis[14] (meningococcus)	Penicillin G	Chloramphenicol[6,10]; cefuroxime[2] cefotaxime[2]; ceftizoxime[2,6]; ceftriaxone[2]; trimethoprim-sulfamethoxazole[6]; a sulfonamide[15]
Gram-positive bacilli		
Bacillus anthracis (anthrax)	Penicillin G	An erythromycin[6]; a tetracycline[12]
Clostridium perfringens (welchii)[16]	Penicillin G	Chloramphenicol[6,10]; metronidazole; clindamycin; a tetracycline[12]
Clostridium tetani[17]	Penicillin G	A tetracycline[12]
Clostridium difficile[18]	Vancomycin	Metronidazole; bacitracin[6]
Corynebacterium diphtheriae[19]	An erythromycin	Penicillin G
Corynebacterium, JK strain	Vancomycin[6]	
Listeria monocytogenes	Ampicillin[6] with or without gentamicin[6]	Trimethoprim-sulfamethoxazole[6]; a tetracycline[12]; an erythromycin
Enteric gram-negative bacilli		
★ *Bacteroides*		
Oropharyngeal strains	Penicillin G[6,20]	Clindamycin; cefoxitin[2]; metronidazole; chloramphenicol[6;10]
Gastrointestinal strains[21]	Clindamycin or metronidazole	Cefoxitin[2]; chloramphenicol[6,10]; mezlocillin, ticarcillin, or piperacillin; imipenem; ticarcillin-clavulanic acid[6]
★ *Campylobacter fetus*, ssp *jejuni*	An erythromycin[6]	A tetracycline[12]; gentamicin[6]; chloramphenicol[6;10]

Table 11.1 (cont'd)

Infecting organism	Drug of first choice	Alternative drugs
**Enterobacter*	Cefotaxime[2,22], ceftizoxime[2,22] or ceftriaxone[2,22]	Gentamicin, tobramycin, netilmicin, or amikacin; carbenicillin[23] ticarcillin[23], mezlocillin[6,23], piperacillin[23], or azlocillin[6,23]; imipenem[22]; trimethoprim-sulfamethoxazole; chloramphenicol[10]
* *Escherichia coli*[24]	Ampicillin with or without gentamicin, tobramycin, netilmicin, or amikacin	A cephalosporin[2,3,22]; carbenicillin[23], ticarcillin[23], mezlocillin[23], piperacillin[23], or azlocillin[23], gentamicin, tobramycin, netilmicin, or amikacin; amoxicillin-clavulanic acid; ticarcillin-clavulanic acid[23]; trimethoprim-sulfamethoxazole; imipenem[22]; a tetracycline[12]; chloramphenicol[10]
* *Klebsiella pneumoniae*[24]	A cephalosporin[2,3,22]	Gentamicin, tobramycin, netilmicin, or amikacin; amoxicillin-clavulanic acid; ticarcillin-clavulanic acid[23]; trimethoprim-sulfamethoxazole; imipenem[22]; a tetracycline[12]; chloramphenicol[10]; mezlocillin[23] or piperacillin[23]
* *Proteus mirabilis*[24]	Ampicillin[25]	A cephalosporin[2,3,22]; carbenicillin[23], or azlocillin[23]; gentamicin, tobramycin, netilmicin, or amikacin; trimethoprim-sulfamethoxazole; imipenem[22]; chloramphenicol[6,10]
* *Proteus*, indole-positive (including *Providencia rettgeri*, *Morganella morganii* and *Proteus vulgaris*)	Cefotaxime[2,6,22], ceftizoxime[2,22], or ceftriaxone[2,22]	Gentamicin, tobramycin, netilmicin, or amikacin; carbenicillin[23], ticarcillin[23], mezlocillin[23], piperacillin[23], or azlocillin[23]; amoxicillin-clavulanic acid[6]; ticarcillin-clavulanic acid[23]; imipenem[6,22]; trimethoprim-sulfamethoxazole; a tetracycline[6,12]; chloramphenicol[6,10]
* *Providencia stuartii*	Cefotaxime[2,22], ceftizoxime[2,22], or ceftriaxone[2,6,22]	Imipenem[6,22]; ticarcillin-clavulanic acid[6,23]; gentamicin[6], tobramycin, netilmicin[6], or amikacin; carbenicillin[6,23], ticarcillin[6,23], mezlocillin[6,23], piperacillin[6,23], or azlocillin[6,23]; trimethoprim-sulfamethoxazole[6]; chloramphenicol[6,10]; cefoxitin[2,22]
* *Salmonella typhi*[26]	Chloramphenicol[10]	Ampicillin; amoxicillin[6]; trimethoprim-sulfamethoxazole[6]
* Other *Salmonella*[27]	Ampicillin or amoxicillin[6]	Chloramphenicol[10]; trimethoprim-sulfamethoxazole[6]
* *Serratia*	Cefotaxime[2,28], ceftizoxime[2,28], or ceftriaxone[2,28]	Gentamicin or amikacin; imipenem[28]; trimethoprim-sulfamethoxazole[6]; carbenicillin[6,29], ticarcillin[6,29], mezlocillin[29], piperacillin[29], or azlocillin[6,29]; cefoxitin[2,6,28]
* *Shigella*	Trimethoprim-sulfamethoxazole	Chloramphenicol[6,10]; a tetracycline[12]; ampicillin
* *Yersinia enterocolitica*	Trimethoprim-sulfamethoxazole[6]	Gentamicin[6], tobramycin[6], or amikacin[6]; a tetracycline[6,12]; cefotaxime[2,6] or ceftizoxime[2,6]
Other gram-negative bacilli		
* *Acinetobacter* (Mima, Herellea)	Imipenem[22]	Tobramycin[6], gentamicin[6], netilmicin[6], or amikacin; carbenicillin[6,23], ticarcillin[6,23], mezlocillin[6,23], piperacillin[23], or azlocillin[6,23]; trimethoprim-sulfamethoxazole[6]; minocycline[12]; doxycycline[12]
* *Aeromonas hydrophila*	Trimethoprim-sulfamethoxazole[6]	Gentamicin[6], tobramycin[6], or netilmicin[6]; imipenem[6]; a tetracycline[6,12]
Bordetella pertussis (whooping cough)	An erythromycin	Trimethoprim-sulfamethoxazole[6]; ampicillin[6]
* *Brucella* (brucellosis)	A tetracycline[12] with or without streptomycin	Chloramphenicol[6,10] with or without streptomycin; trimethoprim-sulfamethoxazole[6]; rifampin[6] with a tetracycline[12]
Calymmatobacterium granulomatis (granuloma inguinale	A tetracycline[12]	Streptomycin

Table 11.1 (cont'd)

Infecting organism	Drug of first choice	Alternative drugs
* *Eikenella corrodens*	Ampicillin[6]	An erythromycin[6]; a tetracycline[6,12]
**Francisella tularensis* (tularemia)	Streptomycin or gentamicin[6]	A tetracycline[12]; chloramphenicol[6,10]
**Fusobacterium*	Penicillin G[6]	Metronidazole; clindamycin; chloramphenicol[6,10]
Gardnerella (Haemophilus) vaginalis[30]	Metronidazole[6]	Ampicillin[6]
* *Haemophilus ducreyi* (chancroid)	Ceftriaxone[2] or an erythromycin[6]	Trimethoprim-sulfamethoxazole[6]
* *Haemophilus influenzae*		
meningitis, epiglottitis, arthritis, and other serious infections	Chloramphenicol plus ampicillin initially[31]	Cefuroxime[2]; cefotaxime[2]; ceftriaxone[2]
Other infections	Ampicillin or amoxicillin	Trimethoprim-sulfamethoxazole; cefuroxime[2]; a sulfonamide, with or without an erythromycin; amoxicillin-clavulanic acid; cefaclor[6]; cefamandole[2]; cefotaxime[2]; ceftizoxime[2]; ceftriaxone[2,6]; a tetracycline[12]
Legionella micdadei (*L. pitts-burgensis*)	An erythromycin[6] with or without rifampin[6,32]	Trimethoprim-sulfamethoxazole[6]
Legionella pneumophila	An erythromycin with or without rifampin[6,32]	Trimethoprim-sulfamethoxazole[6]
Leptotrichia buccalis (Vincent's infection)	Penicillin G	A tetracycline[12]; clindamycin[6]
Pasteurella multocida	Penicillin G	A tetracycline[6,12]; a cephalosporin[2]; amoxicillin-clavulanic acid[6]
* *Pseudomonas aeruginosa*		
Urinary tract infection	Carbenicillin or ticarcillin	Piperacillin, mezlocillin, or azlocillin; ceftazidime[2]; imipenem; gentamicin; tobramycin; netilmicin; amikacin
Other infections	Carbenicillin, ticarcillin, mezlocillin, piperacillin, or azlocillin plus tobramycin, gentamicin, or netilmicin[33]	Amikacin with carbenicillin, ticarcillin, mezlocillin, piperacillin, or azlocillin[33]; tobramycin, gentamicin, netilmicin, or amikacin with ceftazidime[2], imipenem, or cefoperazone[2]
Pseudomonas (Actinobacillus) *mallei* (glanders)	Streptomycin with a tetracycline[6,12]	Streptomycin with chloramphenicol[10]
* *Pseudomonas pseudomallei* (melioidosis)	Trimethoprim-sulfamethoxazole[6]	A tetracycline[6,12] with or without chloramphenicol[10,34]; chloramphenicol[10] plus kanamycin[6], gentamicin, or tobramycin; a sulfonamide[6]
Pseudomonas cepacia	Trimethoprim-sulfamethoxazole[6]	Choramphenicol[10]; ceftazidime[2]; imipenem
Spirillum minus (rat bite fever)	Penicillin G	A tetracycline[6,12]; streptomycin
Streptobacillus moniliformis (rat bite fever; Haverhill fever)	Penicillin G	A tetracycline[6,12]; streptomycin
Vibrio cholerae (cholera[35])	A tetracycline[12]	Trimethoprim-sulfamethoxazole[6]
Vibrio vulnificus	A tetracycline[6,12]	Penicillin G[6]
Yersinia pestis (plague)	Streptomycin	A tetracycline[12]; chloramphenicol[6,10]; gentamicin[6]
Acid-fast bacilli		
Mycobacterium tuberculosis[36]	Isoniazid with rifampin[37]	Ethambutol; streptomycin[10]; pyrazinamide; aminosalicylic acid (PAS); cycloserine[10]; ethionamide[10]; kanamycin[6,10]; capreomycin[10]
Mycobacterium kansasii[36]	Isoniazid[6] with rifampin[6] with or without ethambutol[6]	Streptomycin[6,10]; ethionamide[6,10]; cycloserine[6,10]

Table 11.1 (cont'd)

Infecting organism	Drug of first choice	Alternative drugs
Mycobacterium avium-intracellulare-scrofulaceum complex[36]	Isoniazid[6], rifampin[6], ethambutol[6], and streptomycin[6,10]	Clofazimine[38]; capreomycin[6,10]; ethionamide[6,10]; cycloserine[6,10]; rifabutine (ansamycin)[38]; imipenem[6]; amikacin[6]
Mycobacterium fortuitum complex[36]	Amikacin[6,10] and doxycycline[6]	Cefoxitin; rifampin[6]; an erythromycin[6]; a sulfonamide
Mycobacterium marinum (balnei)[39]	Minocycline	Trimethoprim-sulfamethoxazole[6]; rifampin[6]; cycloserine[6,10]
Mycobacterium leprae (leprosy)	Dapsone[10] with rifampin[6] with or without clofazimine[38]	Acedapsone[10,38]; ethionamide[6,10]; protionamide[38]
Actinomycetes		
Actinomyces israeli (actinomycosis)	Penicillin G	A tetracycline[12]
Nocardia	Trisulfapyrimidines	Trimethoprim-sulfamethoxazole[6]; minocycline[6]; trisulfapyrimidines with minocycline[6], ampicillin[6], or erythromycin[6]; amikacin[6]; cycloserine[6,10]
Chlamydiae		
Chlamydia psittaci (psittacosis; ornithosis)	A tetracycline[12]	Chloramphenicol[10]
Chlamydia trachomatis		
(trachoma)	A tetracycline[12] (topical plus oral)	A sulfonamide (topical plus oral)
(inclusion conjunctivitis)	An erythromycin (oral or IV)	A sulfonamide
(pneumonia)	An erythromycin	A sulfonamide[6]
(urethritis or pelvic inflammatory disease)	A tetracycline[12] or an erythromycin	Sulfisoxazole[6]
(lymphogranuloma venereum)	A tetracycline[12] or an erythromycin[6]	
Mycoplasma		
Mycoplasma pneumoniae	An erythromycin or a tetracycline[12]	
Ureaplasma urealyticum	An erythromycin[6]	A tetracycline[6,12]
Rickettsia — Rocky Mountain spotted fever, endemic typhus (murine), tick bite fever, trench fever, typhus, scrub typhus, Q fever	A tetracycline[12]	Chloramphenicol[10]
Spirochaetes		
Borrelia burgdorferi (Lyme disease)	A tetracycline[6,10,40]	Penicillin G[6] or V[6]; an erythromycin[6]
Borrelia recurrentis (relapsing fever)	A tetracycline[12]	Penicillin G[6]
Leptospira	Penicillin G[6]	A tetracycline[6]
Treponema pallidum	Penicillin G[1]	A tetracycline[12]; an erythromycin
Treponema pertenue (yaws)	Penicillin G[6]	A tetracycline[12]
Viruses		
Herpes simplex (keratitis)	Trifluridine (topical)	Vidarabine (topical); idoxuridine (topical)
(genital)	Acyclovir	
(encephalitis)	Acyclovir[6]	Vidarabine
(neonatal)	Acyclovir[6]	Vidarabine[6]
(disseminated, adult)	Acyclovir[6]	Vidarabine[6]
Influenza A	Amantadine	
Respiratory syncytial virus	Ribavirin	
Varicella-zoster	Acyclovir[6]	Vidarabine

1. Penicillin V is preferred for oral treatment of infections caused by non-penicillinase-producing staphyloccci and other gram-positive cocci but is ineffective for gonorrhea. For initial therapy of severe infections, penicillin G, administered parenterally, is first choice. For somewhat longer action in less severe infections due to Group A streptococci, pneumococci, gonococci, or *Treponema pallidum*, procaine penicillin G, an intramuscular formulation, is administered once or twice daily. Benzathine penicillin G, a slowly absorbed intramuscular preparation, is usually given in a single monthly injection for prophylaxis of rheumatic fever, once for treatment of Group A streptococcal pharyngitis, and once or more for treatment of syphilis.
2. The cephalosporins have been used as alternatives to penicillins in patients allergic to penicillins, but such patients may also have allergic reactions to cephalosporins.
3. For parenteral treatment of staphylococcal or non-enterococcal streptococcal infections, a 'first-generation' cephalosporin such as cephalothin, cephapirin, cephradine or cefazolin can be used; for staphylococcal endocarditis, some Medical Letter consultants prefer cephalothin or cephapirin. For oral therapy, cephalexin or cephradine can be used. The 'second-generation' cephalosporins cefamandole, cefuroxime, cefonicid, ceforanide, cefotetan, and cefoxitin and the 'third-generation' cephalosporins cefotaxime, cefoperazone, ceftizoxime, ceftriaxone, and ceftazidime have greater activity against enteric gram-negative bacilli. Moxalactam, another 'third-generation' cephalosporin, has been associated with serious, sometimes fatal, bleeding disorders, and some Medical Letter consultants now advise against its use; in any case, it should not be used to treat infections caused by gram-positive organisms. With the exception of cefoperazone and ceftazidime, the activity of all currently available (March, 1986) cephalosporins against *Pseudomonas aeruginosa* is poor or inconsistent.
4. For oral use against penicillinase-producing staphylococci, cloxacillin or dicloxacillin is preferred; for severe infections, a parenteral formulation of methicillin, nafcillin, or oxacillin shoud be used. Neither ampicillin, amoxicillin, bacampicillin, cyclacillin, hetacillin, carbenicillin, ticarcillin, mezlocillin, azlocillin nor piperacillin is effective against penicillinase-producing staphylococci. However, the combination of clavulanic acid with amoxicillin or ticarcillin is active against these organisms.
5. Occasional strains of coagulase-positive staphylococci and many strains of coagulase-negative staphylococci are resistant to penicillinase-resistant penicillins; these strains are also resistant to cephalosporins and to imipenem.
6. Not approved for this indication by the U.S. Food and Drug Administration.
7. Occasional strains of Group A streptococci and pneumococci may be resistant to erythromycins.
8. In endocarditis, disk sensitivity testing may not provide adequate information; dilution tests for susceptibility should be used to assess bactericidal as well as inhibitory end points. Peak bactericidal activity of the serum against the patient's own organism should be present at a serum dilution of at least 1:8.
9. Routine antimicrobial susceptibility tests may be misleading. Because of high urine concentrations, ampicillin may be effective in urinary tract infections, even when the organism is reported to be 'resistant.'
10. Because of the frequency of serious adverse effects, this drug should be used only for severe infections when less hazardous drugs are ineffective.
11. In patients allergic to penicillin, an erythromycin is preferred for respiratory infections and chloramphenicol is recommended for meningitis. Rare strains of *Streptococcus pneumoniae* may be resistant to penicillin; these strains are susceptible to vancomycin.
12. Tetracycline hydrochloride is preferred for most indications. Doxycycline is recommended for uremic patients with infections outside the urinary tract for which a tetracycline is indicated. Tetracyclines are generally not recommended for pregnant women, infants, or children eight years old or younger.
13. For more details, see the Medical Letter 1986; 28:23. Some strains of gonococci produce penicillinase and are totally resistant to penicillin G, ampicillin, or amoxicillin; these strains should be treated with ceftriaxone or spectinomycin. Penicillin V, benzathine penicillin G, and penicillinase-resistant penicillins should not be used to treat gonococcal infections.
14. Rifampin is recommended for prophylaxis in close contacts of patients infected by sulfonamide-resistant organisms. Minocycline may also be effective for such prophylaxis but frequently causes vomiting and vertigo. An oral sulfonamide is recommended for prophylaxis in close contacts of patients known to be infected by sulfonamide-sensitive organisms.
15. Sulfonamide-resistant strains are frequent in the USA and sulfonamides should be used only when susceptibility is established by susceptibility tests.
16. Debridement is primary. Large doses of penicillin G are required. Hyperbaric oxygen therapy may be a useful adjunct to surgical debridement in management of the spreading, necrotic type.
17. For prophylaxis, a tetanus toxoid booster and, for some patients, tetanus immune globulin (human) are required.
18. Antibiotic-associated diarrhoea or colitis should be treated by discontinuing the implicated antibiotic and avoiding use of antiperistaltic drugs. When *C. difficile* is involved, vancomycin, metronidazole or bacitracin should be given by mouth. If oral therapy cannot be used (such as with severe ileus or recent surgery), parenteral metronidazole is preferred.
19. Antitoxin is primary; antimicrobials are used only to halt further toxin production and to prevent the carrier state.
20. The proportion of penicillin-resistant *Bacteroides* species from the oropharynx has been increasing recently; for patients seriously ill with infections that may be due to these organisms, or where response to penicillin is delayed, clindamycin is preferred.
21. When infection is in the central nervous system, either i.v. metronidazole or chloramphenicol is recommended.
22. In severely ill patients, some Medical Letter consultants would add gentamicin, tobramycin, netilmicin, or amikacin.
23. In severely ill patients, some Medical Letter consultants would add gentamicin, tobramycin, netilmicin, or amikacin (but see footnote 33).

24. For an acute, uncomplicated urinary tract infection, before the infecting organism is known, the drug of first choice is one of the oral soluble sulfonamides, such as sulfisoxazole, or (for *E. coli* or *Proteus mirabilis*) ampicillin or amoxicillin, or (for *Klebsiella*) a cephalosporin. Trimethoprim or trimethoprim-sulfamethoxazole may also be useful for treatment of urinary tract infections caused by susceptible organisms.
25. Large doses (6 grams or more daily) are usually necessary for systemic infections. In severely ill patients, some Medical Letter consultants would add gentamicin, tobramycin, netilmicin, or amikacin.
26. Ampicillin or amoxicillin may be effective in milder cases. Ampicillin is the drug of choice for *S. typhi* carriers.
27. Most cases of *Salmonella* gastroenteritis subside spontaneously without antimicrobial therapy.
28. In severely ill patients, some Medical Letter consultants would add gentamicin or amikacin.
29. In severely ill patients, some Medical Letter consultants would add gentamicin or amikacin (but see footnote 33).
30. Metronidazole is effective for bacterial vaginosis even though it is not active against *Gardnerella in vitro*. Ampicillin should be used for sepsis.
31. Some strains of *H. influenzae* are resistant to ampicillin and rare strains are resistant to chloramphenicol. Chloramphenicol (75–100 mg/kg/day i.v.) plus ampicillin can be used initially for treatment of meningitis in children more than one month old until the organisms is identified and its antimicrobial susceptibility is determined. Ampicillin is preferred by some Medical Letter consultants for treatment of organisms known to be susceptible.
32. Rifampin should be added only for patients who do not respond to erythromycin alone.
33. Neither gentamicin, tobramycin, netilmicin, nor amikacin should be mixed in the same bottle with carbenicillin, ticarcillin, mezlocillin, piperacillin, or azlocillin for i.v. administration. In high concentration or in patients with renal failure, carbenicillin or ticarcillin may inactivate the aminoglycosides.
34. Seriously ill patients should be treated with both tetracycline and chloramphenicol.
35. Antibiotic therapy is an adjunct to and not a substitute for prompt fluid and electrolyte replacement.
36. Susceptibility tests should be performed by appropriate reference laboratories, but antituberculosis drugs may be effective *in vivo* even when *in vitro* tests show resistance. Some isolates may require vigorous chemotherapy using multiple drugs.
37. Rifampin should be used concurrently with other drugs to prevent emergence of resistance. It is always included in treatment regimens for isoniazid-resistant organisms and is generally used together with isoniazid in the treatment of cavitary and far-advanced pulmonary tuberculosis as well as for extrapulmonary tuberculosis.
38. An investigational drug in the USA.
39. Most infections are self-limited without drug treatment.
40. For treatment of early infection in non-pregnant adults, tetracycline is preferred; for fully developed infection with arthritis or meningitis, i.v. penicillin G is preferred.

GUIDE TO FURTHER READING

1 Marquardt M. Paul Ehrlich. London: Heinemann, 1949.
2 Colebrook L, Kenny M. Treatment with prontosil of puerperal infections. Lancet 1939; 2:1319.
3 Rountree P M, Thomson E F. Incidence of antibiotic-resistant staphylococci in a hospital. Lancet 1952; 2:262.
4 Barber M. Reversal of antibiotic resistance in hospital staphylococcal infection. Br Med J 1960; 1:11.
5 Burns L E. Fatal circulatory collapse in premature infants receiving chloramphenicol. N Engl J Med 1959; 261:1318.
6 Mackowiak P A. The normal microbiological flora. N Engl J Med 1982; 307: 83–93.
7 Engleberg N C, Eisenstein B I. The impact of new cloning techniques on the diagnosis and treatment of infectious diseases. N Engl J Med 1984; 311: 892–901.
8 Mackowiak P A. Microbial synergism in human infections. N Engl J Med 1978; 289: 21–26, 83–87.
9 Johnston R B. Recurrent bacterial infections in children. N Engl J Med 1984; 310: 1237–1243.
10 Keighley M R B. Perioperative antibiotics. Br Med J 1983; 286: 1844–1846.
11 Nichols R L (editorial). Postoperative wound infection. N Engl J Med 1982; 307: 1701–1702.
12 Shapiro M et al. Risk factors for infection at the operative site after abdominal or vaginal hysterectomy. N Engl J Med 1982; 307: 1661–1666.
13 Editorial. Intramuscular or intravenous antibiotics? Lancet 1984; 1: 660–662.
14 Editorial. Plugging the penicillin leak with probenecid. Lancet 1984; 2: 499–500.
15 Editorial. Antimicrobials and haemostasis. Lancet 1983; 1: 510–511.
16 Editorial. Antibiotic antagonism and synergy. Lancet 1978; 2:80–82.
17 Pedler S J, Bint A J K (editorial). Combinations of betalactam antibiotics. Br Med J 1984; 288: 1022–1024.
18 Sanderson P J (editorial). Common bacterial pathogens and resistance to antibiotics. Br Med J 1984; 289: 638–639.
19 Levy S B (editorial). Playing antibiotic pool: time to tally the score. N Engl J Med 1984; 311: 663–664.
20 Levy S B. Microbial resistance to antibiotics. An evolving and persistent problem. Lancet 1982; 2: 83–88.
21 Shapiro M et al. Use of antimicrobial drugs in general hospitals. Patterns of prophylaxis. N Engl J Med 1979; 301: 351–355.
22 Baum M L et al. A survey of clinical trials of antibiotic prophylaxis in colon surgery: evidence against further use of no-treatment controls. N Engl J Med 1981; 305: 795–799.
23 Chiswich M L (editorial). Infection and defences in the neonate. Br Med J 1983; 286: 1377–1378.
24 Wolfson J S, Swartz S W. Serum bactericidal activity as a monitor of antibiotic therapy. N Engl J Med 1985; 312: 968–975.

12

Infection II: Antibacterial drugs

Classification of antibacterial drugs

Antibacterial drugs are most usefully classified according to their molecular structures; members of each group have the same mechanism of action, are usually handled by the body in a similar way and have the same range of adverse effects. The following groups encompass most antibacterial drugs:

Beta-lactams, so called because they contain a β-lactam ring. The major subdivisions are the penicillins whose approved names include and often end in '-cillin' and the cephalosporins and cephamycins, which are recognized by the inclusion of 'cef' or 'ceph' in their approved names.

Aminoglycosides, which contain an amino-sugar and a glycoside. Those that are derived from streptomyces end in '-mycin', for example, tobramycin, streptomycin, neomycin and kanamycin. Others comprise gentamicin (from *Micromonospora purpurea*, which is not a fungus, hence the spelling as '-micin') and the semi-synthetic amikacin and netilmicin.

Sulphonamides are all derivatives of sulphanilamide and usually their names contain 'sulpha' or 'sulfa'.

Tetracyclines, as the name suggests, are four-ringed structures and all approved names contain '-cycline'.

Macrolides contain a macrocyclic lactone ring, for example, erythromycin and spiramycin.

Imidazoles all contain an imidazole ring and the approved names end in '-azole', e.g. metronidazole.

Polypeptides are composed of peptide-linked amino acids and include bacitracin, polymyxin B, colistin and gramicidin.

A number of important antimicrobial agents do not bear a close structural relationship to any of the above groups and these are described individually.

THE BETA LACTAMS

The Penicillins

Penicillin is produced by growing one of the penicillium moulds in deep tanks. According to the variety of fungus and the composition of the medium either benzylpenicillin (penicillin G) or phenoxymethylpenicillin (penicillin V) results.

In 1957, the penicillin nucleus (6-aminopenicillanic acid) was made by fermentation and it became possible to add various side-chains and so to make semi-synthetic penicillins with different properties.

It is important to recognise that all penicillins have not the same antibacterial activity and that it is necessary to choose between a number of penicillins just as between antimicrobials of different structural groups.

Clinically relevant penicillins may be categorised into those that occur naturally and the semisynthetic variants as follows:

Natural penicillins	benzylpenicillin
	phenoxymethylpenicillin
Semisynthetic penicillins	
1. β-lactamase-resistant	methicillin
	oxacillin
	cloxacillin
	flucloxacillin
2. Extended spectrum	
a. aminopenicillins	ampicillin
	ampicillin pro-drugs
	talampicillin
	pivampicillin
	bacampicillin
	ampicillin analogue
	amoxycillin
	(amoxycillin plus clavulanate, Augmentin)
b. amidinopenicillins	pivmecillinam
	mecillinam
c. carboxypenicillins	carbenicillin
	ticarcillin
d. ureidopenicillins	mezlocillin
	azlocillin
	piperacillin

A general account of the penicillins follows and then of the individual members in so far as they differ.

Mode of action is by interference with synthesis of the peptidoglycan layer of the cell wall which normally protects the bacterium from its environment. The β-lactam bond part of the antibiotic is a structural analogue of alanyl-alanine, a constituent of muramic acid, which forms the cross-linkages between peptide chains in the peptidoglycan layer. Defective wall synthesis renders the cell incapable of withstanding the osmotic gradient between the cell and its environment so that it swells and explodes. Penicillins are thus bactericidal and are only effective against multiplying organisms, as resting organisms are not making new cell wall. The main defence of bacteria against penicillins is production of enzymes, β-*lactamases*, which open the β-lactam bond and terminate its activity.

The remarkable safety of penicillin in man is due to the fact that human cell walls are of such different structure that they are unaffected by the drug.

Pharmacokinetics. Some penicillins, notably benzylpenicillin, are destroyed by gastric acid and are unsuitable for oral use. Those that can resist acid (e.g. phenoxymethylpenicillin) are absorbed in the upper small bowel and give a peak plasma concentration within one hour of dosing. The plasma $t_{\frac{1}{2}}$ of penicillins is usually short (see below); they are distributed mainly in the body water (distribution volume approx 18 litres/70 kg).

Penicillins are organic acids and their rapid clearance from plasma is due to secretion into renal tubular fluid by the anion transport mechanism in the kidney. Renal clearance therefore greatly exceeds the glomerular filtration rate (127 ml/min). The excretion rate of penicillin can be usefully delayed by concurrently giving probenecid, which competes successfully for the transport mechanism. Dosage of penicillin may need to be reduced for patients with severely impaired renal function.

Adverse effects. The main hazard with the penicillins is allergic reactions.

After a tonsillectomy, penicillin was administered to a young man who developed a rash. It was decided to change the treatment but, due to an oversight, the patient's name was not removed from the 'penicillin list'. The patient told the nurse of his allergy to penicillin as she was about to give the next injection, but the nurse relied on the list, proceeded to give the injection, and the patient died of anaphylactic shock. All patients should be asked about previous allergy as a routine, and a positive answer should be taken seriously.

A court of law has ruled that the importance of penicillin allergy is such that failure to enquire about previous adverse effects is negligent.

Doctors and nurses who prepare injections carelessly sometimes sensitise themselves to penicillin. Allergies of all kinds occur in up to 10% of patients, principally itching, rashes (eczematous or urticarial), drug fever and angioneurotic oedema. Anaphylactic shock, although rare, can be fatal in 10%. It is more likely if a previous reaction has been of serum-sickness type than if it has been urticarial, and occurs within a few minutes of administration. Allergies are least likely when penicillins are given orally and most likely with topical application of penicillin or with procaine penicillin i.m.

There is *cross-allergy* between all the various forms of penicillin probably due in part to their possession of the 6-aminopenicillanic acid nucleus, and in part to degradation products common to them all. Partial cross-allergy exists between penicillins and cephalosporins which is of particularly concern when the reaction to either group of antimicrobials has been angioneurotic oedema or anaphylactic shock.

When attempting to *predict* whether a patient will have an allergic reaction, a reliable history of a previous adverse response to penicillin or a general tendency to allergic conditions, particularly asthma, may be more useful than tests for hypersensitivity. Immediate-type reactions such as urticaria, angio-oedema and anaphylactic shock can probably be taken to indicate allergy, but interpretation of maculopapular rashes is more difficult. Since alternative drugs can usually be found, penicillins are best totally avoided if there is suspicion of allergy.

When the history of allergy is not clear cut and it is desirable to prescribe a penicillin, *skin tests* for allergy may be used, but fatal anaphylactic shock has been caused even by the tiny amounts used. Intradermal tests are more reliable than the scratch or patch tests, although for allergy caused by topical use, the patch test is a proper approach. The major determinant of reactions to penicillin is the penicilloyl group, which is derived from the β-lactam ring. A number of breakdown products of penicillin including penicillamine and penicilloic acid are referred to as minor determinants of pencillin allergy. Intradermal testing with a preparation containing both major and minor determinants has been successful in predicting allergy to penicillin.* Even with intradermal testing, there is a small risk of anaphylactic shock and an alternative approach is to test the patient's plasma for specific IgE antibodies to penicillin; this is said to correlate with intradermal testing in over 80% of cases.† Testing for allergy to penicillin is best left to those with special experience.

If a minor reaction occurs during a course of therapy, it is sometimes possible to continue with antihistamine (H_1-receptor) and/or adrenal steroid cover, but the latter may be hazardous in the presence of infection because it suppresses inflammation. The features and treatment of *anaphylactic shock* are described elsewhere (see index).

The curious cases of rashes with aminopenicillins (e.g. ampicillin) in lymphoid disease is discussed on p. 216.

Other adverse effects include diarrhoea, which occurs with some penicillins due to alteration in normal intestine flora and may lead to opportunist infection with pseudomonads, *Klebsiella* spp. or *Candida albicans*, although this is uncommon. Neutropenia is a risk if penicillins (or other β-lactam antibiotics) are used in high dose and usually for a period of longer than 10 days.‡ Rarely the penicillins cause anaemia, sometimes haemolytic. Enormous doses cause convulsions.

Penicillins are presented as their sodium or potassium salts, which ions are inevitably taken in significant amounts if high dose is used. The physician should be aware of this unexpected source of sodium or potassium especially in patients with renal or cardiac disease.§

Natural penicillins

Benzylpenicillin (penicillin G; $t_{\frac{1}{2}}$, 30 min; protein binding 60%) is used when high plasma concentration is required; concentrations in acutely inflamed tissues follow approximately the same time course. This is why comfortably spaced doses have to be so large. Only the extraordinary lack of dose-related toxicity of penicillin allows such large fluctuations to be acceptable: sometimes these are ten times above the therapeutic concentration. Benzylpenicillin is very largely eliminated by the kidney, about 80% via the renal tubule,

* Sullivan T J et al. J Allergy Clin Immuno 1981; 68:171.

† Spath P et al. Allergy 1979; 34:405

‡ Editorial. *Lancet* 1985 2:814

§ Baron D N. *Lancet* 1984 1:1113.

and this can be blocked usefully by probenecid, e.g. to treat bacterial endocarditis (when very large doses may be needed), to reduce frequency of injection for small children or for single dose therapy, as in gonorrhoea.

Oral administration is unreliable partly because benzylpenicillin is degraded by gastric acid and partly because absorption from the intestine is incomplete. After i.m. injection, maximum plasma concentrations are reached in 30 to 60 min and the drug is eliminated from plasma in 3–6 h, according to the size of the dose given.

Benzylpenicillin is distributed at varying concentrations throughout the body water; the apparent volume of distribution is 18 litres/70 kg; the drug crosses inflamed membranes quite well but little enters bone and nervous tissue.

Uses: Benzylpenicillin is highly active against *Streptococcus pneumoniae* and the Lancefield group A β-haemolytic streptococci. Viridans streptococci are usually sensitive unless the patient has recently received penicillin. *Streptococcus faecalis* is less susceptible and especially for endocarditis, penicillin should be combined with an aminoglycoside, usually gentamicin. Benzylpenicillin is the drug of choice for infections due to *Neisseria meningitidis* (meningococcal meningitis), *Bacillus anthracis* (anthrax), *Clostridium perfringens* (gas gangrene) and *Clostridium tetani* (tetanus), *Treponema pallidum* (syphilis), *Leptospira* (leptospirosis) and *Actinomyces israelii* (actinomycosis). The sensitivity of *Neisseria gonorrhoeae* varies in different parts of the world, and in some areas resistance is rife. *Staphylococcus aureus* is sensitive except for those strains that produce β-lactamase (penicillinase) and these are many.

Adverse effects. These are uncommon, apart from allergy, which is described above.

Benzylpenicillin is presented as both sodium and potassium salts and each gram contains 2.8 mmol of sodium or 1.7 mmol of potassium. Hence, 20 g, as may be given daily for bacterial endocarditis, will provide an extra 56 mmol of sodium or 34 mmol of potassium. This sodium content may be unwelcome in a patient with cardiac failure. It is usual to administer the potassium salt except for patients with poor renal function, who may develop hyperkalaemia.

Massive doses of penicillin, especially if given to patients with poor kidney function, may cause visual and auditory hallucinations, generalised convulsions and coma. Rarely a specific renal allergy occurs after large doses, which causes interstitial nephritis and renal failure.

Preparations and dosage. It is salutary to reflect that the first clinically useful antibiotic is also the least toxic. Because toxicity is virtually confined to allergy, the dose can be adjusted to the known or assumed sensitivity of the organism. The best antibacterial concentration is five to ten times the minimum inhibitory amounts in culture.

For injection. **Benzylpenicillin** may be given i.m. or i.v. (by bolus injection or by continuous infusion). For a sensitive infection, benzylpenicillin 300–600 mg*, 6-hourly is enough. This is obviously inconvenient in domiciliary practice and 600 mg 12-hourly can be used, but because renal excretion is rapid, the minimum blood concentration will fall below that of the same total dose given at shorter intervals. Thus, the maximum blood concentration rises hugely with a big dose, but the *duration* of effect increases only little. If infrequent dosage is unavoidable, a mixture of benylpenicillin and one of its long-acting variants is used (see below).

For relatively insensitive infections and where sensitive organisms are in avascular tissue (infective endocarditis), 6–18 g (10–30 mega-units) are given daily i.v. in divided doses. For such cases it is useful, especially with children, to block active renal tubular excretion with probenecid (which see), to get higher blood concentrations for a longer time with smaller volumes of injection.

When an infection is subdued, a change may be made from the injected to the oral route (phenoxymethylpenicillin) to avoid the discomfort and labour of injections, but it is unwise to depend on the vagaries of intestinal absorption in the very ill.

Intrathecal administration, see below.

Procaine pencillin is given i.m. only (as a suspension). It is a comparatively stable salt and liberates benzylpenicillin over 12–24 h, according to the dose administered. An average dose would be 300 mg once a day or 12-hourly. There is no

* 600 mg = 10^6 units, 1 mega-unit

general agreement on its place in therapy. It is probably best to use benzylpenicillin in the most severe infections, especially at the outset, as procaine penicillin will not give therapeutic blood levels for some hours after injection. It is used for outpatient treatment of sexually transmitted diseases.

Procaine Penicillin Inj., Fortified is an attempt to combine the advantages of benzylpenicillin (rapid absorption and high peak blood concentration) with that of procaine pencillin (slow absorption with lower but steady blood concentration). It contains 300 mg of the procaine salt to 60 mg of benzylpenicillin in 1 ml.

Benzathine penicillin is another sustained-release or depot preparation that gives low blood concentrations lasting from a few days to four weeks following i.m. injection, and according to dose. It is little used in acute infections because blood concentrations are inadequate, but has a place in chemoprophylaxis; the dose for infection with *Streptococcus pyogenes* is 900 mg (1.2 mega-units) i.m., 2–4-weekly. But even infrequent injections are a nuisance and can cause local discomfort, and the risk of a prolonged adverse reaction is always present. Therefore, unless there is a major problem of compliance, phenoxymethylpenicillin (oral 250 mg b.d.) is preferable for such prophylaxis. Benzathine penicillin is occasionally useful for congenital syphilis in infancy.

For oral use. **Phenoxymethylpenicillin** (250 mg; penicillin V), is resistant to gastric acid and so reaches the small intestine intact and is reliably absorbed. It is less active than benzylpenicillin against *N. gonorrhoeae* and *N. meningitidis*, and so is unsuitable for use in gonorrhoea and meningococcal meningitis. It is a satisfactory substitute for benzylpenicillin against *Strep. pneumoniae*, *Strep. pyogenes* and *Staph. aureus*, especially once the acute infection has been brought under control. The dose is 250–500 mg 6-hourly.

Alternative oral, semi-synthetic, acid-resistant penicillins, each with its slightly varying relative potency against particular organisms include *phenethicillin, propicillin, penamecillin.*

All oral penicillins are best given on an empty stomach to avoid the absorption delay caused by food.

Intrathecal administration is probably never essential, but if a diagnostic puncture gives purulent cerebrospinal fluid, some would advocate injecting benzylpenicillin 6 mg in at least 10 ml of fluid to avoid direct damage to the central nervous system (children 0.1 mg/kg diluted appropriately). Ampicillin (10–40 mg) and cloxacillin (10 mg or more) can also be used intrathecally. Overdose causes convulsions, encephalopathy and death; cases of ignorant or careless administration of a full i.m. dose intrathecally still occur with disastrous results. The intrathecal dose is *one-fiftieth* to *one-hundredth* that given i.m.

Semi-synthetic penicillins

β-lactamase resistant. Certain bacteria produce drug-destroying β-lactamases (penicillinases), which, upon coming in contact with the β-lactam ring that is common to all penicillins, open it and terminate the antibacterial activity. The penicillins that resist the action of β-lactamases do so by their possession of an acyl side-chain, which protects the β-lactam bond by preventing the enzyme getting access to it. These penicillins are specifically indicated for the treatment of infections with β-lactamase-producing *Staph. aureus*, and are invaluable in hospitals, where such organisms are particularly common. The drugs do have activity against other bacteria for which penicillin is indicated, but it is important to remember that benzylpenicillin is *substantially* more effective against these organisms — up to 20 times more so in the cases of pneumococci, β-haemolytic streptococci and neisseria. Hence, when infection is mixed, it may be necessary to give benzylpenicillin as well as a β-lactamase-resistant drug.

Cloxacillin ($t_{\frac{1}{2}}$ 30 min, protein binding 95%) resists degradation by gastric acid and is absorbed from the gut, but food interferes with absorption. Cloxacillin (250, 500 mg) is given by mouth, 500 mg 6-hourly, or 250–500 mg i.m. 4–6-hourly.

Flucloxacillin ($t_{\frac{1}{2}}$ 50 min, protein binding 95%) is more fully absorbed and so gives higher blood concentration than does cloxacillin. An oral dose of flucloxacillin 500 mg achieves a peak serum concentration of 14 mg/l, whereas the same dose of cloxacillin gives a peak concentration of 9 mg/l.

Flucloxacillin (250 mg) is given orally or i.m. 250 mg, 6-hourly.

Methicillin ($t_{\frac{1}{2}}$ 30 min) is destroyed by gastric acid and so must be injected i.m. or i.v. Protein-binding (40%) is much less than that of the other penicillinase-resistant penicillins.

Alternatives include *oxacillin*, *dicloxacillin* and *nafcillin*.

Extended-spectrum penicillins. The activity of these semi-synthetic penicillins extends beyond the Gram-positive and Gram-negative cocci that are susceptible to penicillin, and includes many Gram-negative bacilli. They do not resist β-lactamases and are therefore ineffective against organisms that produce these enzymes.

1. **Aminopenicillins.** As a general rule these agents are rather less active than benzylpenicillin against Gram-positive cocci, but more active than the β-lactamase-resistant penicillins (above). They have very useful activity against *Strep. faecalis* and *Haemophilus influenzae* but it is a cause for concern that β-lactamase-producing strains of *H. influenzae* are now being encountered. *E. coli*, *Proteus mirabilis* and *Klebsiella pneumoniae* are variably sensitive and laboratory testing for sensitivity is important. Pseudomonads and proteus species are resistant. The differences between the various members of the group are pharmacological rather than bacteriological.

Ampicillin (250, 500 mg) ($t_{\frac{1}{2}}$ 75 min, protein binding 20%) is acid-stable and is moderately well absorbed when swallowed. The oral dose is 0.5–2 g, 6–8-hourly; or i.m. 250–500 mg, 4–6-hourly. Approximately one-third of a dose appears unchanged in the urine. The drug is concentrated in the bile, which is valuable in biliary tract infections including typhoid carriers.

Talampicillin is an ester of ampicillin which itself is microbiologically inactive; after oral administration it is de-esterified in the gut mucosa or liver to release ampicillin to the systemic circulation (i.e. it is a prodrug). The ester is better absorbed than ampicillin itself, which results in higher blood concentrations for equivalent doses. Talampicillin might be expected to disturb the bowel flora and so cause diarrhoea less than ampicillin because it is inactive when present in the lumen of the gut, although it is still excreted as ampicillin in the bile and enters the bowel as such.

Pivampicillin and *bacampicillin* are other prodrugs that release ampicillin in vivo.

Amoxycillin (250, 500 mg) ($t_{\frac{1}{2}}$ 60 min, protein binding 20%) is a structural analogue of ampicillin that is better absorbed from the gut (especially after food), and for the same dose achieves approximately double the plasma concentration. Diarrhoea appears to be less frequent with amoxycillin than with ampicillin. The oral dose is 250 mg 8-hourly; a parenteral form is available. Other structural analogues of ampicillin include *epicillin* and *ciclacillin*.

Clavulanate-potentiated amoxycillin (Augmentin). Clavulanic acid is a β-lactam compound produced by *Streptomyces clavuligerus*. The substance has little intrinsic antibacterial activity but is important because it binds to β-lactamases and thereby competitively protects the penicillin, so potentiating it against bacteria that owe their resistance to production of β-lactamases. Clavulanic acid is present in tablets as its potassium salt (equivalent to 125 mg of clavulanic acid in combination with amoxycillin 250 mg), as Augmentin. Other such combinations would appear to be suitable, e.g. with ticarcillin. Clearly, it is necessary for the success of the clavulanate and β-lactam penicillin combination that both components should have similar pharmacokinetic properties, and this seems to be so for clavulanate and amoxycillin. Clavulanate-potentiated amoxycillin is a satisfactory oral treatment for infections due to β-lactamase-producing organisms, notably in the respiratory or urinary tracts. It should be used when amoxycillin-resistant organisms are either suspected or proven by culture. The dose is one tablet 8-hourly.

Adverse effects. Diarrhoea may be troublesome with ampicillin (12%) but the incidence is less with prodrugs of ampicillin and with amoxycillin. Ampicillin and its analogues have a peculiar capacity to cause a maculopapular rash resembling measles or rubella, and usually unaccompanied by other signs of allergy. These rashes are very common in patients with disease of the lymphoid system, notably infectious mononucleosis (and may sometimes declare this diagnosis when used for sore throat) and lymphoid leukaemia. A maculopapular rash does not prove allergy to other penicillins, which tend to cause a true urticarial reaction. Opinion differs as to the safety of subsequent use of penicillins without careful testing for allergy.* Patients with renal failure and those taking allopurinol for hyperuricaemia also seem more prone to ampicillin rashes.

2. **Amidinopenicillins.** This group is closely related to the aminopenicillins.

Mecillinam is active principally against Gram-negative bacteria including *E. coli*, salmonellae and shigellae. It is hydrolysed by β-lactamases.

Mecillinam is not absorbed from the gastrointestinal tract. The plasma $t_{\frac{1}{2}}$ life is 1 h in young adults but 4 h in the elderly. The drug is used in severe infection due to Gram-negative bowel organisms and occasionally in enteric fever and invasive salmonella infection.

The dose is 5–15 mg/kg, every 6–8 h by i.m. injection or slow i.v. injection or infusion.

Pivmecillinam is an ester prodrug that is hydrolysed to mecillinam in the intestinal wall and is suitable for oral therapy. Its main use is in urinary tract infection caused by organisms resistant to other oral antimicrobials.

3. **Carboxypenicillins.** Carboxypenicillins were the first pencillins to have antipseudomonal activity. Broadly, they have the same antibacterial spectrum as ampicillin with the additional capacity to destroy *Pseudomonas aeruginosa*.

Carbenicillin ($t_{\frac{1}{2}}$ 75 min) is active against certain strains of pseudomonads, proteus (indole-positive) and *E. coli*, but is destroyed by β-lactamase. It is poorly absorbed from the gut and must be given parenterally to treat systemic infections.

Carfecillin (carbenicillin phenyl sodium) is absorbed from the gut and is suitable for infection of the urinary tract because the drug is concentrated and eliminated by the kidney but plasma concentrations are too low to treat systemic infections. The place of carbenicillin in the treatment of severe systemic infections has largely been taken over by ticarcillin and the ureidopenicillins. Dosage recommendations vary according to the circumstances: for systemic infection with pseudomonads or proteus, give carbenicilin sodium 5 g, by slow i.v. injection or rapid infusion 4–6-hourly; for urinary tract infections, carfecillin 0.5–1.0 g is given by mouth, 8-hourly.

Ticarcillin is similar to carbenicillin but is four times more active against *Ps. aeruginosa*. It is given by i.m. or slow i.v. injection or by rapid i.v. infusion; for systemic infections 15–20 g are given daily in divided doses, usually at 4–8-hourly intervals; for uncomplicated urinary tract infections, 3–4 g are given daily in divided doses.

Note: both carbenicillin and ticarcillin are presented as disodium salts and each 1 g delivers about 5.4 mmol of sodium — this should be borne in mind when treating patients with impaired cardiac or renal function.

4. **Ureidopenicillins.** The ureidopenicillins were developed in a search for extended-spectrum penicillins with more activity against pseudomonads. They are adaptations of the ampicillin molecule, with a side-chain derived from urea — hence the name ureidopenicillin. These agents efficiently penetrate the bacterial cell wall and inhibit its synthesis but are susceptible to degradation by β-lactamases.

Pharmacokinetics. The ureidopenicillins must be administered parenterally. In common with other penicillins, their principal route of elimination is the urine, which they enter via active secretion by renal tubules. In addition, biliary excretion accounts for 20–30%, so that they are therefore less susceptible than are other penicillins to accumulation in patients with poor renal function. An unusual feature about the kinetics of the ureidopenicillins is that as dose is increased, plasma concentration rises disproportionately, i.e. they exhibit *capacity-limited* (*saturation*) *kinetics* probably due to saturation of the non-renal clearance mechanism. Ureidopenicillins are presented as monosodium salts and on average deliver about 2 mmol of sodium per gram of antimicrobial.

The major advantage of these agents is their effectiveness against *Ps. aeruginosa*; azlocillin, for example, is eight times more active than carbenicillin against this organism. Several strains of klebsiella are also sensitive, which is unique amongst the penicillins.

* See Hoigné R et al. In: Dukes MNG, Meyler's side-effects of drugs. Amsterdam: Elsevier, 1984.

All the anti-pseudomonal penicillins can inactivate aminoglycosides *in vitro* and the two types of drug should not be administered in the same syringe or i.v. infusion bottle.

Azlocillin is very effective against *Ps. aeruginosa* infections but less so than the other ureidopenicillins against other common Gram-negative organisms. It is given by i.v. injection 2 g every 8 h, or in serious infections, by i.v. infusion, 5 g every 8 h.

Piperacillin has the same or slightly greater activity as azlocillin against *Ps. aeruginosa* but is more effective against the common Gram-negative organisms. The dose is 100–150 mg kg/day in divided doses (6–8-hourly) by i.m. injection or i.v. injection or infusion, for uncomplicated infections, increasing to 16 g/day when infection is life-threatening.

Mezlocillin is less active than azlocillin or piperacillin against *Ps aeruginosa* but more active than azlocillin against the common Gram-negative organisms. It is given by i.v. injection 2 g every 6–8 h or by i.v. infusion 5 g every 6–8 h for serious infections.

The Cephalosporins

Cephalosporins were first obtained from a fungus *Cephalosporium* cultured from the sea near a Sardinian sewage outfall in 1945. Their molecular structure is closely related to that of penicillin and the development of many semi-synthetic forms followed. They now comprise a group of antibiotics having a wide range of activity and low toxicity. The term cephalosporins will be used here in a general sense for some are strictly *cephamycins* (cefoxitin) or *oxa-β-lactams* (latamoxef).

Mode of action is similar to the penicillins, since both groups possess the β-lactam ring, that is, the cephalosporins bind to bacterial enzymes that are necessary for the formation of the cell wall. Hence, cephalosporins are bactericidal.

Addition of various side-chains on the cephalosporin molecule confers variety in pharmacokinetic and antibacterial activities of the group. They are susceptible to β-lactamases (penicillinases) though the β-lactam ring can be protected by such chemical manoeuvering, which has resulted in compounds with activity against Gram-negative organisms and new generations of cephalosporins.

Pharmacokinetics. Usually, cephalosporins are excreted unchanged in the urine, but some, including cefotaxime, form a desacetyl metabolite. Many undergo active secretion by the renal tubule, which can be blocked usefully with probenecid, but ceftazidime and latamoxef are not affected by probenecid, being eliminated only by glomerular filtration. In general, the dose of cephalosporins should be reduced in patients with poor renal function.

Cephalosporins have a relative short $t_{\frac{1}{2}}$ (except ceftriaxone, see table), usually less than 60 min and 4-hourly dosing may be necessary for serious infections. Some newer cephalosporins are eliminated more slowly. Latamoxef ($t_{\frac{1}{2}}$ 150 min) may be given 8–12-hourly. Protein binding varies between 15% and 90%. Wide distribution in the body allows treatment of infection at most sites, including bone, soft tissue and muscle. The earlier cephalosporins have no place in the therapy of meningitis but latamoxef, and to some extent cefotaxime, attain CSF concentrations sufficient to treat infections caused by sensitive organisms.

Classification of cephalosporins

By convention the *injectable* cephalosporins have been categorised into *generations* of broadly similar antibacterial and pharmacokinetic properties.

First-generation injectables have useful antistaphylococcal activity and comprise *cephazolin* and *cephradine*, together with cephaloridine and cephalothin, which are now seldom used.

Second-generation injectables have antistaphylococcal activity but certain Gram-negative organisms are also susceptible. They comprise *cefuroxime*, *cefamandole* and *cefoxitin*.

Third-generation injectables are mainly effective against Gram-negative organisms but not against staphylococci. They comprise *cefotaxime*, *cefsoludin* and *latamoxef*.

The orally active cephalosporins can be considered equivalent to the first-generation injectables and comprise *cephalexin*, *cephradine*, *cefaclor* and *cefadroxil*.

The proliferation of cephalosporins shows no signs of abating and there is no guarantee that the

12.1 The cephalosporins

Drug	$t_{1/2}$ (h)	Protein binding (%)	Excretion in urine (%)	Dose (g)	Dose interval (h)	Activity against *Staph. aureus*	*H. influenzae*	Entero-bacteriaceae‡	*Ps. aeruginosa*	*Bacteroides fragilis*
1. *Oral drugs*										
Cephalexin	0.8	20	88	0.25–0.5	6–12	++	0/+	++	0	0
Cephradine	0.7	20	86	0.5–1.0	6–12	++	0/+	++	0	0
Cefadroxil	1.5	20	88	0.5–1.0	12	++	++	++	0	0
Cefaclor	0.7	25	86	0.25	8	++	0/+	++	0	0
2. *Parenteral drugs*										
Cephalothin	0.6	70	50	1.0–2.0	4–6	+++	+++	++	0	+
Cephazolin	1.5	80	90	1.0	6–12	+++	++	++	0	+
Cephamandole	0.8	70	75	0.5–2.0	4–8	+++	+++	+++	0	+
Cefoxitin	0.7	75	90	1.0–2.0	6–8	++	++	+++	0	+++
Cefuroxime	1.4	35	80	0.75	8	+++	+++	+++	0	+
Cefotaxime	0.9	40	50	1.0–3.0	6–12	++	+++	+++	+/++	+/++
† Latamoxef sodium	2.5	40	88	0.25–4.0	8–12	++	+++	+++	+/++	++
Cefsoludin	1.5	35	90	0.5–1.0	6–12	++	++	0	+++	+
⋆ Ceftriaxone	8.5	95	55	1.0	24	+++	+++	+++	+/++	+/0
⋆ Cefoperazone	1.7	90	25	2.0	12	+++	+++	+++/++	+++	++/+
Ceftazidime	1.8	17	88	1.0	8	++	+++	+++	+++	+/0
Cefotetan	3.0	87	80	1.0–2.0	12	++	+++	+++	+	+
Cefotiam	0.75	40	70			+++	+++	+++	0	+/0
Ceftizoxime	1.4	30	90	1.0–3.0	8–12	++	+++	+++	+/++	+/++
Cefmenoxime	0.9	52	70			+++	+++	+++	++	+/++

Note. The data in this table are drawn from various sources but mainly from Wise R. Lancet 1982; 2:140 with permission which is gratefully acknowledged (DRL, PNB).

+++ = 10% of the peak serum concentration attained with this drug exceeds mean MIC (minimum inhibitory concentration)

++ = 50% of the peak serum concentration attained with this drug exceeds mean MIC

\+ = 100% of the peak serum concentration attained with this drug exceeds mean MIC

0 = no useful activity.

⋆ high biliary excretion

† strictly an **oxacephem,** a new class of antibiotic closely related to the cephalosporins.

‡ This family contains the common Gram -ve, fermentative intestinal flora except *Ps. aeruginosa*; certain strains may be considered more resistant.

newer drugs will fit tidily into this classification. Therefore, in the present account the cephalosporins are simply separated into their oral and parenteral forms and their characteristics are tabulated as shown in Table 12.1.

Uses of cephalosporins

Formerly, cephalosporins tended to be quoted as useful alternatives for a number of infections, but increasingly often they can be regarded as drugs of choice. Uses include:

Oral cephalosporins are used to treat urinary tract infections, especially those due to enterobacteria resistant to other agents. Exacerbations of chronic bronchitis also respond when these are caused by *H. influenzae*, including β-lactamase-producing strains.

Parenteral cephalosporins, especially the newer drugs, are effective against many Gram-negative organisms and bear comparison with gentamicin, for they may have a similar antibacterial spectrum and the cephalosporins do not need to be monitored for safety by plasma concentration.

1. A cephalosporin combined with metronidazole is a reasonable best guess initial treatment for severe infection when the likely organisms are enterobacteria, staphylococci and *B. fragilis*.

2. Many biliary infections are due to enterobacteria and parenteral cephalosporins are useful both for prophylaxis in surgery and for treatment of established biliary sepsis.

3. Patients with urinary tract infection due to multiply-resistant bacteria may develop bacteraemia after urinary tract instrumentation; parenteral cephalosporins are used to avoid this.

4. Gonorrhoea due to penicillin-resistant gonococci may be treated with a single i.m. dose of a cephalosporin, e.g. cefotaxime.

A cephalosporin should not ordinarily be used for an infection proven to be due to *Staph. aureus*; narrow-spectrum agents such as flucloxacillin or sodium fusidate are the drugs of choice.

Adverse effects. Cephalosporins have a low frequency of adverse effects in relation to antimicrobials in general. The most usual are *allergic* reactions of the penicillin type, with any of the characteristic manifestations — urticaria, angioedema, anaphylactic shock, drug fever, serum sickness and maculopapular rash. *There is a degree of cross-allergy between penicillins and cephalosporins* and if a patient has had a severe or immediate type of allergic reaction or if skin testing shows response to minor determinants of penicillin allergy (see index), then a cephalosporin should *not* be used.

If cephalosporins are continued for more than 2 weeks, thrombocytopenia, neutropenia, interstitial nephritis or abnormal liver function tests may occur; these resolve, on stopping the drug. Certain other reactions which appear specific to latamoxef include prolongation of the prothrombin time, which is corrected by vitamin K, and a disulfiram type of response after ingestion of alcohol.

The Monobactams

The richest source of β-lactam antibiotics has hitherto been moulds, e.g. *Penicillium*. Recently, a new class of antibiotic has been isolated from *Pseudomonas acidophilia* and *Chromobacterium violaceum*. The singular feature of this class of antibiotic is that its basic chemical structure is a simple β-lactam ring, as opposed to the conventional penicillins and cephalosporins, which consist of a β-lactam ring fused to a thiazolidine ring; thus, the new compounds are called *monobactams*. They are notably resistant to the action of β-lactamases.

Aztreonam is the most extensively tested member of this group, and has activity against a wide range of Gram-negative bacteria, including *E. coli, Klebsiella* spp, *Proteus* spp. and *Ps. aeruginosa*; it may prove effective against resistant or hospital-acquired infection with such organisms. The drug has no significant action against staphylococci, streptococci, pneumonococci or bacteroides.

Other new classes of beta-lactam antibiotic include the *penams, penems, carbapenams and carbapenems*, members of which are undergoing clinical evaluation, e.g. imepenem.

THE AMINOGLYCOSIDES

Streptomycin was the first important antibiotic discovered in the purposeful search that followed the demonstration of the clinical efficacy of penicillin. It is obtained from *Streptomyces griseus*, which was cultured by Waksman in 1944 from a heavily manured field and also from a chicken's throat. It was soon introduced into medicine for its bactericidal activity against *Mycobacterium tuberculosis* and other penicillin-insensitive organisms.

Subsequently, several other aminoglycosides have been developed. They resemble each other in their mode of action, therapeutic and toxic, and pharmacokinetic properties; the main differences in their use reflect variation in their antibacterial activity; cross-resistance within this group is variable.

Mode of action. The aminoglycosides are bactericidal. They act inside the cell by binding to the ribosomes in such a way that incorrect amino acid sequences are entered into peptide chains. The abnormal proteins that result are fatal to the microbe.

Pharmacokinetics. Aminoglycosides are water-soluble compounds and do not readily cross lipoprotein cell walls. Absorption from the intestine is poor, and after intramuscular or intravenous injection, the drugs distribute to the extracellular fluid (distribution volume is approximately 18 l/70 kg). Transfer into the cerebrospinal fluid is poor even when the meninges are inflamed. Pulmonary secretions contain only about half the concentrations present in the plasma. Plasma protein binding is usually 30% or less and the $t_{\frac{1}{2}}$ varies between 2 and 5 h. Aminoglycosides are eliminated unchanged mainly by glomerular filtration (renal clearance is 80–90 ml/min) and achieve high concentrations in the urine. Significant accumulation occurs in the renal cortex unless there is severe renal parenchymal disease. Because of their toxicity, dose adjustment is necessary to compensate for varying degrees of renal impairment, including that of normal ageing, and schemes have been developed to assist in prescribing for these patients* (see also Prescribing for patients with renal disease, p. 561). In addition, antibiotic concentrations should be measured regularly in such patients — indeed, with heavy or prolonged use, the margin between therapeutic and toxic concentrations is sufficiently narrow to warrant routine checking plasma concentration, even if renal function is normal. All aminoglycosides are extracted by haemodialysis and plasma concentration should be monitored in patients who receive such treatment.

* Mawer G E et al. Bri J Clin Pharmacol 1974; 1:45. Dettli L. Clin Pharmocokinet 1976; 1:126.

Antibacterial activity. Aminoglycosides are in general active against aerobic Gram-negative organisms and the drugs are important in serious infections. Individual differences in antibacterial activity are given below.

Bacterial resistance to aminoglycosides is an increasing problem and can develop:

1. through the acquisition of *plasmids* (see p. 201), which mediate the formation of enzymes that inactivate aminoglycosides by adenylating, acetylating or phosphorylating their hydroxyl or amino groups. This is the most important mechanism. There are at least 15 such enzymes, eight of which inactivate gentamicin, tobramycin or netilmicin, but amikacin is inactivated only by one and possibly two others and is therefore useful for resistant organisms.

2. through decreased transport of aminoglycosides into the bacterial cell, a pre-requisite for their effectiveness. This may arise during a course of therapy. Resistance to *Ps. aeruginosa* can come about in this way, and may affect one drug or all members of the group.

Uses of aminoglycosides

Systemic use

1. *Gram-negative bacillary infection, particularly septicaemia, pelvic and abdominal sepsis.* Gentamicin remains the drug of choice because of its proven effectiveness against serious infections, and it has held its place despite evidence that tobramycin and netilmicin are less ototoxic and nephrotoxic. Tobramycin should be preferred for infections caused by *Ps. aeruginosa*. Amikacin has the widest antibacterial spectrum of the aminoglycosides but is best reserved for infection caused by gentamicin-resistant organisms. An aminoglycoside should be included in the best-guess

regimen for treatment of serious septicaemia before the causative organism(s) is identified.

2. *Bacterial endocarditis*. An aminoglycoside, usually gentamicin, should comprise part of the antimicrobial combination for enterococcal, streptococcal or staphylococcal infection of the heart valves, and should be included in the therapy of clinical endocarditis which fails to yield a positive blood culture.

3. *Other infections:* tuberculosis, tularaemia, plague, brucellosis (see streptomycin).

Topical uses

Neomycin, whilst too toxic for systemic use, is effective for topical treatment of infections of the conjunctiva or external ear. Gentamicin should not be applied topically as resistant strains of pseudomonads, enterobacteria and staphylococci readily emerge. Framycetin and neomycin are used in antimicrobial combinations to sterilise the bowel of patients who are to receive intensive immunosuppression therapy.

Adverse reactions

Aminoglycosides can cause serious toxicity, which is of the following types:

1. *Ototoxicity*. *Auditory* impairment appears to be more common with amikacin, neomycin and kanamycin; *vestibular* toxicity with streptomycin, gentamicin and tobramycin, but these differences between drugs are not always precise. Tinnitus may give warning of auditory nerve damage. Early signs of vestibular toxicity include motion-related headache, dizziness or nausea and are indications to stop or to re-adjust the dosing schedule.

Without postural sense, swimming becomes dangerous. Caloric tests of vestibular function may enable vestibular damage to be detected before serious symptoms occur. Factors that predispose to ototoxicity include poor renal function and prolonged duration of treatment; both these may lead to high plasma concentrations of aminoglycoside and, for gentamicin, trough concentrations persistently in excess of 2 mg/l increase the risk. Recent or concurrent treatment with another ototoxic drug (e.g. loop diuretic) may also be damaging. The elderly are most at risk. The use of streptomycin to destroy vestibular function (bilaterally) in the treatment of Meniére's syndrome (unilateral), while interesting as applied pharmacology, is hardly therapeutics.

2. *Nephrotoxicity*. Dose-related changes occur in renal tubular cells where aminoglycosides accumulate. Low blood pressure, loop diuretics, advanced age and previous exposure to nephrotoxic substances such as certain cephalosporins are recognised as risk factors. Neomycin, gentamicin and amikacin are more nephrotoxic than tobramycin and netilmicin.

3. *Neurotoxicity*. Large amounts of streptomycin instilled into the pleural or peritoneal cavities may cause respiratory paralysis due to competitive neuromuscular block (curare-like), particularly in patients who have received muscle relaxants or who have myasthenia gravis. Rarely, this effect has been seen after parenteral use. Vague feelings of paraesthesiae of the lips, headache, lassitude and dizziness may occur after injection of streptomycin.

4. Other reactions include rashes, drug fever with eosinophilia and haematological abnormalities, including marrow depression, haemolytic anaemia and bleeding due to antagonism of factor V.

Individual aminoglycosides

Gentamicin (3 mg/kg/day in three equally divided doses if renal function is normal; 5 mg/kg/day or more in life-threatening infections) is active against aerobic Gram-negative bacilli including *E. coli*, *Enterobacter* spp., *K. pneumoniae*, *Proteus* spp. (indole positive) and *Ps. aeruginosa*. The drug is only moderately effective against streptococci and is inactive against anaerobes. Therefore, in the best-guess treatment of septicaemia, gentamicin should be combined with a β-lactam antibiotic or an anti-anaerobic agent (e.g. metronidazole) or with both. Gentamicin is a drug of choice for serious Gram-negative *septicaemia* and it is effective for abdominal and pelvic sepsis, when combined with an agent effective against *B. fragilis*. An important use of gentamicin is in infection of the *endocardium*; in streptococcal endocarditis it is combined with benzylpenicillin; in staphylococcal endocarditis, gentamicin is given with a specific antistaphylococcal agent and in enterococcal endocarditis, gentamicin and vancomycin are used. Infections in neutropenic patients can be managed initially with gentamicin plus one of the antipseudomonas penicillins until specific sensitivities are known.

Dosing should aim at a peak serum concentration of 8 mg/l, 15 min after i.v. injection (5 mg/l, 1 h after i.m. injection) and a trough concentration of less than 3 mg/l, 15 min before the next injection on an 8-hourly regimen. It may be given intrathecally in meningitis due to Gram-negative bacteria since the drug does not enter the CSF readily. When renal function is normal, urine concentration can reach 50–100 times that in plasma, but less toxic drugs are usually used to treat urinary infection. Penetration into inflamed joints is probably reasonably good, but entry into bile is variable in the presence of biliary obstruction. Gentamicin applied to the eye gives good corneal and aqueous humour levels. Topical applications for skin infections are available but the prolonged use of gentamicin in this form is to be condemned as it may lead to the emergence and spread of resistant organisms.

Tobramycin is broadly similar to gentamicin but may be useful when infection with gentamicin-resistant organisms is thought to have occurred; in particular, it is more active against some strains of *Ps. aeruginosa*. Dosage and recommended plasma concentrations are similar to those for gentamicin.

Amikacin (15 mg/kg/day in two equally divided doses, total course not to exceed 15 g) is mainly of value against gentamicin-resistant organisms. Amikacin is two to four times less potent (efficacy and toxicity) than gentamicin and can be given safely in higher doses. Peak plasma concentrations should be kept below 30 mg/l and trough concentrations below 10 mg/l.

Netilmicin (3–5 mg/kg/day in three equally divided doses) is a semi-synthetic aminoglycoside that is active against some strains of bacteria that resist gentamicin and tobramycin; evidence suggests that it may be less ototoxic and nephrotoxic.

Kanamycin is similar to other aminoglycosides, but it has little efficacy against *Ps. aeruginosa*. It can be used as a reserve drug in tuberculosis.

Sisomicin is similar to gentamicin.

Dibekacin is structurally similar to tobramycin and has similar antimicrobial properties.

Neomycin (500 mg) is principally used *topically* for skin and ear infections and for its antibacterial action in the bowel; in the latter case it is preferred above streptomycin because it is more effective against coliforms (*E. coli*, *Proteus* spp., *Ps. aeruginosa*) and because drug resistance is slower to develop.

Neomycin is the best antibiotic to reduce the bacterial population of the intestine in *hepatic failure*; the total dose is 4–6 g daily. *Enough absorption can occur from both oral and topical use to cause eighth cranial nerve damage* (especially if there is renal impairment) and patients have successfully claimed compensation for such injury after topical use (e.g. in the ear). Diarrhoea may be due to neomycin and prolonged oral use causes malabsorption of both food and drugs with characteristic intestinal mucosal changes.

Framycetin is similar to neomycin in use and in toxicity. It is very ototoxic and enough may be absorbed with topical use on raw surfaces to produce this effect. It is also nephrotoxic.

Streptomycin is a drug of declining importance. Because of its toxicity, it is used only where no other drug will serve. It is used in therapy of tularaemia, plague and possibly brucellosis (combined with a tetracycline), but it also has useful activity against *E. coli*, *Proteus vulgaris*, *Ps. aeruginosa*, *H. influenzae*, and *K. pneumoniae*. In the first-line treatment of tuberculosis, streptomycin has been superseded by rifampicin, isoniazid and ethambutol. Drug-resistant organisms rapidly dominate when streptomycin is used alone.

SULPHONAMIDES AND SULPHONAMIDE COMBINATIONS

The first preparations (1935) were linked to dyes (Prontosil Rubrum and Album) but it was soon discovered that is was the sulphonamide that had the antibacterial effect and that the dye was unnecessary.

One of the first definitive clinical trials was done in 1936 on haemolytic streptococcal puerperal infections. In the five preceeding years, the mortality rate from this infection in hospital had averaged 23%. From January 1936, when the sulphonamide treatment was begun, to August, the mortality was 4.7%. This fall was so dramatic that it was unnecessary and undesirable to delay publication of the results until treatment had continued for a full year as had been intended. The authors admitted that the design of their clinical trial did not exclude as a possible explanation of the result a spontaneous alteration in bacteria virulence, or more remotely, the chance admission to hospital of only mild cases in 1936. They discussed these possibilities but found it 'difficult to resist the conclusion that the treatment has profoundly modified the course of the infection'*. This conclusion was soon amply confirmed.

In 1938, sulphapyridine, widely known as M & B (May & Baker) 693 was introduced and there followed a surfeit of sulphonamides from which to choose.

Mode of action. Sulphonamides illustrate well the important pharmacological principle of *competitive inhibition* (see Fig. 12.1).

Folic (pteroylglutamic) acid is essential for the growth of many bacteria. It is a precursor of purines, which are necessary for the formation of DNA and RNA. Para-aminobenzoic acid (PABA) is a precursor of folic acid and sulphonamides are closely related chemically to PABA, see Fig. 12.1.

Some bacteria (e.g. streptococci) are obliged to synthesise their own folic acid from PABA. Sulphonamides are sufficiently *like* folic acid to be taken up by bacteria, and sufficiently *unlike* to *prevent the bacteria from completing the synthesis to folic acid*. As a result of this dietary and metabolic fraud on the bacteria they are deprived of folic acid and cease to multiply. Sulphonamides are therefore primarily bacteristatic. Man does not synthesise folic acid inside the body: he uses preformed folate from leafy vegetables and his cells are thus unharmed by the metabolic effect of sulphonamides.

The rationale of sulphonamide-trimethoprim combination is as follows: the sulphonamide interferes with the conversion of PABA to folic acid (dihydrofolic) acid and the trimethoprim interferes with the next step, conversion of folic acid to folinic (tetrahydrofolic) acid. The inhibition of successive steps in the synthesis of DNA and RNA converts two bacteri*static* compounds into a bacteri*cidal* combination, an example of pharmacological potentiation in that organisms relatively insensitive to either drug (e.g. Proteus) may be killed by the combination.

The first step (inhibited by sulphonamide) does not occur in man, but the second step (inhibited by trimethoprim) is performed by man. However the sensitivity of the enzyme that is inhibited (dihydrofolate reductase) is 50 000 times greater in bacteria than it is in man, so that the drug is relatively safe. Even so, prolonged therapy with full doses can interfere with haemopoiesis.

Pharmacokinetics. Sulphonamides for systemic use are rapidly *absorbed* from the gut. In the blood, protein binding varies between 20% and 90% according to the compound. Unbound sulphonamide diffuses moderately well throughout the body and enters serous cavities particularly easily if there is inflammation.

Cerebrospinal fluid (CSF) has a lower protein content than blood, so that the proportion of free and bound drug will differ. Concentrations are 40–80% of those in blood. Sulphadiazine enters CSF more readily than others.

Metabolism. The principal path is conjugation with an acetyl group transferred from acetyl coenzyme A. Acetylated sulphonamide has no antibacterial effect but retains its toxicity, and some acetylated forms are less soluble so that they may cause crystalluria. The capacity to acetylate is genetically determined in a bimodal form, i.e. there are slow and fast acetylators (see *pharmacogenetics*) but the differences are insufficient to be of practical importance in therapy.

Excretion. Both the free drug and its acetylated form enter the glomerular filtrate and the urine is the principal mode of excretion. Some undergo renal tubular secretion and tubular reabsorption: the latter is substantial for sulphonamides that arc long-acting, contributing to this property.

In an alkaline urine, sulphonamides are more soluble (except sulphadimidine), more active and at higher concentration (due to less tubular reabsorption). The concentration of the daily dose

* Colebrook L et al. Lancet 1936; 2:1319.

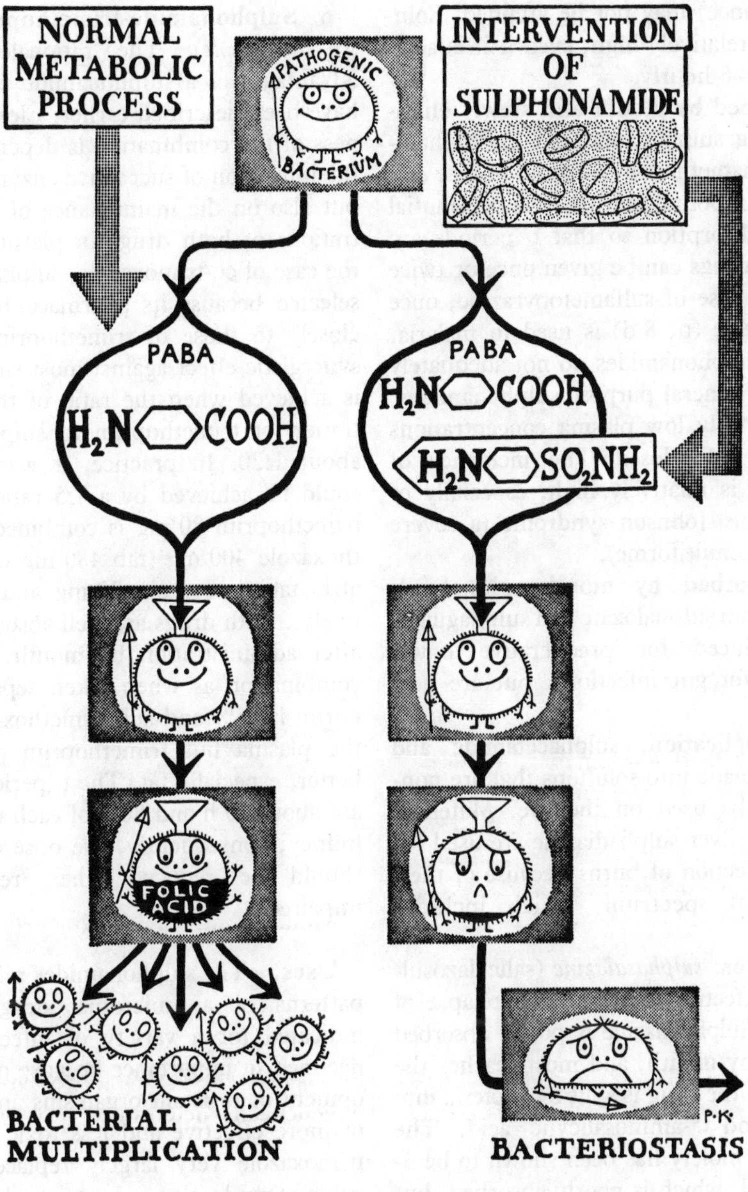

Fig. 12.1 The mode of action of sulphonamides, illustrating the principle of 'competition'

(distributed throughout the body) into about 1.5 l of urine allows high concentrations to be achieved in the urine with doses lower than those required for systemic infections.

Sulphonamides may be classified according to pharmacokinetic properties as follows:

1. **Well absorbed by mouth and rapidly eliminated:**

a. *general purpose*: e.g. sulphadiazine, sulphadimidine (sulphamethazine), and sulphonamide mixtures, e.g. Sulphatriad (sulpha-thiazole, -diazine, -merazine). This group has $t_{\frac{1}{2}}$ periods of 4–15 h; they are given 4–6 hourly.

b. *for urinary infections principally*: e.g. sulphafurazole (sulfisoxazole), sulphamethizole. The $t_{\frac{1}{2}}$ periods are somewhat shorter than the above due to rapid renal clearance, and acetylation is less so that high urinary concentrations of active drug result. But this rapid excretion means that plasma concentrations adequate to treat tissue infection (e.g. renal substance) may not be attained. Solubility in urine is relatively high, even if it is acid. They are given 4–6-hourly.

2. **Well absorbed by mouth and slowly eliminated**: long-acting sulphonamides: e.g. sulphadimethoxine, sulphamethoxypyridazine. These are extensively protein-bound and there is substantial renal tubular reabsorption so that $t_{\frac{1}{2}}$ periods are 30–40 h and the drugs can be given once or twice a day, or, in the case of sulfametopyrazine, once a week. Sulfadoxine ($t_{\frac{1}{2}}$, 8 d) is used in malaria. The long-acting sulphonamides do not adequately substitute for the general purpose sulphonamides, for they provide only low plasma concentrations of free drug at safe doses. The incidence of adverse reactions is relatively high, especially of the serious Stevens–Johnson syndrome (a severe form of erythema multiforme).

3. **Poorly absorbed by mouth**: phthalysulphathiazole, calcium sulphaloxate and sulphaguanidine were produced for preoperative bowel preparation and for gut infections, but are now rarely used.

4. **Topical application**: sulphacetamide and mafenide can be made into solutions that are non-irritant and can be used on the eye. Mafenide (Sulfamylon) and silver sulphadiazine are used for prophylaxis of infection of burns because of their wide antibacterial spectrum, which includes pseudomonads).

5. **Miscellaneous**: *sulphasalazine* (salicylazosulphapyridine) is effective in preventing relapse of ulcerative colitis. Sulphasalazine is poorly absorbed when it is taken by mouth, and most reaches the colon intact; there the drug is split by bacteria into sulphapyridine and 5-aminosalicylic acid. The active therapeutic moiety has been shown to be 5-aminosalicylic acid, which is poorly absorbed, but sulphapyridine is absorbed and there is a good correlation between adverse effects of sulphasalazine and the plasma concentration of sulphapyridine. In effect, therefore, sulphapyridine acts as a carrier to ensure that 5-aminosalicylic acid is liberated within the colon; this has prompted the cynical remark that whereas 5-aminosalicylic acid supplies the benefit, sulphapyridine is there to provide the adverse effects. 5-aminosalicylic acid on its own in special formulation is now used in ulcerative colitis (see index).

6. **Sulphonamide-trimethoprim combination** (*co-trimoxazole*): The rationale and perceived advantages of a sulphonamide plus trimethoprim have been described earlier. Clearly, the effectiveness of the combination is dependent not only on the inhibition of successive enzyme synthetic steps but also on the maintenance of adequate concentrations of both drugs in plasma and tissues. In the case of co-trimoxazole, sulphamethoxazole was selected because its pharmacokinetics correspond closely to those of trimethoprim. The optimum synergistic effect against most susceptible bacteria is achieved when the ratio of the serum concentration of trimethoprim to sulphamethoxazole is about 1:20. In practice, it was found that this could be achieved by a 1:5 ratio of dose; hence, trimethoprim 80 mg is combined with sulphamethoxazole 400 mg (tab 480 mg or 960 mg; paediatric tablets contain 20 mg and 100 mg, respectively). Both drugs are well absorbed from the gut after administration by mouth, as effectively in combination as when taken separately. Trimethoprim is 55% and sulphamethoxazole 34% free in the plasma but trimethoprim penetrates tissues better, especially fat. The $t_{\frac{1}{2}}$ periods of both drugs are about 10 h and 80% of each is excreted by the kidney; consequently, the dose of co-trimoxazole should be reduced when renal function is impaired.

Uses. The sulphonamides reflect the changing patterns of antimicrobial drug use. Formerly indicated for a variety of infections, they have declined in importance because of both the development of resistant organisms and the availability of more effective and less toxic alternatives. Co-trimoxazole very largely replaced the use of a sulphonamide alone. In turn, there is a growing belief that trimethoprim on its own is as effective in many conditions for which the combination has been used, and that it causes fewer adverse reactions.

There is increasing resistance among urinary pathogens to co-trimoxazole; the extent to which this occurs with trimethoprim alone is not yet known.

The position may be assessed as follows:

1. Co-trimoxazole is the *treatment of choice* for pneumonia due to *Pneumocystis carinii*, a life-

threatening infection in immunosuppressed patients. Co-trimoxazole is also indicated for infections with *Nocardia asteroides*.

2. Co-trimoxazole is a useful *alternative* treatment for enteric fever due to chloramphenicol-resistant strains of *Salmonella typhi* and *Salmonella paratyphi* and bacillary dysentery due to strains of shigella resistant to amoxycillin.

3. Co-trimoxazole is being *replaced* by trimethoprim alone for

a. urinary tract infections with susceptible organisms which include *E. coli* and proteus species but not pseudomonads and

b. respiratory tract infections, especially due to the common pathogens *Strep. pneumoniae* and *H. influenzae*.

4. A sulphonamide may be used for the treatment of meningococcal meningitis (sulphadimidine), occasionally for urinary tract infection with suceptible organisms and rarely for respiratory infections.

Dose of co-trimoxazole (960 mg) is twice daily for most infections: i.v. and i.m. formulations are also available.

Doses of some other sulphonamides: sulphadiazine, sulphadimidine (0.5 g) *systemic infections*, loading oral dose 3 g, then 1 g, 6-hourly; *urinary infections*, 1 g, 6-hourly; sulphafurazole (0.5 g) in urinary infection 1 g, 6-hourly: sulphamethizole (100 mg) 200 mg × 5 day.

Adverse effects

Sulphonamides in general. The less serious effects include malaise, headache, nausea or vomiting, diarrhoea, mental depression and rarely cyanosis, which latter is due to methaemoglobinaemia. These may all be transient and are not necessarily indications for stopping the drug.

More serious effects include crystalluria and allergic reactions of many kinds.

Crystalluria occurs particularly with rapidly excreted sulphonamides. It may be symptomless or cause renal colic, haematuria, oliguria and even anuria. If detected before anuria develops, much fluid should be given and the urine made alkaline with potassium or sodium citrate orally or sodium bicarbonate, orally or i.v. according to the state of the patient (particularly regarding renal and cardiac function). The urine should be repeatedly tested to ensure that enough alkali is being given to ensure the pH exceeds 7.0. Ureteric catheterisation or nephrostomy may be necessary.

Allergic reactions due to sulphonamides may include rash, fever, hepatitis, agranulocytosis, purpura, aplastic anaemia, peripheral neuritis, a serum-sickness-like syndrome, polyarteritis nodosa and Stevens–Johnson syndrome.

Co-trimoxazole is generally well tolerated. Rarely, severe skin reactions including erythema multiforme bullosa (Stevens–Johnson syndrome) and toxic epidermal necrolysis (Lyell's syndrome) have been reported. Haemolysis may occur in G-6-PD-deficient subjects. The risk of macrocytic anaemia due to interference with conversion of folic to folinic acid is important with high dose: it can be reversed by giving folinic acid and this will not reverse the antibacterial effect of the trimethoprim since bacteria cannot utilise either preformed folic acid or folinic acid because they do not absorb it. Generally the drug will be withdrawn in preference to continuing it under folinic acid treatment. Co-trimoxazole should not be used in pregnancy because of the possible teratogenic effects of inducing folate deficiency.

TRIMETHOPRIM

Subsequent to its extensive use in combination with sulphonamides, trimethoprim (100 mg; 200 mg) has emerged as a broad spectrum antimicrobial to considerable efficacy on its own. It also has antimalarial efficacy.

The mode of action and pharmacokinetics of trimethoprim are dealt with the foregoing section.

Trimethoprim is active against many Gram-positive and Gram-negative aerobic organisms excepting *P. aeruginosa*. The drug is effective as sole therapy in treating urinary and respiratory tract infections due to susceptible organisms and for prophylaxis of urinary tract infections. The dose is 200 mg twice daily for acute urinary tract or respiratory tract infections.

Adverse effects are fewer than with co-trimoxazole and include skin rash, anorexia, nausea, vomiting, abdominal pain and diarrhoea. Long-term use can interfere with haemopoiesis.

THE TETRACYCLINES

The first tetracycline available for general prescribing was isolated from a soil streptomyces in 1948. This class of antibiotics has broad antimicrobial activity and differences between individual members are small.

Mode of action. Tetracyclines are bacteristatic. They intefere with protein synthesis by binding to ribosomes and preventing access of transfer RNA–amino acid complexes to messenger RNA–ribosome complexes. The mechanism by which they do this is similar in both bacterial and human cells, but bacteria have an active (energy-dependent) transport system that carries tetracyclines against a concentration gradient to achieve high intracellular concentrations. This confers selectivity of action, since human cells do not possess a similar concentrating mechanism, i.e. a blood level that will stop protein synthesis in bacteria is harmless to human cells (but see antianabolic effect, below).

Pharmacokinetics: Most tetracyclines are only partially absorbed from the alimentary tract, enough remaining in the intestine to alter the flora and give rise to troublesome and sometimes dangerous complications such as pseudomembranous colitis. Dairy products reduce absorption to a degree but antacids and iron preparations do so to a much greater extent, probably by chelation to calcium, aluminium and iron.

The tetracyclines are distributed throughout the body but penetrate poorly into the cerebrospinal fluid. Bile concentrations are 5–10 times greater than those in plasma. The drugs cross the placenta; concentration in maternal milk is approximately equal to that in plasma. Tetracyclines are as a rule excreted unchanged in the urine. The $t_{\frac{1}{2}}$ is usually in the range 6–12 h, but when renal function is severely impaired, $t_{\frac{1}{2}}$ may be over 100 h. The antianabolic effect of tetracyclines (see below) raises blood urea and adds to the nitrogen load requiring excretion. Doxycycline and minocycline, exceptionally among the tetracyclines, are subject to non-renal routes of elimination and are sometimes used in patients with impaired renal function because of this property (though they retain antianabolic effect).

Uses. Tetracycline is active against nearly all Gram-positive and Gram-negative pathogenic bacteria except for most strains of proteus and *P. aeruginosa*. It can therefore be used for many common infections, particularly if these are mixed or if therapy must be blind, e.g. bronchitis, bronchopneumonia. Tetracycline does not replace penicillin where the latter is indicated, because penicillin is bactericidal and less toxic.

The **clinical uses of the tetracyclines** are summarised in the table below, which is reproduced with permission of the author and the Editor of the *Lancet*.*

Tetracycline, the therapy of choice	Tetracycline, effective alternative therapy
Brucellosis (in combination with streptomycin)	Bronchitis, acute or chronic
Cholera	Biliary tract infections
Mycoplasma pneumonia	Sinusitis
Rickettsial infections (but chloramphenicol also effective)	Bubonic plague (streptomycin preferred)
Typhus fever	Gonorrhoea
Rocky Mountain spotted fever	Syphilis
Rickettsial pox	Yaws
Q fever	Acintomycosis
Relapsing fever	Anthrax
Tularaemia	Leptospirosis
Psittacosis	*H. influenzae* meningitis
Lymphogranuloma venereum	Eradication of meningococcal carrier state (minocycline only)
Trachoma	Shigella dysentery
Chlamydial salpingitis	*Yersinia enterocolitica* infection
Non-specific urethritis	Rat-bite fever
Chancroid	Whipple's disease
Granuloma inguinale	Falciparum malaria (together with quinine)
Melioidosis	
Acne and rosacea	
Tropical sprue	

Drug resistance is now a common problem in virtually all species of organism. Cross resistance within the group is complete.

An unexpected use for a tetracycline occurs in the treatment of chronic hyponatraemia due to the *syndrome of inappropriate antidiuretic hormone secretion* (SIADH) for which demeclocycline is effective when water restriction has failed. This finding, one of many examples of serendipity in medicine, was made when patients treated with

* Kucers A. Lancet 1982: 2:425.

demeclocycline for acne were found to develop a renal concentrating defect. Demeclocycline produces a state of unresponsiveness to ADH probably by inhibiting the formation and action of cyclic AMP in the renal tubule*. Demeclocycline is convenient to use in SIADH because this action is both dose-dependent and reversible.

Adverse reactions. Heartburn, nausea and vomiting due to gastric irritation, are common. Attempts to reduce this with milk or antacids impair absorption of tetracyclines. Loose bowel movements occur due to alteration of the bowel flora, and this sometimes develops into diarrhoea.

Opportunistic infection may be due to *Candida albicans* (with sore mouth, diarrhoea and pruritus ani), *Proteus* spp., pseudomonads or staphylococci. Withdrawal of the tetracycline as soon as definite diarrhoea occurs is probably the wisest course; spontaneous recovery is then usual.

Disorders of epithelial surfaces, perhaps due partly to vitamin B complex deficiency and partly due to mild opportunistic infection with yeasts and moulds, lead to sore mouth and throat, black hairy tongue, dysphagia and perianal soreness. There is some evidence that administration of vitamin B preparations may prevent or arrest alimentary tract symptoms. It is probably wise to give these vitamins routinely if tetracycline therapy is to be prolonged.

Tetracyclines provide another example (see chloramphenicol) of an important unwanted effect of a drug with valuable actions first being noticed years after widespread clinical use. Being wise after the event provides a pleasantly easy basis for criticism of others, especially if it can be represented as championing the sick or helpless. However, in the following case, the developers of the tetracyclines cannot reasonably be blamed for lack of foresight. Tetracylines are selectively taken up in the *growing bones and teeth* of the fetus and children, due to their chelating properties with calcium phosphate. This causes dental enamel hypoplasia with pitting, cusp malformation, yellow or brown pigmentation and increased susceptibility to caries. The severity and pattern of changes varies with dose of tetracycline and the age of the child.

* Singer I, Rotenberg D. Ann Intern Med 1973; 79:689.

After the 14th week of pregnancy and in the first few months of life, even short courses can be damaging. Prevention of discoloration of the *permanent front teeth* requires that tetracyclines be avoided from the last 2 months of pregnancy to 4 years, and of other teeth until 8 years of age (or 12 years if the third molars are valued). Prolonged tetracycline therapy can also stain the fingernails at all ages.

The effects on the bones after they are formed in the fetus are of less clinical importance because pigmentation has no cosmetic disadvantage and a very short spell of delayed growth may not matter. Whether serious anatomical deformity can result from administration in early pregnancy is not known. No serious growth disorders have yet been reported amongst children with chronic respiratory disease taking tetracycline continuously, though both dentitions can be affected.

Tetracyclines act by inhibiting bacterial protein synthesis but the same effect occurring in man causes blood urea to rise: this is the *antianabolic effect*. The increased nitrogen load can be clinically important in renal failure, in surgical or injured patients, in those with poor general nutrition and in the elderly. Renal damage can occur with high doses.

Tetracyclines also induce photosensitisation and other rashes. Liver and pancreatic damage can occur, especially in pregnancy and with renal disease, when the drugs have been given i.v. Rarely tetracyclines cause benign intracranial hypertension. Minocycline but not other tetracyclines may cause a vestibular disturbance with dizziness, tinnitus and impaired balance, especially in females. The effect disappears when the drug is stopped.

Individual tetracyclines

Tetracycline (250, 500 mg) may be taken as representative of most tetracyclines. It is incompletely absorbed from the gut and significant amounts of the drug are excreted unabsorbed in the faeces; dosing by the i.m. or i.v. routes need be less than half of the oral dose to be similarly effective. Tetracycline is eliminated by the kidney and in the bile and the $t_{\frac{1}{2}}$ is 8 h. The dose is 250 or 500 mg two or four times daily. For *acne*, tetracycline 250 mg is given thrice daily by mouth for 1–4 weeks, followed by twice daily till improvement occurs.

Doxycycline (100 mg) is well absorbed from the gut, even after food. The $t_{\frac{1}{2}}$ is 20 h. It is excreted in the bile, in the faeces, which it re-enters by diffusing across the small intestinal wall, and, to some extent, in the urine. The non-renal mechanisms compensate effectively when renal function is impaired and no reduction of dose is necessary: 100–200 mg may be given once daily.

Minocycline (50, 100 mg) is also well absorbed from the gut, even after a meal. The $t_{\frac{1}{2}}$ is 14 h. Minocycline is partly metabolised in the liver and partly excreted in the bile and urine. When renal function is impaired the dose need not be reduced — it is 200 mg initially followed by 100 mg twice daily.

Other tetracyclines include chlortetracycline, demeclocycline, clomocycline, lymecycline, methacycline, oxytetracycline.

MACROLIDE ANTIBIOTICS

Erythromycin

Erythromycin (250, 500 mg) is the only important member of the macrolide group of antibiotics (other members include spiramycin and oleandomycin). When it was introduced in 1952, the hope was that erythromycin would solve the problem of β-lactamase (penicillinase)-resistant staphylococci, but it was soon found that these and other organisms readily developed resistance if therapy lasted more than a week.

The mode of action of erythromycin is similar to that of the tetracyclines in that is binds to the ribosomes and prevents access of transfer-RNA–amino acid complexes to messenger-RNA complexes, thereby interfering with protein synthesis. It is bacteristatic.

Pharmacokinetics. Absorption after oral administration is incomplete and is best with erythromycin estolate, which form of the drug is well absorbed despite the presence of food in the stomach. The estolate is hydrolysed in the body to release the active erythyromycin, which diffuses readily into most tissues; the $t_{\frac{1}{2}}$ in plasma in 1.5 h and elimination is almost exclusively via the bile and faeces.

Uses

1. Erythromycin is the drug of choice for mycoplasma pneumonia in children, although in adults a tetracycline may be preferred.
2. First choice treatment for infection with *Legionella* spp. (Legionnaires' disease) is erythromycin with or without rifampicin.
3. Erythromycin or a tetracycline is first choice treatment for certain chlamydial infections (see Table 11.1, Antimicrobial drugs of choice), diphtheria (including carriers) and pertussis.
4. In gastroenteritis caused by *Campylobacter jejuni*, erythromycin is effective is eliminating the organism from the faeces, although it does not necessarily reduce the duration of the symptoms.
5. Erythromycin is an effective alternative choice for *penicillin-allergic* patients infected with *Staphylococcus pyogenes*, *Strep. pneumoniae* or *Treponema pallidum*.

Preparations and dosage. The usual oral dose is 250 mg 6-hourly or twice this in serious infection. Tablets are enteric-coated as erythromycin is destroyed by gastric acid.

The ethylsuccinate and stearate esters of erythromycin produce lower plasma concentrations of the active drug than does the same dose of the estolate.

Adverse reactions. Erythromycin is remarkably non-toxic, but the estolate can cause cholestatic hepatitis with abdominal pain and fever which may be confused with viral hepatitis, acute cholecystitis or acute pancreatitis. This is probably an allergy, and recovery is usual, but the estolate should not be given to a patient with liver disease. Other allergies are rare. Gastrointestinal disturbances, particularly diarrhoea, occur but, the antibacterial spectrum being narrower than with tetracycline, opportunistic infection is less troublesome.

IMIDAZOLES

The members of this group of antimicrobials all

contain an imidazole group and their approved names end with '-azole'. They include:

1. Metronidazole and tinidazole (antibacterial and antiprotozoal), which are described here.
2. Ketoconazole and miconazole, which are described under Antifungal Drugs.
3. Nimorazole, which is described under Antiprotozoal Drugs.
4. Mebendazole and thiabendazole, which are listed under Anthelmintic Drugs.

Metronidazole

For years metronidazole was used for trichomoniasis, amoebiasis and giardiasis. The drug was known to be active against anaerobes but its clinical use against these organisms was not pursued since their frequent role in causing infection was not appreciated. Clinical exploitation against anaerobes was encouraged by the report of a dentist whose patient recovered unexpectedly from gingivitis while undergoing treatment for trichomoniasis.

Mode of action. In anaerobic microorganisms (but not in aerobic microorganisms, which it also enters) metronidazole is converted into an active form by reduction of its nitro group: this binds to DNA and prevents formation of nucleic acids.

Pharmacokinetics. The drug is well absorbed after either oral or rectal administration and distributes to achieve sufficient concentration to eradicate infection in liver, gut wall and pelvic tissues (distribution volume 45 l/70 kg). The $t_{\frac{1}{2}}$ in plasma is 4–8 h. Metronidazole is eliminated in the urine, partly unchanged and partly as metabolites.

Uses. Metronidazole is active against a wide range of bacteria including *Bacteroides* spp., anaerobic cocci, *Fusobacterium* spp., *Clostridium* spp. and *Gardnerella vaginalis*. It is also effective against protozoa including *Trichomonas* spp., *Entamoeba histolytica* and *Giardia lamblia*. Its clinical uses are:

1. Treatment of sepsis to which anaerobic organisms are contributing, notably postsurgical infection, intra-abdominal infection, and septicaemia but also wound and pelvic infection, osteomyelitis and abscesses of brain or lung.
2. Prevention of postsurgical infection in which anaerobic bacteria may be expected to play a part, especially after bowel surgery.
3. Trichomoniasis of the urogenital tract in the female and male.
4. Amoebiasis (symptomless carriers of cysts, intestinal and extra-intestinal infection).
5. Giardiasis.
6. Acute ulcerative gingivitis and dental infections.
7. Non-specific vaginitis.

Preparations and dosage. Metronidazole is available as tablets (200, 400 mg), a suspension (200 mg in 5 ml), suppositories (0.5, 1.0 g) and an injection (0.5 g in 100 ml).

Established anaerobic infection is treated with metronidazole by mouth 400 mg, 8-hourly; by rectum 1 g, 8-hourly for 3 days followed by 1 g, 12-hourly; or by intravenous injection 0.5 g 8-hourly; treatment should continue for up to 7 days.

Prophylaxis of anaerobic infection requires the same doses for 2–4 days starting just before the operation.

Details of dosage for protozoal infections appear under the appropriate headings.

Adverse effects. Gastrointestinal disturbances are the chief unwanted effects and include nausea, vomiting, diarrhoea, furred tongue and an unpleasant metallic taste in the mouth. Others are headache, dizziness and ataxia. Rashes, urticaria and angioedema also occur. A disulfiram-like effect is seen with alcohol because metronidazole inhibits alcohol and aldehyde dehydrogenase; patients should be warned appropriately. Peripheral neuropathy and epileptiform seizures have been reported. A metabolite of metronidazole causes the urine to darken.

Large doses of metronidazole are carcinogenic in rodents and the drug is mutagenic in bacteria; however, long-term studies have failed to discover oncogenic effects in humans*.

* Beard C M et al. N Engl J Med 1979; 301:519. Friedman G D. N Engl J Med 1980; 302:519.

Tinidazole (tab 500 mg; infusion 800 mg in 400 ml) is similar to metronidazole but has a longer plasma $t_{\frac{1}{2}}$ (13 h). It is excreted mainly unchanged in the urine. The indications for use and adverse effects are essentially those of metronidazole, although the disulfiram-like reaction with alcohol has not yet been reported with tinidazole. Current practice favours the use of metronidazole because of its satisfactory performance over many years but the longer duration of action of tinidazole may prove to be an advantage; for example, in giardiasis, tinidazole 1.5 g by mouth as a single dose is as effective as a course of metronidazole.

The dose of tinidazole for established anaerobic infection is, by mouth, 2 g on the first day followed by 1 g as a single daily dose or 0.5 g 12-hourly; or intravenously, 800 mg initially, followed by 800 mg as a single daily dose or 400 mg 12-hourly.

CHLORAMPHENICOL

Chloramphenicol was obtained in 1947 from a streptomyces found in a soil sample from a mulched field in Venezuela and from a compost heap in Illinois, USA. It was soon made synthetically.

Chloramphenicol was the first antimicrobial with a wide range of activity against common organisms that was also reliably absorbed from the intestine. It was also dramatically effective against salmonellae and rickettsiae, organisms hitherto invulnerable to drug therapy. Unfortunately, its use in trivial infections soon became widespread, with tragic results for some.

Mode of action. Chloramphenicol interferes with protein synthesis by inhibiting the enzyme that transfers the peptide chain to the new amino acid on the ribosome; it is primarily bacteristatic.

Pharmacokinetics. Chloramphenicol has a bitter taste and is poorly soluble. It is available as the base for oral use in capsules and as two esters (prodrugs); the palmitate, which is tasteless and used as a suspension, and the succinate, which is soluble and is given parenterally. Absorption of the base from the alimentary tract is efficient but the palmitate ester must be hydrolysed by pancreatic lipase before the active chloramphenicol is released and absorbed (patients with cystic fibrosis may require extra pancreatic enzyme to ensure adequate hydrolysis). Distribution is approximately even throughout the body (distribution volume 65 l/70 kg) but concentration in the cerebrospinal fluid and pleural space is about half the plasma concentration. Chloramphenicol succinate, which is usually administered i.v. or i.m. must be hydrolysed to the active chloramphenicol and the capacity to perform this reaction varies greatly between individuals; in serious infections, plasma concentration monitoring may be advisable. Chloramphenicol is inactivated by conjugation with glucuronide in the liver. The $t_{\frac{1}{2}}$ is approximately 2 h in adults. In the *neonate*, the process of hydroxylation and glucuronidation are slow (and the drug is toxic, see below) and plasma concentration are extremely variable; the capacity to the metabolise chloramphenicol increases significantly in the first three weeks of life, which further complicates prediction of the amount of active drug in plasma.

Uses. Chloramphenicol is bactericidal against most strains of *H. influenzae* and *Strep. pneumoniae* and bacteristatic against many other aerobic and anaerobic bacteria; it is also active against mycoplasma, chylamydia and rickettsia, but *Ps. aeruginosa* is resistant. The decision to use chloramphenicol is influenced by its rare but serious toxic effects (see below) and the following points may be made:

1. There is a strong case for initiating treatment of bacterial meningitis with chloramphenicol plus penicillin, until the causal organism is identified. When the organism is *H.influenzea* type b, chloramphenicol should be continued.
2. Similarly, in the initial treatment of brain abscess, chloramphenicol is given with penicillin.
3. Chloramphenicol should be considered for any invasive infection caused by *H. influenzae* in patients allergic to penicillins and cephalosporins, e.g. in the central nervous system or respiratory tract.
4. Chloramphenicol is a treatment of choice for salmonella infections (typhoid fever, salmonella septicaemia) but amoxycillin and co-trimoxazole

are as effective and have less serious adverse reactions.

5. Chloramphenicol penetrates well into the aqueous and vitreous humours after either topical or systemic administration and is effective treatment for ocular infections caused by sensitive organisms.

6. Chloramphenicol is an effective alternative drug for chlamydial or rickettsial infections when first choice agents (erythromycin, tetracycline) cannot be used.

Adverse reactions. Apart from the soreness of the mouth, alimentary tract symptoms due to alteration of normal flora are less common than with tetracyclines because of the more complete alimentary absorption. Rashes are rare. Optic nerve damage occurs but is rare.

The systemic use of chloramphenicol is dominated by the fact that it can cause, though rarely, *fetal aplastic anaemia*; apart from this, it would be a drug of choice for common infections, e.g. bronchitis. The danger is remote enough for a physician habitually to prescribe chloramphenicol for such diseases and yet not to see a case of aplastic anaemia during an entire career. This has led to some to discount the risk (about 1 in 50 000 courses), but to many it is intolerable that trivial disease should be treated with chloramphenicol. 'A girl of four years had an attack of bronchitis with asthma for which she received 1 g chloramphenicol daily for four days. Six months later she developed a sore throat, which was treated with a further course of chloramphenicol, 1 g daily for four days. Three days after completing the course, a purpuric rash appeared and in spite of blood transfusion, she died two weeks later.' Aplastic anaemia was found at necropsy.*

The blood disorder may be thrombocytopenia, granulocytopenia or, worse, aplastic anaemia, any of which may be fatal. It may be detected at an early and recoverable stage by repeated examination of the blood. The danger level is a total leucocyte count below 4.0×10^9 /1 (4 000/mm^3). This may be the only situation in which repeated blood examination offers a real safeguard against unpredictable narrow depression.

Aplastic anaemia is probably of two kinds, an allergy and also a reversible and directly dose-related bone marrow depression that can be regarded as a normal pharmacological effect of the drug. This develops especially if the plasma concentration is greater than 25 μg/ml, if the daily dose is 4.0 g or more, or if therapy is prolonged. The haematological picture is characterized by anaemia, leucopenia, thrombocytopenia, reticulocytopenia and increased plasma iron concentration (chloramphenicol inhibits iron uptake by normoblasts).

Another serious toxic effect of chloramphenicol was discovered as a result of routine use of chemoprophylaxis in premature babies born 24 h or more after spontaneous rupture of the fetal membranes. Their mortality was high and demanded investigation. A controlled experiment seemed the only ethical way to clear up the confusion caused by the uncontrolled introduction of chemoprophylaxis.†

Babies were allocated to four treatment groups:

1. No drug treatment	32 babies, 19% died
2. Chloramphenicol	30 babies, 60% died
3. Penicillin + streptomycin	33 babies, 18% died
4. Penicillin + streptomycin + chloramphenicol	31 babies, 68% died

The cause of death was circulatory collapse (grey syndrome) with high chloramphenicol plasma concentration due to failure of the liver to conjugate, and of the kidney to excrete, the drug. Had the experiment with measurement of plasma concentration been made at the outset, the subsequent experiment, with its loss of life, need never have been made.

Biochemical investigation of the fate of drugs in the immature can alone predict safe dosage schedules. However, it is easy to be wise after an event has occurred, and after the mechanism has been explained.

Dosage. Chloramphenicol (250 mg) 250 to 750 mg may be given orally, 6-hourly. The dose should be as low as is reasonable and medication should not extend beyond 14 days. Parenteral preparations are available.

* Gairdner D. Br Med J 1954; 2:1107.

† Burns L E et al. N Engl J Med 1959; 261:1318.

Topical applications for eye, ear and skin are available and seldom cause allergy. However, bactericidal drugs that are not used for systemic effect, bacitracin, neomycin, polymyxin, chlorhexidine, are generally preferable.

OTHER ANTIMICROBIALS

Clindamycin

Clindamycin (75, 150 mg), a chlorinated derivative of lincomycin, has largely replaced the latter because it has greater antibacterial activity and is better absorbed from the gut. The drug binds to bacterial ribosomes to inhibit protein synthesis, like erythromycin and the tetracyclines. Active transport of clindamycin into leucocytes may explain its effectiveness in septic conditions. Clindamycin has a similar antibacterial spectrum to erythromycin (with which there is partial cross-resistance) and benzylpenicillin but has the useful additional property that it is effective against *B. fragilis*, an anaerobe that is involved in gut-associated sepsis.

Clindamycin is well absorbed from the gut despite the presence of food. It distributes to most body tissues including bone, but only small quantities penetrate the eye and cerebrospinal fluid. The drug is metabolised by the liver and enterohepatic cycling occurs with bile concentrations two to five times those of plasma. Significant excretion occurs by the gut. The $t_{\frac{1}{2}}$ is 3 h.

The *indications* for using clindamycin are:

1. Anaerobic infection caused by penicillin-resistant organisms outwith the nervous system: anaerobic organisms often cause orodental sepsis, aspiration pneumonia and lung abscess and here, clindamycin may prove efficacious should penicillin fail or be contraindicated.

2. Intra-abdominal sepsis and non-sexually transmitted infection of the genital tract in the female, both of which usually involve anaerobes commonly resistant to penicillin: in these circumstances, clindamycin is usually combined with an aminoglycoside.

3. Bone or joint infections, because the drug penetrates these tissues well.

The dose of clindamycin is 150–300 mg 6-hourly.

The most serious *adverse effect* is antibiotic-associated (pseudomembranous) colitis (see p. 202) due to opportunustic infection of the bowel with *Clostridium difficile*, which produces an enterotoxin; clindamycin should be stopped if any diarrhoea occurs.

Sodium fusidate

Sodium fusidate is a steroid antibiotic that is used almost exclusively against β-lactamase-producing staphylococci. These fairly rapidly become resistant and it is commonly given in combination with another antistaphylococcal drug, e.g. flucloxacillin. Sodium fusidate is useless against streptococci, which is unusual in antistaphylococcal drugs.

It is readily absorbed from the gut and distributes widely in body tissues including bone but not in the cerebrospinal fluid. The $t_{\frac{1}{2}}$ is 5 h. The drug is metabolised and very little is excreted unchanged in the urine.

Sodium fusidate is a valuable drug for treating severe staphylococcal infections, especially those due to penicillin-resistant organisms; its effective penetration of bone makes it suitable for osteomyelitis. In an ointment or gel, sodium fusidate is used topically for skin infection and the cream is applied to eradicate the staphylococcal nasal carrier state.

Sodium fusidate (250 mg) is given in a dose of 500 mg 8-hourly by mouth; an i.v. preparation is available.

The drug is well tolerated but mild gastrointestinal upset is not uncommon. Jaundice occurs particularly with the i.v. preparation and the oral route is preferable in patients with abnormal liver function.

Spectinomycin

Spectinomycin is produced by *Streptomyces spectabilis* and is not closely related to any other group of antibiotics. Although the antibacterial spectrum of spectinomycin covers Gram-positive and Gram-negative organisms, its clinical use is confined to *gonorrhoea* in patients *allergic to penicillin* or to infection with gonococci that are penicillin-resistant. The steady growth of resistant gonococci, particularly the β-lactamase-producing type, suggests that spectinomycin will continue to have a significant role in this disease, although resistance is reported.

Spectinomycin is given by single deep i.m. injection, 2 g in males, 4 g in females. The drug may cause nausea, dizziness or urticaria.

Acrosoxacin

Acrosoxacin is related to nalidixic acid and is active against a range of Gram-negative bacteria, but especially *Neisseria gonorrhoeae*. It is not destroyed by β-lactamase. Syphilis and chlamydial infection (non-specific urethritis), which may co-exist with gonorrhoea, are unaffected by the drug. The $t_{\frac{1}{2}}$ in plasma is 4–11 h and it is inactivated by metabolism. The drug is used for acute gonorrhoea, especially when the organism is resistant to or the patient is sensitive to penicillin. A single dose of 300 mg is given by mouth.

Adverse effects include drowsiness, headache, vertigo and lassitude.

Vancomycin

Vancomycin is bactericidal against several species of Gram-negative and Gram-positive cocci. It acts on multiplying organisms by inhibiting formation of the peptidoglycan component of the cell wall. Vancomycin is poorly absorbed from the gut and, there being no satisfactory i.m. preparation, is given i.v. for systemic infections. The drug distributes effectively into body tissues and the $t_{\frac{1}{2}}$ is 6 h; it is eliminated by the kidney. Vancomycin entered clinical use because of its effectiveness against penicillin-resistant staphylococci but ototoxicity has limited its *indications*, which are:

1. Enterocolitis due to *Cl. difficile* or less commonly to staphylococci (pseudomembranous colitis).
2. Serious infection with staphylococci resistant to the usual antistaphylococcal drugs (multiple resistance).
3. Serious staphylococcal infections in individuals who are allergic to penicillins or cephalosporins.
4. Streptococcal endocarditis in patients who are allergic to benzylpenicillin. Here vancomycin should be combined with an aminoglycoside.

The dose for enterocolitis is 0.5 g 6-hourly; the powder (ampoules, 0.5 g) otherwise used for the i.v. route is diluted in water and taken by mouth. Systemic infections require a total of 2 g daily i.v. in divided doses.

Adverse effects. The main disadvantage of vancomycin is damage to the auditory portion of the eighth cranial nerve. Because the drug is eliminated by the kidney, patients whose renal function is impaired are particularly at risk but toxicity should be avoided if the plasma concentration is kept below 30 mg/l by careful monitoring. Tinnitus and deafness may improve if the drug is stopped. Nephrotoxicity and allergic reactions also occur.

Since vancomycin tends to cause thrombophlebitis, the antibiotic should be diluted in isotonic saline 250 ml or glucose 5% and given over 60 minutes, hypotension occurring with rapid infusion. The intravenous infusion site should also be changed more frequently than is usual.

Teicoplanin is structurally related to vancomycin. It inhibits cell wall synthesis and is active against *Strep. pneumoniae*, *Staph. aureus* and enterococci. An unusual feature of the drug is its plasma $t_{\frac{1}{2}}$ of 100 h. The place of teicoplanin in therapy has yet to be established.

Minor antimicrobials

These antibiotics are included because they are effective topically without serious risk of allergy, although toxicity limits or precludes their systemic use.

Novobiocin (1957) is a bacteristatic reserve drug chiefly for treatment of resistant staphylococci. It has lost much of its importance since the introduction of β-lactamase-resistant penicillins.

Mupirocin is produced from *Pseudomonas fluorescens* and is active against both Gram-positive and Gram-negative organisms, including those commonly associated with skin infections. It is available only for topical use against bacterial infections, e.g. folliculitis and impetigo.

Polypeptide antibiotics, which group includes:

Colistin is effective against Gram-negative organisms, particularly *Pseudomonas aeruginosa*. It is used for bowel sterilisation in neutropenic patients, is included in bladder irrigation fluids and topically is given for skin and external ear infections.

Polymyxin B is also active against Gram-negative organisms, particularly *Ps. aeruginosa*. Its principal use now is in bladder irrigation fluids and topically for skin, eye and ear infections.

Bacitracin. In 1943, an antibiotic-producing bacillus was isolated from a compound fracture of the tibia of a 7-year-old girl, Margaret Tracey, during an investigation of the bacterial flora of contaminated accidental wounds. The antibiotic was named after her.

Like the other polypeptide antibiotics, bacitracin is nephrotoxic and now never needs to be given parenterally. It is used topically for skin, ocular and external ear infections, and is included in bladder irrigation fluids.

Gramicidin is used in various topical applications as creams and ointments for skin sepsis, combined with neomycin and framycetin.

NOTE: *Antimicrobials not included in this chapter will be found with the accounts of the diseases they are used to treat.*

GUIDE TO FURTHER READING

1 Editorial. Fifty years of penicillin. Br Med J 1979; 1: 1101–1102.
2 Editorial. Twenty-one years of beating beta-lactamases. Br Med J 1982; 284: 369–370.
3 Beeley L. Allergy to penicillin. Br Med J 1984; 288: 511–512.
4 Wise R. Penicillins and cephalosporins: antimicrobial and pharmacological properties. Lancet 1982; 2: 140–143.
5 Ball A P. Clinical uses of penicillins. Lancet 1982; 2: 197–199
6 Neu H C. Clinical uses of cephalosporins. Lancet 1982; 2: 252–255
7 Wise R, Dyas A. Ampicillin and alternatives. Br Med J 1983; 286: 583–584.
8 Editorial. Moxalactam. Lancet 1981; 2: 23–24.
9 Editorial. Monobactams — antibiotics from the marshes. Lancet 1981; 2:620
10 Phillips I. Aminoglycosides. Lancet 1982; 2: 311–315.
11 Reeves D. Sulphonamides and trimethoprim. Lancet 1982; 2: 370–373.
12 Rubin R H, Swartz M N. Trimethoprim-sulfamethoxazole. N Engl J Med 1980; 303: 426–432.
13 Editorial. Bacterial resistance to trimethoprim. Br Med J 1980; 281: 571–572.
14 Kucers A. Chloramphenicol, erythromycin, vancomycin, tetracyclines. Lancet 1982; 2: 425–429.
15 Bartlett J G. Anti-anaerobic antibacterial agents. Lancet 1982; 11: 478–481.
16 Brown R, Wise R (editorial). Vancomycin: a reappraisal. Br Med J 1982; 284: 1508–1509.
17 Mulhall A et al. Chloramphenicol toxicity in neonates: its incidence and prevention. Br Med J 1983; 287: 1424–1427.

13

Infection III: Chemotherapy of bacterial infections

We live in a world heavily populated by microorganisms of astonishing diversity. Most of these exist in our environment but certain types of microorganism are normally harboured in our bodies. Depending on the circumstances, infectious disease can arise from organisms that are either outside us (exogenous infection) or inside us (endogenous infection) and a knowledge of common pathogens at specific sites provides a good basis for rational initial therapy. Therefore, each of the following accounts begins with a list of the organisms most likely to cause infection in specific tissues. These are based on and printed with the permission of the Chairman of the Editorial Board of the *Medical Letter on Drugs and Therapeutics* (1984), which points out that, although the lists are given in estimated order of frequency in which organisms cause infection, these frequencies are subject to annual, seasonal and geographical variation. Furthermore, organisms not listed may be important causes of infection.

INFECTION OF THE BLOOD

The most likely bacterial pathogens for the following populations are:

Newborn infants

1. *Escherichia coli* (or other Gram-negative bacilli)
2. *Streptococcus* Group B
3. *Listeria monocytogenes*
4. *Staphylococcus aureus*
5. *Streptococcus pyogenes* (Group A)
6. Enterococci
7. *Streptococcus pneumoniae*

Children

1. *Streptococcus pneumoniae*
2. *Neisseria meningitidis*
3. *Haemophilus influenzae*
4. *Staphylococcus aureus*
5. *Streptococcus pyogenes* (Group A)
6. *Escherichia coli* (or other Gram-negative bacilli)

Adults

1. *Escherichia coli* (or other Gram-negative bacilli)
2. *Staphylococcus aureus*
3. *Streptococcus pneumoniae*
4. *Bacteroides*
5. *Streptococcus pyogenes* (Group A)
6. *Staphylococcus epidermidis*
7. *Neisseria meningitidis*
8. *Neisseria gonorrhoeae*

Septicaemia

Septicaemia is a medical emergency. Accurate microbiological diagnosis is of the first importance and blood cultures together with any other relevant specimens should be taken *before* starting antimicrobial therapy. Usually, the infecting organism(s) is not known and treatment must be instituted on the basis of a *best guess*. The clinical circumstances may provide some clues:

1. When septicaemia follows gastrointestinal or genital tract surgery, coliforms, anaerobic bacteria or streptococci are likely pathogens, and the following combinations are effective: gentamicin plus amoxycillin plus metronidazole, or cefuroxime plus metronidazole.
2. Septicaemia related to urinary tract infection usually involves coliforms, enterococci or less commonly, *Pseudomonas aeruginosa*: gentamicin plus ampicillin or cefotaxime alone will be indicated.
3. Neonatal septicaemia is usually due to staphylococci, streptococci or coliforms, occasionally to *Ps. aeruginosa* and cefotaxime either alone or with netilmicin is required.
4. Toxic-shock syndrome is characterised by a generalised erythematous rash, toxaemia, fever, hypotension and is often associated with the use of high-absorbancy vaginal tampons. The toxin responsible is produced by staphylococci, and flucloxacillin is appropriate to eliminate the source.

Antimicrobials should be given *parenterally* in septicaemia.

Septicaemia with circulatory collapse is a special case; it is frequently due to Gram-negative organisms, which produce endotoxins. Indeed, Gram-negative septicaemia is a leading and sometimes unrecognised cause of shock. The pathophysiology is complex but involves capillary damage, reduced plasma volume, compensatory vasoconstriction and tissue anoxia (see hypotensive states).

INFECTION OF EARS AND PARANASAL SINUSES

The most likely bacterial pathogens are:

Ears

Auditory canal

1. *Pseudomonas aeruginosa* (or other Gram-negative bacilli)
2. *Staphylococcus aureus*
3. *Streptococcus pyogenes* (Group A)
4. *Streptococcus pneumoniae*
5. *Haemophilus influenzae* (in children)

Middle ear

1. *Streptococcus pneumoniae*
2. *Haemophilus influenzae* (in children)
3. *Branhamella catarrhalis*
4. *Streptococcus pyogenes* (Group A)
5. *Staphylococcus aureus*
6. Anaerobic streptococci
7. *Bacteroides*
8. Other Gram-negative bacilli (chronic)
9. *Mycobacterium tuberculosis*

Paranasal sinuses

1. *Streptococcus pneumoniae*
2. *Haemophilus influenzae*
3. *Streptococcus pyogenes* (Group A)
4. *Klebsiella* (or other Gram-negative bacilli)
5. Anaerobic streptococci (chronic sinusitis)
6. *Staphylococcus aureus* (chronic sinusitis)

Sinusitis. Although infection of the paranasal sinuses cannot usually be regarded as a threat to life, it does give rise to significant morbidity (and an estimated loss of half a million working days per year in the UK). Since oedema and inflammation of the mucous membrane hinder the removal of pus, a logical first step is to promote normal drainage with a sympathomimetic vasoconstrictor, e.g. ephedrine nasal drops. The common infecting organisms usually respond to amoxycillin with or without clavulanic acid, or possibly doxycycline. In chronic sinusitis, correction of the anatomical abnormalities (polypi, nasal septum deviation) is often important. Very diverse organisms, many of them normal inhabitants of the upper respiratory tract, may be cultured (e.g. anaerobic streptococci, *Bacteroides* spp.) and a judgement is required as to whether any particular organism is acting as a pathogen. Choice of antibiotic should be guided by culture and sensitivity testing; therapy may need to be prolonged.

Otitis media. Mild cases, characterised by pinkness or infection of the eardrum, often resolve spontaneously and need only analgesia and observation. A bulging, inflamed eardrum indicates bacterial otitis media, which is best treated with amoxycillin. Chemotherapy has not removed the need for myringotomy when pain is very severe, and also for later cases, as sterilised pus may not be completely absorbed and may leave adhesions that impair hearing. Deafness may persist long after the infective episode. Chronic infection presents a similar problem to that of chronic sinus infection, above.

INFECTION OF THE THROAT

The most likely bacterial pathogens are:

1. *Streptococcus pyogenes* (Group A)
2. *Neisseria meningitidis* or *Neisseria gonorrhoeae*
3. *Leptotrichia buccalis* (Vincent's infection)
4. *Corynebacterium diphtheriae*
5. *Bordetella pertussis* (whooping cough)
6. *Haemophilus influenzae*

Sore throat may be endemic or epidemic. In the endemic form 50–75%, and in an epidemic 100%, may be due to *Strep. pyogenes*, which is always sensitive to benzylpenicillin. Unfortunately, streptococcal sore throats cannot be clinically differentiated from the non-streptococcal with any certainty. Prevention of complications is more important than relief of the symptoms, which seldom last long.

There is no general agreement whether chemotherapy should be employed in mild endemic sore throat; the disease usually subsides in a few days, septic complications are uncommon and rheumatic fever rarely follows. It is reasonable to withold penicillin unless streptococci are cultured or if the patient develops a high fever. Severe or epidemic sore throat is likely to be streptococcal and benzylpenicillin should be given to prevent these complications. Ideally, it should be continued for 10 days but compliance is bad once the symptoms have subsided and 5 days should be the minimum objective. In a closed community, chemoprophylaxis of unaffected people to stop an epidemic may be considered, for instance with phenoxymethylpenicillin 125 mg orally, twice a day, for a period depending on the course of the epidemic, or a single i.m., injection of benzathine penicillin 900 mg.

In *scarlet fever* and *erysipelas*, the infection is invariably streptococcal and benzylpenicillin should be used even in mild cases, to prevent rheumatic fever and nephritis.

Chemoprophylaxis of streptococcal infection should be undertaken in patients who have had an attack of rheumatic fever. It is continued for at least 5 years, or until aged 20, whichever is the longer period, although some hold that it should continue for life because histological study of atrial biopsies show that the cardiac lesions may progress despite absence of clinical activity. Chemoprophylaxis should be continued for life after a second attack of rheumatic fever.

A single attack of acute nephritis is not an indication for chemoprophylaxis but in the rare cases of nephritis in which recurrent haematuria occurs after sore throats, chemoprophylaxis may be used. It is sometimes used also in the nephrotic syndrome, when recurrent infections are followed by increased proteinuria.

Ideally, chemoprophylaxis should continue throughout the year, but if the patient is unwilling to submit to the routine, it should occur at least in the colder months.

The choice between daily phenoxymethylpenicillin by mouth or 3-weekly benzathine penicillin injections will depend on an assessment of patient preference and likely compliance.

Adverse effects are uncommon. Patients taking penicillin prophylaxis are liable to have pencillin-resistant *Strep. viridans* in the mouth. During even minor dentistry, e.g. scaling, there is a risk of bacteraemia and of infective endocarditis with a penicillin-resistant organism (in those with any residual rheumatic heart lesion). In such a situation chemoprophylaxis must be carried out with another class of drug. The same risk applies with urinary, abdominal and chest surgery, and patients need special chemoprophylaxis (see *endocarditis*, p. 242). Patients taking pencillins are also liable to carry resistant staphylococci.

Pharyngitis may also be due to:

Vincent's infection, which responds readily to benzylpenicillin; a single i.m. dose of 600 mg is often enough except in a mouth needing dental treatment, when relapse may follow. Metronidazole 200 mg by mouth 8-hourly for 3 days is effective.

Diphtheria. Antitoxin 10 000 to 30 000 units i.m. or 40 000 to 100 000 units i.v. in two divided doses 0.5–2 h apart is given according to the severity of the disease. Erythromycin or benzylpenicillin is also used, to arrest toxin production by destroying the bacteria.

Whooping-cough (*pertussis*). Chemotherapy is needed in children who are weak, have damaged lungs or are under 3 years old. Erythromycin is usually recommended at the early catarrhal stage and may curtail an attack if it is given early enough. The drug is not dramatically effective, which is why it is not advocated in every case. Corticosteroids, salbutamol and physiotherapy may be helpful, but there is a need for well-designed clinical trials to establish the efficacy of these.

INFECTION OF THE BRONCHI, LUNGS AND PLEURA

The most likely bacterial pathogens are:

Larynx, trachea and bronchi

1. *Streptococcus pneumoniae*
2. *Haemophilus influenzae*
3. *Streptococcus pyogenes* (Group A)
4. *Corynebacterium diphtheriae*
5. *Staphylococcus aureus*
6. Gram-negative bacilli

Lungs

Pneumonia

1. *Streptococcus pneumoniae*
2. *Haemophilus influenzae*
3. Anaerobic streptococci
4. *Bacteroides* spp.
5. *Staphylococcus aureus*
6. *Mycoplasma pneumoniae**
7. *Klebsiella* spp. (or other Gram-negative bacilli)
8. *Legionella pneumophila*
9. *Streptococcus pyogenes* (Group A)
10. *Rickettsia** spp.
11. *Mycobacterium tuberculosis*
12. *Pneumocystis carinii**
13. *Legionella micdadei L. pittsburgensis*)
14. *Chlamydia psittaci**
15. *Pseudomonas aeruginosa*
16. *Branhamella catarrhalis*

Abscess

1. Anaerobic streptococci
2. *Bacteroides* spp.
3. *Staphylococcus aureus*
4. *Klebsiella* spp. (or other Gram-negative bacilli)
5. *Streptococcus penumoniae*
6. *Actinomyces spp*., *Nocardia* spp.

Pleura

1. *Streptococcus pneumoniae*
2. *Staphylococcus aureus*
3. *Haemophilus influenzae*
4. Gram-negative bacilli
5. Anaerobic streptococci
6. *Bacteroides*
7. *Streptococcus pyogenes* (Group A)
8. *Mycobacterium tuberculosis*
9. *Actinomyces spp*., *Nocardia* spp.

Bronchitis. Most cases of *acute* bronchitis respond well to amoxycillin or trimethoprim. In *chronic* bronchitis, suppressive chemotherapy, generally needed only during the colder months, should be considered for patients with symptoms of pulmonary insufficiency, recurrent acute exacerbations or permanently purulent sputum. Whether therapy should be intermittent or continuous is still uncertain, and so it would seem

* Organisms that are not strictly bacteria but that are suseptible to antibacterial drugs have been included.

reasonable to try intermittent therapy first, and only continuous therapy if it fails. Suitable regimens would be amoxycillin 250 mg by mouth 8-hourly or trimethoprim 200 mg by mouth 12-hourly.

For *intermittent therapy*, the patient is given a supply of the drug and is told to take it in full dose at the first sign of a 'chest' cold, e.g. purulent sputum, and to stop it after 3 days if there is rapid improvement. Otherwise, the patient should continue the drug until recovery takes place. If the illness lasts for more than 10 days, there is a need for reassessment.

The main effect of *continuous therapy* is to reduce the duration of acute exacerbations rather than their number, perhaps because the exacerbations are initiated by virus infection that promotes secondary bacterial invasion.

'Firm insistence that cigarettes will shorten the patient's life and that he must stop smoking is often effective, and will do more for him than years of chemotherapy.'*

If there is airways obstruction, it should be treated by bronchodilators but it may become necessary to consider the use of a corticosteroid, though these are less effective than in asthma. There is no doubt that a corticosteroid can improve ventilation in some bronchitic patients, but benefit tends to diminish with time and there may be an added risk of encouraging infection. If there is not obvious benefit within a week, the corticosteroid should be stopped. It is not a treatment to undertake without strong reason or unless objective measurement of respiratory function is practicable. Disodium cromoglycate helps a minority of such patients.

Pneumonias

The clinical setting is a useful guide to the causal organism and hence to the best-guess choice of antimicrobial.

Pneumonia in previously healthy individuals

Disease that is lobar in distribution is almost certainly *pneumonococcal* and benzylpenicillin is the treatment of choice, or if there is allergy, erythromycin or a cephalosporin. Pneumonia following influenza is often caused by *Staph. aureus*, for which sodium fusidate and flucloxacillin should be used in combination.

Atypical cases of pneumonia may be due to *Mycoplasma pneumoniae*, which may be epidemic, or more rarely *Chlamydia psittaci* (psittacosis or *Coxiella burnetii* (Q fever), when tetracycline or erythromycin should be given. Treatment of ornithosis (psittacosis) should continue for 10 days after the fever has settled, and in mycoplasma pneumonia and Q fever a total of 3-weeks treatment may be needed to prevent relapse.

Pneumonia in individuals with chronic lung disease

Normal commensals of the upper respiratory tract proliferate in damaged lungs, especially following viral infections, pulmonary congestion or pulmonary infarction. Mixed infection is therefore common and, since *H. influenzae* and *Strep. pneumoniae* are often the pathogens, amoxycillin or trimethoprim are reasonable choices. *Klebsiella pneumoniae* tends to cause lung infection in the debilitated elderly and forms abscesses, particularly in the upper lobes. Cefuroxime plus an aminoglycoside is recommended.

In hospitalised patients, *Staph. aureus* should be considered as the cause of pneumonia. *Branhamella catarrhalis*, a commensal of the oropharynx, has recently been recognised as a pathogen in lower-respiratory-tract infections, especially in patients with chronic lung disease, lung cancer, or those taking corticosteroids. Treatment with amoxycillin may fail because about half the strains produce β-lactamase. The organism is also sensitive to cefuroxime, co-trimoxazole or erythromycin.

Pneumonia in immunocompromised patients

Pneumonia is a common infection in those whose humoural or cellular immune systems are defective, e.g. those with acquired immunodeficiency syndrome (AIDS) or who are receiving immunosuppressive drugs. Common pathogenic bacteria may be responsible (*Staph. aureus, Strep. pneumoniae*) but often organisms of lower natural virulence (viruses, fungi) are causal and strenuous efforts should be made to identify the microbe, including, if feasible, bronchial washings or lung

* Editorial. Lancet 1960; 2:1286.

biopsy. *Ps. aeruginosa* may cause pneumonia in the severely ill or immunocompromised patient and another important respiratory pathogen in this group is the protozoon *Pneumocystis carinii*. Until the pathogen is known, the patient should receive broad spectrum antimicrobial treatment, either with an aminoglycoside and amoxycillin or cefuroxime and metronidazole. Pneumocystis infection should be treated with co-trimoxazole (trimethoprim 20 mg/kg/day, sulphamethoxazole 100 mg/kg/day by mouth or i.v. in four divided doses for 14 days); for treatment of pseudomonal infection, see Antimicrobial drugs of choice, p. 206.

Legionnaires' disease

The condition may occur sporadically or in epidemics of various size. Cigarette smokers or debilitated or immunocompromised patients are at increased risk but it may also occur in previously healthy persons. The name derives from an epidemic of pneumonia in 1976 at an American Legion convention in Philadelphia; there were 182 cases of whom 29 died. Comprehensive bacteriological tests failed to produce evidence of infection with any organism known to cause pneumonia until pieces of lung from four fatal cases were injected into guinea pigs and a hitherto unrecognised bacterium grew. The isolation of this bacterium (*Legionella pneumophila*) has given an explanation for several other mysterious outbreaks of respiratory or 'flu-like' disease, including one 11 years before in Washington in which the precaution had been taken to store acute and convalescent sera pending the future discovery of the organism.

Erythromycin 2–4 g i.v. per day in divided doses is the treatment of choice but rifampicin may be added in resistant cases.

Pneumonia due to anaerobic microorganisms

The infection tends to arise following aspiration of material from the oropharynx or in the presence of other lung pathology such as pulmonary infarction or bronchogenic carcinoma, or by transdiaphragmatic spread of intra-abdominal sepsis. The pathogens include anaerobic streptococci, bacteroides and fusobacterium species and the diagnosis may be missed unless anaerobic cultures of fresh material are taken. Treatment with benzylpenicillin and metronidazole should continue for several weeks to prevent relapse, or for months if there has been cavitation.

Pulmonary abscess is treated according to the organism identified and with surgery if necessary.

Empyema is treated according to the organism isolated and with aspiration and drainage. If the pleural fluid is thick with fibrin or pus so that aspiration is difficult and loculation seems likely, surgery is best.

INFECTION OF THE ENDOCARDIUM

The most likely bacterial pathogens are:

1. Viridans group of *Streptococcus*
2. Enterococci (*Streptococcus faecalis*)
3. *Streptococcus bovis*
4. *Staphylococcus aureus*
5. *Staphylococcus epidermidis**
6. Gram-negative bacilli
7. *Streptococcus pneumoniae*
8. *Streptocococcus pyogenes* (Group A)
9. *Corynebacterium* spp.*

When the degree of suspicion is high enough, four blood cultures should be taken in a few hours and antimicrobial treatment should begin. To delay further, e.g. to obtain the results of culture tests, only exposes the patient to the risk of grave cardiac damage or systemic embolism.

The infecting organism(s) differ according to the circumstances and it is useful to *classify infective endocarditis thus*†:

1. **Medical** endocarditis, that is, endocarditis encountered in general medical patients, which is due to viridans streptococci in 80% of cases, enterococci in 10%, and various other organisms in the remainder.

2. **Geriatric** endocarditis, in which *viridans* streptococci are causal in only 50% of cases and *Strep. faecalis* is isolated more commonly than in

* especially with prosthetic valves
† Oakley C M, Darrell J H. Prescribers Journal. 1980; 20(6): 98–106.

younger patients. Gram-negative infections may complicate genitourinary or gastrointestinal disease or investigations.

3. **Narcotic addict** endocarditis results from injections of infected diluent obtained, for example, from the toilet; *Staph. aureus*, streptococci (Group B), and in the USA, *Serratia marcesens* are common causal organisms.

4. **Surgical** endocarditis complicates cardiac surgery. Early in the post-operative period, *Staph. epidermidis*, *Staph. aureus* or a fungus may be pathogens; later, the organisms are those encountered in medical patients except for fungal endocarditis, which may go unrecognised for months.

5. **Culture-negative** endocarditis comprises up to 20% of cases. Failure to grow an organism is usually due to prior antimicrobial therapy or to special culture requirements of the microbe. *Coxiella* or *Chlamydia* spp. are diagnosed by serology tests. It is best to regard culture-negative endocarditis as being due to streptococci and to treat accordingly.

Aspects of the treatment of infective endocarditis

1. *High doses of bactericidal drugs* are needed because the organisms are relatively inaccessible in avascular vegetations and the host reaction (on which cure by bacteristatic drugs depends) is negligible.

2. *Drugs should be given parenterally at least initially* and preferably by intravenous bolus injection, which achieves the necessary high peak concentration to penetrate the relatively avascular valves. The antimicrobial should never be added to the infusion reservoir, whose purpose is only to keep open the route into the vein.

3. *The infusion site* should be changed at least every 2–3 days to prevent opportunistic infection, which is usually with (drug-resistant) staphylococci or fungi. Alternatively, use may be made of a central subclavian venous line sited with careful attention to aseptic technique.

4. *Prolonged therapy* is needed, usually for 4 weeks, and in the case of infected prosthetic valves at least 6 weeks. The patient should be reviewed one month after completing the antimicrobial treatment and blood culture repeated.

5. *Dosage* must be adjusted according to the sensitivity of the infecting organism and therapy may be regarded as adequate if a 1:8 dilution of the patient's plasma kills it. The following regimens are within generally accepted ranges:

*a. Initial treatment** should comprise benzylpenicillin 1.2–2.4 g, 4-hourly plus gentamicin 80 mg, 8- or 12-hourly by i.v. injection; if *Staph. aureus* is suspected, sodium fusidate 500 mg, 8-hourly by mouth should be added. Patients allergic to penicillin should be treated with vancomycin 1 g i.v. over 60 min, 12-hourly.

b. When an organism has been identified, the following is a guide to treatment:

Strep. viridans: benzylpenicillin plus gentamicin i.v. for at least 4 weeks or, if the organism is very sensitive, for 2 weeks followed by amoxycillin 1 g, 8-hourly by mouth for 2 weeks.

Strep. faecalis: benzylpenicillin plus gentamicin i.v. for at least four weeks.

Staph. aureus: flucloxacillin 2 g, 4-hourly by i.v. injection plus either gentamicin 80–120 mg, 8-hourly i.v. or sodium fusidate 500 mg, 8-hourly by mouth.

Staph. epidermidis, which has a predilection for prosthetic valves, should be managed as for *Staph. aureus* if the organism is sensitive but even if this is so valve replacement may be needed.

Coxiella or *Chlamydia*: tetracycline 750 mg 8-hourly by mouth, reducing after 4–6 weeks to 250 mg 12-hourly. Surgery is advised in most cases but some may continue indefinitely on tetracycline.

Fungal endocarditis: amphotericin B plus flucytosine are given.

6. *Culture-negative endocarditis*: benzylpenicillin plus gentamicin are given for 6 weeks.

Prophylaxis of infective endocarditis

Transient bacteraemia is provoked by even minor dental procedures, by surgical incision of the skin, instrumentation of the urinary tract, parturition and even seemingly innocent activities such as brushing the teeth or chewing toffee. Bacteraemia

* Further details appear in Report of a Working Party of the British Society for Antimicrobial Chemotherapy. Lancet 1985; 2:815.

does not always lead to endocarditis, but experience shows that individuals with *acquired* or *congenital* heart defects are at risk from certain procedures and are protected by antimicrobials given prophylactically. The drugs are given as a *short* course in *high* dose at the *time* of the procedure to prevent emergence of resistant organisms.

The recommendations that follow are a summary of a Report of a Working Party of the British Society for Antimicrobial Chemotherapy.* Not every contingency is covered, because antimicrobial prophylaxis may be needed for patients *with cardiac defects* whenever surgery or instrumentation is undertaken on tissue that is heavily colonised or infected and the physician should exercise a clinical judgement that relates to individual circumstances.

1. **Dental procedures**

A. *In general dental practice*

(i) adults should receive amoxycillin 3 g by mouth as a single dose, under supervision, one hour before the procedure. Those who are to have a general anaesthetic should receive amoxycillin 3 g by mouth 4 hours before operation and a further 3 g by mouth as soon as possible after the operation. Children under 10 years should receive half, and those under 5 years should receive one quarter of the adult dose.

(ii) patients allergic to penicillins should receive erythromycin stearate 1.5 g by mouth under supervision 1–2 h before the procedure, followed by 0.5 g 6 h later. Children under 10 years should receive half and those under 5 years should receive one quarter of the adult dose. Patients who require a general anaesthetic should be referred to hospital.

(iii) patients who have received penicillins in the previous month and who would otherwise receive amoxycillin as in (i) above, should receive erythromycin as in (ii) above.

B. *In hospital practice*

Patients who are at special risk or who are to undergo more major dental procedures should be managed in hospital. These comprise:

(i) patients to be given a general anaesthetic who have received penicillins during the previous month.

(ii) patients to be given a general anaesthetic who have a prosthetic valve.

(iii) patients who have had more than one previous attack of endocarditis.

(iv) patients to be given a general anaesthetic who are allergic to penicillins.

Adults in groups (i), (ii) and (iii) should receive amoxycillin 1 g in lignocaine 1% (2.5 ml) plus gentamicin 120 mg i.m. immediately before induction if they are to have a general anaesthetic, or if not, 15 min before the dental procedure. A second dose of amoxycillin 0.5 g i.m. should be given 6 h later. Children under 10 years should receive half the adult dose of amoxycillin and gentamicin 2 mg/kg.

Adults in all groups who are allergic to penicillins should receive vancomycin 1 g by i.v. infusion over 60 min followed by gentamicin 120 mg i.v. immediately before induction of anaesthesia. Children under 10 years should receive by the i.v. route, vancomycin 20 mg/kg and gentamicin 2 mg/kg.

2. **Genitourinary procedures**

(i) Adults who are to have genitourinary procedures under general anaesthesia, and who have no urinary tract infection and are not allergic to penicillins, should receive amoxycillin 1 g in lignocaine 1% (2.5 ml) plus gentamicin 120 mg i.m. immediately before induction, followed by amoxycillin 0.5 g i.m. or orally 6 h later. Children under 10 years should receive amoxycillin 0.5 g and gentamicin 2 mg/kg i.m.

(ii) Adults and children who are allergic to penicillin should receive gentamicin and vancomycin as under 1B (ii) above.

3. **Upper respiratory tract procedures**

Prophylactic antibiotics are required for tonsillectomy or adenoidectomy but not for fibreoptic bronchoscopy, which rarely if ever causes bacteraemia.

(i) Patients who are to undergo surgery or instrumentation of the upper respiratory tract under general anaesthesia, who are not allergic to penicillin and who do not have prosthetic valves, should receive amoxycillin 1 g in lignocaine 1% (2.5 ml) i.m. immediately before induction,

* Report. Lancet 1982; 2:1323 and Simmons N A, et al Lancet 1986; 1:1267.

followed by amoxycillin 0.5 g i.m. 6 h later. Children under 10 years should receive half the adult dose.

(ii) Adults with prosthetic valves should receive amoxycillin 1 g in lignocaine 1% (2.5 ml) plus gentamicin 120 mg i.m. immediately before induction, and amoxycillin 0.5 g i.m. 6 h later. Children under 10 years should receive half the adult dose of amoxycillin and gentamicin 2 mg/kg.

(iii) Patients who are allergic to penicillins should receive vancomycin 1 g by i.v. infusion over 60 min, followed by gentamicin 120 mg i.v. immediately before anaesthesia. Children under 10 years should receive vancomycin 20 mg/kg and gentamicin 2 mg/kg i.v.

INFECTION OF THE MENINGES

The most likely bacterial pathogens are*:

Neonates

1. *Escherichia coli* (and other Gram-negative bacilli)
2. *Streptococcus pyogenes* (Group B)
3. *Staphylococcus aureus*
4. *Listeria monocytogenes*
5. Also — those bacteria that cause meningitis in older children.

Infants and pre-school children

1. *Haemophilus influenzae*
2. *Neisseria meningitidis*
3. *Streptococcus pneumoniae*

School age children and adults

1. *Neisseria meningitidis*
2. *Streptococcus pneumoniae*
3. *Haemophilus influenzae*

Patients with immune deficiency & CNS defects

1. *Streptococcus pneumoniae*
2. Coliform bacteria
3. *Listeria monocytogenes*
4. Other organisms

* After Lambert H P. Br J Hosp Med 1983; 29:128.

Patients with CSF shunts

1. *Staphylococcus aureus*
2. *Staphylococcus epidermidis*
3. Other organisms

Accurate bacteriological diagnosis and speed of initiating treatment are the main factors determining the fate of the patient. Apart from age (above) there may be clinical clues to the infecting organism, for example:

a. A petechial and purpuric rash suggests meningococcal infection.

b. A history of skull fracture, CSF rhinorrhoea or middle ear infection favours pneumococcal meningitis.

c. The presence of congenital nervous system lesions is associated with pneumonococcal or coliform infections.

Notwithstanding the organisms listed at the beginning of this section, there are three common forms of bacterial meningitis, namely:

Meningococcus meningitis: initial treatment is with benzylpenicillin 1.2–2.4 g i.v. 4-hourly. If it is later established that the organism is sulphonamide-sensitive, continuation with sulphadimidine, sulphadiazine or sulphafurazole by mouth is acceptable if repeated parenteral injection is a problem: treatment should last 7–10 days. Chloramphenicol should be given to patients who are allergic to penicillin. Adequate analgesia should be given for headache. Adrenal steroid should be added if there is evidence of adrenocortical insufficiency (Waterhouse–Friderichsen syndrome).

Pneumococcal meningitis: benzylpenicillin 1.2–2.4 g is given i.v. 4-hourly. Treatment should continue for two weeks after the patient has become afebrile and the physician should remember the risk of subsequent relapse.

Haemophilus meningitis: chloramphenicol as the sole antimicrobial is often regarded as sufficient; treatment should initially be i.v. 50 mg/kg daily in divided doses every 6 h and then by mouth 500 mg every 6 h when the patient is well enough to swallow. Some authorities advocate giving amoxycillin with chloramphenicol but resistance to chloramphenicol is at present rare whilst amoxycillin-resistant organisms are becoming more common.

Other types of meningitis: meningitis in neonates and older patients with immune deficiency or nervous system defects tends to be caused by Gram-negative bacilli, e.g. *E. coli, Ps. aeruginosa* or *Klebsiella* spp. An aminoglycoside would normally be the choice in such cases but there is uncertainty that this class of drug achieves adequate concentration throughout the CSF and recent clinical trial evidence suggests that cefuroxime, cefotaxime or latamoxef should be preferred.

Before the infecting organism has been positively identified and its chemotherapeutic sensitivity established, initial therapy should be sufficiently broad to kill all likely pathogens. Thus for:

a. children and adults give benzylpenicillin plus chloramphenicol
b. neonates give cefuroxime plus ticarcillin.

Intrathecal treatment is now in general considered *unnecessary* and it can furthermore be dangerous (encephalopathy with benzylpenicillin).

Chemoprophylaxis. The three common pathogens are spread by respiratory secretions. Asymptomatic nasopharyngeal carriers of the bacteria seldom develop meningitis but they may transmit the pathogens to close personal contacts. Rifampicin is effective at reducing carriage rates.

Meningococcal meningitis is well recognised as occurring in epidemics, in smaller scale outbreaks in closed communities as well as in isolated cases. Close personal contacts of cases should receive rifampicin 10 mg/kg every 12 h for four doses.

Haemophilus meningitis has only more recently been recognised as a contagious disease, with an infectiveness similar to that of meningococcal meningitis. Chemoprophylaxis with rifampicin may be advisable for contacts under four years of age, for they are especially at risk.

Pneumococcal meningitis tends to occur in isolated cases and chemoprophylaxis is not at present recommended.

Tuberculous meningitis. It is essential to use isoniazid and pyrazinamide, which penetrate well into the CSF. Rifampicin enters inflamed meninges well but non-inflamed meninges less so. An effective regimen is isoniazid, rifampicin, pyrazinamide and streptomycin.* Treatment may need to continue for much longer than modern short course chemotherapy for pulmonary tuberculosis.

INFECTIONS OF THE INTESTINES

The most likely bacterial pathogens are:

1. *Campylobacter* spp.
2. *Salmonella* spp.
3. *Escherichia coli*
4. *Shigella* spp.
5. *Yersinia enterocolitica*
6. *Staphylococcus aureus*
7. *Vibrio cholerae*
8. *Clostridium difficile*

Antimicrobial therapy should be reserved for specific conditions having an identified pathogen, which are known to be shortened by drug therapy. Not all acute diarrhoea is infective for it can be caused, for example, by toxins, dietary indiscretions, anxiety and drugs. Even if it is infectious, diarrhoea may be due to viruses, or, if it is bacterial, antimicrobial agents may not reduce the duration of symptoms and may aggravate it by allowing opportunistic infection. Maintenance of hydration, either by i.v. infusion or orally with a glucose-electrolyte solution together with an antimotility drug are the mainstays of therapy in such cases (see also p. 633).

Some specific intestinal infections do benefit from chemotherapy and these are now considered.

Campylobacter jejuni. In less than a decade this obscure avian pathogen has emerged as a leading cause of enteritis in humans. Symptoms range from the relatively mild to severe diarrhoea with passage of blood in the stools and marked abdominal pain. Recovery without antimicrobial drugs is usual. Erythromycin will eliminate the organism from the stools; whether the drug alters the clinical course of the disease is less certain but a 5-day course is worth giving if the illness is severe or protracted.

Shigella. Mild disease requires no specific antimicrobial therapy but toxic shigellosis with

* Parsons M. Br J Hosp Med 1982; 27:682.

high fever should be treated with co-trimoxazole or trimethoprim alone for 5 days unless the local patterns of drug resistance indicate alternative drugs, e.g. ampicillin or nalidixic acid.

Salmonella. The duration of diarrhoea caused by organisms other than *S. typhi* or *S. paratyphi* is not shortened by antimicrobial drugs, which may indeed prolong the stay of organisms in the stools. An antimicrobial should be used for severe salmonella gastroenteritis or bacteraemia or salmonella enteritis in an immunocompromised patient. The choice lies between amoxycillin and co-trimoxazole, according to the sensitivity of the pathogen; chloramphenicol is effective in complicated infections. Unfortunately, use of the drugs as growth promoters in food animals has caused the spread of drug-resistant organisms.

Typhoid fever requires antimicrobial treatment. Chloramphenicol is usually considered to be the drug of first choice. The dose is 50 mg/kg/day for 2 weeks and the i.v. route should be used in severe cases. Severely ill patients may benefit from the addition of dexamethasone 3 mg/kg i.v. initially, followed by 1 mg/kg 6-hourly for 48 h.

Alternative drugs are amoxycillin, 1 g by mouth 6-hourly and co-trimoxazole 960 mg by mouth 12-hourly, in each case for 2 weeks. A longer period of treatment may be required for those who develop complications such as osteomyelitis or abscess.

A *carrier state* develops in a few individuals, who have no symptoms of disease but who can infect others. Organisms reside in the biliary or urinary tracts. Chronic carriage may be more common after typhoid fever has been treated with chloramphenicol. Certainly, this bacteristatic drug should *not* be used to treat the carrier state for there is no local defence reaction to eradicate the immobilised organisms. Amoxycillin in high dose for 3 months may be successful for what can be a very difficult problem.* Cholecystectomy may be needed for chronic infection of the gallbladder followed by amoxycillin for one month.

Esch. coli is a normal inhabitant of the bowel but some *enterotoxigenic* strains do upset bowel function and are frequently a cause of travellers' diarrhoea. Co-trimoxazole or trimethoprim alone may reduce symptoms and shorten the duration of an attack (see Travellers' diarrhoea, p. 635).

Yersinia enterocolitica. Enteritis due to this organism usually does not require an antimicrobial but in severe illness co-trimoxazole or a tetracycline may be used.

Staphyococcus aureus. Staphylococcal enteritis, although rare, may complicate abdominal surgery, shock or antimicrobial therapy. Dehydration, shock and electrolyte imbalance should be treated vigorously. Vancomycin by mouth or flucloxacillin by mouth and i.v. is effective.

Vibrio cholerae. The cause of death in cholera is electrolyte and fluid loss in the stools, which may amount to 0.5–4.5 l/hr. The most important aim of the treatment is rehydration and maintenance of fluid balance with oral or i.v. electrolyte solutions. Tetracycline, doxycycline, co-trimoxazole or chloramphenicol speed the elimination of the organism from the faeces and reduce the amount and duration of diarrhoea. Carriers may be treated by tetracycline by mouth in high dose for 3 days.

Suppression of bowel flora or bowel partial 'sterilisation' prior to colonic surgery in order to prevent post-surgery sepsis has been practised. 'This must be one of the most extraordinary concepts in chemotherapy ever to have gained general currency'.† If the drugs have any effect, this will be to deprive the patient of the flora with which he has an equilibrium. The results of this 'are frequently disagreeable and may be dangerous. The post-operative patient can ill afford to lose his normal bowel flora since it constitutes one of the major protections against occupation by the bowel of undesirable organisms.'† Evidence of benefit from antimicrobials used thus is unconvincing. But *systemic* antimicrobials, e.g. metronidazole plus a cephalosporin started immediately before surgery and continued, confer protection against infection caused by the surgical procedure (see Chemoprophylaxis, p. 199).

Suppression of bowel flora is useful in *hepatic insufficiency*. Here, absorption of products of

* The most famous carrier was Mary Mallon ('Typhoid Mary') who worked as a cook in New York City, using various assumed names and moving through several different households. She caused at least 10 outbreaks with 51 cases of typhoid fever and 3 deaths. To protect the public, she was kept in detention for 23 years; in total she was a carrier for 31 years.

† O'Grady F W. J R Coll Phys Lond 1972; 6:203.

bacterial breakdown of protein (ammonium, amines) in the intestine is believed to lead to cerebral symptoms and even to coma. In acute coma neomycin (6 g daily orally) should be given; as prophylactic, 4 g may be given daily to patients with protein intolerance who fail to respond to dietary protein restriction. Kanamycin is preferable for cases with renal failure because neomycin may cause ototoxicity, the ordinarily negligible amounts that are absorbed becoming important because they are not eliminated.

Sterilisation of bowel may be necessary in preparation for certain forms of intensive anti-leukaemia therapy, which seriously impair natural defences to prevent opportunistic infection. Combinations of drugs are used (e.g. framycetin, colistin, nystatin and amphotericin).

In blind-loop syndrome, it is desired to eliminate bacteria that are using up vitamin B_{12} and altering bile salts so that steatorrhoea results. After an initial course of amoxycillin, therapy can be intermittent, say 3 days a week, to prevent recolonisation.

For similar reasons antimicrobial therapy is used in initial treatment of tropical sprue.

Antibiotic-induced *diarrhoea* is usually assumed to be due to alteration of bowel flora because it occurs more commonly, but not exclusively, with broad-spectrum drugs. Mild cases recover spontaneously when the drug is stopped.

Broad-spectrum antibiotics given by mouth to patients with ulcerative colitis may trigger a relapse and should be avoided.

Antibiotic-associated colitis, see p. 202.

Peritonitis is usually mixed and antimicrobial choice must take account of coliforms, anaerobes and streptococci; a combination of gentamicin, ampicillin and metronidazole or of cefuroxime and metronidazole is usually effective.

INFECTIONS OF THE URINARY TRACT (excluding sexually transmitted diseases)

The most likely bacterial pathogens are:

1. *Escherichia coli*
2. *Proteus* spp.
3. *Klebsiella pneumoniae*
4. *Pseudomonas aeruginosa*
5. *Staphylococcus aureus*
6. Enterococci
7. Micrococci

Urine constitutes a culture medium capable of sustaining a bacterial concentration of 10^9 organisms per ml. It lacks natural defence mechanisms such as lysozymes and immunoglobulin, which are present in other secretions such as tears and saliva.

Identification of the causative organism and its sensitivity to drugs are very important because of the large range of organisms that may be responsible and the prevalence of resistant strains.

In infections of the lower *urinary tract*, it is the concentration of antimicrobial in the urine rather than in the tissues that matters, and as many are concentrated in the urine, an effective dose may be relatively low. However, it is the concentration in the tissues that matters in infections of the *substance of the kidney* and here, the doses needed are those for any systemic infection.

Correction, if possible, of predisposing anatomical abnormalities, such as an enlarged prostate, bladder diverticula, congenital abnormalities of the renal pelvis or ureters, or removal of renal calculi is important for success. If correction is not possible, chemoprophylaxis may help prevent recurrent infections. Indwelling urinary catheters, while sometimes undeniably necessary, also predispose to urinary tract infection, and continued antibiotic treatment in the presence of a catheter will fail.

Elimination of infection is hastened by a urine volume of about 1.5 l/day and by frequent micturition. Relevant antimicrobials are well concentrated in the urine and a moderate diuresis will not significantly diminish their efficacy.

Drug treatment of urinary tract infection falls into several categories.

1. *Lower urinary tract infection.* Initial treatment: trimethoprim, or amoxycillin + clavulanic acid, is usually satisfactory. Therapy should normally last 5 days and may need to be altered once the results of bacterial sensitivity are known.

Single dose therapy: amoxycillin 3 g by mouth in a single dose may be sufficient to cure uncomplicated lower urinary tract infection.

2. *Upper urinary tract infection.* Acute pyelonephritis may be accompanied by septicaemia and it is advisable to start with gentamicin plus amoxycillin or alternatively cefotaxime alone.

3. *Recurrent urinary tract infection* is common. Attacks following rapidly with the same organism may be *relapses* and indicate a failure to eliminate the original infection. Attacks with a longer interval between them and produced by different bacterial types may be regarded as due to *re-infection*, presumably from a source outside the urinary tract. Broadly, relapse implies infection involving the upper urinary tract and re-infection indicates involvement of the lower tract but this distinction is by no means absolute. In treating a relapse it is wise to use a drug capable of achieving high tissue concentrations, e.g. amoxycillin. Repeated short courses of antimicrobials should overcome most recurrent infections but if this fails, 7–14 days of high-dose treatment may be given, following which continuous low-dose prophylaxis may be needed.

4. *Asymptomatic infection* may be found by routine urine testing of pregnant women or patients with known structural abnormality of the urinary tract. Such infection may explain urinary frequency or incontinence in the elderly. Appropriate antimicrobial therapy should be given. Amoxycillin or a cephalosporin are preferred in pregnancy.

5. *Urinary symptoms* without evidence of infection. Recurrent attacks of frequent or painful micturition for women without obvious abnormality of the urinary tract, and failure to find a causative organism, constitute the 'urethral syndrome'. The condition is due probably to proliferation of organisms in the introitus and failure of the urethral defence mechanisms to prevent invasion of the lower urinary tract. Management should include attention to perineal and introital hygiene, cotton as opposed to nylon clothing and a copious fluid intake. Sometimes symptoms are due to anaerobic organisms that require special culture techniques; these respond to erythromycin or amoxycillin rather than to co-trimoxazole.

6. *Prostatitis*. Chronic bacterial prostatitis is believed to be a common cause of recurrent bacteriuria in men whose urinary tracts are otherwise normal. The commonest pathogens are Gram-negative aerobic bacilli. In order to penetrate the prostate in adequate concentration, an antimicrobial needs to be lipid soluble. Both trimethoprim and rifampicin, which may usefully be combined, possess this characteristic; both are also active against Gram-negative aerobic bacilli. Trimethoprim in addition is a weak base and so distributes preferentially to the acidic prostatic fluid (pH 6.2–6.5) by 'ion-trapping' (see p. 115). Trimethoprim plus sulphamethoxazole (co-trimoxazole) has given disappointing results in bacterial prostatitis, which is not altogether surprising for the sulphonamide component is an acid that is trapped in plasma rather than prostatic fluid. Response to a single, short course of antimicrobial is often good, but recurrence is common and a patient can be regarded as cured only if he has been symptom-free and off antimicrobials for a year.

Chemoprophylaxis of urinary infections is sometimes undertaken in patients liable to recurrent attacks or acute exacerbations of ineradicable infection. It may prevent sub-clinical renal damage in schoolgirls who are found to have asymptomatic bacteriuria on routine screening. Nitrofurantoin (0.5–1.0 g/day), nalidixic acid (0.5–1.0 g/day) or trimethoprim 100 mg/day are satisfactory. The drugs are best given as single dose at night time.

Tuberculosis of the genitourinary tract is treated on the principles described for pulmonary infection (p. 253). A satisfactory regimen is rifampicin 450 mg, isoniazid 300 mg and pyrazinamide 1 g daily for 2 months, followed by rifampicin 450 mg and isoniazid 300 mg 3 times a week for a further 2 months, but chemotherapy may need to be continued for longer than this.

Drugs for urinary tract infections

A number of antimicrobial drugs suitable for general use are also appropriate for urinary tract infections. These described elsewhere and include: *amoxycillin (with or without clavulanic acid), trimethoprim, gentamicin, cephalosporins.*

Other *antimicrobials indicated only for infection of the urinary tract* are described here:

Nitrofurantoin (Furadantin) (50, 100 mg) is a synthetic antimicrobial that is active against the majority of urinary pathogens except pseudomonads. The drug is well absorbed from the gastrointestinal tract and although plasma levels are low, it is effectively concentrated in the urine, where about 45% of the drug appears unchanged.

Renal tubular reabsorption occurs but tissue concentrations cannot be sufficiently depended on to render nitrofurantoin a suitable drug for acute pyelonephritis. It is more active, more soluble and more completely excreted in an acid urine. Metabolites may turn the urine dark brown. The $t_{\frac{1}{2}}$ is 30 mins. Excretion is reduced when there is renal insufficiency so the drug is both more toxic and less effective. Nitrofurantoin is taken after food since it is a gastric irritant, in an oral dose of 50–100 mg 6-hourly as therapy or prophylactically in one-quarter to one-half this dose. Since the lower dose is better tolerated, the main use of nitrofurantoin is now for prophylaxis.

Adverse effects include nausea and vomiting, which is claimed to be lessened by combining nitrofurantoin with deglycyrrhinized liquorice (Ceduran), and diarrhoea. Polyneuritis occurs especially in patients with significant renal impairment, in whom the drug is contraindicated. Allergic reactions include rashes, generalised urticaria and pulmonary infiltrations.

Nalidixic acid (Negram) (500 mg), a quinolone, is active against urinary Gram-negative bacilli including *Proteus* spp, but not *Pseudomonas* spp. Its principal use now is for prophylaxis, in an oral dose of 500 mg once or twice daily. Nitrofurantoin causes a false-positive urine test for glucose with Clinitest but not with glucose-specific methods. The drug may cause disturbance of sensory perception and allergic skin reactions: in infants benign intracranial hypertension may be induced.

Newly developed quinolones, e.g. *norfloxacin*, *ciprofloxacin*, are very active against Gram-negative organisms including enterobacteria and may prove effective for systemic infection of this type.

INFECTION OF THE GENITAL TRACT

The most likely bacterial pathogens are:

Female genital tract

Vagina

1. *Neisseria gonorrhoeae*
2. *Streptococcus pyogenes* (Group A)
3. *Gardnerella vaginalis*
4. *Treponema pallidum*

Uterus

1. Anaerobic streptococci
2. *Bacteroides* spp.
3. *Neisseria gonorrhoeae* (cervix)
4. *Clostridia* spp.
5. *Escherichia coli* (or other Gram-negative bacilli)
6. *Streptococcus pyogenes* (Group A)
7. *Streptococcus* (Groups B and C) spp.
8. *Treponema pallidum*
9. *Staphylococcus aureus*
10. Enterococci
11. *Chlamydia trachomatis**
12. *Mycoplasma hominis**

Fallopian tubes

1. *Neisseria gonorrhoeae*
2. *Escherichia coli* (or other Gram-negative bacilli)
3. Anaerobic streptococci
4. *Bacteroides*

Urethra (female and male)

1. *Neisseria gonorrhoeae*
2. *Chlamydia** spp.
3. *Treponema pallidum*
4. *Ureaplasma urealyticum*

Male genital tract

Seminal vesicles

1. Gram-negative bacilli
2. *Neisseria gonorrhoeae*

Epididymis

1. *Chlamydia** spp.
2. Gram-negative bacilli
3. *Neisseria gonorrhoeae*
4. *Mycobacterium tuberculosis*

Urethra
(see above)

A general account of orthodox literature is given below, but treatment is increasingly the prerogative of specialists, who, as is so often the case in many areas, get the best results.

Gonorrhoea. There are several treatments for uncomplicated gonococcal infections in both men

* Organisms that are not strictly bacteria but that are susceptible to antibacterial drugs have been included.

and women. The problem of resistant gonococci is increasing, and selection of a particular drug will depend on sensitivity testing and a knowledge of resistance patterns in different geographical locations. Effective treatment requires exposure of the organism briefly to a high concentration of the drug. Single dose regimens are practicable as well as being obviously desirable for social reasons, including compliance. The following schedules are effective:

Uncomplicated anogenital infections

1. Procaine penicillin 1.4–2.8 g i.m. with probenecid 1.0 g by mouth. Two injection sites may be used for the higher dose.

or

2. Benzylpenicillin, 3 g dissolved in 5 ml of a solution of lignocaine 5%, administered i.m. and preceded by probenecid 1.0 g by mouth. This regimen avoids the possibility of adverse reaction to procaine.

3. Amoxycillin 3.0 g by mouth in a single dose, with probenecid 1.0 g by mouth.

4. Alternatively, if the organism is resistant to or the patient is allergic to penicillins, the following may be used:

Spectinomycin, 2 g i.m. in men, 4 g i.m. in women,

or

tetracycline 0.5 g 6-hourly by mouth for 5 days,

or

co-trimoxazole 1.92 g 12-hourly for 2 days (or 2.4 g followed by another 2.4 g 8 h later),

or

cefuroxime 1.5 g i.m.,

or

acrosoxacin 300 mg as a single dose by mouth.

All oral treatments should be witnessed by the doctor or nurse to ensure compliance.

Complicated gonorrhoea (e.g. pelvic infection) requires more vigorous and prolonged therapy.

Pharyngeal gonorrhoea responds less well to the single dose regimens above, and tetracycline in high doses is needed for 7 days.

Gonococcal conjunctivitis (see Eye Infections, p. 253).

Co-existent infection. Chlamydia trachomatis is frequently present with *Neisseria gonorrhoea* and the use of tetracycline will limit the incidence of chlamydial urethritis.

Whilst benzylpenicillin treatment of acute gonorrhoea at current doses may cure a simultaneously contracted syphilis, it may also mask it so that the primary infection is not seen and a disastrous late syphilis occurs. This may be more a theoretical than a practical risk but a serological test for syphilis should be done 3 months after treating gonorrhoea. Co-trimoxazole and acrosoxacin do not mask syphilis.

Non-gonococcal urethritis. The vast majority of cases of urethritis with pus in which gonococci cannot be identified is due to sexually transmitted non-specific urethritis (NSU). Most of these are caused by *Chlamydia trachomatis* and some by *Ureaplasma urealyticum*. Indeed, chlamydial infection is probably the commonest sexually transmitted disease in developed countries.

Tetracycline 500 mg by mouth, 6-hourly for 14 days is effective for most infections, but 21 days treatment may be needed for complicated cases.

Chlamydia conjunctivitis (see Eye Infections, p. 253).

Syphilis. *Treponema pallidum* never becomes resistant to penicillin.

Primary and *secondary* syphilis is effectively treated by procaine penicillin 600–1200 mg i.m. daily for 15 days. If it is suspected that the patient may not comply with the requirements of this course, a single i.m. injection of benzathine penicillin 1.8 g may be given.

Patients who are allergic to penicillin should receive tetracycline 0.5 g by mouth, 6-hourly for 2 weeks, or alternatively, erythromycin 1 g by mouth, 12-hourly for 2 weeks, which is preferred in pregnancy when tetracycline is contraindicated.

Tertiary syphilis should have the same treatment prolonged to 3 weeks. The cerebrospinal fluid does not return to normal for months, and sometimes never. A second course of penicillin is advisable if the spinal fluid is still abnormal after 6 months.

Congenital syphilis in the newborn may be treated with benzylpenicillin for 10 days at least. Topical application of hydrocortisone to the eyes helps to reduce interstitial keratitis.

A pregnant woman with syphilis should be

treated as for primary syphilis (in each pregnancy, some advocate), in order to avoid all danger to children. Therapy is best given between the third and sixth month, as there may be a risk of abortion if it is given earlier.

Results of treatment of syphilis with penicillin are excellent; virtually 100% cure is achieved in seronegative cases, but the cure rate is lower in seropositive cases.

Follow-up of all cases is essential, for 5 years if possible, with annual serological tests and a final examination of the cerebrospinal fluid. Relapses are rare and it is hard to distinguish these from re-infections. One study found the relapse rate amongst patients on identical treatment to be related to social status, which suggests that most relapses are really re-infections.

Chemoprophylaxis of syphilis may be practised with an orally active penicillin, but there is a risk of contracting an infection, the early signs of which may be suppressed. Masking of gonorrhoea does not occur. Chemoprophylaxis is not to be recommended under normal social conditions. Patients who are known to have been exposed to syphilis recently may be treated as though they had syphilis, but there is no agreement as to the clinical merits of this, although social requirements may occasionally demand it.

The Herxheimer (or Jarisch–Herxheimer) reaction may be due to the massive slaughter of spirochaetes, resulting in the release of toxic substances. As pyrexia, it is common during the few hours after the first penicillin injection; other features include tachycardia, headache, myalgia and malaise, which last up to a day. It cannot be prevented by giving graduated doses of penicillin. An adrenal steroid may stop it and should probably be given in advance if a reaction is specially to be feared, e.g. in a patient with syphilitic aortic valve disease. Start 2 days before and continue for 1 day after antibiotic is given (prednisolone 30 mg/day by mouth will serve).

Chancroid is characterised by painful necrotic genital ulceration that is caused by *Haemophilus ducreyi*. The recommended drug therapy is erythromycin 0.5 g by mouth 6-hourly, or co-trimoxazole 960 mg twice daily for 14 days.

Granuloma inguinale, is caused by a Gram-negative bacillus. The treatment of choice is a tetracycline (see p. 205) (amoxycillin is an alternative) for 3 weeks.

Vaginal infections

Bacterial vaginal infections are treated according to general principles of chemotherapy. Resistant infections sometimes respond if a small dose of an oestrogen is given orally for a month. Local allergy to vaginally applied drugs is common and may be difficult to distinguish from exacerbation of the infection. There are numerous causes of failure to cure and numerous practical details of therapy that are beyond the scope of this book, but which are vital for success. Gynaecological sources should be consulted.

Non-specific vaginitis is a common form of vaginal inflammation in which neither *Trichomonas vaginalis* nor *Candida albicans* can be isolated. There is now good evidence that associates the condition with the presence of *Gardnerella vaginalis* and anaerobic organisms, especially *Bacteroides* spp., the latter being responsible for the characteristic odour of the vaginal discharge. The condition responds well to metronidazole 2 g orally as a single dose; both the female patient and her sex partner(s) should be treated.

Candida vaginitis (see p. 269)

Trichomonas vaginitis (see p. 277)

INFECTIONS OF THE EYE

The most likely bacterial pathogens are:

1. *Neisseria gonorrhoeae* (in newborn)
2. *Haemophilus aegyptius*
3. *Streptococcus pneumoniae*
4. *Haemophilus influenzae*
5. *Moraxella lacunata*
6. *Staphylococcus aureus*
7. *Pseudomonas aeruginosa*

Superficial infections are treated by a variety of antimicrobial drops (1- to 2-hourly or every few minutes in severe cases) and ointments where drops are inconvenient, e.g. at night: neomycin, chloramphenicol, framycetin, tetracycline, polymyxin are superior to sulphonamides (usually sulphacetamide). They are often used in conjunction with hydrocortisone or prednisolone, but this combination is risky, as the steroid may mask the progress of the infection, and should it be applied with an antimicrobial to which the organism is resistant (bacterium or virus) may make the disease worse. Local chemoprophylaxis is used to prevent secondary bacterial infection in virus conjunctivitis.

Local allergy may be confused with persisting infection and treatment uselessly continued.

Intra-ocular infections are treated by systemic and subconjunctival injection. The latter provides high intraocular concentration by direct diffusion.

*Ocular infections in the newborn.** Pus from the eye should be stained and cultured. Neomycin 0.5% ointment applied to both eyes four times daily after feeds is effective for most bacteria but not for chlamydial or gonococcal infection.

Gonococcal conjunctivitis in the newborn. Infection is indicated by the finding of intracellular Gram-negative diplococci. When the organism is *pencillin-sensitive*, flood the eyes with aqueous benzylpenicillin solution, 600 mg/ml, repeat 15 min later, and again after each feed for 3 days; for systemic treatment give procaine penicillin 90 mg i.m. daily for 3 days.

When the organism is *penicillin-resistant*, flood the eyes with sulphacetamide 30% solution; repeat 15 min later, and again after each feed for 3 days; for systemic treatment give cefuroxime 100 mg/kg i.m. daily for 3 days.

Chalmydial conjunctivitis in the newborn. The diagnosis should be suspected if conjunctivitis persists despite neomycin and no bacteria are found on staining and culture; chlortetracycline eye ointment 1% four times daily after feeds should then replace neomycin. When the diagnosis is confirmed, local treatment may be discontinued in favour of erythromycin suspension 50 mg/kg per day by mouth in four divided doses before feeds for 14 days.

Chlamydial conjunctivitis in adults. In the developed world, the genital (D-K) serotypes of the organism are responsible and the reservoir and transmission is maintained by sexual contact.

* Dunlop EMC. Br J Hosp Med 1983; 29:6. Dunlop EMC. Update 1985; 31:339.

Endemic trachoma in developing countries is usually caused by serotypes A, B and C. In either case, tetracycline 500 mg 6-hourly for 14 days (or for 21 days in complicated cases) is effective. Alternatively, pregnant or lactating women may receive erythromycin 500 mg daily for 14 days.

Herpes keratitis, see p. 266.

MYCOBACTERIAL INFECTIONS

Pulmonary tuberculosis

The general principles of treatment are *three* — rest, chemotherapy and prolonged follow-up.

Drug therapy has transformed tuberculosis from a disease with a near-fatal prognosis into one in which almost 100% cure is obtainable. There are several chemotherapeutic regimens for the treatment of respiratory tuberculosis. The general principles on which these schemes are designed are:

1. *Initial* treatment with several drugs followed by:
2. *Continuation* treatment with a reduced number of drugs.

The *reasons* for this are that:

a. resistance develops against all antituberculosis drugs if they are used singly, but is delayed or prevented by using more than one drug.
b. initial resistance to two of the standard drugs is rare.
c. bacterial sensitivity tests take 6–8 weeks, or longer in the case of an unusual organism.

Three main types of antituberculosis drug regimen have evolved, namely:

1. *Conventional continuous chemotherapy* was established during the 1950s and 1960s, lasting for a standard 18–24 months. An initial phase of 2–3 months *triple* drug therapy (isoniazid plus streptomycin plus aminosalicylic acid [PAS]), followed by a continuation phase of *double* drug therapy (isoniazid and PAS), administration being supervised where practicable during the initial phase and reliance being placed on self-administration in the later phase. In some third world countries, thiacetazone has replaced PAS.

The principle guiding the continuation phase is to use a companion drug that prevents the emergence of isoniazid-resistant organisms and to use these two until the infection is eradicated.

This regimen is very effective but its length creates problems. First, patient non-compliance can be as high as 25% and is liable to increase with the passage of time, especially as the patient may be feeling perfectly well for the greater part of the course. Failure to take drugs, even though the patient may collect them daily from the clinic, is the chief reason for failure of antituberculosis chemotherapy. Secondly, a long treatment regimen imposes organisational and financial strain on the health service that has to deliver it.

2. **Intermittent chemotherapy** under full supervision was developed to improve compliance. Most intermittent dosing schemes begin with a period of daily treatment. Chronic toxicity is usually less with intermittent dosing, for the *total* weekly doses are significantly less, even though the *individual* doses are higher.

Twice-weekly regimens: if the strain of mycobacterium is initially sensitive to the drugs used, about 94% of patients treated twice-weekly with isoniazid (oral) and streptomycin (i.m.) respond successfully within 12 months. Concentrations of isoniazid achieved in the body with this scheme are maintained above the therapeutic concentration irrespective of whether the patient is a fast or slow acetylator and both types respond equally well.

Once-weekly regimens: isoniazid plus streptomycin once weekly gave an unsatisfactory result in one study* and rapid acetylators (56% success) fared worse than slow acetylators (76% success). With dosing at intervals of seven days, isoniazid falls below the therapeutic concentration towards the end of the week. The concentration could be maintained by giving a larger dose of isoniazid but the amount required to do this runs an unacceptable risk of producing convulsions at peak concentrations. Better results have been achieved with other weekly regimens; once-weekly isoniazid plus rifampicin given for 12 months to patients in Singapore was completely successful in slow acetylators (but still 5% of rapid acetylators responded unsatisfactorily).† The choice between daily and intermittent chemotherapy will depend on a variety of factors including patient attitude and availability of supervision in hospital or home.

* Tuberculosis Chemotherapy Centre, Madras. WHO Bull 1970; 43:143.

† Singapore Tuberculosis Service/British Medical Research Council. Lancet 1975; 2:1105

3. **Short course continuous chemotherapy** was designed to overcome the drawbacks of the long standard course without sacrificing efficacy. These regimens involve a number of drugs and the theory of their use is as follows.

a. Tubercle bacilli vary in their metabolic activity. Those that metabolise actively are killed by isoniazid. Others, called 'persisters', lie semi-dormant, often within cells, in conditions of low oxygen tension and pH. Pyrazinamide has a special capability for eliminating organisms in an acid environment and rifampicin rapidly kills those that metabolise only briefly and sporadically.

b. Initial drug resistance or the development of resistance during therapy is very low if ethambutol or streptomycin are included in an initial intensive phase.

Various short course schemes differ in the components of the initial phase, but all rely on continuation with isoniazid and rifampicin. Following extensive clinical trials, the British Thoracic Society‡ recommends any of these regimens:

a. isoniazid and rifampicin daily for 6 months, with added streptomycin and pyrazinamide for the first 2 months.

b. isoniazid and rifampicin daily for 6 months, with added ethambutol and pyrazinamide for the first 2 months.

c. isoniazid and rifampicin daily for 9 months with added ethambutol for the first 2 months.

The drugs are given as follows: (when by mouth, as single doses)

isoniazid:	300 mg daily by mouth.
rifampicin:	660 mg daily by mouth (or 450 mg if the patient weighs less than 50 kg).
streptomycin:	0.75 g i.m., 6 days a week.
pyrazinamide:	1.5 g daily by mouth if the patient weighs < 50 kg.
	2.0 g daily by mouth if the patient weighs 50–74 kg.
	2.5 g daily by mouth if the patient weighs > 75 kg.
ethambutol:	15 mg per kg by mouth daily.

‡ British Thoracic Society. Br J Dis Chest 1984; 78:330.

These are all highly effective regimens with relapse rates in the region of 1–2% in those who continue for 6 months; even if patients default after say, 4 months, tuberculosis can be expected to recur in only 10–15%.

Special problems

Resistant organisms may be evidenced by deterioration in the chest radiograph or the continued presence or reappearance of bacilli in the sputum. While it is desirable to confirm sensitivity by bacteriological testing, the about 8-week delay in obtaining this information means that decisions have often to be made on clinical grounds alone.

Initial drug resistance is seen in about only 4% of patients (usually to isoniazid), but rarely to rifampicin or ethambutol. By contrast, atypical mycobacteria are usually resistant to most standard drugs but happily they are of low virulence and usually are sensitive to erythromycin.

Preventive treatment or *chemoprophylaxis* may be either *primary*, i.e. the giving of antituberculosis drugs to uninfected individuals, which is seldom justified, or *secondary*, which is the treatment of infected but symptom-free individuals, e.g. those known to be in contact with the disease and who develop a positive tuberculin reaction. Secondary chemoprophylaxis may be justified in children under the age of three because they have a high risk of disseminated disease; isoniazid alone may be used since there is little risk of resistant organisms emerging.

Non-respiratory tuberculosis. The principles of treatment — rest, chemotherapy and prolonged follow-up — are the same as for respiratory tuberculosis. In only a few cases is surgery now necessary. It should always be preceded and followed by chemotherapy. Whether the short-course regimens for respiratory tuberculosis are also effective for non-respiratory infection is not established, although evidence from lymph node* and urinary tract tuberculosis suggests they may be. A 12–18 month continuation phase usually with rifampicin and isoniazid is advised until the position is clear.†

* British Thoracic Society Research Committee. Br Med J 1985; 290:1106.

† Cooke N J. Editorial. Br Med J 1985; 291:497.

Many chronic tuberculosis lesions may be relatively inaccessible to drugs as a result of avascularity of surrounding tissues and treatment frequently has to be prolonged, and dosage high, especially if damaged tissue cannot be removed by surgery, e.g. tuberculosis of bones.

Renal tuberculosis: see Infections of the urinary tract (p. 249).

Meningeal tuberculosis: see Infection of the meninges (p. 245).

Skin tuberculosis, particularly lupus vulgaris, usually responds well. Some physicians have given isoniazid alone but it is preferable to give two drugs.

Adrenal steroids and tuberculosis. In pulmonary tuberculosis a corticosteroid should be given to severely ill or moribund patients. It reduces the reaction of the body to tuberculoprotein and buys time for the chemotherapy to take effect. They also cause the patient to feel better much more quickly.

In the absence of effective chemotherapy, an adrenal steroid will cause tuberculosis to extend *and it should never be used alone, e.g. for another disease, if tuberculosis is suspected.*

Antituberculosis drugs

Antituberculosis drugs, with some exceptions, tend to be used exclusively for that condition and are therefore described here.

Isoniazid (INH, INAH, isonicotinic acid hydrazide)

Isoniazid was introduced as a tuberculostatic agent in 1952. Its development was the result of attempts to combine the known antituberculosis effects of nicotinamide and thiosemicarbazones.

Isoniazid is selectively effective against *Mycobacterium tuberculosis* and has little or no activity against other bacteria: the drug probably acts by interfering with bacterial respiration. It is either bacteristatic or bactericidal, according to concentration and temperature. Isoniazid is active against intracellular organims.

Pharmacokinetics. Isoniazid is well absorbed from the alimentary tract and is distributed throughout the body water, easily crossing tissue barriers and entering cells and cerebrospinal fluid; the distribution volume is 40 l/70 kg. It should always be given in cases where there is special risk of meningitis (miliary tuberculosis and primary infection).

Isoniazid is inactivated by acetylation, i.e. conjugation with an acetyl group. There are great differences in the rate at which people acetylate the drug and it has been found that this depends on a single gene (see Pharmacogenetics). People are either slow acetylators (autosomal homozygous recessive) or rapid acetylators (heterozygotes and homozygous dominants). After the initial peak concentration, which is similar in both slow and fast acetylators, the steady state plasma concentration in fast acetylators is less than half that in slow acetylators. The $t_{\frac{1}{2}}$ of isoniazid in slow acetylators is 2.5–3 times that in fast acetylators (i.e. 65 min against 170 min).

Carefully controlled trials have shown that those individuals who acetylate and thus inactivate the drug rapidly fare worse than those who acetylate slowly when isoniazid is used in intermittent dosing regimens; on a once-daily treatment regimen with isoniazid alone, both fast and slow acetylators respond equally well.

The usual oral *dose* of isoniazid (50, 100 mg) is 300 mg daily. It can be given i.m.

Adverse effects. Isoniazid is well tolerated but it does interfere with pyridoxine metabolism by inhibiting the formation of the active form of the vitamin; pyridoxine output in the urine is increased.

The principal effect of this is peripheral neuropathy with numbness and tingling of the feet; pain, touch and temperature are mostly affected but seldom deep sensation. Motor involvement is less common but there may be muscle weakness and loss of deep tendon reflexes. Neuropathy is unusual in well-nourished patients treated with standard doses of isoniazid, although there is a greater risk in slow acetylators and malnourished individuals; states of mild pyridoxine deficiency may also be aggravated, e.g. pregnant women, the elderly, those with liver disease and alcoholism. Pyridoxine 10 mg per day by mouth prevents neuropathy and does not interfere with the therapeutic effect, so it is not necessary to adjust the dose according to acetylator status. Other adverse effects include mental disturbances, incoordination, optic neuritis and convulsions.

Liver damage may occur, varying from moderate elevation of hepatic enzymes to severe hepatitis with fatal outcome. This appears to be due to the production in the liver of a chemically reactive metabolite of isoniazid. Both fast and slow acetylators are affected. Most cases of hepatitis usually develop within the first 8 weeks of receiving isoniazid and liver function tests should be monitored during this period at least.

Isoniazid may precipitate epilepsy. It also inhibits the metabolism of phenytoin, rising concentration of which causes symptoms of overdose. Patients taking carbamazepine develop excessive sedation if isoniazid is added. If an alternative antiepileptic drug is not an option, then the dosage of phenytoin or carbamazepine should be reduced and plasma concentration monitored, if practicable.

Rifampicin

Rifampicin (rifampin) is one of the group of rifamycin antibiotics that were isolated from *Streptomyces mediterranei*. Its potent bactericidal activity against the tubercle bacillus (comparable to that of isoniazid) and its suitability for oral administration have made it a drug of choice for the treatment of tuberculosis. It also has a rapid bactericidal effect on *Mycobacterium leprae* and is used in leprosy (see index).

The drug has a wide range of antimicrobial activity and other uses include the treatment of leprosy, severe Legionnaire's disease (with erythromycin) and prostatitis (with erythromycin), and the chemoprophylaxis of meningococcal meningitis.

Rifampicin kills bacteria by binding to DNA-dependent RNA polymerase and inhibiting RNA synthesis; it is particularly effective against mycobacteria that lie dormant within cells.

Pharmacokinetics. The drug is well absorbed after administration by mouth. The $t_{\frac{1}{2}}$ is 3.5 h after initial doses, but shortens to 2.5 h on repeated dosing because rifampicin is an effective *enzyme inducer* and increases its own metabolism (as well as that of several other drugs — see below). It penetrates well into most tissues, sometimes giving concentrations higher than those in the plasma at the same time. The distribution volume is 60 l/70 kg.

Entry into the CSF when meninges are inflamed is sufficient to maintain therapeutic concentrations at normal oral doses but transfer is reduced as inflammation subsides in about one or two months. Being a lipid-soluble drug, rifampicin crosses cell membranes and so can attack intracellular bacilli.

Deacetylation takes place in the liver but this form retains antibacterial activity; most of the antibacterial activity in bile is due to this metabolite. Enterohepatic recycling takes place, and eventually about 60% of a single dose is eliminated in the faeces. Urinary excretion of unchanged drug also occurs.

Dosage of rifampicin (150, 300 mg) is as follows; adults approximately 10 mg/kg body weight/day; children up to 20 mg/kg body weight/day to maximum of 600 mg. The drug should be taken as a single dose on an empty stomach 30 min before breakfast to ensure high blood concentrations. Combined rifampicin and isoniazid tablets are available (Rimactazid).

Adverse effects. Rifampicin rarely causes serious toxicity. Some adverse reactions relate to intermittent dosing, others occur whether dosing is daily or intermittent.

Intermittent dosing either as part of a regimen or through poor compliance causes effects that probably have an immunological basis; namely:

1. *An influenza-like syndrome*, with malaise, headache and fever, may occur in 50% of patients on once-weekly regimens of 25 mg/kg or more. Some patients also experience shortness of breath and wheezing.

2. *Acute haemolytic anaemia* may occur within 2–3 h of a dose of rifampicin but is rare.

3. *Acute renal failure* may occur, sometimes with haemoloysis, sometimes without. It is an indication to stop rifampicin immediately and never give it to the patient again.

Intermittent or daily dosing is associated with the following:

1. Hepatitis. This is usually attributed to rifampicin, although almost all patients with it are also taking other antituberculosis drugs. The reaction is characteristically mild, but if the onset of hepatitis is early after starting rifampicin, the course tends to be more severe. Patients with pre-existing liver disease, alcoholism, or elderly subjects appear to be more at risk. A mild liver reaction is not necessarily an indication for stopping the drug, as raised liver enzyme concentrations in the plasma and abnormal histology can return to normal despite continued use of rifampicin.

2. Thrombocytopenia, which is closely associated with the presence of circulating IgG and IgM antibodies, which fix complement to platelets when rifampicin is present. It is a sign that rifampicin should be discontinued and never again given to the patient.

3. Cutaneous reactions, principally flushing and itching with or without a rash.

Other effects. Rifampicin is a powerful inducer of hepatic drug metabolising enzymes and speeds the inactivation of numerous drugs, including warfarin, oral contraceptives, narcotic analgesics, oral antidiabetic agents and dapsone. Appropriate increase in dosage is required to compensate for increased drug metabolism.

Red discolouration of urine, tears and sputum occurs, which is harmless, and is a useful check that the patient is taking the drug. Rifampicin also causes an orange discolouration of soft contact lenses.

Ethambutol

Ethambutol is a synthetic compound that is less active than isoniazid, rifampicin and streptomycin, and should be used only in combination. Its antibacterial spectrum is limited to mycobacteria and only growing cells are affected, possibly by inhibiting mycobacterial RNA synthesis.

Pharmacokinetics. Over 75% of the drug is absorbed from the gastrointestinal tract, and treatment by mouth is satisfactory. It enters most body tissues and appears to be well concentrated in the lung. Only insignificant amounts of ethambutol cross into the CSF if the meninges are not inflamed, but in tuberculous meningitis sufficient may reach the CSF to inhibit mycobacterial growth. The $t_{\frac{1}{2}}$ is 5 h. Excretion is mainly by the kidney, the high renal clearance (400 ml/min) indicating tubular secretion as well as glomerular filtration. The dose should be reduced when renal function is impaired and when creatinine clearance reaches 10 ml/min an alternate day regimen or a daily dose of 5 mg/kg is indicated.

Dosage of ethambutol (100, 400 mg) is 15 mg/kg/day administered as a single dose by mouth; for re-treatment, 25 mg/kg/day is used, reducing after two months to 15 mg/kg/day to avoid ocular toxicity. Intermittent therapy, 45–50 mg/kg twice weekly, or 90 mg/kg once weekly has also been used successfully.

Adverse effects. In recommended doses, which take account of any reduced renal function, ethambutol is relatively non-toxic. The main problem is ocular damage (retrobulbar neuritis) with loss of visual acuity, central scotomata, occasionally also peripheral vision loss and red–green colour blindness. These effects are dose-related, and have been estimated to be 2% or less in patients receiving 25 mg/kg/day. The changes reverse if treatment is stopped promptly but colour vision defect may recover only slowly. If the drug is not stopped the patient may go blind. It is prudent to get baseline tests of vision before starting treatment with ethambutol. Ocular toxicity may effect one eye only, so the eyes should be tested independently. Patients can be told to make a point of reading small print in newspapers and so to detect and report adverse ocular effects at an early stage. Routine specialist sight testing is not necessary if this is done.

Ethambutol reduces renal urate clearance, which leads to elevation of plasma uric acid concentration. Peripheral neuritis occurs but is rare.

Pyrazinamide

Pyrazinamide is a derivative of nicotinamide and is included in first-choice combination regimens because of its particular ability to kill 'persisters', that is, mycobacteria that are dormant, often within cells. It is well absorbed from the gastrointestinal tract and metabolised in the liver, very little unchanged drug appearing in the urine. The $t_{\frac{1}{2}}$ is 9 h.

The *dose* of pyrazinamide (500 mg) is 20–30 mg/kg by mouth to a maximum of 3 g daily.

Adverse effects are of two principal types:

1. Arthralgia, which is relatively frequent with daily but less so with intermittent dosing. The condition is associated with raised plasma uric acid concentration, but unlike gout, affects both large and small joints. Hyperuricaemia is caused by pyrazinoic acid, the principal metabolite of pyrazinamide, which inhibits renal tubular secretion of uric acid. Symptomatic treatment with aspirin is usually sufficient and it is rarely necessary to discontinue pyrazinamide because of arthralgia.

2. Hepatitis, which was particularly associated with the high doses (40–50 mg/kg) formerly used; this is not a problem with modern short-course schedules (20–30 mg/kg daily). The complaint of anorexia and nausea provide a warning that hepatitis may be developing.

Aminosalicylic acid (sodium* aminosalicylate, para-aminosalicylic acid, PAS)

Although no longer a first-line drug in the management of tuberculosis, PAS can still be used in the event of bacterial resistance to other drugs. PAS is used in many developing countries with a tuberculosis problem, but in richer countries its bulk, unpleasant taste and adverse effects have caused it to be replaced by ethambutol.

Pharmacokinetics. PAS is effective when taken by mouth but the drug irritates the gastrointestinal mucosa and hence it is best taken with food or an antacid. The drug is metabolised in the body; half of a dose appears in the urine as the acetylated form. Isoniazid, which is also acetylated, achieves higher blood concentrations with PAS than when it is given alone, because both drugs compete for the same metabolic path. Elimination of PAS depends both on the rate of metabolism and on the rate of renal excretion. The $t_{\frac{1}{2}}$ is 30 min.

* The calcium salt can be used where sodium is unwanted, e.g. in cardiac disease, but it is less well absorbed.

The *dose* of PAS is 10–20 g daily by mouth in divided doses.

Adverse effects are seldom serious, although nausea, vomiting and diarrhoea due to local irritation are common, and in some cases, malabsorption may result. These reactions are less with the sodium salt than with the free acid. Other adverse effects include crystalluria, agranulocytosis, thrombocytopenia and allergies (especially fever, rash, enlarged lymph nodes) and encephalitis. It is prudent to stop PAS if anything more serious than a mild rash occurs. Goitre with hypothyroidism, diabetes, hepatitis and hypokalaemia also occur.

Streptomycin

Streptomycin is described under the Aminoglycosides (p. 223).

Thiacetazone

Thiacetazone has tended to replace PAS in antituberculosis regimens in certain developing countries because of its low cost. It is usually combined with isoniazid.

Pharmacokinetics. The drug is sufficiently absorbed from the gastrointestinal tract to be suitable for oral administration. About one third is eliminated unchanged in the urine and the remainder is metabolised. The $t_{\frac{1}{2}}$ is 13 h.

Adverse reactions include gastrointestinal symptoms, blurred vision, conjunctivitis and vertigo. More serious effects are erythema multiforme, haemolytic anaemia, agranulocytosis, cerebral oedema and hepatitis. Patients with liver disease should not be given thiacetazone; neither should those with reduced renal function, for there is only a small difference between a therapeutic and a toxic dose.

Alternative or reserve drugs are used where there are problems of drugs intolerance and bacterial resistance. They are in this class because of either greater toxicity or of lesser efficacy. Selection and management is best left to specialists. Drugs include: *ethionamide* (gastrointestinal irritation, allergic reactions) and *prothionamide*, which is similar; *capreomycin* (nephrotoxic); *cycloserine* (CNS toxicity); and *kanamycin*.

Leprosy

Effective treatment of leprosy is complex and requires much experience if the best results are to be obtained. As with tuberculosis, prolonged treatment is required. The drugs used include:

Dapsone, a bacteristatic sulphone has for many years been the standard drug for the treatment of all forms of leprosy but irregular and inadequate duration of treatment with a single drug have allowed the emergence of resistance, both primary and secondary. This is now a major problem in control of the disease. There are parallels with tuberculosis. Dapsone may cause allergic reactions such as erythema nodosum leprosum.

Rifampicin (see also p. 256) is bactericidal and has the advantage that it is safe and effective when given once-monthly, for all human cultures recognise months, whether calendar or lunar. Monthly contact between patients and health workers is feasible in most countries and boosts compliance, for the swallowing of medicines by the patient can be witnessed.

Clofazimine posseses a leprostatic action and its anti-inflammatory effect prevents erythema nodosum leprosum. It causes reddish discolouration of the skin and other cutaneous lesions, which may persist for months after the drug had been stopped.

Other drugs used against leprosy are *ethionamide* and *prothionamide*.

The problems of drug-resistant leprosy now require that multiple drug therapy be used and the following **regimens** are recommended:*

Multibacillary leprosy

Rifampicin 600 mg by mouth, monthly and supervised, plus dapsone 100 mg by mouth, daily and unsupervised, plus clofazimine 50 mg by mouth daily and unsupervised, plus 300 mg monthly and supervised. (Ethionamide or prothionamide 250–375 mg by mouth daily may be substituted should skin pigmentation render clofazimine unacceptable).

* WHO Study Group Report. WHO Tech Rep Ser 1982; no. 675.

Treatment should continue for 2 years of ideally until slit skin smears are negative. Further follow up for as long as 8 years may be necessary.

Paucibacillary leprosy

Rifampicin 600 mg by mouth, monthly and supervised, plus dapsone 100 mg by mouth, daily and unsupervised.

Treatment should continue for 6 months with follow up for 4 years to check for recurrence of disease.

Thalidomide (see index), despite its notorious past, still finds a use in the control of allergic lepromatous reactions by immunosuppression.

OTHER BACTERIAL INFECTIONS

Burns. Infection may be substantially reduced by compresses of silver nitrate solution (0.5%), silver sulphadiazine or by mafenide. Substantial absorption can occur from any raw surface and use of aminoglycoside (e.g. neomycin) preparations can cause ototoxicity.

Gas gangrene. The skin between the waist and the knees is normally contaminated with anaerobic faecal organisms. However assiduous the skin preparation be for orthopaedic operations or thigh amputations, it will not kill the spores. Surgery done for vascular insufficiency where tissue oxygenation may be poor is likely to be followed by infection. *Clostridium perfringens* (*welchii*) is sensitive to benzlypenicillin, which should be used for prophylaxis immediately before such operations.

Wounds. Systemic treatment is necessary for several days at least in dirty wounds where sutures have to be left below the skin, and in penetrating wounds of body cavities. Benzylpenicillin is probably best, but in the case of penetrating abdominal wounds, metronidazole should be added i.v. (see also tetanus). For antiseptics suitable for topical use see p. 735.

Abscesses and infections in *bone* and *serous cavities* are treated according to the antimicrobial sensitivity of the organism concerned but require high doses because of poor penetration. Local instillation of the drug may be needed.

In *osteomyelitis*, early treatment is urgent to prevent bone necrosis. Bacteriological identification is of great importance and blood for culture (50% of cases are positive) should be taken before therapy begins; indeed, aspiration of the bone to get the organism has been advocated.

As the organism is commonly *Staph. aureus*, flucloxacillin and sodium fusidate should be used. Treatment is required for weeks. Surgery is often needed in late cases; in early cases its place is controversial.

Skin carriers of staphylococci may be treated with mupirocin ointment 2% or with hexachlorphane (liquids or soaps). Excessive use of strong preparations of hexachlorophane can lead to absorption of enough to damage the CNS in infants.

Brucellosis responds to tetracycline (2 g/day for 3 weeks) plus, in severe cases, streptomycin (1 g/day for 2 weeks). Co-trimoxazole is an alternative to tetracycline. Relapses are treated similarly. Mild Herxheimer reactions may occur at the start of treatment.

Actinomycosis. The organism is sensitive to a range of drugs but access is poor because of granulomatous fibrosis. High doses of benzylpenicillin, 3 to 6 g/day are given for several weeks. Surgery is likely to be needed.

Leptospirosis. To be effective, chemotherapy should be started within 4 days of the onset of symptoms. Benzylpenicillin 600 mg 6-hourly for 7 days is recommended.

General supportive management is important, including attention to fluid balance and observation for signs of hepatic, renal or cardiac failure.

GUIDE TO FURTHER READING

1 Sheagren J N. Staphylococcus aureus. The persistent pathogen. N Engl J Med 1984; 310: 1368–1373, 1437–1442.
2 Bluestone C D. Otitis media in children: to treat or not to treat? N Engl J Med 1982; 306: 1399–1404.
3 Feigin R D. Editorial. Otitis media: closing the information gap. N Engl J Med 1982; 306: 1417–1418.
4 Editorial. Aerobic infections of the lung. Lancet 1983; 2: 800–801.
5 Kaye S B. Editorial. Pneumocystis pneumonia. Br Med J 1983; 286: 499–500.
6 Lockley M R, Wise R. Editorial. Pneumococcal infections. Br Med J 1984; 288: 1179–1180.
7 Johnson NMcI. Editorial. Pneumonia in the acquired immune deficiency syndrome. Br Med J 1985; 290: 1299–1301.
8 Editorial. Infective endocarditis. Lancet 1984; 1: 603–604.
9 Morris G K. Editorial. Infective endocarditis: a preventable disease? Br Med J 1985; 290: 1532–1533.
10 Swartz M N. Editorial. Bacterial meningitis. More involved than just the meninges. N Engl J Med 1984; 311: 912–914.
11 Nelson J D. Editorial. How preventable is bacterial meningitis? N Engl J Med 1982; 307: 1265–1267.
12 Lambert H P. Editorial. Prophylaxis in haemophilus meningitis. Br Med J 1984; 288: 739.
13 Symonds J. Editorial. Campylobacter enteritis in the community. Br Med J 1983; 286: 243–244.
14 Candy D C A. Editorial. Diarhoea, dehydration and drugs. Br Med J 1984; 289: 1245–1246.
15 Editorial. Antibiotic-associated colitis — the continuing saga. Br Med J 1981; 282: 1913–1914.
16 Schachter J. Chlamydial infections. N Engl J Med 1978; 298: 428–435, 490–495, 540–549.
17 Taylor-Robinson D, McCormack W M. The genital mycoplasmas. N Engl J Med 1980; 302: 1003–1010, 1063–1067.
18 Britigan B E et al. Gonococcal infection: a model of molecular pathogenesis. N Engl J Med 1985; 312: 1683–1694.
19 Editorial. Chronic bacterial prostatitis. Lancet 1983; 1: 393–394.
20 Komaroff A L. Acute dysuria in women. N Engl J Med 1984; 310: 368–375.
21 Gould I M, Wise R. Pseudomonas aeruginosa: clinical manifestations and management. Lancet 1985; 2: 1224–1226.
22 Joint Tuberculosis Committee of the British Thoracic Society. Control and prevention of tuberculosis: a code of practice. Br Med J 1983; 287: 1118–1121.
23 Glassworth J et al. Tuberculosis in the 1980s. N Engl J Med 1980; 302: 1441–1449.
24 Fass R J. Editorial. The quinolones. Ann Int Med 1985; 102(3): 400–402.

14

Infection IV: Chemotherapy of viral, fungal, protozoal and helmintic infections

CHEMOTHERAPY OF VIRAL INFECTIONS

Antiviral agents are most active when viruses are replicating. Therefore, the earlier that treatment is given, the better the results. An important difficulty is that a substantial amount of viral multiplication has often taken place before symptoms occur. Apart from primary infection, viral illness is often the result of reactivation of latent virus particles in the body. In both cases, patients whose immune systems are compromised suffer particularly severe illness.

Since viruses are intracellular parasites and participate in the metabolism of host cells, they present a more difficult problem of chemotherapy than do bacteria. Nevertheless, differences between viral and human metabolism have been identified and this has opened the way for substantial progress in the development of specific antiviral drugs. An account follows of those that are of proven usefulness.

Acyclovir

Acyclovir is a prodrug; it is a purine nucleoside analogue that, when converted to acyclovir triphosphate, inhibits DNA synthesis. The enzyme responsible, thymidine kinase, is present in both virus particles and human cells but the viral form binds acyclovir more avidly and forms the triphosphate a million times more rapidly, which accounts for the successful antiviral activity and relative freedom from toxicity of acyclovir.

The drug is sparingly soluble and only 20% is absorbed from the gut, but this is sufficient for the systemic treatment or prophylaxis of genital herpes. It distributes widely in the body, although the concentration in cerebrospinal fluid is approximately half that in plasma, and the brain concentration may be even less. These differences are taken into account in dosing for viral encephalitis. The drug is excreted in the urine by glomerular filtration and tubular secretion. The $t_{\frac{1}{2}}$ is 3 h.

Acyclovir is active against herpes simplex and varicella-zoster virus infections and is used for:

1. *Immunocompromised patients*: treatment of herpes simplex or primary or recurrent varicella-zoster infections. The i.v. route should be used. In severely immunocompromised patients, the drug may be given prophylactically.
2. *Non-immunocompromised patients* with severe or complicated varicella-zoster infections.
3. *Primary treatment or prophylaxis for recurrent genital herpes simplex*. The oral route is adequate in non-immunocompromised patients; topical therapy may encourage the emergence of resistant strains.
4. *Herpes simplex keratitis* as an ophthalmic ointment; H. labialis as a cream.
5. *Herpes simplex encephalitis*: evidence indicates that acyclovir is effective i.v. and when a presumptive diagnosis of herpes simplex encephalitis is made the drug should be started immediately and continued for 10 days or until another diagnosis is made.*

Treatment should begin as early as possible in the following doses:

i.v. 5–20 mg/kg are given 8-hourly for 5–10 days, depending on the severity of the infection.

* Whitley R J et al. N Engl J Med 1986; 314:144.

oral: 200 mg (one tablet) 5 times daily for at least 5 days.

topical: 3% ointment is applied to the eye 5 times daily until three days after complete healing. Cream (5%) is applied to the skin.

Adverse effects are remarkably few. Patients whose serum creatinine is raised experience nausea or vomiting. Administration by rapid i.v. injection has resulted in crystal formation in renal tubules, but this can be avoided by ensuring good urine flow and infusing the drug over 1 h. Acyclovir has a pH of 11.0 in its infusion fluid (water or isotonic saline), and extravasation causes severe local inflammation. Topical application gives rise to a mild transient stinging sensation. A diffuse superficial punctate keratopathy develops in about one-fifth of patients; this clears when the drug is stopped.

Vidarabine

Vidarabine was first introduced as an anticancer agent. It is a purine analogue that acts principally by inhibiting DNA polymerase and is effective against DNA viruses.

The drug is poorly soluble and is infused in dilute solution over 12 h. In the body it is rapidly converted to hypoxanthine arabinoside, which is more soluble but has less antiviral activity than vidarabine. Hypoxanthine arabinoside distributes preferentially to tissues; cerebrospinal fluid concentrations equal those in plasma. The $t_{\frac{1}{2}}$ is 3.5 h.

About half the daily dose of vidarabine appears in the urine within 24 h as hypoxanthine arabinoside, and negligible amounts as the parent drug.

Vidarabine has a spectrum of activity that covers varicella zoster virus, vaccinia and herpes virus. The drug is more toxic than acyclovir, which, having similar antiviral activity, is usually preferred. Vidarabine may be used for:

1. ***Immunocompromised patients*** with varicella-zoster infections, especially if it is begun when new lesions are forming.
2. ***Herpes keratoconjunctivitis***.
3. ***Neonatal herpes***.

Adverse effects. The large volume of fluid in which vidarabine must be given may be a disadvantage in patients with encephalitis and cerebral oedema. Gastrointestinal upsets occur in about one-fifth of patients, some days after therapy has started, but these usually lessen in severity even though the drug is continued. Toxic neurological effects occur in one-tenth or less of patients, but these include parkinsonian tremor, ataxia, myoclonus, hallucinations, confusion and coma. High doses induce pancytopenia and megaloblastosis. Vidarabine has been shown to cause chromosomal damage in human cells and there should be careful assessment of its expected benefits before the drug is used in women of childbearing potential.

Idoxuridine

Idoxuridine was found in 1962 to benefit herpes keratitis and became the first widely used antivirus drug. It is an analogue of thymidine, which it replaces in DNA, thereby preventing viral multiplication, but, of course, it also interferes with mammalian cells, notably bone marrow, liver and kidney. Toxicity precludes the systemic use of idoxuridine, but it is effective topically.

Idoxuridine is primarily active against herpes simplex virus and varicella-zoster virus. It is used in the following conditions:

1. *Herpes zoster* (shingles) responds best if treated within the first 3 days of onset of the rash.* Idoxuridine is placed on the lesions four times daily for 4 days; in mild cases, a 5% solution dissolved in dimethylsulphoxide (DMSO) is used, in severe cases, a 40% solution is applied on lint and changed every 24 h. DMSO, in addition to solubilising idoxuridine, is bacteristatic and reduces the risk of secondary infection. It is important to remember that shingles follows the nerve root distribution and idoxuridine should be applied to the whole *sensory dermatome*, not merely to the vesicles. Adequate treatment may reduce postherpetic neuralgia.

2. *Herpetic keratitis* (simplex) is the principal communicable cause of blindness in developed countries. Idoxuridine is applied to the eye as a

* The rash and pain of this condition give rise to its evocative description as 'a belt of roses from Hell'.

solution every hour during the day, and every 2 h at night or as an ointment is placed in the conjuctival sac five times a day. Secondary bacterial infection may need treatment. Best results are achieved with early treatment of acute dendritic ulcers.

Adverse effects of idoxuridine are few except from stinging when it is applied to the lesions, but DMSO causes reddening of the skin due to histamine release, and occasionally blisters, which may be confused with viral lesions.

Amantadine

Amantadine is active against RNA viruses, notably influenza A. Its mode of action is not fully known but it probably prevents uncoating of the virus and release of nucleic acid into the target cell.

Amantadine is absorbed effectively from the gastrointestinal tract and is eliminated in the urine. The $t_{\frac{1}{2}}$ is 12 h in young adults and double this in the elderly.

Amantadine is *used* for the prevention and treatment of infection with influenza A (but not B) virus. The earlier the drug is started, the better. The people most likely to benefit include the elderly, the debilitated, those with respiratory disability and people living in crowded conditions, especially during an influenza epidemic.

The dose is 100 mg (one capsule) 12-hourly, usually for 5–7 days.

Adverse reactions are mild and include dizziness, nervousness, lightheadedness and insomnia, which appear within 3–4 days of starting the drug and disappear when it is stopped. Drowsiness, hallucinations, delirium and coma also occur, more commonly with patients with impaired renal function. Convulsions may be induced, and amantadine should be avoided in epileptic patients. Amantadine causes other adverse effects when it is taken for longer duration for the treatment of Parkinson's disease (see p. 379).

Rimantadine is similar to amantadine and may have fewer adverse effects.

Interferons

Virus infection stimulates the production of protective glycoproteins (interferons, discovered 1957) in a wide variety of cells in the body. Interferons released from these cells act on other cells, triggering protective mechanisms that resist viral invasion. They also modify other cell-regulatory mechanisms and inhibit neoplastic growth. Plainly such substances have potential to prevent and to treat virus diseases as well as potential against some cancers.

Interferons comprise numerous proteins and are classified (α, β, γ) according to their antigenic and physicochemical properties.

Human α-interferon is manufactured on an industrial scale by infecting (with a parainfluenza virus) human lymphoblastic cells in suspension culture (Namalwa cells, from a lymphoma in a patient of that name), producing a mixture of more than 17 α-interferon subtypes (Wellferon); or by implanting into bacteria (*E. coli*) a gene code for interferon protein and culturing the organism in enormous tanks to produce a single α-interferon subtype (Intron-A), or a β-subtype.

Clinical success with α-interferon (i.m. or s.c.) has been achieved particularly in an uncommon chronic leukaemia (hairy cell), in myeloma, Kaposi's sarcoma, and malignant melanoma, also in prevention (by nasal spray) of the common cold (rhinovirus) and the treatment (by topical application) of herpes simplex lesions and genital warts. Prospects for interferon therapy include chronic active hepatitis, and non-Hodgkin's lymphoma, etc., alone or in combination with other modes of therapy (acyclovir, radiotherapy). Interferon therapy may need to be prolonged (months).

Injected interferon causes an influenza-like syndrome (maybe the symptoms of natural flu are due to endogenous interferon production); tolerance to this may develop with repeated administration; the syndrome is mitigated by paracetamol.

Transient bone marrow suppression (leucocytes, platelets) occurs.

Inosine pranobex mediates an antiviral activity by stimulating proliferation of lymphoid B and T cells, and interferon. The drug is a complex of inosine, which as a purine intermediate is a natural cell constituent, and of para-acetamidobenzoate. It is suitable for administration by mouth but must be given in frequent doses as it is rapidly metabolised and excreted. Inosine pranobex appears to be effective in the management of mucocutaneous infections with herpes simplex (type 1 and/or type 2). Claims that it is useful in a number of other viral illnesses have yet to be substantiated.

Other antiviral agents include: phosphonoformate, trifluorothymidine, ribavirin, zidovudine (azidothymidine, AZT), see p 278.

Treatment of viral infections

A summary follows of viral infections that are amenable to drug treatment.* The case of immunocompromised patients is considered separately in view of their special susceptibility to latent or acquired viral infection.

Herpes zoster (shingles)
Non-immunocompromised patient
1. Idoxuridine applied to the affected dermatome until no new vesicles appear.
2. Prednisolone in the acute phase reduces the incidence and duration of postherpetic neuralgia.
3. Acyclovir i.v. for complicated cases.

Immunocompromised patient
Acyclovir i.v. and vidarabine are effective especially if given within 3 days of onset, and diminish cutaneous dissemination and neuralgia: acyclovir is preferred, since it is safer; interferon-α seems to be effective but needs more evaluation.

Varicella (chicken pox)
Non-immunocompromised patients
Usually a mild illness but acyclovir may be used if there are serious complications, e.g. pneumonitis.
Immunocompromised patient
1. Prophylaxis: zoster immunoglobulin (ZIG) or acyclovir
2. Treatment: acyclovir, vidarabine and interferon have similar therapeutic efficacy if given early but acyclovir is the most acceptable.

Labial or mucocutaneous herpes simplex
Non-immunocompromised patient
Acyclovir may provide benefit.
Immunocompromised patient
1. Prophylaxis: acyclovir orally, or i.v. as cover for intense immunosuppression.
2. Treatment: acyclovir (preferred) or vidarabine.

* This is drawn from various sources but substantially from Nicholson K G. Lancet 1984; 2:617, 677, 736, whom we thank, DRL, PNB.

Genital herpes simplex
Primary
Acyclovir topically, by mouth or i.v. depending on severity.
Recurrent
Prophylaxis: acyclovir by mouth. Treatment: antiviral therapy has not been effective.

Herpes simplex keratitis
Topical acyclovir or trifluorothymidine are preferred; vidarabine or idoxuridine

Neonatal herpes simplex
Vidarabine or acyclovir.

Herpes simplex encephalitis
Acyclovir i.v.; dexamethasone.

Influenza A
Prophylaxis; amantadine or rimantadine. Treatment: amantadine or rimantadine, started within 48 h will reduce the duration of illness by one-third.

CHEMOTHERAPY OF FUNGAL INFECTIONS

Widespread use of immunosuppressive chemotherapy has led to a rise in the incidence of opportunistic infection and chemotherapy of the mycoses has correspondingly assumed greater importance.

Polyene antibiotics

The polyene antibiotics act by binding tightly to certain sterols present in membranes of fungal, protozoal and mammalian, but not of bacterial, cells. The resulting deformity of the membrane allows leakage of intracellular ions such as potassium and enzymes, causing cell death. Those polyenes that have useful antifungal activity (amphotericin B, nystatin) bind selectively to ergosterol, the most important sterol in fungal (but not mammalian) cell walls; not unexpectedly, those that bind to cholesterol, found in mammalian cell walls, are unacceptably toxic.

Amphotericin

Amphotericin is poorly absorbed from the gut and must be given by i.v. infusion. It is relatively insoluble in water and the parenteral form is a micellar* suspension with the bile salt desoxycholate from which the active drug separates in the body; about 95% of the drug in the plasma is bound to serum lipoproteins. The drug penetrates well into tissues but poorly into body fluids and serous cavities — hence intrathecal, intravesical or intra-articular administration may be necessary. It is metabolised and little unchanged drug appears in the bile or urine. The $t_{\frac{1}{2}}$ is about 15 days and it is not surprising that after stopping treatment, drug persists in the body for several weeks.

Uses. Amphotericin B is at present the drug of choice for most systemic fungal infections, including candidiasis, aspergillosis, coccidioidomycosis and histoplasmosis.

Because amphotericin B has significant adverse effects, the decision to undertake treatment is an important one and the diagnosis of systemic mycotic infection must be firmly established. The apparent presence of fungus may be due to a contaminated i.v. needle, or in the urine due to an indwelling catheter. Tissue biopsy may be necessary to confirm the diagnosis.

A conventional course of *treatment* lasts 6–12 weeks, in which time 2–3 g of amphotericin is given by daily i.v. infusion.

Adverse effects. Gradual escalation of the dose will limit the appearance of adverse effects but toxicity may have to be accepted in life-threatening infection. Renal impairment invariably accompanies treatment with amphotericin B, and a 40% fall in glomerular filtration rate may be expected, although treatment need not be stopped until serum creatinine has reached 200 μmol/l. The same dose may be resumed in 3–5 days but it may be months before renal function is normal again. Other adverse effects include anorexia, nausea, vomiting, malaise, abdominal, muscle and joint pains, loss of weight, anaemia, hypokalaemia (due to distal renal tubular acidosis), hypomagnesaemia and fever. Symptoms may be alleviated by aspirin, an antihistamine (H_1 receptor) or an antiemetic. Severe febrile reactions are alleviated by hydrocortisone 25–50 mg before each infusion.

Amphotericin B is irritant to veins and heparin 100 units added to the infusion may limit thrombophlebitis.

Nystatin

Nystatin (susp. 100 000 units/ml; tab. 500 000 units) derives its names from the New York State Department of Health. It is too toxic for systemic use. The drug is not absorbed from the alimentary canal and is used for prevention or treatment of superficial candidiasis of the mouth, oesophagus or intestinal tract, as pessaries for vaginal candidiasis and as cream or powder for cutaneous infection. The dose for candidiasis of the alimentary tract is one tablet or 5 ml of the suspension, 6-hourly.

Imidazoles

The antibacterial, antiprotozoal and antihelmintic members of this group are described in the appropriate sections. The antifungal imidazoles probably act by more than one mechanism. They inhibit formation of ergosterol, an important constituent of the fungal cell wall, which thus becomes permeable to intracellular constituents. Imidazoles also interfere with enzymes that generate and inactivate hydrogen peroxide, the intracellular concentration of which rises, causing death by autodigestion.

The group includes drugs used to treat infection with bacteria (metronidazole), protozoa (nimorazole) and helminths (mebendazole, thiabendazole); those used to treat fungal infections (ketoconazole, miconazole) are described below.

Ketoconazole

Ketoconazole (200 mg) is sufficiently well absorbed from the gut to permit systemic antifungal treatment by oral administration. The drug is widely distributed in tissues but concentrations in cerebrospinal fluid and urine are low. Absorption of ketoconazole from the gut is impaired by drugs or diseases that reduce secretion of gastric juice. Its action is terminated by metabolism and the $t_{\frac{1}{2}}$ is 8 h.

* Micelles are molecular aggregates.

Table 14.1 Treatment or systemic mycoses

Disease	*Treatment*	*Notes*
Candidiasis		
Systemic	Amphotericin B (± flucytosine)	Flucytosine acts synergistically with amphotericin B; flucytosine may be used alone for urinary candidosis. Ketoconazole by mouth may be used for prophylaxis in immunosuppressed patients. Surgery may be needed for endocarditis.
Chronic mucocutaneous	Ketoconazole	
Aspergillosis		
Systemic	Amphotericin B	
Pulmonary aspergilloma with haemoptysis	Surgery ± amphotericin	Conservative management if symptomless.
Allergic bronchopulmonary aspergillosis	Corticosteroid	
Histoplasmosis	Amphotericin B	Ketoconazole is an alternative. Surgical excision may be indicated for the localised pulmonary form.
Cryptococcosis	Amphotericin B + flucytosine	
Coccidioidomycosis	Amphotericin B	Ketoconazole is an alternative.
Paracoccidioidomycosis	Ketoconazole	Amphotericin B is an alternative.
Blastomycosis	Amphotericin B	Ketoconazole is an alternative.
Mucormycosis	Amphotericin B	
Sporotrichosis		
Cutaneous	Potassium iodide by mouth.	
Disseminated	Amphotericin B	

Uses. Ketoconazole is effective by mouth for the treatment of *superficial* mycoses. It is the drug of choice for chronic mucocutaneous candidiasis and it will eradicate dermatophyte infections of skin, nails and hair. Serious liver toxicity must, however, call into question the systemic use of ketoconazole for superficial mycoses when alternative remedies exist.

The place of ketoconazole in the management of *systemic* mycoses is being established; paracoccidioidomycosis improves dramatically and it is also effective for coccidioidomycosis and histoplasmosis.

The usual *dose* for superficial and deep mycoses is 200 mg daily, or 400 mg daily in resistant cases.

An unexpected, non-mycotic use for ketoconazole is for advanced prostatic cancer, the bone pain of which may be substantially improved in some cases.

Adverse reactions following systemic use include nausea, giddiness, headache, pruritus and photophobia. Of greater concern is *liver damage*, which ranges from transient elevation of hepatic transaminases and alkaline phosphatase to severe derangement of liver function and death. Liver damage may progress despite discontinuing ketoconazole.

The cortisol response to exogenous corticotrophin is reduced with as little as 400 mg of ketoconazole and replacement corticosteroid may be needed when the drug is used in high dose to treat advanced prostatic carcinoma.

Miconazole

Miconazole differs from ketaconazole in that it is sparingly soluble and incompletely absorbed from the gut; it must be given i.v. for systemic treatment, solubilised with polyethoxylated castor oil. The drug penetrates poorly into the cerebrospinal fluid.

Miconazole is *used* topically to treat fungus infections of the skin and mucous membranes (yeasts, dermatophytes). Following oral dosing blood concentrations appear to be adequate for prophylaxis against fungus infection in suseptible, e.g. immunosuppressed, individuals.

The drug is also advocated for various systemic mycoses and appears useful in coccidioidomycosis and candidiasis; but the necessity for i.v. administration and the toxicity of the preparation are significant disadvantages.

Adverse effects associated with miconazole are probably in the main due to the castor oil vehicle; these include phlebitis, pruritus, nausea, chills and rash.

Clotrimazole proved unsuitable for systemic use but is an effective topical agent for dermatophyte, yeast, and other fungal infections (intertrigo, athletes' foot, ringworm, pityriasis versicolor, fungal nappy rash). A variety of formulations serve these needs.

Econazole is a similar broad-spectrum topical antifungal drug.

Isoconazole is effective as a single-dose topical therapy for vaginal candidiasis.

Griseofulvin

Griseofulvin (125, 500 mg) was the first drug to be effective, taken by mouth, against superficial fungus infections in man. It was isolated in 1939 from *Penicillium griseofulvum* from the soil underneath conifers in an English county (Dorset), but was not introduced into clinical practice until 1958 because big doses are toxic to animals, although it had been used some years earlier to control moulds on vegetables grown in glasshouses. Its great insolubility had seemed a bar to clinical efficacy.

Action. The precise modes of its antifungal activity are complex, but the usefulness of griseofulvin depends on its remarkable ability to bind to keratin as it is being formed in the cells of the nail-bed, hair follicles of skin, for dermatophytes specifically infect keratinous tissues. Griseofulvin does not kill fungus already established, it merely prevents infection of new keratin so that the duration of treatment is governed by the time that it takes for infected keratin to be shed — on average, hair and skin infection should be treated for 4–6 weeks while toe nails may need a year or more. Reinfection will occur if treatment is stopped while infected keratin is still in the body. Local hygiene therefore remains important. Treatment must continue for a time after both visual and microscopic evidence have disappeared.

Pharmacokinetics. Fat in a meal assists absorption of griseofulvin. It is metabolised in the liver and induces hepatic enzymes. The $t_{\frac{1}{2}}$ is 36 h.

Uses. Griseofulvin is effective against all superficial ringworm (dermatophyte) infections but it is ineffective against pityriasis versicolor, superficial candidiasis and all systemic mycoses.

The *dose* is 0.5–1.0 g (but not less than 100 mg/kg body weight) once daily after a meal.

Adverse effects include gastrointestinal upset, headache in up to 50% of patients, and various central nervous system disturbances. Allergic skin reactions may occur but are not usually severe. Griseofulvin interferes with porphyrin metabolism; the drug is contraindicated in acute intermittent porphyria and is best avoided in other forms of porphyria.

Flucytosine

Flucytosine (5-fluorocytosine) interferes with fungal nucleic acid synthesis and is useful for certain systemic mycotic infections. It is efficiently absorbed from the gut, very little is protein-bound and almost all is excreted unchanged in the urine. Flucytosine penetrates effectively into body fluid. The $t_{\frac{1}{2}}$ is 4 h.

Uses. Flucytosine appears particularly effective for chromomycosis, cryptococcosis (with amphotericin B) and may be used in localised candidiasis (e.g. cystitis).

Both oral and i.v. forms are available; the daily dose needs to be reduced for patients with impaired renal function.

Adverse effects. The drug is well tolerated but transient nausea, vomiting, diarrhoea and skin rashes occur with treatment.

Potassium iodide is given by mouth to treat cutaneous sporotrichosis.

Treatment of fungal infections

Superficial mycoses

Dermatophyte infections. Longstanding remedies such as compounds of benzoic and salicylic acids are still acceptable for mild tinea infections, but a topical imidazole (miconazole, clotrimazole, econazole), which is also effective against candida, may be preferred if the diagnosis is not clear. Griseofulvin should be used for extensive tinea infection.

Candida infections of the skin and oral mucous membrane are generally treated satisfactorily with topical nystatin, amphotericin B, clotrimazole, econazole or miconazole. Local hygiene is also important. An underlying explanation should be sought if a patient fails to respond to these measures, e.g. diabetes, the use of a broad-spectrum antibiotic or of immunosuppressive drugs.

Vaginal candidiasis is treated by clotrimazole, econazole, miconazole or nystatin as vaginal suppositories (pessaries) or tablets, or cream, inserted once or twice a day with cream or ointment on surrounding skin. Failure may be due to a concurrent intestinal infection causing reinfection and nystatin tablets may be given by mouth 8-hourly with the local treatment. The male sex partner may use a similar antifungal ointment for his benefit and for hers (re-infection).

Systemic mycoses

A detailed account for treatment is beyond the scope of this text but the principal features are summarised in Table 14.1*.

* The Medical Letter on Drugs and Therapeutics, 1984. Cohen J. Lancet 1982; 2:532.

CHEMOTHERAPY OF PROTOZOAL INFECTIONS

Malaria

It is necessary to know the principal features of the life cycle of the malaria parasite in order to understand its therapy. Successful treatment requires that the parasite be eradicated from both the liver and the blood. Drug resistance is a very real problem and varies with geographical location. The correct choice of drug is therefore vital.

History. Quinine as cinchona bark was introduced into Europe from South America in 1633. It was used for all fevers, amongst them malaria. Further advance in the chemotherapy of malaria was delayed until 1880, when Laveran† finally identified the parasites in the blood. His views were not generally accepted and 6 years later, Osler‡, at a meeting in the USA expressed grave doubts of the relevance of Laveran's 'bodies'. The subsequent discussion so impressed him that he put off his holiday in Canada to investigate the blood of malarial patients. He saw the parasites and said that he 'had been taught the folly of scepticism based on theoretical considerations'.

The mode of spread of malaria was still uncertain when, in 1894, Manson§, while walking along Oxford Street, London, told Ross‖ to 'look for the parasite's dung in the mosquito's stomach'. Ross returned to India with a microscope, followed his advice and soon provided the final link in the malarial parasite's life cycle.¶

Quinine was the principal antimalarial drug available until 1930, when, as a result of research based on Ehrlich's work on dyes (see chemotherapy), mepacrine (quinacrine), a dye derivative, was introduced. It did not supersede quinine until, in 1942, the Japanese armies captured South East Asia and the Pacific Islands, which had supplanted South America as the source of

† Charles Louis Alphouse Laveran (1845–1922), Professor of Medicine, Paris (France) (Also winner of Nobel Prize).
‡ William Osler (1849–1919), Professor of Medicine at McGill University (Canada), Johns Hopkins University (USA), Oxford University (UK).
§ Patrick Manson (1844–1922), physician and parasitologist.
‖ Ronald Ross (1857–1932), physician and investigator.
¶ Russel P F. Lancet 1953; 2:944.

quinine. The withdrawal of quinine supplies from the Allied forces precipitated a military crisis and mepacrine was hastily manufactured to meet it. The proper use of mepacrine reduced the malaria rate amongst Australian troops in New Guinea from 740 cases per thousand per annum in November 1943, to 26 cases per thousand per annum one year later. So important was the prevention of clinical malaria to the prosecution of the war that the daily taking of mepacrine was made a matter of military discipline. Fairley* writes how some soldiers with malaria were found to have low plasma concentration of mepacrine and how, after having excluded other causes, the 'suggestion' that they would be kept 'in the North' until their malaria stopped was followed by a dramatic rise of mepacrine plasma concentration and cessation of clinical malaria.

It was vital that the dosage of mepacrine necessary to enable troops to fight in hyperendemic areas without serious casualties from malaria should be found quickly. At a base in North Queensland, Australia, extensive experiments were carried out. Physical stress is believed to promote malarial relapses and so the trials of mepacrine were carried out on volunteers under conditions simulating those of jungle warfare. Volunteers were first exposed to the bites of infected mosquitoes. They were then injected with adrenaline or insulin, put half-naked into, and kept immobile in a refrigerator at −9 °C for one hour or 'worked or exercised in tropical climate at the hottest time of the year to a point verging on physical exhaustion'. Some were 'taken over hills for 6–10 miles, induced to swim against a stream until they were tired out, and were then walked back over the hills at as fast a pace as possible by a specially trained sergeant major'. Others marched 80–85 miles over mountains in 3 days or were put into a decompression chamber. Mepacrine was an effective prophylactic under all these conditions.†.

Since this time, numerous antimalarial drugs have been made, and there is a choice of remedies.

* Neil Hamilton Fairley (1891–1966), Australian physician: demonstrated that the wider gape of the viper's jaw enabled it to inject more venom than other snakes.

† Fairley N H, Trans R. Soc Trop Med Hyg 1945; 38:311.

Life cycle of malaria parasite and sites of drug action (Fig. 14.1 overleaf)

Female anopheles mosquitoes require a blood meal for egg production and in the process of feeding inject salivary fluid containing sporozoites into humans. Since no drugs are effective against sporozoites, infection with the malaria parasite cannot be prevented.

Hepatic cycle (site 1 in the diagram). Sporozoites enter liver cells and usually after 5–16 days but sometimes after months or years are released into the circulation as merozoites. *Plasmodium falciparum* is an exception in that it has no persistent hepatic cycle. Primaquine, proguanil and pyrimethamine (*tissue schizontocides*) act at this site and are used for:

1. *Radical cure* — an attack on persisting hepatic forms (hypnozoites) once the parasite has been cleared from the blood; this is most effectively accomplished with primaquine.

2. *Preventing* the hepatic cycle from becoming established is called *causal prophylaxis*. Primaquine is effective but too toxic for prolonged use. Pyrimethamine combinations (below) have slight efficacy.

Erythrocyte cycle (site 2 in the diagram). Merozoites reproduce asexually in red cells and are released when the cells burst giving rise to the clinical attack. The parasite re-enters red cells and the cycle is repeated after 48 h with *P. vivax* and *P. ovale* (benign tertian malaria), after 36 h with *P. falciparum* (subtertian malaria) and after 72 h with *P. malariae* (quartan malaria). Chloroquine, proguanil, pyrimethamine, quinine and tetracyclines (*blood schizontocides*) kill the asexual forms. Drugs that act on this stage in the cycle of the parasite may be used:

1. To *treat* acute attacks of malaria;

2. To *prevent* attacks by early destruction of the erythrocytic forms. This is called *suppressive prophylaxis*

Sexual forms (site 3 in the diagram). Some merozoites differentiate into male and female gametocytes in the erythrocytes and can only develop further if they are ingested by a mosquito.

Quinine, chloroquine and primaquine (*gametocytocides*) act on sexual forms and *prevent transmission* of the infection because the patient becomes

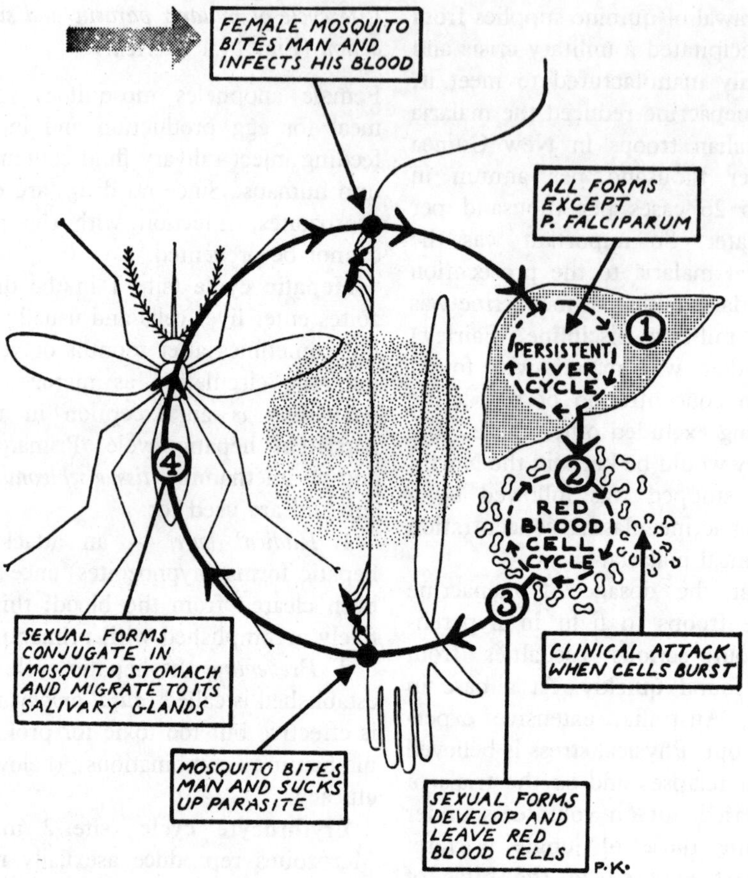

Fig. 14.1 Life cycle of the malaria parasite. The numbers are referred to in the text.

non-infective and the parasite fails to develop in the mosquito (site 4 in the diagram).

In summary, *drugs may be selected*:

1. To *treat* clinical attacks
2. To provide *radical cure*
3. To *prevent* clinical attacks

Drug-resistant malaria

Drug-resistant parasites constitute a persistent problem. Chloroquine-resistant *P. falciparum* occurs in South-East Asia, East Africa and Central and South America. Resistance to dihydrofolate reductase inhibitors such as proguanil and pyrimethamine occurs in all common species of plasmodium, particularly in Africa. Fortunately, resistance to quinine is uncommon, and pyrimethamine acts synergistically with sulphadoxine or dapsone to provide an effective treatment for drug-resistant strains. Mefloquine appears to be a satisfactory alternative. The physician who is not familiar with the resistance pattern in the locality from which the patient has come or to which the patient is going is well advised to check the current position.*

Antimalarials and immunity

Repeated attacks of malaria confer partial immunity and the disease often becomes no more than an occasional inconvenience. Unfortunately, a reliable vaccine to confer active immunity has yet to be developed and prevention depends on drugs and on casually acquired immunity.

* Many countries provide advice centres. In the UK they are listed in the British National Formulary.

The *partially immune* should as a rule not take a prophylactic. The reasoning for this is that they will slowly lose their immunity because of the resulting absence of the red cell cycle; should they then cease to use the prophylactic they are left highly vulnerable to the disease. There are however exceptions to this general advice and the partially immune may or should use a prophylactic:

1. if it is virtually certain that they will never abandon its use,
2. if they go to another malarial area where the strains of parasite may differ,
3. during the last few months of pregnancy in areas where *P. falciparum* is prevalent, to avert the risk of miscarriage.

The *non-immune* should receive continuous prophylaxis in malarial areas. Drugs will be chosen in the light of local knowledge of drug-resistant strains.

Notes on individual drugs

Chloroquine. This 4-aminoquinoline is concentrated within parasitised red cells where it complexes with plasmodial DNA, interferes with the ability of the parasite to digest haemoglobin and deprives it of essential amino acids, so causing its death. It is also effective in amoebiasis.

Pharmacokinetics. The drug is readily absorbed from the gut, is about 50% plasma protein bound, and is concentrated several-fold in various tissues — liver, spleen, heart, kidney and the eye (cornea and retina). The $t_{\frac{1}{2}}$ after a single weekly dose is about 3 days. However, with daily administration and resulting accumulation in tissue from which it is slowly released, the $t_{\frac{1}{2}}$ increases to more than twice that time, and some drug remains in the body for months after administration has ceased. Because of the diversion into tissues and of plasma protein binding, a priming dose is used in order to achieve adequate free plasma concentration. Chloroquine is mainly inactivated by metabolism but about one-quarter is excreted unchanged in the urine.

Adverse effects are infrequent at doses normally used for malaria treatment and prophylaxis, but toxicity is more common with the higher or prolonged doses given for resistant malaria or for rheumatoid arthritis or lupus erythematosus (see index).

Corneal deposits of chloroquine may be asymptomatic or may cause halos around lights or photophobia. These are not a threat to vision and reverse when the drug is stopped. But retinal toxicity is more serious and may be irreversible; it generally occurs at doses in excess of 250 mg/day. Hyperpigmentation of the retina may be seen and the functional defect can take the form of scotomas, photophobia, defective colour vision and decreased visual acuity resulting, in the extreme case, in blindness. Other adverse reactions include mental disturbances, proximal myopathy, peripheral neuropathy and interference with cardiac rhythm, the latter especially if the drug is given i.v. in high dose (it has a quinidine-like action). Rashes, bleaching of hair and gastrointestinal symptoms also occur.

Hydroxychloroquine and *amodiaquine* are similar.

Mefloquine, an amino alcohol, acts in a manner similar to chloroquine. Its $t_{\frac{1}{2}}$ is 17 days and this is the result of both tissue (e.g. liver) storage and of enterohepatic circulation. It may be an effective alternative for chloroquine-resistant strains especially in combination with other drugs; mefloquine plus sulfadoxine plus pyrimethamine is being evaluated. Patients with glucose-6-phosphate dehydrogenase deficiency appear to tolerate the drug.

Primaquine is an 8-aminoquinoline and, though structurally so close to the 4-aminoquinolines, acts not on the erythrocytic but on the hepatic forms of the parasite, apparently by affecting mitochondrial function.

Primaquine is well absorbed from the gastrointestinal tract, is only moderately concentrated in the tissues and is rapidly metabolised. Adverse effects include abdominal cramps, methaemoglobinaemia and haemolytic anaemia, especially in patients with genetic deficiency of erythrocyte glucose-6-phosphate dehydrogenase. In such persons, the risk of haemolytic anaemia is greatly reduced by giving primaquine at weekly intervals for 8 weeks.

Pyrimethamine and **proguanil** inhibit the enzyme that converts folic to folinic acid (dihydrofolate reductase), having an affinity for it in the parasite far greater than for the same enzyme in man. Trimethoprim is similar, but its selectivity is greatest for bacterial enzyme (see co-trimoxazole) although it also has antimalarial activity. Cognoscenti use the term 'antifols' for these drugs. They can also be potentiated by sulphonamides for malarial therapy, e.g. pyrimethamine plus sulfadoxine (Fansidar), pyrimethamine plus dapsone (Maloprim).

Proguanil (chloroguanide), a biguanide, is moderately well absorbed from the gut. The drug is extensively bound to plasma protein, but little to the tissues, so it is not stored in the body and must be given daily when used as prophylaxis. *Pyrimethamine* ($t_{1/2}$ 3 days; a diaminopyrimidine) has similar kinetics, except that tissue binding is stronger and once weekly administration is enough for prophylaxis.

Apart from alimentary-tract symptoms, adverse reactions are uncommon despite their 'antifol' activity, though depression of haemopoiesis can occur.

Quinine is obtained from the bark of the Cinchona tree. It appears to interfere with the ability of the parasite to digest haemoglobin, thus depriving it of essential nutrients. As an antimalarial, quinine is less effective than the synthetic alternatives except in chloroquine-resistant cases. It is also used for myotonia and muscle cramps because it prolongs the muscle refractory period. Dilute solutions are included for their bitter taste in tonics and aperitifs. Quinine stimulates the pregnant uterus and is well known to the public as an abortifacient, but it is unreliable as such even in lethal doses.

Pharmacokinetics. Quinine is well absorbed from the alimentary tract although it is a strong irritant and causes vomiting by local gastric effect as well as by stimulating the vomiting centre. It is almost completely metabolised in the liver and the $t_{1/2}$ is 11 h.

Adverse effects. Some toxic effects of quinine are common to quinidine, salicylates and cinchophen and the term 'cinchonism' is used to describe them. They consist of interference with the auditory nerve causing tinnitus, deafness, nausea, vomiting and vertigo, and of ocular disturbances, notably constriction of the visual fields. Even complete blindness, the onset of which may be very sudden, may develop when large amounts are taken, e.g. to induce abortion or in attempted suicide. The cause of this is disputed; it is probably due to direct toxicity on the retinal cells and not to vascular spasm. In addition, quinine causes rashes, diarrhoea with abdominal pain, fever, hypotension, convulsions and respiratory depression. Quinine can disturb atrioventricular conduction (it is an optical isomer of quinidine) and careful minitoring is needed for any patient with a pre-existing abnormality of cardiac rhythm who must receive the drug. High parasitaemia and the use of quinine i.v. are associated with hypoglycaemia.

Dosage schedules for treatment of an overt attack of malaria* (oral unless otherwise stated)

Infection with P. falciparum

A. *Mild to moderate severity*

1. In areas of 4-aminoquinoline sensitivity give:

	day 1	*day 2*	*day 3*
Chloroquine (base)†	900 mg in 2–3 doses	300 mg	300 mg
or			
Amodiaquine (base)†	600–800 mg in 2–3 doses	400 mg	400 mg

2. In areas of sensitivity to antifolate-sulphonamide combinations but insensitivity to 4-aminoquinolines, give sulphadoxine‡ 1.5 g plus pyrimethamine 75 mg (Fansidar, 3 tablets) in a single dose. This is a useful combination to carry for emergency treatment.

In more severe case, give quinine 600 mg,. 8-hourly for 3–9 doses.

3. In areas of insensitivity to both 4-

* Based on WHO Tech Rep Ser 711, 1984

† The active component of many drugs, whether acid or base, is relatively insoluble and this present a problem in formulation. The problem is overcome by using a soluble salt, i.e. by adding an acid to a base or vice versa. Hence the base quinine is available as quinine sulphate (with sulphuric acid, MW 98) or quinine hydrochloride (with hydrochloric acid, MW 37). The weight of the salt differs according to the acid component, i.e. quinine base 100 mg ≡ quinine sulphate 121 mg ≡ quinine bisulphate 169 mg ≡ quinine hydrochloride 122 mg. The amount of drug prescribed is therefore expressed as the weight of the active component, the *base*, to avoid confusion as to how much quinine is actually being given.

‡ See sulphonamides.

aminoquinolines and antifolate sulphonamide combinations, give quinine 600 mg 8-hourly for 3 days, or for 7 days for cases from South-East Asia, where there may be reduced sensitivity to quinine. Tetracycline 1–2 g per day may be added to this regimen for extra security.

B. *Severe infection when the patient is unable to take medication by mouth*

Quinine (base) 10 mg/kg body weight, is administered by i.v. infusion in dextrose 5% (as hypoglycaemia may occur) over 2–4 h, every 8–12 h until the patient is able to take oral medication.

Note:

1. Provided it is certain that the patient has not taken prior medication, a priming dose of quinine 20 mg/kg may be given as above.
2. Dexamethasone is *contraindicated* for cerebral malaria.
3. Monitor blood glucose.

Infection with P. vivax or P. ovale

Chloroquine or amodiaquine are given as described for sensitive *P. falciparum* infections, followed by primaquine, 15 mg (base) on days 4–17 for radical cure if the patient is not to be further exposed to infection. Patients who are deficient of glucose-6-phosphate dehydrogenase may receive primaquine 30–45 mg (base) weekly for 8 weeks.

Dosage schedules for suppressive prophylaxis

Warning. Fansidar or amodiaquine **for prophylaxis** have become suspect because serious blood disorders and skin reactions are increasingly reported. Maloprim seems acceptable on present evidence (BNF 1986).

1. *In areas with chloroquine-sensitive strains give*:

Chloroquine or amodiaquine* 300 mg (base) weekly

Prophylaxis should begin the day before travel to a malarial area to ensure that blood and tissue concentrations of drug are adequate* on entry. The first dose should be repeated on the second day of prophylaxis, which should be continued weekly.

Prophylaxis should be continued 6 weeks after leaving the endemic area to kill parasites that are acquired about the time of departure and are still incubating in the liver.

2. *In areas with low-grade chloroquine resistance* there are particular issues that may require specialist advice. The rationale for treatment is that chloroquine or amodiaquine are safe and efficacious and that sensitive plasmodial species (*P. malariae, P. ovale, P. vivax*) and even strains of *P. falciparum* may co-exist with resistant parasite within a geographical location. Therefore for:

a. short-term travellers (3 weeks or less) give: *chloroquine or amodiaquine* as above, but Maloprim or Fansidar, 3 tablets, should be kept in readiness and taken if the traveller develops a febrile illness and professional medical advice is not readily available. Prophylaxis with weekly chloroquine or amodiaquine should continue after such presumptive use of Fansidar.

b. long-term travellers may consider prophylaxis with chloroquine plus Maloprim taken weekly but the decision to do so will be influenced by local factors including living conditions and availability of medical advice, and must be balanced against the possibility of serious adverse reaction to Fansidar.

3. *In areas with highly chloroquine-resistant, sulfadoxine/pyrimethamine-resistant P. falciparum, with P. vivax also present, give*:

Maloprim, Fansidar or amodiaquine 300 mg (base).

These doses should be taken weekly.

Children: alternative treatment and prophylaxis schedules should be consulted.

Amoebiasis

Infection occurs when mature cysts are ingested and pass into the colon where they divide into trophozoites; these forms either enter the tissues or reform cysts. Amoebiasis occurs in two forms, both of which need treatment.

* The advice to begin prophylaxis 1–2 weeks before exposure to infection 'in order to get the plasma concentration up' is based on misconceptions of the pharmacokinetics of drugs that can reduce the parasitaemia of acute malaria in 24 h; though it may be sensible to emphasise the importance of prophylaxis and to instil a good habit in advance.

Bowel lumen amoebiasis is asymptomatic and trophozoites (non-infective) and cysts *infective* are passed into the faeces. Treatment is directed at eradicating cysts with a luminal amoebicide (diloxanide).

Tissue-invading amoebiasis gives rise to dysentery, amoebic hepatitis and abscess. Drugs effective against trophozoites must be used (metronidazole, tinidazole, chloroquine).

Treatment with tissue amoebicides should always be followed by a course of therapy with a luminal amoebicide to eradicate the source of the infection.

Metronidazole (200, 400 mg) (see p. 231) has potent amoebicidal activity. It is well absorbed and reaches sufficient tissue concentration to eradicate infection in liver and gut wall. Metronidazole is therefore the agent of first choice for the treatment of symptomatic amoebiasis but it is ineffective for chronic intestinal amoebiasis in which cystic forms persist in the bowel lumen.

Tinidazole is (see p. 232) also an effective amoebicide.

Chloroquine (see p. 273) is effective solely in hepatic amoebiasis as it attains sufficient concentration to be active only at this site. The drug is less effective and slower in its action than metronidazole, with which it may be used in combination.

Emetine, an alkaloid of ipecacuanha and *dehydroemetine* have been largely superseded by metronidazole in the treatment of amoebic infections, as the latter is equally effective, less toxic and also effective orally. Emetine has a place in patients who cannot tolerate or do not respond to metronidazole. The drug is toxic to the myocardium and the ECG should be monitored; patients should be kept in bed during treatment and should not take vigorous exercise for a further three weeks. If conduction defects, cardiac dysrythmias or tachycardia occur, the drug should be stopped. Dehydroemetine is as effective but is less cumulative and cardiotoxic effects are less frequent.

Emetine (as ipecacuanha) retains the use implied by its name in the management of oral self-poisoning (p. 178).

Diloxanide furoate is useful only in eradicating the cystic forms from the bowel lumen. The drug is well tolerated, the commonest adverse effect being flatulence.

Tetracyclines act indirectly by modifying the intestinal flora necessary for amoebae to survive in the bowel lumen. *Paromomycin* has a direct amoebicidal action. They are indicated in combination with metronidazole or emetine in severe amoebic dysentery with extensive ulceration.

Treatment of amoebiasis

Acute amoebic dysentery should be treated with metronidazole 800 mg × 3/day for 5 days followed by diloxanide furoate 500 mg × 3/day for 10 days.

Hepatic amoebiasis requires metronidazole 800 mg × 3/day for 5 days followed by diloxanide furoate 500 mg × 3/day for 10 days. Hepatic abscesses may require to be drained.

Asymptomatic passage of cysts in the faeces: give diloxanide furoate 500 mg × 3/day for 10 days.

Toxoplasmosis

Toxoplasmosis is treated with *pyrimethamine* and *sulphadiazine* for several weeks or alternatively with *spiramycin*.

Giardiasis

Chronic infection with *Giardia lamblia* is treated with *metronidazole* 2 g daily for 3 days or 400 mg × 3/day for 7 days.

Trypanosomiasis

African form. In early cases without CNS involvement *suramin* or *pentamidine* are used parenterally. They are ineffective in the late stages of the disease when the brain is involved, as they do not enter the central nervous system. Pentamidine is also used prophylactically in areas where the disease is endemic. In cases with involvement of the central nervous system, the arsenical *melarsoprol* (too toxic for use in less severe cases) is the drug of choice.

South American form (Chagas' disease). *Nifurtimox*, a nitrofuran, is effective both in the acute and chronic states of the disease. Therapy has to be given for 3–4 months.

Leishmaniasis

Leishmaniasis, whether visceral (kala-azar), mucocutaneous or cutaneous, is treated with sodium stiboglucanate (*pentavalent antimony*). Amphotericin B or pentamidine is used for resistant cases.

Trichomoniasis

Trichomonas vaginitis (and urethritis) is treated with metronidazole 400 mg by mouth, 12-hourly for 7 days or 2 g by mouth as a single dose. Apparent relapses may be reinfections and so it is wise to inspect the sex partner. If there are

Table 14.2 Drugs for helmintic infections

Infection	Drug	Comment
Ascariasis *Ascaris lumbricoides*	levamisole or mebendazole or pyrantel	Piperazine is an alternative
Cutaneous larva migrans	thiabendazole	
Dracontiasis *Dracunculus medinensis* (guinea worm)	niridazole	Metronidazole is an alternative
Enterobiasis *Enterobius vermicularis* (pinworm)	mebendazole or piperazine or pyrantel	Treat all members of the family
Filariasis		
Wucheria bancrofti	diethylcarbamazine	Corticosteroid and antihistamine (H_1-receptor) may be needed for allergic manifestations
Onchocerca volvulus (river blindness	diethylcarbamazine	Follow with suramin to kill adult worms. Ivermectin appears an effective alternative
Hookworm		
Ankylostoma duodenale	tetrachloroethylene	Avoid alcohol and fatty foods after treatment
Necator americanus	bephenium	Probably more effective against *A. duodenale*. Mebendazole and thiabendazole are also used
Schistosomiasis		
Schistosoma haematobium	praziquantel	Metrifonate is an alternative.
S. japonicum	praziquantel	
S. mansoni	praziquantel	Oxamniquine is an alternative.
Strongyloidiasis *Strongyloides stercoralis*	thiabendazole	
Tapeworms		
Diphyllobothrium latum (fish) *Taenia saginata* (beef) *Taenia solium* (pork)	niclosamide or praziquantel	
Echinococcus granulosus (hydatid disease)	surgery for cysts	Mebendazole may be used when cysts rupture.
Cysticercus cellulosae (cysticercosis)	praziquantel	Surgery may be needed.
Trichinosis *Trichinella spiralis*	thiabendazole	Corticosteroid for severe symptoms. Mebendazole is an alternative.
Trichuriasis *Trichuris trichiura* (whipworm)	mebendazole	
Visceral larva migrans	diethylcarbamazine or thiabendazole	

repeated occurences he should be treated even if he appears to be free from infection. Co-existing gonorrhoea or candidiasis are causes of failure of treatment. Nimorazole is an alternative.

CHEMOTHERAPY OF HELMINTIC INFECTIONS

Helminths have complex life-cycles, special knowledge of which is required by those who treat infestations. Table 14.2 will suffice here. Drug resistance has not so far proved to be a clinical problem, though it has occurred in animals on continuous chemoprophylaxis.

ADDENDUM

Zidovudine (azidothymidine, AZT) (Retrovir) $t_{\frac{1}{2}}$, 1 h) is a prodrug for an inhibitor of the human immunodeficiency virus (HIV) which causes the autoimmune deficiency syndrome (AIDS). Short-term oral use has resulted in partial restoration of immune function and clinical improvement.

GUIDE TO FURTHER READING

1 Sharpe A H, Fields B N. Pathogenesis of viral infections. N Engl J Med 1985; 312: 486–497.
2 Hirsch M S, Schooley R T. Treatment of herpesvirus infections. N Engl J Med 1983; 309: 963–970, 1034–1039.
3 Corey L, Spear P G. Infection with herpes simplex viruses. N Engl J Med 1986; 314: 686–91, 749–57.
4 Nicholson K G. Properties of antiviral agents. Lancet 1984; 2 503–506, 562–564.
5 Douglas R G, Editorial. Amantadine as an antiviral agent in influenza. N Engl J Med 1982; 307: 617–618.
6 Jeffries D J. Clinical use of acyclovir. Br Med J 1985; 290: 177–178.
7 Lemon S M. Type A viral hepatitis. New developments in an old disease. N Engl J Med 1985; 313: 1059–1067.
8 Cohen J, Antifungal chemotherapy. Lancet 1982; 2: 532–537.
9 Hay R J, Editorial. Ketoconazole: a reappraisal. Br Med J 1985; 290: 260–261.
10 Peters W, Hall A P, Editorial. The treatment of severe falciparum malaria. Br Med J 1985; 291: 1146–1147.
11 Wyler D J, Malaria — resurgence, resistance and research. N Engl J Med 1985; 308: 875–878, 934–939.
12 Bruce-Chwatt L J. Recent trends of chemotherapy and vaccination against malaria: new lamps for old. Br Med J 1985; 291: 1072–1076.
13 Public Health Laboratory Malaria Reference Laboratory. Prevention of malaria in pregnancy and early childhood. Br Med J 1984; 289: 1296–1297.
14 Most H. Treatment of parasitic infections of travellers and immigrants. N Engl J Med 1984; 310: 298–304.
15 Editorial. Ivermectin in onchocerciasis. Lancet 1984; 2: 1021.
16 Bell D, Editorial. Onchocerciasis now. Br Med J 1985; 290: 1450–1451.
17 Editorial. The lymphatic filariases. Lancet 1985; 1: 1135–1136.
18 Editorial. Albendazole: worms and hydatid disease. Lancet 1984; 2: 675–676.
19 Yarchoan R, Broder S, Development of antiretroviral therapy for the acquired immunodeficiency syndrome and related disorders. N Engl J Med 1987; 316: 557–564.

15

Inflammation and non-steroidal anti-inflammatory drugs: Arthritis

INFLAMMATION

The classical signs of inflammation have long been recognised; the tissues become *red, swollen, tender* or *painful*, there is local *heat* and the patient may be *febrile*. At a microscopic level the capillaries become more permeable and fluid and other elements from the blood leak into the tissue spaces, leucocytes and other phagocytic cells migrate into the area, and rupture of cell lysosomes releases lytic enzymes into the tissues. The inflammatory response in rheumatoid arthritis is manifested by an acute inflammatory exudate of neutrophil leucocytes into the synovial space and chronic inflammation of the synovial tissues. The former appears to involve an antigen–antibody interaction with complement; leucocytes are attracted into the synovial space to phagocytose the antigen–antibody–complement complexes and liberate lysosomal enzymes that damage tissues, including cartilage. Macrophages in the hypertrophied synovial tissue are stimulated to produce proteases and collagenases, which contribute to the destruction of collagen and bone.

Pharmacological interest in inflammation has been stimulated by the discovery that the process is accompanied by the local liberation of a number of chemical mediators that include histamine, 5-hydroxytryptamine, bradykinin, leukotrienes and prostaglandins. Individual mediators may differ in their importance to various types of inflammation; histamine, for example, is necessary for the type of response seen in urticaria but not that of rheumatoid arthritis and H_1-receptor antihistamines are effective in the former but not the latter. It is apparent, nevertheless, that most types of inflammation involve *prostaglandins*, as is illustrated by their capacity to reproduce the classical features of inflammation when injected into tissues. This is now discussed.

Erythema and oedema can be induced in cutaneous vessels by prostaglandins of the E and I series in the minute quantities likely to be produced during inflammation.

Hyperalgesia and pain are caused by the intradermal or i.m. injection of prostaglandins of the E and F series. Normally painless stimuli become painful and this suggests that prostaglandins may sensitise nerve endings and lower the pain threshold, which then allows other mediators to produce pain at concentrations that would normally be innocuous. Thus in pain, prostaglandins appear to act as modulators, capable of increasing or decreasing response, rather than as mediators. This is further considered on p. 304.

Fever. The fine balance between generation and loss of heat by the body is controlled by the hypothalamus and set at a particular point that we recognise as normal body temperature (37° C).

Fever may be regarded as disorder of thermoregulation in which the set point is displaced upwards and the result is elevation of body temperature. It may be caused by a variety of types of tissue damage (malignancy, infarction, inflammation) and by microorganisms. The condition is mediated by an endogenous pyrogen named *interleukin-1*, which is produced peripherally and carried in the systemic circulation to specific sites in the hypothalamus where it acts through local production of prostaglandin E_2. Prostaglandins used therapeutically to induce abortion (dinoprost, dinoprostone) may cause transient pyrexia. Fever due to resetting of the body's thermostat should be distinguished from the hyperpyrexia that results from excessive heat gain or production, as in sunstroke or malignant hyperpyrexia.

NON-STEROIDAL ANTI-INFLAMMATORY DRUGS

Several types of drug influence the inflammatory process or its manifestations and they do so by a variety of actions. These include the adrenal glucocorticoid steroids, immunosuppressive agents, colchicine, chloroquine, penicillamine and gold salts; these drugs are described elsewhere, see index. The class of drug described here, of which aspirin is the prototype (non-steroidal anti-inflammatory drugs, NSAIDs), is worthy of separate consideration, for its members, although structurally heterogenous, possess a single common mode of action which is *to block prostaglandin biosynthesis* by inhibiting the conversion of arachidonic acid to precursor cyclic endoperoxides by the enzyme cyclo-oxygenase. This action is reflected in the range of effects, both beneficial and adverse, which the individual members share, as is now discussed (see diagram p. 716).

Analgesia: NSAIDs are effective against pain of mild-to-moderate intensity. Their maximum efficacy is much lower than that of the opioids but they do not cause dependence.

Anti-inflammatory action is useful in a variety of conditions including rheumatoid arthritis, osteoarthritis, musculoskeletal disorders and pericarditis.

Antipyretic action: NSAIDs effectively lower fever.

Platelet function is reduced because formation of thromboxane is prevented; thromboxane is derived from prostaglandins and causes platelets to aggregate. This action is used to protect against vascular occlusion (see p. 579).

Prolongation of gestation and labour: prostaglandin synthesis by the uterus increases substantially in the hours before parturition. This has led to the suggestion that an inhibitor of prostaglandin synthesis, e.g. indomethacin, might inhibit premature labour, but the possibility of premature closure of the fetal ductus arteriosus (see below) precludes this use, certainly beyond brief periods.

Patency of the ductus arteriosus is maintained by prostaglandins and when the ductus remains patent after birth, an attempt may be made to close it by giving indomethacin, for the alternative is surgical ligation.

Primary dysmenorrhea is associated with the production of large quantities of prostaglandin in the uterus and with uterine hypercontractility; this is the rationale for its treatment with an inhibitor of prostaglandin synthesis, e.g. mefenamic acid.

Gastric or intestinal mucosal damage is the commonest adverse effect of the NSAIDs. Mucosal prostaglandins inhibit acid secretion and further appear to exert a cytoprotective effect by promoting the secretion of mucus and by strengthening the mucosa against back-diffusion of acid from the gastric lumen to the sub-mucosal tissues where it causes damage. Inhibition of prostaglandin biosynthesis is believed to account for the erosions, ulceration and bleeding caused by NSAIDs. Thus therapeutic and adverse effects are due to the same mechanism. These drugs are therefore administered with food or, to avoid the oral route, per rectum. In patients admitted to hospital with acute upper gastrointestinal haemorrhage, aspirin may be a causative factor in up to 50% of cases, and other NSAIDs in 20%. There can be no doubt that these drugs cause loss of life from gut haemorrhage. NSAID use is also associated with an increasing incidence of perforated peptic ulcer, notably in the elderly.

Urticaria, severe rhinitis and asthma occur in susceptible individuals (e.g. with nasal polyposis) who are exposed to NSAIDs, notably aspirin; the mechanism is not understood but is thought to involve inhibition of synthesis of bronchodilator prostaglandins.

Fluid and electrolyte balance may be upset in a variety of ways, all of which appear to be mediated through inhibition of synthesis of the renal prostaglandins, which have an important influence in salt and water homeostasis. NSAIDs cause sodium retention and oedema; if water retention is disproportionate, hyponatraemia may result; hyperkalaemia may be caused by inhibition of the renin–angiotensin–aldosterone system. These actions result in reduction of the diuretic, natriuretic and antihypertensive effects of diuretic drugs; NSAIDs also counteract the antihypertensive effect of β-adrenoceptor antagonists, probably by their action on renal prostaglandin synthesis.

Analgesic nephropathy. Mixtures (rather than single agents) of NSAIDs taken repeatedly over years can cause grave and often irreversible renal damage, notably chronic interstitial nephritis, renal papillary necrosis and acute renal failure; these effects appear to be due at least in part to ischaemia through inhibition of locally produced vasodilator prostaglandins. The condition is most common in people who take high doses repeatedly over years, e.g. for severe chronc rheumatism and in patients with personality disorder. The latter have been described as characteristically sallow, middle-aged women who smoke heavily, cannot sleep without sedatives, have recurrent ill-health and who have 'suffered dreadfully' from headaches for as long as they can remember.* They have frequently had a broken marriage and may have attempted suicide. The disease manifests itself as renal symptoms, particularly nocturia and renal colic; anaemia and hypertension are common; proteinuria may be only slight; sterile pyuria is common. Whilst analgesic nephropathy appears to be associated with long-term abuse of NSAID mixtures, mounting evidence that phenacetin was particularly responsible has rendered this drug obsolete.†

Notwithstanding the above range of actions of the NSAIDs, there are important differences between individual members of the group. These are most readily reflected in their anti-inflamma-

* Kincaid-Smith P. Prescribers' Journal 1970; 10:8

† *Phenacetin abuse and toxicity*. Although phenacetin was introduced in 1887, it was not until 1953 that suspicion was aroused that it might cause renal damage. Certainty was not easily attained because, as well as the difficulties of interpreting associations discovered by retrospective enquiry, phenacetin was almost never used alone and it is hard to separate the effects of the several ingredients of mixtures. These mixtures have been widely abused, particularly on the European mainland, being used for any trivial discomforts. The remarkable extents to which people can become dependent on them is shown by events in a Swedish town, which also illustrate that drug abuse has emotional and social as well as pharmacological aspects.

During the influenza pandemic of 1918 a physician to a big factory in the town prescribed a powder containing phenacetin (0.5 g), phenazone (0.5 g) and caffeine (0.15 g). There was substantial mortality from the epidemic, but survivors thought they felt fitter and reinvigorated during convalescence if they took the powder. They continued to take it after recovery, in the expectation of becoming stronger and 'more nimble of finger', so that they would earn more in the factory.

Use of the powder, which could be got without prescription, spread through the town. Consumption increased and 'many families,' 'could not think of beginning the day without a powder'. It became almost almost as usual to offer a powder as a cigarette. When visiting friends in hospital, a powder 'was as welcome as flowers, fruit or chocolate, whatever the nature of the illness. Attractively wrapped packages of powder were often given as birthday presents.' Doctors regarded the habit as 'something of a joke'.

The phenacetin consumption of the town was about ten times as great as in a similar Swedish town. The deaths from renal insufficiency rose in the phenacetin town, but not in the control town, and in the decade of 1952–61, they were more than three times as many.

An investigation was resisted by the factory workers and there was even an instance of organised burning of a questionnaire on powder-taking. It was eventually discovered that most of those who used powders did so, not for pain, but to maintain a high working pace, from 'habit', or to counter fatigue.

There is no reason to think phenacetin or phenazone effective for these, but each powder contained enough caffeine to give a noticeable effect, and as many as 10–12 a day were sometimes taken. The workers developed a considerable emotional dependence on the powders in the exact form in which they were accustomed to taking them. Any slight change in the appearance of the powder rendered it, they thought, useless. Along with warnings of the danger of renal damage, a clinic was set up to help people break their habit. At first those who went to it were subject to 'persecution or derision' by their colleagues, but eventually the rising death rate brought home to the consumers the gravity of the affair, something that has yet to be achieved for cigarette smoking.

In 1961, phenacetin was withdrawn from sale to the public in Sweden and could be obtained only by prescription. The devotees of the powder changed to a phenazone, caffeine formula. When asked, they usually replied 'that it was quite useless, but that one had nonetheless to take a few now and then'. Sales of this powder, however, remained about the same as those of the original phenacetin-containing powder.

Sudden withdrawal demonstrated that there was no physical dependence on the mixture and the emotional dependence was probably a social rather than a pharmacological phenomenon, though the latter remains possible. (Grimlund K. *Acta Med Scand* 1963; 174: suppl. 405.))

tory effect, which provides a clinical basis for their classification as follows:

1. **Drug with analgesic and with weak anti-inflammatory effect**. Aniline derivative: *Paracetamol* is the only member of this group now used (phenacetin being obsolete).

2. **Drugs with analgesic and with mild-to-moderate anti-inflammatory effect**

a. Propionic acid derivatives: *fenbufen, fenoprofen, flurbiprofen, ibuprofen, indoprofen, ketoprofen, naproxen, suprofen, tiaprofenic acid*.

b. Fenamic acid derivative: *mefenamic acid*.

3. **Drugs with analgesic and marked anti-inflammatory effect**

a. Salicylic acid derivatives: *aspirin, benorylate, choline magnesium trisalicylate, diflunisal, salsalate, sodium salicylate*.

b. Pyrazolone derivatives: *azapropazone, phenylbutazone*.

c. Acetic acid derivatives: *diclofenac, etodolac, fenclofenac, indomethacin* (*indometacin*), *sulindac, tolmetin*.

d. Oxicam derivative: *piroxicam*.

The above is not a rigid classification since effect also depends on the dose used and there is some overlap of the groups, but it generally holds true.

Drug with analgesic but with weak anti-inflammatory effect

Paracetamol (acetaminophen, Panadol) (500 mg) is a popular 'home medicine'. Worldwide the annual consumption of paracetamol exceeds 25 000 tons and in the UK its sales are greater than those of aspirin. Its analgesic efficacy is equal to that of aspirin but in clinical doses it has no useful anti-inflammatory effects, i.e. it inhibits prostaglandin synthetase in the brain but hardly at all in the periphery. Thus, where inflammation is contributing to pain, as it often is, aspirin is preferred. Paracetamol is effective in mild-to-moderate pain such as that of headache or dysmenorrhoea and it is also useful in patients who should avoid aspirin because of gut intolerance, a bleeding tendency or allergy.

Pharmacokinetics. Paracetamol is well absorbed from the alimentary tract. About 50% of the drug is bound to plasma proteins and the $t_{½}$ is 2 h. The drug is conjugated principally as glucuronide and also as sulphate in the liver and these products are inactive. Minor metabolites of paracetamol are also formed, of which one oxidation product, N-acetyl-benzoquinoneimine, is highly reactive chemically. This substance is normally rendered harmless by conjugation with SH-(*thiol*) groups of glut*athione*. However, the supply of hepatic glutathione is limited and if the amount of metabolite formed is greater than the availability of glutathione, then the metabolite is available to react with cellular macromolecules, e.g. key enzymes, and so to cause cell death. This explains why paracetamol, normally a safe drug, can give rise to hepatic necrosis in overdose. Indeed, severe hepatic damage can result from 10 g (20 tablets) taken at once, which is only 2.5 times the recommended maximum daily clinical dose (4.0 g). Patients whose hepatic metabolising enzymes are induced as a result of taking drugs or alcohol may be especially at risk in minor overdose as their livers may form more of the toxic metabolite.

The dose is 0.5–1 g every 4–6 h to a maximum of 4 g in a day.

Adverse effects are few. The drug may rarely cause skin rash and allergy. It is well tolerated by the stomach because the peripheral effect is weak.

Acute paracetamol overdose. As is explained above, the liver is the organ most at risk but acute renal tubular necrosis also occurs partly in association with fulminant hepatic failure and partly because the kidney also contains the oxidising enzymes that form the toxic metabolite. Plasma bilirubin, hepatic enzymes (e.g. aspartate aminotransferase) prothrombin time and plasma creatinine should be monitored. The clinical signs (jaundice, abdominal pain, hepatic tenderness) do not become apparent for 24–48 h, and liver failure, when it occurs, does so within 2–7 days of the overdose. It is vital that this delay be remembered, for lives can only be saved by effective anticipatory action.

In addition, the plasma concentration of paracetamol is of predictive value; if it is below 200 mg/l (1.32 mmol/l) at 4 h after ingestion, or below 50 mg/l (0.33 mmol/l) at 12 h, then serious hepatic damage is unlikely. The patient's estimate of the quantity ingested is notoriously unreliable, especially in cases of deliberate self-poisoning.

The general principles for treating drug overdose apply (Ch. 10). If the patient is seen early, activated charcoal by mouth can reduce further absorption, but the decision to use it must take into account its capacity to bind an oral antidote (methionine). Hepatic failure should be managed along conventional lines with neomycin, lactulose, vitamin K, and i.v. fluids including glucose.

Specific therapy is directed to supplying compounds containing SH-(thiol) groups and to replenishing the store of liver glutathione, which is available to conjugate with and inactivate the toxic metabolite, and second may reduce the oxidised thiol groups that are responsible for inactivating essential enzymes. Glutathione itself cannot be used as it penetrates cells poorly, but N-acetylcysteine (NAC) and methionine* are effective as they are precursors for the synthesis of glutathione. NAC appears to be more effective because its conversion into glutathione requires fewer enzymes. Clearly the earlier such therapy is instituted the better, to limit the effect of the toxic metabolite. Methionine seems to be effective for 8–9 h after overdose but NAC probably benefits for at least 12 h. Once the liver and the kidney are seriously damaged, NAC and methionine are likely to be ineffective and run the risk of precipitating hepatic coma. Therefore:

a. in cases in which plasma concentration in relation to time after the overdose indicates likelihood of significant liver damage give *NAC* (Parvolex) i.v. 150 mg/kg in 200 ml dextrose 5%, over 15 min, then 50 mg/kg in dextrose 5%, 500 ml over 4 h, then 100 mg/kg in dextrose 5%, 1000 ml over 16 h, to a total of about 300 mg/kg in 20 h.

b. in cases in which significant liver damage appears unlikely, give *methionine* by mouth 2.5 g 4-hourly, up to 10 g total.

Chronic overdose. Whereas nephropathy is well known to occur in analgesic abusers, renal damage has not to date been firmly associated with taking paracetamol alone. Also chronic use has not been shown convincingly to cause liver damage. Nonetheless long-term use of the drug in high dose should be discouraged.

* A paracetamol-methionine ester (Pamaton) has been produced, the methionine content ensuring that hepatic glutathione levels are maintained when the drug is used in therapeutic (and over) dose.

Drugs with analgesic and mild to moderate anti-inflammatory effect

Propionic acid derivatives

Ibuprofen (Brufen) (200, 400, 600 mg) was the first drug of this class to be widely used; it can be regarded as typical of the group. It is well absorbed after an oral dose to give maximum plasma concentrations 1–2 h later; the $t_{\frac{1}{2}}$ is 2 h. Ibuprofen is largely metabolised and the products are eliminated principally in the urine and also via the bile. No unchanged drug appears in the urine. Binding to plasma proteins is 99% but interaction due to displacement with other extensively bound drugs, e.g. coumarin anticoagulants or oral hypoglycaemics, does not appear to be a problem.

The dose is 600–1200 mg/day in 3–4 divided doses: maximum dose 2400 mg/day.

Others of this group include *fenbufen, fenoprofen, flurbiprofen, indoprofen, ketoprofen, naproxen* and *tiaprofenic acid*. They all have similar properties and are most used in painful conditions not accompanied by prominent inflammation, e.g. mild rheumatoid disease and musculoskeletal disorders. Naproxen (Naprosyn) appears to perform marginally better than the others in comparative trials but patients prefer individual members of the group and this is more apparent than consistent differences between the drugs. Naproxen ($t_{\frac{1}{2}}$, 13 h) and fenbufen ($t_{\frac{1}{2}}$, 10 h) are suitable for twice-daily dosing.

The main advantage over aspirin is a lower incidence of *adverse effects*. Those that occur are usually related to the gut and range from epigastric discomfort to activation of peptic ulcer and bleeding. Ibuprofen, particularly at low dosage, appears to be less toxic to the gastrointestinal tract than others in this class. Headaches, dizziness, fever and rashes also occur.

Ketoprofen elevates methotrexate plasma concentrations when both drugs are used together.

Fenamic acid derivative

Mefenamic acid (Ponstan) (250, 500 mg) is slowly absorbed from the small intestine to give maximum plasma concentration at 2–4 h. The $t_{\frac{1}{2}}$ is 3 h. It is eliminated partly unchanged and partly as metabolites in the urine; 20% is excreted in the faeces. Mefenamic acid is used for mild-to-moderate pain where inflammation is not marked, e.g. muscular, dental and traumatic pain and headache; it is also used for dysmenorrhoea and menorrhagia due to uterine dysfunction. The dose is 500 mg × 3/day after food. The principal adverse effects are haemolytic anaemia, upper abdominal discomfort, peptic ulcer and diarrhoea. Elderly patients who take mefenamic acid may develop non-oliguric renal failure especially if they become dehydrated, e.g. by the diarrhoea, which it also causes; the drug should be avoided or used with close supervision in the elderly. Competition with coumarin anticoagulants for plasma protein binding sites may increase anticoagulant effect.

Drugs with analgesic and marked anti-inflammatory effect

Salicylates and derivatives, principally aspirin

Willow bark contains salicin from which salicylic acid is derived. It was used for fevers in the 18th century as a cheap substitute for imported cinchona (quinine) bark. Willow bark was thought worthy of testing because both willow trees and fevers occurred in marshy places and, according to the 'doctrine of signatures', where a disease was found so there would be a remedy nearby provided by a beneficient Nature. This success is regarded now as the result of chance, though it was then considered to provide evidence in favour of the hypothesis of 'signatures'. The latter half of the 19th century saw the first use of sodium salicylate in acute rheumatism and the preparation and introduction in 1899 of acetylsalicylic acid (aspirin).

Over 40 000 tons of aspirin are consumed in the world each year. 'The British eat about two thousand tons (> 2 million kg) of aspirin yearly. This makes 6000 million tablets, or two tablets weekly for every citizen. In Connecticut, USA, 37% of all bottles of blood collected came from donors who had recently eaten aspirin.'*

Aspirin (acetylsalicylic acid) is rapidly hydrolysed to salicylic acid in the plasma. Both substances act by inhibiting prostaglandin synthesis, although by different mechanisms. Salicylic acid is irritant to the stomach and is administered either as aspirin or as sodium salicylate, both of which rapidly achieve effective tissue concentrations. Aspirin and salicylate have the effects listed below. This account refers generally to salicylate but cites aspirin or sodium salicylate when the information refers particularly to these drugs. Aspirin is by far the commonest form in which salicylate is taken.

The principal effects of salicylates are listed below:

1. Analgesia
2. Antipyresis
3. Anti-inflammatory effect
4. Respiratory stimulation
5. Metabolic effects
6. Uricosuric effect
7. Reduced platelet adhesiveness
8. Hypoprothrombinaemia

1. *Analgesic effect* is mild, being less than that of codeine. There is no evidence of any central effects on the psychic reaction to pain that plays so important a part in the action of the opioid analgesics. Analgesia seems to be due to both central and peripheral action. Salicylate is most effective against mild pain of somatic as opposed to visceral origin.

2. *Antipyresis.* Salicylate acts in the hypothalamus to place at a lower level the set point of temperature control, which is elevated by fever. Though sweating is usual, it is not essential to the antipyretic effect. Paradoxically salicylate poisoning can cause hyperpyrexia (see below). Nowadays, when antipyretics are seldom used for the purpose implied by their name, there is less interest in this effect†, but before antimicrobials existed phys-

* Editorial. Lancet 1972; 1:477.

† There is a moderately strong suspicion that aspirin may be a cause of the rare Reye's syndrome (encephalopathy, liver injury) in children and teenagers recovering from febrile viral infections (respiratory, varicella). Paracetamol is preferred in such illnesses. Parents should be educated about this as most such administration is on their own initiative, not prescribed.

icians could often do nothing else to show their power over the disease. The efforts previously devoted to reducing fever are now turned more profitably to removing its cause.

3. *Anti-inflammatory* (antirheumatic) effect (see *mode action* above).

4. *Respiratory stimulation* is a characteristic of salicylate intoxication. It occurs both directly as a result of action on the respiratory centre and indirectly through increased CO_2 production (see below). In severe poisoning, serious depression of respiration can occur.

5. *Metabolic effects* are important and understanding them aids the management of poisoning. As the plasma salicylate concentration rises, the following sequence of events occurs:

a. *Increased peripheral O_2 consumption* due to stimulation of cellular metabolism (uncoupling of oxidative phosphorylation), with increased CO_2 production, leads to increased respiration.

b. *Respiratory alkalosis* results from (a) and from 4 (above).

c. Because of (b), *blood pH tends to rise* and is compensated by renal loss of bicarbonate, which is necessarily accompanied by sodium and potassium ions as well as water, and dehydration and hypokalaemia result. The reduction of plasma bicarbonate deprives the body of one of its buffering systems so that it becomes particularly vulnerable to metabolic acidosis.

d. *Metabolic acidosis* is contributed to by several factors including: accumulation of lactic and pyruvic acids due to toxic interference with Kreb's cycle enzymes; stimulation of lipid metabolism causing increased production of ketone bodies; salicylic acid in the blood; renal insufficiency due to vascular collapse; and dehydration (no fluid intake, hyperpnoea, hyperpyrexia).

There is also late toxic respiratory depression causing CO_2 retention.

Carbohydrate metabolism. Salicylate can lower the *blood sugar*, by increasing peripheral utilisation of glucose (and has been used in diabetes mellitus). With heavy doses, however, hyperglycaemia may occur, perhaps due to depression of aerobic glycolysis, increased hepatic glycogenolysis and increased adrenal cortical activity.

6. *Renal tubular reabsorption of urate* is reduced and salicylate can be used to deplete gouty patients of uric acid. However, high doses (5–8 g/day) are needed, and few patients can tolerate these. The uricosuric effect is greater in an alkaline urine. Low doses of salicylate (less than 2 g/day) cause urate retention (see gout).

Salicylate antagonises the action of uricosuric drugs, which all act by decreasing tubular reabsorption of urate (by competing in the organic acid transport system as does probenecid).

7. *Reduction of blood platelet adhesiveness* follows irreversible inhibition (by acetylation) of platelet cyclo-oxygenase by aspirin and reduced production of thromboxane (see index). The result is prolongation of the bleeding time. This action of aspirin may be valuable in occlusive arterial disease. It may also enhance any bleeding condition including anticoagulant use.

8. *Hypoprothrombinaemia* occurs with large doses; it is unlikely at less than 5 g of aspirin or sodium salicylate a day. The effect may be due to competition between salicylate and vitamin K for it is preventable and reversible by vitamin K_1. Severe haemorrhage is rare.

Pharmacokinetics. Aspirin is well absorbed from the gastrointestinal tract, partly from the stomach for, being an acid, it is un-ionised and lipid soluble at gastric pH, but mainly from the upper small intestine, which has an enormous surface area. The rate of absorption from the gut is influenced by gastric emptying, by the pH at the mucosal cell surface and by pharmaceutical factors such as the rate of disintegration and dissolution of the tablet. Aspirin (acetylsalicylic acid) has a $t_{\frac{1}{2}}$ of 15 min, being converted into salicylic acid, which also inhibits prostaglandin synthesis. Salicylic acid is 80%–95% bound to plasma protein; it distributes mainly into the extracellular fluid and the distribution volume is 10 l/70 kg.

Salicylic acid is inactivated by conjugation with glycine. At low therapeutic doses this reaction proceeds by first-order kinetics, salicylic acid has a $t_{\frac{1}{2}}$ of 5 h and less than 10% of the drug can be recovered as unchanged salicylic acid in the urine. However, the conjugation saturates at high therapeutic doses and in overdose, i.e. salicylic acid exhibits zero-order elimination kinetics and most of the drug in the body and over 80% of that in the urine is present as salicylic acid. The problem in overdose therefore is the removal of salicylic acid, which is achieved by alkalinising the urine (see below).

A reasonably steady plasma concentration can be maintained if salicylate is given 6-hourly by mouth but if a high dose is given repeatedly there is risk of accumulation to toxic amounts as elimination becomes zero order. The complaint of tinnitus is a useful warning sign but the plasma concentration should be monitored during high and continuous dosing.

Uses. Salicylates relieve mild-to-moderate pain of non-visceral origin, e.g. headache, osteoarthritis, myalgia and also dysmenorrhoea. The anti-inflammatory action is valuable for conditions in which an inflammatory reaction is prominent. Despite the introduction of many new NSAIDs, aspirin and variants of salicylates remain standard drugs for inflammatory arthropathies including rheumatoid disease, Still's disease and acute rheumatic fever.

Preparations and dosages. Aspirin remains a valuable drug, and there is still no adequate substitute; because it is free from patent restrictions and because pharmaceutical formulation is unusually important in reducing gastric toxicity, there is a plethora of commercial preparations, plain, buffered, soluble, effervescent, enteric coated.

A properly compounded *Aspirin Tablet, Dispersible* (300 mg; single dose 300–900 mg) and a reliable *enteric-coated* preparation will suffice for most patients. The dispersible tablet contains aspirin, citric acid and calcium carbonate. When it is put in water the citric acid reacts with the calcium carbonate to form calcium citrate solution, and this dissolves the aspirin to form calcium acetylsalicylate. The reason for this roundabout approach is that the shelf life of calcium acetylsalicylate is dependent on storage conditions. It is hygroscopic and, unless protected from moisture, the drug is hydrolysed. Badly stored (damp) aspirin hydrolyses to salicylic and acetic acids, and the latter is readily recognised by its smell.

There are many tablets containing mixtures of aspirin, paracetamol, codeine and caffeine. Details can be found in any formulary.

Benorylate (Benoral) (750 mg) is an ester of aspirin and paracetamol which, being non-ionic and lipid soluble, is well absorbed from the gut. It is also less irritant to the stomach and causes less blood loss from it than does aspirin. When benorylate is hydrolysed in the liver and plasma, paracetamol and aspirin are released. It is an alternative to aspirin. The dose is 4–8 g/day divided between 2–3 doses.

Diflunisal (Dolobid) (250, 500 mg) is a fluorophenyl derivative of salicylic acid. It is eliminated largely as conjugates in the urine. The drug is 98% bound to plasma proteins and the plasma $t_{\frac{1}{2}}$ is 10 h. The dose is 250–500 mg twice daily for pain relief; it is also uricosuric, possibly more so than aspirin.

Diflunisal compares favourably with aspirin in the treatment of osteoarthritis and it may cause fewer gastric adverse effects, although diarrhoea is more common. There may be cross allergy with aspirin.

Aloxiprin (Palaprin) is a condensation product of aspirin and aluminium hydroxide: it is an alternative to soluble aspirin.

Salsalate (disalcid) is an ester that is hydrolysed to salicylic acid in the blood.

Methyl salicylate (oil of wintergreen) is too irritant to be used internally. It is used in counter-irritant liniments. Its smell sometimes attracts children; if they drink it, treatment is urgent.

Adverse reactions are in general those described earlier for NSAIDs but some aspects merit further comment.

a. *Salicylism* results from use in high dose and is expressed as tinnitus and hearing difficulty, dizziness, headache and confusion.

b. *Allergy*. Aspirin is a common cause of allergic symptoms and signs. It is debatable whether an antigen–antibody reaction is involved and the term 'aspirin intolerance' or 'pseudoallergy' may be preferred. Patients exhibit severe rhinitis, urticaria, angioedema, asthma or shock. Those who already suffer from recurrent urticaria or asthma are more susceptible.

c. *Congestive heart failure or pulmonary oedema*

may occur in those with acute rheumatic fever and carditis. The explanation appears to be increaased plasma volume (of uncertain cause) and increased peripheral oxygen uptake necessitating greater cardiac output. The risk is greater if sodium salicylate is used in full dose because of the extra sodium load.

d. *Pregnancy*. During pregnancy, continuous use causes anaemia and there is increased incidence of prolonged gestation, ante- and post-partum haemorrhage and caesarian section (see above for likely mechanisms).

e. *Analgesic nephropathy*. Long term abuse of analgesic mixtures (which may include salicylate) leads to nephropathy, but there is evidence that aspirin used as the sole treatment for rheumatoid arthritis for many years has no general adverse effect on renal function.

f. *Gastrointestinal disorders*. About 1 in 15 of the population cannot take aspirin without risking symptoms (heartburn, epigastric distress, vomiting). If a particle of aspirin is placed on human buccal mucosa, within 30 min the mucosa becomes white, opaque and wrinkled and a slough that readily peels away is formed. Gastroscopic studies in man reveal congested, haemorrhagic areas where particles are lodged, and these may occur in the absence of symptoms. Aspirin does not act merely as a local chemical irritant but also increases gastric mucosal cell shedding (so do alcohol and mustard). The normal stomach mucosa sheds 0.5 million cells/min and it is not surprising that interference with such an active process causes trouble. The characteristic aspirin-induced lesion is a superficial erosion and bleeding from this will be enhanced by the effects on platelets (7, above).

Occult blood loss (usually 5 ml/day above control value of 0.7 ml) occurs in most people taking aspirin continuously. Sometimes larger amounts of blood are lost and iron-deficiency anaemia occurs, especially in those predisposed (women who menstruate). The site of blood loss is predominantly the stomach and it seems that anything that reduces the concentration of aspirin applied to the mucous membrane or increases ionisation (so that it is less lipid soluble and less will penetrate gastric mucosal cells) lessens the liability to bleed and/or the amount of blood lost. Therefore, pharmaceutical ingenuity can reduce the risk, and a rapidly disintegrating (dispersing) tablet, or one that makes a buffered solution and is then swallowed with much fluid, is least likely to cause trouble (e.g. Alka-Seltzer),* though most preparations do not have enough buffering power to be useful. None of these preparations, except perhaps Alka-Seltzer, which contains a large amount of sodium bicarbonate, is free from irritant effect, and in some subjects they are no safer than ordinary aspirin. Enteric-coated aspirin causes less blood loss, for the small intestine is less affected than the stomach, but absorption is delayed for 6 or more hours, so that this preparation is unsuitable for occasional analgesia, though well suited for long-term medication, as in rheumatoid arthritis.

A history of taking aspirin recently is more common in patients with *overt gastroduodenal haemorrhage*, particularly those with acute erosions. The risk seems to be greatest in those who take aspirin regularly or in large dose but some patients suffer profuse gastric haemorrhage as a result of taking a single dose of aspirin. The latter appears to be an idiosyncratic response and such individuals may have a minor abnormality in the haemostatic mechanism. Any patient with evidence of a mild defect in haemostasis, e.g. prolonged bleeding after tooth extraction, should be advised to treat aspirin with particular caution.

Alcohol increases gastric haemorrhage from ordinary aspirin but the effect is negligible with adequately buffered aspirin.

Gastric ulcer is associated with the regular use of aspirin but the frequency of the relationship is not clear.

Salicylate is plainly best avoided in patients with disease of the upper gastrointestinal tract, particularly with a history of peptic ulcer, but any proposal that the drug should be abandoned in favour of newer analgesics ignores the fact that it

* Alka-Seltzer contains aspirin 324 mg: citric acid 965 mg: sodium bicarbonate 1625 mg; the tablet is big. In water it forms a solution of sodium acetylsalicylate, sodium citrate and sodium bicarbonate. Storage in a damp atmosphere allows the chemical reaction to take place.

has been used successfully for decades by the public and the medical profession despite these effects. Considering that thousands of tons are eaten annually, serious adverse effects from salicylate are uncommon. However if aspirin were being introduced now it seems unlikely that any regulatory authority would have the hardihood to allow general sale to the public.

Overdose. The typical clinical picture of moderate overdose (plasma salicylate 500–700 mg/l) consists of nausea, vomiting, epigastric discomfort, tinnitus, deafness, hyperpnoea, headache, sweating, hypokalaemia, restlessness and mental confusion. With a big overdose (plasma salicylate > 750 mg/l) these symptoms may be followed by hyperpyrexia, pulmonary oedema, mania, convulsions and coma with severe dehydration and ketosis.

Despite the fact that aspirin reduces platelet activity and salicylates cause hypoprothrombinaemia and adverse effects on the stomach, gastric erosions and bleeding are uncommon after aspirin overdose.

Metabolic changes have an important bearing on therapy (see 5, above) and arterial blood gases and pH should be monitored in serious cases.

Adults who have taken a single large quantity usually develop a *respiratory alkalosis* but when poisoning is severe a *metabolic acidosis* follows; commonly a mixed acid–base disturbance is found.

Children under 4 years tend not to exhibit the respiratory alkalosis but readily develop severe metabolic acidosis, sometimes even after salicylate has been used in high therapeutic doses.

The reason for this disparity is unknown; it may be a true age difference in response, or it may be due to the different circumstances in which poisoning occurs, whether as a single large amount or during prolonged therapy.

A single serum salicylate concentration is not a reliable guide to the severity of poisoning because it gives no indication of the course of the poisoning before it was measured. A concentration above 400 mg/l can be taken as confirming the diagnosis, and if it is above 750 mg/l in a patient who took the drug hours previously, the case is severe. Serial measurements give more information.

The general measures described in Chapter 10 apply to management but the following are relevant specifically for salicylate overdose.

a. Gastric lavage (or therapeutic emesis with syrup of ipecacuanha in children) is worth undertaking for up to 24 h after overdose, for tablets may lie as an insoluble mass in the stomach. Activated charcoal may be worth giving as it adsorbs both salicylate that has not been absorbed from the gut and also drug that diffuses from the blood into the gut.

b. Hypoprothrombinaemia may be treated by giving vitamin K_1 i.v.

c. Fluid and electrolyte repair. Correction of dehydration, which can be severe due to sweating, vomiting and overbreathing, is of the first importance. The i.v. route should be used for moderate or severe poisoning. As hypokalaemia is usual and hypoglycaemia is common, dextrose 5% with added potassium will often be indicated. Reduction of hyperpyrexia by sponging helps to reduce fluid loss.

d. Acid–base disturbance. Patients showing alkalosis or mixed alkalosis/acidosis with normal blood pH need no therapy directed to changing the blood acid–base balance but calcium gluconate may be given i.v. if hyperventilation and alkalosis cause tetany. Sodium bicarbonate is used to correct metabolic acidosis (blood pH < 7.2) and to alkalinise the urine to remove salicylate (below). Its administration should be controlled by plasma standard bicarbonate and blood pH measurements, because hypokalaemia may be aggravated. Pulmonary oedema may result from sodium overload. A low plasma bicarbonate content does *not* alone indicate acidosis, and if sodium bicarbonate is given, the patient may develop severe alkalosis. Lack of facilities to measure these and/or of ability to interpret the results, greatly increases the dangers of salicylate poisoning.

e. Removal of salicylate from the body by alkalinising the urine is rational (see Ch. 10). Salicylic acid becomes ionised and lipid insoluble in the tubular fluid, it thus cannot diffuse into the tubular cells and remains in the lumen. The technique has been used successfully even in alkalotic adults. An adequate urine flow is desirable but diuresis induced by large volumes of i.v. fluid and frusemide does not aid salicylate clearance and can be dangerous. The essence of treatment is to keep the urine alkaline, ideally at pH 8, by infusing bicarbonate i.v. (sodium bicarbonate 1.4% is a convenient strength). *The practical importance of pH is shown by the fact that the amount of salicylate in urine at pH 8 is four times that at pH 7.* A high plasma salicylate concentration may be halved in about 8 h by this procedure. Replacement infusions of fluid, glucose and electrolytes may be interspersed with those of sodium bicarbonate, according to the patient's needs and blood and urine pH.

f. Haemodialysis or haemoperfusion can be done in specially equipped centres and are indicated when the plasma salicylate exceeds 900 mg/l. Exchange transfusion can be used for children. The decision to use these techniques should not be left until the patient is moribund. Patients, particularly children, poisoned by salicylate, can die in a very few hours.

Cautionary tale. A child who swallowed its mother's *enteric-coated* aspirin died because monitoring was not continued long enough; he was discharged from hospital prematurely.

Pyrazolone derivatives

Drugs of this group induce hepatic drug metabolising enzymes.

Azapropazone (Rheumox) (300, 600 mg) has anti-inflammatory, analgesic, antipyretic and uricosuric effects. It is well absorbed from the gut and maximum plasma concentration is attained within 4–6 h. The drug is 95% bound to plasma proteins, the $t_{\frac{1}{2}}$ is 20 h and over 60% is excreted as the unchanged drug in urine. Azapropazone is used to treat pain and inflammation in rheumatoid disease and other musculoskeletal disorders.

The dose is 1.2 g/day in 2 or 4 divided doses. Those taking the drug long-term should take a smaller dose; the elderly should take 300 mg in the morning and 300–600 mg at night.

Adverse effects include dyspepsia and gastrointestinal bleeding, headache, vertigo, oedema and allergic skin rashes. Interaction with coumarin anticoagulants, tolbutamide and phenytoin occurs, increasing the effect of these drugs.

Phenylbutazone, widely used for inflammatory arthropathies in the past, has been withdrawn from general availability on prescription in the UK because of toxicity, notably fluid retention (sufficient to cause cardiac failure), aplastic anaemia and agranulocytosis. It is still licenced to treat ankylosing spondylitis under specialist supervision. Oxyphenbutazone, which is similar, remains available as an ointment for ocular inflammation, e.g. iridocyclitis.

Phenazone (antipyrine) it is now obsolete as an antipyretic and analgesic but its pharmacokinetic properties (well absorbed, distributed throughout the body water, only 10% protein bound and 95% metabolised) render it useful as a research tool to measure differences in hepatic drug metabolising capacity.

Acetic acid derivatives

Indomethacin (indometacin, Indocid) (25, 50 mg) is a highly effective anti-inflammatory, analgesic and antipyretic agent. After oral administration, absorption from the gut is rapid and almost complete. The drug is 90% bound to plasma proteins. It is inactivated by the formation of metabolites, some of which undergo enterohepatic cycling and some drug is eliminated unchanged by the kidney. The $t_{\frac{1}{2}}$ is 7 h but can be variable because of enterohepatic recycling. Indomethacin is used to relieve moderate to severe pain and inflammation due to rheumatoid disease, acute musculoskeletal disorders and gout. It is also effective for pain due to pericardial inflammation after myocardial infarction.

The dose is 25–50 mg two or three times daily to a maximum of 200 mg in a day; a sustained-release formulation (75 mg) is available; a suppository of 100 mg at night is effective for relief of morning stiffness.

Adverse effects of indomethacin relate to its strong anti-inflammatory effect and include gastric irritation with ulcer formation, bleeding and perforation. Dyspeptic symptoms can be reduced if the drug is taken with food or as a suppository. Symptoms and signs of infection may be masked by indomethacin. Headache is common, often similar to migraine, and is attributed to cerebral oedema; it usually occurs soon after beginning treatment and can be limited by starting at a low dose and increasing only gradually. Vomiting, dizziness and ataxia may follow. Indomethacin may aggravate pre-existing renal disease. Thus the drug is best avoided when there is gastroduodenal, renal or central nervous system disease or in the presence of infection; it is not recommended for children. Allergic reactions occur and there is cross-reactivity with aspirin. Indomethacin may cause salt and fluid retention; it reduces the effectiveness of diuretic drugs (and may cause renal failure with triamterene) and counteracts the antihypertensive action of β-adrenoceptor antagonists, possibly by inhibiting renal prostaglandin synthesis. Concurrent use of probenecid raises indomethacin plasma concentration. Indomethacin may potentiate the effect of oral anticoagulants.

Sulindac (Clinoril) (100, 200 mg) is structurally related to indomethacin. It is a prodrug, i.e. the substance itself is relatively inactive but it is converted into an active sulphide metabolite in the body and by the gut flora (ileostomy patients have lower plasma concentrations of the sulphide). Unusually among the NSAIDs, the active (sulphide) metabolite of sulindac does not inhibit *renal* prostaglandin synthesis (see below). After an oral dose of sulindac, the plasma concentration of the sulphide metabolite reaches a peak about 3 h later and declines with a $t_{\frac{1}{2}}$ of 18 h. Both sulindac and its sulphide metabolite are more than 90% bound to plasma proteins.

Sulindac is used for pain and inflammation in rheumatoid disease, musculoskeletal disorders and in gout.

The dose is 50–200 mg twice daily with food.

Adverse effects. The anti-inflammatory action of sulindac is less than that of indomethacin, but so is its toxicity. In common with other NSAIDs, there are gastric effects, ranging from dyspepsia to peptic ulcer. The central nervous system effects described for indomethacin (above) also occur. Adverse effects on the kidney may be less likely as renal prostaglandin synthesis is not affected. Sulindac potentiates the effect of warfarin.

Diclofenac (Voltarol) appears to be similar in efficacy to the propionic acid derivatives. The drug is more than 95% bound to plasma proteins and the $t_{\frac{1}{2}}$ is 2 h. It is used for moderate pain and inflammation due to rheumatoid disease and musculoskeletal disorders. Gastrointestinal and central nervous system and other adverse effects occur in common with other members of this group. Diclofenac elevates plasma lithium concentration by interfering with its renal excretion.

Tolmetin has an anti-inflammatory action that is greater than aspirin but less than indomethacin. The drug is readily absorbed from the gastrointestinal tract, is 99% bound to plasma proteins and the $t_{\frac{1}{2}}$ is about 3 h. It is used to relieve pain and inflammation in rheumatoid disease and musculoskeletal disorders. Adverse effects and interactions are those of the NSAID group and may cause 10% of patients to discontinue the drug. Allergic or pseudoallergic reactions appear to be more common with tolmetin and may occur in those who are not allergic to aspirin or other NSAIDs.

Etodolac is extensively protein bound and the $t_{\frac{1}{2}}$ is 7 h. The pharmacokinetics do not appear to differ as between the young and the elderly. The drug is used in rheumatoid disease. It appears to be well tolerated.

Oxicam derivative

Piroxicam (Feldene) (20 mg) has anti-inflammatory action that is approximately equal to that of indomethacin. It is completely absorbed from the gastrointestinal tract and 99% is plasma protein bound. Enterohepatic cycling helps to maintain the plasma concentration and the $t_{\frac{1}{2}}$ is 48 h. Steady-state plasma concentrations appear not to alter significantly with age. Piroxicam is used for rheumatoid disease, musculoskelatal disorders and gout. The dose is 10–30 mg daily in single or divided doses. Adverse effects are those to be expected with NSAIDs, gastrointestinal and central nervous system complaints being the commonest.

DRUG TREATMENT OF RHEUMATOID DISEASE

Rheumatoid disease is characterised by a proliferative, invasive, destructive inflammation of synovial membrane, associated with systemic disturbance. It affects 1–3% of the population of Europe and North America. Best results are obtained with early treatment, physiotherapy, and drugs.

The first aim of drug therapy is to relieve pain and muscle stiffness using NSAIDs. If these measures do not control the symptoms and there is radiological evidence of progressive joint destruction or of extra-articular disease (e.g. vasculitis, rheumatoid lung), other drugs may be used in an attempt to modify the course of the disease or to induce its remission.

Relief of pain and muscle stiffness and suppression of inflammation

a. When the disease is mild, a reasonable course is to start with a *proprionic acid derivative* (fenbufen, fenoprofen, flurbiprofen, ibuprofen, indoprofen, ketoprofen, naproxen, suprofen, tiaprofenic acid) since these drugs are less toxic to the stomach than those with more prominent anti-inflammatory action, but they may also have less therapeutic efficacy. It may be necessary to try several within the group to find one that suits an individual patient; any drug selected should be used for 1–2 weeks before abandoning it. *Paracetamol* may be added if further analgesia is required.

b. More often the inflammation is rather more severe and a NSAID with more pronounced anti-inflammatory effect is needed. Some prefer *aspirin* (2–6 g/day) but the high dose needed (just below that which induces tinnitus) means that gastric intolerance is common. Salicylate plasma concentrations of 250 mg/l in adults or 300–350 mg/l in children are usually required but it is not routinely necessary to measure plasma concentrations as relief of symptoms is an adequate guide to therapy. Other forms of aspirin, e.g. benorylate, aloxiprin, may suit individual patients better. Alternatively, one of the other major anti-inflammatory drugs such as *indomethacin* or *piroxicam* may be used instead of aspirin. If nocturnal pain or morning stiffness is a problem, indomethacin given either orally (sustained release) or as a suppository at night may benefit because its duration of action is sufficiently long ($t_{\frac{1}{2}}$, 7 h).

Modification of the disease process

The decision to embark on treatment with disease-modifying drugs should be undertaken only by a physician with special experience of their use.

a. **Gold salts** appear to reduce immune responsiveness by inhibiting the migration of mononuclear cells into areas of inflammation; they may also stabilise lysosomal membranes and thus prevent the release of enzymes that damage cartilage.

Sodium aurothiomalate injection is commonly used but an oral form, *auranofin*, has been developed and is under evaluation. Distribution of gold is complex, it binds extensively to plasma albumin and is also distributed to inflamed synovium, kidney and liver. After a single dose the $t_{\frac{1}{2}}$ is about one week but it may be several weeks or months after long-term dosing. It is eliminated mainly by the kidney and to a lesser extent in the faeces, which it probably enters following biliary excretion. The drug is given by weekly (deep i.m.) injections, the objective of the therapeutic regimen being gradually to build up the amount of gold in the body to an effective concentration and then to deliver a maintenance dose until the disease becomes inactive. If there is no response within 4 months, it is probably best to change to another treatment.

Gold is used in patients with active, progressive disease, as shown by early deformities or radiological bone changes, in whom anti-inflammatory analgesics have failed and in whom it is wished to avoid beginning an adrenal steroid or to reduce steroid dosage. Evidence indicates that radiographic progression of the disease is slowed. Gold or penicillamine (see below) are probably the most effective agents for preventing progression of the arthritis, best results being obtained in early cases. In the event of failure to respond to gold, penicillamine should be tried and vice versa (but not together); 80% of patients will respond to one or other.

Adverse effects occur in about one-third of patients and in some gold may have to be discontinued. They include pruritus, dermatitis, glossitis and stomatitis, most commonly, and also blood disorders, hepatic and renal damage, peripheral neuritis and encephalopathy. The patient should be warned to report any untoward symptoms at once. Serious effects are rare if the patient is carefully observed and the drug stopped at the earliest sign of toxicity. The urine should be examined for protein before each injection. Gold should be stopped at once on the appearance of any toxic effect and should not be given again unless the reaction was trivial, in which case it may be recommenced at lower dose after the toxic effect has disappeared, but not before 6 weeks have passed. Any serious effect, or one that does not subside rapidly, should be treated with a chelating agent; dimercaprol is probably preferable to penicillamine, an adrenal steroid may be useful, as at least some of the toxicity is due to allergy.

b. **Penicillamine** (Distamine) may benefit rheumatoid arthritis by modifying immune processes; it interferes with the activation of complement and suppresses immunoglobulin production. The drug also chelates a number of metals (including gold), which action is valuable in poisoning (see Ch. 10). It is well absorbed following administration by mouth; after a single oral dose the $t_{\frac{1}{2}}$ is 60 h but when chronic dosing is discontinued, plasma concentration falls with a $t_{\frac{1}{2}}$ of 176 h, suggesting that the drug is being released from a tissue store. It is eliminated in the urine. The indications for using penicillamine are those described for gold (above). Adverse effects are also frequent with penicillamine. They may cause one-third of patients to discontinue the drug but can be reduced if the dose is raised only at monthly intervals. A number of patients experience gastrointestinal upset (anorexia, nausea, vomiting, diarrhoea) and dose-related impairment of taste is common; the latter usually recovers despite continuation of treatment. Thrombocytopenia is frequent but resolves when the drug is withdrawn unless it is an indication of the more serious aplastic anaemia that penicillamine may also cause. Allergic reactions, including rashes and fever, tend to occur during the early stages of treatment. Proteinuria may develop during the sixth and 12th month of treatment; it appears to be dose-related and if it is heavy, penicillamine should be stopped, for nephrotic syndrome may develop if it is not. All patients who receive penicillamine should be closely supervised and blood and urine must be monitored.

Captopril, which was introduced for its cardiovascular effects as an angiotensin converting enzyme inhibitor, has a structural similarity to penicillamine and is being evaluated for treating rheumatoid disease.

c. **Antimalarials** of the chloroquine group were tried in rheumatoid arthritis following improvement of the arthritis of discoid lupus erythematosus during antimalarial treatment of its skin manifestations. They offer an alternative to gold, penicillamine and other immunosuppressive drugs as they are less toxic, but they are also less effective.

Chloroquine is described with other antimalarials in Chapter 14. In rheumatoid arthritis benefit is not seen for about 4 weeks; up to 50% of patients may respond usefully. Chloroquine accumulates in many organs, including the eye, where it can cause retinal damage that may be irreversible; this is the principal disadvantage of its use in rheumatoid disease, which must necessarily be long-term. Serious ocular damage should be avoided if the dose of chloroquine is below 3.5 mg/kg (hydroxychloroquine 6.5 mg/kg) but patients should have an ophthalmological examination before starting, and every 6 months during therapy.

An attempt should be made to withdraw the drug slowly in less than a year. Omission of the drug for 3 months every 4–6 months (drug holiday) may allow prolonged therapy with safety.

Hydroxychloroquine is an alternative that may cause less adverse effects.

d. **Sulphasalazine** has recently been reintroduced for the treatment of rheumatoid arthritis, a condition for which it was first used in 1940. The drug is poorly absorbed from the gastrointestinal tract so that most reaches the colon where it is split into sulphapyridine and 5-aminosalicylic acid. The active part is probably sulphapyridine, which reduces antigen absorption from the gut; the mild anti-inflammatory action of 5-aminosalicylic acid is likely to make a limited contribution at most. Sulphasalazine is further described in Chapter 32, for its main use is to control inflammatory bowel disease. Its therapeutic efficacy in rheumatoid disease appears to equal that of gold; the doses necessary to achieve this are greater than those normally used for ulcerative colitis and adverse effects, notably dyspepsia, can be troublesome. Treatment can however be continued indefinitely.

e. **Immunomodulator drugs** may be justified for they can produce improvement in severe rheumatoid arthritis. The rationale for their use is not completely clear, for the group includes drugs that both suppress and stimulate the immune system.

Azathioprine (Imuran) is an immunosuppressive that is as effective as gold or pencillamine and like these drugs it can be used for its corticosteroid-sparing effect in patients who have received excessive corticosteroid. Marrow suppression may develop and regular blood counts should be performed. Alementary disturbance also occurs. Other immunosuppressives such as *cyclophosphamide* and *chlorambucil* are more effective but carry a greater risk of toxicity and should be reserved for cases resistant to less toxic drugs. Radiographic evidence indicates that cyclophosphamide retards joint destruction. Immunosuppressives are carcinogenic and the magnitude of this risk, which is particularly important in younger patients with a long life expectancy, is uncertain; they are also mutagenic and teratogenic, so that precautions to avoid reproduction whilst taking the drugs are essential for both sexes. *Chlorambucil* and *methotrexate* have also been tried with some success, as indeed have total lymphoid and total body irradiation.

Levamisole, first used as an anthelmintic, is also immunostimulant, bringing lowered immune responses to normal (not above). It appears to be as effective in rheumatoid arthritis as are gold and penicillamine but adverse effects limit its use.

The use of adrenal steroids

A systemic adrenal steroid may be used for a patient who has failed to respond to several second rank agents or if these drugs produce intolerable adverse effects. Furthermore, since the therapeutic benefit of second rank drugs may take several weeks to develop, a corticosteroid may be combined with these agents to provide interim relief of inflammatory symptoms.

Instead of the usual daily therapy, a single enormous dose, e.g. methylprednisolone 1 g i.m. monthly for 1–3 months is sometimes used for convenience. It is also appropriate to use a corticosteroid when it is known that the duration of the course will be short, as in the case of a rheumatoid patient who is terminally ill with another condition. Apart from indications such as these, however, most rheumatologists are reluctant to start systemic corticosteroids for rheumatoid disease because of the danger of unwanted effects. There is no doubt that, say, prednisolene 20–40 mg/day, will very effectively suppress inflammation that is inordinately severe (e.g. with vasculitis or rheumatoid lung) and indeed prednisolone administered over a period of months may actually slow down aggressive or rapidly progressing disease. The object of using a systemic corticosteroid is to reduce inflammation in affected joints at a dose that is sufficiently low to administer with safety over a long period. When the decision to use systemic corticosteroid is taken the total daily maintenance dose should not exceed prednisolone 7.5 mg or its equivalent of other steroids and once-daily administration at 08:00 may minimise adrenal suppression. Corticotrophin (see index) may be used instead of an oral corticosteroid to manage a particularly acute exacerbation of the disease. The dose of tetrocosactrin should not exceed 1 mg per week, and preferably the total course of corticotrophin should not exceed 2–3 weeks.

Intra-articular injection of corticosteroid (e.g. triamcinolone, hydrocortisone, prednisolone, dexamethasone) is very effective when one joint is relatively more affected than others. Benefit from one injection may last many weeks (shorter in active cases). Aseptic precautions must be extreme, for the steroid will suppress inflammatory response and any introduced infection may spread destructively and dramatically. With repetition, enough may be absorbed into the blood to cause adrenal suppression. The placebo effect of intra-articular injection is great. Too frequent resort to corticosteroid injection may actually promote joint damage by removing the protective limitation conferred by pain; such injections should not exceed two or three per year.

Choice of drugs in rheumatoid arthritis can be summed thus:

1. *NSAIDs* should be used first, usually a propionic acid derivative, and the choice of any particular drug will depend on the amount of pain or inflammation present and on patient tolerance.

When inflammation is prominent, a NSAID with high-efficacy anti-inflammatory action, e.g. *indomethacin* or *piroxicam*, is justified. *Local* injections of *corticosteroid* are valuable for individual joints that are more severely affected.

2. *Disease-modifying drugs* should be used when inflammatory symptoms persist and when radiological evidence indicates progression of joint damage. Evidence suggests that these drugs slow the progress of the disease although they may not reduce the ultimate degree of deformity and disability. There is now a tendency to employ them earlier, sometimes within three months of onset of the disease. *Gold*, *penicillamine* and *sulphasalazine* appear to have a similar therapeutic efficacy, but sulphasalazine is significantly the least toxic; the *immunosuppressives* are more effective and more toxic; the *antimalarials* are less effective and less toxic.

3. *Systemic corticosteroids* tend to be reserved for cases with inflammation so severe that it cannot be controlled by the second rank (disease modifying) drugs.

Other aspects of the treatment of this disease are important but are outside the scope of this book.

Rheumatic fever

So effective are salicylates in relieving pain and inflammation in rheumatic fever that failure to respond within 48 h throws doubts on the diagnosis. From their introduction into therapeutics, adrenocortical steroids have also been used. They provide dramatic relief but should be reserved to replace salicylates in patients with severe carditis. Neither salicylate nor adrenal steroid prevent the development of late cardiac complications.

In the acute stage, soluble aspirin in a dose of about 100 mg/kg/day should be given. Sodium salicylate should be avoided because the extra sodium intake adds to the risk of cardiac failure (below). In the adult a plasma salicylate concentration of 250 mg/l is usually effective but in children levels up to 350 mg/l may be required. Dosing in the individual patient will be adjusted according to the tolerance of salicylate and relief of symptoms. In most mild cases treatment is continued for 6 weeks.

When there is evidence of carditis with cardiac enlargement or pericarditis, a corticosteroid should be used instead of salicylate since the latter may precipitate cardiac failure (by raising plasma volume and increasing peripheral uptake of oxygen, which necessitates greater cardiac output). Prednisolone 10–15 mg/day is usually sufficient and specific therapy for cardiac failure may also be necessary. A 10-day course of benzylpenicillin should be given to kill any streptococci. For prophylaxis see Chapter 13 (Infection of the throat).

Osteoarthritis

Any NSAID may be used, depending on the amount of pain and inflammation experienced by the patient, and on the tolerance of adverse effects. There is no general case for using intra-articular corticosteroid in osteoarthritis but local injection of triamcinolone can provide relief for a single periarticular tender spot or for a knee joint that is acutely inflamed.

Ankylosing spondylitis

Indomethacin is effective and may also be needed at night to treat stiffness the next morning. Adrenal steroids are rarely used. Phenylbutazone is very effective but it is also toxic.* In severe cases, where it gives relief but causes gastrointestinal toxicity, suppositories may be substituted for oral therapy. The value of radiotherapy is controversial. Physical methods of treatment including active exercises are the first importance to prevent deformity.

DRUGS AND GOUT

Gout is characterised by acute attacks of arthritis due to chronic deposits (tophi) of monosodium

* In the UK phenylbutazone is available only through hospitals, i.e. general practitioners are not trusted to use it with restraint. This may be thought extraordinary and has, not surprisingly, annoyed general practitioners. Phenylbutazone *was* a first choice NSAID until the ingenuity of industrial drug developers produced effective alternatives that are less toxic. Patients are inconvenienced by being unable to get supplies from their general practitioner.

urate in and about cartilage and kidneys and by urate nephrolithiasis. The condition affects about 0.25% of the population of Europe and North America. Drugs are effective in the management of gout but some drugs can precipitate the disorder.

Some physiology and pathophysiology

Uric acid is a constituent of purine bases (guanine, adenine) that take part in the formation of nucleic acids. The urate pool in a normal man on a purine-free diet is about 1200 mg and in a woman about half that. Patients with gout but no visible tophi have a urate pool that is two or three times normal and since this exceeds the amount that can be carried in solution in the extracellular fluid, microcrystalline deposits form; patients with tophi have a urate pool that may be 15–26 times normal. Urate is mainly excreted by the kidney and the following processes are relevant: being only 5% bound to plasma proteins, it is freely filtered by the glomerulus and then reabsorbed from the tubule lumen and also secreted from the blood into the lumen; the urate that appears in the urine represents the excess of secretion over reabsorption, which are both active, energy-requiring processes that can be affected by drugs.

Two phenomena are necessary for an attack of gout: (a) crystals of monosodium urate are deposited from hyperuricaemic body fluids (the detailed factors that start this process are still largely obscure) and (b) a local inflammatory response to the presence of the crystals with phagocytosis (of the crystals). It is known that actively phagocytic leucocytes produce lactic acid, and this promotes urate crystallisation, for urates are less soluble in an acid medium. With more crystallation there is more inflammation and more phagocytosis with more lactic acid production, and a self-propagating, self-stimulating inflammatory reaction results. Inflammation is also enhanced by digestive enzymes released from leucocyte lysosomes.

Hyperuricaemia and gout may therefore result from two principal processes.

1. *Underexcretion of urate* due to
   a. a primary renal abnormality
   b. drugs that interfere with the tubular handling of urate; these include all diuretics (except spironolactone), aspirin (in low dose, see below), pyrazinamide, nicotinic acid, and alcohol (which increases urate synthesis and also forms lactic acid that inhibits tubular secretion of urate).
2. *Overproduction of urate* due to
   a. various enzyme defects that increase purine biosynthesis.
   b. excessive cell destruction releasing nucleic acids, as occurs when myeloproliferative or lymphoproliferative disorders are treated by drugs or radiotherapy.

Drugs that are effective in the management of gout are as follows:

A. *Drugs that suppress the symptoms — anti-inflammatory drugs with or without analgesic effect*: azapropazone, diclofenac, indomethacin, naproxen, piroxicam and sulindac; colchicine; adrenal steroids and corticotrophin.

B. *Drug that prevents urate synthesis*: allopurinol.

C. *Drugs that promote elimination of urate — uricosurics*: probenecid, sulphinpyrazone.

Anti-inflammatory and analgesic drugs

Except for colchicine, those listed above in this category are described earlier in the chapter or elsewhere.

Colchicine (0.5 mg) is an alkaloid from the autumn crocus. It is an antimitotic agent obsolete in neoplastic disease, but valuable in gout, in which it relieves the pain and inflammation in a few hours. Such rapid relief is considered to confirm the diagnosis because non-gouty arthritis is unaffected, though failure does not prove the patient has not gout. The precise reason for the curious specificity of colchicine in relieving the pain of gout is not certainly known but the likely explanation is that colchicine inhibits the migration of leucocytes into the inflamed area and thus it interrupts the inflammatory cycle described above.

Colchicine is absorbed from the gut, some is metabolised in the liver and some is excreted unchanged in the bile and reabsorbed from the gut. This enhances its gut toxicity. The $t_{\frac{1}{2}}$ is 20 min.

In acute gout colchicine 1 mg may be given by mouth, followed by 0.5–1 mg 2-hourly until either relief or adverse effects occur. Benefit is usually felt in 2–3 h and is marked within 12 h. The total needed is usually 3–6 mg and it is unwise to exceed 10 mg. Once the effective dose is known, patients can take this total at once when they feel an attack coming on, and then 0.5 mg hourly.

Colchicine is an effective suppressant prophylactic against gout in doses of 0.5–1 mg per day, or on alternate days. Colchicine is also the mainstay of therapy for familial Mediterranean fever; it prevents both the disabling febrile attacks and the amyloidosis to which these patients are prone.

Adverse effects may be severe, with abdominal pain, vomiting and diarrhoea, which may be bloody. It is probably due to inhibition of mitosis in the rapidly reproducing cells of the intestinal mucosa. Renal damage can occur, and, rarely, blood disorders. Large doses cause muscular paralysis.

Blockade of uric acid synthesis

Allopurinol (Zyloric) (100 mg) inhibits xanthine oxidase, the enzyme that converts xanthine and hypoxanthine to uric acid. Patients taking allopurinol excrete less urate and more xanthine and hypoxanthine in the urine; these compounds are both more readily excreted in renal failure and are more soluble than urate so that xanthine stones rarely form. Allopurinol was first used in leukaemia therapy to prevent the oxidation of the active 6-mercaptopurine to an inactive metabolite, and its effect on uric acid synthesis was noticed. If an ordinary dose of 6-mercaptopurine be given to a patient whose gout is being treated with allopurinol, dangerous potentiation occurs.

Allopurinol is readily absorbed from the gut, it is metabolised in the liver to alloxathine, which is also a xanthine oxidase inhibitor; it is excreted unchanged and as alloxanthine by the kidney. The $t_{\frac{1}{2}}$ is 5 h.

Allopurinol is indicated where there is renal failure, where urate lithiasis has occurred or where tophi are extensive, in blood diseases in which there is spontaneous hyperuricaemia, and during treatment of myeloproliferative disorders when cell destruction creates a high urate load. Allopurinol prevents hyperuricaemia due to diuretics. It can be combined with a uricosuric agent.

During about the first two months of therapy there is increased risk of acute gout, despite a reduction in blood urate. This may be due to a falling and fluctuating plasma urate concentration encouraging the solution and perhaps intermittent recrystallisation of urate from tophi. A NSAID or colchicine should be used as a suppressant during this period, and patients should be warned of the possibility, for it can create an unfavourable impression if the patient, who has been told only that the drug will prevent gout, promptly has a severe attack.

A single daily dose of 300 mg by mouth is usually adequate but up to 600 mg or even more in total may be given in severe cases.

Adverse effects apart from the precipitation of acute gout (above) are rare and include allergies of various kinds, leucopenia, gut upsets and liver damage.

Uricosurics

Probenecid (Benemid) (0.5 g) is a uricoscuric agent. It is not an analgesic. Probenecid was introduced when penicillin was in very short supply and there was a need for agents that would prevent its active excretion by the renal tubule and so enable high plasma concentration to be maintained by small doses. Probenecid does this effectively, but as penicillin has become so cheap and freely available, the objective is usually achieved now by simply increasing its dose. Probenecid is, however, occasionally used in infections where exceptionally high penicillin plasma concentration is desired, as in some cases of infective endocarditis, in children in whom large and frequent injections are specially unpleasant, and where the maximum effect is needed from a single dose treatment, e.g. in gonorrhoea, when patient default is common.

Probenecid inhibits the transport of organic acids across various epithelia of which the most important is the kidney tubule. The effect depends on the dose given: a small dose prevents tubular secretion and actually prevents urate loss but an adequate dose inhibits reabsorption of urate from the tubular lumen and has a useful uricosuric effect.

Probenecid is 90% bound to plasma proteins, partly metabolised and partly excreted unchanged in the urine. The $t_{\frac{1}{2}}$ depends on the dose and varies from 5 to 8 h.

The dose to prevent gout is probenecid 0.5 g by mouth per day for the first week, rising to 1–2 g total/day. The blood urate concentration falls rapidly at first, and then levels off about two thirds of the original concentration. As the initial loss is high, crystals of urate may appear in the urine unless it is maintained at pH 6 or above for the first month of probenecid (or any other uricosuric) administration (e.g. with Potassium Citrate Mixture 12–24 g/day with water or Sodium Bicarbonate Powder 5–10 g/day with water). A high fluid intake (3 l/day) should also be taken to avoid the dangers of mechanical obstruction or stone formation. During sleeping hours the urine may be kept both alkaline and dilute by taking a single tablet of acetazolamide 250 mg on retiring. Patients who have renal insufficiency should be carefully supervised (and potassium citrate may cause dangerous hyperkalaemia). Probenecid should not be used if there is renal failure (see allopurinol): it may be ineffective and may worsen renal damage.

Probenecid causes gastrointestinal upset in a few patients and allergy occasionally. It blocks renal tubular excretion and prolongs the effect of organic acids in addition to the penicillins (above) and these include cephalosporins, naproxen, indomethacin, methotrexate and sulphonylureas.

Sulphinpyrazone (Anturan) (100 mg) is related to phenylbutazone and acts like probenecid. It is a highly effective uricosuric and alkalinisation of the urine and high fluid intake (see below) are necessary at first to avoid crystalluria. For this reason dosage may begin with 50 mg by mouth 12-hourly, rising to 100 mg 6-hourly over a few weeks. It may be possible to reduce to half that dose later. Sulphinpyrazone causes gastric upset and is contraindicated in peptic ulcer.

Sulphinpyrazone has also been tested for prevention of myocardial reinfarction. In a large, randomised double-blind trial* in patients treated for a year after myocardial infarction, the death rate from cardiac causes was 4.9% in the sulphinpyrazone group as compared with 9.5% in the placebo group. The effect may be related to its action of reducing platelet adhesiveness and aggregation.

Aspirin and salicylates should be avoided in gout (the patient should be warned of the ubiquity of aspirin in proprietary preparations) because small doses inhibit urate secretion, causing urate to be retained (see *probenecid* above).

DRUG TREATMENT OF GOUT

Acute gout. NSAIDs are highly effective in acute gout, terminating the attack in a few hours. It is important to begin treatment as early as possible. Indomethacin is a first choice and may be given in a dose of 25–50 mg orally three times a day with a fourth (sometimes larger) dose at night. Gastrointestinal symptoms are reduced if the drug is taken with food. The bed time dose can be given as a suppository (100 mg). Naproxen, diclofenac, sulindac, piroxicam and azapropazone are effective alternatives. Colchicine is traditional and may be used when patients cannot tolerate NSAIDs. It may be the drug of first choice in a *first* attack of severe monarticular arthritis, as a good response helps make the diagnosis, which can be difficult. Other anti-inflammatory drugs are non-selective.

If these drugs fail, prednisolone may be used starting with 40 mg per day and reducing as quickly as symptoms allow. Withdrawal may be followed by relapse and it may be prudent to add colchicine to cover this stage.

Useless agents. It requires only a moment's thought to appreciate that uricosurics and allopurinol are useless in *acute* attacks.

Recurrent and progressive gout may be prevented by:

a. persuading the patient to avoid debauchery (see below), and

b. allopurinol or a uricosuric drug if the serum urate consistently exceeds 0.6 mmol/l and the patient has had three or more attacks of acute gout.

Therapy should begin in a quiescent period. Allopurinol is usually preferred and is the treatment of choice if the patient has impaired renal function (see above). Allopurinol may be combined with uricosurics. *Salicylates must not be given concurrently with other uricosurics* as they interfere

* The Anturane Reinfarction Trial Research Group. N Engl J Med 1978; 298:289.

with their action (see above). Paracetamol may be used as an analgesic without interfering with therapy.

Colchicine also prevents gout, probably by suppressing acute attacks at their inception. It has no effect on urate excretion.

Rapid lowering of plasma urate by any means may precipitate acute gout, probably by causing the dissolution of tophi. It is therefore usual to give prophylactic suppressive treatment with indomethacin during the first two months of treatment with allopurinol or uricosurics, and with the latter the urine should be made alkaline and the volume maintained high to avoid crystalluria.

Benefit from the lowered plasma urate will not be noticeable for some weeks. Medication should be adjusted to keep the plasma urate in the normal range. It can seldom be abandoned. Colchicine or indomethacin prophylaxis alone is undesirable, for the plasma urate remains high, allowing the disease process to continue (tophi, renal damage).

Chronic tophaceous gout. Tophi can sometimes be reduced in size and even removed by the use of allopurinol and uricosuric agents and allopurinol.

Acute *pyrophosphate arthropathy* responds similarly to acute gout.

Precipitation of gout by diuretics. Any vigorous diuresis may precipitate acute gout by causing volume depletion, which results in increased reabsorption of all substances that are normally reabsorbed in the proximal renal tubule, including urate. Furthermore most diuretics are organic acids that may compete with urate for secretion by the renal tubule; this effect is antagonised by allopurinol and uricosurics.

Diet, alcohol and gout

Gouty patients tend also to be overweight and loss of weight lowers the plasma urate. However, obese patients on starvation treatment may develop gout due to ketosis causing precipitation of urate (due to acidity) in tissues, and some advocate allopurinol at this time.

Knowledge that alcohol induces acute gout is of long standing, and has been celebrated in verse:

A taste for drink, combined with gout,
Had doubled him up for ever.
Of *that* there is no manner of doubt —
No probable, possible shadow of doubt —
No possible doubt whatever.*

But the poet did not know of the mechanisms. Alcohol increases the liability to acute gout by raising urate production and by causing lactic acidosis (which causes urate to precipitate in tissue and blocks its excretion by the renal tubule).

* W S Gilbert (1836–1911). *The Bab Ballads: The Highly Respectable Gondolier*.

GUIDE TO FURTHER READING

1 Nuki G. Non-steroidal and anti-inflammatory agents. Br Med J 1983; 287: 39–43.
2 Editorial. Non-steroidal anti-inflammatory drugs: Have we been spoilt for choice? Lancet 1984; 1: 141–142.
3 Clive D M, Stoff J S. Renal syndromes associated with nonsteroidal antiinflammatory drugs. N Engl J Med 1984; 310: 563–572.
4 Editorial. Patent ductus and indomethacin. Lancet 1981; 1:877.
5 Balali-Mood M et al. Mefenamic acid overdose. Lancet. 1981; 1: 1354–1356.
6 Taha A et al. Non-oliguric renal failure during treatment with mefenamic acid in elderly patients: a continuing problem. Br Med J 1985; 291: 661–662.
7 Zimran A et al. Incidence of hyperkalaemia induced by indomethacin in a hospital population. Br Med J 1985; 291: 107–108.
8 Pullar T et al. Which component of sulphasalazine is active in rheumatoid arthritis? Br Med J 1985; 290: 1535–1538.
9 Iannuzzi L et al. Does drug therapy slow radiographic deterioration in rheumatoid arthritis? N Engl J Med 1983; 309: 1023–1028.
10 Editorial. Oral gold for rheumatoid arthritis. Br Med J 1984; 289: 858–895.
11 Editorial. Penicillamine nephropathy. Br Med J 1981; 282: 761–762.
12 Fleck B W et al. Screening for antimalarial maculopathy in rheumatoid clinics. Br Med J 1985; 291: 782–785.
13 Wright V. Treatment of severe rheumatoid arthritis. Br Med J 1986; 292: 431–432.
14 Gardner D L. The nature and cause of osteoarthritis. Br Med J 1983; 286: 418–424.
15 O'Hare J P et al. Observations on the effects of immersion in Bath spa water. Br Med J 1985; 291: 1747–1751.
16 McCarthy D J. Editorial. Treating intractable rheumatoid arthritis. N Engl J Med 1981; 305: 1009–1010.
17 Prockop D J et al. Biosynthesis of collagen and its disorders. N Engl J Med 1979; 301: 13–23, 77–85.

18 Editorial. Interleukin-1 in defence of the host. Lancet 1985; 1: 536–537.
19 Million R et al. Long-term study of management of rheumatoid arthritis. Lancet 1984; 1: 812–816.
20 Boss G R et al. Hyperuricaemia and gout. Classification, complications and management. N Engl J Med 1979; 300: 1459–1468.
21 Scott T J. Editorial. Food, drink and gout. Br Med J 1983; 287: 78–79.
22 Somerville K et al. Non-steroidal anti-inflammatory drugs and bleeding peptic ulcer. Lancet 1986; 1: 462–464.

16

Central nervous system I: Pain and analgesics: Drugs in terminal illness

Pain is the commonest symptom that takes a patient to a doctor. The fact that a patient has a pain does not mean a drug is required, but analgesics play a major role in the management of pain whether or not the patient's problem, e.g. trauma, pleurisy, osteoarthrosis will be resolved, or better managed, by non-drug therapy. Optimal management of a disease or symptom requires that the clinician should have a conceptual framework for what is happening to the victim, and this is very true of pain. The choice and use of analgesics and adjuvant drugs in acute and in chronic pain need to be based on concepts of what is happening in the patient's body and mind.

One of the greatest services doctors can do their patients is to acquire skill in the management of pain.

. . . For what avails
Valour or strength, though matchless, quelled with pain,
Which all subdues, and makes remiss the hands
Of mightiest? Sense of pleasure we may well
Spare out of life perhaps, and not repine,
But live content — which is the calmest life;
But pain is perfect misery, the worst
Of evils, and, excessive, overturns
All patience.*

Definitions

Pain is an unpleasant sensory and emotional experience associated with actual or potential tissue damage, or described in terms of such damage.† The word 'unpleasant' comprises the whole range of disagreeable feelings from being merely inconvenienced to misery, anguish, anxiety, depression and desperation, to the ultimate cure of suicide.‡

Analgesic drug. A drug that relieves pain due to multiple causes (e.g. aspirin, paracetamol, morphine). Drugs that relieve pain due to a single cause or specific pain syndrome only, e.g. gastric antacids, ergotamine (migraine), carbamazepine (neuralgias), glyceryl trinitrate (angina pectoris), are not classed as analgesics; adrenocortical steroids that suppress pain due to inflammation of any cause are also not classed as analgesics despite their extensive use to relieve pain.

Analgesics are classed as **narcotic** (which act in the central nervous system and cause drowsiness, i.e. opioids) and **non-narcotic** (which act chiefly peripherally, e.g. paracetamol, aspirin).

Adjuvant drugs or co-analgesics are those used alongside analgesics in the management of pain; they are not themselves analgesics, though they

* John Milton (1608–1674). Paradise Lost. Book 6. 456–464.
† Merskey H et al. Pain terms: a list with definitions and notes on usage. Pain 1979; 6:249.
‡ Melzack R, Wall P. The challenge of pain. London: Penguin. 1982.

may modify the perception or the concomitants of pain that make it worse (anxiety, fear, depression*), e.g. psychotropic drugs, or they may modify underlying causes, e.g. spasm of smooth or of voluntary muscle.

The phenomenon of pain

It used to be thought that pain was explicable by a physiologically simple concept. Tissue injury or disease activated specific pain receptors that passed impulses to a 'pain centre' in the central nervous system where they entered consciousness as pain. Treatment consisted of removing the causes, of suppressing the pain impulses so that they did not enter consciousness or, failing that, of depressing consciousness; morphine both suppressed the impulses and altered consciousness and was good for severe pain; codeine and aspirin were suitable for milder pain.

The chief inadequacies of this oversimple picture are *four*; lack of recognition, (a) that pain could occur without tissue injury or evident disease and could persist after injury had healed, (b) that serious tissue injury could occur without pain, (c) that emotion (anxiety, fear, depression) was an inseparable concomitant of pain, that it could modify both its intensity and the victim's behavioural response and, (d) that there is important processing of afferent nociceptive (see below) and other impulses in the central nervous system (spinal cord and brain).

Appreciation that pain is both a sensory and an emotional (affective) experience has allowed clinicians to realize that automatically to meet a complaint of pain of any sort with a prescription alone is not an adequate response, for 'There is always more to analgesia than analgesics',† and that pain that is not the subject of a simple analysis by the clinician (and explanation to the patient) may be inadequately relieved because of lack of understanding, which also causes lack of resoluteness and tenacity in management. That doctors often do not provide adequate relief of severe pain (post-surgical, terminal care of advanced cancer) by bad choice and by overusing and, also important, underusing drugs, and defective relations with their patients, has been, and still is, a justified and shaming criticism.

Pain is not simply a perception, it is a complex phenomenon or syndrome, only one component of which is the sensation actually reported as pain.

Pain has four major components present to varying extent in any one case:

1. *Nociception*‡ is a consequence of tissue injury (physical trauma, disease): nociceptors are specialized nerve endings serving their own afferent fibres (A-delta and C); nociception is not due to overstimulation of touch or other receptors.

2. *Pain* is a result of nociceptive input plus a pattern of impulses of different frequency and intensity from other peripheral receptors, and of their processing in the central nervous system; but pain can occur without nociception (some neuralgias§) and nociception does not invariably cause pain; pain is a psychological state though most pain has an immediately antecedent physical cause.

3. *Suffering* is a consequence of pain and of lack of understanding by patients of the meaning of the pain; it comprises anxiety and fear (particularly in acute pain) and depression (particularly in chronic pain), which will be affected by patients' personalities and beliefs about the significance of the pain, e.g. merely a postponed holiday, or death, or a future of disability with dependence on others. Depression makes a major contribution to suffering; it is treatable, as are the other affective concomitants of pain.

4. *Pain behaviour* comprises consequences of the above, it includes behaviour that is interpreted by others as signifying pain in the victim, e.g. such immediate and obvious aspects as facial expression, restlessness, seeking isolation (or company), medicine-taking, as well as, in chronic pain, the development of querulousness, depression, despair and social withdrawal.

The clinician's task is to determine the significance of these items for each patient and to direct therapy accordingly. Analgesics may, but not necessarily will, be the mainstay of therapy; adjuvant

* Tricyclic antidepressants may reduce morphine requirement in terminal care without noticeably altering mood.

† Twycross R G. J R Coll Physicians Lond 1984; 18:32.

‡ Latin: *noxa*: injury.

§ *Neuralgia* is pain felt in the distribution of a nerve.

(non-analgesic) drugs may be needed, as well as non-drug therapy (radiation, surgery).

It is also useful to distinguish between *acute pain* (an *event* whose end can be predicted) and *chronic pain* (a *situation* whose end is commonly unpredictable, or will only end with life itself).

Acute pain with major nociceptive input (physical trauma, pleurisy, myocardial infarct, perforated peptic ulcer) is seen by patients as a transient, though sometimes severe threat and they react accordingly. It is a symptom that may be dealt with unhesitatingly and effectively with drugs at the same time as the causative disease is assailed. The accompanying anxiety will vary according to the severity of the pain, and particularly according to its meaning for the patient, whether termination with recovery will soon occur, major surgery is threatened, or there is prospect of death or invalidism. The choice of drug will depend on the clinician's assessment of these factors. Morphine by injection has retained a pre-eminent place for over 100 years because it has highly effective antinociceptive and anti-anxiety effects; modern opioids have not rendered morphine obsolete, or even obsolescent, for acute severe pain.

Acute pain without nociceptive input (some neuralgias) is less susceptible to drugs unless consciousness is also depressed, and any frequently recurrent acute pain (e.g. trigeminal neuralgia) poses management problems that are more akin to chronic pain.

Chronic pain is better regarded as a syndrome* rather than as a symptom (see above). It presents a depressing future to the victim who sees no prospect of release from suffering, and poses long-term management problems that are different from acute pain. Suffering and affective disorders can be of overriding importance and the consequences of poor management may be prolonged and serious for the patient. Analgesics alone are often insufficient and adjuvant drugs as well as non-drug therapy gain increasing importance. Even when they are effective in chronic pain, the high-efficacy opioids (morphine, pethidine) alter mood and carry a substantial risk of dependence that will have adverse consequences in the long term. Continuous use of these drugs is best avoided in chronic pain, *except* that of terminal care. But the lower efficacy opioids (codeine, dextropropoxyphene) may often be needed.

Sedative-hypnotic drugs, e.g. benzodiazepines, may be needed for anxiety but may induce depression.

Antidepressants can often be useful.

Chronic pain syndrome is a term used for persistence of pain when detectable disease has disappeared, e.g. after an attack of low back pain. It characteristically does not respond to standard treatment with analgesics. Whether the basis is neurogenic, psychogenic or sociocultural it should not be managed by intensifying drug treatment. Opioid analgesics, which may be producing dependence, should be withdrawn and the use of psychotropic drugs, e.g. antidepressants or neuroleptics, and non-drug therapy, including psychotherapy, should be considered.

Further considerations of the causes and management of pain, and on the choice and use of analgesics

1. *Tissue injury* causes a diverse pattern and intensity of impulses to enter the spinal cord, where complex processing occurs. Pain is triggered when the input exceeds a critical level and impulses pass up to the brain where they are processed in the reticular and limbic systems particularly, and whence modulating inhibitory impulses pass down to regulate/inhibit the continuing afferent input. There is no 'pain centre' in the brain.

2. *Endogenous opioid neurotransmitter mechanisms* (endorphins, dynorphins, enkephalins) in the spinal cord and brain constitute an inhibitory system that is activated by nociceptive and other input, including treatments such as transcutaneous nerve stimulation and acupuncture. Administered opioids (morphine) produce analgesia by their selective action on the specific opioid receptors of this system. The fact that there are several types of receptor (mu, delta, kappa, epsilon, sigma) explains the differing patterns of actions of opioids and gives hope that selective new high-

* A set of symptoms and signs that are characteristic of a condition though they may not always have the same cause (Greek: *syn* together, *dramein* to run)

efficacy analgesics free from the disadvantages of the existing opioids may be designed.

Naloxone (competitive opioid antagonist or receptor blocker) can oppose the effects of endogenous opioids, at least to some degree, and has been found, as expected, to worsen (dental) pain.* Naloxone does not induce hyperalgesia or spontaneous pain because the opioid paths are quiescent until activated by nociceptive and other afferent input. Interestingly, naloxone has been found (in some studies) to reduce placebo effect.

In addition to these opioid mechanisms, non-opioid mediated pathways are important in pain. There is suggestion that opioid pathways are more important in acute severe pain, and non-opioid paths in chronic pain, and that this may be relevant to choice of drugs.

3. When a tissue is injured (any cause), or even merely stimulated, *prostaglandin synthesis* in that tissue increases. Prostaglandins have two major actions: they are mediators of inflammation and they also sensitise nerve endings, lowering their threshold of response to stimuli, mechanical (tenderness of inflammation) and chemical, allowing the other mediators of inflammation, e.g. histamine, serotonin, bradykinin, to intensify the activation of the sensory endings.

Plainly, a drug that prevents the synthesis of prostaglandins is likely to be effective in relieving pain due to inflammation of any kind, and this is indeed how aspirin and other non-steroidal anti-inflammatory drugs (NSAIDs) act. This discovery was made in 1971, aspirin having been extensively used in medicine since 1899.†

4. *The mechanism* by which paracetamol, aspirin and other non-steroidal anti-inflammatory drugs (NSAIDs) relieve pain is by *cyclo-oxygenase* (*prostaglandin synthetase*) *inhibition* thus:

Arachidonic acid (an essential fatty acid) is derived from fatty acids and animal cell membranes in the diet. It is (in an esterified form) a constituent of phospholipids of cell walls and other compound physiological lipids; there is thus plenty of it in the body and it is released from cell walls (which can be regarded as a store) by a phospholipase A_2.‡ The arachidonic acid is then oxidized by cyclo-oxygenase to cyclic endoperoxides, which are converted enzymically to a range of prostaglandins mediating inflammation and pain (above) and including prostacyclin and thromboxane, which have important vascular actions (see diagram on p. 716).

With this mode of action it is evident that these drugs (NSAIDs) will relieve pain when there is some peripheral tissue injury with consequent inflammation, as there almost always is with pain. They also act in the central nervous system (prostaglandins are synthesized in all cells§ except erythrocytes) and there is probably some central component to the analgesic effect of NSAIDs; aspirin in therapeutic doses does alter the EEG, though the significance of this is unknown.

But, it has to be said that analgesic and anti-inflammatory effects are not parallel, e.g. aspirin relieves pain rapidly at doses that do not significantly reduce inflammation and the onset of its anti-inflammatory effect at higher doses may be slow. Paracetamol is an effective analgesic for mild pain but has little anti-inflammation effect in arthritis, though substantial effect on post-dental extraction swelling. Other NSAIDs show a different mix of action against pain and inflammation.

An account of individual non-steroidal anti-inflammatory drugs will be found in Chapter 15.

5. *The pain threshold is lowered* by anxiety, fear, depression, anger, sadness, fatigue, insomnia, and it is *raised* by relief of these (by drugs or by non-drug measures) and by successful relief of pain.

Since emotion is such an important factor in pain, it is no surprise that dummy tablets or injections (placebos) have long been known to alleviate pain, giving relief usually to about 35% of cases, but with the added disadvantage that they rapidly lose effect with repetition.

* Naloxone also appears to cause pyrovats (practitioners of religious firewalking ceremonies) to quicken their pace over the hot coals.

† Propagandists for complementary (alternative) medicine allege that orthodox scientific medicine will not recognize any therapy (e.g. complementary medicine) unless its mode of action is known. This is untrue. Validated empirical observation, i.e. scientific evidence, is and always has been accepted.

‡ Inhibition of this phospholipase is the basis of the anti-inflammatory action of adrenocortical steroids.

§ Which shows the undesirability of naming substances with reference to their, often chance, mode of discovery.

6. The importance of *the meaning of pain* to its victim is illustrated by injuries of war and of civilian life: 'To the wounded soldier who had been under unremitting shell fire for weeks, his wound was a good thing (it meant the end of the war for him) and was associated with far less pain than was the case of the civilians who considered their need for surgery a disaster.'* The desire for analgesics was less amongst victims of battle injuries than amongst comparable civilian injuries.† On the other hand, morphine has been found to be relatively ineffective against experimental pain in man, probably because it acts best against pain that has emotional significance for the patient.

New analgesics have been successfully developed by *animal testing*, possibly because the emotional response to experimental pain in an animal is akin to the human response to disease or accidental injury. This emotional response does not generally occur in a subject who has volunteered to undergo laboratory experiments that can be stopped at any time, and it probably accounts for the fact that a placebo gives relief in only 3% of these cases; also for the fact that experimental pain in man has proved to be of small value in assessing the clinical value of potential analgesics that may act on the psychic response, with the possible exception of intraperitoneal bradykinin‡, which has been used in healthy volunteers and which no doubt arouses emotion when the volunteer actually realises what he has agreed to experience; but this is hardly suitable for routine drug testing. The same applies to non-steroidal anti-inflammatory analgesics though assiduous investigators are now getting better results.§

7. In *acute pain* of limited duration analgesics may be given according to need as the pain returns, for the pain will not last long and the situation is changing; standard doses are used and adjuvant drugs are usually unnecessary; there should be no hesitation about using injection rather than the oral route; sedation is acceptable.

In *chronic pain* analgesics should be given to forestall or prevent pain, for the situation is relatively stable and the return of pain can be predicted; dose is adjusted (titrated) to suit the individual, gradually increasing until the patient is pain free; adjuvant drugs are frequently necessary; therapy should be oral if possible; sedation is unacceptable.

8. *Corticosteroids* diminish inflammation of all kinds by preventing prostaglandin synthesis (the phospholipase A_2 that releases the arachidonic acid that is required for such synthesis is inhibited, see above). Short-term use may be valuable; long-term use poses many problems (see Ch. 34); in general the corticosteroid should be withdrawn after one week if there is no benefit.

Clinical evaluation of analgesics

When a drug has been found to raise the threshold of response to the measured application of heat, electric shock or local pressure in animals, and is thought to have reasonable prospect of being an improvement on existing analgesics (or at least not worse) it must be evaluated in man by trial on patients suffering from the pain of disease.

Therapeutic trials in *acute pain* are often conducted on patients who have undergone abdominal surgery or third molar tooth extraction, and in *chronic pain* on chronic rheumatic conditions. Only the patients can say what they feel and pain is best measured by a *questionnaire* or by a *visual analogue scale*; a line, 10 or 20 cm long, one end of which represents pain 'as bad as it could possibly be' (which patients identify as 'agonising') and the other end 'no pain'; patients mark the line on the point they feel represents their pain between these two extremes. Such techniques are amazingly reproducible.

Adverse effects are, of course, simultaneously recorded and taken into account when deciding its clinical utility. Since what is being measured is how patients *say* they feel, careful precautions must be taken if a reliable result is to be obtained. The trial must be double-blind, or made double-blind as soon as possible. Observers who interrogate the patients for relief (intensity and duration) and adverse effects must be constant and trained. It has been found, for example, that if asked by a personable young woman, a higher proportion of patients admit to pain relief than if the same question is put by a man.

* Beecher H K. Pharmacol Rev 1957; 9:59.
† Beecher H K. JAMA 1956; 161:1609.
‡ Lim R K S et al. Clin Pharmacol Ther 1967; 8:521.
§ Stacher G et al. Br. J. Clin. Pharmacol 1986; 21:35

The necessity for the utmost care in design of drug trials and the interpretation of the results is well shown by the following experiment.*

One physician, using the double-blind technique, treated patients suffering from joint pain with aspirin and with dummy tablets. The patients filled in report cards after two weeks, analysis of which showed that they could not distinguish between the effect of aspirin and the dummy (or placebo). A second physician performed a similar study, also double-blind, in which the patients were interviewed by an observer at their bedside, who recorded the development of analgesic effect. The analysis of the records of this experiment showed that the patients distinguished between aspirin and the dummy tablets, and that these results were 'highly significant statistically', that is, the results were unlikely to be due to chance, which is what this phrase means. It does not mean that the results *cannot* be due to chance. The question now arises which result should be accepted. The second may be taken as reliable, partly because it accords with general clinical experience over 50 years, although this is by no means infallible, and partly because it is well known that memory for pain is bad, so that recollection of pain that occurred days or weeks ago for comparison with pain felt in the present cannot be, and is not, reliable, whereas comparison of the present with, say, half an hour ago, can give very consistent results. If a trial of the first kind were done on a new analgesic there would be a risk of missing a useful drug. No amount of care in recording results, no expertise by the statistician, can compensate for such a fault in design, responsibility for which lies with the clinician.

The *reliability of clinical methods* of measuring analgesic efficacy has been well shown. When one new analgesic was being tried, it was found that the dose required to produce a given amount of relief increased steadily with the age of the drug sample. Enquiry of the maker whether the drug was chemically stable was met by an assurance that it was. The clinical experiments were repeated with the same result, and further chemical investigation revealed that the compound was indeed not stable.

Other support for the reliability of these techniques comes from the fact that similar results are obtained with the same drugs in different centres and that workers have identified 'unknown' coded samples.†

Despite all the activity of chemists producing new compounds and of physicians in testing them with increasing accuracy, the alkaloids of opium and aspirin (1899), remain pre-eminent in the treatment of pain.

The choice of analgesics

1. *Ranking of analgesics for clinical efficacy.*‡

Mild pain. Non-narcotic (non-opioid) analgesics or non-steroidal anti-inflammatory drugs (NSAIDs), e.g. aspirin, ibuprofen, and paracetamol§. Where these fail after using the full dose range, proceed to:

Moderate pain.

a. Narcotic (opioid) analgesics, low-efficacy opioids, e.g. codeine, dihydrocodeine, dextropropoxyphene, pentazocine.

b. Combined therapy of NSAIDs plus low-efficacy opioid, *not* necessarily as a fixed-dose formulation, many of which have an inadequate dose of one or other ingredient (see below) so that separate administration is commonly preferable though less convenient. Where these fail proceed to:

Severe pain.

a. High-efficacy opioids, e.g. morphine, diamorphine, methadone, dextromoramide, phenazocine, dipipanone, pethidine, levorphanol, buprenorphine.

b. An added NSAID is useful if there is a substantial tissue-injury component, e.g. gout, bone metastasis.

Overwhelming pain. High efficacy opioids plus

* Modell W et al. JAMA 1958; 167:2190.

† Beecher H K Pharmacol. Rev. 1957; 9:59.

‡ Based on Twycross R G In: Saunders Cicely M, ed. The management of terminal disease. London: Arnold. 1978. The work of this author contributes much to this chapter.

§ Paracetamol is sometimes not classed as an NSAID because its anti-inflammatory pattern differs substantially from most, i.e. it is weak in rheumatoid arthritis.

a sedative/anxiolytic (diazepam) or a phenothiazine tranquilliser, e.g. chlorpromazine, methotrimeprazine (which also has analgesic effect).

Note: adjuvant drugs may be useful in all grades of pain.

2. *Some good advice: 'Keeping it simple'**

'The three basic analgesics are aspirin, codeine and morphine†. The rest should be considered alternatives of fashion or convenience. Appreciating this helps to prevent the doctor "kangarooing" from analgesic to analgesic in a desperate search for some drug that will suit the patient better. If non-narcotic or weak narcotic preparations such as aspirin–codeine, paracetamol–dextropropoxyphene, fail to relieve, it is usually best to move directly to a small dose of morphine (the author refers to chronic cancer pain) than, for example, to prescribe dihydrocodeine [i.e. change to an analgesic of higher efficacy rather than to another of similar efficacy].

'It is necessary to be familiar with one or two alternatives for use in patients who cannot tolerate the standard preparation. The individual doctor's basic analgesic ladder, with alternatives, should comprise no more than nine or ten drugs in total. It is better to know and understand a few drugs well than to have a passing acquaintance with the whole range.'

3. *Simultaneous use of two analgesics* of different modes of action is rational, but two drugs of the same class/mechanism of action are likely to be unprofitable unless there is a difference in emphasis, analgesia versus anti-inflammatory action; or a patient taking a NSAID with a long $t_{\frac{1}{2}}$, e.g. naproxen, is benefited by having available an additional drug of shorter $t_{\frac{1}{2}}$ to be taken for an acute exacerbation, e.g. ibuprofen, aspirin. Aspirin plus paracetamol is widely used and although aspirin (certainly) and paracetamol (probably) act by blocking prostaglandin synthesis there are substantial (and unexplained) differences between them.

A *low*-efficacy opioid can reduce the action of a *high*-efficacy opioid by excluding the latter from receptors (by competition).

Partial agonist (agonist/antagonist) opioids will antagonize other opioids e.g. heroin, and may even induce the withdrawal syndrome in dependent subjects, see p. 316.

4. *Fixed-ratio analgesic combinations*. Large numbers of these are available. They are particularly offered as bridging the efficacy gap between aspirin or paracetamol and morphine. Many have an inadequate dose of one or other ingredient, e.g. codeine 5 mg, caffeine 10 mg. Doctors should consider the formulae of these preparations before adding them to their therapeutic weaponry.

Caffeine has been shown to enhance the analgesic effect of aspirin and of paracetamol and to accelerate the onset of effect, but at least 30 mg and probably 60 mg are needed (a cup of coffee averages about 80 mg and tea averages one third of this).

Tablets containing paracetamol (325 mg) plus dextropropoxyphene (32.5 mg) (co-proxamol, Distalgesic), in a dose of 1–2 tablets, provide an effective dose of both drugs. There is controversy about the merit (benefit:risk) of this formulation, which has been extremely popular with both prescribers and patients. Clinical trials are inconclusive as to whether it has efficacy superior to either drug alone and its popularity may be influenced by a mild euphoriant effect of the opioid, to which dependence can occur. A major objection to it is that in (deliberate) overdose death may occur within one hour due to the rapid absorption of the dextropropoxyphene and combination with alcohol appears seriously to add to hazard. There has been enormous debate about this popular product, the passion with which it is conducted demonstrating that reliable data are lacking. Regulatory authorities are in a position to tell the manufacturer to obtain definitive data, but they seem reluctant to do so.

We do not make recommendations from amongst the many preparations available because they are so unsatisfactorily formulated; separate administration (theoretically) is to be preferred despite its lesser convenience.

Pain syndromes

In general, pain (acute or chronic) arising from *somatic structures* (skin, muscles, bones, joints)

* Twycross R G. J Roy Coll Physicians Lond 1984; 18:32. The author is a leading authority on pain control and the management of terminal disease.

† None of these has been introduced in the present century.

responds to analgesics such as aspirin and paracetamol (non-narcotic), which do not alter psychic function and do not induce serious dependence (addiction). But pain arising from *the viscera* is most readily reduced by morphine* (narcotic), which alters both the pain threshold and the psychic reaction to pain and induces serious dependence. This distinction is not, of course, absolute and a high-efficacy opioid is needed for severe somatic pain. Mild pain from any source may respond to the non-narcotic analgesics and these should always be tried first.

Pain due to spasm of visceral smooth muscle, when severe, requires large doses of morphine, pethidine or buprenorphine. These drugs themselves cause spasm of visceral smooth muscle and so have a simultaneous action tending to increase the pain. Papaveretum may be less prone to do this as it contains other opium alkaloids. Phenazocine and buprenorphine are less liable to cause spasm. An anticholinergic drug such as atropine may be given simultaneously to antagonise this effect. Mild pain due to spasm can sometimes be relieved by atropine-like drugs, alone or in combination with a non-narcotic analgesic or pentazocine.

Spasm of striated muscle is often a cause of pain, including **chronic tension headache**. Treatment is directed at reduction of the spasm in a variety of ways, including psychotherapy, sedation and the use of a centrally acting muscle relaxant as well as non-narcotic analgesics, e.g. orphenadrine plus paracetamol (Norgesic), baclofen or diazepam. Local injections of lignocaine are sometimes effective as are alcoholic drinks.

Neuralgias, such as *post-herpetic neuralgia*, *trigeminal neuralgia* or *causalgia*, can present almost insoluble problems. Analgesics may play only a subsidiary part in their management. In severe cases very high doses of non-narcotic analgesics with low-efficacy opioid are often reached with little benefit and an almost inevitable demand for high-efficacy opioid follows, with the risk of serious dependence as well as of inefficacy at doses that leave consciousness unimpaired. Psychotropic drugs may be useful adjuvants.

It has been accidentally discovered that an antiepileptic, *carbamazepine* (Tegretol) (200 mg), structurally related to imipramine, is effective in trigeminal neuralgia, probably by reducing excitability of the trigeminal nucleus. It supplants other drug therapy. A start should be made with a low dose, which should be adjusted to suit individuals, who generally soon learn to alter it themselves during remissions and exacerbations. It is not used for prophylaxis. The daily dose is 200–1600 mg orally, in divided doses. It is sometimes possible to withdraw the drug gradually over several months without relapse.

In this and in other forms of neuralgia, drugs worth trying in resistant cases include *phenytoin* (it raises the threshold of nerve cells to electrical stimulation), *baclofen* and *antidepressants* or *tranquillisers*, which may potentiate analgesics and also have an independent effect.

Phenytoin may sometimes help tabetic pain when other measures fail.

Sedation during the acute stage of herpes zoster in patients over 55 years may perhaps help to prevent *post-herpetic neuralgia*, a horrible condition.

Phantom limb pain is commonly resistant to analgesics. Prolonged relief may follow transient changes in sensory input; *decrease* (local anaesthetic to sensitive spots in the stump); *increase* (vibration).

Thalamic pain e.g. following a cerebrovascular accident, commonly fails to respond to analgesics. Chlorpromazine is worth trying, and carbamazepine, and other adjuvant drugs.

The pain of inflammation (see above) responds to NSAIDs (aspirin is an NSAID although some talk as though it is not), but may need added low-efficacy opioid.

Arthritis, see above and Ch. 15.

The pain of **minor trauma**, e.g. many sports injuries, is commonly treated by local skin cooling (spray of chlorofluoromethanes) or counter irritants (see index).

The pain of severe trauma usually needs narcotic analgesics; for **post-surgical pain** see p. 439.

The pain of peripheral vascular insufficiency should be treated with non-narcotic analgesics. Low efficacy opioids may be needed eventually.

* Surgeons are rightly concerned that diagnosis of the acute abdomen be not hindered by a large dose of morphine administered with humane intent by the primary care doctor who first sees the patient.

Vasodilator drugs may help but also may be quite ineffective.

The pain of malignant disease requires the full range of analgesics *and* adjuvant drugs (see above, and terminal care, below).

Bone pain requires NSAIDs alone and with opioids.

Headache originating inside the skull may be due to traction on or distension of arteries arising from the circle of Willis, or to traction on the dura mater. Headache originating outside the skull may be due to muscle spasm* or arterial inflammation or distension. It may be also be a referred pain from, for example, the teeth, neck or nasal sinuses. Treatment by drugs is directed to relieving the muscle spasm, producing vasoconstriction or simply administering analgesics, beginning, of course, with the non-narcotics, paracetamol and aspirin.

Vascular headaches: a. **Migraine** (classical and common). Whether or not migraine has a neurological basis, there are detectable changes in the blood platelets and vasculature that allow some purposeful basis for therapy.

Migraine is triggered by a variety of factors, including stress (exertion, excitement, anxiety, fatigue, anger) and by food containing vasoactive amines (chocolate, cheese), by food allergy and also by hormonal changes (menstruation and oral contraceptives) and hypoglycaemia. Most, perhaps all, of these precipitating factors are associated with increased release in the body of vasoactive monoamines, adrenaline, noradrenaline, and also of arachidonic acid (precursor of prostaglandins, including thromboxane). These substances increase blood platelet aggregation and adhesion to vessel walls.

At the time of an attack of migraine the blood platelets have a low concentration of monoamine oxidase and consequently higher-than-usual serotonin content: this they also release more readily than normal platelets on aggregation.

The serotonin (and the adenine nucleotides ADP and ATP) released from platelets cause vasoconstriction which, in the small arteries of the cerebral cortex, results in ischaemia that induces the visual defects and other sensory changes characteristic of the aura of classical migraine.

These active substances (autacoids†) also act on most cells causing release of histamine and of proteolytic enzymes (which change inactive plasma kininogens to active kinins, e.g. bradykinin), so that yet more potentially pain-producing substances are generated. This concentration of autacoids lowers the threshold of nociceptive nerve endings in the vascular walls (not only arteries) so that the afferent input to the spinal cord is increased sufficiently to induce pain. Then, as the plasma concentration of serotonin falls, there is vasodilatation in both intra and extracerebral vessels and the sensory aura passes off. The pulsation of the arteries causes throbbing pain, as does cough (stretching of venous sinuses), in vessels with sensitised receptors.

Nausea and vomiting with gastric stasis are usual, and if drugs are not vomited, their absorption becomes slow and erratic.

If this story, despite its evident inadequacies, is even approximately true, the therapy of migraine can be seen to have some rational basis.

The *acute migraine attack* should be treated as early as possible with an oral soluble analgesic formulation so that it may be absorbed before there is vomiting and gastric stasis: aspirin (600 mg) is effective and its antiaggregatory action on the platelets may add to its advantage; paracetamol (1.0 g; no action on platelets) is an alternative.

Metoclopramide (10 mg orally) is a useful antiemetic that also promotes gastric emptying and has been shown to enhance aspirin absorption. But plainly, if vomiting and gastric stasis already exist, it may not be absorbed and should be given i.m. (10 mg). Prochlorperazine (rectally), cyclizine and buclizine are alternative antiemetics.

Sedation (with a benzodiazepine) is useful especially if the attack has been triggered by emotional stress, and sleep is an important remedy in migraine. Efficient use of an analgesic, an antiemetic‡ and a sedative is adequate for 90% of

* As in *tension headache* or frontal headache from 'eyestrain.'

† *Autacoid* is a generic term for endogenous active substances that are not classifiable as neurotransmitters or hormones.

‡ Patients seem enthusiastic about combinations of antiemetic (metoclopramide or buclizine) and aspirin or paracetamol, sometimes with small amounts of codeine or docusate sodium, e.g. Migraleve, Migravess, Paramox.

acute attacks. The remaining 10% need ergotamine.

Severe migraine attacks require *ergotamine*, which will benefit about 60% of those treated. Ergotamine has α-adrenoceptor agonist (vasoconstrictor) and anti-serotonin effect. It must be handled cautiously. Mild overdose causes nausea and vomiting and can worsen headache (ergot has the complex agonist/antagonist action characteristic of ergot derivatives, p. 713) and this can lead patients and incautious doctors to think the migraine is uncontrolled and to increase the dose, with disastrous consequences.

Ergotamine constricts all peripheral arteries (an effect potentiated by concomitant β-adrenoceptor block), not just those affected by the migraine process, and overdose can cause peripheral gangrene; paraesthesiae in hands or feet give warning. Because ergotamine has complex actions on receptors and its binding is relatively stable, vasoconstriction is best antagonized by a non-selective vasodilator such as sodium nitroprusside (rather than by an α-adrenoceptor blocker). Subjects of vascular disease, coronary and peripheral, are particularly at risk from ergotamine (angina pectoris, gangrene).

Another reason for giving close attention to dosage is that, though ergotamine has a $t_{\frac{1}{2}}$ of 2 h, effect on arteries (due to tissue binding) persists as long as 24 h, i.e. repeated doses lead to cummulative effects long outlasting the migraine attack.

Ergotamine may be given orally (to be swallowed: crushed tablets), sublingually (bypassing gastric stasis), rectally, or by inhalation.

With *enteral* forms ergotamine, total dosage in an acute attack should not exceed 6 mg (if there is no benefit from the first 2 mg, see below, the likelihood of higher dose being effective is small), and the maximum in one week should not exceed 10 mg.

By *inhalation* (360 μg per puff of metered aerosol), a puff every 5 min for up to 6 puffs (2.2 mg in an attack), and in one week 15 puffs (5.4 mg) maximum.

In one case of overdose a doctor overprescribed ergotamine and the dispensing pharmacist did not query the prescription. A court of law found both doctor and pharmacist to have been negligent, i.e. to have failed to take reasonable care in circumstances where it was foreseeable that such failure was likely to cause injury. The court ordered doctor and pharmacist to share a payment of compensation to the patient, who had suffered peripheral gangrene.

Ergotamine is a powerful oxytocic and is dangerous in pregnancy. It may precipitate angina pectoris, probably by increasing cardiac pre- and afterload (venous and arterial constriction) rather than by constricting coronary arteries.

Caffeine enhances absorption of ergotamine (both speed and peak blood concentration) and is often combined with it (though it may prevent sleep).

Preparations of ergotamine for the acute attack (see above for maximal doses) include:

Tablet (to swallow, crushed) ergotamine 1 mg + caffeine 100 mg (Cafergot); two tablets at onset and then one every 30 min if necessary (maximum 6).

Tablet (to swallow, crushed) ergotamine 2 mg + cyclizine 50 mg + caffeine 100 mg (Migril); one or two at onset then 30 min intervals (maximum 4).

Tablet (sublingual) ergotamine 2 mg (Lingraine); one tablet at onset and then one every 30 min if necessary (maximum 4).

Suppository ergotamine 2 mg + caffeine 100 mg (Cafergot); one at onset and then about hourly if necessary (maximum 3).

Inhalation by metered aerosol (Medihaler-ergotamine), for dose see above.

Ergotamine should not be used for prophylaxis.

Carbon dioxide inhalation (cerebral vasodilator) can sometimes stop an attack if given during the aura (cortical vasoconstriction). The most convenient technique is to rebreathe into a bag until dyspnoea occurs.

Dihydroergotamine is less effective than ergotamine.

Drug prophylaxis of migraine should be considered when, after adjustment of lifestyle, diet, etc. there are still two or more attacks per month. Benefit may be delayed for several weeks.

Options (which may help up to 60% of patients) include:

Aspirin continuously, e.g. 300 mg × 2/day, which blocks synthesis of thromboxame (aggregatory factor) in platelets. Higher doses will also block synthesis of prostacyclin (platelet antiaggregatory factor) in arterial walls and may make migraine worse. *If* this is the true mode of action in prophylaxis, much lower doses of aspirin may be effective.

β-*adrenoceptor block* by propranolol (the d-isomer, which lacks β-blocking action though it has membrane stabilizing effect, also prevents migraine) and atenolol, timolol and metoprolol (which are not partial agonists) but not alprenolol, acebutolol and pindolol (which are partial agonists). Plainly β-adrenoceptor block is not the prime therapeutic action.

If ergotamine (for acute attack) is given to a patient taking propranolol for prophylaxis there is risk of additive vasoconstriction (block of β-receptor dilatation with added α-receptor constriction).

The effective dose of propranolol is variable, 80–240 mg/ day orally.

Calcium entry blockers, e.g. verapamil, have been found to be effective.

Pizotifen blocks serotonin (5-HT) receptors as well as having some H_1-antihistamine and anticholinergic actions (it is structurally related to cyproheptadine and to tricyclic antidepressants).

Clonidine (25 μg) in a special low-dose formulation (Dixarit), not to be confused with the high-dose formulation (100 μg) used for hypertension (Catapres).

Methysergide (an ergot derivative) blocks serotonin receptors but it has a grave rare adverse effect, an inflammatory fibrosis, retroperitoneal (causing obstruction to the ureters), subendocardial, pericardial and pleural. Drug 'holidays', i.e. withdrawal for 1–2 months each 6 months, are a prudent safeguard. Because of this risk, methysergide cannot be a drug of first choice.

Other drugs for which efficacy has been claimed include amitriptyline (tricyclic) and MAOI antidepressants.

After six months it is worth trying slow withdrawal of the prophylactic drug.

Attention to detail in the treatment of migraine is well repaid. General aspects of treatment are often more important than are drugs, e.g. psychotherapy, modification of way of living. *Premenstrual migraine* may respond to a diuretic.

b. **Cluster headaches** may be treated as for migraine, but use of ergotamine may need to be more prolonged. If used over weeks, two days in each week should be ergot-free to avoid toxicity. Since bouts of headache tend to be of limited duration (e.g. a few weeks) short courses of methysergide are justified in intractable cases; pizotifen can be beneficial.

Headache of intracranial pressure responds to dexamethasone, which reduces the pressure, and non-opioid analgesics.

Nerve compression can be relieved by corticosteroid (prednisolone), nerve block (local anaesthetic); **nerve destruction** can be achieved by alcohol, phenol, chlorocresol.

Dysmenorrhoea, see p. 712.

Miscellaneous. Inhalation of trichloroethylene or nitrous oxide and oxygen, as in obstetrics, may be used temporarily for severe intermittent pain when other drugs fail, in, for instance *urinary lithiasis*, *trigeminal neuralgia* and during *postoperative chest physiotherapy*.

The general principle that the best treatment of a symptom is the removal of its cause is well exemplified in the routine treatment of the pain of peptic ulcer, for which analgesics are not used, but the principle is harder to apply successfully in the pain of irritable bowel syndrome.

Self-administered pain relief: on demand analgesia

Patient-controlled analgesia. It is obviously more satisfactory if patients can manage their own analgesics rather than be dependent on others. In mild and moderate pain it is easy to provide tablets for this purpose, but in severe chronic and acute recurrent pain, e.g. post-surgical, obstetric, myocardial infarction and terminal illness, other routes are needed to provide speedy relief just when it is needed, and a range of apparatuses has been developed, from the familiar (in obstetrics) inhalation devices to patient-operated pumps for i.v., i.m., s.c. and epidural routes.

There are obvious problems (e.g. training patients, supervision, preventing overdose) in achieving the objectives, better patient satisfaction with reduced (or, at least, not increased) demand on nurses' time, or allowing the patient to die comfortably at home.

TERMINAL ILLNESS

Symptom control and the quality of life

It is a general truth that we are all dying; the difference between individuals is the length and quality of the time that remains.* Terminal illness means that period (generally weeks) when active treatment of disease is no longer appropriate and the emphasis of care is on providing the maximum quality of life during these final weeks. This means that symptom control becomes the priority because, 'One cannot adequately help a man to come to accept his impending death if he remains in severe pain, one cannot give spiritual counsel to a woman who is vomiting, or help a wife and children say their goodbyes to a father who is so drugged that he cannot respond.'†

As the scope of life contracts, so the quality of what remains becomes more precious. Symptoms should not be allowed to destroy it. Drugs are pre-eminent in symptom control.

A remarkable instance of success in terminal care is provided by 'an elderly gentleman with obstructing carcinoma of the esophagus who was a keen gardener. He remained at home, free from pain, attended a garden show on Saturday, worked in his garden on Sunday, and died on Monday'.‡ He was treated with continuous subcutaneous heroin (diamorphine) infusion (heroin has a higher solubility than morphine and so is more suitable for such use). Whilst the randomized controlled trial provides a major basis for therapeutic advance, telling us what *generally does* happen, the clinical anecdote yet has value, telling us what *can* happen, and providing examples for us to emulate.

Such an ideal course as the above example is too much to expect always. But with intelligent use of drugs, which follows from informed analyses of objectives, doctors can enable their patients to depart from life in peace§ and with dignity, i.e. *true euthanasia*.‖

While the skilful use of drugs can provide incalculable relief and deserves careful study, this must not hide the fact that the manner, attentiveness, and human feeling of the attendants are dominant factors once any grosser physical and mental aberrations have been controlled by drugs. The needs of the dying have been summarised as security, companionship, symptomatic treatment, and medical nursing and domestic care. Nearly half of the deaths in England and Wales occur in the patient's own home.

1. *Pain*. The considerations already discussed apply, but there are some aspects that deserve special attention.

Analgesics should be given regularly (adjusted to the patient's need, often 3- to 4-hourly) to *prevent* pain and not only to suppress it. Suppression of existent pain requires larger doses, particularly where the pain has generated anxiety and fear. When it is certain that pain will return, it is cruel to allow it to do so when the means of prevention exist.

It is kind to leave a dose of analgesic accessible to patients, especially at night, when unnecessary suffering may result from reluctance to call a nurse or disturb a relative. In terminal illness, the question of whether or not the patient will become dependent on opioids ceases to be a matter of importance (but see below) and the ordinary precautions against dependence need not be rigorously followed.

Control of severe pain without objectionable sedation can be achieved in terminal illness by morphine (given orally) in up to 90% of patients. Oral use preserves patients' independence (they do not have to rely on another person to give the next dose) as well as reducing the unpleasantness of frequent injections and the use of nursing time.

Full relief can only be achieved by attention to detail. This is sadly, too often, neglected. We therefore provide a detailed account of morphine use in this most important area of medical care

* Mack R M. Lessons from living with cancer. N Engl J Med 1984; 311:1640. Recommended reading: a personal account by a surgeon who had lung cancer with metastases.

† Dr. Mary Baines, St. Christopher's Hospice, London.

‡ Russell P S B. N Engl J Med 1984; 311:1634.

§ . . .; and for many a time
I have been half in love with easeful Death,
Call'd him soft names in many a mused rhyme,
To take into the air my quiet breath;
Now more than ever seems it rich to die,
To cease upon the midnight with no pain.
(John Keats: 1795–1821).

‖ *Euthanasia* (Greek: *eu* gentle, easy; *thanatos* death) is the objective of all. It does not mean deliberately killing people peacefully, which is *voluntary* euthanasia.

where thoughtful attention to detail is so rewarding to patients, families and indeed to doctors themselves.

Oral morphine in the pain of terminal care

a. Use a *simple aqueous solution**, the strength of which is adjusted to give a volume of 5–10 ml per dose, e.g. begin with 1 mg/ml.

b. The usual oral *starting dose* is 5–10 mg 4-hourly (2.5 mg in the frail elderly): it can also be used by buccal or sublingual route (lower dose).

c. *Peak plasma concentration* is reached in 1½–2 h.

d. If the *first dose* is not more effective than previous medication, increase the second dose.

e. If the pain is not more than 90% controlled in the first 24 h *increase* the dose by 50%. After that adjust dose 24 hourly as in (i) below.

f. *Dose*: most patients get satisfactory pain control at 5–30 mg 4-hourly (a few will need more than 200 mg, but rarely 500 mg has been required): arbitrary fixed dosage is inappropriate: doses and frequency are adjusted to meet the patients' need.

g. *Change to morphine from other high-efficacy opioids*; higher starting doses of oral morphine will be needed.

h. A *larger dose at night* (1.5–2 × daytime dose) or an added hypnotic may allow the patient to pass the night without waking in pain (and so to omit one night dose).

i. *Dosage increments* of oral morphine given 4–hourly:
- below 15 mg, add 5 mg
- up to 30 mg, add 10 mg
- up to 90 mg, add 15 mg
- up to 180 mg, add 30 mg
- above 180 mg, add 60 mg

j. *Constipation will occur*, see below; it is essential to manage it.

k. *Initial drowsiness* (a few days) and confusion (in the elderly) are common and usually pass off: this should be explained to the patient ('You may feel sleepy or a little muddled'): if unpleasant sedation persists then small doses of amphetamine may be used.

l. *Initial nausea* and vomiting may occur: an antiemetic controls it (e.g. prochlorperazine 2.5–5 mg, orally, 6–8 hourly) and can generally be withdrawn after 4–5 days.

m. When there are *problems with 4-hourly* administration of the liquid preparation, a slow-release oral formulation (8- to 12-hourly) is an alternative, as are suppositories or buccal (sublingual) formulations (the latter route bypasses the first-pass or pre-systemic elimination and does not require such high doses as if swallowed).

n. *Breakthrough pain*: an additional dose of morphine or other agonist opioid analgesic (*not* an agonist/antagonist) provided for self-administration is valuable, not least because it gives the patient confidence. An NSAID can also be used.

o. *Respiratory depression* is seldom a problem with morphine used in this way and unpleasant sedation and vomiting are transient.

p. *Dependence*, both physical and psychological, occurs, but the latter to only a small degree compared with drug abuse or other chronic pain syndrome; the social, psychological and medical aspects of morphine use in terminal care are so different from that of drug abuse that comparisons are inappropriate; dose reduction, when required, e.g. after relief of pain by palliative radiotherapy or nerve block, should, of course, be gradual, but abrupt withdrawal (accidental) has been found to cause only mild withdrawal syndrome.

q. *Tolerance* is dealt with by increasing the dose.

r. *To transfer from oral morphine to injection*, e.g. due to difficult swallowing, vomiting, the injected dose should be half the oral dose (if heroin is substituted, then one third): most patients can be managed without injections, which limit independence, are unpleasant, prodigal of nursing time and are more difficult to provide at home where most patients will prefer to die.

s. *Phenothiazines* are antiemetic, antianxiety and sedative agents and they may change the affective response to pain (particularly methotrimeprazine).

t. *Tricyclic antidepressants* have a morphine-sparing effect even in the absence of an effect or mood.

* Solutions of morphine deteriorate once they are opened (exposed to air), and if exposed to light (keep in dark) and heat, they lose potency over as few as 2–4 weeks; competent pharmaceutical advice and preparation is required. The taste of morphine is bitter and patients may choose their own concomitant drink to mask it. Tablets may be used.

u. *Other adjuvant drugs* should be used concurrently as appropriate, e.g. antidepressants, amphetamine (elevates mood and enhances analgesia), hypnotics.

v. *Routine addition of other drugs such as cocaine, chlorpromazine and alcohol* has no merit.

2. *Anorexia* is common in patients with widespread cancer; prednisolone 15–30 mg daily and/or alcohol in the patient's preferred form before meals, may help, or carbonated or other drink for which the patient has a taste.

3. *Confusion* may not need treatment unless it is accompanied by restlessness: haloperidol in emergency: thioridazine (does not cause much sedation): chlorpromazine (if sedation is desired): chlormethiazole for insomnia.

4. *Constipation* is usual in dying patients, whether due to opioid analgesic (see above) or to inadequate intake of food and fluid, and physical inactivity. It can be exceedingly troublesome, and management should begin early to forestall the need for the major unpleasantness and humiliations of manual removal of faeces and the lesser ones of enemas. Dietary measures should be used where practicable. A stimulant laxative and faecal softener (danthron plus poloxamer: Dorbanex) is commonly effective: suppositories (e.g. glycerol or bisacodyl) are useful. Good advice from St. Christopher's Hospice: if the bowels have not been opened for three days, perform a rectal examination and if the rectum is found to be loaded insert a suppository.

5. *Convulsions*: sodium valproate orally is preferred to phenytoin as the latter interacts extensively with other drugs (p. 376): where oral use is impracticable use phenobarbitone i.m.: for status epilepticus see p. 374.

6. *Cough*: see p. 596.

7. *Diarrhoea*: see p. 633.

8. *Dyspnoea*. Chronic dyspnoea (not due to respiratory failure) may be relieved by an opioid (respiratory centre depression reducing its sensitivity to chemical stimuli), but when there is respiratory failure due to pulmonary disease any sedation may cause serious respiratory depression; oxygen is used as appropriate: a benzodiazepine reduces the anxiety of dyspnoea: dexamethasone reduces inflammation around obstructive tumours that cause dyspnoea. Accumulations of mucus that the patient is too weak to expel cause 'death rattle'; this terminal event, often more distressing to others than to the patient, may be eliminated by (further) drying up the secretions with an anticholinergic drug (hyoscine or atropine 4- to 8-hourly).

9. *Emergencies* such as major haemorrhage, pulmonary embolus, severe choking, fracture of large bone: give morphine 10 mg plus hyoscine 0.4 mg i.m.: this combination provides acute relief and some desirable short term retrograde amnesia which, with luck, will extend to the whole unpleasant episode.

10. *Hiccup* (due to diaphragmatic spasm): where this is intractable and exhausting, chlorpromazine or metoclopramide may help.

11. *Insomnia*: temazepam or chlormethiazole (which may be less prone to cause confusion in the elderly.)

12. *Intestinal obstruction* can be managed without surgery* (which only adds to the distress of dying); it is done by giving loperamide (or diphenoxylate) and/or hyoscine (or atropine) sublingually or s.c., for colic, antiemetics (sometimes combining two having different sites of action), and a faecal softener (without added laxative, which would increase peristalsis) for as long as obstruction is incomplete; there may be an inflammatory element in tumour obstruction that can be relieved by substantial doses of corticosteroid (prednisolone 15 to 30 mg/day). When obstruction is complete the patient may vomit once or twice a day without great distress, but oral therapy may become impracticable; to avoid injections in an emaciated patient, drugs may then be given by suppository (opioid plus antiemetic).

13. *Itch*: see p. 737.

14. *Lymphoedema*, e.g. due to pelvic cancer, that causes pain may be helped by prednisolone (15–30 mg/day).

15. *Mental distress* may be helped by alcohol–opioid mixtures, antidepressants or tranquillisers, according to circumstances.

Patients may too easily be drugged into uncomplaining silence, but it does not follow that they are not still in deep distress:

* A detailed account is given by Baines M et al. Lancet 1985; 2:90.

'. . . the grief that does not speak
Whispers the o'er-fraught heart, and bids it break'.*

And this unpleasant way of ending life can be avoided by discerning choice and, particularly, careful dosage of drugs.

16. *A mouth* that is dry and painful may be due to candidiasis (treat with nystatin), to dehydration (rehydrate the patient where this can be done orally, otherwise the symptom can be managed by frequent small drinks or crushed ice to suck plus assiduous mouth hygiene to prevent unpleasant infection), or to anticholinergic drugs including some antidepressants (withdraw the drug or adjust its dose).

17. *Nausea and vomiting*, whether due to disease or to opioid drug, cause great distress and can be more difficult to manage than pain; two drugs acting by different mechanisms may be needed when a single agent fails, e.g. phenothiazine plus anticholinergic, or either plus metoclopramide, see p. 622. For vomiting of *hypercalcaemia*: use an antiemetic and treat the cause (p. 755).

18. *Night sweats*: can be distressing and cause insomnia: indomethacin helps.

19. *Restlessness* in terminal illness that has no obvious cause (e.g. pain, full bladder) may be treated with methotrimeprazine (a phenothiazine tranquilliser with analgesic effect) by injection: it may be combined with morphine (or diamorphine), which are tranquillisers as well as analgesics: diazepam is useful for muscle twitching.

20. *Swallowing* of solid-dose forms may not only be difficult but they may stick in the oesophagus in weak recumbent patients, especially if adequate fluid is not taken with the dose (at least two big gulps or 100 ml with the patient's trunk vertical); potassium chloride and emepronium are known especially to ulcerate the oesophagus.

21. *Urinary frequency, urgency and incontinence*: flavoxate, emepronium (anticholinergics) may be useful: the pain of an indwelling catheter may be benefitted by diazepam. Anticholinergics may cause retention of urine if there is anatomical obstruction.

* William Shakespeare (1564–1616). *Macbeth*, Act 4, Scene 3.

NARCOTIC OR OPIOID† ANALGESICS

'Among the remedies which it has pleased Almighty God to give to man to relieve his sufferings, none is so universal and so efficacious as opium.'
Thomas Sydenham, physician, 1680.

It is not known when opium was first procured and used as a drug, but it was certainly in prehistoric times, and medical practice still leans heavily on its alkaloids, using them as analgesic, tranquilliser, antitussive and in diarrhoea. Opium is obtained by incising the seed heads of the opium poppy, allowing the exuded juice to dry for 24 h and then collecting it. A good yield of opium requires greater sunshine than is usual in Britain, although the plant will grow here.

Crude opium alone was used in medicine until 1803, when the principal active ingredient was isolated by Friedrich Sertürner, who tested the separate fractions he extracted from it on animals and proceeded to try pure morphine on himself and three young men. He observed that the drug caused cerebral depression and spasms of the extremities and that it relieved toothache. He named it after Morpheus.‡

Opium contains many alkaloids, but the only important ones are *morphine* (10%) and *codeine*, although two others, noscapine (narcotine) and papaverine, are occasionally used. In general, morphine is used now where opium was used in the past; its effects differ little from those of opium. However, purified preparations of mixtures of opium alkaloids (e.g. papaveretum, Omnopon) are available.

Mode of action

Endogenous opioid peptides (endorphins, dynorphins, enkephalins), discovered in 1975, have been termed 'the brain's own morphine'. At last

† The term opi*ate* has been used for the natural alkaloids of opium, and opi*oid* for other agents having similar action. The distinction is neither generally observed nor particularly useful. We here use *opioid* for all receptor-specific substances.

‡ In classical mythology Morpheus was son of Somnus, the infernal deity who presided over sleep. He was generally represented as a corpulent, winged boy holding opium poppies in his hand. His principal function seems to have been to stand by his sleeping father's black-curtained bed of feathers, on watch to prevent his being awakened by noise.

the question why the brain has opioid receptors when there are no opioids in the body can be dismissed. These opioids are neurotransmitters in complex pain-inhibitory systems (see p. 303). They attach to specific opioid receptors (about five classes), and it is on these receptors that administered opioids also act. Opioid drugs may be agonist to one class of opioid receptor, and antagonist (blocker) to another, which explains the differing patterns of action seen amongst opioids. A drug may also have dual agonist/antagonist effect on a single receptor (which will result in a limited ceiling of therapeutic efficacy, and antagonism if it is given in the presence of a high efficacy opioid, i.e. it will precipitate a withdrawal syndrome in subjects dependent on morphine or heroin). In addition, a weak (low-efficacy) agonist (codeine) will compete with a high-efficacy opioid for receptors and so reduce the receptor occupany, and therefore the therapeutic efficacy of the latter, i.e. a weak agonist partially antagonizes a strong agonist. It is no surprise that there are differences between drugs in emphasis or pattern of the many actions of opioids.

Some of the endorphins, dynorphins and enkephalins are about as active as morphine and some are more effective; some are short and some are long-acting. The discovery of the role of natural opioid mechanisms in physiology and pathology opens up possibilities for major developments in pain management, and indeed, wider, for peripheral opioid mechanisms may play a role in shock, for example.

The continuing unravelling of opioid mechanisms has not yet provided an explanation of opioid tolerance and dependence; ideas include suppression of endogenous opioid production with rebound on withdrawal and hypersensitivity of receptors; tolerance and dependence may be mediated by different mechanisms.

Morphine

Morphine will be described in some detail and other opioid analgesics in so far as they differ from it.

The principal *acute* actions of morphine may be summarised:

On the central nervous system:

Depression, leading to:
- analgesia
- respiratory depression
- depression of cough reflex
- sleep

Stimulation, leading to:
- vomiting
- miosis
- hyperactive spinal cord reflexes, some only convulsions (very rare)

Changes of mood, euphoria or dysphoria

Dependence; affects other systems too.

Smooth muscle stimulation:
- Gastrointestinal muscle spasm (delayed passage of contents with constipation)
- Biliary tract spasm: Bronchospasm
- Renal tract spasm: dubious, see below.

Cardiovascular system: dilatation of resistance (arterioles) and capacitance (veins) vessels.

These items will be discussed:

Morphine on the central nervous system. Morphine is the most generally useful high-efficacy opioid analgesic; it eliminates pain and also allows subjects to tolerate pain, i.e. the sensation is felt but is no longer unpleasant. It both stimulates and depresses the central nervous system. It induces a state of relaxation, tranquillity, detachment and well-being (euphoria), or occasionally of unpleasantness (dysphoria), and causes sleepiness, inability to concentrate and lethargy, always supposing that this pleasant state is not destroyed by nausea and vomiting, more common if the patient is ambulant. Excitement can occur but is unusual; it is said that women are more prone to it than men, though there is now evidence against this, and it seems to be 'another of those interesting myths that textbook writers are fond of repeating without evidence down through the years.'* However, there is no doubt that morphine excites cats and horses, though it is illegal to put this to practical use in horse or cat racing. Generally, morphine has useful hypnotic and tranquillising actions and there should be no hesitation in using it in full dose in appropriate circumstances, e.g. acute pain and fear, as in myocardial infarction or road traffic accidents.

* Lasagna L. Pharmacol Rev 1964; 16:47.

Morphine *depresses respiration* principally by reducing sensitivity of the respiratory centre to rises in blood carbon dioxide tension. With therapeutic doses there is a reduced minute volume due to diminished rate and tidal volume. With higher doses carbon dioxide narcosis may develop.

Morphine is dangerous when the respiratory drive is at all impaired by disease, including CO_2 retention from any cause, emphysema, or raised intracranial pressure.

In *asthmatics*, in addition to the effect on the respiratory centre, it may cause thickening of bronchial secretions, which, with depression of cough and bronchospasm (see below) will increase small airways resistance.

In postoperative patients morphine may promote pulmonary atelectasis by discouraging deep breathing, but abdominal or thoracic pain discourages it also.

Morphine is useful in the emergency relief of paroxysmal nocturnal dyspnoea, relieving mental distress by tranquillising, cardiac distress by reduction of sympathetic drive (see below) and respiratory distress by rendering the centre insensitive to afferent stimuli from the congested lungs. Morphine also suppresses *cough* by a central action. It stimulates the third nerve nucleus causing *miosis* (pin-point pupils are characteristic of poisoning, acute or chronic; at therapeutic doses the pupil is merely smaller): it can obscure valuable pupillary changes in changing neurological states, e.g. head injury.

The chemoreceptor trigger zone of the *vomiting centre* is stimulated, causing nausea (40%) and vomiting (15%), a side-effect which, in addition to being unpleasant, can be dangerous in patients who have had gastric operations, a cataract removed, or myocardial infarction. A preparation of morphine plus an antiemetic, e.g. cyclizine (Cyclimorph) reduces this liability. Some spinal cord reflexes are also stimulated and so morphine is unsuitable for use in tetanus and convulsant poisoning; indeed, morphine can itself cause convulsions.

Morphine causes *antidiuresis* by releasing antidiuretic hormone, and this can be clinically important.

Morphine on smooth muscle. Alimentary tract. Morphine activates receptors on the smooth muscle of both large and small bowel, causing it to contract. Peristalsis (propulsion) is reduced and segmentation increased. Thus, although morphine 'stimulates' smooth muscle, constipation occurs, with the intestine in a state of tonic contraction. The central action of the drug probably also leads to neglect of the urge to defaecate. Delay in the passage of the intestinal contents results in greater absorption of water and increased viscosity of faeces, which contributes to the constipation. The management of opioid-induced constipation is an important aspect of terminal care.

Morphine causes high intra-sigmoid pressures, which in colonic diverticular disease may result in the diverticula blowing up and becoming obstructed and failing to drain into the colon. Pethidine neither produces these high pressures nor prevents drainage, and so is preferable for the pain of acute diverticulitis if it should be severe enough to demand a narcotic analgesic. Morphine may also endanger anastomoses of the colon immediately postoperatively and it should not be given in intestinal obstruction (excepting in terminal care).

Intrabiliary pressure may rise substantially after morphine, due to spasm of the sphincter of Oddi. Sometimes biliary colic is made worse by morphine, presumably in a patient in whom the dose happens to be adequate to increase intrabiliary pressure, but insufficient to produce more than slight analgesia. In patients who have had a cholecystectomy this can produce a syndrome sufficiently like a myocardial infarction to cause diagnostic confusion. The electrocardiograph may be abnormal and the serum transaminase may rise. Naloxone may give dramatic symptomatic relief. Another result of this action of morphine is to dam back the pancreatic juice and so to cause a rise in the serum amylase concentration. Morphine is therefore best avoided in pancreatitis; but buprenorphine has less of this effect.

Urinary tract. Any contraction of the ureters is probably clinically unimportant. Retention of urine may occur (particularly in prostatic hypertrophy) due to a mix of spasm of the bladder sphincter and to the central sedation causing the patient to ignore afferent messages from a full bladder.

Bronchial muscle is constricted, partly due to histamine release, but so slightly as to be of no importance, *except in asthmatics* in whom morphine is best avoided anyway because of its respiratory depressant effect.

When morphine is used and the *smooth muscle effects are objectionable*, atropine may be given simultaneously to antagonise spasm. Unfortunately it does not always effectively oppose the rise of pressure induced in the biliary system, nor does it restore bowel peristalsis. Glyceryl trinitrate will relax morphine-induced spasm.

Uterus. Labour is prolonged, but this may be the result of central psychological effects reducing patient cooperation rather than to an action on the uterus.

Cardiovascular system. Morphine, by a central action, impairs sympathetic vascular reflexes (causing veno- and arteriolar dilatation) and stimulates the vagal centre (bradycardia); it also releases histamine (vasodilatation). These effects are ordinarily unimportant, but they can be beneficial in acute heart failure (reduced cardiac workload as well as tranquillisation), though they are sometimes harmful in patients taking antihypertensives, in acute myocardial infarction and with low blood volume; excessive bradycardia can be blocked by atropine.

Other effects of morphine include sweating, pruritus and piloerection.

Chronic use of morphine and other opioids is marked by acquired *tolerance* to the depressant agonist effects, e.g. analgesic action and respiratory depression (the fatal dose is higher), but not to some stimulant agonist effects, e.g. constipation and miosis, which persist.

Opioids that have mixed agonist/antagonist actions induce tolerance to the agonist but not to the antagonist effects; naloxone (a pure antagonist) induces no tolerance to itself.

There is a cross-tolerance between opioids. (For dependence and withdrawal see below).

Acquired tolerance develops over days with continued frequent use and passes off (variably for different actions) over a few days to weeks. Children have been said to be naturally intolerant (i.e. responsive to low doses) of morphine, but this is not so and it is valuable in acute heart failure in children (s.c. 0.2 mg/kg). Infants and the aged are intolerant.

Pharmacokinetics. Give s.c. (particularly) or i.m., morphine is rapidly absorbed when the circulation is normal, but in circulatory shock absorption will be delayed and it is best given i.v. Oral morphine is subject to extensive pre-systemic or first-pass metabolism (conjugation; gut wall and liver) and only about 20% of a dose reaches the systemic circulation; the oral dose is about twice the injected dose. The buccal route (the tablet is placed between lip and gum) or the sublingual route are also practicable and there is no first-pass metabolism; it is comparable to i.m. injection.

Morphine in the systemic circulation is metabolised by both liver and kidney; the conjugated metabolites include the pharmacologically active morphine-6-glucuronide. Elimination of morphine (10%) and metabolites is largely renal, but data conflict on whether action is prolonged in renal failure; it probably is not.*

Other routes of administration used by specialists are epidural (obstetrics) and intrathecal.

The plasma $t_{1/2}$ is 2–4 h and the duration of useful analgesia is 4–6 h (shorter in younger than in older subjects).

Morphine crosses the placenta and depresses respiration in the fetus at brith.

Dosage. Given s.c., i.m. or i.v. 10 mg is usually adequate; with 15 mg unwanted effects increase more than does analgesia. For oral dosage see terminal care p. 313. Continuous pain suppression can be achieved by morphine orally 4-hourly and s.c. 3-hourly or by continuous s.c. infusion using a battery-powered pump attached to the patient, who may even be ambulant.

The important uses of morphine and its allies are:

1. To relieve *severe pain* (but beware of masking useful diagnostic signs, e.g. in the acute abdomen and pupillary signs in neurology).
2. To relieve *anxiety* in serious and frightening disease, e.g. circulatory shock, severe haemorrhage, accidents.
3. To relieve *dyspnoea* in acute left ventricular failure (paroxysmal nocturnal dyspnoea).

* Woolner, D. F. *et al* (1986) *Brit. J. Clin. Pharmacol.* **22**, 55.

4. *Premedication* for surgery.

5. Symptomatic control of acute non-serious *diarrhoea*, e.g. travellers' diarrhoea (codeine, loperamide).

6. To suppress *cough*.

7. To control *acute restlessness* (rarely).

8. To produce *euphoria* as well as pain relief in the dying.

Any of the desired effects may be interfered with by opioid-induced nausea, vomiting and dysphoria.

Hazards

Morphine and disease. Morphine has long been a standard tranquilliser for shocked patients, but there may be such intense peripheral vasoconstriction that s.c. absorption is delayed for hours. A second or even third dose may therefore be injected before the patient has absorbed the first and so lead to poisoning when the vasoconstriction passes off. In such cases morphine should be given i.m. or slowly i.v.

In hepatic failure small doses can cause coma (see *drugs and the liver*), and it may be dangerous in hypothyroidism (slow metabolism). Serious hypotension can occur in myocardial infarction and with antihypertensive drugs, also vagal bradycardia (treatable by atropine 0.3 to 0.6 mg i.v.).

In respiratory insufficiency (emphysema, asthma, raised intracranial pressure) it is dangerous, see above; also in diverticulitis, pancreatitis and after cholecystectomy, see above.

Interactions. Morphine is potentiated by neostigmine, chlorpromazine (perhaps) and MAOIs and tricyclic antidepressants. Any central nervous system depressant will have additive effects.

Adverse effects have been mentioned and discussed. Dependence and overdose are treated below. Opioid use in obstetrics requires special care (p. 454).

Opioid dependence. It is now known that physical dependence begins to occur within 24 h if morphine is given 4-hourly, and after surgery some patients may be unwittingly subjected to a withdrawal syndrome that passes for general post-operative discomfort.

Acquired tolerance may rapidly reach a high degree, an exceptional addict taking 600 mg or more several times a day. An average addict is more likely to take about 300 mg. Duration of tolerance after cessation of administration is variable for different actions, from a few days to weeks. Thus, an addict who has undergone withdrawal and lost his tolerance, and who later resumes his opioid career may overdose himself inadvertently.

Morphine dependence is more disabling physically and socially than is opium dependence. It is said, and there is reasonable support for it, that the use of opium by Eastern peoples presents about as serious a social problem as the use of alcohol by Western peoples. All are agreed, however, that dependence on the pure alkaloids has results so detrimental to society as well as to the individual that their supply as social drugs in the same manner as alcohol and tobacco cannot be permitted.

The typical *acute withdrawal syndrome in opioid (morphine) dependence* consists largely of effects that are opposites to the normal actions.*

'When an addict misses his first shot, he senses mild withdrawal distress ("feels his habit coming on") but this is probably more psychological than physiological, for fear plays a considerable role in the withdrawal syndrome. At this stage a placebo may give relief. During the first 8–16 h of abstinence the addict becomes increasingly nervous, restless and anxious; close confinement tends to intensify these symptoms. Within 14 h (usually less) he will begin to yawn frequently; he sweats profusely and develops running of the eyes and nose comparable to that accompanying a severe head cold. These symptoms increase in intensity for the first 24 h, after which the pupils dilate and recurring waves of goose flesh occur. Severe twitching of the muscles (the origin of the term "kick the habit") occurs within 36 h and painful cramps develop in the backs of the legs and in the abdomen; all the body fluids are released copiously; vomiting and diarrhoea are acute; there is little appetite for food and the addict is unable to

* There is increasing evidence that the acute opioid withdrawal syndrome is due to noradrenergic 'storm' as a consequence of abrupt release from opioid suppression: central physiological regulation of the noradrenergic system may depend on endogenous opioid mechanisms.

sleep. The respiratory rate rises steeply. Both systolic and diastolic blood pressure increase moderately to a maximum between the third and fourth day; temperature rises an average of about 0.5°C, subsiding after the third day; the blood sugar content rises sharply until the third day or after; the basal metabolic rate increases sharply during the first 48 h. These are the objective signs of withdrawal distress which can be measured; the subjective indications are equally severe and the illness reaches its peak within 48–72 h after the last shot of the opioid, gradually subsiding thereafter for the next 5–10 days. Complete recovery requires from 3–6 months with rehabilitation and, if needed, psychiatric treatment. The withdrawal syndrome proper is self-limiting and most addicts will survive it with no medical assistance whatever (this is known as kicking the habit "cold turkey"). Abrupt withdrawal is inhumane, but with the development of such drugs as methadone, it is possible to reduce the distress of withdrawal very considerably',* for though there is cross-tolerance, exception, see before. It is impossible to rule on morphine or heroin withdrawal. For further discussion see under *drug dependence*.

It is usual to cover the acute withdrawal period (about 10 days) of injected morphine or heroin with an opioid taken orally and having a long $t_{\frac{1}{2}}$ (e.g. methadone; $t_{\frac{1}{2}}$, 48 h), perhaps supplemented with chlorpromazine or a benzodiazepine. Central noradrenergic mechanisms are depressed by continuous opioid exposure and withdrawal results in rebound hyperactivity, which is responsible for many of the acute manifestations. Clonidine (0.1 mg × 4/day, reducing over about 4 days) can reduce these effects usefully by its agonist action on central presynaptic α_2-adrenoceptors that results in inhibition of sympathetic autonomic outflow; hypotension may occur.

A withdrawal syndrome occurs in the newborn of dependent mothers. Opioids with mixed agonist/antagonist actions will precipitate a withdrawal syndrome in dependent subjects, as will naloxone (it is unkind, because it is unnecessary, to use naloxone as a diagnostic test in suspected addicts). Complete recovery of normal physiology after withdrawal may take weeks.

There is a risk of making patients seriously dependent if prolonged or frequent treatment of pain with a high-efficacy opioid is undertaken (the more widely the doses are spaced, the less the risk), e.g. for trigeminal neuralgia, migraine or recurrent urinary lithiasis. Terminal care is an exception, see before. It is impossible to rule on how quickly a patient can become seriously dependent, but it is generally a matter of weeks or months, though detectable physical dependence can occur in a day if the drug is given intensively.

Overdose. Death from overdose (of all opioids, low and high efficacy: agonist or agonist/antagonist) is due to respiratory depression. Blood pressure is usually well maintained, if the patient is supine, until anoxia causes circulatory failure. At this point the pupils, whose small size is a useful diagnostic indicator, may dilate (also if there is hypothermia). Correct diagnosis is vital for naloxone is a selective competitive antagonist. Naloxone does not have any of the actions of morphine, i.e. it has no agonist effects (coma, repiratory depression, miosis). Therefore it is safe to give naloxone as a therapeutic test in an unconscious or drowsy patient suspected of opioid overdose. The $t_{\frac{1}{2}}$ of naloxone (1 h) is shorter than most opioids and repeated doses or infusion will be needed. The guide to therapy is the state of respiration, not consciousness. Patients with opioid overdose should be watched for recurrence of ventilatory depression, which is an indication for further naloxone. (For details of naloxone use see p. 325.) Apart from naloxone the general treatment is the same as for overdose by any cerebral depressant.

Addicts often take overdoses, whether accidentally or not, and naloxone, as well as reversing the life-endangering respiratory depression, will induce an acute (noradrenergic) withdrawal syndrome. Close cardiovascular monitoring is necessary, with use of peripheral adrenoceptor blocking agents or perhaps clonidine (see above), according to need.

Preparations of opium and morphine

There is a large number of obsolescent and obsolete formulations of opium.

Small doses of opium can be used for the symp-

* From Maurer D W, Vogel V H. Narcotics and narcotic addiction. Springfield, I U.: Charles C. Thomas. 1962. Courtesy of Authors and Charles C. Thomas, publisher, Springfield, Ill.

tomatic control of the milder diarrhoeas, e.g. Opium Tabs, Kaolin and Morphine Mixture; and for cough, e.g. Opiate Squill Linctus (Gee's Linctus; squill, obtained from a bulbous plant, contains emetic glycosides that are also supposedly expectorant; its preferred use is as a rat poison, for rats cannot escape by vomiting). These and other preparations may be used by those who have a mind to and they have the efficacy of the opium they contain.

The only preparation of opium that remains in widespread use is *papaveretum* (Omnopon), a mixture of purified opium alkaloids chiefly used in pre-anaesthetic medication.

Morphine salts are used by injection, and by the oral, buccal, sublingual and rectal routes. Sustained-release formulations, oral (MST Continus) and i.m. (Duromorph, a microcrystalline form), are available.

The opioids discussed below are considered in relation to morphine ($t_{1/2}$ does not necessarily indicate duration of useful analgesia, which is related to affinity of the opioid for receptors: but $t_{1/2}$ gives useful information on accumulation).

Classification of opioids by analgesic efficacy

Low-efficacy for mild and moderate pain	*High-efficacy for severe pain*
codeine	morphine
dihydrocodeine	diamorphine (heroin)
dextropropoxyphene	pethidine (meperidine)
pentazocine	papaveretum
nalbuphine	methadone
	phenazocine
	buprenorphine
	levorphanol
	dextromoramide
	dipipanone
	meptazinol

Notes:

1. The division into two classes is not absolute and some drugs listed for moderate pain can be used for severe pain by injection.

2. Fentanyl, alfenatil, phenoperidine and piritamide are high-efficacy opioids used for surgery/anaesthesia.

3. Etorphine is a high-efficacy opioid used in veterinary practice.

Agonist/antagonist opioids (partial agonists) were developed in the unrealized hope of eliminating the potential for abuse, they include pentazocine, buprenorphine, butorphanol, meptazinol and nalbuphine; they may induce psychotomimetic reactions, and nalorphine is no longer used as an antagonist because of this. They are less liable to induce dependence and to cause respiratory depression than are the pure agonists.

Codeine (methylmorphine) (15, 30 mg) is a low-efficacy opioid; it has a $t_{1/2}$ of 3 h and 10% is converted to morphine (i.e. it cannot control severe pain) but most of its other actions are about one-tenth that of morphine. It also has a qualitative difference from morphine in that large doses cause excitement. Dependence occurs but much less than with morphine.

Its principal uses are for mild and moderate pain and cough (long-term use is accompanied by chronic constipation) and for the short-term symptomatic control of the milder acute diarrhoeas. The dose of codeine alone is 10–60 mg orally 4-hourly: and by injection up to 30 mg. There are numerous formulations for cough (e.g. Codeine Linctus) and for pain, in which it is commonly combined with aspirin and/or paracetamol (Aspirin and Codeine Tabs: Aspirin, Paracetamol and Codeine Tabs).

Pethidine (meperidine, Demerol) (50 mg) was introduced in 1939. It was discovered during a search for smooth muscle relaxants acting like atropine. Structurally, it is not obviously related to either morphine or atropine, though it is said that cognoscenti can discern resemblances to both. When given to mice it caused the tail to stand erect (Straub phenomenon) a characteristic of morphine-like drugs due to spasm of the anal sphincter. This attracted attention and pethidine was examined for analgesic effect.

Pethidine cannot relieve such severe pain as can morphine (i.e. lower therapeutic efficacy) but is effective against pain beyond the reach of codeine. Despite its substantial structural dissimilarity to morphine, pethidine has many similar properties including that of being antagonised by naloxone.

Pethidine differs from morphine in the following ways:

It does not suppress cough usefully.

It does not constipate, but its effect in the upper small intestine is similar to morphine and there is spasm of the sphincter of Oddi.

It is less likely to cause, urinary retention and to prolong childbirth.

It has little hypnotic effect.

Duration of analgesia is substantially shorter (2–3 h).

Pethidine causes vomiting about as often as does morphine; it has atropine-like effects, including dry mouth and blurred vision (cycloplegia; and sometimes mydriasis though usually miosis). Overdose or use in renal failure can cause central nervous system stimulation (myoclonus, convulsions) due to the major metabolite norpethidine, which is excreted by the kidney.

There is disagreement on the extent to which pethidine depresses respiration. It is probable that in equianalgesic doses it is as depressant as morphine.

Pethidine dependence occurs with some tolerance, especially to the the side-effects, but its psychic effects are less constant and less marked than those of morphine. Pethidine has evident advantages over morphine for pain that is not very intense, and it is widely used. It is usually given orally (50–100 mg) or i.m. (25–100 mg), when its effects last 2–3 h). The solution is irritant and so it is not given s.c. Given i.v. (25–50 mg) it is used sometimes in anaesthetic practice to provide a state of 'general analgesia'. It is widely used in obstetrics because it does not delay labour like morphine; but it enters the fetus and can depress respiration at birth.

Pethidine ($t_{\frac{1}{2}}$, 3 h) is metabolised in the liver and 5% is excreted unchanged in the urine. The latter is substantially greater if the urine is acid and this can be put to practical use in obtaining evidence in suspected cases of pethidine dependence (levorphanol and methadone behave similarly). In overdose it is not worthwhile to acidify the urine since naloxone is convenient and effective.

Methadone (Physeptone) (1946) (5 mg) is a synthetic drug structurally and pharmacologically similar to morphine. Vomiting is fairly common (though somewhat less than with morphine) especially if the patient is ambulant, and sedation is less. 5–10 mg are given about 6–12 hourly, orally or s.c. But since it has a long $t_{\frac{1}{2}}$ of wide range, 20–80 h, accumulation will occur, especially in the aged. Analgesia may last for as long as 24 h. If used for chronic pain in terminal care (12-hourly) an opioid of short $t_{\frac{1}{2}}$ may be provided for breakthrough pain rather than an extra dose of methadone.

Dependence occurs but this is less severe (slower onset and less severe withdrawal syndrome) than with morphine and heroin, and addicts to these drugs (by injection) are often transferred to oral methadone as part of their treatment.* Addicts who are cooperative enough to take oral methadone will feel less 'kick/buzz/rush' from i.v. heroin or morphine should they be unable to resist temptation, because their opioid receptors are already occupied by methadone and the i.v. drug must compete.

Methadone is also useful for severe cough, *Levorphanol* (Dromoran) is similar to methadone.

Diamorphine (heroin) is a semisynthetic drug first made from morphine at St. Mary's Hospital, London in 1874. It was introduced in 1898 as a remedy for cough and for morphine addiction and is very effective against both. Some years passed, however, before it was appreciated that it 'cured' morphine addiction by substituting itself as the addicting agent. Since then it has become a popular opioid with addicts and has achieved such a reputation that it is difficult now to discover whether abusers are attracted to it because it is pleasanter or because of its reputation, plus its ready availability from drug peddlers. It is rapidly (in minutes) converted to morphine in the body.

It is commonly stated that heroin is the 'most potent' of all dependence-producing drugs. Weight-for-weight it is certainly more potent than morphine, and this is of importance in illicit traffic as heroin takes up less space, but in so far as efficacy in inducing dependence is concerned there is doubt. Indeed, it has been reported that some addicts have voluntarily preferred methadone to heroin.

In almost every country the manufacture of heroin, even for use in medicine, is now illegal. The first to try this prohibition as a remedy for

* In the UK a special *Methadone Mixture 1 mg/ml* (the concentration is part of the official title) and coloured green is specially provided for the management of opioid addicts; it is × 2½ the strength of Methadone Linctus, for cough (yellow or brown); they must not be confused.

widespread drug addiction was the USA, which banned heroin manufacture in 1924, provoked by the magnitude of their addiction problem and not yet discouraged by their experience of this type of approach with alcohol prohibition (1919 to 1933).

An effort was made in 1953 to achieve a world-wide ban on heroin in medicine (so that any heroin, whenever it was found *must* be illegal) and most countries agreed. The UK did not agree because legitimate supplies for medicine were not then getting into illicit channels (it has since remained available but is not exported).

Many clinicians have long thought and some have passionately believed that heroin has unique therapeutic properties (euphoria, analgesic efficacy, lack of adverse effects) but research, as opposed to clinical impressions, has shown these beliefs in the superiority of heroin to be unfounded, *except* that heroin is more soluble than morphine to a useful degree* when continuous pain control in terminal care can no longer be achieved by enteral morphine (oral, buccal, suppository) for any reason. The greater solubility of heroin is then a real advantage in wasted subjects requiring multiple injections (or continuous infusion) of high doses.

Pharmacokinetics. Diamorphine (heroin) given parenterally has a plasma $t_{\frac{1}{2}}$ of 3 min, being metabolised to the two active substances 6-acetylmorphine and morphine ($t_{\frac{1}{2}}$, 2–4 h). When given orally heroin is subject to complete pre-systemic or first-pass metabolism and has all been converted to morphine by the time it reaches the systemic circulation. It has been pointed out that oral heroin is essentially a pro-drug and 'may be considered a relatively inefficient means of providing systemic morphine'†. It may be that the greater weight-for-weight potency of heroin (1 mg heroin ≡ 1.5 mg morphine) is due to the metabolite 6-acetylmorphine and to the common use of morphine as sulphate and heroin as hydrochloride.

Heroin is *used* for pain (above) and for severe cough (Diamorphine Linctus).

Pentazocine (Fortral, Talwin) (1967) is an opioid antagonist/agonist; it can induce a withdrawal syndrome in addicts (antagonist effect); it can also induce psychological and physical dependence (agonist effect), and this can be severe. It has not proved to be the solution to separating the property of potent analgesia from that of producing dependence as was thought initially, though it is a distinct advance.

Its *analgesic efficacy* approximates to that of morphine, but its *potency* (weight for weight) is about one-third of morphine. Its $t_{\frac{1}{2}}$ is about 3 h.

Adverse effects include: nausea, vomiting, dizziness, sweating, hypertension, palpitations, tachycardia, central nervous system disturbances (euphoria; dysphoria, psychotomimesis), and all are more likely with the higher peak plasma concentrations achieved after injection.

Uses are those of morphine (excepting in diarrhoea), and also for lesser and chronic pain for its liability to induce dependence is less than morphine.

Dosage. Pentazocine Tabs (25, 50 mg), 25–100 mg, 3–4-hourly: Pentazocine Inj, 30–60 mg, i.m., 3–4-hourly.

Pentazocine compared with morphine

Dependence liability: less, but definitely occurs.
Effect on opioid dependence: induces withdrawal syndrome.
Respiratory depression and sedation: less.
Duration of action: shorter. *Psychotominetic effects*: more.
Overdose respiratory depression: naloxone effective against both.
Nausea and vomiting: similar.
Constipation: less.
Cardiovascular effects of high doses: (chiefly important in myocardial infarction)
- *morphine*: hypotension, bradycardia.
- *pentazocine*: hypertension (systemic and pulmonary), tachycardia; so avoid in cardiovascular disease

Phenazocine (Narphen) is a high-efficacy agonist used particularly in biliary colic for it has less capacity than other opioids to cause spasm of the sphincter of Oddi.

Buprenorphine (Temgesic) (200 μg) is a high-efficacy agonist/antagonist with a duration of action of 6–8 h (and a single dose $t_{\frac{1}{2}}$ of only 3 h due to rapid tissue uptake); it has less liability to

* *Solubility* in water: morphine sulphate 1 in 21: heroin hydrochloride 1 in 1.6.
† Inturrisi C E et al. N Engl J Med 1984; 310:1213.

induce dependence and respiratory depression than pure agonists; it has little effect on the cardiovascular system and may spare the sphincter of Oddi (from induced spasm).

Buprenorphine is tenaciously bound to opioid receptors (i.e. has a high affinity) and so the respiratory depression of overdose is only partially reversed by the competitive antagonist naloxone; a non-specific respiratory stimulant (doxapram) may be needed, or assisted respiration. Because of extensive pre-systemic elimination when swallowed, buprenorphine is given by the buccal (sublingual) route (200–400 μg) or by i.m. or slow i.v. injection (300–600 μg).

Dextropropoxyphene (Doloxene) is structurally close to methadone and differs in that it is less analgesic, antitussive, and less dependence-producing. Its analgesic usefulness approximates to that of codeine. It is rapidly absorbed and has a $t_{\frac{1}{2}}$ of about 12 h. In overdose the rapidity of absorption is such that respiratory arrest may occur within one hour, so that many subjects die before reaching hospital. Combination with alcohol (common with self-poisoning) enhances repiratory depression. Some critics think this disadvantage outweighs the benefits of the drug and wish to see it withdrawn. Dextropropoxyphene is commonly combined with paracetamol (co-proxamol, Distalgesic) and with aspirin (Doloxene Cpd) (see also p. 307).

Dihydrocodeine (DF118) (30 mg) is a low-efficacy opioid, but, curiously, it can make post-operative dental pain worse. It is not known how many agonist opioids can make pain worse, but naloxone (antagonist) can do this. It may be that where endogenous opioid pathways are highly activated by afferent nociceptive input, a weak agonist, by competitively replacing the more active endogenous opioid, acts as an antagonist. Whatever the explanation, such observations remind us of the importance of placebo-controlled studies in real-life situations and that assumptions that one pain is like another and so will respond similarly to drugs cannot be relied on. The investigators in this study remarked that placebo-controlled studies have 'been criticized on legal, ethical and practical grounds. In particular, critics have questioned the probity of investigators who subject patients to placebos when they anticipate that the active drug will be effective. When we embarked on this trial, we expected to observe an analgesic effect — probably greater than aspirin or paracetamol — with dihydrocodeine. The demonstration of hyperalgesia would have been impossible without a placebo and vindicates our approach to clinical studies of the efficacy of analgesics.'* Dosage is 30–60 mg orally: 25–50 mg deep s.c.

Dextromoramide (Palfium) and *dipipanone* (Diconal is dipipanone plus cyclizine, an antiemetic) are less sedating and shorter acting than morphine; they are suitable for acute attacks of pain, e.g. breakthrough pain in terminal illness.

Other opioids include: butorphanol, ethoheptazine, meptazinol, oxycodone, alphaprodine.

Opioids used particularly during and after surgery:

Fentanyl (Sublimaze) has higher efficacy than morphine, analgesia lasts 30–60 min (single dose) and $t_{\frac{1}{2}}$ is 6 h; it is used i.v. for neuroleptanalgesia (see index); the difference between the short duration of analgesia and the relatively long $t_{\frac{1}{2}}$ suggests that the termination of effect of a single dose is the result of distribution of the drug, not of elimination; fentanyl is also used in combination with *droperidol* (a butyrophenone neuroleptic; Thalamonal).

Phenoperidine (Operidine) ($t_{\frac{1}{2}}$, 30 min) is similar.

Alfenatil (Rapifen) ($t_{\frac{1}{2}}$, 1.5 h) given i.v., provides maximum analgesia in 90 sec, which lasts about 10 min from a single dose; it is used for brief painful operations.

Nalbuphine (Nubain) is an agonist/antagonist given by injection.

Opioids (*non-analgesic*) *used for cough* include pholcodeine, dextromethorphan, noscapine (narcotine).

Opioids (*non-analgesic*) *used for antimotility effect* on the gut include loperamide and diphenoxylate (p. 635).

Miscellaneous

Papaverine differs from the more important opium alkaloids in that its only useful effect is relaxation of smooth muscle throughout the body, especially in the vascular system when injected. Oral prep-

* Seymour R A et al. Lancet 1982; 2:1425.

arations exist. It is occasionally injected into an area where local vasodilatation is desired, especially into and around arteries and veins to relieve spasm during vascular surgery and when setting up i.v. infusions.

Nefopam (Acupan) is neither an opioid nor an NSAID; it is effective against moderate and severe pain; its mode of action is unknown. Since it lacks the disadvantages of opioids (constipation, repiratory depression) and has greater efficacy than NSAIDs, it provides an alternative. It is not antagonised by naloxone.

Opioid antagonists

Naloxone (Narcan) is a (pure) competitive opioid antagonist at ordinary doses. It antagonises both agoinst and agonist/antagonist opioids (though it may not be sufficient alone in buprenorphine overdose since this drug binds particularly tenaciously to receptors).

Pharmacokinetics. Naloxone has high presystemic elimination when swallowed and is not used by this route. Given i.v., reversal of respiratory depression begins in 1–2 min, reversal of other effects — analgesia, depressed consciousness — can be slower. A prompt marked improvement in respiration has diagnostic value in opioid overdose, but poor or no response may occur because insufficient has been given, or with buprenorphine (above) or due to cerebral hypoxia or to hypothermia in severe cases.

Naloxone acts for about one hour, which happens to be about the $t_{\frac{1}{2}}$, though the peak effect on depressed respiration may be as brief as 10 min. Opioid analgesics act for much longer than their $t_{\frac{1}{2}}$ (due to tissue uptake; see above) and either repeated i.v. doses of naloxone will be needed, or continuous i.v. infusion; given s.c. or i.m. onset of action is slower and duration is longer.

Dosage in suspected opioid overdose is as follows: initially 0.4–1.2 mg (some advocate up to 2 mg) i.v.; the patient is closely observed (respiration, pupils, consciousness) for 3 min; if response occurs but is inadequate, give a second dose; if there is no response but the history of opioid overdose is strong (accident in hospital, known heroin abuser) then repeat doses until there is a response or until 10 mg has been given.

Infusion i.v. may be up to 5 mg/hour and may be required for days with opioids having a long $t_{\frac{1}{2}}$ (methadone). In overdose in opioid-dependent subjects, naloxone will quickly induce an acute withdrawal syndrome (see p. 320).

Naloxone is also used to counter excess opioid effects after surgical analgesia or childbirth.

Now that it is known or suspected that physiological opioid mechanisms are not confined to analgesia, and may play a physiological detrimental role in vascular shock (suppression of adrenergic responses), in non-opioid comas, and in some psychological disorders, naloxone has been tried in a wide range of conditions, but in none has it yet found a definitive role.

Naltrexone is similar to naloxone but longer acting.

Other opioid antagonists include nalorphine, levallorphan, cyclazocine and naltrexone, but these all have some agonist activity. They are inappropriate for treatment of opioid overdose, but the long-acting member, naltrexone, ($t_{\frac{1}{2}}$, 10 h; duration of action up to 24 h) may find a use (orally daily or by s.c. implantation monthly) in cooperative opioid abusers, for it can block the 'kick' of i.v. injection and also opioid euphoria.

GUIDE TO FURTHER READING

1 Beecher H K. Measurement of pain. Pharmacol Rev 1957; 9:59.

2 Modell W et al. Factors influencing clinical evaluation of drugs with special reference to the double-blind technique. JAMA 1958; 167:2190.

3 Beecher H K. Control of suffering in severe trauma. JAMA 1960; 173:534.

4 Lasagna L. The psychophysics of clinical pain. Lancet 1962; 2:572.

5 Bellville J W et al. The respiratory effects of codeine and morphine in man. Clin Pharmacol Ther 1968; 9:435.

6 The controversy over the proposal to ban heroin from medicine in Britain which throws light on human nature more, perhaps, than on human pharmacology, may be followed in:
Br Med J 1955; 1:1264.
Br Med J 1955; 2:1319, 1375, 1437, 1453, 1507, 1626.
Br Med J 1956; 1:298.
Lancet 1955; 1:1277, 1311.

7 Editorial. Heroin for cancer: a great non-issue of our day. Lancet 1984; 1:1449.

8 Lasagna L et al. The optimal dose of morphine. JAMA 1954; 156:230.

9 Twycross R. Relief of terminal pain. Br Med. J. 1975; 2:212.
10 Editorial Narcotic analgesics in terminal care. Lancet 1975; 2:694.
11 Evans J M et al. Degree and duration of reversal by naloxone of effects of morphine in conscious subjects. Br Med J 1974; 2:589.
12 Dige-Petersen H et al. Subclinical ergotism. Lancet 1977; 2:65.
13 Twycross R. Value of cocaine in opiate-containing elixirs. Br Med J 1977; 2:1348.
14 Isbell H. The search for a non-addicting analgesic: has it been worth it? Clin Pharmacol Ther 1977; 22:377.
15 Säive I et al. Oral morphine in cancer patients. Br J Clin Pharmacol 1985; 19:495.
16 Sriwatanakuly K et al. Evaluation of current clinical trial methodology in analgesimetry based on experts' opinions and analysis of several analgesic studies. Clin Pharmacol Ther 1983; 34:277.
17 Loch W E E et al. Local aspirin analgesia in the oral cavity. Clin Pharmacol Ther 1983; 33:642.
18 Tokola R A et al. Effect of migraine attacks on paracetamol absorption. Br J Clin Pharmacol 1984; 18:867.
19 Seymour R A et al. Dihydrocodeine-induced hyperalgesia in postoperative dental pain. Lancet 1982; 1:1425.
20 Rosen A. Patient controlled analgesia. Br Med. J. 1984; 289:640.
21 Inturrisi C E et al. The pharmacokinetics of heroin in patients with chronic pain. N Engl J Med 1984; 310:1213.
22 Thompson J W. Opioid peptides. Br Med J 1984; 288:259.
23 Laska E M et al. Effect of caffeine on acetaminophen analgesia. Clin Pharmacol Ther 1983; 33:498.
24 Jersell T M. Pain. Lancet 1982; 2:1084.
25 Kiser R S et al. Acupuncture relief of chronic pain syndrome correlates with increased plasma met-enkephalin concentrations. Lancet 1983; 2:1394.
26 Larson A G et al. The who and why of pain; analysis by social class. Br Med J 1984; 288:883.
27 Mondzac A M. Compassionate pain relief; is heroin the answer? N Engl J Med 1984; 311:530.
28 Angell M. The quality of mercy. N Engl J Med 1982; 306:98.
29 Pearce J M S. Migraine: a cerebral disorder. Lancet 1984; 2:86.
30 Creditor M C. Me and migraine. N Engl J Med 1982; 307:1029.

17

Central nervous system II: Sleep and hypnotics: Anxiety and anxiolytic sedatives

Definitions: drugs that depress the central nervous system

The following terms are commonly used:

Narcotic: a drug that induces drowsiness, sleep, or stupor (dazed state: state of helpless amazement), especially with analgesia (from Greek *narkosis*, state of being benumbed).

Hypnotic: a drug that induces sleep.

Anaesthetic: a drug that induces absence of sensation: anesthetics may be general or local.

Sedative: a drug (or dose of a drug) that calms or soothes without inducing sleep though it may cause sleepiness: a small dose of a hypnotic or tranquilliser often suffices for this.

Tranquilliser: a drug that will quieten a patient without significantly impairing consciousness. The ideal tranquilliser would allay pathological anxiety (i.e. be an **anxiolytic**) and nervous tension without altering any other cerebral functions; especially it would not cause sleepiness; in fact there is no clear distinction between tranquillisers and sedatives. It would also suppress mania and psychotic overactivity. The term **ataractic** is sometimes used; it is derived from a Greek word meaning impassiveness or indifference. **Neuroleptic** is another imprecise term generally used for the more powerful tranquillisers used for antipsychotic effect.

Psychotropic: a drug that alters mental function.

Analgesic: a drug that relieves pain.

Anticonvulsant: a drug that prevents and suppresses convulsions.

It is evident that the above terms describe the *uses* of drugs and are not based on any pharmacological classification; one drug may be correctly described as hypnotic, sedative or tranquilliser according to how and with what intent it is used, e.g. some benzodiazepines.

No group is more indefinite than the tranquillisers, which are a heterogeneous assemblage arbitrarily considered to include only the more recently introduced substances and to exclude the barbiturates and other hypnotics, although these are effective as tranquillisers in practice. There is some justification for this because transquillisers such as chlorpromazine do not, even at high doses, induce the relatively harmless and readily reversible unconsciousness characteristic of hypnotics.

SLEEP AND HYPNOTICS

Sleep is an active (not merely a passive, see below), circadian, physiological depression of consciousness. It is characterised by cyclical electroencephalographic (EEG) and eye movement changes, measures of which are used to describe sleep stages because they are convenient and seem to correlate with the fundamental physiological changes in neurotransmitter (noradrenaline, dopamine, serotonin, acetylcholine) functions that are inaccessible in clinical situations. Since these neurotransmitters are involved in psychiatric disorders it is no surprise that sleep disturbances are associated with mental disease.

Normal sleep (categorised by eye movements) is of two kinds:

1. **NREM** (non-rapid eye movement), **orthodox**, forebrain or slow-wave EEG **sleep**; awakened subjects state they were 'thinking': heart rate, blood pressure and respiration are steady or decline and muscles are relaxed; growth hormone secretion is maximal.

2. **REM** (rapid eye movement); **paradoxical**, hindbrain or fast-wave EEG **sleep**; awakened subjects state they were 'dreaming': heart rate, blood pressure and respiration are fluctuant, cerebral blood flow increases above that during wakefulness, the penis is erect (unless there is dream anxiety), skeletal muscles are profoundly relaxed though body movements are more pronounced.

A normal night begins with a sleep latency period as the subject passes from wakefulness into NREM sleep. An initial hour of NREM sleep is followed by about 20 min REM sleep, after which cycles of NREM sleep (about 90 min) abruptly alternate with REM sleep (about 20 min) for the rest of the night (i.e. about four cycles). Both kinds of sleep seem to be necessary for health (REM sleep especially to alleviate fatigue). *Hypnotics* in full doses can disrupt the normal sleep pattern, suppressing REM sleep, though tolerance may develop. Benzodiazepines and chloral do this least. No hypnotic can be said to induce natural sleep.

On *withdrawal* of a drug that has suppressed REM sleep there is a rebound increase in this kind of sleep, as though the body requires to recover what has been lost; nightmares occur with severe rebound; abnormal sleep patterns may persist for weeks after withdrawal.

It has not been conclusively shown that the kind of abnormality induced by hypnotics is harmful. But there is some evidence that deprivation of REM sleep may be responsible for emotional disorder so that hypnotics should not be used without good reason. That hypnotics are extensively prescribed, and indeed overprescribed, is well known.* In one study† of 7500 patients registered in an industrial general practice, 97 (1.3%) were receiving repeat prescriptions for hypnotics. They tended to be over 60 years with a preponderance of widows. The original indications were: (1) *medical* (48 patients): the prescribing began for some general medical or surgical disorder, particularly musculoskeletal pain; (2) *psychiatric* (30 patients): depressive-anxiety reactions, e.g. bereavement; (3) *onset insomnia* (19 patients): difficulty in getting to sleep; this was associated with neurotic personality disorder. Twenty per cent of patients started taking hypnotics in hospital. Only 6 of the 97 patients agreed to immediate withdrawal of the hypnotic. The others were dependent to varying degrees, chiefly mild, in that they considered adequate sleep would not be possible without drugs and that they would develop anxiety if withdrawal were attempted. The authors modestly suggest that a more critical attitude to hypnotic prescribing is required.

Non-hypnotic drugs and sleep. A range of other drugs have effects *on eye movement pattern* similar to hypnotics, when given in sufficient dose, e.g. heroin, morphine, alcohol, tricyclic and MAOI antidepressants, amphetamine and other appetite suppressants (though not fenfluramine). But effects on onset and duration of sleep differ.

The evaluation of hypnotics‡ in man is planned to throw light on the effects that will concern prescribers and patients. Evaluation begins with single dose studies in healthy volunteers in the morning, after a normal night's sleep. Tests to evaluate alertness, cognitive function, manual dexterity, coordination, reaction time, memory, etc. are administered. Then the drug is given at night to assess nocturnal effects, and residual effects the next day (hangover). The drug is then used in patients suffering insomnia (this presents particular ethical problems since the most suitable patients are those with chronic insomnia, in whom the clinical objective is to get them off all drugs rather than to encourage them to take new drugs).

* '. . . many times, reaching for the prescription pad and writing something out is a way the doctor says "Get lost! I don't want to hear you". It is a way of terminating the encounter.' Leo Hollister; Prof. of Medicine, Psychiatry and Pharmacology, Stanford University, USA.

† Johnson J et al. Br Med J 1968; 4:613. Later studies confirm this general pattern.

‡ Guidelines for the clinical investigation of hypnotic drugs Copenhagen: WHO Regional Office for Europe. 1983.

Assessment is by questionnaires, with particular interest in sleep latency (time taken to go to sleep), number of nocturnal awakenings, time of final awakening and quality of sleep (including dreaming); subsequent daytime effects (hangover) are of particular concern.

Sleep laboratory studies with EEG, eye movement and electromyographic (under the jaw) recording are conducted on a small number of subjects (they are expensive to do in terms of facilities, staff and skills).

It is also desirable to determine whether tolerance, and/or dependence occur, whether the drug is safe in long-term use, interactions with other drugs (including alcohol) and dosage in the old and in subjects with impaired elimination.

Hangover. The effects of hypnotics, including ordinary doses of some benzodiazepines (e.g. nitrazepam) taken at ordinary bedtime carry over into the afternoon of the following day. Often patients are aware of drowsiness, but even when they are not, impaired psychomotor performance occurs as shown by reaction time, tapping speed, attentiveness, ability speedily to cross out all examples of a single letter on a printed page, and ocular flicker fusion. This is not surprising since the half-life of nitrazepam is about 20 h. Discussion of drug effects on skilled tasks, especially car driving, is on p. 430. Patients who have accidents and who have not been warned of the hazards of sedation during the day are likely to have a valid claim for compensation for any injury due to the negligence of the prescriber.

Termination of action of a *single* dose of a drug having a long $t_{\frac{1}{2}}$ is often determined by distribution into tissues where it has no action (e.g. fat, muscle) rather than by metabolism or elimination, so that the duration of action of a single dose may be satisfactorily free from hangover despite a long $t_{\frac{1}{2}}$ (e.g. nitrazepam). But when a drug with a long $t_{\frac{1}{2}}$ is used nightly, there will be accumulation (of drug or of active metabolites) until a steady state is reached (at about five half-lives) and daytime impairment of performance may then become unacceptable. Thus, the $t_{\frac{1}{2}}$ gives useful knowledge, but it is not the only factor in determining duration of action; tissue concentrations and receptor binding (affinity) are also important.

As a general guide, drugs with a $t_{\frac{1}{2}} < 8$ h may, and those with a $t_{\frac{1}{2}} > 16$ h will have residual effects the following day.

Timing of hypnotic administration. Patients should be advised. Generally a hypnotic is best taken on going to bed or a few minutes before. In bed, the subject may read a suitable book that provides interest but no excitement (arousal), e.g. most biographies, a textbook (the size of this book, or smaller) or a book having a high moral tone. If the hypnotic was taken on an empty stomach, sleep latency will commonly be about 20 min. Some people are suited by taking the hypnotic (e.g. a slowly absorbed benzodiazepine) one hour before going to bed, but for others this can carry a risk of going to sleep prematurely and even in a potentially hazardous or unpleasant situation, e.g. in the bath.

Occasionally it is appropriate to advise a patient who suffers intermittent insomnia or is being weaned from chronic drug use, to go to bed, read a suitable book (above) and to take a short half-life drug (e.g. triazolam) if still wakeful after one or two hours; the availability of a single dose at the bedside* for use if needed, gives confidence and may itself increase the ability to do without it. (Availability of a bottle of tablets at the bedside traditionally carries risk of inadvertent repeated self-administration; no doubt the risk of this is low, but it cannot be dismissed.)

Dependence. It can be assumed that all hypnotic induce tolerance and dependence, with sudden withdrawal effects ranging from insomnia, even to convulsions (where dosage has been high and prolonged). *Withdrawal* from chronic users should always be gradual; the longer the use the slower should be the withdrawal (over weeks, reducing both dose and frequency); if symptoms (anxiety, insomnia, nightmares) occur then consumption should be stabilized until the symptoms disappear (a β-adrenoceptor blocker may assist by allaying somatic symptoms of anxiety); obviously, withdrawal symptoms are less acute with drugs (and metabolites) having a long $t_{\frac{1}{2}}$ (slow fall in drug concentration giving time for adap-

* A single overdose may be followed by disturbed sleep for weeks even in unhabituated subjects.

tation). The subject should be warned of the possibility of symptoms and counselled that they will pass away; if confidence is lost, withdrawal will be unsuccessful.

INSOMNIA

Insomnia deserves special attention; its successful management involves much more than merely prescribing drugs, which should be regarded as temporary expedients only (see also above). *Insomnia is defined* as a belief or feeling on the part of the patients that they are not getting enough sleep. Poor sleepers tend to overestimate the time it takes them to fall asleep (sleep latency) and to underestimate the time they stay asleep. When awakened during NREM (orthodox) sleep, subjects who complain of insomnia may claim they were not asleep. But some studies have found that nurses are liable to overestimate patients' sleep.

Kales* usefully classifies insomnia as either (1) failure to fall asleep within 45 min or (2) difficulty in staying asleep (six or more awakenings per night, or less than 6 h sleep): either of these at least four nights a week.

Types of insomnia include:

1. Tense people who lie awake in bed for hours unable to relax, and then sleep well.
2. Exhausted people who, because they sleep early in the evening wake early in the morning. They probably need no drug, but a midday rest.
3. People who wake repeatedly throughout the night, for no obvious reason.
4. People who wake repeatedly from physical discomfort or pain and who need treatment of that condition plus a hypnotic (temporarily).
5. Depression, in which sleep is shorter (early waking), less sound, interrupted and restless; patients need treatment for depression, not hypnotics.
6. Caffeine can cause difficulty getting to sleep, which increases with age, and alcohol, though it can help people to get to sleep can cause early waking (minor withdrawal symptoms).
7. Overuse of hypnotics with development of tolerance (3–14 days) and withdrawal syndrome when attempts to abstain are made.

A hypnotic is most often needed in:

1. *Transient and situational insomnia*, e.g. acute emotional disturbance, bereavement, domestic conflict, noisy hotel, to help the patient cope with brief episodes.
2. *Persistent insomnia*, which may have no apparent cause or may follow on after the passing of an acute situation; it also occurs in states of chronic anxiety and unhappiness. The objective is to restore the sleep habit by brief use of a drug. Where use is prolonged beyond a few days, insomnia due to withdrawal may be interpreted by patients as demonstrating a need to continue the drug, which can cause great difficulty, especially if the doctors have not adequately counselled the patients and got their own objectives clear. It is all too easy to follow the indulgent path of repeat prescriptions.

Thus in both the above situations there is danger that emotional and physical dependence on the drug will occur. It is important not to allow prescription of hypnotics and sedatives to become a means of evading the patient's real problem. 'Unfortunately, some patients use the sedative hypnotics as a crutch to help them in the struggle against the everyday pressure of living,'† and sadly, even the best doctor sometimes surrenders to patient demand.

Oswald‡ concludes that a prescription for a hypnotic is fully justified for a few nights or weeks to combat insomnia due to anxiety *provided* there is good reason to expect the cause to be removed either by changes in environment or by treatment (e.g. antidepressant drug or electric convulsions or other non-drug treatment). But where there is chronic insomnia or a long-standing personality disorder he does not consider prescription justified because: (1) tolerance develops, (2) dependence is likely, (3) sleep is not natural.

'At a very rough reckoning about one night's sleep in every ten in this country is hypnotic induced. . . . People seem to want to turn consciousness on and off like a tap. . . . While it is time-consuming to take a careful clinical

* Kales J et al. Clin. Pharmacol. Ther 1971; 12:691.

† Friend D G. Clin. Pharmacol Ther 1960; 1:5

‡ Oswald I. Pharmacol Rev 1968; 20:274.

history, to conduct a full clinical examination and to give wise advice, it takes only a moment to write a prescription and this does please and often satisfies the patient. . . . We do not always draw a clear distinction between the patients' *wants* and what we think are his *needs*, and it is regrettable how much we accede to the patients' demands in order to placate them and to save ourselves time and trouble.'*

Sedatives and hypnotics are also used in many other situations — in hypertension, with analgesics, before surgery and endoscopies and in conjunction with psychotherapy.

Choice of a hypnotic. The **benzodiazepines** are now overwhelmingly the first choice† because they:

1 alter sleep pattern least
2 are safer than other drugs in overdose and
3 do not significantly induce drug metabolising enzymes that cause unwanted interactions.

There are numerous members to choose between. *The principal factors that determine selection are pharmacokinetic*:

a. speed for absorption and passage into the central nervous system (i.e. lipid solubility)
b. half-life of the drug.
c. presence of active metabolites in sufficient amounts to have effect.
d. half-life of any active metabolites

Taking these factors into account, *a choice may be offered* as follows:

temazepam: $t_{\frac{1}{2}}$, 6–8 h, inactive metabolites; insignificant accumulation with repeated daily use, but may sometimes be too short acting for subjects of early waking.

triazolam: $t_{\frac{1}{2}}$, 2–4 h with active metabolites of $t_{\frac{1}{2}}$, 7 h; no accumulation with repeated daily use: the short $t_{\frac{1}{2}}$ of the drug may be associated with rebound (withdrawal) during the night and so it is less suitable for early waking, or may even cause it.

lormetazepam: $t_{\frac{1}{2}}$, 9 h with inactive metabolites; insignificant accumulation with daily use.

The above are all absorbed reasonably fast: *lorazepam* and *oxazepam* are absorbed rather too slowly for use when rapid onset is important.

benzodiazepines with long $t_{\frac{1}{2}}$ and/or with metabolites of long $t_{\frac{1}{2}}$ (e.g. diazepam, nitrazepam, flurazepam) are satisfactory as hypnotics for single, but not for daily doses. The action of a single dose is terminated by distribution in the body, not by metabolism. With repeated daily doses there will be accumulation over about the $t_{\frac{1}{2}}$ (parent drug plus active metabolites) × 5, i.e. over days (an important active metabolite of many benzodiazepines is desmethyldiazepam, $t_{\frac{1}{2}}$, about 65 h).

The long $t_{\frac{1}{2}}$ drugs (and active metabolites) may be used if subsequent day-time sedation is desired in anxious subjects. Speed of onset, duration of effect and incidence of hangover depend on the dose and on the patient almost as much as on the choice of drug.

Benzodiazepines are numerous. Those not discussed here may give satisfactory results, but clinicians should decide what they want to achieve and consider the kinetics of the drug and its metabolites before using it.

Barbiturates. There is an increasing consensus that barbiturates are unsuitable as hypnotics because

1. Barbiturates have a low therapeutic index, i.e. relatively small overdose (× 10 therapeutic dose) endangers life, with unconsciousness and respiratory depression.

2. Barbiturates illicitly obtained are popular drugs of social abuse.

3. Physical dependence occurs, with severe withdrawal syndrome sometimes including convulsions.

4. Barbiturates are potent inducers of hepatic drug metabolising enzymes and so are a source of drug interactions.

Alcohol (ethanol) cannot be recommended as a hypnotic (rebound awakening in early morning hours, dependence, diuresis, enzyme induction), though we would not wish to condemn its use as a nightcap by those who are determined that they will be unable to sleep without it.

Safety of hypnotics. Benzodiazepines are the

* Dunlop D. Br Med Bull 1970; 26:236.
† The insomnia of depression, often early waking, is better treated by a sedative antidepressant.

safest, i.e. minimal enzyme induction and minimal hazard in overdose, including hazard to inquisitive children imitating their parents/grandparents pill-swallowing proclivities.

Other hypnotics are more hazardous in overdose.

Interactions. All hypnotics synergise with alcohol and other cerebral depressants.

Non-benzodiazepine hypnotics are hepatic enzyme inducers. Benzodiazepines are hypnotics of first choice in patients taking warfarin (a drug with a narrow therapeutic range and particularly prone to pharmacokinetic interaction).

Age. In the elderly it is normal for sleep requirement to become less, and nocturnal awakenings to become more frequent. An aging person who complains of this should obviously not be treated with a hypnotic; any persistent demands should be resisted for the most likely result will be that they will spend the rest of their lives taking a hypnotic to no advantage and to potential disadvantage. Sleep disturbance in dementia may demand a hypnotic with or without a tranquilliser, e.g. promazine.

The *elderly* are less tolerant of hypnotics and shoud generally not receive long $t_{\frac{1}{2}}$ drugs, and should start with half the usual dose.

The old, particularly those with organic brain failure, may become confused with hypnotics and an occasional patient becomes excited or has nightmares on a particular drug. Confusion is more likely if a patient who has taken a full dose of hypnotic is kept awake by pain; adequate analgesia should accompany the hypnotic. The need to micturate may result in drugged old people hazardously wandering around the house.

Children: a benzodiazepine, chloral hydrate or promethazine is used.

Irritant drugs (chloral hydrate) are obviously unsuitable for peptic ulcer patients. In cases where it is especially desired to avoid any respiratory depression, e.g. in severe asthmatics or in head injury, even benzodiazepines in ordinary doses can impair ventilation.

*Food as an aid to sleep.** A *small* meal of milk and cereal promotes less restless sleep and there is experimental support for the popular belief that milk-cereal drinks do the same. The effect persists into the later night, suggesting that the cause is not only psychological expectation resulting from folklore and advertising, though these doubtless assist.

Since broken sleep increases with age it may be worth recommending the adoption of a pre-bed snack or drink before prescribing hypnotics to older patients with mild insomnia.

Snoring implies a risk of sleep apnoea, from which the subject needs to wake up. Hypnotics are contraindicated.

* Brezinova V. et al. Br Med J 972; 2:431.

ANXIETY

Anxiety in moderation is an appropriate and even useful response to life events and situations provided it stimulates achievement that may mitigate or remove the cause. But inappropriate or excessive or chronic anxiety is disabling, especially where the cause cannot be removed.

Yet anxiety may also occur without apparent exogenous cause, and subjects of this free-floating anxiety need and deserve help. Non-drug therapy may be best for many, but drugs are often useful for patients having a high level of anxiety. Doctors should not be over-ready to prescribe drugs, but neither should they be over-timid, for anxiety can be a curse that destroys the quality of life.

In the first half of this century, sedative doses of barbiturates and bromides were used to reduce the activity of the CNS in patients who complained of anxiety, then came neuroleptics such as chlorpromazine (1952), for which the term *tranquilliser* was coined because the drug could reduce excitement without notably impairing consciousness, and then meprobamate (1957), which had a great success probably because the term 'tranquilliser' was already coined and it sounded better than the familiar 'sedative', which it, in fact, is.

In 1960 chlordiazepoxide (Librium) the first *benzodiazepine* was introduced, and this group of drugs now dominates anti-anxiety medication.

But anxiety does not manifest itself only as a psychic or mental state, there are also somatic or physical concomitants, e.g. consciousness of the action of the heart (palpitations), tremor, diarrhoea, which are associated with increased activity of the sympathetic autonomic system. These symptoms are not only due to anxiety but also add to the feeling of anxiety (feedback loop). In patients whose complaints are primarily of somatic symptoms of anxiety rather than of anxiety itself a β-*adrenoceptor blocking drug* can give benefit; but it will generally not help where there is, for example, tachycardia that is not causing symptoms.

Somatic symptoms of sympathetic overactivity accompany the performance of stressful tasks, car racing or driving in busy traffic, stage fright, e.g. acting, public speaking, playing a musical instrument, surgery and other sports such as ski-jumping (requiring skill without maximum output of work), bowling, shooting, sitting examinations, and β-adrenoceptor block allows the subject to feel calmer and so can improve performance.

Even in experienced surgeons a rise in heart rate begins as soon as scrubbing-up for an operation session is begun. In one study* (8 surgeons) mean *maximum* heart rates were 137/min with mean heart rate 121/min (peak rates above 150/min were reached by two surgeons) regardless of the nature of the operation and regardless of seniority. Tachycardia of this degree corresponds to physical work that cannot be sustained for more than 10 min without extreme fatigue. Those people who cannot conceal their emotional state will be interested to know that 'if anything, those surgeons who were outwardly the most calm experienced the highest heart-rates'.* The mean heart-rate of surgeons operating after taking a β-adrenoceptor blocking drug (oxprenolol 40 mg orally) was 84/min. But it has not been shown that the surgeons actually operated better or were less fatigued.

Choice and mode of use of anxiolytic agents

1. *Benzodiazepines*, e.g. diazepam, oxazepam, are a first choice.
2. A β-*adrenoceptor blocker*, e.g. propranolol, where there are somatic symptoms.
3. A *sedative anti-depressant* where there is depression with anxiety, e.g. amitriptyline.
4. Other agents, e.g. chlormethiazole, may particularly suit the aged, alcoholics.

Use of low doses of neuroleptics, e.g. chlorpromazine, for anxiety, has been superseded by benzodiazepines. Neuroleptics can be effective but are liable to have too many autonomic side-effects.

Brief use is preferred. Benzodiazepines are liable to induce dependence and patients in acute high-level anxiety states should be counselled that treatment will be brief (days or a few weeks). But in low level and chronic anxiety, particularly where the causes can be seen to be irremovable, long-term therapy may seem inescapable although there is evidence that brief non-specialized counselling is as effective. After the drug has been taken for 4–6 months, efforts should be made to withdraw it; but this can be impossible and indefinitely prolonged therapy sometimes becomes obligatory as the lesser of two evils. This is why counselling should be preferred to the use of a drug at the outset.

Some *tolerance* to benzodiazepines occurs but anxiolytic efficacy has been shown to last 6 months.

Benzodiazepines with a long $t_{\frac{1}{2}}$ (of parent drug and/or active metabolite) are preferred for smooth effect. Either a single nocturnal dose (where there is also insomnia), which will give anxiolytic effect the next day, or small divided doses (to minimise peaks of effects) during the day. The less lipid-soluble drugs give smoother effect (slower absorption and slower entry into the CNS).

Where there are somatic symptoms, a β-adrenoceptor blocker may be effective alone or in combination with a benzodiazepine.

HYPNOTICS AND ANXIOLYTIC SEDATIVES

Benzodiazepines

History. Benzodiazepines were discovered by serendipity†. In the mid-1950s the clinical successes of chlorpromazine, reserpine and meprobamate suggested that tranquillisers were more than just general cerebral depressants. Industrial

* Foster S E et al. Lancet 1978; 1:1323.

† *Serendipity* is the faculty of making fortunate discoveries by general sagacity or by accident: the word derives from a fairy tale about three princes of Serendip (Sri Lanka) who had this happy faculty.

chemists (of Hoffman–LaRoche*) were encouraged to produce novel compounds of kinds that would lend themselves to molecular manipulation. An extensive biological screening programme was undertaken. Eventually, other problems seeming more important, the project lost priority and chlordiazepoxide was left lying around for two years before it was eventually studied. In animal tests it was superior to existing tranquillizers, including a marked taming effect in monkeys. Priority regained, some 16 000 patients were soon treated and the drug was licenced for general use in 1960. Since then thousands of benzodiazepines have been synthesized, hundreds tested and many tens have been marketed.

Actions and uses. Benzodiazepines have *hypnotic*, *sedative*, *anxiolytic*, *anticonvulsant* and (central) *muscle relaxant* actions. They bind to specific receptors in the central nervous system, the natural ligand (binding substance) for which remains unidentified. The result is to enhance the effects of gamma-aminobutyric acid (GABA; an important inhibitory neurotransmitter that probably acts by opening chloride ion channels into cells). There are several sub-types of benzodiazepine receptor, which raises the possibility of separating the various actions of the benzodiazepines by molecular manipulation so that, for example, anxiolytic effect may be achieved without concomitant sedation, which would be an important advance (there is some selectivity in this area between existing drugs).

Benzodiazepines may act largely on the brain reticular activating system (reducing sensory input), the limbic system (affect), the median forebrain bundle (reward and punishment systems) and the hypothalamus.

In addition, as expected, there exist antagonist or blocking benzodiazepines for which clinical uses might be found (termination of agonist effect after use, e.g. endoscopies and in overdose).

There are also benzodiazepines that have opposite (not merely blocking) actions, i.e. excitation, and these are called inverse agonists. The full possibilities for scientific discovery and therapeutic use of benzodiazepines in behaviour modification have yet to be explored.

Benzodiazepines also have effect on the function of other neurotransmitters (catecholamines, serotonin, etc.), which may have relevance to their use in mental disorders.

Occasionally the agonist (sedative) compounds in current use cause paradoxical effects, e.g. uncovering of depression, excitement, rage; interactions with GABA are being found to be increasingly complex.

Benzodiazepines shorten the time taken to go to sleep (sleep latency), decrease intermittent awakening and increase total sleep duration. Choice of drug as hypnotic is determined by pharmacokinetic properties (see, *choice of a hypnotic*, above). The choice as anxiolytic sedative is also largely determined by pharmacokinetic properties (see Table 17.1, p. 335); slow absorption and long $t_{\frac{1}{2}}$ give smooth effect. Selectivity between anxiolytic and sedative effects is low, though some trials suggest it, e.g. clorazepate may be less sedative than diazepam for equal anxiolytic effect, but no definitive recommendations can be made. Diazepam remains the standard member of the group, having a $t_{\frac{1}{2}}$ of 30 h with an active metabolite (desmethyldiazepam) with a $t_{\frac{1}{2}}$ of 65 h or even longer. A single dose before going to bed provides quick hypnotic effect and anxiolytic effect with less sedation throughout the next day. If a dose is needed during the day the rapid absorption of diazepam may cause undesirable sedation (which can be mitigated by using several small doses though that adds incovenience). The more slowly absorbed oxazepam may be preferred.

A detailed list of *conditions in which benzodiazepines may be useful* includes:

anxiety (without or with psychotic states), panic attacks, insomnia, alcohol withdrawal states, night terrors and somnambulism (children), muscle spasm due to a variety of causes, including tetanus and cerebral spasticity; epilepsy; anaesthesia and sedation for endoscopies and cardioversion.

Curiously, perhaps, benzodiazepines are extensively prescribed by primary care doctors for depression; but they are *not* antidepressant (except

* Sternbach L H. In: Costa E, ed. The benzodiazepines. New York: Raven Press. 1983.

perhaps alprazolam when anxiety is dominant in a mixed anxiety/depression). The reason is obscure but may be related to complaints of side-effects from the usual antidepressants.

Tolerance occurs with chronic use.

Anterograde amnesia (e.g. telephone number recall) occurs with high doses, e.g. i.v. for endoscopy, dental surgery (with local anaesthetic), cardioversion, and in these situations it can be regarded as a blessing. But embarrassing amnesia can also occur with oral use.

Elderly and/or troubled people arrested for *shoplifting* frequently claim that their crime was caused by chronic benzodiazepine (or other) therapy. Whilst it is natural to regard such claims with suspicion, those of us (not taking a benzodiazepine) who have nearly walked out of a self-service shop carrying goods we have neglected to present for payment will not be over-ready to dismiss the possibility (though amnesia selective for payment must arouse scepticism). A useful way of looking at the matter is to consider, not whether the drug caused an involuntary act of shoplifting (which is unlikely), but whether it might have made a contribution to absentmindedness so that the necessary conscious intent to steal (required by law) was not formed. When the circumstances of the particular case are known, the question may be asked whether it is *safe* to convict the person, i.e. that it is beyond reasonable doubt* that the drug was irrelevant. Many doubtful and pathetic instances are recorded in the newpapers; doctors are often asked to given evidence in Court; they will seek to be neither credulous nor callous.

Dependence, as shown by occurrence of withdrawal symptoms, is usual with therapeutic doses used beyond a few weeks, though it is commonly mild. Dependence occurs earlier with the short-acting members and withdrawal symptoms occur sooner and are more severe.

Withdrawal symptoms are maximal after 3–7 days (depending on the $t_{\frac{1}{2}}$ of the drug) and pass off over 2–4 weeks. They are greatly affected by expectation and personality, e.g. symptoms are passive-dependent traits.†

Symptoms include anxiety, agitation, irritability, confusion, depersonalisation, sleep disturbance, tremor, headache, muscle twitching or aches, sweating, diarrhoea, etc. convulsions and psychotic reactions may occur in severe cases. But patients have commonly been prescribed a benzodiazepine for similar symptoms and there is doubt in many cases just how much is a recrudescence of previous disorder and how much is evidence of true pharmacological dependence. Accounts of supposed withdrawal symptoms lasting for several months should be interpreted with caution. *Withdrawal* of benzodiazepines should be gradual after as little as 3 weeks use, but for long term users it should be very slow, e.g. one-sixth of the dose every 2 weeks, aiming to complete it in about 12 weeks. Withdrawal should be slowed if marked symptoms occur (milder symptoms may be controlled by β-adrenoceptor block). Towards the end of the withdrawal of a short $t_{\frac{1}{2}}$ drug it may be useful to substitute a long $t_{\frac{1}{2}}$ drug (diazepam) to minimize rapid fluctuations in plasma concentrations.‡ In difficult cases withdrawal may be assisted by concomitant use of a sedative antidepressant. Dependence will be minimized by critical prescribing using low doses for short periods or intermittently. Only in exceptional cases should use exceed a few weeks.

Interactions. There are additive effects with CNS *depressants*, including alcohol, which also speeds benzodiazepine absorption. *Cimetidine* may increase plasma concentrations of diazepam and chlordiazepoxide by as much as 50% (delayed metabolism and clearance); this does not happen with oxazepam and lorazepam. High caffeine intake reduces the anxiolytic effect.

Overdose. Benzodiazepines are remarkably safe in acute overdose and the therapeutic dose × 10

* The criterion of proof used in the Court of Law is:
civil cases — balance of probabilities.
criminal cases — beyond reasonable doubt.
Shoplifting is a crime because it is prohibited by law under penalty.

† The difficulty of assessing symptoms is shown by a study in which patients on long-term diazepam therapy experienced symptoms when they thought the drug was being withdrawn but in fact dosage remained the same. Tyrer P et al. Lancet 1983; 2:1402.

‡ For a detailed account see Higgitt A C et al. Clinical management of benzodiazepine dependence. Br Med J 1985; 291:688.

Table 17.1 Data on some benzodiazepines. *Long* $t_{1/2}$ drugs/metabolites are appropriate for anxiety. Short $t_{1/2}$ drugs/metabolites are appropriate *hypnotics*.

Names	Plasma $t_{1/2}$ (h)	Metabolites($t_{1/2}$)	Remarks
Alprazolam (Xanax)	14	inactive	May have antidepressant as well as sedative effect when anxiety is dominant.
Bromazepam (Lexotan)	12	inactive	—
Chlordiazepoxide (Librium)	17	active (14, 40) desmethyldiazepam (65) [see *note* 5]	Steady state reached about 3 day
Clobazam (Frisium)	18	active (42)	Used in epilepsy as well as anxiety
Clonazepam (Rivotril)	30	inactive	Used in epilepsy
Clorazepate (Tranxene)	pro-drug	desmethyldiazepam (65)	—
Diazepam (Valium)	30	active (10) desmethyldiazepam (65)	High lipid solubility so quickly effective
Flunitrazepam (Rohypnol)	20	active (minor)	—
Flurazepam (Dalmane)	pro-drug (1)	active (6) desmethyldiazepam (65)	Effect depends on metabolites
Ketazolam (Anxon)	pro-drug (1.5)	active (30) desmethyldiazepam (65)	Partly metabolized to diazepam
Loprazolam (Dormonoct)	7	Active (7)	Insignificant accumulation
Lorazepam (Ativan)	15	inactive	See text
Lormetazepam (Lobramet, Noctamid)	9	inactive	Insignificant accumulation
Medazepam (Nobrium)	pro-drug (1.5)	desmethyldiazepam (65)	—
Midazolam (Hypnovel)	2	inactive	Injected as adjunct in anaesthesia for endoscopies, dentistry, etc.
Nitrazepam (Mogadon)	24	inactive	Remaining popular as a hypnotic: superseded because of long $t_{1/2}$
Oxazepam (Serenid)	10	inactive	Slowly absorbed and distributed (lower lipid solubility)
Prazepam (Centrax)	pro-drug	desmethyldiazepam (65)	Effect depends on metabolites
Temazepam (Euhypnos)	8	inactive	Insignificant accumulation
Triazolam (Halcion)	2	active (7)	Rebound/withdrawal effect may occur during night due to short $t_{1/2}$

Notes:
1. The use of official (generic) names to stress *similarity* and proprietary names to stress *difference* is well shown.

2. The $t_{\frac{1}{2}}$ variability in individuals is very wide indeed though only a single figure is given the table; benzodiazepines are extensively bound to plasma proteins.
3. Formation of active metabolites does not necessarily mean they play a major role, especially with single doses.
4. Steady state will be reached in about $t_{\frac{1}{2}} \times 5$ of parent drug and active metabolites when present (but some have only a minor role in clinical effect).
5. The principal active metabolite having a long $t_{\frac{1}{2}}$ (65 h, but with range 30–200) and common to many members is *desmethyldiazepam* (nordiazepam); drugs having this metabolite are suitable as anxiolytics. There is no point in changing a patient from one agent having desmethyldiazepam as a major metabolite to another drug of the same kind. Generally agents that are conjugated have inactive metabolites, and those that are oxidised have active metabolites.
6. Liver disease may prolong $t_{\frac{1}{2}}$ up to × 3.
7. Duration of action is prolonged in the elderly and additive effects with alcohol are important.

induces sleep from which the subject is easily aroused. It is said that there is no reliably recorded case of death from a benzodiazepine taken alone by a person in good *physical* health, which is a remarkable tribute to their safety (high therapeutic index); even if the statement is not absolutely true, death must be extremely rare. But deaths have occurred in combination with alcohol (which combination is quite usual in those seeking to end their own lives). There is not, at present, a clinically available specific antidote to benzodiazepines and treatment is according to general principles.

Benzodiazepines in pregnancy. The drugs are not certainly known to be safe, and indeed diazepam is teratogenic in mice*. The drugs should be avoided in early pregnancy as far as possible. It should be remembered that safety in pregnancy is not only a matter of avoiding prescription after a pregnancy has occurred, but that individuals on long-term therapy may become pregnant. In late pregnancy benzodiazepines cross the placenta and can cause fetal cardiac arrhythmia, muscular hypotonia and poor suckling. Impairment of behavioural development in the newborn is possible.

Social aspects of benzodiazepine use cause concern, and this is natural with up to 2% of the population taking the drugs chronically because they cannot sleep, they feel anxious or worried, or they are unhappy. The enormous demand for these drugs (met by the medical profession) makes it hard to doubt that they relieve an immense amount of misery (as do tobacco and alcohol, which seem to be far more toxic both to the individual and to society). But increasingly there is criticism of lavish prescribing of these drugs and it is impossible to view with equanimity the continuous long-term use by numerous individuals of benzodiazepines over years. The possible social consequences of blunting of cognition and emotion remain undefined. The suggestion that benzodiazepines should be sold directly to the public without a doctor's prescription has not found favour.

* Determined investigators can devise experiments in animals so that either fetal hazard or fetal safety is implied and it may not be obvious which predicts to man.

Adverse effects. Dependence and sedation causing hazard with car driving or operating any machinery (warn the patient). Additive effects occur with alcohol, which is best avoided, though this will be a counsel of perfection in habitual alcohol users. Paradoxical behaviour effects — aggression, excitement, confusion — occur occasionally. Headache, giddiness, alimentary tract upset, skin rashes and reduced libido can occur.

Suggestions that long-term use can cause organic brain damage are not firmly substantiated.

Doses as hypnotic (oral)

Temazepam capsules (10, 20 mg)	10–30 mg orally
Triazolam Tabs (125, 250 μg)	125–250 μg orally
Lormetazepam Tabs (500 μg, 1 mg)	500 μg–1 mg orally

The elderly should be started on half the above doses. Sudden withdrawal can cause confusion.

Doses as anxiolytic sedative

Diazepam Tabs (2, 5, 10 mg), 2 mg × 3/day increasing to a total daily dose of 30 mg if really necessary (it may take 2 weeks to reach a steady state at each dose) *or* use 5–30 mg at night if there is insomnia and take advantage of anxiolytic effect the next day.

Oxazepam Tabs (10, 15, 30 mg), 10–30 mg × 3/day.
Suppositories are available, e.g. diazepam (5, 10 mg).

Injectable preparations

Intravenous formulations, e.g. diazepam 10–20 mg, given at 5 mg/min into a *large* vein (antecubital fossa) to minimise thrombosis: the dose may be repeated in 30–60 min for status epilepticus or in 4 h for severe acute anxiety or agitation: *midazolam* is a shorter acting alternative for endoscopies, etc. The dose should be titrated according to response, e.g. drooping eyelids, speech response, response to commands.

Intramuscular injection of *diazepam* is absorbed erratically and may be slower in acting than an oral dose: *lorazepam* and *midazolam* are absorbed rapidly.

The elderly should receive half doses.

Other benzodiazepines. Camazepam, clotiazepam, cloxazolam, delorazepam, estazolam, etizolam, fosazepam, fludiazepam, halazepam, haloxazolam, mexazolam, nimetazepam, oxazolam, pinazepam, quazepam, tetrazepam, etc.

It is profusion of this amount that gives rise to circiticism of both the pharmaceutical industry who produce the drugs (each company hoping that its product will indeed be an advance, but marketing it all the same if it is not) and regulatory bodies who permit it. It is good to have a choice, but there is such a thing as too much.

Lorazepam differs from other members sufficiently to warrant description. It has a plasma $t_{\frac{1}{2}}$ of about 15 h. It is less lipid soluble than others (diazepam) and so penetrates and leaves the CNS more slowly so that onset and offset of effect is smoother. Its $t_{\frac{1}{2}}$ means that it is not undesirably accumulative. Lorazepam is metabolised (conjugated) to inactive metabolites, a process that is less influenced by age than is the oxidation of other members, e.g. diazepam. These properties render it more suitable as an anxiolytic than as a hypnotic. Unfortunately it appears to have a peculiar capacity to induce dependence and withdrawal of the drug can be particularly difficult, a substantial disadvantage.

Given i.v. as a sedative, e.g. in intensive care, and as premedication for surgery and endoscopies, the onset of effect (15 min) is slower than with diazepam and midazolam (2 min), which are more lipid soluble; but it acts for longer and may induce more amnesia, for which many patients may be thankful.

Given i.m. it is absorbed more speedily than diazepam, which means that it is more suitable than diazepam for status epilepticus, when i.v. injection is impracticable.

Other hypnotics

Chloral hydrate (1869) (500 mg) was the first synthetic hypnotic to be introduced and was a welcome alternative to opium and alcohol. Chloral hydrate is a solid and is usually given orally in solution because it is so irritant to the stomach; it tastes horrible; a capsule is available.

Chloral induces sleep in about half an hour, lasting 6–8 h with little hangover. Chloral is a prodrug. It is rapidly metabolised by alcohol dehydrogenase into the active hypnotic *trichloroethanol* ($t_{\frac{1}{2}}$, 8 h). This is conjugated with glucuronic acid to an inert form. The ultimate metabolites are excreted in the urine and give a positive result in urine tests for reducing substances, but not, of course, for glucose oxidase (enzyme) tests. Chloral is dangerous in serious hepatic or renal failure, and may be bad for peptic ulcer.

The oral hypnotic dose of chloral hydrate is 500 mg to 2 g.

Interaction with ethanol is to be expected since chloral shares the same metabolic path (alcohol dehydrogenase).

Trichloroethanol is a competitive inhibitor of the conversion of ethanol to acetaldehyde so that plasma ethanol concentration is higher than it would otherwise be; *thus ethanol is potentiated by chloral*.

Ethanol delays conjugation of trichloroethanol with glucuronic acid to an inert form, and it also induces the enzyme alcohol dehydrogenase, which converts chloral to trichloroethanol; *thus chloral is potentiated by ethanol*.

If chloral has been taken for several days, ingestion of alcohol may induce vasodilatation, hypotension and tachycardia that cannot be explained by a simple potentiation.

Interaction with anticoagulants: competition for plasma proteins.

Triclofos (Tricloryl) (500 mg) is a stable ester of trichloroethanol ($t_{\frac{1}{2}}$, 8 h), see above. The oral dose is 1–2 g.

Dichloralphenazone (Welldorm) (650 mg) is less irritant to the gut. The oral dose is 650 mg–1.3 g. Phenazone is an analgesic, obsolete because of adverse reactions, but this complex has proved satisfactory. The phenazone renders the complex a potent enzyme inducer.

Paraldehyde (1882) has had long use as a safe (little respiratory depression), oral hypnotic and, by injection, for control of mania, alcohol withdrawal, status epilepticus and tetanus. But it has major disadvantages, it smells unpleasant and is partly excreted unchanged via the lungs (75% is metabolised: $t_{\frac{1}{2}}$, 5 h). It is an irritant and so unpleasant to swallow and causes painful muscle necrosis when injected i.m. When subject to light and heat it decomposes to acetic acid and deaths due to corrosive poisoning by decomposed paraldehyde have occurred. As the drug is used less, the hazard that stored drug is old and decomposed increases. For these reasons and because of the availability of benzodiazepines and phenothiazines, paraldehyde may be deemed obsolete. But it is cheap and may be chosen for that reason. The dose is 5–10 ml by oral, i.m. (larger doses should be divided between two sites) or rectal (dilute × 10 in 0.9% NaCl solution) administration. It dissolves plastic syringes.

Chlormethiazole (Heminevrin) is structurally related to vitamin B_1 (thiamine), though this seems to be irrelevant to its particular recommended use in alcohol withdrawal syndromes (started at a high dose and withdrawn over 6 or 7 days), but not for patients who continue to drink, and in senile psychosis and confusion; it is a hypnotic, sedative and anticonvulsant (used in status epilepticus but not for maintenance). Dependence occurs and use should always be brief. When taken orally, it is subject to extensive hepatic first-pass metabolism (which is defective in the old who get higher, as much as × 5, peak plasma concentrations), and the plasma $t_{\frac{1}{2}}$ is 4 h (with more variation in old than young). It is available as a *syrup*, 5 ml of which (250 mg chlormethiazole edisylate) is equivalent to one *capsule*. (192 mg chlormethiazole base): it is also available as an i.v. infusion. The hypnotic dose is 1 or 2 capsules or 5 or 10 ml syrup.

Phenothiazines. *Promethazine* (Phenergan) is a useful long-lasting hypnotic, especially in children. It is an antihistamine (H_1-receptor); other antihistamines having sedative action are also used as hypnotics.

Trimeprazine (Vallergan) is used for short-term sedation and hypnosis in children.

Other hypnotics and anxiolytic sedatives of no particular merit include: meprobamate (Miltown), chlormezanone (Trancopal), methyprylone (Noludar).

Barbiturates (1903). Although their use as hypnotics and sedatives is increasingly deplored (low therapeutic index, social abuse, dependence, enzyme induction), use, and abuse, continues. Therefore a general account is retained here. Knowledge of how to handle overdose remains important. Death may follow as little as × 10 the therapeutic dose.

The development of organic chemistry in the 19th century led to the testing on animals of many compounds in the search for an ideal hypnotic drug. Because urethane was known to be a hypnotic, although weak and unreliable, other urea derivatives were investigated. Derivatives of barbituric acid* (malonyl urea) were found to be effective and in 1903 barbitone was introduced. Since then a huge number of barbiturates has been tested and many are used to provide depression of the central nervous system ranging from *mild sedation* to *surgical anaesthesia*. For use as hypnotics and sedatives, depressant barbiturates have qualitatively similar actions; but they differ in the rate and method of disposal in the body, which has a bearing on their clinical use, and phenobarbitone and methylphenobarbitone have a greater *anticonvulsant* effect relative to the hypnotic effect. The *mode of action* may be similar to benzodiazepines, but with much less selectivity.

Results of experiments vary with drug and dose, but in general barbiturates impair *intellectual func-*

* Reputedly named by the original synthesiser after 'a charming lady named Barbara'. Miller L C. JAMA 1961; 177:27.

tions less than sensory-motor functions. In doses of 100–300 mg they impair learned behaviour; both sustained attention and distractability are reduced, and so are some conditioned response.

Simulated motor driving becomes less efficient (quinalbarbitone 100 mg) and judgement is distorted (swimmers thought they had done unusually well when they had really performed badly).

Elation and decreased motor activity may occur (quinalbarbitone 50 mg). Visual perception is reduced and the duration of auditory stimuli is underestimated — time seems to be 'flying' (quinalbarbitone 200 mg).

Analgesia. Hypnotics do not affect pain selectively, but they probably interfere with its perception; patients are less concerned about their pain. By reducing the anxiety associated with pain and its anticipation they can be useful in management provided an analgesic is given too. Unless this is done a full hypnotic dose may cause restlessness and mental confusion.

There is also evidence that barbiturates can antagonise analgesics and this may be borne in mind when they are used in patients with pain.

Respiration. A hypnotic dose of a barbiturate in a patient with marked respiratory insufficiency, e.g. severe pulmonary emphysema or asthma, will depress respiratory minute volume and arterial oxygen saturation. Benzodiazepines, paraldehyde and chloral are less objectionable in this respect.

Cardiovascular function. Barbiturates lower blood pressure at hypnotic and anaesthetic doses by reducing cardiac output, probably by reducing venous return to the heart due to peripheral venous pooling. Compensatory vascular reflexes are depressed.

Toxic doses may depress the myocardium and also reduce the peripheral resistance by blocking the sympathetic nerves.

Alimentary tract. Prolonged barbiturate sedation constipates.

Tolerance. When 18 former addicts were given 0.4 g pentobarbitone or quinalbarbitone daily for 90 days, tolerance began to develop within 14 days. They showed significant decrease in hours of sleep, in signs of clinical intoxication and in peformance in psychomotor tests. Tolerance probably occurs to all hypnotics, but it is less marked than with opioids. With barbiturates and meprobamate the tolerance is at least partly due to *enzyme induction*, and this can enhance adrenal steroid metabolism enough to reduce efficiency of steroid therapy.

Emotional and physical dependence occur with regular dosage of 0.4 g/day, or more, of barbiturate. If the dose exceeds 0.6 g/day the subject generally shows clinical signs of intoxication — impairment of mental ability, regression, confusion, emotional instability, nystagmus, dysarthria, ataxia and depressed somatic reflexes.

The withdrawal syndrome begins in 8–36 h and passes off over 8–14 days. It comprises, in approximate order of appearance, anxiety, twitching, intention tremor, weakness, dizziness, distorted vision, nausea.

There is now enough evidence that the traditional *classification* of barbiturates as long, medium and short acting, derived from experiments on animal anaesthesia, does not apply to their clinical use and so it should be abandoned. However, for overdose, rates of metabolism and excretion do have some relevance (see below). Duration of hypnotic effect is similar for drugs previously classified into each group, being about 8 h. Incidence of hangover is similar, and it is common after a placebo, being more closely related to the patient than to the drug.

Pharmacokinetics. Absorption after oral administration is rapid: plasma protein binding is variable, those with longer half-lives being less protein bound than those with shorter half-lives. Half-lives are the result of renal excretion and of metabolism in those used as hypnotics and sedatives. For those used as i.v. anaesthetics (see index), redistribution is a major factor in *plasma half-life of* initial doses.

Plasma $t_{\frac{1}{2}}$:

85 h: phenobarbitone.
24–48 h: pentobarbitone, quinalbarbitone (secobarbital), amylobarbitone, butobarbitone.
12–24 h: cyclobarbitone, reptabarbitone.

Distribution is throughout the body with rather more in the central nervous system than elsewhere.

Metabolism and excretion. For most barbiturates metabolism is chiefly hepatic with a little urinary excretion and, from the point of view of safety, the more rapidly metabolised barbiturates may be preferred. Those most rapidly metabolised are quinalbarbitone, pentobarbitone and cyclobarbitone, followed by amylobarbitone and butobarbitone. The most persistent is phenobarbitone (about 25% excreted unchanged by the kidney).

The reason why there is little renal excretion of most barbiturates is not that they do not appear in the glomerular filtrate, but because barbiturate that appears in the glomerular filtrate, if unionised, diffuses back into the circulation through the renal tubule. This diffusion will be less if the drug is ionised, and, being weak organic acids, ionisation will be maximal at a high (alkaline) pH. This has been used successfully in the *treatment of overdose* by *phenobarbitone*, which has a pK_a of 7.2, and raising the urine pH to 7.5–8.5 achieves a substantial shift of un-ionised drug to the ionised and lipid-insoluble state. Urinary elimination may be more than doubled. Other barbiturates have higher pK_a (nearer 8) and so alkalinisation of the urine by sodium bicarbonate does not have useful effect. This mechanism is explained on p. 115.

Important features of severe overdose include *prolongation of* $t_{\frac{1}{2}}$ of the barbiturate with prolonged coma (days); *hypotension* due to CNS and cardiac depression, which is treated by restoring central venous pressure and so cardiac output, by use of i.v. fluid and, if that fails, using a drug with cardiac inotropic effect (dobutamine); *elimination* of the drug is promoted by ensuring a good urine volume (e.g. 200 ml/h) and rendering it *alkaline* for phenobarbitone (see above); *active elimination* by haemoperfusion or dialysis may be needed in particularly severe and complicated cases (renal failure, pneumonia); the use of a diuretic to enhance elimination makes management more difficult and risky without adequate benefit to compensate for this. *Respiratory stimulant* (doxapram) is only useful to sustain respiration until mechanical assistance can be set up. After overdose *sleep pattern* may be abnormal for weeks even in unhabituated subjects.

Contra-indications to barbiturates. In severe pulmonary insufficiency, e.g. emphysema, even hypnotic doses of barbiturates depress respiration (see general account above).

Hepatic failure potentiates barbiturates (except barbitone, which is not metabolised).

Attacks of porphyria (see index) are induced in predisposed people.

The principal barbiturates have been listed under half-life, above: see also *anaesthesia* for i.v. barbiturates and *epilepsy*.

Uses. Obsolete as *hypnotics* and *sedatives*, see above. The choice of drugs in *convulsive states* is discussed below. For *anaesthesia* no drug has been shown to be superior to thiopentone. For oral use the barbiturate or its more soluble sodium salt can be used, it matters little; but for parenteral administration a sodium salt is required. Soluble barbiturates may be injected i.m or s.c., when the dose is similar to that given orally. For i.v. injection the drug is given slowly (except thiopentone) and the dose judged by results. It is dangerous to give the more slowly metabolised and excreted drugs i.v.

Acute adverse effects of barbiturates are almost entirely those of overdose: coma and respiratory and circulatory failure, leading to renal failure. Allergic reactions occur occasionally, particularly with phenobarbitone, rashes being the most common (bullae in acute poisoning can be of diagnostic use), but severe fatal reactions have rarely been recorded. See also *contra-indications* and *interactions*, above.

Dependence is now recognised as a serious problem: see above.

Bromides (1875) are now obsolete (not particularly effective and $t_{\frac{1}{2}}$ of 4 weeks) not only for epilepsy and as general sedatives but also for night screaming in children, townswomen who are going out of their minds, 'frightful imaginings' in late pregnancy, seasickness, somnambulism, nymphomania, and spermatorrhoea consequent on 'undue indulgence in bed'*.

* Ringer S, Sainsbury H. A handbook of therapeutics. London: H K Lewis. 1897.

GUIDE TO FURTHER READING

1 Osward I. Sleep studies in clinical pharmacology. Br J Clin Pharmacol 1980; 10:317.
2 Greenblatt D J et al. Toxicity of nitrazepam in the elderly: a report from the Boston Collaborative Drug Surveillance Program. Br J Clin Pharmacol 1978; 5:407.
3 Adam K et al. Do placebos alter sleep? Br Med J 1976; 1:195.
4 Kales A et al. Evaluation, diagnosis, and treatment of clinical conditions related to sleep. JAMA 1970; 213:2229.
5 Johns M W et al. (1970). Sleep habits and symptoms in male medical and surgical patients. Br Med J 1970; 2:509.
6 Sellers E M et al. Interaction of chloral hydrate and ethanol in man: 1. metabolism; 2. hemodynamics and performance. Clin Pharmacol Ther 1972; 13:37, 50.
7 Smith G M. Increase sensitivity of measurement of drug effects in expert swimmers. J Pharmacol Exp Ther 1963; 139:114.
8 Pawer K G et al. Controlled study of withdrawal symptoms and rebound anxiety after six week course of diazepam for generalised anxiety. Br Med J 1985; 290:1246.
9 Catalan J et al. Benzodiazepines in general practice, time for a decision. Br Med J 1985; 290:1374; and subsequent correspondence.
10 Symposium. Benzodiazepines: a clinical review. Br J Clin Pharmacol 1981; 11: 1S–119S.
11 Amrein R et al. Pharmacokinetic and clinical considerations in the choice of a hypnotic. Br J Clin Pharmacol 1983; 16:55.
12 Hockings N et al. Hypnotics and anxiolytics. Br Med J 1983; 286:1949; and subsequent correspondence.
13 Adam K et al. Sleep helps healing. Br Med J 1984; 289:1400.
14 Jochemsen R et al. Kinetics of five benzodiazepines in healthy subjects. Clin Pharmacol Ther 1983; 34:42.
15 Greenblatt D J et al. Current status of benzodiazepines. N Engl J Med 1983; 309:354, 410.
16 Aurell J et al. Sleep in the surgical intensive care unit: continuous polygraphic recording of sleep in nine patients receiving postoperative care. Br Med J 1985; 290:1029.
17 James I et al. Beneficial effect of nadolol on anxiety-induced disturbances of performance in musicians. Am Heart J 1984; 108:1150.
18 Batter M et al. Cross-national study of the extent of anti-anxiety/sedative drug use. N Engl J Med 1974; 290:769.
19 Drew P J J et al. The effect of acute beta-adrenoceptor blockade on examination performance. Br J Clin Pharmacol 1985; 19:783.
20 Braestrup C et al. Anxiety. Lancet 1982; 2:1030.
21 Editorial. Beta-blockers in situational anxiety. Lancet 1985; 2:193.
22 Nicholson A N et al. Sleep after transmeridian flights. Lancet 1986; 2:1205.

ADDENDUM

Buspirone (Buspar) is not structurally related to other antianxiety drugs. It does not appear to impair intellectual performance, nor to add to the cerebral depression caused by other drugs including alcohol. Clinical trials have shown short-term efficacy in anxiety. It may cause generally minor nervous system and gut symptoms.

18

Central nervous system III: Drugs and mental disorder: Psychotropic or psychoactive drugs

Background to the use of drugs in mental disorder

'Writing prescriptions is easy, understanding people is hard'

(Franz Kafka, 1883–1924).

In the debate whether there is a physical or a psychological basis for psychiatric disturbance it might seem that the two hypotheses are irreconcilable. But the ultimate experience of mental activity involves electrochemical changes in transmission in the brain, and whether the initiating factors are primarily psychological or physical (biochemical) the use of a chemical to alter function beneficially can be appropriate. Most psychiatrists would seek for precipitating psychological and social events and endeavour to modify these as a part of therapy. They would do this despite their knowledge that there are important biochemical changes in the brain, but they would also seek to modify these with drugs.

Undue reliance on drugs could lead to an undesirable reduction in the vital role of trained staff operating in a positive therapeutic environment, but neuroleptics can be a valuable means of enabling these staff to make psychological contact with and work alongside disturbed patients.

Drugs are cheaper to supply than are trained staff. But drugs are not a substitute for trained staff.

But with the increasing recognition of mental illness as a major cause of disability, interest in the possibilities of drug therapy has naturally increased. Chemists have responded by making innumerable substances for investigation, hoping that some of them may prove to be medicines. One snag is the difficulty of predicting therapeutic efficacy from the animal experiments that must necessarily precede clinical trial; another is how to determine by clinical trial whether a genuine therapeutic effect has occurred and, if so, whether it was in fact due to the drug. It is not surprising that no exact animal parallels for human mental disorders exist and that, as a result, 'the major problem of replicating in the laboratory the actions of potential tranquillisers in human psychoses and neuroses remains almost completely unsolved'.*

* Riley H et al J Pharm, (Lond.) 1958; 10: 657. This remains true.

Thus major advances in drug therapy must be largely dependent on luck until any biochemical characteristics of normal and abnormal mental function are defined. Paul Ehrlich wrote that '*we must learn to aim, learn to aim with chemical substances*'. But in order to aim we must have targets to aim at, and if benefits are to be obtained without unwanted effects, the targets must be precisely defined. In mental disorder the targets are increasingly being defined, though they currently have a tendency to disappear or change, or, to alter the metaphor, 'Though there have been many apparent breakthroughs, time and again they have been like elephants' footprints in the mud, making a large initial impression but quickly fading into the background. Evidence is accumulating of biochemical abnormalities in psychiatric disorder: the main difficulty lies in interpretation'.*

It may be that there is greater likelihood of therapeutic success from drugs in the psychoses in which behaviour differs from normal in *kind*, than in psychoneuroses in which it differs from normal mainly in *amount*.

Psychotropic drugs (i.e. drugs that alter mental function) act by altering chemotransmitter systems that pass nerve impulses at synapses, i.e. from the ending of one neurone across the synaptic cleft to the next neurone, e.g. noradrenaline, dopamine, 5-HT (serotonin), acetylcholine, gamma-aminobutyric acid (GABA), histamine, endorphins, prostaglandins. Plainly the formation, storage, release and the occupation of receptors by these active substances offer opportunities for intervention with appropriately designed chemicals (drugs).

Localisation of function (via these transmitters) within the brain, suggests **three main anatomical sites of action**† of drugs in mental disease:

a. *reticular activating system*: attention, arousal, anxiety.
b. *limbic system*: affect or emotional content.
c. *hypothalamus*: control of autonomic nervous system: pituitary–endocrine control.

There is a complex range of interrelationships, e.g. the locus coeruleus interconnects the reticular formation, hypothalamus and cortex, also utilising these transmitters. But the transmitters are not confined to these sites, and so non-selective drugs will be expected to cause unwanted (adverse) effects, as indeed they do.

Enough is now known to allow the formulation of crude provisional **schemes of drug action** and adverse reaction that begin to give the kind of understanding that may help clinicians to use psychotropic drugs more effectively than would be the case if they merely followed routine instructions as they do in cooking. What follows is *not* a definitive account, it cannot be, but it is offered to show the kind of approaches and interpretations that are currently being made.

SCHIZOPHRENIC SYNDROME

There is reason to think the schizophrenic syndrome and schizophrenic symptoms are associated with increased dopaminergic activity in the limbic structures of the brain. This may be due to increased sensitivity or number of dopamine receptors (postsynaptic), or to overproduction of dopamine or reduced destruction due to enzyme abnormalities or deficiencies. Drugs that benefit schizophrenia, e.g. phenothiazines, butyrophenones or thioxanthenes, are competitive antagonists of dopamine, i.e. dopamine receptor blockers, and a precursor of dopamine, levodopa, predictably exacerbates symptoms of schizophrenia. But dopaminergic neurones are not confined to the limbic system. They occur also in the nigrostriatal (extrapyramidal) system and elsewhere (e.g. controlling hypothalamic hormone-releasing factors). Thus a non-selective dopamine antagonist (e.g. chlorpromazine) would be expected to benefit schizophrenia but also to cause extrapyramidal movement disorders and endocrine changes, e.g. prolactin release. And this is indeed the case, all these effects occur with chlorpromazine, which has in addition α-adrenoceptor and cholinergic blocking activity. Indeed it was given the proprietary name 'Largactil' because it has such a large number of actions. Despite this lack of selectivity, chlorpromazine, the first (1951) neuroleptic or antipsychotic drug, was a major advance in therapeutics. Since there is no animal model of schizo-

* Editorial. Lancet 1978; 1:422.
† After Hollister L E Clinical Pharmacology of psychotherapeutic drugs. 2nd Ed. Edinburgh: Churchill Livingstone. 1983.

phrenia, the fact that chlorpromazine produced parkinsonism in man (along with relief of schizophrenic symptoms) and a cataleptic state in animals led to use of this effect in animals as a screening or predictive laboratory test for potential anti-schizophrenia action. Thus an unwanted effect was used as the basis for predicting a wanted effect. But, despite this built-in selection for unwanted effects, drugs that are more selective for dopamine receptors in the limbic system than they are for receptors in the nigro-striatal system have been found (e.g. clozapine*).

In general drugs benefit the *positive symptoms* of schizophrenia (hallucinations, delusions) rather than the *negative symptoms* (apathy).

It is now possible to begin to explain the mechanism of the troublesome *adverse effects* of dopamine-receptor blocking neuroleptics, and such knowledge is useful in management of patients. It may be summarised:

1. *Extrapyramidal motor disorders*: tremor, dystonia, akathisia, akinesia and/or a parkinsonian syndrome are to be expected. Natural parkinsonism is due to underactivity or deficiency in dopaminergic neurones causing imbalance between dopaminergic and cholinergic systems (see Parkinson's disease). Evidently a dopamine receptor blocker will mimic this disease.

These adverse reactions are generally best treated by withdrawing or reducing the dose of the drug. But this may not be practicable since valuable benefit may be lost. In such cases it is necessary to treat the motor disorder with another drug. An anticholinergic drug should be used, but routine prophylactic use is not justified. Many phenothiazines also have anticholinergic effects and these are less liable to cause these extrapyramidal disorders because they mitigate the adrenergic/cholinergic imbalance.

Levodopa (converted to dopamine in the brain) is inappropriate because it will either be ineffective in the presence of a dopamine receptor blocker or if it is effective it will also antagonise the therapeutic effect in the limbic system.

2. *Tardive dyskinesia* (from Latin *tardus*, slow or late-coming) is a disorder of involuntary movements (choreoathetoid movements of lips, tongue, face, jaws, and of limbs and sometimes trunk). It occurs generally after 2–5 years use of a dopamine receptor blocker and is due, paradoxically, to increase dopamine-sensitivity or activity. It particularly affects patients with organic brain disease and the elderly. It occurs in about 5% of mixed psychiatric patients, but up to 40% of long-term institutionalised schizophrenics. It may be permanent.

A hypothesis of causation is as follows: released synaptic transmitter from nerve endings passes across the synaptic cleft and is normally taken up by post-synaptic receptors on the receiving neurone. But there are also presynaptic receptors on the transmitting neurone, the function of which is to modulate the release of transmitter, i.e. there is a feedback mechanism. When the post-synaptic dopamine receptors are blocked then the released dopamine activates the pre-synaptic receptor to increase the synthesis and release of dopamine in an 'attempt' to overcome the block; and there is also formation of new post-synaptic receptors (also an 'attempt' to restore function to its previous state). The result of this is that dopaminergic transmission may be restored to 'normal' despite the presence of the blocking drug. When this happens the extrapyramidal reactions (above) may disappear. But sometimes the restored dopaminergic activity passes above normal despite the continued presence of the blocking drug, and this hyperactive dopaminergic state becomes the cause of tardive dyskinesia, i.e. the patient has passed from a state of drug-induced reduction of dopaminergic activity to an indirectly drug-induced excess of dopaminergic activity. If this state continues then damage to the pre-synaptic membrane may result so that the pre-synaptic receptors become supersensitive and the condition is permanent (irreversible).

If the neuroleptic is suddenly withdrawn, tardive dyskinesia may become worse because of the sudden accessibility to transmitter of the previously blocked but now more numerous receptors.

Also, anticholinergics, which are useful where there is a deficiency of dopaminergic activity (extrapyramidal disorders, above, and parkinsonism), since they restore the dopaminergic/cholinergic balance, will exacerbate tardive dyskinesia by increasing the imbalance that has already risen.

* Curiously clozapine is liable to cause agranulocytosis in Finns.

Rational treatment of tardive dyskinesia, if the hypothesis is correct, implies:

a. Use of minimum effective dose of neuroleptic.

b. Alteration of neuroleptic medication (increase of dose may, by blocking more dopamine receptors, cause transient improvement but may ultimately worsen the condition). Slow withdrawal of the drug is likely to be followed by recovery in early cases (occurring in the first year of therapy) but in only half of later onset cases, who remain permanently affected. This is a serious matter.

c. Depletion of dopamine (catecholamine) stores, e.g. by tetrabenazine or reserpine, though risk of mental depression probably contraindicates the latter.

d. Increasing cholinergic activity by withdrawing any anticholinergic drug being given against extrapyramidal reactions. Enhancement of cholinergic activity by giving precursors of acetylcholine (deanol, choline) has been only marginally effective, and anticholinesterases have transiently modified the condition.

e. Increase GABA-inhibitory action by using a benzodiazepine; there is a complex interrelation of GABA with dopaminergic/cholinergic balance.

f. Miscellaneous: lithium, valproate or baclofen have been found beneficial in individual cases.

Generally, drug therapy is unsatisfactory and the most rewarding approach may be by **drug-holidays**, say one month in six, though there is risk of therapeutic relapse, and by early detection (tongue movements) by frequent observations, when the condition is likely to be reversible.

The introduction of chlorpromazine in 1951 stimulated research and now there are large numbers of neuroleptics of several different kinds: *see classification* below.

There is evidence that β-*adrenoceptor blocking drugs* that readily enter the central nervous system (lipid soluble) may benefit some cases of schizophrenia and low doses may benefit *neuroleptic akathisia*.

DEPRESSION

The first drug to be found effective in elevating mood in endogenous depression was amphetamine (developed in the late 1930s). But it was soon found only to be useful in mild cases and to be prone to abuse. Amphetamines release noradrenaline stored in nerve endings and prevent its re-uptake into those same nerve endings by inhibiting the amine pump mechanism (see below).

In 1951, iproniazid (developed as an antituberculosis agent) was noticed to elevate mood, an effect associated with inhibition of the enzyme monoamine oxidase (MAOI). It was soon replaced in tuberculosis by isoniazid which did not inhibit MAO.

In 1954 reserpine was found to cause depression and to prevent the normal storage of noradrenaline (a substrate for MAO) in nerve endings.

Thus a drug that inhibited metabolism of monoamines (noradrenaline and 5-HT) and allowed them to accumulate in nerve endings (MAOI) relieved some cases of depression, and a drug that depleted nerve endings of their catecholamine stores (reserpine) caused depression.

Research was directed to monoamine metabolism, storage and release.

At about this time (1957) the development of further tricyclic neuroleptics derived from chlorpromazine led to the synthesis of a tricyclic iminodibenzyl derivative (imipramine), which, though it differed structurally only slightly from chlorpromazine, had no useful neuroleptic action but was found in clinical trials to have a useful antidepressant effect (i.e. luck remains an important factor in therapeutic discovery). When noradrenaline is released from a nerve ending into the synaptic cleft, its action on post-synaptic receptors is terminated not by destruction, as is the case with acetylcholine, but by diffusion away from the synaptic cleft and by re-uptake (by amine pump) into the nerve ending, where it is stored, and its metabolism is regulated by MAO (which is wholly inside the nerve ending). Tricyclics block the amine pump.

Thus all the drugs affecting depression were concerned with amine storage, release, or uptake.

It is no surprise that an *amine hypothesis of depression* appeared, i.e. endogenous depression was due to deficiency of CNS noradrenergic or serotonergic (5-HT) transmission, and MAOIs rectified this by preventing amine destruction, and tricyclics by preventing re-uptake (inhibition of amine pump) so that the concentration in nerve endings and at post-synaptic receptors was enhanced. Differences in clinical effect were attributed to differences in pattern of MAO inhibition (MAO-A or MAO-B, see below) or by differences in the ratio of inhibition of noradrenaline to 5-HT re-uptake.

But this 'amine hypothesis' in its simplest form must be inadequate, for there are now in use antidepressants that inhibit the amine pump (cell uptake) for noradrenaline only (viloxazine), for 5-HT only (clomipramine) and for neither (mianserin, iprindole). But it is also possible that some drugs, e.g. mianserin, block a negative feed-back effect mediated by pre-synaptic receptors, so causing an increased release of transmitter.

Noradrenaline and other neurotransmitters including histamine (the 'first messengers') combine with post-synaptic receptors on the outside of the cell membrane, activating the enzyme adenylate cyclase on the inside of the cell membrane. This enzyme mediates an increase in intracellular cyclic-AMP (the 'second messenger'), which induces the physiological response.

Thus it could be that antidepressants (mianserin, iprindole) without effect on the amine pump could have antidepressant effect if they blocked histamine-induced changes (H_2-receptors) in adenylate cyclase, instead of noradrenaline or 5-HT activity, and this they do.

The delay in onset of antidepressant effect (7–14 days) may represent the time needed to overcome compensatory feedback changes (if it is not due to inadequate initial dosage). Severe depression requires electroconvulsive therapy, which works quickly and may forestall suicide.

In summary:

'There is some evidence that current antidepressant drugs act by increasing the availability of transmitter to the receptor, thereby increasing the size of the post-synaptic response. Thus, L-tryptophan increases 5-HT synthesis, monoamine-oxidase inhibitors prevent amine degradation, and tricyclic antidepressants block the inactivation of the transmitter by re-uptake into the nerve ending. Our hypothesis is that ECT [electroconvulsive therapy] also produces an increased post-synaptic effect but by increasing the post-synaptic response to the same amount of released transmitter. Considering the similarity in the various antidepressant treatments in altering monoamine function, it would be surprising if the increase in functional activity of brain monoamines produced by repeated electroconvulsive shock [in animal studies] did not have something to do with its therapeutic effect in depression'.*

MANIA

Mania may be accompanied by overactivity of catecholamine tramission (i.e. the opposite of depression) and drugs that enhance transmission can cause mania (MAOIs, tricyclics, levodopa). *Lithium* may give benefit by enhancing destruction of amines in nerve endings so that less are released, or it may reduce the sensitivity of the post-synaptic receptors. Its exact mode of action currently remains uncertain. Because its onset of action is slow it is not suitable sole treatment during the severe manic phase which will require a neuroleptic for control. Lithium is adequate for mild cases, but its chief use is prevention of relapse. Mania has also been modified (reduced) by the amino acid precursor of serotonin, L-tryptophan, i.e. serotonin deficit may be 'permissive' for both depression (above) and mania, and catecholamine excess or deficiency determines which it shall be.† Increased cholinergic activity (physostigmine) also can transiently reduce mania.

PREVENTION OF ENDOGENOUS DEPRESSION (a phasic or relapsing disorder)

When the oscillation is between normal mood and depression (unipolar depression) tricyclic antidepressants may prevent relapse and are more effective than lithium.

Prevention of manic-depressive disorder. In this condition oscillation is between states both above and below normal mood (bipolar) and lithium is effective in prophylaxis of both the manic and depressive phases.

ANXIETY. See Ch. 17.

* Grahame-Smith D G et al Lancet 1978; 1:254.
† Foster G E et al. Lancet 1978; 1:1323.

CLINICAL EVALUATION

Clinical evaluation is done by recording changes in behaviour, performance of tasks and psychomotor tests, and opinions of the patient himself as well as of his family, nurses and doctors. There is a large number of rating scales, inventories, questionnaires and check lists to measure, anxiety, depression, guilt, etc. and they can be applied by observers or by the patient himself.

Biochemical techniques, e.g. study of chemotransmitters and metabolites and accessible tissues, e.g. platelets, are being developed, but the evidence they give is indirect and precise reliable correlations with clinical state will have to be established if they are to be useful. The final court of appeal must always be the patient's clinical condition. Controlled trials in psychiatry also require to take into account important environmental factors or life events, e.g. attitudes of relatives, bereavement, etc.

Not only is quantitative evaluation extraordinarily difficult in psychiatry, but there are also problems of diagnosis.

Psychiatric diagnosis is not only less precise than that in most other branches of medicine, but it has been suggested that the usual criteria of what constitutes a 'disease' may not be applicable in psychiatry. The performance of well-designed clinical trials in psychiatry also presents many difficulties, in the use of the double-blind technique, assessment of results and avoidance of interference by factors other than the drug under investigation. Unfortunately, many published clinical studies, even a majority, are so designed that no conclusion can legitimately be drawn as to the value of the drug, although a conclusion commonly is drawn nonetheless. '. . . totally uncontrolled studies of the effects of a new drug, especially when the dependent variable is something as amorphous and elusive as anxiety, can be misleading. A striking testimonial to the validity of this statement is the way in which the popularity of new drugs typically runs through the well-documented cycle of panacea, poison, pedestrian remedy. The high incidence of uncontrolled studies is not a feature confined to drugs affecting behaviour. It seems characteristic of clinical research. . . . When one considers that the principles of the controlled experiment were written about by Bacon, in 1620, and Pascal in 1648 . . ., an examination of the literature in 1958 can be somewhat discouraging'.[*] It has got only a little better since.

Some of the hazards of uncontrolled studies have been demonstrated. In one case patients and hospital staff were told that two new drugs were to be tried, an 'energiser' and a 'tranquilliser'. The tablets were orange and yellow respectively, and were available in 25 mg and 50 mg 'sizes'. Improvement was reported in 53% of patients taking the 'energiser' and in 80% of those taking the 'tranquilliser'. In fact both 'drugs' were lactose, made to taste bitter with quinine.[†]

Even where a careful double-blind technique is used successfully, bias due to the personality and beliefs of the physicians about the remedies can still affect the result. In a study on relief or anxiety by two active drugs and a placebo, the results varied according to which of two physicians was treating the patients.

Dr. A. was youngish in appearance, he expected no difference between the three treatments and his attitude to the patients was non-committal. No difference between the treatments was found.

Dr. B. had greying hair and a fatherly appearance and he expected that the pharmocologically active substances would prove superior to the placebo. Patients reported that he was 'helpful' and 'dependable'. A difference in favour of one of the active drugs appeared in his patients.

When both groups were added together there was no significant difference.[‡]

It is probable that effects of doctors' personalities and opinions can influence even the best conducted studies, and this may be more likely to happen where the drug is an adjuvant and not the mainstay of therapy. The fact that endeavours to eliminate bias are not always completely successful has been used as an argument against attempting controlled techniques in psychiatric comparisons. The logic of this is obscure. The special problems

[*] Laties V G et al. J Chronic Dis 1958; 7:500.
[†] Loranger A W et al. JAMA 1961; 176:920.
[‡] Uhlenhuth E H et al. Am J Psychiatry 1959; 115:905.

of assessing therapy in psychiatry will continue to be debated for a long time, for they will not be easily or quickly solved.

The enthusiasm with which drugs are welcomed by patients and used by doctors should make us pause. 'Is it not possible that the use of these drugs represents a modern version of the "furor therapeuticus" — a traditional "occupational disease" of the physician? The last several decades have brought us, in rapid succession, various forms of "shock treatments", psychosurgery, and lastly, the tranquillising drugs. All have in common the fact that they provide socially sanctioned patterns of medical action and thus help the physician to do something when he is faced with a psychiatric problem'.*

The physician is not necessarily treating only the patient when he gives a drug. He may be treating himself, or he may be using himself to treat the patient and employing the drug as a symbol of this.

CLASSIFICATION OF PSYCHOTROPIC† DRUGS

'Drugs are available which will increase the overall output of patients with too little behaviour, and other drugs are available which reduce the output of patients with too much behaviour'.‡ This bald statement usefully emphasises the depth of ignorance which is the most prominent feature of the background to the use of drugs to influence behaviour.

So little is known about the biochemical basis of mental disorder that no definitive classification based on mechanisms of action can be offered. Drugs are classified provisionally according to the symptoms they are used to relieve, but there is no general agreement and the following will have to serve. The main headings are those used by a World Health Organization Scientific Group.§

* Szasz T S. Arch Neurol Psychiat 1957; 77:86.

† Psychotropic = affecting the mind.

‡ Dews P B In: Drill V, ed. Pharmacology in medicine. New York: McGraw-Hill, 1958.

1. **Neuroleptics** (antipsychotics) are drugs with therapeutic effect on psychoses, they cause emotional quietening, indifference and psychomotor slowing.

a. **Phenothiazines classed by clinical effects.**

Name	*Sedation*	*Anti-cholinergic effects*	*Extra pyramidal effects*
Class 1			
Chlorpromazine (Largactil)			
Methotrimeprazine *Veractil*	strong	moderate	moderate
Promazine (Sparine)			
Class 2			
Pericyazine (Neulactil)			
Pipothiazine *Piportil*	moderate	pronounced	slight
Thioridazine (Melleril)			
Class 3			
Fluphenazine (Modecate)			
Perphenazine (Fentanyl)			
Prochlorperazine (Stemetil)	slight	slight	pronounced
Thiethylperazine (Torecan)			
Thiopropazate (Dartalan)			
Trifluoperazine (Stelazine)			

b. **Butyrophenones** are similar to Class 3 phenothiazines (see above). The group includes benperidol (Anquil), droperidol (Droleptan), haloperidol (Serenace), trifluperidol (Triperidol). The **diphenylbutylpiperidines,** closely related to the *butyrophenones*: fluspirilene (Redeptin), pimozide (Orap).

c. **Thioxanthenes**: chlorprothixene (Taractan), flupenthixol (Depixol), clopenthixol (Clopixol).

d. **Miscellaneous**: tetrabenazine (Nitoman), clozapine, loxapine, oxypertine (Integrin), sulpiride (Dolmatil).

2. **Anxiolytic sedatives** and other drugs used in anxiety, see Ch. 17.

§ World Health Organization WHO Tech Rep Ser 1967; 371.

3. **Antidepressants.**

a. **Tricyclic and related agents**

Name	*Class*	*Remarks*
Amitriptyline (Tryptizol)	tricyclic	Sedative: may be cardiotoxic (sudden death), e.g. in the elderly, rather more than other tricyclics
Butriptyline (Evadyne)	tri-	Less sedative
Clomipramine (Anaframil)	tri-	Less sedative
Desipramine (Pertofran)	tri-	Less sedative
Dothiepin (Prothiaden)	tri-	Sedative
Doxepin (Sinequan)	tri-	Sedative
Imipramine (Tofranil)	tri-	Less sedative
Iprindole (Prondol)	tri-	Less sedative
Lofepramine (Gamanil)	tetra-	Less sedative
Maprotiline (Ludiomil)	tetra-	Less sedative
Mianserin (Bolvidon)	tetra-	Sedative: lacks interaction with antihypertensives characteristic of tricyclics and may carry less cardiac risk in the elderly.
Nortriptyline (Aventyl)	tri-	Less sedative
Protriptyline (Concordin)	tri-	Stimulant
Tofenacin (Elamol)	mono-	Metabolite of orphenadrine: low efficacy
Trazodone (Molipaxin)	other	Sedative: rarely causes priapism.
Trimipramine (Surmontil)	tri-	Sedative
Viloxazine (Vivalan)	bi-	Less sedative

Notes

1. Tolerance to sedation may occur.
2. Hypnotics and anxiolytic sedatives may be combined as necessary.
3. Another antidepressant or neuroleptic should not be combined without special reason.
4. Anticholinergic side-effects are common and tolerance may develop with continued treatment.

b. **Monoamine oxidase inhibitors**: phenelzine (Nardil), isocarboxazid (Marplan), tranylcypromine (Parnate).

c. **Miscellaneous**: *Tryptophan* (Optimax, has added vitamins), a catecholamine precursor: *flupenthixol* (Fluanxol), a thioxanthene neuroleptic: *alprazolam* (Xanax), a benzodiazepine that may have antidepressant effect.

4. **Psychostimulants** increase the level of alertness and/or motivation.

a. *amphetamines*: also *methylphenidate* (Ritalin): *pemoline* (Ronyl): *fencamfamin* (Reactivan, has added vitamins): *prolintane* (Villescon, has added vitamins). This group is obsolete except for occasional special use, e.g. amphetamine in terminal care.

b. *caffeine*

5. **Psychodysleptics** (hallucinogens, psychedelics, psychotomimetics) produce mental phenomena, particularly cognitive and perceptual: see non-medical drug use.

6. **Lithium** for mania and manic-depressive psychosis.

7. **Combinations** of psychotropic drugs are sometimes useful. Initially at least, the drugs should be given separately, e.g. first an anti-anxiety agent and then a phenothiazine added and the dose adjusted to suit the patient. Fixed-dose combinations are unsatisfactory, chiefly because of this need to adjust the dose; but patients are less likely to take two separate drugs reliably. Though there is evidence that mild-to-moderate mixed anxiety-depression (such as is seen in general practice and seldom finds a way to a psychiatrist) may benefit from, e.g. a mix of tricyclic + neuroleptic (Motival, Triptafen) or tricyclic + benzodiazepine, etc. These preparations are frequently condemned by specialists but prescribed by family doctors; they should be further studied.

The first fixed-dose combination to be introduced was barbiturate + amphetamine (e.g. Drinamyl); it is an effective euphoriant and so is particularly liable to dependence and abuse: it is, or should be, obsolete.

DOSAGE OF PSYCHOTROPIC DRUGS

Because of the difficulty in measuring responses in psychiatry, and the variability caused by environmental factors, drugs are commonly given in arbitrarily fixed, or at least crudely adjusted, doses. This militates substantially against precise clinical evaluation and against achievement of optimum therapeutic effect, unless plasma concentrations are measured and can be related to therapeutic effect (see Ch. 8).

In the case of *tricyclic antidepressants*, standard doses may produce steady-state plasma concentrations varying by a factor of ten or more. The ideal therapeutic response may occur at intermediate plasma concentrations, falling off as the concentration rises above an optimum, i.e. there is a 'therapeutic window.' It is plain that when a patient does not respond, knowledge of plasma concentration will be valuable in order to allow a decision whether this is a true therapeutic failure or whether the dosage is wrong, etc. This information is at present seldom available.

Once-daily dosage (at night) is commonly satisfactory, with increments at intervals appropriate to the plasma $t_{\frac{1}{2}}$, which indicates when a steady state will have been reached, i.e. about five half-lives.

For *neuroleptics* (which are difficult to measure) also, individual variation is great and drug $t_{\frac{1}{2}}$ ranges from 10 to 50 h. Injectable depot formulations, given at intervals of several weeks, are widely used.

DETAILS OF THE DRUGS BY CLASS

Neuroleptics

Phenothiazines: see also Table, p. 349.

Chlorpromazine. As a result of investigation of phenothiazine compounds for possible anthelmintic effect, first promethazine, the useful sedative and antihistamine, was discovered, and then chlorpromazine (1951). This illustrates what is still so often the case, that useful drugs are commonly found accidentally.

Chlorpromazine has a large number of actions. Practical therapeutics might be better served if they were distributed amongst three or four drugs instead of being concentrated in one. They include:

Central nervous system. The term *neuroleptic* was introduced to describe the characteristic emotiona quietening, indifference and psychomotor slowing induced by chlorpromazine. It blocks dopamine receptors.

There is evidence that chlorpromazine acts in the hypothalamus and brain-stem reticular formation. In animals chlorpormazine quietens wild and angry monkeys. It has a remarkable ability to control hyperactive and hypomanic states without seriously impairing consciousness, and it modifies abnormal behaviour in schizophrenic states. It is ineffective against depression unless this is accompanied by agitation and indeed may make it worse. Normal people often feel sleepy, apathetic and indifferent to the environment after taking chlorpromazine and it also induces some indifference to pain. In large doses chlorpromazine causes dystonias. In moderate doses it controls the muscle spasm of tetanus, but very large doses may make it worse. This is probably an effect on the reticular formation where stimulation of one area activates, and of another depresses, spinal reflexes. Chlorpromazine also reduces muscle spasticity due to other neurological lesions. Epilepsy may be precipitated in predisposed people, but the drug has been used with success in epileptics with schizophreniform illness.

Chlorpromazine is an *anti-emetic* effective against both drug and disease-induced vomiting, but ineffective against motion sickness.

The *α-adrenoceptor blocking effect* is moderately strong, and postural hypotension may occur. The peripheral vasodilatation induced by this action of chlorpromazine causes heat loss, and body temperature may fall, as with other long-acting vasodilators, especially if the patient is anaesthetised or is old. Some central effect on the temperature regulating mechanism is also probable. The use of the term 'artificial hibernation' in connection with the use of chlorpromazine, with or without other drugs, is particularly inappropriate for there is no general slowing down of bodily processes; if anything the circulation is more, not less, active.

Potentiation of other drugs. Chlorpromazine potentiates all cerebral depressants including alcohol, analgesics, hypnotics, and anaesthetics, and curare. These effects can have clinical importance, but usually only if the drugs are being used in large doses.

Miscellaneous actions. Chlorpromazine has weak *anticholinergic* (atropine-like) antihistamine, ganglion-blocking and quinidine-like actions (it can produce ECG changes). It is a local anaesthetic, but in solution it is very irritant.

Pharmacokinetics. Chlorpromazine has a $t_{\frac{1}{2}}$ of about 25 h; there is substantial hepatic first-pass effect and drug action is terminated by metabolism. However, therapeutic effect on behaviour may be delayed for as long as 4 weeks; benefit may last months after cessation, and hepatic metabolites may be excreted for months.

Chlorpromazine is used in mental disorders, as an antiemetic and to aid the production of hypothermia. It is used in severe pain, both to potentiate other drugs and to induce indifference to pain by altering the emotional response. It may relieve the abdominal pain of porphyria, but use should be brief to avoid causing liver damage. It is worth trying in persistent pruritis. It can also be tried against intractable *hiccup*, as may a very wide variety of drugs including carbon dioxide, haloperidol, pethidine, phenytoin, methamphetamine, hyoscine, quinidine, orphenadrine, amitriptyline and metoclopramide, which indicates that the physiology of hiccough is not understood.

Dosage varies widely. Starting doses may be 25 mg orally, i.m. (not s.c. as it is irritant) 4- to 6-hourly; dosage may be increased every 3 to 4 days.

Adverse reactions include drowsiness and lethargy (though the patient remains rousable), postural hypotension, hypothermia in the elderly, dry mouth, and acute dystonia and the parkinsonian syndrome (which is amenable to anticholinergic antiparkinsonian drugs, e.g. benztropine, which can be given i.v. if necessary). In addition, an acute dystonia can mimic tetanus and misdiagnosis has resulted. Akathisia (an irresistable urge to move about) occurs and may be helped by a benzodiazepine. These are very frightening to the patient. For tardive dyskinesia see above. Phenothiazines should not be used for minor conditions.

Galactorrhoea (with amenorrhoea) occurs due to block of the dopamine-mediated prolactin-inhibiting path in the hypothalamus (plasma prolactin concentration is raised).

Blood disorders and rashes, sometimes photosensitive, occur, and with prolonged use there may be permanent pigmentation. Fits may occur and, rarely, lens opacities.

The most serious effect is obstructive jaundice, in which cellular damage is generally trivial, the principal impact being on the bile canaliculi, which show cellular infiltration and biliary stasis. Jaundice most commonly occurs 2–4 weeks after starting therapy but relapse can occur at once on restarting it in a patient who has had chlorpromazine jaundice. This and its irregular occurrence suggest that it is an allergic reaction. Recovery is almost invariably complete within a few weeks, but permanent liver damage has been reported. Hepatic biopsy has revealed lesions in patients taking chlorpromazine who are free from jaundice. The possibility of liver damage or blood disorder is sufficiently high to make casual use of chlorpromazine reprehensible. Great care is necessary if there is a history of alcoholism.

Fluphenazine decanoate, i.m. injection (in oil) is used at intervals of 2–6 weeks.

Other phenothiazines. There is a great variety available. Although most of those advocated in psychiatry represent attempts to improve on chlorpromazine, none has been shown definitely to be an all-round improvement. Their effect are similar to those of chlorpromazine although they differ in emphasis, see Table, p. 349.

Table 18.1 Some phenothiazine neuroleptics

Classification by side chain	Proprietary name and tablet size in mg	Total oral daily dose in mg (2–4 doses)*
Dimethylaminopropyl		
chlorpromazine	Largactil (10, 25, 50, 100)	50–1500*
promazine	Sparine (25, 50, 100)	50–600*
Piperazine		
trifluoperazine	Stelazine (1, 5)	3–45*
perphenazine	Fentazin (2, 4, 8)	6–48*
Peperidine		
thioridazine	Melleril (10, 25, 50, 100)	60–600*

* Milder cases treated as out-patients generally receive dosage at the lower end of this range.

Butyrophenones: *haloperidol* is pharmacodynamically similar to phenothiazines (Class 3 in the table on p. 349), it has a $t_{\frac{1}{2}}$ of about 18 h.

Thioxanthenes are also pharmacodynamically similar to the phenothiazines. *Flupenthixol* particularly is used, often as a depot i.m. injection of the decanoate (in oil) every 2–4 weeks. It also has antidepressant action.

Rauwolfia alkaloids (reserpine, etc.) are obsolete in psychiatry.

Tetrabenazine (Nitoman) is a synthetic drug, the actions of which resemble reserpine; it is worth trying in severe dyskinesias, e.g. Huntington's chorea.

Injectable depot (sustained-release) neuroleptics. Since about 40% of schizophrenics do not take tablets prescribed and even in hospital 20% of patients may not actually swallow the tablet given to them, it is useful to have neuroleptics that can be given i.m. at long intervals (2–6 weeks) for maintenance therapy. Use of these preparations has three advantages. The default rate is halved, and defaulters are identifiable, and absence of a hepatic first-pass metabolism (that accompanies oral use) may allow control that is unobtainable with oral use.

Extrapyramidal syndromes are common (2 days after injection and lasting for 5 days) and can be controlled by anticholinergic antiparkinsonian drugs (e.g. benzhexol, orphenadrine). Severe depression can occur, and sometimes excitement (flupenthixol).

Preparations include the decanoate of fluphenazine (Modecate) and the enanthate (Moditen Enanthate). Flupenthixol decanoate (Depixol) has been shown to have less depressant effects and in small doses is used as an antidepressant.

Neuroleptic malignant syndrome is a rare condition clinically similar to anaesthetic malignant hyperthermia (which is caused by a genetic idiosyncracy). The condition can occur early or late in therapy, developing over about 2 days; it has a fatality rate of about 20%. Treatment is urgent and dantrolene is the drug of choice. Haloperidol and fluphenazine may be the commonest precipitants but other neuroleptics and also some antidepressants may also do so. The condition may not be distinguishable from a severe Parkinsonian reaction, at least early in its development, and an anticholinergic drug, i.v. has been recommended (e.g. procyclidine).

Antidepressants*

Tricyclic, and the related **mono-**, **bi-** and **tetracyclic** antidepressants (See Table, p.350) are structurally related to the phenothiazines and initially were synthesised during a search for new tranquillisers. Tricyclics prevent the active reuptake into cellular stores of released noradrenaline. This action probably contributes to their potentiating effect on injected adrenaline and noradrenaline (negligible with isoprenaline) and to their antagonism of antihypertensives that act via the sympathetic autonomic system (but not β-adrenoceptor blockers) and to their cardiotoxicity in overdose. They also have anticholinergic and anti-5HT effects. Therapeutic effect is delayed for 7–14 days.

Pharmacokinetics. Tricyclic antidepressants are well absorbed and have a high apparent volume of distribution (see index) implying that they are concentrated in some tissues and indeed they have been found to be concentrated in the myocardium. Steady-state plasma concentrations show great individual variation but are correlated with therapeutic effect and so measurement of plasma concentration can be useful, especially if there is apparent failure of response. Tricyclics are metabolised in the liver. The $t_{\frac{1}{2}}$ varies from 15 to 100 h, with imipramine at the lower end and protriptyline at the upper.

Adverse effects include those characteristic of anticholinergic action (dry mouth, etc.), and there is a risk to glaucomatous and prostatic patients. There also occur postural hypotension, tremors, hallucinations, confusion, excitement, precipitation of epilepsy and jaundice, and there may be cardiac hazard (sudden death) in using tricyclics in patients with any cardiac disease and perhaps even in those with apparently healthy hearts (but see mianserin below). *Poisoning* causes cardiac dysrhythmias, hypertension and convulsions, which are treated by antidysrhythmic drugs, α- or β-adrenoceptor block and anticonvulsants (e.g. diazepam). Life-threatening anticholinergic effects can be reversed by physostigmine. Acidosis may occur and can be treated with sodium bicarbonate. Overdose should be taken extremely seriously, especially in children; cardiac monitoring should be used whenever practicable.

The physician may find himself in the curious position of warning a patient who has expressed a desire to end his own life of the hazards of the drug, i.e. of the importance of keeping his drug in a place safe from children and of refraining

* Classification of drugs by therapeutic use can be misleading, e.g. antidepressants can be useful in some cases of anxiety, panic attacks and nocturnal enuresis.

from overdose to himself. Nevertheless, the common anticholinergic effects should be mentioned (dry mouth, constipation, altered ocular focusing) because they almost always occur and add to the burden of worry in a depressed patient if he is unaware of their origin and that they do not herald disaster; they also promote non-compliance.

Abuse is not a problem with tricyclics since their immediate effects are not noticeably pleasant, but some dependence does occur and sudden withdrawal may be followed by unpleasantly increased dreaming.

Non-tricyclic antidepressants (maprotiline, mianserin) may have a higher risk of convulsions and of serious allergic hepatic and haematological adverse reactions.

Interactions. Catecholamines and other sympathomimetics are potentiated. This is important and even the amounts of adrenaline or noradrenaline in dental local anaesthetics may produce a serious rise in blood pressure. Severe toxicity, resembling atropine overdose, can occur if full doses are combined with an MAO inhibitor. Such combination is sometimes used clinically, but great caution is needed.

Tricyclics antagonise adrenergic-neurone-blocking antihypertensives by preventing their uptake into the adrenergic nerve ending, which is their site of action. The tetracyclic, mianserin, does not do this.

Neuroleptics inhibit metabolism of tricyclics. Enzyme induction (e.g. anticonvulsants) can even halve plasma concentration of tricyclics.

Effects of alcohol may be increased.

Choice of tricyclic or allied antidepressant. Choice is largely made on secondary psychotropic actions — sedative, less sedative or stimulant members (see Table, p 350).

In the presence of cardiac disease and old age, mianserin may be preferred as safer than others.

Use. Antidepressants are commonly given two or three times a day. But it is often satisfactory, particularly for the sedative drugs, to give a single evening dose; the half-lives of most are long enough to render this appropriate, and peak plasma concentrations occur during the night; the stimulant drugs may increase insomnia. Slow-release formulations of drugs with a long $t_{\frac{1}{2}}$ are unnecessary and illogical.

Dose. A general scheme* that takes account of the need for quick response as well as the accumulative properties (long $t_{\frac{1}{2}}$) of some tricyclics is as follows.

Amitriptyline (10, 25, 50 mg) single daily dose 3 h before bedtime, or imipramine (10, 25 mg) in the morning:

Day 1.	50 mg	*Day 2.*	75 mg
Days 3–6.	100 mg	*Days 7–14.*	150 mg

After 14 days, if response is inadequate, add 25 mg increment every 2–3 days up to a maximum daily dose of 300 mg. *Day 28*. Re-evaluate: if no response reconsider diagnosis or change to different drug. Obviously, the patient will be closely supervised and the increments ceased or dosage lowered at any sign of intolerance.

Comparable regimens can be devised for other drugs having different dose ranges.

With such regimens there may be some accumulation of drug and once therapeutic effect is established the dose may be gradually lowered to the minimum that will maintain benefit.

There is some evidence that tricyclic antidepressants have a therapeutic range of concentration both below *and* above which efficacy is lost. Thus if a patient does not respond, or loses response, it may be because his plasma concentration is too high or too low. This need not astonish, for drugs at high concentrations may antagonise their own actions by a variety of mechanisms, e.g. activating or blocking receptors for which affinity is low at low concentrations. This phenomenon, named *therapeutic window*, is of clinical importance, and plainly will complicate patient management.

Duration and withdrawal. Therapy may be continued three to six months and the drug withdrawn over about 6 weeks (to avoid an unpleasant acute withdrawal syndrome of headache, nausea and anxiety) or else, if there is established cyclic (unipolar) depression it may be continued at low dose for long-term prophylaxis (25–50 mg daily). Relapse of depression may be delayed for about 2 months, so follow up of patients is essential.

* Based on Hollister, L E (1978) (1983) *Clinical Pharmacology of Psychotherapeutic Drugs*. Edinburgh: Churchill Livingstone.

Other uses include *nocturnal enuresis* and *chronic pain. Pathological laughing and weeping* such as occurs with bilateral forebrain disease (e.g. multiple sclerosis) may respond to low dose amitriptyline.

Other drugs listed in the classification above can give satisfactory results. They vary in minor respects and there is hope that some may be less cardiotoxic in overdose, e.g. mianserin.

Warnings. Benefit from antidepressants may be delayed for 7–14 days and patients should be told this for it is quite time for a person who is already minded to end his life to take a firm decision and to act on it. Electroconvulsive therapy acts quicker and may be needed as initial therapy, and there need be no delay in starting the drug.

Epilepsy. Drugs of this group being liable to precipitate fits. Treated epileptics are likely to require higher doses to compensate for hepatic enzyme induction by the anticonvulsants.

Monoamine oxidase inhibitors (MAOI)

In 1951 iproniazid (related to isoniazid) was tested for clinical antituberculosis activity and it was noticed that it stimulated the central nervous system. Early trials in psychiatry proved negative, but in 1958 a favourable report of its effect in chronically regressed and withdrawn patients precipitated a flood of therapeutic trials; in the three years 1959–62 over 1300 reports were published on this group of drugs.

Iproniazid inhibits monoamine oxidase, an enzyme present in the central nervous system, in adrenergic and dopaminergic nerve endings, in the liver and gut wall, and which is concerned in the breakdown of serotonin (5-hydroxytryptamine, 5-HT) and catecholamines (adrenaline, noradrenaline, dopamine). Many compounds with this effect and less toxicity have since been made; the structure of some resembles that of amphetamine.

Actions. Drugs of this group have been found to have, to varying degrees, the following actions:

1. MAO inhibition (other enzymes too); inhibition is irreversible, i.e. they are 'hit and run' drugs.
2. Sympathomimetic effect (some only, see below).
3. Sympathetic blocking effect.

Their actions and interactions are as complicated as is to be expected from these facts.

When monoamine oxidase is unselectively inhibited, there is an increase of 5-HT and catecholamines in the central nervous system. In man, substances that inhibit the enzyme have powerful mental effects, ranging from feelings of well-being and increased energy to frank psychosis.

There is also an increase in catecholamine stores in adrenergic and dopaminergic nerve endings. It is evident that there will be *potentiation of sympathomimetics* that act indirectly (i.e. by releasing stored noradrenaline) and of sympathomimetics that are substrates for MAO (present in the gut wall and liver). But important potentiation of administered adrenaline, noradrenaline and isoprenaline is not to be expected since these substances are chiefly destroyed by catechol-O-methyltransferase in the blood, and in any case MAO is not the chief factor in terminating effects of these substances at receptors. This is done by diffusion away from the area and by reuptake into nerve endings. In this respect, adrenergic endings differ from cholinergic endings.

It is plain, both from experimental pharmacological studies and from fatal accidents during therapy, that *sympathomimetics can be highly dangerous* to patients taking MAO inhibitors.

Some MAO inhibitors (tranylcypromine) also have direct sympathomimetic activity similar to that of amphetamine, i.e. releasing stored noradrenaline, unrelated to enzyme inhibition. Thus, hypertensive attacks are to be expected; when they occur, they resemble the hypertensive attacks of phaeochromocytoma.

MAO inhibitors can, by themselves, also cause hypotension and it is uncertain whether this is related to MAO inhibition. There is probably a direct blocking action on the peripheral sympathetic system, partly on ganglia and partly due to reduced release of the transmitter (noradrenaline) at postganglionic endings. The hypertensive interactions mentioned above will still take place in the presence of hypotensive effect, so that a patient might suffer from postural hypotension, eat a meal of cheese (see below) and die in a hypertensive crisis.

Symptoms of hypertensive crises are severe throbbing headache with slow palpitation. If headache occurs without hypertension it may be due to histamine release.

Treatment of hypertensive crisis. The mechanism is excessive stimulation of α-adrenoceptors as in a phaeochromocytoma. The rational and effective treatment is an α-adrenoceptor blocker (phentolamine, 5 mg, i.v.). Should excessive tachycardia occur after the phentolamine, a β-adrenoceptor blocker may be added. A vasodilator is also effective but other kinds of antihypertensive are irrational and some can even potentiate sympathomimetics.

Selective MAO inhibition. There are at least two types of MAO, A and B. *Both types* use as substrate *dopamine, tyramine* and tryptamine. But *MAO-A* metabolises *noradrenaline* and *serotonin*, and MAO-B does not (it metabolises phenylethylamine). Noradrenaline may be important in depression, and is important in the notorious dietary interactions with tyramine-containing foods (tyramine discharges stored noradrenaline from nerve endings).

Thus selective inhibition of MAO-B by *selegiline* (deprenyl) will be free from these dietary interactions because MAO-A remains available to metabolise sympathomimetics, e.g. tyramine, in the gut wall and liver, and to metabolise noradrenaline in adrenergic nerve endings. But the corpus striatum of the brain (site of the defect in parkinsonism) contains mainly MAO-B so that selegiline will reduce dopamine destruction there and benefit parkinsonism (see index). Selective inhibition of MAO-A (by clorgyline) seems unlikely to find a clinical use.

Adverse effects also include irritability, apathy, sadness, insomnia, fatigue, ataxis, tremulousness, restlessness, impotence, difficult micturition, sweating, hyperpyrexia, gastro-intestinal disturbances, leucopenia, oedema, rashes, convulsions, jaundice. Optic nerve damage occurs with some. Appetite may increase.

Pharmacokinetics. MAO inhibitors are taken orally; they are *hit and run* drugs, i.e. their effects greatly outlast their detectable presence in the body because they inhibit the enzyme irreversibly and termination of effect is dependent on synthesis of fresh enzyme, which takes weeks. Thus adverse interactions may occur as long as 2–3 weeks after therapy has been withdrawn.

The hydrazine group (see below) is acetylated (like isoniazid) and the population is divided into slow and fast acetylators.

Interactions with *sympathomimetics* are discussed above. Patients must be warned not to indulge in *self-medication* of any kind, for many trivial remedies sold direct to the public, e.g. for coughs and colds, contain sympathomimetics. Unfortunately some *foods* contain substantial amounts of sympathomimetics, largely tyramine, which act by releasing tissue-stored noradrenaline. These substances are normally inactivated by MAO in the intestine wall and liver (presystemic elimination), where large amounts of enzyme occur. Patients are therefore deprived of this protection, so that, as well as having larger stores in nerve endings (waiting to be released), they absorb more of the sympathomimetics.

The first food interaction with MAO inhibitors was reported in 1963 and concerned cheese. It might be thought that, as cheese has been known to contain tyramine for at least 60 years, the danger might have been predicted, but it was not, and the association of hypertensive headache with evening meals of cheese was made by clinical acumen of a pharmacist whose wife was taking an MAOI.

Responses are variable, but *any food subjected to microbial decomposition* during preparation may contain pressor amines due to decarboxylation of amino acids.

The following foods either can produce, or may be expected to be capable of producing, dangerous hypertensive effects; cheese, especially if well matured (the amines are produced from the amino acids of casein by bacteria, e.g. tyramine from tyrosine); yogurt; some pickled herrings; broad bean pods (contain dopa, a precursor of adrenaline); yeast extracts (Marmite); meat extracts (Bovril); wines (especially red), beers; flavoured textured vegetable protein. This list may be incomplete and there is a large number of anecdotal case reports supposedly implicating a wide range of foods. Any partially decomposed food may cause a reaction. It is plain that patients must receive detailed instructions about their diet. They may cautiously try some of the above items to discover whether they are safe for themselves, and, if they are, they should not assume that the same food from different sources is harmless.

Interactions with drugs other than sympatho-

mimetics. The following substances that are not metabolised by MAO may be *potentiated*:

Other antidepressants: excitement and hyperpyrexia with tricyclics and allied drugs, especially clomipramine.

Narcotic analgesics: if *pethidine* is given to a patient taking an MAO inhibitor there is liable to be respiratory depression, restlessness, even coma, and hypotension. This is probably due to inhibition of the hepatic enzyme that demethylates pethidine. Interaction with other opioid occurs but is milder. If an opioid analgesic is essential, start with one tenth of the usual dose.

Central nervous system depressants, barbiturates, tranquillisers, antihistamines, alcohol (probably), antiparkinsonian drugs, but not inhalation anaesthetics, carbamazepine. Because of the use of numerous drugs during and around elective surgery, a MAOI is best withdrawn 2 weeks before.

Antihypertensives (but hypertension and excitement may occur with methyldopa).

Insulin and oral hypoglycaemics.

Bee venom (perhaps): an environmental hazard.

The mechanisms of many are obscure, perhaps they are due to inhibition of other drug-destroying enzymes. Reactions can be very severe and even fatal.

Use of MAO inhibitors. It is plain that patients taking these drugs are at risk in a number of ways and that, in the absence of specific indications for them, as well as of any evidence that they are superior to tricyclic and allied antidepressants, they are not drugs of first choice, though they may be found to suit some patients best. They are more effective in reactive than in endogenous depression and may have a place as adjuvants in severe phobic states (claustrophobia, agoraphobia) resistant to other forms of treatment, e.g. deconditioning or behaviour therapy. So numerous are the necessary precautions, and so important is it that it be known, in the event of accident, that the patient is taking a MAO inhibitor, that patients should be supplied with a printed card with appropriate warnings.

The *therapeutic effects* of MAO inhibitors occur in from a day or two to 2 weeks, and may persist for as long as 2–3 weeks after stopping treatment because they inhibit MAO irreversibly so that enzyme activity can only be restored by synthesis of fresh enzyme.

Anxiety and agitation may be made worse and depressed patients may even become hypomanic. Chlorpromazine can reduce this, given cautiously in low dose.

Other antidepressant drugs should not generally be commenced until 2 weeks after stopping the MAO inhibitor, because of the slow resynthesis of MAO.

Overdose can cause hypomania, coma, and hypotension or hypertension. General measures are used as appropriate with minimal administration of drugs (chlorpromazine for restlessness and excitement: phentolamine for hypertension: no vasopressor drugs for hypotension, because of risk of hypertension, use posture and plasma volume expansion).

This group of drugs includes:

Hydrazine group: phenelzine (Nardil); isocarboxazid (Marplan); iproniazid (Marsilid). Jaundice is more common than with non-hydrazines.

Non-hydrazine group: tranylcypromine (Parnate); the member most likely to cause hypertension: selegiline (deprenyl, Eldepryl) for parkinsonism.

Lithium

Lithium had some use in the 19th century for gout and as the bromide for sedation and against epilepsy.

In the 1940s lithium chloride was used as a salt substitute in low-salt diets for patients with cardiac failure. The toxicity of lithium was discovered and some patients died.

In 1949, during a search for biologically active substances in the urine of manic patients by injecting it into rats, it was found that the rats were affected by the large amounts of urea. Lithium urate, which is highly soluble, was selected to conduct investigations into urate toxicity. It was found to be sedative and to protect against manic urine toxicity. It was tried in manic patients, was found to be effective in the acute state and, later, to prevent recurrent attacks.*

The *mode of action* of lithium is uncertain; it

* Cade J F J The story of lithium. In Ayd F J, Blackwell B, eds. Biological Psychiatry. Philadelphia: Lippincott. 1970.

affects amine (noradrenaline, dopamine, serotonin) functions in the central nervous system, somewhat opposite to the effect of MAOIs, and it alters sodium and potassium fluxes across cell membranes.

Knowledge of *pharmacokinetics* of lithium is important for successful use since the therapeutic plasma concentration is close to the toxic concentration. Lithium is a small ion that, given orally, is rapidly absorbed throughout the gut. High peak plasma concentration can be avoided by using slow-release formulations. At first the distribution is throughout the extracellular water, but with continued administration it enters the cells and is distributed throughout the total body water with a somewhat higher concentration in brain (white matter), bones and thyroid gland. The apparent volume of distribution is about 50 l in a 70 kg man (whose total body water is about 40 l) which is compatible with the above. Lithium is not bound to plasma or other proteins.

Lithium is easily dialysable from the blood but the concentration gradient from cell to blood is not great and intracellular concentration (which determines toxicity) falls slowly. Lithium enters cells about as readily as does sodium but does not leave as readily (mechanism uncertain).

Lithium is eliminated in the urine; the ion is filtered at the glomerulus and reabsorbed in the renal tubule by diffusion along with sodium. Intake of sodium and water are the principal determinants of lithium elimination. In sodium deficiency lithium is retained in the body, thus *concomitant use of a diuretic* can reduce lithium clearance by as much as 50%, and precipitate toxicity. Lithium toxicity is treated by giving sodium chloride and water.

With chronic use the $t_{\frac{1}{2}}$ of lithium is 15–30 h. With such a $t_{\frac{1}{2}}$ and the need to maintain a plasma concentration close to the toxic level it is important to avoid unnecessary fluctuation (peak and trough concentrations). Lithium is therefore usually given 12 hrly and slow-release formulations, if reliable, are welcome and allow once daily administration.

A steady-state plasma concentration will be attained after 4–5 half-lives, i.e. about 5–6 days in patients with normal renal function. Old people and patients with impaired renal function will have a longer half-life so that steady state will be reached later and dose increments must be adjusted accordingly.

*Dosage regimen.** Give 600 mg orally (or 900 mg in large people), measure plasma concentration 24 h later, and calculate the dose required to raise the plasma concentration to the therapeutic range, 0.6–1.4 mmol/l (mEq/l) for early response in mania or 0.5–1.2 mmol/l (mEq/l) for maintenance.

An alternative, for those who dislike making calculations, is to give the priming dose of 600–900 mg (in 3 doses on the first day) increasing to 1200–1800 mg on the second day and measure the steady-state plasma concentration 5 days later. Various other regimens will serve.

The dose is adjusted to keep the plasma concentration constant (variable, 600–3600 mg total per day), and it should be measured weekly for 4 weeks and then 4–6 weekly.

It is evident that lithium therapy requires as much attention as insulin.

Uses. Lithium may be used alone to control mild mania, but benefit is delayed for days and in severe cases a neuroleptic will be needed for immediate effect.

Lithium is the most effective drug in prophylaxis of manic depressive disorder. Duration of use is likely to be indefinite; reliable criteria for safe (i.e. slow) withdrawal without relapse have not been defined.

It has been used in a variety of other conditions, drug dependence, including alcoholism, and aggressive behavioural disorders, but there is insufficient evidence to make it a treatment of choice.

Adverse effects and overdose. Adverse effects become common as the plasma concentration exceeds 1.5 mmol/l (mEq/l). Over 2.0 mmol/l adverse effects begin to be serious (central nervous system) and at 4.0 mmol/l dialysis should be considered.

Early effects that may not interfere with treatment include nausea and mild diarrhoea.

As the plasma concentration rises, central nervous system effects become prominent (coarse

* Lithium carbonate 400 mg = 10.8 mmol Li^+.
Lithium citrate 564 mg = 6 mmol Li^+.

tremor, drowsiness, giddiness, ataxia, tinnitus, blurred vision, dysarthria, muscle twitching), and now intervention is required. Oedema can occur. In severe overdose the patient may be unconscious and develop cardiac arrhythmias.

Prolonged use can cause hypothyroidism. Nephrogenic diabetes insipidus (at therapeutic plasma concentrations) can occur with even brief use; the distal renal tubule becomes refractory to antidiuretic hormone. Renal cellular injury may occur with use prolonged beyond 3–5 years.

Overdose is treated by alkaline diuresis using water and, if appropriate, an osmotic diuretic, and administration of sodium bicarbonate. *A sodium-losing diuretic must not be given* (see above)!

Precautions. Knowledge of renal and thyroid function is desirable before starting therapy. Patients should be warned of the common first symptoms of overdose, i.e. nausea, vomiting, diarrhoea, coarse tremor. They can then stop taking lithium immediately, and usually long before there is an opportunity to measure the plasma concentration. Prolonged use (years) should only be practiced if it is certain that benefit warrants it.

Lithium toxicity may be precipitated by water and electrolyte changes (sodium) as by diuretics, diarrhoea, vomiting and renal disease.

Interactions. Neuroleptics are potentiated: diuretics, see above: prostaglandin synthetase inhibitors (NSAIDs) may potentiate lithium (reduced elimination).

Pregnancy. Lithium may cause fetal cardiac abnormality. If lithium must be used, close monitoring of plasma concentration is needed because of the physiological pregnancy changes in body water and electrolytes. The newborn infant may be hypotonic and breast feeding is best avoided.

SUMMARY OF CHOICE OF DRUGS IN MENTAL AND BEHAVIOURAL DISORDERS

Notes

1. Non-drug therapies are not discussed here. This is not because they are unimportant, but because they are outside the scope of a book on pharmacology.

2. Patients often get better without drugs, and sometimes in spite of them.

Warning. A patient with 'endogenous depression' became very much better during 3 or 4 weeks following prescription of an antidepressant drug. The physician reminded her of the importance of continuing therapy despite the improvement. The patient smiled and said 'Oh, doctor, the tablets did not agree with me, so I stopped taking them after the first two or three days'.* **N.B.** (a) antidepressants require about 10 days to produce benefit; (b) there is a great deal more to treating most diseases than simple prescribing drugs, and this is particularly true of psychological disorders; (c) when a patient improves following a prescription, it cannot be assumed that it is because of the prescription.

3. Psychotropic drugs provide symptomatic or suppressive treatment only; they do not eliminate disease processes, but it is possible that by reducing a symptom a vicious cycle may be broken, and in severe cases drugs may allow the patient to re-establish contact with his environment and thus to become accessible to social and psychotherapy.

The effects of all drugs acting on mental processes vary greatly with the circumstances and the dose and the attitude of the prescriber.

In **psychotic states** (severe *manic or depressive illness* and *schizophrenia*) neuroleptics or antidepressants (tricyclic or allies) are given in rapidly increasing doses at first, with longer intervals between increases later.

Withdrawal should be gradual to avoid sudden and dangerous relapse. Duration of treatment is impossible to predict; no attempt at withdrawal should be made until 6–8 weeks after apparent recovery from an acute episode and two thirds of chronic cases need treatment for 3–4 years, in which cases a long-acting i.m. formulation may be preferred.

Severe intercurrent illness may reduce drug requirement.

In general, as with all potentially toxic drugs, the lowest effective doses should be used,

* Merry J Lancet 1972; 1:1175.

especially in patients living at home. Resistant cases may be admitted to hospital to receive high dosage.

Manic states. *Acute severe mania* may be controlled by chlorpromazine (50–100 mg i.m.) or by haloperidol (5–10 mg i.m.) repeated as necessary, with transfer to oral therapy for longer term management.

If the patient is in a single room, accompanied by a suitable nurse, smaller doses of neuroleptic drug will be needed, for excitement tends to subside sooner under these circumstances than it does in the presence of other patients, or if the patient is left entirely alone. Some manic patients are not quietened even by large doses of depressants, until they suddenly collapse with respiratory depression. Lithium can be used in milder cases where there is no haste.

The traditional remedies, morphine, hyoscine and paraldehyde, are effective in acute cases, but are now obsolescent.

Lithium requires 2–3 weeks to work (see above).

Depression. The place of drugs in treatment remains controversial. Most cases eventually recover spontaneously and most drugs take a week or two to act, so that careful controls are needed if credit for recovery is to be correctly allotted. Antidepressants can precipitate epilepsy in those with a family history of epilepsy, who have had previous ECT, or organic brain damage.

Reactive (exogenous) depression: see under psychoneuroses below.

Endogenous depression: the tricyclic or allied group is the first choice, and a sedative or stimulant member is chosen according to individual need (see Table, p 350). But ECT may be needed if depression is severe or if a quick effect is needed. A combination of a tricyclic and ECT may be ideal in severe cases, and the drug may reduce the number of shocks needed.

In very agitated depression a phenothiazine (chlorpromazine) may be a useful adjunct to a tricyclic antidepressant. Benzodiazepines are contraindicated (but see alprazolam).

It is important not to withhold ECT when a tricyclic fails. In one trial* half the patients who failed to respond to imipramine in 4 weeks benefited from ECT.

At the first sign of overdose of antidepressant, the drug should be withdrawn and chlorpromazine given.

Insomnia of depression (characteristically, early waking) may be relieved by an antidepressant drug and not require a hypnotic.

Prophylaxis of manic depressive illness: lithium, see above.

The schizophrenias. Neuroleptics are the most important drugs and they can greatly reduce aggression, hyperactivity, delusions and hallucinations. When the acute phase has subsided (days/weeks), maintenance therapy may be needed to prevent relapse, especially if the patient's family is critical or emotional as it often is, understandably. Additional treatments, e.g. an antidepressant (tricyclic) or ECT, may be needed. Acute episodes may respond at once, but in chronic states response may be delayed for 3 weeks or more.

Chlorpromazine, flupenthixol (also has antidepressant effect) and pimozide (particularly for apathetic, withdrawn patients) are drugs of choice.

Organic brain syndromes, progressive senile dementias in which patients are uncooperative and disturbed are sometimes helped by a neuroleptic, promazine or thioridazine. Anxiolytic sedatives (benzodiazepines) are best avoided lest slightly agitated patients who can conduct their personal toilet are converted to tranquil patients who cannot. These patients are commonly intolerant of drugs and a low dose should be used initially. Nocturnal delirium may be made worse by barbiturates and helped by caffeine taken as strong tea. No doubt the familiar tea ritual also plays its part in helping the British patient to keep a normal relationship with the environment.

Toxic confusional states, e.g. delirium tremens or post-operative confusion, may be benefited by diazepam, chlorpromazine or chlormethiazole. Paraldehyde is also often satisfactory. Correction of any accessible biochemical, toxic or anoxic abnormality is of the first importance.

Psychoneuroses. Drugs are less useful than in psychotic states, as the environment is relatively more important. They are best confined to short periods, to help patients over a bad phase of

* Medical Research Council Br Med J 1965; 1:881.

illness. Prolonged drug therapy is seldom rewarding. It must be admitted that this view is not unanimously held, some physicians believing that drug therapy is of great value in the routine treatment of psychoneuroses. Only the collection of scientific data in carefully designed and conducted therapeutic experiments can resolve this difference.

Reactive depression is commonly associated with *anxiety* and is best treated by an anxiolytic sedative or a tricyclic antidepressant. A MAO inhibitor may be used if these fail. See also *pain*. See also *combinations of psychotropic drugs*, above.

For *anxiety and tension* a benzodiazepine or other anxiolytic sedative may be used (see Ch. 17). Neuroleptics are best avoided in milder cases. Alcohol is, of course, highly effective, as the many neurotics who have become addicted testify. *Obsessional* and *hysterical* states are helped little, if at all, by drugs, but anxiolytic sedatives and antidepressants (clomipramine) may be tried.

Severe chronic phobic anxiety that has resisted other treatment sometimes responds to an MAOI despite the absence of depression.

Drugs may also be used to remove peripheral effects of anxiety or tension that add to it by causing distress, e.g. a centrally acting muscle relaxant for excessive voluntary muscle tone or a β-adrenoceptor blocker for tachycardia.

Panic attacks are treated acutely by a benzodiazepine; recurrent attacks may be preventable by an antidepressant.

Aids to psychotherapy. Apart from the above uses, i.v. drugs are occasionally given for *narco-analysis* or *abreaction*, and *psychodysleptics* have not found a role.

Anorexia nervosa: drugs are adjuvant only; chlorpromazine is useful, and cyproheptadine (Periactin) may be tried as an appetite stimulant.

In both **anorexia** and **bulimia nervosa** patients dread obesity and take active measures to keep their weight down, e.g. by self-inducing vomiting. They may abuse the readily available mixture of ipecacuanha (used as an emetic to treat poisoning) even to taking several doses per day; such chronic overdose of the active principle (emetine) causes myocardial toxicity and peripheral myopathy. The patients may also abuse diuretics and purgatives (with accompanying electrolyte disturbances) and appetite suppressants.

Narcolepsy is benefited by activating noradrenergic mechanisms with amphetamine, dexamphetamine, methylphenidate, mazindol or fencamfamin. A tricyclic antidepressant may be tried.

Hyperkinetic syndrome in children (attention deficit disorder) responds to adrenergic activation by dexamphetamine (or methylphenidate or pemoline). The child becomes less active and is more able to sustain attention. If these drugs fail, an antidepressant may be tried. Drug therapy should be as brief as possible (3 weeks to 3 months) and confined to children above 5 years. There is risk that growth may be diminished by disruption of the sleep pattern and so of the circadian rhythm of growth hormone secretion. This is especially important at the period of closure of the epiphyses, when drugs should be withheld if possible.

There have been complaints, with seeming justification, that merely naughty active children who are a nuisance at school or in the home or whose behaviour is the result of parental marital problems are being misdiagnosed and made into drugged family scapegoats.

Enuresis in children can often be controlled by a tricyclic antidepressant (imipramine), but relapse on ceasing its use is usual. There is a very real hazard of accidental poisoning and parents must be made to understand the risk of leaving the drug accessible in the home of small children. Attractively tasty syrups are hazardous; tablets should be used, but only after non-drug approaches have failed, say after 7 years of age, not before.

Behaviour control. The fact that drugs can be used to quell inconvenient behaviour of mental defectives, the demented or psychotics, and as a cheap substitute for skilled staff in institutions, including prisons, is a matter for concern. Similar use on persons deemed by authority to be social or political deviants is also something to be feared; there is little doubt that it has occurred.

Excessive sex drive in men may be reduced by oestrogen or by antiandrogen (cyproterone). The breasts may enlarge sufficiently to require surgical removal. These treatments may be indicated in abnormal personalities with pronounced sexual aggression. They raise particularly powerful ethical issues where the choice is between therapy with liberty, or loss of liberty, e.g. repeated sexual assaults on children. Benperidol (a butyrophenone) can also be effective.

The foregoing account of the use of drugs in mental and behavioural disorders is so inadequate in relation to the dominating importance of the subject that it is worth pointing out that knowledge is in its infancy. In relation to drug therapy, virtually nothing is known about the causes of mental disease or about how many drugs may work to relieve symptoms, though many pharmacological *facts* are known (see above). The frequent references to alterations of monoamine function illustrate this. In addition, there is a dearth of well-designed therapeutic trials such as are essential to determine what drugs can do.

Suicide and prescribed drugs

It is not uncommon to have to prescribe drugs for potentially suicidal patients living at home. In such cases it is usual to prescribe minimal doses for short periods and, when the danger seems serious, to hand over the supply of drugs to a responsible person rather than to the patient. Benzodiazepines are the sedatives and hypnotics of choice in such patients as heavy overdose is most unlikely to kill the patient.

Some antidepressants may be less cardiotoxic in overdose than others, see above.

An ingenious formulation of paracetamol containing enough methionine to protect the liver in overdose has been devised.

PSYCHOSTIMULANTS

Amphetamines

Amphetamine (racemic) and *dexamphetamine* (dextro: the laevo-form is relatively inactive) are the principal drugs of this group used as psychostimulants; their use in depression is obsolete. Amphetamine will be described, and its allies only in the ways in which they differ. Amphetamine acts by releasing noradrenaline stored in nerve endings in both the CNS and the periphery. As with all drugs acting on the central nervous system, the psychological effects vary with mood, personality and environment as well as with dose. The difference in response between children and adults is well illustrated by amphetamine and ephedrine, for in *children* these drugs are generally sedative, not excitant. The following description can thus only be approximate.

Subjects become euphoric and both mentally and physically more active and fatigue is postponed. They may be more confident and show more initiative, better satisfied with a performance which has, in fact, deteriorated in accuracy as well as being more speedily accomplished. On the other hand there may be anxiety and a feeling of nervous and physical tension, especially with large doses, and subjects may show tremors and confusion, and feel dizzy. Time seems to pass with greater rapidity. The sympathomimetic effect on the heart, causing palpitations, may intensify discomfort or alarm.

Amphetamine increases peripheral oxygen consumption, and this, together with vasoconstriction and restlessness leads to hyperpyrexia in overdose.

Acute poisoning is manifested by excitement and peripheral sympathomimetic effects; convulsions may occur; also, in acute or chronic overuse, a state resembling hyperactive paranoid schizophrenia with hallucinations. Hyperpyrexia occurs (see above) especially if the subject exercises, with cardiac dysrhythmias, vascular collapse and death. Treatment is chlorpromazine with added hypotensive (e.g. labetalol) if necessary. Urinary acidification greatly enhances renal elimination.

Pharmacokinetics. Amphetamine is readily absorbed by any usual route and is largely eliminated unchanged in the urine. Urinary excretion is pH dependent; being a basic substance, elimination will be greater in an acid urine. To achieve useful effect in overdose (i.e. pH less than 5.5), 7.0 g of ammonium chloride orally in a single dose is needed and subsequent doses according to urine pH. This is unpleasant to take and may be resented or vomited (see *alteration of urinary pH*).

Since the plasma $t_{\frac{1}{2}}$ of amphetamine is about

12 h and sedation and use of α- and β-adrenoceptor blocking drugs to control cardiovascular effects is usually sufficient, it will generally not be important to alter urinary pH. As with any convulsant, environmental stimuli should be reduced to a minimum. Urinary acidification can also be used to obtain evidence in cases of suspected misuse.

It is of interest that in mice the lethal dose of amphetamine is higher if the mice are caged separately than if they are caged in groups, probably due to a higher environmental temperature in the latter case.

Dependence on amphetamine and similar sympathomimetics occurs; it is chiefly emotional, but there is an abstinence syndrome, suggesting physical dependence; tolerance occurs.

Mild dependence on prescribed amphetamines has long been common, particularly amongst people with unstable personalities, depressives, and tired, lonely housewives. In the 1960s, adolescents began to turn to amphetamines for occasional use to keep awake to have 'fun' and then as an aid to the challenges normal to that period of life. Unfortunately, drugs provide only the temporary solution of avoidance and postponement of these challenges, retarding rather than assisting progress to maturity.

As well as oral use, i.v. administration (with the pleasurable 'flash' as with opioids) is employed. Severe dependence induces behaviour disorders, hallucinations and even florid psychosis which can be controlled by haloperidol. Withdrawal is accompanied by lethargy, sleep, EEG changes, desire for food and sometimes severe depression, which leads to a desire to resume the drug.

Appetite suppression, see below.

Amphetamine has had multifarious **uses**, but its potential for abuse is such that it should only be used where essential, and this rare:

1. *Narcolepsy*: patients pass directly into REM sleep; amphetamine delays onset of REM sleep.

2. In some *hyperactive children* with abnormal EEG.

3. As an *analeptic* in poisoning by hynotics if facilities for controlled respiration are not available.

4. *Miscellaneous*: against fatigue (seldom justified); appetite suppression (alternatives are preferable): use in sport is abuse.

Dexamphetamine is similar to amphetamine.

Methamphetamine (Methedrine) is similar to amphetamine but central nervous system effects are greater.

Phenmetrazine (Preludin) is similar to amphetamine and is chiefly used to reduce appetite. Dependence occurs. *Phentermine* (Duromine) is similar as is *diethylpropion* (Tenuate) and there are others. There is, of course, a lot more to the treatment of obesity than merely giving drugs.

Methylphenidate (Ritalin) (10 mg) has effects similar to amphetamine. It is sometimes useful in parkinsonism. The oral dose is 20–60 mg total/day in divided doses.

Pemoline (Kethamed) and *meclofenoxate* (Lucidril) see under *intellectual function*.

Barbiturate-amphetamine combinations. Many years ago clinicians had thought concomitant use, whether taken separately or in a fixed-close formulation, useful in depression and pharmocologists vaguely disapproved of what they considered a naive approach. Eventually the mixture was investigated scientifically, and it is now known that such combinations can produce effects not elicited with either drug alone. For instance, the mixtures enhance the spontaneous exploratory behaviour of rats when placed in new environments, which ordinarily inhibit such activity. It is possible that this is because amphetamine increases activity, and the barbiturate reduces fear.*

In normal man the mixtures induce elation and sociability, and the exercise of simple skills is impaired less than with the barbiturate alone.

The therapeutic values of barbiturate and amphetamine is questionable, but the potential for abuse is not and they should only be prescribed together after this risk has been carefully considered.

Tablets of one combination, because of their distinctive triangular shape and colour, became

* Rushton R et al. Br J Pharmacol 1963; 21:295.

known as 'purple hearts', and an extensive illicit trade developed, particularly amongst adolescents. In 1964 one manufacturer changed the tablet to an inconspicuous round blue tablet in an attempt to discourage misuse.

A typical combination contains dexamphetamine 5 mg plus amylobarbitone 30 mg.

Obesity, appetite suppression and stimulation

It was noticed casually in 1937 that patients receiving amphetamine tended to lose weight. This was investigated in animals and man and found to be due to a reduction in voluntary food intake. Dogs would starve in the presence of food when given amphetamine, although they still showed interest in being fed and jealousy of the dog being fed before them. It was only when food was actually placed in their cage that enthusiasm abated. Tolerance to the anorexiant effect occurs. Drugs play only a minor adjuvant and transient role in the management of that complex social behavioural condition, obesity. Suppression of appetite or of satiety is likely to help only that minority of patients who are driven to eat by excessive hunger.

Sympathomimetics with pronounced psychostimulant effects suppress appetite, but the effect is transient, being as short as 2–3 weeks (use should not exceed 3–6 months); dependence occurs. They should only be used briefly, if at all, as and aid to dietary re-education.

Fenfluramine (Ponderax) (20, 40 mg) is structurally related to amphetamine, but it causes release of serotonin from nerve stores, rather than noradenaline. It is sedative rather than stimulant to the CNS and it may induce satiety rather than suppress appetite. There may be some elevation of mood at the outset of therapy. Some physical dependence to fenfluramine does occur and sudden withdrawal is followed by depression, especially marked after 4 days; it is best to withdraw the drug gradually.

Fenfluramine also has some peripheral effects on carbohydrate and lipid metabolism and it is uncertain whether these promote weight reduction.

Interactions. Fenfluramine does not antagonise antihypertensive therapy as do the amphetamines, indeed there may be some potentiation. Hypertension may occur with MAOIs. Sedatives and antidiabetics may be potentiated.

Adverse effects include sleepiness, depression, diarrhoea, impotence, and increased dreaming. There is some potential for abuse.

Heavy overdose can cause central nervous system stimulation and cardiac dysrhythmias.

Fenfluramine is probably the drug of choice for obesity (when a drug is needed), and certainly so in hypertensives. It may be given for 3 months and slowly withdrawn. It should not be necessary to give drug therapy indefinitely for obesity, and it will be ineffective anyway. Abrupt withdrawal can cause depression.

The oral dose of fenfluramine is: for mild obesity 20 mg twice daily, increased to thrice after a week; for severe cases increase this gradually over 4 weeks to 160 mg total/day in three doses.

Mazindol (Teronac) is structurally unrelated to amphetamine. But it potentiates sympathomimetics and may reverse the effect of antihypertensives.

Biguanide antidiabetics reduce intestinal carbohydrate absorption and may induce weight loss without reducing blood glucose concentration. But their use is probably best confined to diabetics.

Bulk preparations, e.g. methylcellulose or sterculia, are used to fill the stomach with non-nutrient material and induce a feeling of satiety*. Their use is probably based on a wrong physiological concept (unless enormous amounts are taken). Animals eat for calories, not bulk; it it possible to feel hungry in the absence of a stomach. Patients might as well be invited to eat flavoured toilet paper.

Thyroxine (T_4; or tri-iodothyromine, T_3) are probably beneficial only when a diet so restricted as to amount to starvation has diminished the normal conversion of T_4 to T_3, a rare situation. Otherwise administration of T_4 or T_3 suppresses normal hormone production by the familiar feedback mechanism, and should not be used in the usual weight-losing regimens.'

* This approach has been carried to the extreme of inflating a balloon in the stomach.

Appetite stimulation. Cyproheptadine (Periactin) (Periactin) blocks serotonin and histamine H_1-receptors. It has the unusual effect of increasing appetite, probably via an action on serotonin receptors in the hypothalamus. It is sometimes used as adjuvant therapy in anorexia nervosa. In general, little or nothing is gained by stimulating appetite by drugs.

Cyproheptadine also reduces corticotrophin release by blocking the serotonergic path controlling corticotrophin releasing factor and it has been used with variable success in Cushing's syndrome.

Insulin increases appetite by reducing blood dextrose concentration.

Cannabis may induce hunger.

The xanthines and xanthine-containing drinks

(caffeine, theophylline, theobromine)

These three compounds are obtained from plants. They are qualitatively similar but differ markedly in potency. *Tea* contains caffeine and theophylline. *Coffee* contains caffeine, and *cocoa* contains caffeine and theobromine. The cola nut ('cola' drinks) contains caffeine. Theobromine is weak and is of no clinical importance. Theophylline is relatively insoluble and is made more soluble by combining it with other substances as in *aminophylline*, a combination with ethylenediamine, etc.

Mode of action. Caffeine and theophylline have complex and incompletely elucidated effects on intracellular calcium, on adenosine receptors (block) and on noradrenergic function; their action as an inhibitor of phosphodiesterase, the enzyme that breaks down cyclic-AMP (formation of which is stimulated by adrenoceptor agonists), so that bronchodilatation is enhanced (especially by theophylline), only occurs significantly at concentrations higher than those reached in therapeutic use. When theophylline is used alongside salbutamol in asthma their actions add up to increased *benefit* to the bronchi, but increased *risk* to the heart.

Pharmacokinetics. Absorption of xanthines after oral or rectal administration varies with the preparation used. It is generally good but can be erratic. The $t_{\frac{1}{2}}$ is 5 h (perhaps as long as 10 h in some people). Xanthines are metabolised largely by xanthine oxidase; they are not converted to uric acid and so need not be prohibited in gout.

For further details of theophylline see *asthma*.

Actions on the central nervous system. Caffeine is more potent than theophylline, but both drugs stimulate mental activity where it is below normal; they do not raise it above normal; thought is more rapid and fatigue is removed or its onset delayed. The effects on mental and physical performance vary according to the state and personality of the subject. Reaction-time is decreased. Performance that is inferior because of excessive anxiety may become worse.

The effects of caffeine and amphetamine on performance and mood have been compared.*

There is no doubt that both amphetamine and caffeine can improve *physical performance* both in tasks requiring more physical effort than skill (athletics) and in tasks requiring more skill than physical effort (monitoring instruments and taking corrective action in a mock aeroplane cockpit). These tasks are affected by both physical ability and mental attitude. It is uncertain whether the improvement consists only of restoring to normal performance that is impaired by fatigue or boredom, or whether the drugs can also enable the subject to improve on his normal maximum performance. The drugs may produce their effects by altering both physical capacity and mental attitude. There are various differences between them, perhaps the most obvious being their effect on hand steadiness; this is decreased by caffeine and increased by amphetamine. Large doses of amphetamine before athletic effort can be dangerous.

There is insufficient information on the effects on *learning* to be able to give any useful advice to students preparing for examination other than that *intellectual performance* may be improved when it has been reduced by fatigue or boredom.

Effects on *mood* vary greatly amongst individuals and according to the environment and the task in hand. In general, caffeine and amphetamine induce feelings of alertness and well-being, euphoria or exhilaration. Onset of boredom,

* Weiss B et al Pharmacol Rev. 1962; 14:1.

fatigue, inattentiveness and sleepiness is postponed. Overdose can cause anxiety, tension and tremors and will certainly reduce performance. The regular, frequent use of caffeine-containing drinks to obtain their effects is part of normal social life; ill-effects are rare and seldom serious when they occur (see below). However, the use of amphetamine in the way that caffeine is generally used carries the danger of serious dependence and, eventually, of psychotic states.

That the effects of caffeine are generally desired is shown by the remarkable popularity of caffeine-containing drinks throughout the world. Habitual tea and coffee drinkers are seldom willing to recognise that they have an emotional drug dependence, however.

Respiratory stimulation occurs with large single doses.

Sleep. Caffeine affects sleep of older more than it does of younger people and this may be related to the fact that older people show greater catecholamine turnover in the central nervous system than do the young. Onset of sleep (sleep latency) is delayed, bodily movements are increased, total sleep time is reduced, there are increased awakenings. Tolerance to this effect does not occur, as is shown by the provision of decaffeinated coffee in some restaurants; the caffeine is extracted (most, but not all) by trichloroethylene.

Skeletal muscle. Metabolism is increased, and this may play a part in the enhanced athletic performance mentioned above.

Cardiovascular system. Both drugs directly stimulate the myocardium and cause increased cardiac output, tachycardia and sometimes ectopic beats and palpitations. This effect occurs almost at once after i.v. injection and lasts half an hour. Theophylline effectively relieves acute left ventricular failure. There is peripheral (but not cerebral) vasodilatation due to a direct action of the drugs on the blood vessels, but stimulation of the vasomotor centre tends to counter this. Changes in the blood pressure are therefore somewhat unpredictable, but 250 mg caffeine usually causes a transient rise of blood pressure of about 14/10 mm Hg in occasional coffee drinkers, but no additional effect in habitual drinkers. The cerebral circulation responds differently; the vessels constrict, with consequent reduction of blood flow. Increased coronary artery blood flow may occur but increased cardiac work counterbalances this in angina pectoris. When given i.v. (aminophylline) slow injection is essential because high peak concentrations are equivalent to acute overdose (below).

Smooth muscle (other than vascular muscle, which is discussed above) is relaxed. The only important clinical use for this action is in asthma (theophylline). Therapeutic effect is unpredictable but can be excellent.

Kidney. Diuresis occurs in normals chiefly due to reduced tubular reabsorption. The drugs are not used for this purpose as superior agents are available.

Miscellaneous effects. Gastric secretion is increased by caffeine given as coffee (by decaffeinated coffee too) more than by caffeine alone, and the basal metabolic rate may increase slightly (see skeletal muscle, above).

Acute overdose, e.g. aminophylline i.v., can cause convulsions, hypotension, cardiac dysrhythmia and sudden death. *Chronic overdose*, see below.

Preparations and uses of caffeine and theophylline

Caffeine alone is not used in therapeutics. It is included in analgesic tablets, where it is thought to potentiate non-narcotic analgesics, and it is used in migraine (enhances ergotamine absorption) Theophylline is valuable in asthma.

The most generally useful preparation is **aminophylline** (100 mg) which is a salt of theophylline with ethylenediamine. Aminophylline is irritant and because of this is often given i.v. (250–500 mg over about 10 min in 20 ml of water), although sudden death may occur if it is given fast: a special formulation is available for i.m. use. $t_{\frac{1}{2}}$ is 3–13 h (the longer time occurs with high plasma concentrations, i.e. saturation kinetics). Patients are liable to vomit if given more than 300 mg orally three times a day. Aminophylline suppositories are more reliable than tablets, but can cause proctitis, especially if used more than twice a day. When given i.v. some of the observed respiratory stimulation is due to the ethylenediamine.

Attempts to make non-irritant orally reliable preparations of theophylline have resulted in *choline theophyllinate* (oxtriphylline, Choledyl; 100,

200 mg), which is reasonably effective. The dose is 100–400 mg orally 6-hourly. It is used to relieve bronchospasm, and with dubious effect in angina pectoris. Numerous theophylline variants are available, e.g. acepifylline (Etophylate), etamiphylline, diprophylline, proxyphylline, oxpentifylline. Sustained-release formulations are convenient for asthmatics and are numerous. Suppositories and rectal solutions are available.

The principal uses of aminophylline are:

Asthma. In severe asthma when β-adrenoceptor agonists fail (often given i.v.); and orally to provide a background bronchodilator effect.

Other uses are *paroxysmal nocturnal dyspoea* (i.v. for immediate effect), to terminate an attack, and, rarely, in severe heart failure where diuretics and digoxin fail, aminophylline may increase cardiac output and therefore renal blood flow to allow a diuresis to start.

In the dying patient aminophylline i.v. may cause brief and unrepeatable but socially useful recovery of consciousness and coherence.

In angina pectoris the value of aminophylline or its allies is doubtful, and there are better drugs.

Xanthine-containing drinks (see also above)

Cocoa never hurt anybody, probably because nobody has ever drunk enough of it, but tea and coffee in excess can make people tense and anxious as well as cause exacerbation of peptic ulcer. Small children are not usually given tea and coffee because they are less tolerant of the central nervous system stimulant effect, but cola drinks irrationally escape this prohibition. At different times coffee has incurred disapproval of stricter elements of both Islamic and Christian religions. It is possible to make an imposing list of diseases which may be caused or made worse by caffeine-containing drinks, but there is no conclusive evidence to warrant any general prohibitions. High doses of caffeine in animals damage chromosomes and cause fetal abnormalities; but studies in man suggest that normal consumption poses no risk. Epidemiological studies suggest increased risk (× 2–3) of coronary heart disease in heavy coffee consumers (> 5 cups/day). A link with carcinoma of the pancreas has been proposed but has not been confirmed.

Dependence. Slight tolerance to the effects of caffeine (on all systems) occurs. Withdrawal symptoms, attributable to psychological and perhaps mild physical dependence occur in habitual coffee drinkers (5 or more cups/day) 12–16 h after the last cup; they include headache, irritability, jitteriness; they may occur with transient changes in intake, e.g. high at work, lower at the weekend.

Overdose. Excessive prolonged consumption of caffeine causes anxiety, restlessness, tremors, insomnia, headache, cardiac extrasystoles and confusion; diarrhoea may occur with coffee and constipation with tea. The cause can easily be overlooked if specific enquiry into habits is not made. A heavy user may be defined as one who takes more than 300 mg caffeine/day, i.e. four cups of 150 ml of brewed coffee, each containing 80 ± 20 mg caffeine per cup or five cups (60 ± 20) for instant coffee. The equivalent for tea would be ten cups at approx 30 mg caffeine per cup. Plainly caffeine drinks brewed to personal taste of consumer or vendor must have an extremely variable concentration according to source of coffee or tea, amount used, method and duration of brewing. There is also great individual variation in the effect of coffee both between individuals and sometimes in the same individual at different times of life, see sleep, above.

Decaffeinated coffee contains about 3 mg per cup; cola drinks contain 8–13 mg caffeine/100 ml; cocoa as a drink, 4 mg per cup; chocolate (solid) 6–20 mg per 30 g.

Allergy to tea and coffee doubtless occurs. A careful history to distinguish this somewhat dubious condition from overdose is essential.

Blood lipids. Cessation of coffee drinking can reduce serum cholesterol concentration in hypercholesterolaemic men.

Ginseng is the root of two plants of the same family (oriental, *Panaz ginseng*: Siberian, *Eleutherococcus senticosis*). It contains a range of biologically active substances including saponins and sterols. It has been used as a tonic or stimulant for thousands of years. Ginseng doubles the time that mice placed in water can swim before becoming exhausted; it appears to have antifatigue effects in various other tests in mice (climbing up a rope that is moving downwards) and to increase sexual activity. In man, ginseng has been claimed to benefit performance of (Russian) athletes and astronauts, and to reduce absenteeism due to respiratory illness in mining and steel workers and truck drivers. Oriental soldiers at war have used ginseng.

Despite accumulating evidence and wide use by the public, the medical profession in Western countries remains sceptical of the value of this 'tonic'. A range of side-effects is reported, including oedema, hypertension, rashes, sleeplessness and oestrogen-like effects.

INTELLECTUAL FUNCTION AND DRUGS

With ageing populations becoming more and more forgetful, investigators and drug developers are turning to the possibilities of improving mental function, especially *memory*, in the old. Experiments on memory in rats are easy to do and numerous drugs appear to have some effect, e.g. endorphins and naloxone, corticotrophin and vasopressin (peptides), adrenergic and cholinergic agents. The locus coeruleus of the brain is known to be concerned with memory regulation, and these drugs can be shown to increase its neuronal firing.

No drugs have been shown to reliably and substantially improve impaired or normal memory in man over long periods.

But there is evidence of some effect for meclofenoxate, pemoline and co-dergocrine. It is unlikely that vasodilatation has any effect, and any benefit of such drugs is likely to be due to brain cell actions.

Prescribers who seek to help their senile or other patients' memory with drugs will do well to remember that whilst benefits will be limited at best, it is quite easy to impair the fragile intellectual function of the old with ill-chosen, uncritical, unmonitored prescribing.

Alzheimer's disease is characterised by decline in memory and is associated with defective cholinergic activity in the brain. At least some benefit occurs with agents that enhance cholinergic function, e.g. the centrally acting anticholinesterase agent, tetrahydroaminoacridine (THA).

Learning. Studies in animals have shown that drugs that modify cholinergic and adrenergic mechanisms in the central nervous system or alter the synthesis of RNA can enhance learning. It will be time to take this topic seriously in medicine when efficacy has been demonstrated in a resistant human population such as medical students.

GUIDE TO FURTHER READING

1 Van Putten T. Why do schizophrenic patients refuse to take their drugs? Arch Gen Psychiat 1974; 31:67.
2 American Psychiatric Association. The current status of lithium therapy: report of the APA Task Force. Am J Psychiat 1975; 132:997.
3 Boston Collab. Drug Surveillance Program. Clinical depression of the central nervous system due to diazepam and chlordiazepoxide in relation to cigarette smoking and age. N Engl J Med 1973; 288:277.
4 Greden J F. Anxiety or caffeinism: a diagnostic dilemma. Am J Psychiat 1974; 131:1089.
5 Goldberg L. Monoamine oxidase inhibitors: adverse reactions and possible mechanisms. JAMA 1964; 190:456.
6 Rogers S C et al. A statistical review of controlled trials of imipramine and placebo in the treatment of depressive illness. Br J Psychiat 1975; 127:599.
7 Tonks C M Lithium intoxication induced by dieting and saunas. Br Med J 1977; 2:1396.
8 Goel K M et al. Amitriptyline and imipramine poisoning in children. Br Med J 1974; 1:261.
9 Moir D C et al. Cardiotoxicity of amitriptyline. Lancet 1972; 2:561
10 George K A et al. Relative amnesic actions of diazepam, flunitrazepam and lorazepam in man. Br J Clin Pharmacol 1977; 4:45.
11 Lader M H. Human pharmacology of antidepressives. Br J Clin Pharmacol 1977; 4:135S.
12 Creek R A, Lader M H, eds. Symposium. New approaches to diagnosis and treatment of affective disorders. Br J Clin Pharmacol 1984; 19: Supp. 1.
13 Nicholson A N et al. eds. Symposium. Psychotropic drugs and performance. Br J Clin Pharmacol 1984; 18: Suppl. 1.
14 Guzé B H et al. Neuroleptic malignant syndrome. N Engl J Med 1985; 313:163.
15 Iversen L L. Neurotransmitters and CNS disease: introduction. Lancet 1982; 2:914.
16 Bloom F E. Neurotransmitters and CNS disease: the future. Lancet 1982; 2:1381.
17 Thompson T L et al. Psychotropic drug use in the elderly. N Engl J Med 1983; 308: 134, 194.

18 Morgan H G. Do minor affective disorders need medication. Br Med J 1984; 289:783.
19 Anonymous. A schizophrenic describes his recovery. Lancet 1983; 2:562.
20 Biederman J et al. Psychopharmacology in children. N Engl J Med 1984; 310:968.
21 Skegg K et al. Incidence of self-poisoning in patients prescribed psychotropic drugs. Br Med J 1983; 286:841.
22 Orme M L'E. Antidepressants and heart disease. Br Med J 1984; 289:1.
23 Guzé B H et al. Neuroleptic malignant syndrome. N Engl J Med 1985; 313:163.
24 Graboys T B et al. Coffee, arrhythmias, and common sense. N Engl J Med 1983; 308:835.
25 Levy M et al. Caffeine metabolism and coffee attributed sleep disturbances. Clin Pharmacol Ther 1983; 33:770.
26 Gilliland K et al. Ad lib caffeine consumption, symptoms of caffeinism, and academic performance. Am J Psychiat 1981; 138:512.
27 Thelle D S et al. The Tromsø heart study: does coffee raise serum cholesterol? N Engl J Med 1983; 308:1454.
28 La Croix A Z et al. Coffee consumption and the incidence of coronary heart disease. N Engl J Med 1986; 315:977.
29 Editorial. Akathisia and antipsychotic drugs. Lancet 1986; 2:1131.
30 Davis K L et al. Cholinergic drugs in Alzheimer's disease. N Engl J Med 1986; 315:1286.

19

Central nervous system IV: Epilepsy: Parkinsonism: Tetanus

EPILEPSY AND ANTIEPILEPSY DRUGS

Bromide (1857) was the first effective antiepileptic drug, but is now obsolete. When phenobarbitone was introduced in 1912 it was found to control patients resistant to bromides and to be far superior to barbitone, which had been available since 1903. It became clear that minor differences in molecular structure were clinically significant and that, in the barbiturate series, there was prospect of separating hypnotic from anticonvulsant effects. But these possibilities could not be exploited without animal models that include fits induced by drugs, electroshock and light (the photosensitive Senegalese baboon).

The first success was the discovery of phenytoin, which is structurally related to the barbiturates, in 1938. Since then many drugs have been discovered, but phenytoin remains a drug of choice in the treatment of major epilepsy.

Epilepsy comprises sudden, excessive depolarization of groups of cerebral neurones, which may remain localized (focal epilepsy) or which may spread to cause a generalized seizure.

Mode of action. Antiepilepsy (anticonvulsant) drugs inhibit the neuronal discharge or its spread, and do so by altering cell permeability to ions and by enhancing the activity of natural inhibitory neurotransmitters such as gamma-aminobutyric acid (GABA), which induces hyperpolarization.

Whilst general anaesthetics suppress all neuronal activity and can be used to stop fits in an emergency, useful antiepileptics and drugs that suppress the attacks selectively with minimal or no sedation.

Drug treatment of epilepsy

As more effective anticonvulsants become available the possibility of dramatic advances naturally becomes less, so that it is important to be able to detect even small improvements in therapeutic effect. This means that therapeutic trials have to be designed and conducted more carefully and accurately than before.

Measurement of therapeutic effect includes careful recording of attacks (by patient or other), provision to ensure that patients who do not take the drug as instructed are detected (measurement of plasma concentrations is best), avoidance or control of environmental interfering factors (e.g. stress, alcohol), knowledge of pharmacokinetics of drugs under test. For ethical reasons initial trials are generally on patients taking orthodox therapy who are not well controlled, though this adds to the problems of measuring comparative efficacy. Also trials must be prolonged for months to allow for spontaneous variations in seizure frequency.

General principles in the treatment of epilepsy

1. Treatment of causative factors, e.g. cerebral neoplasm.
2. Avoidance of precipitating factors, e.g. alcohol, stress.
3. Anticipation of natural variations, e.g. fits may occur only at night or shortly after waking.
4. Antiepileptic drugs.

The **principles of drug therapy of epilepsy** are simple and illustrate many of the principles of drug therapy in general:

1. Therapy should start with a single well-tried and relatively non-toxic drug *The majority of patients can be and should be controlled on one drug.*

2. Dosage should be adjusted according to known pharmacokinetic properties and with measurement of plasma (or saliva) concentrations (if practicable) where any problems of efficacy or adverse reactions arise (see below). In the absence of facilities for measurement of plasma concentration then it may be necessary to establish the maximum tolerated dose (see below).

3. Attention to detail, including measurement of plasma (or salivary) concentrations, allow the majority of patients, 80% or more, to be managed on a single drug. Few patients benefit from more than two drugs.

4. If the first drug fails to give complete control there is a choice between withdrawing it completely (*slowly*, if it has had any useful effect at all) and *substituting* a drug of a different chemical group, or else of *adding* a second drug of a different chemical group. A third drug is needed only rarely.

5. Effective therapy must never be stopped suddenly either by the doctor (carelessness) or by the patient (carelessness, intercurrent illness or ignorance), or status epilepticus may occur. But if sudden withdrawal is imposed by occurrence of toxicity, a substantial loading dose of another antiepileptic should be given at once.

6. This trial of drug after drug should be continued *until the epilepsy is controlled*, or until there are no more drugs to try. Up to 3 months may be needed to try a drug thoroughly in an individual patient.

7. In cases where fits are liable to occur at a particular time of day, dosage should be adjusted to achieve *maximal drug effect at that time*.

Starting drug therapy. Start with about one-third of the expected maintenance dose and increase it weekly to reach the maintenance dose in 3 to 4 weeks, by which time any enzyme induction will have occurred and a steady state reached after the most recent dose increment. In the case of phenytoin a substantial loading dose may be used, following by the lower maintenance dose. If plasma concentration measurements are available, a blood sample, taken at the end of the longest interval between doses, i.e. trough or minimal concentration (usually, and inconveniently, early morning), provides useful background information for further dose adjustment.

If fits continue the dose should be adjusted upwards until fits cease or adverse effects occur.

Plasma concentration monitoring is useful in the following circumstances:

1. About 4 weeks after commencing therapy (see below)
2. When fits occur with standard dosage: the patient may be non-compliant or compliant and simply need more drug
3. When adverse effects occur
4. When sodium valproate is added to another drug (pharmacokinetic interaction)
5. When another antiepileptic drug is withdrawn in the presence of sodium valproate
6. In pregnancy
7. When there is hepatic or renal disease.

Routine monitoring of plasma concentration is not necessary and wastes expensive resources.

Note. Monitoring is particularly useful with *phenytoin* (which shows saturation kinetics) and is seldom really useful with other drugs unless there is a specific problem to be solved.

Results of drug treatment: duration: withdrawal. 60%–95% of patients with treatable epilepsies (i.e. patients with fits but who are otherwise normal) can be completely relieved within 1 year. Plainly it is undesirable in principle to continue drug therapy for the rest of the patient's life if it can be safely withdrawn for, apart from general concerns about long-term drug therapy, there is evidence suggestive of adverse effects on behaviour and cognitive function that must be a particular cause for disquiet during childhood (development and education).

After at least 2 years (perhaps rather 3 or 4 years) of complete freedom from attacks, withdrawal of medication should be considered. In adult epilepsy, drug withdrawal is associated with about 20% relapse during withdrawal and a further 20% relapse over the following 5 years, after which relapse is unusual.*

* In children, prognostic factors for successful withdrawal of therapy have been defined. Shinnar S et al. New Engl J Med 1985; 313:976.

Relapse is more likely when the epilepsy has been severe and prolonged.

Relapse is more likely with major than with minor epilepsies.

Withdrawal should be slow, over about 6 months. If a fit occurs, full therapy must be resumed again for 2–3 years.

Sudden withdrawal may result in status epilepticus and patients must be counselled about the need for compliance. If patients lose their drug they must urgently obtain a further supply.

Pregnancy and epilepsy

1. *Pharmacokinetics* are altered due to two physiological changes (a) an increase in body water (concentration of drug falls) and (b) a reduction in plasma albumin. This latter leads to a decrease in the amount of protein-bound drug and to an increase in the amount of free drug. It is the latter that has therapeutic effect. But the increased free drug is accompanied by an increase in metabolism (when first order kinetics apply) and the end result is unpredictable, e.g. the total plasma concentration (free plus bound drug) may fall and although the *percentage* of free drug may rise, the *absolute* concentration of free drug may be insignificantly changed. This would be easy to monitor if measurement of plasma concentration was of free drug only, but it is not, it is of total (free plus bound) drug*. Since what is important therapeutically is the concentration of free drug, and what is measured is the concentration of the free plus bound drug (total drug), it is evident that an acceptance of the total plasma concentration as a guide to therapy when protein binding has changed can be misleading. Drug metabolism may be increased. Erratic fluctuations in plasma concentrations may occur.

In practice, the patient is closely watched clinically and the dose of drug increased if seizures occur more often than expected. After delivery the pharmacokinetics reverts to pre-pregnancy state over a few days.

Antiepileptic drugs pass into breast milk, but the total quantities ingested by the baby are small and breast feeding may be considered safe. Though there is slight possibility of sedation of the baby the advantages of breast feeding outweigh this.

2. *Fetal abnormality*. Children of mothers taking antiepileptic drugs show an approximately × 3 increased rate of malformations at birth, especially cleft palate and lip, and heart abnormalities. This is probably due to the drugs rather than to the disease. Withdrawal of effective therapy during early pregnancy cannot be recommended (except perhaps in cases of minor epilepsy, when consciousness is not lost). Women of reproductive age should be treated with the simplest possible regimen (one drug at minimum effective dose, which will be assisted by measuring plasma concentration). Folate deficiency due to altered folate metabolism also occurs with hydantoin and barbiturate anticonvulsants and is a suspected cause of fetal neural tube defects, so that a folate supplement seems sensible in a woman who wishes to become, as well as who has become, pregnant.

It is not possible to rank the anti-epileptic drugs for teratogenicity, but very tentatively it may be suggested that phenobarbitone, carbamazepine and clonazepam may be less teratogenic than phenytoin and sodium valproate. A curious multiple syndrome has been tentatively named 'fetal hydantoin syndrome', and sodium valproate may be particularly associated with spina bifida.

Newborn babies of mothers taking antiepileptics sometimes have reduced clotting factors, prothrombin, etc., remediable by giving vitamin K antenatally; it is attributed to the drugs, perhaps by enzyme induction.

Contraception. Because of induction of steroid metabolising enzymes by some antiepileptic drugs, with possible failure of contraception, it is prudent either to prescribe the higher dose oestrogen-containing oral contraceptives (at a level that avoids breakthrough bleeding, e.g. 40, 50 μg oestrogen) or, perhaps better, use a different mode of contraception.

Fits in children are treated as in adults, but children may respond differently and become irritable, e.g. with sodium valproate or phenobarbitone. If febrile convulsions have occurred, a

* Measurement of free drug alone, rather than total drug, is technically difficult as a routine.

drug used for major epilepsy may be given continuously until the child is 5 years old, when fits with fever become less likely. Giving the drug intermittently whenever fever occurs, as has been suggested (e.g. oral or rectal diazepam) can fail to protect, since to obtain adequate plasma concentrations at the outset when they are most needed would require the early administration of a substantial loading dose, and this is hardly practicable. Early administration of an antipyretic (paracetamol) by parents is a sensible precaution at first evidence of fever.

It remains uncertain whether antiepileptic drugs interfere with development and education and it is certainly unwise to assume they do not. The sensible course is to control the epilepsy with minimal doses and attention to precipitating factors, with drug withdrawal when it is deemed safe to attempt it (see above).

Anaesthesia and surgery in treated epileptics requires careful consideration of the way in which plasma concentrations of the drug(s) will be kept in the therapeutic range, employing various routes of administration as commonsense and pharmacokinetic considerations counsel. Sodium valproate may interfere with blood coagulation (inhibits platelet aggregation). Some anaesthetics (ether, methohexitone, ketamine) may induce convulsions. Reduction in hepatic metabolic capacity may occur indirectly (reduced blood flow, hypoxia) or directly (halothane liver damage) with a rise in plasma concentration of antiepileptic drug (e.g. phenytoin). Therefore plasma concentrations of drugs are best kept in the lower part of the therapeutic range.

A possible beneficial side-effect. Use of phenytoin, carbamazepine and barbiturate is associated with a rise in the blood of high-density lipoprotein (HDL), which has an inverse relationship with mortality from ischaemic heart disease. A 29% reduction in mortality from this cause in epileptics treated with these, but not with other antiepilepsy drugs has been suggested by a case control study.*

* Muvronen A et al. Br Med J 1985; 291:1481.

Drugs of choice in the epilepsies (Table 19.1)

Generalized epilepsies
Major seizures (grand mal or tonic-clonic)
First choice: sodium valproate, phenytoin
Second choice: carbamazepine, phenobarbitone
Minor seizures (petit mal or absence epilepsy)
First choice: ethosuximide
Second choice: sodium valproate, clonazepam (or clobazam)
Myoclonic: sodium valproate, clonazepam (or clobazam)

Focal or partial epilepsies
Definitive ranking is controversial: carbamazepine, phenytoin, phenobarbitone, primidone

Status epilepticus: diazepam, phenytoin, phenobarbitone

Prophylaxis of post-injury or post-neurosurgery epilepsy: as for major seizures above.

Frequency of administration. In general, taking into account convenience as well as pharmacokinetics, two equal daily doses morning and evening are recommended for routine practice. It is practicable to use once-daily administration with some drugs (having regard to the $t_{\frac{1}{2}}$) but there will be higher peaks of plasma concentration and the consequences of a forgotten dose will be greater; sustained-release formulations are available.

Interval between dose increments. If fits are infrequent it is obviously difficult to adjust dosage by therapeutic response. With phenytoin a useful plan is to get the plasma concentration into the therapeutic range (measure it 7–10 days after instituting therapy and make appropriate adjustment) or, where this is not available, raise the dose gradually at 1–2 week intervals until an unwanted effect (nystagmus, dysarthria, ataxia) occurs and then reduce it slightly (maximum tolerated dose) (but control may be achieved below this dose). Attention to patient compliance is obviously of great importance.

A fit or series of fits in a known epileptic often presents to a doctor who has never seen the patient before. It is important to consider the cause, whether it is non-compliance (which can be due to intercurrent disease), an inadequate drug regimen or an advance in the severity of the disease. Obviously drug plasma concentrations will help. It is important to avoid casual or impulsive alterations of regimen of drugs, which take a week or more to reach a steady state (long $t_{\frac{1}{2}}$), in the absence of accurate diagnosis.

Status epilepticus: a treatment of choice is *diazepam* i.v. 10 mg over 2 min. It can be repeated as necessary, or an i.v. infusion (40 mg in 500 ml dextrose 5% or saline)* max. rate 20 mg/hr can be used. Hypotension and respiratory depression (particularly if other antiepileptics have been used) may occur. If i.v. injection is impracticable give a *solution* per rectum. Aborption from i.m. injection is slow and erratic. Alternatives include: clonazepam i.v. (see below): phenytoin i.v. 150–250 mg at up to 50 mg/min in patients who have not been taking it orally: sodium phenobarbitone i.m. 200 mg: paraldehyde i.m. 5–10 ml: general anaesthesia with or without neuromuscular block may be necessary. Once the emergency is over, exploration of the reason for the episode and reinstitution of therapy, guided if possible by plasma concentrations, is required. Chlormethiazole i.v. is used for the fits of pre-eclamptic toxaemia of pregnancy.

Pharmacology of individual drugs: *for choice and some data see above.*

Hydantoins: Phenytoin (diphenylhydantoin, Epanutin, Dilantin) (1938) alters ionic fluxes (Na, K, Ca) across cell membranes; it is said to have a membrane stabilizing action, which may prevent the initiation and spread of epileptic discharges. Phenytoin orally is well absorbed but there have been pharmaceutical bioavailability problems in relation to the nature of the diluent in the capsule (see bioavailability). Phenytoin provides a major example of the importance of knowledge of *pharmacokinetics* for successful prescribing. Phenytoin is about 90% bound to plasma albumin so that quite small changes in binding (e.g. a drop to 80%) will have a major effect on the concentration of *free* drug (see pharmacokinetics in pregnancy above). Drugs that may *interact* by competition

* This solution will retain full potency for about 6 h.

Table 19.1 Data on principal antiepileptic drugs

Drug	Usual total daily maintenance oral dose range (mg in 2 doses; tab. size — mg)	Plasma $t_{\frac{1}{2}}$ (h)	Therapeutic range: plasma* conc. in mg/l (monitoring often unnecessary)
Phenytoin (Epanutin)	300–400 (25, 50, 100)	10–60†	10–20
Phenobarbitone (Luminal)	100–300 (15, 30, 60, 100)	100	15–35
Ethosuximide (Zarontin)	1000–2000 (250)	50	50–100
Carbamazepine (Tegretol)	800–1800 (100, 200, 400)	35, 20‡	6–10
Sodium valproate (Epilim)	1000–2500 (100, 200, 500)	10	50–100
Clonazepam (Rivotril)	4–8 (0.5,2)	40	

* Many patients are controlled with plasma concentrations *below* the lower limit of the therapeutic range, and substantial diurnal fluctuations may occur.
† Phenytoin shows saturation (zero-order) kinetics, see below.
‡ Carbamazepine $t_{\frac{1}{2}}$ is less with chronic treatment.

with phenytoin for plasma proteins include sodium valproate, sulphonamides, aspirin (high dose), oral hypoglycaemics, clofibrate, warfarin, tricyclic antidepressants. Simple displacement interaction is generally not clinically important when first-order kinetics applies (metabolism increases in proportion to the rise in free drug concentration) but when there is saturation (zero-order kinetics) or, in addition, metabolising enzyme inhibition, toxicity may result.

Phenytoin is hydroxylated in the liver and this process becomes saturated at about the doses needed for therapeutic effect. Thus phenytoin at low doses shows first-order kinetics but this changes to saturation kinetics or zero-order kinetics as the therapeutic plasma concentration is approached, i.e. smaller dose increments at longer intervals are needed to obtain the same proportional rise in plasma concentration. This is discussed in Chapter 8.

A clinically meaningful single plasma half-life can be quoted only for a drug that is subject to only first-order kinetics. At low doses, giving sub-therapeutic plasma concentrations, the $t_{\frac{1}{2}}$ of phenytoin is 10–15 h. But a higher doses, giving therapeutic plasma concentrations (enzyme has become saturated), the $t_{\frac{1}{2}}$ can be > 60 h. This has major implications for patient care, e.g. the time taken to reach a steady-state plasma concentration after a dose increment (about five half-lives) is 2–3 days at low dose and about 2 weeks at high doses. Thus dose increments should become smaller and less frequent as dosage increases (this is why there is a 25 mg capsule). Plainly serial plasma concentration measurement will help the prescriber.

Enzyme induction. Phenytoin is a potent inducer of hepatic metabolising enzymes affecting itself, other drugs and natural endogenous substances. The consequences of this are; a slight fall of steady-state phenytoin level over the first few weeks of therapy, though this may not be noticeable if dose increments are being given; enhanced metabolism of other drugs including other antiepileptics, warfarin, steroids (adrenal and gonadal) thyroxine, tricyclic antidepressants, antirheumatics, doxycycline; naturally this can also work in reverse, and introduction of other enzyme inducers may lower phenytoin concentrations when there is capacity for increase in enzyme induction, e.g. ethanol; the occurrence of osteomalacia in epileptic patients after years of therapy is attributed to enhanced metabolism of vitamin D, as is folate deficiency.

Inhibition of phenytoin metabolism either by competition for the enzyme or by direct inhibition of enzyme activity can occur; plasma concentration of phenytoin rises. A prime example is sulthiame, a minor antiepileptic, the efficacy of which is probably due to this effect rather than to intrinsic activity of the drug. Sulthiame, added to phenytoin, increases phenytoin plasma concentration after an interval of 1–3 weeks, suggesting a mechanism more complex than simple competition for a metabolic path. Other drugs that inhibit phenytoin metabolism are cimetidine, co-trimoxazole, isoniazid, chloramphenicol, azapropazone, disulfiram, phenothiazines. There is a considerable body of mediocre and contradictory data, the lesson of which is that *possible interaction should be in the mind wherever other drugs are prescribed to a patient taking phenytoin.*

Adverse effects of phenytoin, many of which can be very slow to develop, include a considerable variety of central nervous system effects, from sedation to delirium to acute cerebellar disorder to convulsions; peripheral neuropathy; rashes (dose related); gum hyperplasia (perhaps due to inhibition of collagen catabolism) more marked in children and when there is poor gum hygiene; coarsening of facial features; hirsutism; Dupuytren's contracture, pseudolymphoma; megaloblastic anaemia that responds to folate (perhaps partly due to increased folate requirements; folate is a co-factor in some hydroxylations that are increased as a result of enzyme induction by phenytoin); anaemia probably only occurs when dietary folate is inadequate, but some degree of macrocytosis is common.

Overdose (cerebellar symptoms and signs, coma, apnoea) is treated according to general principles. The patient may remain unconscious for a long time because of zero-order kinetics, but will recover if respiration and circulation are sustained.

Other uses. The membrane-stabilising effect of phenytoin is used in cardiac dysrhythmias and, rarely, in resistant pain, e.g. trigeminal neuralgia.

Preparations, as well as capsules for oral use, phenytoin is available for i.v. injection; it should not be given i.m. if this can be avoided as the pH of the solution has to be high to render it soluble; the fall in pH in the muscle leads to precipitation of the drug with slow absorption.

Ethotoin (Peganone) is an alternative hydantoin.

Barbiturates (see index). Anticonvulsant members include phenobarbitone, ($t_{\frac{1}{2}}$, 85 h), methylphenobarbitone and primidone (Mysoline), which is largely metabolised to phenobarbitone (i.e. it is a prodrug).

Sodium valproate (Epilim) may act by inhibiting the enzyme responsible for the breakdown of the inhibitory neurotransmitter, GABA (i.e. it inhibits GABA transaminase).

Pharmacokinetics. Valproate is about 90% bound to plasma albumin. It is metabolised in the liver and has a plasma $t_{\frac{1}{2}}$ of about 10 h.

Valproate inhibits the metabolism of phenobarbitone. It displaces phenytoin from plasma albumin but the rise in free phenytoin is accompanied by increased phenytoin elimination and so the total phenytoin plasma concentration falls, but the concentration of free phenytoin is not much changed (when first-order kinetics apply).

Valproate does not induce drug metabolising enzymes but its metabolism is enhanced by induction due to other antiepileptics.

Adverse effects are generally minor, e.g. nausea, but can include the following: liver failure (risk maximal at 2–12 weeks) and liver function tests are advised during the first 6 months of therapy; transient rise in liver enzymes may occur without sinister import, but such patients should be closely monitored until the biochemical measures return to normal; pancreatitis; coagulation disorder due to inhibition of platelet aggregation (coagulation should be assessed before surgery); increased alertness and appetite, with weight gain. A curious effect is temporary hair loss following which regrowth may be curly; 'We thought the change might be welcomed by the patients, but one girl preferred her hair to be long and straight, and one boy was mortified by his curls and insisted on a short hair cut.'* False positive may occur in urine testing for glucose.

Carbamazepine (Tegretol) is structurally related to imipramine. Because another antiepileptic (phenytoin) is sometimes beneficial in trigeminal neuralgia, carbamazepine was tried in this condition, for which it is now the drug of choice (see neuralgias).

Pharmacokinetics. Carbamazepine induces drug metabolising enzymes and its $t_{\frac{1}{2}}$ falls from about 35 h to about 20 h over the first few weeks of therapy; it enhances the metabolism of warfarin and oral contraceptives.

Adverse effects include CNS symptoms, gut symptoms, skin rashes and blood disorders (blood counts are advised during early months of treatment); and liver and kidney dysfunction. Rarely, carbamazepine can worsen fits in children.

Clonazepam (Rivotril) is a benzodiazepine used for routine control of a variety of epilepsies (see above); *clobazam* is an alternative. Other benzodiazepines have antiepileptic action, but only at doses causing unacceptable sleepiness. The plasma $t_{\frac{1}{2}}$ is 40 h. For *status epilepticus* clonazepam (1 mg initially in special freshly made dilution) may be given i.v. slowly (30 sec); it should not be given i.m. lest absorption be as slow as **diazepam** i.m. when peak plasma concentration can be delayed as long as 2 h, which is useless for the urgent control needed in this medical emergency and complicates any other therapy given in the interval. *Lorazepam*, i.m. is somewhat more rapidly absorbed.

Succinimides: Ethosuximide (Zarontin) has a plasma $t_{\frac{1}{2}}$ of 50 h. Adverse effects include gastric upset, CNS effects, including dyskinesias, and allergic reactions including eosinophilia and other blood disorders, and lupus erythematosus.

Oxazolidinediones, e.g. troxidone (trimethadione, Tridione) used for petit mal, are obsolescent largely because of unpleasant and serious adverse reactions.

Sulthiame (Ospolot) is a sulphonamide that has weak antiepileptic effect; much of the efficacy attributed to it may be due to its inhibitory effect on the metabolism of phenytoin and phenobarbitone given concurrently.

Acetazolamide (Diamox) is a carbonic anhydrase inhibitor that, by producing acidosis, sometimes benefits minor motor epilepsy as does a ketogenic diet.

PARKINSONISM

Dr James Parkinson described this condition in his 'Essay on the Shaking Palsy' in 1817. The drug management has evolved partly through serendipidy (*anticholinergics*) and partly rationally from an understanding of the pathophysiology of the disease (*dopaminergics*). Drugs do not cure but can confer considerable benefit.

Background

Two balanced systems are important in the extrapyramidal control of motor activity at the level of the corpus striatum and substantia nigra; in one the neurotransmitter is *acetylcholine*, in the other

* Jeavons P M et al. Lancet 1977; 1:359.

it is *dopamine*. In Parkinson's disease the nigrostriatal pathway is defective (see also MPTP Parkinsonism, p. 396) and the striatal concentrations of dopamine are very reduced, so that the cholinergic system is dominant. The essential dysfunction appears to be in the dopamine neurone and dopamine receptor. There is now evidence for the existence of two types of dopamine receptor. D_1 receptors are linked to a dopamine-sensitive adenylate cyclase and their activation results in an increase in cyclic AMP concentrations; they are found in the corpus striatum. D_2 receptors are independent of adenylate cyclase and exist in the terminals of the nigrostriatal and corticostriatal neurones as well as in the corpus striatum itself. While the full functional significance of the individual subtypes is not yet understood, evidence suggests that Parkinson's disease probably arises from dysfunction of D_2 receptors. There are two approaches to restoring the dopaminergic/cholinergic balance:

1. to **reduce** cholinergic activity by anticholinergic drugs, and
2. to **enhance** dopaminergic activity by dopaminergic drugs which may:

a. *replete* neuronal dopamine through giving levodopa (L-dihydroxyphenylalanine), which is a natural precursor. Administration of dopamine itself is ineffective as it does not pass into the brain from the blood.

b. *release* dopamine from stores and inhibit its re-uptake (amantadine).

c. *prolong* the action of dopamine through selective inhibition of its metabolism (selegiline).

d. act as *dopamine agonists* (bromocriptine, lisuride, pergolide).

Both approaches are effective in therapy and may usefully be combined. It therefore comes as no surprise that drugs which prolong the action of acetylcholine (anticholinesterases) or drugs which deplete dopamine stores (reserpine) or block dopamine receptors (neuroleptics, e.g. chlorpromazine or haloperidol) will all exacerbate the symptoms of parkinsonism or induce a Parkinson-like state. Other parts of the brain in which dopaminergic systems are involved include the medulla (induction of vomiting), the hypothalamus (suppression of prolactin secretion) and certain paths to the cerebral cortex. Different effects of dopaminergic drugs can be explained by activation of these systems, namely emesis, suppression of lactation (mainly bromocriptine) and occasionally psychotic illness. Drugs used to manage psychotic behaviour, e.g. phenothiazines, may act by blockade of dopaminergic paths and, as is to be expected, they are also anti-nauseant, may sometimes cause galactorrhoea, and may induce parkinsonism. Neuroleptic-induced parkinsonism is alleviated by anticholinergics, but not by levodopa or amantadine, probably because the neuroleptics block dopamine receptors on which these drugs act. But many neuroleptics also have some anticholinergic activity; those with greatest potency in this respect, e.g. thioridazine, are the least likely to cause parkinsonism.

Drugs used to treat Parkinson's disease

Dopaminergic drugs

Levodopa (250, 500 mg) is a natural amino acid precursor of dopamine. The latter cannot be used because, being poorly lipid soluble, it is not well absorbed from the gut and it does not usefully penetrate the CNS. Levodopa is absorbed from the small intestine by active transport and has a $t_{\frac{1}{2}}$ of about 30 min. The drug can traverse the blood-brain barrier and within the brain it is decarboxylated to the neurotransmitter dopamine. But a major disadvantage is that levodopa is also extensively decarboxylated to dopamine in peripheral tissues and only about 5% of an oral dose of levodopa reaches the brain. (Dopamine formed in peripheral tissues does not enter the brain because it is not lipid soluble.) Thus large quantities of levodopa have to be given and the drug and its metabolites cause significant adverse effects, notably nausea but also cardiac dysrhythmia and postural hypotension. This problem has been solved party by the development of decarboxylase inhibitors, which do not enter the *central nervous system*, so that they prevent only the *extracerebral* metabolism of levodopa. The inhibitors are given in combination with levodopa and there are two preparations with little to choose between them; *benserazide with levodopa* in a 1:4 ratio (Madopar: 12.5 + 50 mg; 25 + 100 mg; 50 + 200 mg) and *carbidopa with levodopa* in a 1:10 ratio (Sinmet: 10 + 100 mg; 25 + 250 mg: also a 1:4 ratio as Sinemet Plus [25 + 100 mg], useful when only a small total dose of levodopa is required). The same brain concentrations are produced as with levodopa given alone, but only 25% of the dose of levodopa is required with the combinations. Consequently the incidence of adverse effects is lowered, especially nausea, which occured in about 80% of patients starting on levodopa but in less than 15% on the combination.

Interactions: Dopamine is a substrate for MAO and is also converted to noradrenaline by dopamine β-oxidase: thus dangerous hypertension may occur if a monoamine oxidase inhibitor is given. Reserpine depletes cerebral dopamine and antagonises the effect of levodopa. Tricyclic antidepressants are safe. Metabolites of dopamine interfere with some tests for phaeochromocytoma.

Dopa-decarboxylase is a pyridoxine-dependent enzyme and concomitant use of pyridoxine (e.g. in self-medication with a multivitamin preparation) can reverse the benefits of levodopa used alone, but does not reverse the now usual levodopa-decarboxylase inhibitor (above).

Adverse effects: Postural hypotension occurs. Nausea may be a limiting factor if the dose is increased too rapidly; it may be helped by cyclizine 50 mg taken 30 min before food. Levodopa-induced involuntary movements may take the form of general restlessness or head, lip or tongue movements or choreoathetosis. Mental changes may be seen: these include depression, which is common (best controlled with a tricyclic antidepressant) and hallucinations. Agitation and confusion also occur but it may be difficult to be sure whether these are due to drug or to disease. Cardiac dysrhythmias are a rare feature. Increased sexual activity may occur and may or may not be deemed an adverse effect. It is probably due to improved motility and resulting enthusiasm rather than to a pharmacodynamic effect of levodopa.

Amantadine (100 mg) is an antiviral drug which, given for influenza to a parkinsonian patient, was noticed to be beneficial. The two effects are probably unrelated. It appears to act by increasing synthesis and release of dopamine, and by diminishing re-uptake. The drug is much less efficacious than levodopa, whose action it will slightly enhance; it is more useful than anticholinergic drugs, with which it has an additive effect. Advantages include simplicity of use (initial oral dose 100 mg daily, increasing to twice or thrice daily, but rarely more than this) and relative freedom from adverse effects, which, however, include ankle oedema, postural hypotension, livedo reticularis and central nervous system disturbances — insomnia, hallunications and, rarely, fits.

Bromocriptine (Parlodel) (2.5, 10 mg) is a derivative of ergot that has dopamine agonist activity. The drug is rapidly absorbed; the $t_{\frac{1}{2}}$ is 1.5 h, so that its action is smoother than that of levodopa, which can be an advantage in patients who develop end-of-dose deterioration on levodopa. Dosing should start at 1.25 mg orally nightly, increasing at approximately weekly intervals and according to clinical response to 10–80 mg per day taken in three divided doses with food. This is much more than the dose that is necessary to suppress lactation.

Nausea and vomiting are the commonest adverse effects; these may respond to domperidone but tend to become less marked as treatment continues. Postural hypotension may cause dizziness or syncope. In high dose confusion, delusions or hallucinations may occur.

Selegiline (Eldepryl) is a selective inhibitor of monoamine oxidase (MAO) type B. MAOs have an important function in modulating the intraneuronal content of neurotransmitter. The enzymes exist in two principal forms, which have specific substrates, inhibitors and locations in particular tissues. MAO-A deaminates serotonin, noradrenaline, tyramine and dopamine and is present in the intestine and lungs. The MAO-B is chiefly in the substantia nigra and corpus stratum, where its physiological role is the metabolism of dopamine. Selegiline, because it inhibits MAO-B, delays the breakdown specifically of nigrostriatal dopamine, prolonging its effect. Thus its principal therapeutic benefit is to extend the action of levodopa in those patients who experience end-of-dose deterioration. It appears to be ineffective against the on-off swings in motor activity that occur with levodopa.

The importance of the distinction between type

A and type B MAOIs becomes further apparent when potential adverse reactions are considered (p. 355).

Selegiline, because it is a MAO-B inhibitor, does *not* create the risk of a hypertensive 'cheese reaction', since tyramine is metabolised as it traverses the gut wall by MAO-A, which is still active. Levodopa, given to a patient who is receiving selegiline, does not cause a hypertensive crisis, as that fraction of the drug which is converted to dopamine and then noradrenaline is metabolised by MAO-A in the periphery (e.g. lungs).

The oral dose of selegiline is 5 mg twice daily. Its adverse effects are those of increased dopamine activity (see above).

Anticholinergic drugs

Anticholinergics act by blocking acetylcholine in the central nervous system, thereby partially redressing the imbalance created by decreased dopaminergic activity. Their use originated when hyoscine was given to parkinsonian patients in an attempt to reduce sialorrhoea, and it then became apparent that they had other beneficial effects in this disease. Synthetic derivatives are now used. These include *benzhexol*, *orphenadrine*, *benztropine*,and *procyclidine*.

There is little to choose between these. Anticholinergics produce modest improvements in tremor, rigidity, sialorrhoea, muscular stiffness and leg cramps, but not in akinesia.

Unwanted effects include dry mouth, blurred vision, constipation, urine retention, glaucoma, hallucinations, toxic confusional states and psychoses (which should be distinguished from pre-senile dementia).

Treatment of Parkinson's disease

The main features that require alleviation are *tremor*, *rigidity*, and *hypokinesia*.

General measures are always important. These include the encouragement of regular physical activity and specific help such as physiotherapy and speech therapy. Encouragement of a positive attitude to the disease may help to maintain independence.

Drug therapy plays an important role.

Initial treatment. Drugs should be started only when symptoms interfere with activities that are important to the patient. Tremor is usually an early complaint that *anticholinergics* relieve. This class of drug also alleviates sialorrhoea but less so the rigidity and they are ineffective for hypokinesia. Anticholinergic drugs should be avoided in patients with glaucoma, difficulty in micturition, constipation and psychiatric disturbance.

Amantadine may be effective in the early stages of the disease, either alone or in combination with an anticholinergic.

Long-term treatment at some stage will involve dopamine replacement with *levodopa* (combined with a decarboxylase inhibitor) to replace CNS dopamine. Rigidity and hypokinesia respond best to this but the combination is less effective in relieving tremor. Levodopa restores normal or near — normal activity in more than 75% of patients. Indeed, failure to respond should prompt the physician to question whether the patient has another basal ganglia defect (multi-system atrophy, cerebrovascular disease) or whether other drugs, e.g. phenothiazines, are involved. Dosage is best increased gradually, e.g. weekly or fortnightly, using the smallest quantity that is effective. The optimum dose varies from patient to patient and within each patient with passage of time. The preparation Sinemet Plus contains relatively more carbidopa to ensure that there is adequate decarboxylase inhibition when a small dose of levodopa is required. The varying amounts of levodopa in the Sinemet and Madopar preparations (above) permit flexibility in dose adjustment and small alterations may be beneficial. Eventually, the progress of the disease demands that the total dosage be increased to the level at which adverse effects become troublesome. It is then of advantage to reduce each individual dose and increase the frequency of administration. After six years, on average 25% of patients will still derive substantial or moderate benefit from levodopa and experience an almost normal life expectancy. About 50%, however, fail to sustain the effect or find they cannot tolerate its adverse effects.

One of the main problems with long-term treatment is fluctuation in response to levodopa. This is often a gradual process beginning with:

1. *early morning akinesia* progressing to
2. *peak dose dyskinesia* and
3. *end-of-dose deterioration*, then the most severe form
4. *the 'on-off' phenomenon.*

This latter term describes random fluctuations from mobility to dyskinesia or to parkinsonian immobility. Severe dystonic muscle cramps of hand or foot may accompany the dyskinesia. In some patients, fluctuations are related to the timing of drug administration, when peak plasma concentrations coincide with the dyskinetic phase and low plasma concentrations with immobility, but other patients swing between states of mobility and akinetic mutism without apparent relation to the timing of doses. After receiving levodopa for 10 years, over 50% of patients experience such swings.

Management of problems with long-term levodopa is difficult; it may involve the following:

1. gradual and partial substitution of levodopa with selegiline, which delays dopamine breakdown. This is effective for end-of-dose akinesia in about 40% of patients but it is not successful at alleviating severe on-off fluctuations. Substitution of levodopa with bromocriptine has also been advocated because the latter has a longer duration of action, but this drug is more likely to produce adverse effects than is selegiline.

2. Shortening the interval between doses of levodopa to hourly or less. Timing of dose in relation to meals is important for these interfere with absorption of the drug, especially when the protein content is high.

Drug-induced parkinsonism due to dopamine-receptor blocking drugs should be distinguished from idiopathic Parkinson's disease. In one series* of 95 new cases of parkinsonism referred to a department of geriatric medicine, 51% were associated with prescribed drugs and half of these required hospital admission. The clinical features of the drug-induced disease were very similar to those of idiopathic parkinsonism. After withdrawal of the offending drug most cases resolved completely in 7 weeks. Amongst the neuroleptic phenothiazines the commonest agent was prochlorperazine (Stemetil), usually given for vague postural instability and which no longer seemed indicated in any case. 'One old lady who had received trifluoperazine (for a minor fright and anxiety) for 5 weeks, took 36 weeks to recover from the drug-induced parkinsonism but never managed to get home again.'

* Stephen P J, Williamson J. Lancet 1984; 2:1082.

Other disorders of movement

Tremor may be physiological, in which case it is rarely disabling and will have a removable underlying cause such as thyrotoxicosis, anxiety or a sympathomimetic drug, but if immediate symptomatic relief is required, then a β-*adrenoceptor blocker* is usually effective.

Essential tremor is often, and with justice, called benign, but a few individuals may be incapacitated by it. *Alcohol*, through a central action, helps about 75% of patients but is plainly unsuitable for long-term use and a β-*adrenoceptor blocker* will benefit about 50%, while *primidone* appears to improve some sufferers.

Drug induced dystonic reactions are seen:

1. As acute responses, often of the torsion type occur following administration of phenothiazines, butyrophenones or metoclopramide. An anticholinergic drug, e.g. benztropine given i.v. over 24–48 h, provides relief.

2. In some patients who are receiving levodopa for Parkinson's disease when inversion of the foot and pain in the leg and foot are the common form (see levodopa).

3. In patients on long-term neuroleptic treatment, who develop *tardive dyskinesia* (see p. 345).

Chorea from whatever cause may be alleviated by drugs that reduce the effect of dopamine; perphenazine or fluphenazine have been shown to give benefit.

Tics can often be suppressed voluntarily but other repetitive, spasmodic contractions may benefit from drugs, e.g. chlorpromazine for intractable *hiccup*, haloperidol for *stuttering*.

Spasticity results from lesions of various types and sites within the central nervous system. It is useful to view spasticity as having positive features, such as flexor spasms and negative features such as weakness and loss of dexterity. Drugs used include baclofen, dantrolene and diazepam (see Index).

TETANUS

Whilst only the pharmacology of the convulsions can be strictly considered appropriate to this book, the practical immunological aspects of tetanus are also discussed as they form a perennial and common clinical problem.

Active immunisation provides the best and safest protection against tetanus. If all wounded patients were known to be actively immune there would be no need for passive protection. Since this ideal situation does not exist, many wounded patients need *passive protection* by immunoglobulin (antitoxin) or sometimes by antibiotic.

Prevention of tetanus*

Surgical toilet

Surgical toilet is of prime importance, since removal of foreign bodies and of tissues that are dead or likely to die renders the wound less suitable for the growth of tetanus bacilli. Provided careful surgical toilet is practised, patients with wounds that are less than 6 hours old, clean, non-penetrating, and with negligible tissue damage do not need human tetanus immunoglobulin, even if the patient is not actively immune to tetanus. This point requires emphasis since *human antitoxin should not be given throughtlessly to every wounded patient who consults his doctor; the material is expensive and supplies probably cannot be increased indefinitely.*

Human tetanus immunogobulin (*antitoxin*)

Human tetanus immunoglobulin provides passive immunity against tetanus. It is generally accepted that immunity requires the maintenance of a serum concentration of antitoxin greater than 0.01 unit/ml until toxin production ceases in a wound. Human antitoxin concentrations in the blood fall at a slower rate than equine antitoxin concentrations; consequently, an injection i.m. of only 250 units of human tetanus immunoglobulin may be relied on to give a serum concentration of antitoxin that remains above 0.01 unit/ml for about 4 weeks. There seems to be no risk of an early immune elimination, as sometimes occurs with equine anti-toxin, and a 250-unit dose is recommended for all ages (bacteria do not produce less toxin when infecting a child). If the wound remains unhealed at 4 weeks a second dose should be given.

Minor adverse reactions sometimes follow the injection of human immunoglobulin and a few severe reactions, sometimes resembling anaphylactic shock, have been described. These usually occur in patients given repeated injections for treatment of hypogammaglobulinaemias, but severe reactions are extremely unlikely to occur in healthy patients who receive human immunoglobulin only for tetanus prevention. A trial dose of immunoglobulin to predict the occurrence of anaphylactic shock is therefore unnecessary, just as it is in the case of vaccines used for routine immunisation. Nevertheless, as with any immunisation procedure, adrenaline should be immediately available whenever immunoglobulin is given.

Toxoid

Active immunisation. For active immunisation *adsorbed* toxoid is recommended — that is, toxoid containing an aluminium adjuvant (Adsorbed Tetanus Vaccine B. P.). Adsorbed toxoid is effective when given at the same time as antitoxin (but into a different limb), stimulates a higher, longer-lasting antitoxin response than plain toxoid, and is satisfactory for boosting immunity in wounded people. Plain toxoid is therefore not recommended.

A complete basic course comprises three spaced doses of toxoid, with for example, 6 to 12 weeks between the first and second doses and 4–12 months between the second and third.

The period for which antitoxin is found in the blood of actively immunised people after a complete basic course of adsorbed tetanus toxoid is uncertain, but evidence is accumulating that immunity usually lasts for 10 years, though it is less durable after plain toxoid. After a booster dose of adsorbed toxoid, immunity is believed to last even longer, but until it is established that this is almost invariably the case, booster doses are recommended at 10-year intervals.†

* By permission after Smith J W G et al. Br Med J 1975; 3:455.

† *Routine* booster doses are probably unnecessary. Mathias, R G. et al. (1985). Lancet. 1:1089

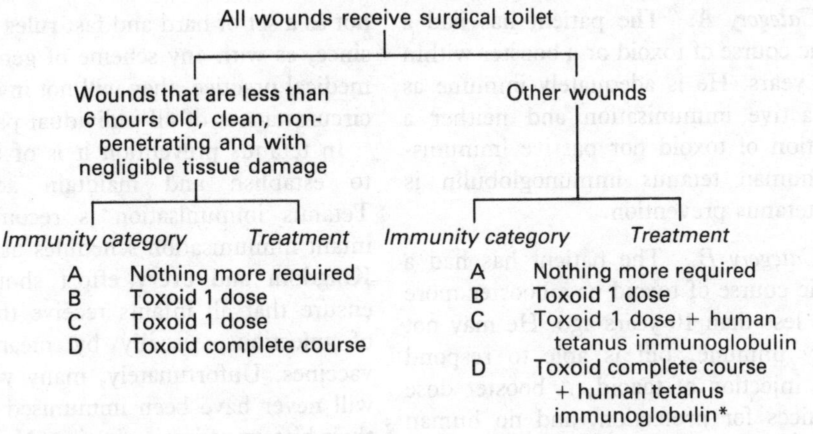

A Has had a complete course of toxoid or a booster dose within the past 5 years
B Has had a complete course of toxoid or a booster dose more than 5 and less than 10 years ago
C Has had a complete course of toxoid or a booster dose more than 10 years ago
D Has not had a complete course of toxoid or immunity status is unknown

* Where human immunoglobulin is not available or restricted, the choice for additional prophylaxis lies between horse antitoxin and antibiotics. Both have serious disadvantages. Horse antitoxin: allergy and rapid immune elimination. Antibiotics (penicillin, erythromycin, tetracycline): ineffective against toxin already formed: penicillin destroyed by concurrent wound infection with penicillinase-producing bacteria. Antibiotic should be given for a minimum of 4 days in the less contaminated wounds treated early and for longer in other cases, up to 4 weeks.

Fig. 19.1 Recommendations for prevention of tetanus in the wounded. Adrenaline injection (*B.P.*) should be available during prophylactic procedures for treatment of anaphylactic shock (in adults 0.5–1 ml intramuscularly).

Role of the booster dose at injury. The recommendation that a booster dose is given at injury to those immunised or boosted between 5 and 10 years previously is made for three reasons. First, it is desirable to stimulate an increase in the blood antitoxin when the patient may be faced with the challenge of toxin production in a wound. Secondly, there is the possibility that some people may have responded inadequately to the tetanus toxoid given earlier, and may thus lack circulating antitoxin at the time of injury. This is most likely in those who were immunised with plain toxoid, and since adsorbed toxoid was introduced in the UK only in 1963, there will still be many such people. Thirdly, it is desirable to take the opportunity of boosting the patient's immunity to ensure that he will remain actively immune for many years. The booster dose of toxoid for wounded patients immunised more than 10 years earlier is recommended for similar reasons but, owing to the longer time interval, there is a greater possibility that circulating antitoxin may be absent in such patients, particularly since many of them will have been immunised with plain toxoid. Moreover, their booster response may be slow — that is, tetanus toxin might be produced in a wound before antitoxin appears in the circulation; for this reason human tetanus immunoglobulin is recommended.

Adverse reaction to tetanus toxoid. Adverse reactions — usually pain at the site of injection — may occur, particularly when tetanus toxoid is given frequently to boost immunity, as for example in factory workers receiving minor wounds. Unnecessary booster doses of toxoid should therefore be avoided.

Immunity categories

The measures to be recommended for tetanus prevention in a wounded patient depend on whether or not he has been actively immunised and on the degree of immunity he is likely to possess. It is therefore necessary to evaluate the immunity of each patient and we suggest that the following four categories be used.

Immunity Category A. The patient has had a complete basic course of toxoid or a booster within the past five years. He is adequately immune as a result of active immunisation and neither a booster injection of toxoid nor passive immunisation with human tetanus immunoglobulin is required for tetanus prevention.

Immunity Category B. The patient has had a complete basic course of toxoid or a booster more than five and less than 10 years ago. He may not be adequately immune, but is able to respond rapidly to an injection of toxoid. A booster dose therefore suffices for protection, and no human tetanus immunoglobulin is needed.

Immunity Category C. The patient has had a complete basic course of toxoid or a booster dose more than 10 years ago. The immunity of such patients may be inadequate and some may not respond quickly enough to a toxoid booster. Thus, if the wound is not a minor one human tetanus immunoglobulin should be given. An injection of adsorbed toxoid should also be given simultaneously, but into a different limb.

Immunity Category D. The patient has not had a complete basic course of toxoid, or his immunisation status is not known. He is therefore not actively immune, or is not known to be. Thus, human tetanus immunoglobulin may be needed for immediate protection; it should be given simultaneously (but into a different limb) with a first injection of toxoid, which should be followed later by second and third injections to complete the basic course. Patients who are known to have had only one or two injections of toxoid may also be regarded for practical purposes as falling into this category.

Discussion

The measures to be taken for tetanus prevention in an individual wounded patient are decided on the basis of a knowledge and understanding of the pathological process of tetanus, the mode of action and limitations of the various preventive measures available, and the nature of the patient's wound and his history of tetanus immunisation. The recommendations should therefore be regarded not as a set of hard and fast rules but as guidelines since, as with any scheme of general guidance on medical practice, they will not invariably cover the circumstances of all individual patients.

In tetanus prevention it is of basic importance to establish and maintain active immunity. Tetanus immunisation is recommended in the infant immunisation schedules used in the United Kingdom and every effort should be made to ensure that all infants receive the proper course of injections, usually by means of combined vaccines. Unfortunately, many wounded patients will never have been immunised or do not know their history of immunisation. Nevertheless, measures should be taken to ensure that such patients become actively immunised, and it is for this purpose that their recommended treatment at the time of injury includes an injection of toxoid, given as the first of a full course of injections. If this policy is adopted in time fewer patients should require human immunoglobulin for temporary protection at injury. The doctor should explain the significance of active immunisation to his older patients so that increasing numbers of the population will come to realise the advantage of being immunised and of knowing their immunity status.

Wounded patients may require an antimicrobial for treatment or prevention of sepsis, and there is evidence that such treatment may sometimes usefully support the action of antitoxin in preventing tetanus. But, with the availability of human tetanus immunoglobulin, antimicrobials should now mainly revert to their former role of dealing with sepsis generally rather than the prevention of tetanus specifically; the use of antimicrobials has therefore not been included in our recommendations.*

Treatment of clinical tetanus: the objectives can be summarised:

1. To immediately neutralise with antitoxin any bacterial toxin that has not yet become attached irreversibly to the central nervous system.
2. To kill the tetanus bacteria by chemotherapy.

* By permission after Smith J W G et al. Br Med J 1975; 3:455.

3. To control the convulsions whilst maintaining respiratory and cardiovascular function (which latter may be disordered by the toxin, see below).

4. To prevent intercurrent infection (usually pulmonary).

5. To prevent electrolyte disturbances and to maintain nutrition.

Clinical trials have shown that 10 000 I.U. (i.v.) of equine antitoxin are almost certainly enough. Obviously human antitetanus immunoglobulin is preferable, but definitive trials have not been done and it is reasonable to suppose that the same dose would be appropriate. The objective is to provide high blood levels of antitoxin which outlast the infection.

If equine antitoxin only is available there is plainly a problem of possible rapid immune elimination in patients who have had equine antitoxin before. In these circumstances a higher dose is needed (say 20 000 I.U.) to ensure therapeutic effect since the antitoxin must neutralise the patients' antibodies as well as the bacterial toxin.

Since large amounts of toxin may be present in the tissues surrounding the wound, local infiltration of severe tetanus-prone wounds with 3000–4000 I.U. of antitoxin is advisable.

There is evidence from animals that antitoxin given i.v. has greater efficacy than when given i.m. But i.v. injection is more likely to cause adverse reactions (anaphylaxis in the case of equine antitoxin). Human immunoglobulin should be given i.m. because given i.v. the aggregated molecules of immunoglobulin can cause anaphylactoid reaction, though this is less likely if the preparation is diluted × 2 in 0.9% sodium chloride solution.

If equine antitoxin is used a test for allergy should be made by putting a drop of antitoxin on the skin and pricking obliquely through it to the full depth of the epidermis (with saline control) and read in 15 min. If there is no reaction, 10 000 I.U. may be given i.v.

If there is a reaction to the test, treatment will depend on its kind and severity (see *drug allergy*). However, it is still necessary to proceed, under antihistamine (say, diphenhydramine 50 mg orally or 25 mg i.m.) and hydrocortisone (100 mg i.v.) cover, to give 20 000 I.U. equine antitoxin. Unfortunately there are no reliable data to guide the technique.

Drugs for treating severe reactions should be ready in syringes at the bedside (see *anaphylactic shock*).

A recurrence of anaphylaxis within a few hours of an attack is unlikely.

In the unlikely event of an actively immunised person getting tetanus, an injection of toxoid may be given but the large therapeutic dose of antitoxin may interfere with it.

Chemotherapy with penicillin, metronidazole or tetracycline will stop further production of toxin. It is often continued as prophylaxis against pneumonia, but there is no certainty whether it is better to do this and risk pneumonia from antibiotic-resistant organisms or to stop the antibiotic after the wound had healed and start it again if infection occurs. In any case a severe wound may require prolonged chemotherapy, so that this choice does not always arise.

Convulsions may be controlled by diazepam or phenobarbitone. Both have the disadvantage that adequate dosage may lead to loss of consciousness for long periods and so promote respiratory failure and pneumonia, though this is least with diazepam, which is probably the drug of first choice, though it may not control severe cases. Chlorpromazine controls convulsions without causing loss of consciousness, but may fail in the most severe cases. An excess of chlorpromazine may make the convulsions worse, probably by stimulating the brain stem reticular formation. Morphine or pethidine have no useful anticonvulsant effect; either may stimulate the spinal cord.

The dosage and route of administration can only be decided when confronted with the patient. A regimen which should control convulsions of almost any severity would be diazepam 3.0 mg/kg/day (orally or parenterally) or chlorpromazine 1–1.5 mg/kg 4–6 hourly plus phenobarbitone 0.5 mg/kg intermittently (between the chlorpromazine doses) as required, usually parenterally. It may be impossible to avoid abolishing consciousness at times.

An alternative is to paralyse the patient with tubocurarine or gallamine (on theoretical grounds these are preferable to depolarising agents) and provide artificial respiration and enough sedation to impair awareness and memory. This requires skill and much equipment, with facilities for measuring blood pH, electrolytes and gases as well as ability to understand the meaning of the results. Unfortunately this limits its applicability, particularly in the countries where tetanus is common, so that it is especially difficult to know whether results are superior to the more conservative anticonvulsant regimens. This treatment reduces the mortality in severe cases of tetanus neonatorum, though not in those cases classified as mild or moderate, but results in adults remain equivocal, though a similar effect is likely. Treatment by paralysis need only be considered at present in very severe cases, and these are a minority. Unfortunately it is not easy to know which cases are going to become severe. Paralysis and artificial respiration should be seriously considered in all cases with laryngospasm, respiratory failure, severe chest infection and spasms so severe that they can only be controlled by making the patient unconscious. The action of the toxin in the CNS may cause *overactivity of the sympathetic autonomic system* (tachycardia, hypertension), which may be sufficient to require administration of α- and β-adrenoceptor blocking drugs. Attacks of hypotension can also occur.

Anticonvulsant therapy may be needed for 2 weeks or more and so attention to nutrition and body electrolytes is vital right from the start. Nursing care, in avoiding convulsions and pneumonia, is at least as important as drug therapy.

An attack of tetanus does not confer immunity and if the patient has had horse serum it is particularly important that he be actively immunised.

GUIDE TO FURTHER READING

1 Mucklow J C et al. Compliance with anticonvulsant therapy in a hospital clinic and in the community. Br J Clin Pharmacol 1978; 6:75.
2 Tyrer J H et al. Outbreak of anticonvulsant intoxication in an Australian city. Br Med J 1970; 4:271.
3 Petereit L B et al. Effectiveness of prednisolone during phenytoin therapy. Clin Pharmacol Ther 1977; 22:912.
4 Christiansen C et al. Actions of vitamins D_2 and D_3 and 25-OHD_3 in anticonvulsant osteomalacia. Br Med J 1975; 2:363.
5 Shorvon S D et al. Reduction in polypharmacy for epilepsy. Br Med J 1979; 2:1023.
6 Chadwick D et al. When do epileptic patients need treatment? Starting and stopping medication. Br Med J 1985; 290:1885.
7 Perucca A et al. Comparative study of the relative enzyme inducing properties of anticonvulsant drugs in epileptic patients. Br J Clin Pharmacol 1984; 18:401.
8 Fischbacher E. Effect of reduction of anticonvulsants on wellbeing. Br Med J 1982; 285:423.
9 Editorial. New drugs for epilepsy. Lancet 1985; 1:198
10 Tsanaclis L M et al. Effect of valproate on free plasma phenytoin concentrations. Br J Clin Pharmacol 1984; 18:17.
11 Delgado-Escueta A V et al. The treatable epilepsies. N Engl J Med 1983; 308:1508, 1576.
12 Delgado-Escueta A V et al. Management of status epilepticus. N Engl J Med 1982; 306:1337.
13 Editorial. Teratogenic risks of antepileptic drugs. Br Med J 1981; 283:515.
14 Mattson R M et al. Comparison of canbamazepine, phenobarbital, phenytoin, and primidone in partial and secondarily generated tonic-clonic seizures. N Engl J Med 1985; 313:145.
15 Marsden C D. Basal ganglia disease. Lancet 1982; 2: 1141–1146.
16 Curtis L et al. Effect of L-dopa on course of Parkinson's disease. Lancet 1984; 2: 211–212.
17 Editorial. MPTP parkinsonism. Br Med J 1984; 289: 1401–1402.
18 Editorial. Parkinson's disease, 1984. Lancet 1984; 1: 829–830.
19 Nutt J G, Woodward W R, Hammerstad J P, Carter J H, Anderson J L. The 'On-off' phenomenon in Parkinson's disease. N Engl J Med 1984; 310: 483–488.
20 Mayeux R, Stern Y, Mulvey K Cote L. Reappraisal of temporary levodopa withdrawal ('drug holiday') in Parkinson's disease. N Engl J Med 1985; 313: 724–728.
21 Young R R, Delwaide P J. Spasticity. N Engl J Med 1981; 304: 28–34, 96–99.
22 Hern J E C. Tremor. Br Med J 1984; 288: 1072–1073.
23 Lader M H, Editorial. Neuroleptics and abnormal movements. Br Med J 1982; 285:463.
24 Editorial. The management of dystonias. Lancet 1985; 1: 321–322.
25 Domenighetti G M et al. Hyperadrenergic syndrome in severe tetanus: extreme rise in catecholamines responsive to labetalol. Br Med J 1984; 288:1483.
26 Vakil B J et al. A comparison of the value of 200,000 I.U. tetanus antitoxin (horse) with 10,000 I.U. in the treatment of tetanus. Clin Pharmacol Ther 1968; 9:465.
27 Hopkins A. Prescribing in pregnancy. Epilepsy and anticonvulsant drugs. Br Med J 1987; 294:497.

20

Central nervous system V: Non-medical use of drugs: Drug dependence: Tobacco, alcohol and cannabis

The enormous social importance of the major topics of this chapter justifies the detailed treatment.

'All the naturally occurring sedatives, narcotics, euphoriants, hallucinogens, and excitants were discovered thousands of years ago, before the dawn of civilisation . . . By the late Stone Age man was systematically poisoning himself. The presence of poppy heads in the kitchen middens of the Swiss Lake Dwellers shows how early in his history man discovered the techniques of self-transcendence through drugs. There were dope addicts long before there were farmers.'*

The drives that persuade or compel a person more or less mentally healthy to resort to drugs to obtain 'chemical vacations from intolerable selfhood'† will be briefly considered here, as well as some account of the pharmacological aspects of drug dependence.

'That humanity at large will ever be able to dispense with Artificial Paradises seems very unlikely. Most men and women lead lives at the worst so painful, at the best so monotonous, poor and limited that the urge to escape, the longing to transcend themselves if only for a few moments, is and has always been one of the principal appetites of the soul'†. The dividing-line between legitimate use of drugs for social purposes and their abuse is indistinct for it is not only a matter of *which* drug, but of *amount* of drug and of whether the effect is directed antisocially or not. 'Normal' people seem to be able to use alcohol for their occasional purposes without harm but, given the appropriate degree of mental abnormality or environmental adversity, many may become dependent on it, both emotionally and physically. But *drug abuse is not primarily a pharmacological problem, it is a social problem with important pharmacological aspects*.

The discussion in this chapter is largely confined to psychotropic drugs, i.e. drugs that alter mood, consciousness or other psychological or behavioural factors; they include opioids, sedatives, hypnotics, tranquillisers, stimulants and hallucinogens. But it also includes 'substance' abuse and the wider range used, or misused, in sport.

Abuse potential of a drug is related to its capacity to produce *immediate* satisfaction (e.g. amphetamine and heroin give immediate effect, anti-depressants do not) and to its route of administration in descending order, inhalation/i.v.; i.m./s.c., oral.

* Huxley A. Ann N Y Acad Sci 1957; 67:677.
† Huxley A. The doors of perception. London: Chatto and Windus, 1954.

Some terms used

Drug abuse.* What constitutes abuse is determined by the opinions generally held in a particular society. Thus, in Britain, temperate use of tobacco and alcohol to insulate from environmental stress and anxiety and to ease social intercourse, a form of *self-medication*, is generally accepted; a substantial minority do not consider occasional taking of cannabis to be abuse; a small minority do not consider all use of LSD or heroin to be abuse. Thus, **non-medical (non-prescription or social) drug use** (i.e. all drug use that is not on generally accepted medical grounds) may be a term preferable to abuse. Non-medical use means the continuous or occasional use of drugs by the individual, whether of his own choice or under feelings of compulsion, to achieve his own well being, or what he conceives as his own well being (see motives below).

Drugs used for non-medical purposes are often divided into two groups, **hard** and **soft**. Hard drugs are those that are liable seriously to disable the individual as a functioning member of society by inducing severe emotional and, in the case of cerebral depressants, physical dependence. The group includes heroin, morphine and analogues.

Soft drugs are less dependence-producing. There may be emotional dependence, but there is little or no physical dependence except with heavy doses of depressants (alcohol, barbiturates). The group includes sedatives and tranquillisers, amphetamines, cannabis, hallucinogens, alcohol, tobacco.

As with many attempts to make convenient classifications, this fails, for it does not recognise individual variation in drug use. Barbiturates can be used in heavy, often i.v., doses that are gravely disabling and induce severe physical dependence with convulsions on sudden withdrawal; i.e. for the individual the drug is 'hard'. But there are many middle-aged people mildly dependent on them as hypnotics and sedatives who retain their position in home and society. Similarly, amphetamines can be used in ways that cause doubt whether they should be described as 'hard' or 'soft'.

The terms **hard-use** where the drug is central in the user's life and **soft-use** where it is merely incidental, are of assistance in making this distinction, i.e. what is classified is not the drug but the effect it has or the way it is used by the individual.

Non-medical drug use has two principal forms:

1. *Continuous use*, when there is a true dependence, e.g. opioids, alcohol, barbiturates.
2. *Intermittent or occasional use* to obtain an experience, e.g. LSD, cocaine, cannabis, solvents, or to relieve stress, e.g. alcohol.

Both uses commonly occur in the same subject, and some drugs, e.g. alcohol, are used in both ways, but others, e.g. LSD or cannabis, are virtually confined to (2).

The motives for non-medical (or non-prescription) drug use† include:

1. Relief of anxiety, tension and depression; escape from personal psychological problems; detachment from harsh reality.
2. Search for self-knowledge and for meaning in life, including religion. The cult of 'experience' including aestheticism and artistic creation, sex and 'genuine', 'sincere' interpersonal relationships, to obtain a sense of 'belonging'.
3. Rebellion against or despair about orthodox social values and the environment.
4. Fear of missing something, and conformity with own social subgroup.
5. Fun, amusement, recreation, excitement, curiosity.

Two claims for the non-medical use of psychotropic drugs may be mentioned, (1) that there is

* The World Health Organization adopts the definition of the United Nations Convention on Psychotropic Drugs (1971). Drug abuse means the use of psychotropic substances in a way that would 'constitute a public health and social problem'.

† Reliable datas on drug abuse/misuse by *medical students* are scarce. In one study in the USA (995 questionnaires with 48% usable response) the results were: students (%) had *tried* the following drugs (% classifying themselves as *users*): *Marijuana* 62.5%(27.4%): *cocaine* 33(10.8): *stimulants* 26.3(6.9): *tranquillizers* 20.2 (9.9). Since some students may have been multiple drug users, the *total* percentage of *users* will be less than the sum of the figures given. (Epstein R et al. N Engl J Med 1984; 311:923). No doubt figures will differ from place to place, but these should cause concern both amongst students and the profession.

such a thing as a '**drug-culture**', and (2) that drugs provide **mystical or religious experience**.

The phrase 'drug culture' implies that drugs can provide the spiritual, emotional and intellectual experiences and development that are the basis for a way of life that can be described as a 'culture'.

It is inherently unlikely that chemicals could be central to a constructive culture and no support for the assertion has yet been produced. (That chemicals might be central to a destructive culture is another matter.) That like-minded people practising what are often illegal activities will gather into closely knit sub-groups for mutual support, and will feel a sense of community, is to be expected, but that is hardly a 'culture'. Even when drug-using sub-groups are accepted as representing a culture (or sub-culture), it may be doubted if drugs are sufficiently central to their ideology to justify using 'drug' in the title, i.e. drug use is a secondary associated, and not a primary phenomenon. But claims for the individual and social value of drug experience must surely be tested by the criterion of fruitfulness for the individual and for society,* and the judgement of the individual concerned alone is insufficient; it should be confirmed by others. The results of illegal drug use do not give encouragement to press for a large-scale experiment in this field. To justify such an experiment (as with any other clinical trial) it would seem necessary to show reason to believe that what are universally agreed to be good human qualities, e.g. love of neighbour expressed in effective, practical action are either likely to be promoted, or at least unlikely to be diminished by a drug. (Love of neighbour is incompatible with driving a car over him.) That drugs, including alcohol, can induce states of vague benevolence and feelings of spirituality is undoubted, but the test is not only how a person feels, but what he does in response to the feeling.

The other claim is that drugs provide **mystical experience** and that this has valid religious content, so that it has great value and importance for the individual. If mysticism is to be discussed at all, it must be defined. *Mystical experience* is perhaps best defined by listing its characteristics; these are feelings of:

1. Unity: a sense of oneness with nature and/or God.
2. Ineffability: the experience is beyond the subject's power to express or describe.
3. Joy, peace, sacredness.
4. Knowledge: insight into truths of life and values, illuminations, revelations of enormous significance.
5. Transcendence of space and time.

Mystical states are both transient and passive (the subject feels his will is in abeyance).

When such states do occur there remains the question whether they tell us something about a reality outside the individual or merely something about the mind of the person having the experience.

There are three *forms of mysticism*†:

1. *Nature mysticism*: 'an intuition, which is sometimes so vivid as to appear to be a vision, of reality and unity in the world "outside" the mind . . . it is associated with natural beauty and sublimity, or with a quasi personified "nature" as its object.'

2. *Soul mysticism*: the soul or spirit strives to enter, not into communion with God or Nature, but into a state of complete isolation from everything other than itself. The chief object is the quest of a man's own self and of knowledge about it.

3. *God mysticism*: the spirit is absorbed into the essence of God or achieves some form of union with God. There is an inexpressible knowledge and love of God or of religious truth.

Naturally such experience is attractive, so that there is a demand for any easy means to deliver it. But it must be stressed that there can be no guarantee that a mystical experience will occur with any drug.

Mystical experience is not a normal dose-related pharmacodynamic effect of any drug, its occur-

* This criterion is not new: St. Matthew's Gospel; 7:5. St. Paul's Epistle to the Romans; 12: 4–5.

† Definitions from:
Knowles D. What is Mysticism. London: Sheed and Ward. 1971.
Happold F C. Mysticism. Harmondsworth: Penguin Books. 1963.

rence depends on many factors, the subject (personality, mood) and his environment, and any preparation he may have undergone. The drug *facilitates* the experience, it does not *induce* it; drugs can facilitate unpleasant as well as pleasant experiences. It is not surprising that mystical experience can occur with a wide range of drugs that alter consciousness:

'. . . I seemed at first in a state of utter blankness . . . with a keen vision of what was going on in the room around me, but no sensation of touch. I thought that I was near death; when, suddenly, my soul became aware of God, who was manifestly dealing with me, handling me, so to speak, in an intense personal, present reality . . . I cannot describe the ecstasy I felt'. This experience occurred in the 19th century* with chloroform, which is not a drug recommended by contemporary mystics.

There is no good evidence that drugs can produce experience that passes the test of *results*, i.e. fruitfulness (above). Indeed, reliance on repeated drug experience may even inhibit the development of independence from the material things of this world, which is vital for anything that deserves to be described as freedom of spirit.

Whether a single administration of a drug can be used to initiate or trigger experiences that may result in an individual gaining beneficial insight is unproved. If emotional shock is acceptable in religious conversion there seems no obvious reason why a drug should not also be used once after careful preparation. Plainly there is a risk of the experience becoming an end in itself rather than a means of development.

It is interesting that the *double-blind controlled trial* has been attempted in the field of spiritual experience and knowledge where, it has been pointed out, the passion with which a belief is defended is commonly in inverse proportion to the strength of the evidence that can be adduced for it.

Twenty well-prepared Christian theological students received, by random allocation, either psilocybin (a hallucinogen) or nicotinic acid (as an 'active' placebo). They attended a Good Friday church service lasting $2\frac{1}{2}$ h and wrote accounts of their feelings, completed questionnaires and were interviewed to elicit evidence of mystical experience (see above). It was concluded that psilocybin facilitated mystical experience.† While such work is of interest it may be remembered that religious experience 'means the whole of life interpreted, rather than isolated feelings. A religious man is not one who has "experiences" . . . but one who takes all life in a religious way . . . religious experience . . . is not the isolated outbreak of abnormal phenomena in this or that individual (though to read some psychological treatments of religious experience one would suppose so)'.‡

Conclusions on non-medical use of drugs for valuable experience

The above brief discussion does little more than raise issues that deserve consideration. Drug-induced experience can only be discussed in terms of attitudes and beliefs held by the individual as to the nature of man, his purpose (if any), his obligations (if any) and his relationship to a transcendent being or God (if any). An author in this field has a choice of attempting an impartiality that is almost certainly spurious, or of openly allowing his views to obtrude. The latter course seems preferable, as less misleading. The writers' views on the **three major areas of non-medical drug use** are as follows:

1. *For relaxation, recreation, protection from and relief of stress and anxiety; relief of depression*: moderate use of some 'soft' drugs may be accepted as part of our society provided they do not detract from living fully, loving fully, and striving for good.

2. *For spiritually valuable experience*: justification is doubtful.

3. *As basis for a 'culture' in the sense that drug experience* (a) can *be, and* (b) should *be central to*

* Quoted in James W. Varities of religious experience. Harlow: Longmans. 1902. Many subsequent editions of this classic.

† Pahnke W N In: Aaronson et al., eds. Psychedelics: the uses and implications of hallucinogenic drugs. London: Hogarth Press. 1970.

‡ Dodd C H. The authority of the Bible. London: Fontana. 1960.

an individually or socially constructive way of life: a claim without validity.

Legalisation of drugs for non-medical use

The decision whether a drug is acceptable in medical practice is made after an evaluation of its safety in relation to its efficacy. The same principle should be used for drugs for non-medical or social use. But the usual medical criteria for judging efficacy against disease or discomfort are hardly applicable. The reasons why people want to use cannabis or other drugs for non-medical purposes are listed above. None of them can carry serious weight if the drug is found to have serious risks to the individual* or to society, with either acute or chronic use. Ordinary prudence dictates that any such risks should be carefully defined before a decision on legalisation is made.

But there are other indirect effects of drug use, including loss of education or employment. The autocratic implementation of laws that are not widely accepted in the community can lead to corruption in the police and alienation of reasonable people who would otherwise be an important stabilising influence in society. Lack of discrimination by the law may lead to progression by association from the less to the more harmful drugs, since similar illegal behaviour is needed to obtain all.

But though written laws are so often inflexible and group together what would best be separated, informal judicial discretion under present law may be permitting more experimentation than would recurrent legislative debate leading to substitution of one written law for another written law. It is recognised that this untidy approach, which may be best for the time being, cannot satisfy the extravagant advocates either of licence or of repression.†

A suggested intermediate course for cannabis is that penalties for possession of small amounts for personal consumption should be removed (i.e. decriminalization as opposed to legalization), whilst retaining penalties for suppliers.

* Hazard to the individual is not a matter for the individual alone if it also has consequences for society.

† See, for an excellent discussion, Hawks D. The law relating to cannabis 1964–73: how subtle an ass? In: Graham J D P, ed. Cannabis and health, London: Academic Press. 1976.

Drugs and sport

The rewards of competitive sport, both financial and in personal and national prestige, are the cause of determination to win at (almost) any cost. Drugs are used optimistically to enhance performance though efficacy is largely undocumented. Detection can be difficult when the drugs or metabolites are closely related to physiological substances, and when the drug can be stopped before the event without apparent loss of efficacy, e.g. anabolic steroids. It will be interesting to see if the extensive and expensive resources currently being deployed to unmask the unsportsmanlike ultimately will prove to have been well spent.

Drugs may be used in the following ways:

1. For events in which *body weight and brute strength* are the principal determinants (weight lifting, rowing, shot putting): *anabolic steroids*. There is evidence that, taken together with a high-protein diet and exercise, they increase lean body weight (muscle), but any effect on performance is less certain.

There is a low risk of liver damage (cholestatic), especially if the drug is taken intermittently, which is certainly insufficient to deter 'sportsmen', who may be more inclined to take more seriously the fact the anabolic steroids suppress pituitary gonadotrophin, and so testosterone production; there seem to be no controlled data on women.

Sportsmen who have to run even a little (e.g. javelin throwing) are more likely to be handicapped by increased weight.

2. For events in which *output of energy is explosive* (*100 m sprint*) *or prolonged at a high level* (bicycling, marathon running): *stimulants*. They have probably caused death in bicycle racing (continuous hard exercise with short periods of sprint) due to hyperpyrexia in metabolically stimulated vasoconstricted subjects exercising maximally under a hot sun. Fencamfamin (effects probably similar to amphetamine) has also been used in team games (e.g. by footballers) and no doubt also all other central nervous system stimulants.

3. For events in which *steadiness* is essential (pistol, rifle shooting): β-*adrenoceptor blockers*.

4. For events in which *body pliancy* is a major factor (gymnastics), delaying puberty in child gymnasts by endocrine techniques.

5. *Miscellaneous*. Minor injuries are usual during athletic training and these may be suppressed by drugs (corticosteroids, NSAIDs) to allow the training to proceed maximally.

Generally, owing to recognition of natural biological differences most competitive events are sexually segregated. In many events men have a natural biological advantage and the (inevitable) consequence has been that women have been virilised (by administration of androgens) so that they may outperform their sisters.

It seems safe to assume that anything that can be thought up to gain advantage will be tried by competitors eager for immediate fame.

Accurate data are difficult to obtain in these areas. No doubt placebo effects are important, i.e. beliefs as to what has been taken and what effects ought to follow.

The dividing line between what is and what is not acceptable practice is hard to draw.

Caffeine can improve physical performance and it illustrates the difficulty of deciding what is 'permissible' or 'impermissible'. A cup of coffee is part of a normal diet, but some consider taking the same amount of caffeine in a tablet, injection or suppository to be 'doping'.

The problem raised by use of local anaesthetic, anti-inflammatory analgesics and adrenal steroids for strains, hormonal adjustment or suppression of menstruation, drugs for anxiety, etc., are ethical rather than medical, as is the use of hypnosis in the reported competition success of a swimmer who, it is alleged, had been persuaded under hypnosis into the belief that he was being pursued by a shark.

DRUG DEPENDENCE

Drug dependence is a state arising from repeated, periodic or continuous administration of a drug, that results in harm to the individual and sometimes to society. The subject feels a desire, need or compulsion to continue using the drug and feels ill if deprived of it (abstinence or withdrawal syndrome).

Drug dependence is characterised by the following phenomena:

1. **Emotional (psychic) dependence**: the first to appear: there is emotional distress if the drug is withheld.

2. **Physical dependence**: follows emotional dependence in some cases: there is a physical illness if the drug is withheld.

3. **Tolerance**: this also occurs to many drugs that do not induce dependence, e.g. LSD.

It was once customary to divide regular continuous drug abuse into two categories, 'addiction' and 'habit'. Attempts to draw firm distinctions between the graver addiction and the less serious habit have been unsuccessful. It was said that in addiction subjects had a 'compulsion' to take the drug, that they became both emotionally and physically dependent on it and that this resulting state was detrimental not only to the subject but to society. It was more serious than drug habit, in which the subject merely had a 'desire' for the drug, on which his dependence was solely emotional, and the evil effects were virtually confined to the individual. The distinction failed because of the impossibility of distinguishing between 'desire' and 'compulsion', the absence of any important physical dependence with cerebral stimulants (cocaine, amphetamine), which were generally agreed to be drugs of addiction, and the difficulty of separating damage to the individual from damage to society. Also the same drug could form a minor habit in one individual and be the subject of gross addiction in another. Alcohol is an obvious example. It provides an occasional pleasure or solace for some, it is taken regularly by others, who feel unhappy if they are deprived of it, and a minority of people disintegrate socially through its effects and are physically dependent to such a degree that they become gravely ill if they cannot get it.

In 1964 the World Health Organization Expert Committee on Addiction-producing Drugs recommended that the term **drug dependence** should be substituted for both 'addiction' and 'habit'. The various drug dependences have some common features. It may well be that personality disorders and the socio-economic environment are the important determinants of whether dependence occurs and of the drug that is chosen (which is also influenced by availability, see 'substance' abuse below). Drug dependence is not solely, or even mainly, a problem of pharmacology. This is supported by the fact that there are sometimes sudden changes in the drug of choice amongst drug-abusing groups, and there is evidence that rats which are offered morphine and choose to take it develop greater dependence and a readiness to revert to it after withdrawal than do rats to which morphine is arbitrarily administered.

The pharmacological properties of the chosen drug, the dose used and the frequency of administration are all important factors in determining the speed of onset of and the degree of dependence, emotional and/or physical.

The use of the term 'addict' or 'addiction' has not been completely abandoned in this book because the new and sensible terminology can be cumbersome, especially when referring to drug-dependent individuals, and in distinguishing the severer forms of dependence, which present a problem as grave as dependence on tea-drinking is trivial. But the use of the term *drug dependence* is welcome, because it removes a distinction that was never a true difference, and it renders irrelevant arguments about whether some drugs, e.g. tobacco, are addictive or merely habit-forming.

The mechanisms of physical dependence on drugs and development of tolerance are ill-understood. Physical dependence and tolerance imply that adaptive changes have taken place in body tissues so that when the drug is withdrawn these adaptive changes are left unopposed, resulting generally in a rebound overactivity. The discovery that the CNS employs morphine-like substances (endorphins) as neurotransmitters allows speculation that exogenously administered opioid may suppress endogenous production of endorphins by a feed-back mechanism so that when administration of opioid is suddenly stopped there is an immediate deficiency of endogenous opioid, which thus causes the withdrawal syndrome. **Tolerance** could result from a compensatory biochemical cell response to continued exposure to opioid. In short, both physical dependence and tolerance may result from the operation of homeostatic adaptation to continued high occupancy of opioid receptors. Changes of similar type may occur with GABA transmission.

Physical dependence develops to a substantial degree with cerebral depressants, but is minor or absent with stimulant drugs.

The distinction between physical and emotional dependence is not always clear, for the mental misery of the deprived heavy tobacco smoker may manifest itself in physical symptoms, such as digestive disturbances and tremors.

There is commonly **cross-tolerance** between drugs of similar, and sometimes even of dissimilar, chemical groups, e.g. barbiturates, alcohol and benzodiazepines.

Although 'no drug possesses mysterious powers to subjugate a human being',* there is danger in experimenting with the more potent agents. It is said that a feeling of pleasure on first experience of a drug can be an index of 'addiction proneness', and this was evidently so for that famous addict, Thomas de Quincey, who, in 1804, suffering from facial pain, 'met a college acquaintance who recommended opium'. He purchased some tincture and went home. '. . . I took it; and in an hour, O heavens! what a revulsion! what a resurrection, from its lowest depths, of the inner spirit! . . . That my pains had vanished, was now a trifle in my eyes; this negative effect was swallowed up in the immensity of those positive effects which had opened before me, in the abyss of divine enjoyment thus suddenly revealed. Here was a panacea . . . for all human woes; here was the secret of happiness, about which philosophers had disputed for so many ages, at once discovered; happiness might now be bought for a penny, and carried in the waistcoat-pocket; portable ecstasies might be had corked up in a pint-bottle; and peace of mind could be sent down by the mail'.† Or, as a modern American addict has more succinctly, though less elegantly, put it, 'The all think they

* Maurer D W, Vogel V H. Narcotics and narcotic addiction. Springfield: Thomas, 1962.

† De Quincey T. Confessions of an English opium eater. Many editions since 1821.

can take just one joy-pop but it's the first one that hooks you'.[†]

On the other hand many people experience nothing but unpleasantness with the opium group of drugs. In case these quotations should give an impression that there is anything amusing or romantic about severe opioid dependence, it may be categorically stated that it is, in virtually all cases, a ruinous, degrading and sordid state not only for the addict, who is a sociopath, but for his family and friends. Unfortunately the subject cannot decide for himself that his dependence will remain mild. The opinion of de Quincey is unsound, and his career as an addict was quite exceptional.

Despite the fact that the sale of opium to the public in Britain was not closely restricted by law until 1923, there was never a large body of opium addicts in the country. Restriction was inevitable, however, because of the ease with which morphine can be extracted from it, a standing temptation to unscrupulous people who in some countries promote addiction, even amongst juveniles, for gain. The argument of de Quincey in 1821, 'what a man may lawfully seek in wine, surely he may lawfully find in opium' does not now arouse the sympathy of more than a small minority. Nor are we as surprised as he was that 14 insurance offices in succession 'repulsed me as a candidate . . . on that solitary ground of having owned myself to be an opium-eater'.[*]

Emotional dependence occurs to any drug that alters consciousness however bizarre, e.g. muscarine (see index) and to some that, in ordinary doses, don't, e.g. non-narcotic analgesics, purgatives, diuretics; these latter provide problems of psychiatry rather than of psychopharmacology.

Emotional dependence can occur merely on a tablet or injection, regardless of its content, as well as to particular drugs. Mild dependence does not require that a drug should have important psychic effects, the subject's beliefs as to what it does are as important (e.g. purgative and diuretic dependence in people obsessed with dread of obesity). We are all physically dependent on food, and some develop a strong emotional dependence and eat too much.

[*] De Quincey T. Confessions of an English opium eater. Many editions since 1821.

[†] Maurer D W, Vogel V H. Narcotics and narcotic addiction. Springfield: Thomas. 1962.

General pattern of non-medical drug use

Any age: alcoholism: mild dependence on hypnotics and tranquillisers: occasional use of LSD, and cannabis.

20–35 years old: hard-use drugs, chiefly heroin, morphine (imported illicitly) and synthetic analogues, e.g. dipipanone, dextromoramide, methadone (diverted prescriptions): amphetamine (injected).

Under 16 years: volatile inhalants e.g. solvents of glues, aerosol sprays, vapourised (by heat) paints: 'solvent or substance' abuse: 'glue-sniffing'.

Some topics

Multiple drug misuse (hypnotics, sedatives, amphetamines, opioids, cocaine) is now a marked feature and the pattern of drugs used changes frequently.

Supply of drugs to addicts. In the UK, heroin or cocaine may only be prescribed for maintenance of an addict (during treatment or after cure has failed) by specially licensed doctors. Addicts so treated must be notified to the Home Office, as must any patient addicted to any opioid, natural or synthetic. The decision to prescribe is entirely in the hands of the licensed doctor. Initially there was a tendency to supply (by National Health Service prescription) both drugs and sterile injection equipment (to minimise infection which, with overdose, is a chief cause of the high mortality in illicit i.v. users). But now the policy is to use, whenever practicable, an oral methadone formulation[‡] this is made specially to discourage use by injection; it occupies opioid receptors and so reduces the kick of any subsequent i.v. injection. It is considered the lesser evil to supply pure drug to known people who remain in touch with responsible physicians.[§]

If this procedure were not used it is thought

[‡] A bright green syrupy liquid.

[§] But alternative drugs may legally be supplied by any doctor and some have found themselves under great pressure (even threats of physical violence) from drug abusers who may also sell what they get.

that the illicit market would expand even more than it is doing. The need for money to finance the market would cause the price to be high and addicts would turn to persistent crime to pay for their addiction. The matter remains speculative, but as the amount of injectable drugs prescribed for addiction declined over one period of 10 years, the price of illicit heroin (usually injected) rose 15–35 times.

When injectable drugs are prescribed there is currently no way of assessing the truth of the addict's statement that he needs *x* mg of heroin (or other drug) and the dose has to be assessed intuitively by the doctor. This has resulted in addicts obtaining more than they need and selling it, sometimes to initiate new users. The use of oral methadone or other opioid for maintenance by prescription is devised to mitigate this problem.

Withdrawal syndrome in opioid dependence. Whilst this can undoubtedly be very unpleasant (described on p. 319) the notion that once 'hooked' the addict continues to seek the drug *primarily* to avoid the unpleasantness of withdrawal may be false. The high relapse rate after full withdrawal suggests this; also addicts are reported as seeking 'supernormality' rather than normality as well as the intense pleasurable 'kick' or 'high', so that even after complete withdrawal the psychopathic or neurotic subject is left with unrealised expectations, which cause him to seek relief in drugs.

Treatment of severe pain in an opioid addict presents a special problem. High-efficacy opioids may be ineffective (tolerance) or overdose may result; Low-efficacy opioids will not only be ineffective but may induce withdrawal symptoms, especially if they are agonist/antagonists, e.g. pentazocine. This leaves aspirin as a drug of choice. But an opioid addict is liable to despise what he regards as trivial and commonplace and so exhibit a 'negative placebo' response. Aspirin can be offered can be offered in one of its various proprietary disguises and combinations, e.g. Paynocil (aspirin 600 mg plus aminoacetic acid 300 mg). Nefopam is a non-opioid analgesic that may relieve severe pain.

Route of administration and effect. With the i.v. route, much higher peak plasma concentrations can be reached than with oral administration. This accounts for the 'kick' or 'flash' that abusers report and which many seek, likening it to sexual orgasm or better. As an addict over-dramatically said 'The ultimate high is death'* and it has been reported that when hearing of someone dying of an overdose, some addicts will seek out the vendor since it is evident he is selling 'really good stuff'.* Addicts who rely on illegal sources are inevitably exposed to being supplied diluted or even inert preparations at high prices. North American addicts who have come to the UK believing themselves to be accustomed to high doses of heroin, have suffered acute poisoning when given, probably for the first time, pure heroin at an official UK drug dependence clinic.

Mortality. Young illicit users by i.v. injection (heroin, barbiturates, amphetamine) have a mortality up to × 40 normal. They die of overdose and of septicaemia, endocarditis, hepatitis, AIDS, gas gangrene, tetanus, pulmonary embolism, etc. from the contaminated materials used without aseptic precautions.

Escalation. A variable proportion of subjects who start with cannabis and amphetamine eventually take heroin. This disposition to progress from occasional soft use of drugs through to hard use, when it occurs, is less likely to be due to pharmacological actions, than to psychological and social factors.

De-escalation also occurs as users become disillusioned with drugs as they get older.

Miscellaneous. Any drug that alters consciousness is liable to abuse, even antiparkinsonian drugs (levodopa, anticholinergics) have been employed.

Substance abuse. Seekers of the 'self-gratifying high'† also inhale any volatile substance that may affect the central nervous system, adhesives ('glue-sniffing'), lacquer-paint solvents ('huffing')†, petrol, nail varnish, any pressurised aerosol and butane liquid gas (which latter especially may freeze the larynx, allowing fatal inhalation of food, drink or gastric contents, or even flood the lungs); solids, e.g. paint scrapings, solid shoe polish, may be volatilised over a fire. These substances are

* Bourne P. Acute drug abuse emergencies. New York: Academic Press, 1976.

† Editorial. A-huffin' and a-puffin', a-sniffin' and a-suckin'. Lancet 1974; 2:876.

particularly abused by the very young (schoolchildren), no doubt largely because they are accessible at home and in ordinary shops and they cannot easily buy alcohol.* The solvents and propellants are toxic and deaths have occurred. If the substance is put in a plastic bag from which the user takes deep inhalations, or is sprayed in a confined space, e.g. cupboard, there is particularly high risk.

'A 17-year-old boy was offered the use of a plastic bag and a can of hair spray at a beach party. The hair spray was released into the plastic bag and the teenager put his mouth to the open end of the bag and inhaled . . . he exclaimed, "God, this stuff hits ya fast!" He got up, ran 100 yards and died.†

'Designer drugs'.‡ This 'unfortunate name' means molecular modifications produced in secret for profit by skilled and criminally minded chemists. Manipulation of fentanyl has resulted in compounds of extraordinary potency.

In 1976 a too-clever 23-year-old addict seeking to manufacture his own pethidine 'took a synthetic shortcut and injected himself with what was later with his help proved to be two closely related byproducts; one was MPTP' (methylphenyltetrahydropyridine).§ Three days later he developed a severe parkinsonian syndrome that responded to levodopa. MPTP selectively destroys melanin-containing cells in the substantia nigra. Further such cases have occurred from use of supposed synthetic heroin. MPTP has since been used in experimental research on parkinsonism.

What the future holds for individuals and for society in this area can only be imagined.

Treatment of drug dependence

Treatment consists of:

1. **Withdrawal** of the drug, which, whilst obviously important, is only a step on what can be a long and often disappointing journey to psychological and social rehabilitation (e.g. 'therapeutic communities'). In the case of drugs that cause physical dependence, withdrawal may be gradual (over about 10 days or more) or sudden, provided that in the latter case steps are taken to control the abstinence syndrome.

This may be done by judicious use of the same drug, but some prefer to use alternative drugs, generally, though not always, of similar kind; for instance a *heroin* addict can be given methadone, an *alcoholic* may be given chlormethiazole, diazepam or chlordiazepoxide. A *barbiturate* addict may be given 30 mg phenobarbitone for every 100 mg of other barbiturate used per day (with max dose 400 mg phenobarb/day) and this withdrawn over 2–3 weeks. If a patient is in very poor physical condition, withdrawal should be postponed until he is better. Sympathetic autonomic overactivity can be treated with a β-adrenoceptor blocker (or clonidine).

2. **Maintenance**. Relapsed addicts who live a fairly normal life are sometimes best treated by supplying drugs under supervision. There is no legal objection to doing this in Britain (see above) but naturally this course, which abandons hope of cure, should not be adopted until it is certain that cure is virtually impossible. A less harmful drug by a less harmful route may be substituted, e.g. oral methadone for i.v. heroin. Addicts are often particularly reluctant to abandon the i.v. route, which provides the 'immediate high' that they find, or originally found, so desirable.

Biochemical techniques for identification of most drugs, including opioids, in blood and urine are available. They facilitate management.

Testing new drugs for power to induce serious dependence

The occurrence of physical dependence is an important indicator. Drugs are given regularly to animals (monkeys, dogs) for about 4 weeks and then withdrawn suddenly to see if an abstinence syndrome occurs. In the case of opioids physical dependence can also be shown by giving an antagonist (naloxone). Power of a drug to suppress an abstinence syndrome is also evidence that it may itself induce serious dependence.

New drugs have sometimes been tested similarly in volunteer ex-addicts.

* In the U.K. sale of alcohol to anyone under 18 years is illegal and the vendor may lose his valuable licence to trade if he is convicted of breaking this law.
† Bass M. Sudden sniffing death. JAMA 1970; 212:2075.
‡ Lancet 1985; 2:1179.
§ Williams A. Br Med J 1984; 289:1402. Davis G C et al. Psychiatry Res 1979; 1:249.

Types of drug dependence: the World Health Organization recommends that drug dependence be specified by 'type' when under detailed discussion.

Morphine-type:
- emotional dependence severe
- physical dependence severe; develops quickly
- tolerance marked
- cross-tolerance with related drugs
- naloxone induces abstinence syndrome

Barbiturate-type:
- emotional dependence severe
- physical dependence very severe; develops slowly at high doses
- tolerance less marked than with morphine
- cross-tolerance with alcohol, chloral, paraldehyde, meprobamate, glutethimide, methyprylone, chlordiazepoxide, diazepam, etc.

Amphetamine-type:
- emotional dependence severe
- physical dependence slight: psychoses occur during use
- tolerance occurs

Cannabis-type:
- emotional dependence, some
- physical dependence dubious; no characteristic abstinence syndrome
- tolerance slight

Cocaine-type:
- emotional dependence severe
- physical dependence absent (or slight)
- tolerance absent

Alcohol-type:
- emotional dependence severe
- physical dependence with prolonged heavy use
- cross-tolerance with other sedatives

Tobacco-type:
- emotional dependence strong
- physical dependence slight

Drug mixtures:

Barbiturate–amphetamine mixtures induce a characteristic alteration of mood that does not occur with either drug alone
- emotional dependence strong
- physical dependence occurs
- tolerance occurs

Heroin-cocaine mixtures: similar characteristics

Prevention of drug dependence after medical use of drugs

Addicts who claim that their state is the result of misprescription of drugs by their medical attendants are sometimes not speaking the truth, but seeking to shift their feeling of guilt to other shoulders.

The risk of addicting a normal person to narcotic analgesics during therapeutic use is small if drugs are handled properly, but it exists in chronic recurrent painful conditions. It is wise to withhold drugs of addiction from such people as long as possible and then, if they must be used, to space the doses as widely as possible. It may also sometimes be wise to conceal the nature of the drug, especially if the patient is mentally abnormal or unstable.

In patients who have only a brief expectation of life the production of dependence is of little importance and need not generally be taken into consideration when planning therapy (see *terminal illness*).

TOBACCO

Tobacco was introduced to Europe from South America in the 16th century. For some time smoking* attracted a good deal of opprobrium and was forbidden by both Church and State, but this did not stop it and soon the State found that tobacco was a habit-forming drug of sufficient power to bear heavy taxation without causing habitués to abandon it, and yet of insufficient power to cause unacceptable disruption of the community. Both Church and State soon found that their objections were not, after all, so important. This applies to alcohol as well, and it has been pointed out that so excellently habit-forming are they in fact, from the Government's point of view, that these two drug dependencies can now be made to pay for two-thirds of the National Health Service in the UK, including

* 'A habit . . . dangerous to the lung.' King James I, 1604.

both its vast hospital services and general practitioner network. In the USA, the Federal Government spends in subsidies to tobacco farmers larger sums than it does on telling people not to smoke.

The composition of tobacco smoke is complex (about 500 compounds have been identified in it) and varies with the type of tobacco and the way it is smoked. The chief pharmacologically active ingredients are *nicotine* (acute effects) and *tars* (chronic effects).

Smoke of *cigars and pipes* is *alkaline* (pH 8.5) and nicotine is relatively un-ionized and lipid soluble so that it is readily absorbed in the mouth. Cigar and pipe smokers thus obtain nicotine without inhaling (they also have a lower death rate from lung cancer).

Smoke of *cigarettes* is *acidic* (pH 5.3) and nicotine is relatively ionized and insoluble in lipids. Desired amounts of nicotine are only absorbed if it is taken into the lungs, where the enormous surface area for absorption compensates for the relative lipid insolubility. Cigarette smokers therefore inhale (they have a high rate of death from lung cancer). The amount of nicotine absorbed from tobacco smoke varies from 90% in those who inhale to 10% in those who do not.

Tobacco smoke contains 1–5% *carbon monoxide* and habitual smokers have 3–7% (heavy smokers as much as 15%) of their haemoglobin as carboxyhaemoglobin, which cannot carry oxygen. This is sufficient to reduce exercise capacity in patients with angina pectoris. The plasma $t_{\frac{1}{2}}$ of caboxyhaemoglobin is about 4 h so that heavy smokers with angina pectoris who reduce their cigarette consumption by only a few cigarettes a day will not achieve any useful reduction in carboxyhaemoglobin. Chronic carboxyhaemoglobinaemia causes polycythaemia.

Substances (polycyclic hydrocarbons and N-nitroso compounds) carcinogenic to animals have been identified in tobacco smoke condensates from cigarettes, cigars and pipes. They may be responsible for the hepatic *enzyme induction* that occurs in smokers.

Tobacco dependence. The reasons people habitually smoke tobacco are certainly complex and 'it is no easy matter to reach a simple and reasonable conclusion concerning the mental health aspects of smoking. The purported benefits on mental health are so intangible and elusive, so intricately woven into the whole fabric of human behaviour, so subject to moral interpretation and censure, so difficult of medical evaluation and so controversial in nature that few scientific groups have attempted to study the subject'.*

A critic's prejudices will largely decide whether this 'pharmacologic aid in (man's) search for contentment'* is viewed as acceptance of a genial social and solitary pleasure or as a humiliating surrender to self-indulgent vice.

The following *notes* throw a little light on the subject here and there.

The *satisfaction* of smoking is due to nicotine, but also to tars, which provide flavour.

Whilst there is no substantial and clear-cut *personality* difference between smokers and non-smokers, cigarette smokers tend to be more extraverted, less rigid and more prone to antisocial tendencies than non-smokers. Pipe smokers are notably introverted.

Smoking is not specially associated with neuroticism or with increased liability to psychiatric illness.

Psychoanalysts have made a 'characteristic contribution to the problem. "Getting something orally", one asserts . . . "is the first great libidinous experience in life"; first the breast, then the bottle, then the comforter, then food and finally the cigarette'.† The common sight of a pipe-smoker with an empty or unlit pipe in his mouth or manually fondling it would seem to lend support to this. Some who give up smoking substitute other oral activities — nail-biting, gum chewing and eating.

Sigmund Freud was a life-long tobacco addict. He suggested that some children may be victims of a 'constitutional intensification of the erotogenic significance of the labial region', which, if it persists, will provide a powerful motive for smoking.‡

* US Dept. Health, Education and Welfare. *Smoking and Health*. 1964.

† Scott R B. Br Med J 1957; 1:671.

‡ Quoted in Roy. Coll. Phys. (1977). *Smoking or Health*. London: Pitman.

In 1929 Freud posed for a photograph holding a large cigar prominently. 'He was always a heavy smoker — twenty cigars a day were his usual allowance — and he tolerated abstinence from it with the greatest difficulty'. Jones E. *Sigmund Freud: life and work*. London: Hogarth Press. 1953.

Starting to smoke may be linked with 'self-esteem and status needs', but probably not to adolescent rebellion.*

There is no difference in intelligence between smoking and non-smoking children, but the former are less academically successful, as are university students who smoke. Criteria for determining whether an observed association is causal are discussed later in this chapter.

Progression of tobacco use*

In most cases, learning to smoke occurs in adolescence and the subject's smoking status is confirmed by age 20 years.

Initially the factors are entirely psychosocial, pharmacodynamic effects being unpleasant. But under psychosocial pressures the subject continues, learns to limit and adjust nicotine intake, and the pleasant pharmacological effects of nicotine develop, as does tolerance. Thus to the psychosocial pressure is now added pharmacological pleasure. Consumption rises and inhalation deepens. With developing maturity the psychosocial aspects diminish in importance and the desire and need for nicotine become dominant. If the nicotine intake becomes high, the drive for relief and avoidance of withdrawal symptoms produces the 'chain-smoker', whose objective is to maintain plasma nicotine ($t_{\frac{1}{2}}$ 2 h) concentration.

Thus, most people who began to smoke because they wanted to look 'tough' or 'grown up' or because most of their friends smoke, outgrow these immature drives and smoke because they are dependent on nicotine.

The extraordinary power of this 'pleasure-drug', nicotine, has been summed up,

'And a woman is only a woman, but a good cigar is a Smoke.'†

Emotional stress is associated with heavier smoking amongst smokers rather than with starting to smoke by non-smokers.

Social environment plays a large part in determining smoking, and the offering and accepting of tobacco, as of alcohol, is important in the development of personal relations in business and in private life.

When considering the significance of the association of smoking with mental states and personality characteristics it is particularly important to avoid assuming explanations for which there is really no evidence, e.g. the fact that when under emotional stress a person smokes more may be because stress is relieved by smoking — which is widely believed — or because smoking is merely an expression of stress.

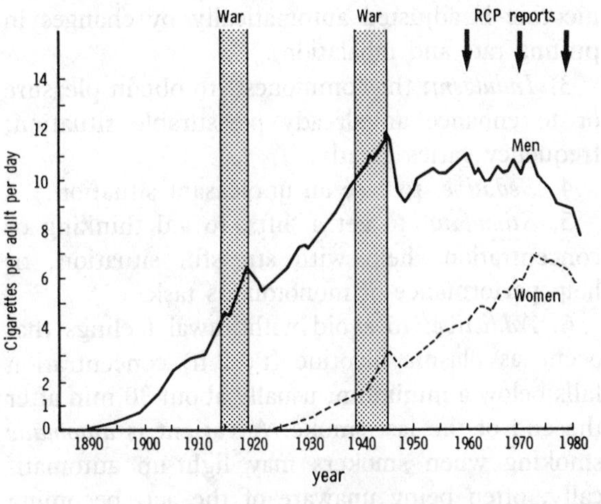

Fig. 20.1 Tobacco consumption in the UK 1890 to 1981, given as average number of cigarettes per adult per day for men and women separately, irrespective of whether they smoke or not. The arrows indicate the dates of the three previous Royal College of Physicians (ROP) reports. Data from Tobacco Research (now Advisory) Council. By permission, Royal College of Physicians, from *Health or Smoking*? London: Pitman, 1983.

Types of smoking‡

A. **Non-pharmacological**

1. *Psychosocial*: uses symbolic value of the act to increase social confidence, status and self-esteem.

2. *Sensorimotor*: to obtain oral, sensory and manipulatory satisfaction.

B. **Pharmacological** (plasma concentration of

* US Dept. Health, Education and Welfare. *Smoking and Health*. 1964.

† Rudyard Kipling (1865–1936).

‡ After Royal College of Physicians. *Smoking or Health*. London: Pitman 1977.

nicotine is adjusted automatically by changes in puffing rate and inhalation).

3. *Indulgent*: the commonest: to obtain pleasure or to enhance an already pleasurable situation; frequency varies greatly.

4. *Sedative*: to ease an unpleasant situation.

5. *Stimulant*: to get a 'lift', to aid thinking or concentration, help with stressful situation, or help performance of monotonous task.

6. *Addictive*: to avoid withdrawal feelings that occur as plasma nicotine ($t_{\frac{1}{2}}$, 2 h) concentration falls below a minimum, usually about 30 min after the end of the last smoke. A variant is *automatic* smoking when smokers may light-up automatically, often being unaware of the act, becoming aware only if a cigarette is not at hand.

Note:

a. obviously, non-pharmacological motivations may apply to all types under B.

b. degree of dependence advances from psychological in 1 and 2 to psychological and physical in 6.

Characteristics of dependence: psychological dependence is extremely strong and tolerance and some physical dependence occur. Transient withdrawal effects include EEG and sleep changes and impaired performance in some psychomotor tests and disturbance of mood, and increased appetite, though it is difficult to disentangle psychological from physical effects in these last, and cardiovascular and gastrointestinal changes.

Acute effects of smoking tobacco can be summarised:

Increased airways resistance occurs due to the non-specific effects of submicronic particles, e.g. carbon particles less than 1 μm across. The effect is reflex. Even inert particles of this size cause bronchial narrowing sufficient to double airways resistance. This is insufficient to cause dyspnoea, though it might affect athletic performance. Four to five-fold increase in resistance is necessary to cause noticeable dyspnoea and ten to twenty-fold increase to cause severe dyspnoea such as can occur in asthma.

Nicotine inhalations of concentration comparable to that reached in smoking do not increase airways resistance.

Ciliary activity, after transient stimulation, is depressed, and particles are removed from the lungs more slowly.

Carbon monoxide absorption is physiologically insignificant in healthy young adults, but may be significant in the presence of coronary heart disease (see above).

Nicotine: *pharmacokinetics*. Nicotine is absorbed through mucous membranes in a highly pH-dependent fashion (see above). The plasma $t_{\frac{1}{2}}$ is 2 h. It is largely metabolised to inert substances though some is excreted unchanged in the urine (pH dependent).

Pharmacodynamics. Nicotine can both stimulate and depress nervous tissue function, depending on the dose and the interval between doses, and the psychological state of the subject; it can relieve anxiety or boredom.

No definitive statement can be made relating the pharmacodynamics of nicotine to the pleasure experienced by the smoker. Smokers who become more alert tend to take a lower dose of nicotine than do smokers who become more tranquil. In doses used in smoking, nicotine causes release of catecholamines in the hypothalamus and antidiuretic hormone from the posterior pituitary.

In *large doses** nicotine stimulates directly the ends of peripheral cholinergic nerves whose cell bodies lie in the central nervous system, i.e. it acts at autonomic ganglia and at the neuromuscular junction. This is what is meant by the term 'nicotine-like' or 'nicotinic' effect. Higher doses paralyse at the same points. The central nervous system is stimulated, including the vomiting centre, both directly and via the carotid body; tremors and convulsions may occur. As with the peripheral actions, depression follows stimulation.

* Fatal nicotine poisoning has been reported from smoking, from swallowing tobacco, from tobacco enemas, from topical application to the skin and from accidental drinking of nicotine insecticide preparations. In 1932 a florist sat down on a chair, on the seat of which a 40% free nicotine insecticide solution had been spilled. Fifteen minutes later he felt ill (vomiting, sweating, faintness, and respiratory difficulty, followed by loss of consiousness and cardiac irregularity). He recovered in hospital over about 24 h. On the fourth day he was deemed well enough to leave hospital and was given his clothes which had been kept in a paper bag. He noticed the trousers were still damp. Within one hour of leaving hospital he had to be readmitted suffering once again from nicotine poisoning. He recovered over three weeks, but for persistent ventricular extrasystoles [Faulkner J M. JAMA 1933; 100:1663].

In *low doses* such as are taken in ordinary smoking, the effects of nicotine on viscera are probably largely reflex, from stimulation of sensory receptors (chemoreceptors) in the carotid and aortic bodies, pulmonary circulation and left ventricle. Some of the results are mutually antagonistic. The following account tells what generally happens after one cigarette, from which about 1 mg nicotine is absorbed, although much depends on the amount and depth of inhalation and on the duration of end-inspiratory breath holding.

On the cardiovascular system the effects are those of sympathetic stimulation. There is vasoconstriction in the skin and vasodilatation in the muscles, tachycardia and a rise in blood pressure of about 15 mm Hg systolic and 10 mm Hg diastolic, and increased noradrenaline in the blood. Ventricular extrasystoles may occur. Cardiac output, work and oxygen consumption increase. Coronary vascular resistance decreases and blood flow increases in men aged 20–50 years. However if the resistance is fixed by atherosclerosis, flow does not increase, though work and oxygen consumption do. This may be a mechanism of tobacco-induced angina pectoris. It is possible that nicotine stimulates the myocardium by releasing noradrenaline stored in it, but at present it seems likely that this effect only occurs with higher doses.

Nicotine increases fatty acid concentration in the blood, and also platelet stickiness, effects that may be clinically significant in atheroma and thrombosis.

On the gastrointestinal tract there are no important effects either on movement or secretion. Nausea and vomiting occur in the novice, probably due to stimulation of the vomiting centre.

Appetite increases when smokers stop. The mechanism is uncertain.

It is well known that *tolerance* develops to nicotine and that a first experience commonly causes nausea and vomiting, which quickly ceases with repetition of smoking.

Conclusion: the pleasurable effects of smoking are derived from a complex mixture of multiple pharmacological and non-pharmacological factors.

In this account *nicotine* is represented as being the major (but not the sole) determinant of tobacco dependence after the smoker has adapted to the usual initial unpleasant effects. But there remains some uncertainty as to its role, e.g. the failure of i.v. nicotine to fully substitute for smoking. Plainly it is important to analyse its exact place if less harmful alternatives to smoking, such as nicotine chewing gum, are to be exploited.

Effects of chronic tobacco smoking

The Royal College of Physicians of London feels it has a duty to pronounce 'on a question of public health when action is required'. In 1725 it offered advice 'concerning the disastrous consequences of the rising consumption of cheap gin', and in 1962, 1977 and 1983, on the effects of smoking on health.* Its published reports are models of clarity and brevity.

The US Public Health Service has also published extensive reports.

The evidence for an association of smoking with various diseases consists both of retrospective surveys, in which the smoking habits of those who were ill were compared with those of a chosen control group, and of prospective surveys (fewer, because more difficult to do), in which the habits of a population sample were recorded and they were then followed up and their fate determined. Retrospective studies are open to objection because of the risk of bias in selection of subjects and of controls to match them with, and it is therefore desirable that they should be supported by propective studies to obtain convincing evidence as to whether an association is really one of cause and effect.

Statistical methods cannot, of course, provide proof of causal relationship. The causal significance of an association is a matter of judgement which goes beyond any statement of statistical probability. *To decide whether an observed association is causal*, several criteria, no one of which alone is sufficient, must be satisfied. These include:

1. *Consistency* of association — diverse methods of approach should give the same answer.

* It is not intended to imply that the College was unconcerned about public health for over a century. This account relies heavily on these reports and on those of the US Public Health Service.

2. *Specificity* and *strength* of association — specificity means the precision with which the presence of, say, chronic bronchitis or lung cancer, can be used to predict that the victim smokes and vice versa — also the size of effect should be sufficient not to be obscured by any associated but non-causal factors, e.g. alcohol consumption, and a correlation of effect (disease) with dose (amount smoked) is also important.

3. *Temporal* association — the supposed cause *smoking*, must operate before any evidence of the disease appears.

4. *Coherence* of association — the associated event should fit in with all known facts of the natural history of the disease.

General

The importance of finding out just what smoking does or does not do is shown in this table:

Percentage of men aged 35 who may expect to die before the age of 65

Non-smokers	15%
Smokers of 1–14 cigarettes a day	22%
Smokers of 15–24 cigarettes a day	25%
Smokers of 25 or more cigarettes a day	40%

The average loss of life of a smoker of 25 cigarettes/day is about 5 years (UK and US studies).

The time by which a habitual smoker's life is shortened is about 5 min per cigarette smoked.

The extra risk of death (compared with that of life-long non-smokers) declines after a smoker ceases to smoke and returns to about that of non-smokers over 10–15 years.

The above applies to ordinary cigarettes (see *safer smoking* below).

Induction of hepatic drug metabolising enzymes occurs, probably from the polycyclic hydrocarbons (tar) in smoke.

An important prospective survey was that of Doll and his colleagues, who in 1951 sent a questionnaire on smoking habits to all British doctors. Their evaluation after 20 years* of the 34 440 men (69%† of the possible response) who replied to the original questionnaire revealed:

1. 10 072 deaths had occurred.
2. Death rate of cigarette smokers was × 2 that of life-long non-smokers.
3. Smoking caused death chiefly by:
   a. heart disease
   b. lung cancer
   c. chronic obstructive lung disease
   d. various vascular diseases

'The distinctive features of this study were the completeness of the follow-up, the accuracy of death certification, and the fact that the study population as a whole reduced its cigarette consumption substantially during the period of observation. As a result lung cancer grew relatively less common as the study progressed, but other cancers did not, thus illustrating in an unusual way the causal nature of the association between smoking and lung cancer'.

General practitioners smoke 37% more cigarettes than do hospital physicians and surgeons and have a commensurately higher death rate from smoking-related diseases‡.

We are grateful for permission to base the following account on *Smoking or Health* (Royal College of Physicians of London, 1977) and on *Health or Smoking*? (Royal College of Physicians of London, 1983).

Smoking and cancer

Lung cancer accounted for over 37 000 deaths in the UK in 1974, 14 500 of these occurring in people under the age of 65. In men under 65 the death-rate is now falling, but it is still rising in women (except the youngest age group). These facts are compatible with the inevitable 20–40 year lag before changed habits affect the incidence of disease. The risk of death from lung cancer is related to the number of cigarettes smoked and the age of starting, and is reduced by smoking

* Doll R et al. Br Med J 1976; 2:1525.

† Plainly any survey that fails to achieve almost 100% response is open to criticism that those who did not respond, in this case 31%, are a self-selected group that, had they responded, would have radically changed the conclusions drawn. This criticism would have substantial weight if it were not for the mass of confirmatory data from other investigations.

‡ Doll R et al. Br Med J 1977; 1:1433.

filter-tipped cigarettes. Giving up smoking reduces the risk of death relative to that of the non-smoker, and after 10 years the risk approximates to that of the life-long non-smoker. Direct evidence for this comes from the long-term prospective study of British male doctors. Most of the smokers among them have given up smoking and deaths from lung cancer have dramatically declined,* whilst other men have been slower to give up smoking and deaths from lung cancer only began to decline later.

Pipe and cigar smokers suffer much smaller risks than cigarette smokers, probably because they inhale less.

Lung cancer is also increased by exposure to certain chemicals used in industry.

It has been suggested that the close relation of smoking to lung cancer is not causative but due to the coexistence in individuals of susceptibility to lung cancer and to the desire to smoke, and that these two factors are inherited together. This 'genetic hypothesis' is rejected on the basis of the changing pattern of incidence of lung cancer in the two sexes during the last 70 years, the decline of lung cancer among doctors in the UK associated with their giving up smoking, and because the other known causes of lung cancer cannot thus be accounted for. There may nevertheless be a genetic factor that determines which smokers are most likely to develop lung cancer.†

If the whole population were to follow the example of professional men in cutting down smoking, and cigarettes were made less harmful (lower tar content), deaths from lung cancer could fall by 80% within 20 years, for this is a largely preventable disease.

Other cancers. The risk of smokers developing cancer of the mouth and throat is 5–10 times greater than that of non-smokers. It is as great for pipe and cigar smokers as it is for cigarette smokers. Cancer of the pancreas, kidney and urinary tract are also commoner in smokers.

Mechanism. Smoking can cause changes in DNA, and it seems likely that such an effect is causally relevant.

Smoking and diseases of the heart and blood vessels

Coronary heart disease (CHD) is now the leading cause of death in many developed countries. In the UK about 30% of these deaths could be attributed to smoking. **Under the age of 65, smokers are about twice as likely to die of CHD as are non-smokers, and heavy smokers about $3\frac{1}{2}$ times as likely**. The mortality of women from CHD and their consumption of cigarettes are both rising. Sudden death may be the first manifestation of CHD and, especially in young men, is related to cigarette smoking. Smoking may induce chest pain on exertion (angina) from CHD and reduce ability to take vigorous exercise.

Among the conditions that contribute to CHD the most important are increased cholesterol in the blood, high blood pressure, and cigarette smoking. If more than one factor is present the risk is correspondingly increased. Thus smoking is especially dangerous for people in whom these other risk factors are present, and they should be firmly warned not to smoke.

Atherosclerotic narrowing of the *smallest* coronary arteries is enormously increased in heavy and even in moderate smokers; the increased platelet adherence caused by smoking increases the readiness with which thrombi form. The carboxyhaemoglobinaemia of habitual smokers

* Between 1954 and 1971, the proportion of male doctors smoking cigarettes halved (43% to 21%), while that for all men in England and Wales remained about the same. Over this period the death rate in men from lung cancer fell by 25% in doctors while in the general population it increased by 26%.

† A curious by-way is a study of lung cancer in Seventh Day Adventists, in the USA. It appears that members of this religious sect, which prohibits smoking, have an incidence of lung-cancer one-eighth of that of non-members. Indeed the only two men with lung cancer were converts who had smoked cigarettes until middle-age. In respect of cancer of sites not associated with smoking there was no difference from the control group, so that Seventh Day Adventists evidently have no general immunity from cancer. Therefore, to accommodate this evidence to the hypothesis of a genetic cause of both smoking and lung cancer, it would be necessary to stipulate that those born into the sect, but not those converted to it, inherit a low susceptibility to lung cancer (Wynder E L et al. Cancer 1959; 12:1016).

'To many it will come as no surprise to learn that the benefits of religious observances are by no means restricted to the future life. But not often before can the evidence have been put on such a sure statistical basis.' (Editorial Br Med J 1959; 2:1465.

(see above) is enough to cause polycythaemia, which increases blood viscosity.

Stopping smoking reduces the excess risk of CHD in people under the age of 65, and after about 10 years of abstinence the risk approximates to that of non-smokers.* Smokers who stop after a heart attack are less likely to have further attacks than those who go on smoking. **The investigation of British doctors already referred to has shown that in comparison with a rising rate of deaths from CHD in men under 65 there has been a steady fall in doctors of the same ages as a result of their having given up smoking.***

Pipe and cigar smokers run little or no excess risk of CHD provided they are not heavy smokers and do not inhale. Heavy cigarette smokers who change over to pipe or cigar smoking often continue to inhale and thereby fail to reduce their risk.

Disease of the arteries of the leg is even more closely related to smoking, over 95% of patients with this condition, which causes pain on walking, being smokers. In many gangrene sets in and amputation is required. Death from aneurysm of the aorta is about five times commoner in smokers: there is also an association, though less marked, between smoking and strokes.*

Chronic lung disease

The adverse effects of cigarette smoke on the lungs may be separated into two quite distinct conditions.

1. *Chronic mucus hypersecretion*, which causes persistent cough with phlegm and fits with the original definition of simple *chronic bronchitis*. This condition arises chiefly in the large airways, usually clears up when the subject stops smoking and does not on its own carry any substantial risk of death.

2. *Chronic obstructive lung disease*, which causes difficulty in breathing due to narrowing of the air passages in the lungs. This condition originates chiefly in the small airways, includes a variable element of destruction of peripheral lung units (emphysema), is progressive and largely irreversible and may ultimately lead to disability and death.

Although both conditions may be produced by smoking and can co-exist in a given individual, they are distinct, not least in that the obstructive condition is responsible for much disability and death, whereas the mucus hypersecretion does not of itself influence life expectancy. Patients with either condition do, however, share a strong tendency to suffer from acute infective illnesses for which the term 'bronchitis', implying as it does infection in the bronchial tree, is frequently used and not inappropriate. These infective illnesses are substantial causes of discomfort and of absence from work through sickness. Airways obstruction is often more severe during an infective episode but recovery is usual, and these episodes do not seem to accelerate the progression of chronic obstructive lung disease.

The obstructive syndrome is as specifically related to smoking as is lung cancer, and in one prospective survey of the effects of smoking on mortality (that among British doctors) the relative risk for chronic obstructive lung disease was even more extreme than that for lung cancer. Despite this, in discussing the health effects of tobacco, there has generally been far more emphasis on lung cancer than on this more disabling, but equally fatal disorder.

The onset of the disease, the mechanism of which is unknown, is perhaps best characterised

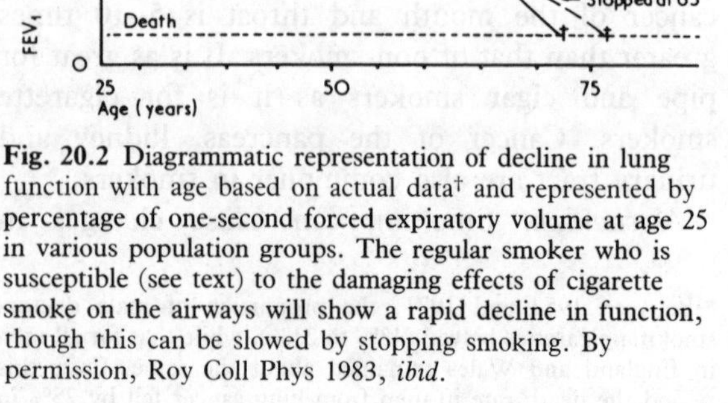

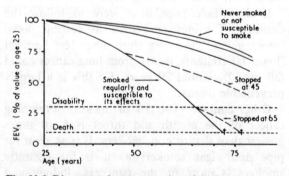

Fig. 20.2 Diagrammatic representation of decline in lung function with age based on actual data† and represented by percentage of one-second forced expiratory volume at age 25 in various population groups. The regular smoker who is susceptible (see text) to the damaging effects of cigarette smoke on the airways will show a rapid decline in function, though this can be slowed by stopping smoking. By permission, Roy Coll Phys 1983, *ibid.*

* Hypertensives who smoke are more liable to develop accelerated (malignant) phase which runs a rapid course.

† Fletcher C M et al. Br Med J 1977; 1:1645.

by patterns of change in the lung function test known as the one-second forced expiratory volume (FEV_1). These are outlined in Figure 20.2, where for simplicity FEV_1 is expressed as a percentage of what it would have been at age 25. FEV_1 loss is typically a slow process, spread out over several decades, rather than a sudden change from normality to disease. Moreover, it tends to be largely irreversible and once FEV_1 falls to about one litre the subject is usually disabled. Among non-smokers the normal range of rates of loss of FEV_1 is narrow and almost all non-smokers reach the age at which they die from another cause long before becoming disabled by obstructed airways. Among smokers, however, the range of rates of loss of FEV_1 is much wider. For reasons that are still obscure, some smokers do not suffer a particularly rapid rate of loss of FEV_1 as a result of their smoking. By contrast, some 'susceptible' smokers suffer such unusually rapid rates of loss of FEV_1 that if they continue to smoke they will be first disabled and then killed by their obstructive lung disease. Among these 'susceptible' smokers the effects of stopping smoking are of critical importance. If such people stop smoking their FEV_1 will not recover, but their subsequent rate of loss of FEV_1 will usually revert to about that seen in non-smokers (Figure 20.2). Thus *if susceptible smokers stop well before they are disabled, they will not die from chronic obstructive lung disease, but if they do not stop until they are disabled, then they are likely to die from it within a few years.* Indeed, because progressive respiratory disability may cause people to stop smoking, deaths from this disease tend to occur not in continuing smokers but among people whose disease has led them to stop smoking a few years previously.

As with all the main tobacco-related diseases, however, the chief problem is no longer whether tobacco causes the disease or not, but rather what can be done to avoid these effects of tobacco. The best way is to cease smoking, and the next to reduce the amount smoked.

Other conditions: Gastric or duodenal ulcers are twice as common and twice as likely to cause death in smokers as in non-smokers, probably because smoking delays healing of the ulcers and increases the relapse rate. Diseases of the teeth and gums are also commoner in smokers.

Non-smokers are on average slightly heavier than smokers, and gain in weight may be a problem to some after giving up; but this disadvantage is outweighed by the overall benefits of stopping.

Cigarette smoke depresses immunity in animals and in man, and this may contribute to their increased liability to infection.

Other conditions commoner in smokers than in others include pulmonary tuberculosis, a rare form of blindness, certain skin rashes, and chest complications after surgical operations.

General physical fitness is diminished by smoking, which impairs the function of the heart, lungs, and blood.

Benefits of smoking

There are a few illnesses that smokers are less liable to develop than are non-smokers; among these are toxaemia of pregnancy, pulmonary embolus after operation, Parkinson's disease and possibly ulcerative colitis. The questions whether these associations are causal or casual remain controversial. Smoking appears to increase the metabolism of oestrogens by enzyme induction, so that incidence of oestrogen-induced endometrial cancer falls slightly and severity of post-menopausal osteoporosis is increased. It must be emphasised, however, that in all cases the risks of regular cigarette smoking are vastly greater than are these minor benefits.

The psychological benefits (relief from stress and boredom) have not been quantified and for most people, no doubt, they may be attained in other less harmful ways.

Women and smoking

Few women smoked before World War II. After that time the habit became increasingly popular, so that by 1956 some 42% of women aged 16 and over were smokers. Until the mid-1970s the figure remained relatively constant — fluctuating between 40% and 45%. There is, however, a recent indication of a definite decline in the proportion of women smoking. Anecdotally, women, like men, in managerial posts are often heavy smokers. More reliable information comes from the health care professions. Whilst smoking is on the decline among doctors this has not been so evident among nurses. They have one of the highest smoking rates in the professional classes, at just under 50%. An additional factor may be stress. Nurses in psychiatric units and certain intensive care units where stress can be considerable have higher smoking rates than nurses in less stressful posts such as community care.

Support for the concept that smoking may be used by women (as well as men) as a means of coping with the stresses of life, comes also from the observations that women who smoke both drink more and take more mood-changing drugs than non-smoking women. A formal attempt to evaluate this was made by rating a smoker's desire to smoke in situations ranging from stressful to boring. Women showed a greater desire to smoke in circumstances of emotional strain or anxiety, whilst men, though more likely than women to smoke under all circumstances, showed the greatest need for cigarettes in circumstances producing boredom or fatigue.

Fertility. Women who smoke are more likely to be infertile or take longer to conceive than women who do not smoke. In addition, smokers are more liable to have an earlier menopause than are non-smokers. These observations point to smoking adversely affecting ovarian function, though how it does this remains unclear.

Complications of pregnancy. Smokers who become pregnant have a small increase in the risk of spontaneous abortion, bleeding during pregnancy and the development of various placental abnormalities. In New Zealand, Ireland and the US there is something like a twofold increased risk of spontaneous abortion in women smoking 20 or more cigarettes a day, and this is quite independent of socio-economic, marital or other factors. On the other hand, women who smoke have a lowered incidence of toxaemia of pregnancy though the advantages of this do not offset the disadvantages of smoking during pregnancy. The placenta is heavier in smoking than non-smoking women and its diameter larger. The enlarged placenta and placental abnormalities may represent adaptations to lack of oxygen due to smoking, secondary to raised concentrations of circulating carboxyhaemoglobin.

The unborn child. The offspring of women who smoke are approximately 200 g lighter than the offspring of women who do not smoke. The mechanism of the retardation of intrauterine growth is probably due to a direct effect of some constituent of tobacco smoke, such as carbon monoxide, rather than to an indirect effect such as nutritional deficiency in smoking women.

The offspring of smoking women also have a small increased risk of death in the period around birth.

This risk of smoking is independent of other variables such as social class, level of education, age of mother, race or extent of antenatal care. The increased risk rises to twofold or more in heavy smokers and appears to be entirely accounted for by the increased incidence of placental abnormalities and the consequences of low birthweight.

Suggestions that the risk of congenital abnormalities are increased have not, in general, been confirmed, nor have reports that the offspring of women smokers are less physically or mentally active at the time of birth. However, there is considerable evidence that the children of mothers who smoke have certain disadvantages even up to the age 11 years. It is not clear whether these are due to the long-term effects of the mother smoking during pregnancy or are the consequence of the mother or parents continuing to smoke as the child grows up.

Ex-smokers and women who give up smoking in the first 20 weeks of pregnancy have offspring whose birthweight is similar to that of the children of women who have never smoked.

The *placentas* of smokers show more abnormal DNA than those of non-smokers.

Contraception. Women who smoke tend to favour the Pill as a method of contraception and they too bear the brunt of its ill-effects. The risk of myocardial infarction, stroke and other cardiovascular diseases in young women is increased approximately three- to four-hold by either oral contraceptive use or by smoking. But when the two are combined the risks multiply together leading to an approximately tenfold increase in risk overall. This effect is more marked in those over 45 years of age and somewhat less in those under 35 years.

Starting and stopping

Some children begin to smoke at 5 years of age, and it has been found that about one-third of adult regular smokers began before they were 9. About 80% of children who smoke regularly continue to do so when they grow up. The earlier in life a person starts to smoke regularly, the greater is the risk of early death.

Children of social classes 4 and 5* are more likely to smoke than those from the other social classes. If parents smoke, their children are liable to follow their example. Short courses of teaching about the effects of smoking have been of little use, but longer term, well-designed teaching methods can be helpful. Smoking has been found to be less common among boys at schools where the head-master is a non-smoker: anyone who reaches the age of 20 without smoking is unlikely to begin. The main reasons for starting are social pressure from friends who smoke and what has been called 'anticipation of adulthood'; the main deterrents are parental disapproval and the danger of lung cancer.

Contrary to what is widely believed it is not generally difficult to stop, only 14% finding it 'very difficult'. But ex-smoker status is unstable and the success rate of a smoking withdrawal clinic is rarely above 30%. The situation is summed up by the witticism, 'Giving up smoking is easy, I've done it many times'. That persons in social classes 1 and 2*, and especially doctors, are most likely to stop suggests the importance of intelligent recognition of the health risks.

Though they are as aware of the risks of smoking as men, *women* find it harder to stop. They make attempts to stop as often as men and try as many different methods — but they consistently have lower success rates. This trend crosses every age group and occupation. Even when initial success rates are encouraging, women find it twice as difficult as men to remain committed non-smokers. Women left in the home whilst their husbands are out at work and children at school seem to find giving up cigarettes especially difficult. The reasons for these depressing observations are not known. Women express concern about weight gain after stopping smoking†, feel they have greater stresses to combat, or need to keep their emotions in check with smoking.

There are *special aids*: group therapy, snuff, graded cigarette holders, hypnosis, acupuncture and nicotine chewing gum. None of them has a very high success rate and, apart from nicotine gum, no one emerges as strikingly more effective than any other. Nicotine chewing gum, when used casually without special attention to technique, has proved no better than other aids, but if used carefully as recommended it has been found to achieve higher success rates. All of these aids are capable of helping some smokers, but none is a substitute for the will and resolve of the individual to give up.

If the patient is heavily tobacco-dependent and anxiety and tension are concomitants of attempts to stop smoking, then a sedative or tranquilliser may be useful for a short time, but it is important to avoid substituting one drug-dependence for another.

Various astringents are used in the mouth to make the smoke taste bad.

In short, drugs have little place, and 'the weaponry which may help the patient to hurdle his

* *Social Classes in the UK* (Registrar General's classification).
1. *Professional*, etc. occupations, including doctors, lawyers, chemists.
2. *Intermediate* occupations, including managers, Members of Parliament, administrators, teachers.
3. *Skilled* occupations, manual and non-manual, including foremen, cooks, typists, shop assistants.
4. *Partly skilled* occupations, including bus conductors, telephone operators.
5. *Unskilled* occupations, including office cleaners, labourers.
(The classification gives most weight to occupational skill and time spent in formal education.)

† This is a real phenomenon. Smoking 24 cigarettes a day increases overall energy expenditure by 10% (there is concomitant 20% increase in mean heart rate and 45% increase in urinary noradrenaline; effects attributable to nicotine). Subjects who stop smoking (24 cigs/day) may expect a weight gain of up to 10 kg if their calorie intake is unchanged (Hofstetter A et al. N Engl J Med 1986; 314:79).

habit'* is divided between 'appeals to sense and the psyche' and so is beyond the scope of this book.

Tobacco-dependence is more an emotional than a physical dependence. Patients are prone to solace themselves with food on abandoning the habit, and to gain weight in consequence. If an appetite suppressant is used, the patient may become dependent on it.

Whether a patient should give up smoking depends on numerous factors, including the amount of evidence that smoking causes or aggravates disease in people in general and in the patient in particular, and the patient's attitude to his habit. Some people are so miserable without tobacco that the risk of disease is the lesser evil. To smoke, or not to smoke, is not primarily a problem of pharmacology, and this also applies to alcohol. There is ample evidence to warrant strong advice against starting to smoke, but doctors are not consulted on this by individuals. The problem with, say, the chronic bronchitic dependent on tobacco is different. Persuasion will be adapted to his personality but over-hasty and unreasonable prohibitions of patients' pleasures or vices do no good. The pliable patient is made wretched, but most are merely alienated, as was D G Rossetti (1828–82), who wrote,

My doctor's issued his decree
That too much wine is killing me,
And furthermore his ban he hurls
Against my touching naked girls.
How then? Must I no longer share
Good wine or beauties, dark and fair?
Doctor, goodbye, my sail's unfurled,
I'm off to try the other world.

Safer smoking

Despite all that has been done by education and propaganda, people continue to smoke cigarettes. In setting out to examine the claims for less dangerous forms of smoking, we wish to underline from the outset that the top priority is to persuade smokers to give up smoking. Smoking cessation is indeed possible for very large numbers of people. There are at least eight million ex-smokers in the UK and 33 million in the USA. Yet some smokers cannot give up and others will not. Thus, though falling short of the ideal of a smoking-free society, it is worth-while considering ways in which the smokers can have the tobacco he craves in a less dangerous form.

Smoking pipes or cigars might be one way of achieving this end. The total death rates among men who have smoked only pipes are not significantly greater than those of non-smoker, and cigar smokers have only a modest increase in risk of premature death. The most likely explanation of this relative immunity is that nicotine is absorbed from the alkaline smoke in the mouth so that smokers of pipes need not inhale. But a switch from cigarettes to pipes would benefit only some smokers, for once smokers have experienced the special pattern of nicotine absorption that comes from inhaling cigarette smoke, they usually continue to inhale after switching to pipes or cigars, and consequently would probably derive little benefit from the change. It would not be easy, nor would it indeed be desirable in any way to persuade children who take up smoking to adopt a form of smoking different from that of adults.

To substitute a smokeless way of taking tobacco, e.g. **dry snuff**† for smoking cigarettes would be another possible solution for a few individuals, since snuff takers absorb nicotine from their noses in a pattern not very different from that of cigarette smokers from their lungs. Unfortunately, although there are said to be 500 000 snuff takers in Britain, no survey has yet been made of any diseases to which they may be liable. Since there are carcinogens in snuff there might be an excess of nasal cancer. It is certainly recognised that those who **chew tobacco** or hold **wet snuff** (in a porous sachet) in their mouths (snuff dipping) have an increased risk of cancer of the mouth. From a practical viewpoint, however, even if the adverse effects were only slight, it is hard to believe that a massive switch

* Sprague H B. Monthly scientific publication of the American Heart Association, Inc., October 1964.

† **Snuff** is powdered tobacco mixed with other substances. Prolonged use causes atrophy of the nasal mucous membrane with replacement of ciliated columnar by squamous epithelium. Some kinds used in Africa may be locally carcinogenic.

from cigarette smoking to snuff taking could be brought about, or that it would be acceptable to smokers.

Since the role of cigarette tars in the causation of cancer of the lung has for long been much clearer than the role of any component of cigarette smoke in causing cardiovascular or respiratory diseases, attention has been concentrated on developing lower tar cigarettes. This has been done by using different varieties of tobacco, by curing it in different ways, by the use of filters, and by increasing the porosity of the paper so that the smoke is diluted by air taken in as the smoker draws on his cigarette. Loss of flavour of the smoke can be compensated for by adding flavouring to the cigarettes (though there is no means of predicting whether or not this too might be hazardous to health). How far the total risk of premature death has been reduced by the smoking of lower tar/nicotine cigarettes is uncertain. A worthwhile reduction in the young smoker's risk of lung cancer has already occurred, which suggests that reductions will eventually appear throughout middle and old age. There is also an encouraging reduction in deaths from chronic obstructive lung disease which may, at least in part, be due to lower yields of tar and nicotine*. However, there is no evidence that deaths from coronary heart disease, the major killer among smoking-related diseases, have been affected, and no evidence has been produced relating to risks to the children of smoking mothers.

It is debatable how much further this approach can proceed. In view of the potential for tar as well as nicotine to cause cigarette dependence, any further lowering of tar delivery may simply lead to a compensatory increase in the amount smoked.

Passive smoking

Many non-smokers are exposed to tobacco smoke. At home, at work, on public transport and in public places, they can scarcely avoid breathing air contaminated by other people's smoke. This mode of smoke inhalation is not actively sought: it may therefore be called *involuntary or passive smoking.*

Passive smoke exposure has achieved prominence not only as a source of annoyance, but because of fears concerning possible health hazards. It is difficult to measure the extent of the risk to health from passive smoke exposure. Consequently, there is as yet no sure way of relating these anxieties to actual disease.

Mainstream and sidestream smoke. Smoke drawn through the tobacco and taken in by the smoker is known as mainstream smoke. Smoke which arises from smouldering tobacco and passes directly into the surrounding air, whence it may be inhaled by smokers and non-smokers alike, is known as sidestream smoke. Mainstream and sidestream smoke differ in composition, partly because of the different temperatures at which they are produced. Some substances are found in greater concentrations in undiluted side-stream smoke than in undiluted mainstream smoke, including nicotine (×2.7), carbon monoxide (×2.5), ammonia (×73), and some carcinogens (e.g. benzo-a-pyrene ×3.4). However, whereas the smoker is exposed to undiluted mainstream smoke, the sidestream smoke, to which the passive smoker is exposed, is diluted by room air to a variable extent depending on distance from the smoking source and the amount of ventilation. The room air itself contains smoke that has been inhaled and then exhaled into the air. The composition of this smoke depends on whether or not the smoker takes it into his lungs, where some constituents will be retained and others exhaled again. The concentrations of the various components of tobacco smoke breathed by the non-smoker from a smoky atmosphere are therefore extremely variable and largely unpredictable.

Smoked in a standard way, the average 1982 cigarette in the UK yields about 16–17 mg of *carbon monoxide* in the mainstream and about 40 mg in the sidestream smoke. Cigars, both regular and small, produce more carbon monoxide than cigarettes. It is a gas that mixes readily with ambient air.

The concentration of carbon monoxide produced by smoking has been measured under experimental conditions in rooms of various size and in

* Evidence from Finland suggests that low-tar cigarettes are not safer than medium-tar cigarettes. Rimpla A H et al. Br Med J 1985; 290:1461.

everyday social conditions. Smoke-free air contains about 2.0 parts per million (ppm) of carbon monoxide. Examples of concentrations found in smoky conditions include, 7–9 ppm at parties, 8–33 ppm in a conference room, 40 ppm in a submarine, 15–60 ppm in a room, and 12–110 ppm in a car. The concentrations reached depend very much on the degree of ventilation. Under ordinary social conditions with good ventilation, levels are usually below 10 ppm when smokers are present and below 3 ppm when they are not.

Unlike carbon monoxide, some of the *nicotine* derived from cigarette smoke will settle out of the air in a room. Nicotine concentrations in the blood and urine of people exposed experimentally to smoky atmospheres and in submarines are increased, but are much lower than those found in smokers. About half of the non-smokers living in cities have nicotine in their blood, and most have nicotine in their urine. The health consequences of this are unknown.

Not enough is known about *lung disease* in adult passive smokers to allow any definitive statements. But smoking by parents directly affects the health of their children. Children whose parents smoke have more respiratory symptoms and are more prone to respiratory infections than the children of non-smokers. The association is particularly marked in the first year of life, when bronchitis and pneumonia are more than twice as common in infants whose parents smoke than when this is not so. There is a clear link between the number of cigarettes smoked by parents and the frequency of such illnesses, which cannot be explained in terms of perinatal illness, breast feeding or poor housing or social conditions. Maternal smoking habits are more important than paternal, and the effect is lost by three years of age, indicating that close contact is required. Children who suffer such infections have clear evidence of impaired lung function by five years of age and children of smoking parents are, on average, shorter than other children at primary school age by up to 1 cm, after adjusting for other factors.

Disadvantages may persist even longer: at the age of 11, intellectual performance as revealed by reading comprehension and mathematical ability is behind that of children of non-smoking mothers by a span of 6 to 7 months. It is not clear whether this is solely a consequence of parental smoking as the child grows up, or whether it could be a delayed effect of maternal smoking during pregnancy.

*Medical students and smoking**

Although medical students smoke less now than they did 10 years ago, male students smoke about the same as the general public of the same age and social classes (1 and 2), i.e. the decline in smoking is related to social class and not to specialised knowledge or to any feeling of obligation to set an example to others in this serious health issue. But, amongst women medical students, the smoking rate is only 50% that of the female general public of the same age and social classes. No doubt the obvious interpretation of this difference is the correct one.

Hospital nurses are the sole health professional group in which smoking prevalence is not very much lower than in the general population.

Tobacco amblyopia is rare. It may be due to nicotine induced retinal vasoconstriction. There is a characteristic centrocecal scotoma, particularly to red and blue. Nutritional deficiency may promote it and it is commonest in pipe and cigar smokers. Slow recovery is usual provided tobacco is abandoned. Hydroxocobalamin to bind any cyanide absorbed from smoke, plus a vasodilator, may help. But its relation to smoking remains uncertain.

The demonstrable and suspected deleterious effects of heavy tobacco smoking are quite enough without there being any necessity for those who disapprove of the habit on moral grounds to invent others, as has been done in the past. 'An old dresser of mine at the hospital, of the name of Bain, who was an amiable attentive pupil, but never very efficient, smoked, I have since heard, a good deal when at the hospital, but after he left he was smoking nearly all day long. His debility was now so great that he was obliged to have a glass of bitter beer in the morning before he could

* Lester E. Br Med J 1977; 2:1630, and subsequent correspondence 1978; 1:175.

rise. He was not addicted to drinking . . . The whole of his ailments were produced by tobacco-smoke'.*

ETHYL ALCOHOL (ETHANOL)

> 'The services rendered by intoxicating substances in the struggle for happiness and in warding off misery rank so highly as a benefit that both individuals and races have given them an established position within their libido-economy. It is not merely the immediate gain in pleasure which one owes to them, but also a measure of that independence of the outer world which is so sorely craved . . . We are aware that it is just this property which constitutes the danger and injuriousness of intoxicating substances . . .'†

Although the importance of alcohol in therapeutics is small, its social significance is so big that a fuller account of its pharmacology is warranted than would otherwise be appropriate.

The history of alcohol is part of the history of civilisation 'ever since Noah made his epoch-making discovery'.‡ Perhaps its main use in therapeutics has been with opium as an analgesic and surgical anaesthetic before the introduction of ether.

Alcohol acts on the central nervous system in the manner of the inhalation anaesthetics.

Pharmacokinetics: *absorption* of alcohol taken orally is rapid, for it is highly lipid soluble and diffusible, some from the stomach, but most from the small intestine. With moderate amounts, the highest blood concentration, as might be expected, is reached with stronger solutions.

However, solutions above 20% are absorbed more slowly because high concentrations of alcohol inhibit gastric peristalsis and cause pylorospasm, thus delaying the arrival of the alcohol in the small intestine. Large doses taken in very dilute solution are absorbed relatively slowly because of the large amount of water.

Absorption is delayed by food, especially milk, the effect of which is probably due to the fat it contains. But this is not simply an effect of any fat, for suet and olive oil are less effective. Carbohydrate also delays absorption of alcohol and so alcohol in beer is absorbed more slowly than a simple solution. Habitual drinkers may absorb alcohol more rapidly than others. They excrete it at normal rates, but metabolism is faster due to *enzyme induction*, though it can also *inhibit* metabolism of other drugs (see below).

After absorption, alcohol is rapidly *distributed* throughout the body water (distribution 0.7 l/kg men: 0.6 l/kg women) and is not selectively stored in any tissue. It enters fat relatively slowly and *women* have higher blood concentrations when taking the same dose per kg as men, because they have a higher proportion of fat to lean body mass. If food is taken simultaneously alcohol disappears from the blood more rapidly than otherwise; it is not known how this happens.

Maximum *blood concentrations* after oral alcohol therefore depend on numerous factors including the total dose, the strength of the solution, the time over which it is taken, the presence or absence of food, the time relations of taking food and alcohol and the kind of food eaten, as well as on the speed of metabolism and excretion. A single dose of alcohol, say 60 ml (48 g; equivalent to 145 ml whisky, five to six 'whiskies', or *units*, see Figure 20.3) taken over a few minutes on an empty stomach will probably produce maximal blood concentration at from 1 to $1\frac{1}{2}$ h and will not all be disposed of for 6–8 h or even more. There are very great individual variations. About 90% of absorbed alcohol is *metabolised*, the remainder being excreted in the breath, the urine and the sweat; convenient methods of estimation of alcohol in all these are available.

Alcohol follows first-order kinetics only after the smallest doses. Once the blood concentration exceeds about 10 mg/100 ml the enzymic elimination processes are saturated and elimination rate no longer increases with increasing concentration but becomes steady at 10–15 ml per hour in occasional drinkers. Thus as the blood concentration rises the $t_{\frac{1}{2}}$ gets longer, with potentially major consequences for the individual. Thus alcohol is subject to *dose-dependent kinetics*, *saturation kinetics* or *zero-order kinetics*. For further details of pharmacokinetics see p. 108.

* Solly S. Lancet 1857; 1:176.

† Freud S. *Civilisation, war and death, Psycho-analytic epitomes, No.* 4. Hogarth Press, 1939,

‡ *Genesis*; 9:21; Huxley A. Ann N Y Acad Sci 1957; 67:675.

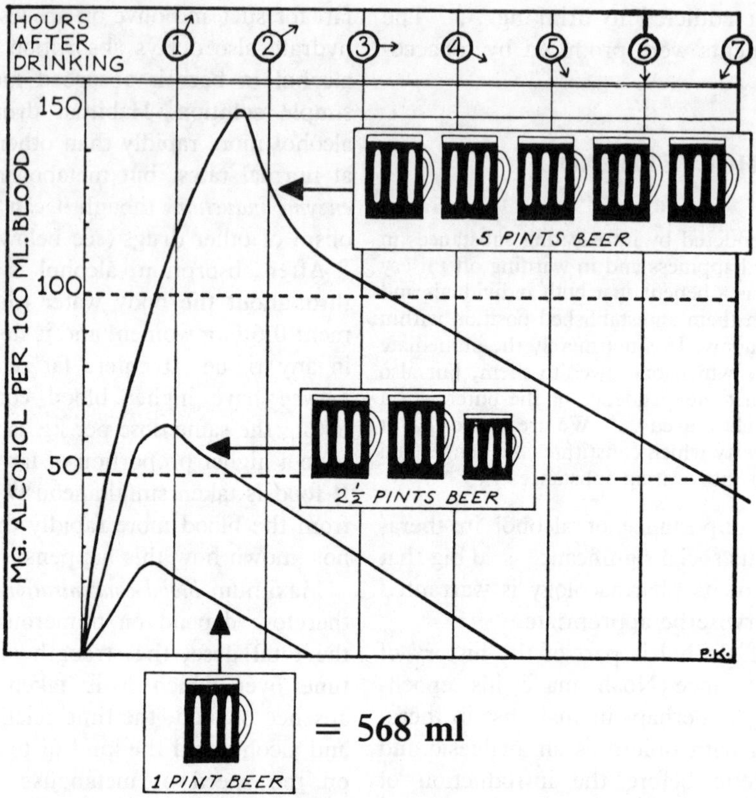

Approximate blood concentrations after three doses of alcohol.

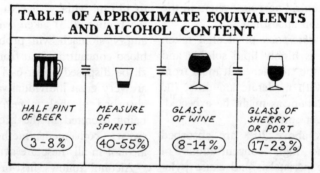

Fig. 20.3 Four standard **UNITS** of drink (in which social consumption is measured): a *unit* contains approx. 10 ml (8 g) of alcohol.
(Knowledge of blood alcohol level does not allow a reliable estimate of how much has been consumed.)

In tolerant individuals metabolism is faster due to hepatic enzyme induction, but this is not the sole explanation of tolerance, which is also a tissue tolerance.

Alcohol is *metabolised* (oxidised) by enzyme systems in the liver, first, by the enzyme alcohol dehydrogenease, into acetaldehyde and then to acetate, which is metabolised to carbon dioxide and water. Some chemicals, for instance disulfiram (Antabuse), block the conversion of acetaldehyde to acetate so that the acetaldehyde accumulates and makes the subject feel ill. Metabolites are responsible for organ damage in chronic overconsumption; acetaldehyde in the liver and probably fatty ethyl esters in other organs.

Blood concentration of alcohol has great medicolegal importance. *Alcohol in alveolar air* is in equilibrium with that in pulmonary capillary blood and reliable, easily handled devices have been developed to measure it, for this avoids 'assaulting' the subject with a needle and can be used by police at the roadside.

Actions. The most important actions of alcohol are on the central nervous system, which it depresses like other anaesthetic agents. It is not a stimulant; hyperactivity, when it occurs, is due to removal of inhibitory effects. The concept of higher levels of the central nervous system dominating lower levels is naive, and it is now known that there is a complex interdependence of the various parts, so that changes at one 'level' affect function at other 'levels', 'higher' or 'lower'. Alcohol, in ordinary doses, may act chiefly on the arousal mechanisms of the brain stem reticular formation. Direct cortical depression probably only occurrs with high doses.

With increasing doses the subject passes through all the stages of general anaesthesia and may die of respiratory depression.* Psychic effects are the most important socially, and it is to obtain these that the drug is habitually used in so many societies, to make social intercourse not merely easy but even pleasant. They have been admirably described by Sollmann; 'The first functions to be lost are the finer grades of judgement, reflection, observation and attention — the faculties largely acquired through education, which constitute the elements of the restraint and prudence that man usually imposes on his actions. The orator allows himself to be carried by the impulse of the moment, without reflecting on ultimate consequences, and as his expressions become freer, they acquire an appearance of warmth, of feeling, of inspiration. Not a little of this inspiration is contributed by the audience if they are in a similar condition of increased appreciation. . . . Another characteristic feature, evidently resulting from paralysis of the higher functions, is the loss of power to control moods'.†

Environment, personality, mood and dose of alcohol are all relevant to the final effect on the individual.‡

These and other effects that are characteristic of alcohol, have been celebrated in verse.§

Ho! Ho! Yes! Yes! It's very all well,
You may drunk I am think, but I tell you I'm not,
I'm as sound as a fiddle and fit as a bell,
And stable quite ill to see what's what.
I under *do* stand you surprise a got
When I headed my smear with gooseberry jam:
And I've swallowed, I grant, a beer of lot —
But I'm not so think as you drunk I am.

Can I liquor my stand? Why, yes, like hell!
I care not how many a tossed I've pot,
I shall stralk quite weight and not yutter an ell,
My feech will not spalter the least little jot:
If you knownly had own! — well, I gave him a dot,
And I said to him, 'Sergeant, I'll come like a lamb—
The floor it seems like a storm in a yacht,
But I'm not so think as you drunk I am.'

For example, to prove it I'll tale you a tell—
I once knew a fellow named Apricot—
I'm sorry, I just chair over a fell—
A trifle — this chap, on a very day hot—
If I hadn't consumed that last whisky of tot!—
As I said now, this fellow, called Abraham—
Ah? One more? Since it's you! Just a do me will spot—
But I'm not so think as you drunk I am.

ENVOI

So, Prince, you suggest I've bolted my shot?
Well, like what you say, and soul your damn!
I'm an upple litset by the talk you rot—
But I'm not so think as you drunk I am.

There is good reason to believe that, in general, efficiency, both mental and physical, is reduced by alcohol in any amount worth taking for social purposes. There is an important exception; the person who is so disabled by anxiety or nervous tension that performance is gravely impaired may improve with the correct dose of alcohol. The alleviation of great anxiety may improve performance more than the alcohol depresses it. Such people, mentally abnormal, are more liable to become alcohol addicts. Another exception is a

* Loss of consciousness occurs at blood concentrations around 300 mg/100 ml.

† Sollmann T. Manual of pharmacology. 8th ed. Philadelphia: Saunders, 1957.

‡ That which hath made them drunk hath made me bold.' Lady Macbeth in *Macbeth*, Act 2, Scene 2. W. Shakespeare.

§ By Sir J C Squire (1884–1958). Quoted, by permission, R H A Squire. To be properly appreciated, this poem should be read aloud.

minority of introverted people; it is referred to below.

Innumerable tests of physical and mental performance have been used to demonstrate the effects of alcohol. Results show that alcohol reduces visual acuity and delays recovery from visual dazzle, it impairs taste, smell and hearing, muscular co-ordination and steadiness and prolongs reaction time. It also causes nystagmus and vertigo. At the same time the subjects commonly have an increased confidence in their ability to perform well when tested and underestimate their errors, even after quite low doses. Attentiveness and ability to assimilate, sort and quickly take decisions on continuously changing information input, decline. This results particularly in inattentiveness to the periphery of the visual field, which is important in motoring. All these are evidently highly undesirable effects when a person is in a position where failure to perform well may be dangerous.

The effects of alcohol and psychotropic drugs on *motor driving* (Figure 20.4) have been the subject of well-deserved attention, and many countries have made laws designed to prevent motor accidents caused by alcohol. The problem has nowhere been solved. In general it can be said that the weight of evidence points to a steady deterioration of driving skill and an increased liability to accidents, which begins with the entry of alcohol into the blood and steadily increases with blood concentration.

'Alcohol brings disaster on the road less because of lack of skill than because of *defective judgement in relation to skill*. . . . Furthermore, let us recognise that the danger may be less from the few who have imbibed a lot than from the many who have taken a little'.*

Unfortunately it is not possible to observe and make measurements of driving skill in subjects who are both unaware that they are under observation and who are yet driving under normal traffic conditions. The undoubted tendency of alcohol to increase distractability, proneness to take risks and carelessness has not therefore been measured under normal conditions; in experimental conditions the well-known ability of alcoholics to 'pull themselves together' and to perform well temporarily when they know they are being tested will tend to give an unduly favourable picture of the effects of alcohol, but despite this, the evidence that its effects on driving are wholly evil is impressive.

In one study on city bus drivers, all of whom were recipients of awards for safe driving, it was found that even with these experienced professionals there was no 'safe' blood-alcohol level below which it was certain that no impairment of judgement would occur.

The drivers were invited to estimate through what gaps they *thought* they could drive their bus, were then given a driving test to determine the smallest gap through which they would *actually attempt* to drive and finally were told to drive through gaps regardless of their opinions. The main conclusion was that 'the performance of the drivers deteriorated, they were involved in great hazards, and they displayed a false confidence in their driving ability'.†

In another study using a motor driving trainer it was found that alcohol even in small doses caused drivers to move away from the kerb and to tolerate steering swings towards the road centre but not towards the kerb, also steering wheel movement increased and its timing became more faulty. An attempt to correlate these responses with personality suggested that extraverts were not worried by the stress imposed by taking alcohol, they did not alter their speed greatly but were much less accurate. Introverts however appeared to try to compensate for the alcohol effect, earnestly striving to show that they were efficient, with the result that they over-reacted to the situation, moving the steering wheel more and changing speed, some slowing right down and others seemingly trying to show how quickly they could drive. In the introvert group, two out of nine subjects made fewer errors. No extravert made fewer errors.‡

There can be little doubt that alcohol plays a huge part in causing motor accidents, being a factor perhaps in as many as 50%. Youth is also

* Cohen J. In *Alcohol and road traffic*. London: British Medical Association, 1963.

† Cohen J et al. Br Med J 1958; 1:1438.

‡ Drew G C et al. Br Med J 1958; 2:993.

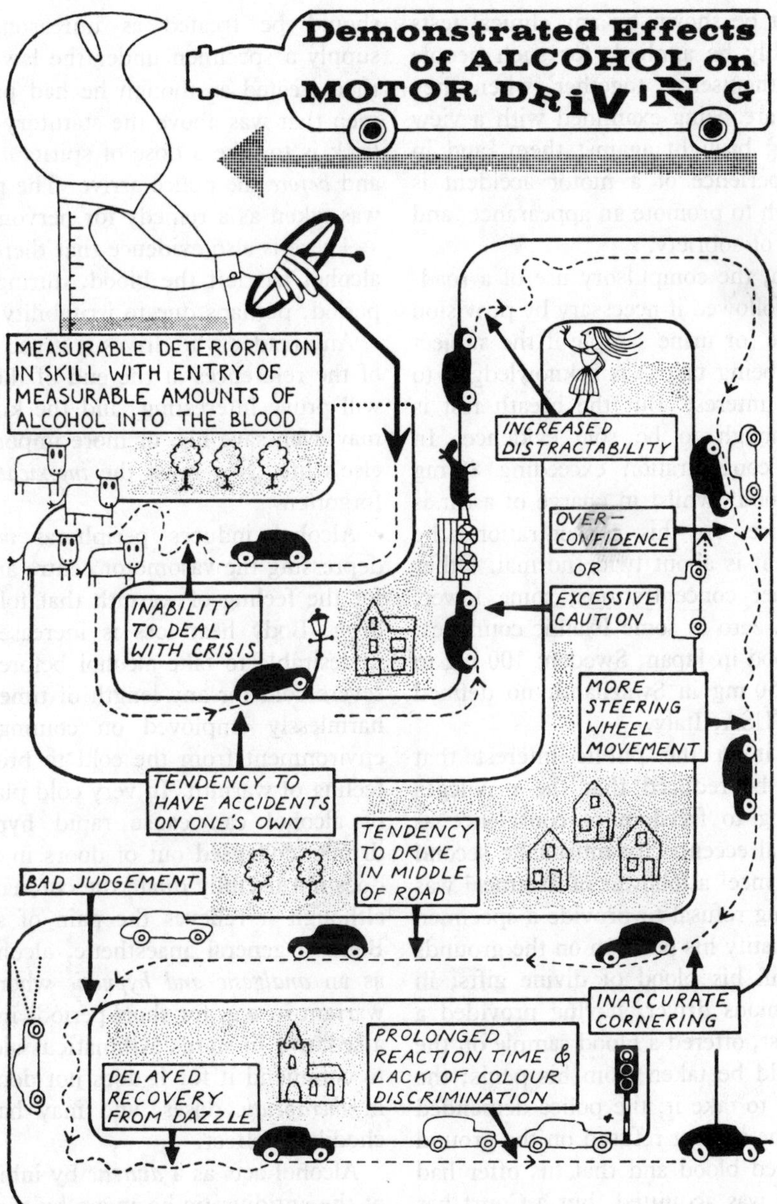

Fig. 20.4 See also the text.

associated with increased liability to road accidents. The adolescent who drives after drinking is a grave menace. Alcohol adversely affects the prognosis of head injuries. Increasingly, for public safety, stress is laid on measuring blood or breath concentrations of alcohol, and these are likely to be more widely employed as the serious impairment of judgement caused by even small amounts of alcohol is recognised and the consequences condemned by society. Schemes for clinical examinations for 'intoxication' usually consist of general observations on behaviour and simple tests for physical inco-ordination. But the carelessness or lack of vigilance which follows even very small amounts of alcohol and which is probably a far commoner cause of accidents than is physical incoordination cannot be shown by any clinical tests that can reasonably be applied, for such people can easily 'pull themselves together' when they realise that they are being examined with a view to a charge being brought against them, and in any case the experience of a motor accident is often quite enough to promote an appearance, and indeed a feeling, of sobriety.

For this reason, the compulsory use of a roadside breath test, followed if necessary by provision of a blood sample (or urine sample if the subject objects of blood being taken) is acknowledged to be in the public interest. But the breath test is now accurate enough to be sole evidence. In Britain a blood concentration exceeding 80 mg alcohol/100 ml blood* whilst in charge of a car is a statutory offence. At this concentration, the liability to accident is about twice normal. Other countries set other concentrations, some lower, some higher, e.g. zero in some Islamic countries: 50 mg/100 ml blood in Japan, Sweden: 100 mg in some of USA: 150 mg in Swaziland: no defined limit in much of USA, Italy.

So clearly is it in the public interest that drunken driving be reduced that the privileges normally attaching to freedom of conscience as well as to personal eccentricity must take second place. In one instance† a follower of Mesmer‡ was convicted following refusal to provide a specimen after seeking to justify his position on the grounds of the presence in his blood of divine gifts; in another, an ingenious driver, having provided a positive breath test, offered a blood sample on the condition it should be taken from his penis; the physician refused to take it; the police demanded a urine sample; the subject refused on the ground that he had offered blood and that his offer had been refused. He was acquitted, but a Court has since decided that the choice of site for blood-taking is for the physician, not for the subject, and that such transparent attempts to evade justice should be treated as unreasonable refusal to supply a specimen under the law. The subject is then treated as though he had provided a specimen that was above the statutory limit.† Another trick is to take a dose of spirits *after* the accident and *before* the police arrive. The police are told it was taken as a remedy for nervous shock.

There is also evidence that there is danger after alcohol has left the blood, during the 'hangover' period, perhaps due to irritability and fatigue.

Any reader who drives is urged to consult some of the references at the end of the chapter. They will prove interesting, and the knowledge gained may even save his, or more important, somebody else's life. Nor must the *intoxicated pedestrian* be forgotten.

Alcohol induces peripheral *vasodilatation* by depressing the vasomotor centre and this accounts for the feeling of warmth that follows taking the drug. Body heat loss is increased so that it is undesirable to take alcohol before going out into severe cold for any length of time, but it may be harmlessly employed on coming into a warm environment from the cold to provide a pleasant feeling of warmth. In very cold places the overuse of alcohol can cause rapid hypothermia, e.g. drunks collapsed out of doors in winter. Alcohol does not usefully dilate the coronary blood vessels although it relieves the pain of angina pectoris. Being a general anaesthetic, alcohol can be used as an *analgesic and hypnotic* when circumstances warrant it, e.g. for short periods in the elderly. As a sedative in status asthmaticus alcohol has much to commend it for it does not depress respiration in *therapeutic* doses, and may have some bronchodilator effect.

Alcohol acts as a *diuretic* by inhibiting secretion of the antidiuretic hormone by the posterior pituitary gland. The reason it is useless as a diuretic in heart failure is that the diuresis is of water, not of salt.

Alcohol injures the *gastric mucosa* with back diffusion of acid and increased cell shedding. It has little effect on gastric secretion (contrary to previous belief). After an acute binge the mucosa

* Approximately equivalent to 35 μg alcohol in 100 ml expired air (or 107 mg in 100 ml urine). In practice, prosecutions are only undertaken when the concentration is significantly higher to avoid arguments about biological variability and instrumental error. Urine concentrations are little used since the urine is accumulated over time and does not provide the immediacy of blood and breath.

† Br Med J 1974; 2:620.

‡ Friedrich Anton Mesmer (1733–1815) developed a theory that a healing occult force akin to magnetism permeated the universe, though concentrated in men and especially in himself.

shows erosions and petechial haemorrhages (recovery may take three weeks) and up to 60% of chronic alcoholics show chronic gastritis. Alcohol has no proven important influence on peptic ulcer disease.

The *vomiting* which is so common an accompaniment of acute alcoholism is not primarily due to gastric irritation, for the incidence of vomiting at equivalent blood alcohol levels is similar following oral or i.v. administration. This is not to deny that very strong solutions and dietary indiscretions accompanying acute and chronic alcoholism can cause vomiting by local gastric effects. That the emetic blood alcohol concentration is below that which induces coma may be one of the reasons for the rarity of deaths from acute alcoholism and for the fact that when death occurs, it is commonly due to suffocation from inhaled vomit.

Glucose tolerance: alcohol initially increases the blood glucose, due to reduced uptake by the tissues. This leads to increased *glucose metabolism*. A substantial dose of alcohol may cause slight hyperglycaemia due to activity of the sympathetic autonomic.

Alcohol inhibits gluconeogenesis, and in a person whose hepatic glycogen is already low (e.g. a person who is getting most of his calories from alcohol or who has not eaten adequately for 3 days), this can result in hypoglycaemia that can be severe enough to cause irreversible brain damage. The hypoglycaemia is commonly at its maximum 6–18 h after taking the alcohol. It can be difficult to recognise clinically in a person who has been drunk, and this adds to the risk.

Hypoglycaemia is also enhanced by exaggeration of the normal insulin response to carbohydrate ingestion, and by exercise.

Hyperuricaemia occurs (with precipitation of gout) due to accelerated degradation of adenine nucleotides resulting in increased production of uric acid and its precursors. Only at high alcohol concentrations does alcohol-induced high blood lactate compete for renal tubular elimination and so diminish excretion of urate.

Acute effects on sexual function. Nothing really new has been said since William Shakespeare wrote that alcohol 'provokes the desire, but it takes away the performance.' Performance in other forms of athletics is also impaired. Prolonged substantial consumption lowers plasma testesterone concentration at least partly as a result of hepatic enzyme induction; feminisation may be seen.

As a *source of energy* (rather than a food) alcohol may be very useful in debilitated patients. It is rapidly absorbed from the alimentary tract without requiring digestion and it supplies 7 calories* per gram as compared with 9 from fat and 4 from carbohydrate and protein. Heavy doses cause hyperlipidaemia in some people.

Tolerance to alcohol can be *acquired* and Gaddum has made the practical point that it costs the regular heavy drinker two-and-a-half times as much to get drunk as it would cost the average abstainer.† This is probably due both to enzyme induction and to adaptation of the central nervous system. There are also racial differences in *natural tolerance*; whites are more tolerant than Mongolians.

Acute alcohol poisoning is a sufficiently familiar condition not to require detailed description. It is notorious that the behaviour changes, mental confusion, inco-ordination and even coma, which are characteristic, can be due to numerous other conditions and diagnosis can be extremely difficult if a sick or injured patient happens to have taken alcohol as well. Alcohol can cause severe hypoglycaemia (see above). Anyone who is liable to find himself called upon, especially by the police, to diagnose drunkenness, or rather perhaps to exclude other causes as responsible for a person's behaviour, should consider his procedure very carefully. When applying clinical tests for drunkenness it is worth remembering that habitual physical skills can be retained to an advanced stage and that the results of performance tests cannot always be interpreted unambiguously.

'One evening a motorist, whose speech was slurred and who was excited, brought to my house a cyclist he had knocked over. I told him he had had too much to drink and advised him to leave his car and walk home. He was very incensed at this and demanded that I should call a policeman as I had insulted him. I rang up the police station,

* 1 calorie ≈ 4.2 joules

† Gaddum J H. In *Lectures on the Scientific Basis of Medicine*, 1954–55. London: Athlone Press, 1956.

and asked the constable who arrived to persuade him to go home quietly without his car. The constable got him outside on the pavement, and after testing his walking, told him that he would be wise to follow my advice but that he was at liberty to make his own choice.

'The driver thereupon got into his car, started off at a fast speed down a hill, mounted the pavement on the opposite side of the road, returned to his own side, crossed the pavement there, and collided with the wall bordering the churchyard. He had no explanation to offer for this driving. He was arrested, brought back to my house, and I was asked to certify him. I refused to do this, and he was examined later at the station by a colleague who told me the rest of the story. After submitting the defendant to various inconclusive tests and fortified by the history, he told him he was drunk. He was then asked by the motorist: "Doctor, could a drunk man stand up in the middle of this room, jump into the air, turn a complete somersault, and land down on his feet?" My colleague was injudicious enough to say, "Certainly not" — and was then and there proved wrong'.* The introduction of the breathalyser has largely eliminated such professional humiliations.

When a person is behaving in an excited or violent fashion due to alcohol it is dangerous to attempt to control him with sedatives or opioids because of the risk of inducing severe respiratory depression as a result of synergism of the drugs. But if sedation is essential, chlorpromazine, diazepam or paraldehyde in low dose are least hazardous. In patients who are comatose, the stomach may be emptied by tube; emesis, either therapeutic or due to the alcohol, is dangerous in any patient with impaired consciousness. Respiratory stimulants, e.g. doxapram, or controlled respiration are used as required: circulatory failure may occur. Alcohol dialyses well, but dialysis will only be used in extreme cases.

Large doses of *fructose* (laevulose)† i.v. enhance alcohol metabolism but also induce lactic acidosis. Claims that a dose of fructose swallowed during and/or at the end of an evening's drinking can render a subject who is unfit to drive, fit to do so, are dangerously misleading.

Acute hepatitis, which can be extremely severe, can occur with extraordinarily heavy acute drinking bouts. The serum transaminase rises after alcohol in alcoholics but not in others. The single case report that after a binge the cerebrospinal fluid tasted of gin remains unconfirmed.

Chronic alcohol consumption. The effects described above will occur, but also, with heavy continuous drinking there will be malnutrition (subjects take all the calories they need from alcohol, see above, and cease to eat adequately) with deficiency of B group vitamins particularly. The malnutrition complicates the long-term effects of alcohol itself. Chronic *heavy* alcohol use is associated with organ damage due to metabolites of alcohol (see metabolism, above); hepatic cirrhosis; deteriorating brain function (psychotic states, dementia) peripheral neuropathy and, separately, myopathy; cancer of the upper alimentary and respiratory tracts (many alcoholics smoke heavily, and this contributes), and hepatic carcinoma; chronic pancreatitis; cardiomyopathy; bone marrow depression, including megaloblastosis (due to the alcohol and to alcohol induced folate deficiency); deficiency of vitamin K dependent blood clotting factors (due to liver injury); multiple effects on the hypothalamic/pituitary/endocrine system (endocrine investigations should be interpreted cautiously).

In general, reversal of all or most of the effects is usual in early cases if alcohol is abandoned. In more advanced cases, the disease may be halted but in severe cases it may continue to progress. Stopping drinking improves survival only in early cases. When wine rationing was introduced in Paris in the 1939–45 war, deaths from hepatic cirrhosis dropped to about one-sixth the previous level; 5 years after the war they had regained their previous level. A similar, though lesser, effect was seen during alcohol prohibition in the USA (1919–33).

Alcohol dependence syndrome‡ (chronic alcoholism): general aspects of dependence are discussed

* Worthing C L. Br Med J 1957; 1:643.

† Sucrose is hydrolysed to dextrose (glucose) and fructose in the intestine, but this takes time.

‡ A World Health Organization report prefers this term to 'alcoholism'.

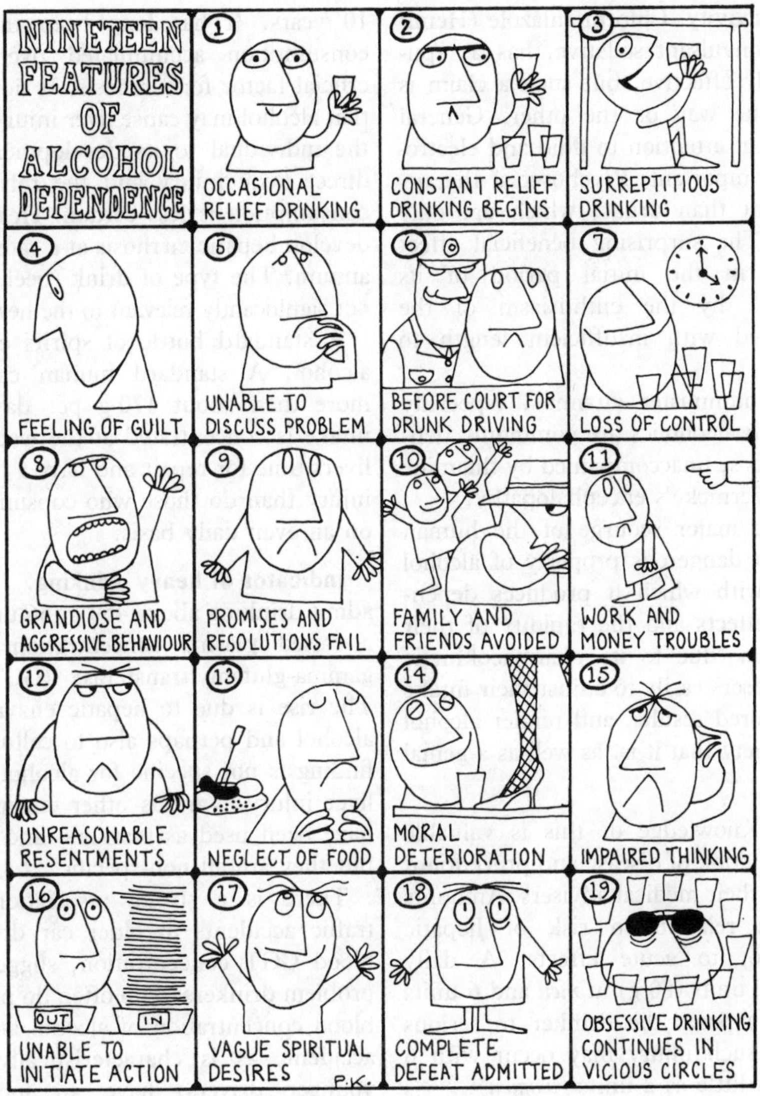
NINETEEN FEATURES OF ALCOHOL DEPENDENCE
1
OCCASIONAL RELIEF DRINKING
2
CONSTANT RELIEF DRINKING BEGINS
3
SURREPTITIOUS DRINKING
4
FEELING OF GUILT
5
UNABLE TO DISCUSS PROBLEM
6
BEFORE COURT FOR DRUNK DRIVING
7
LOSS OF CONTROL
8
GRANDIOSE AND AGGRESSIVE BEHAVIOUR
9
PROMISES AND RESOLUTIONS FAIL
10
FAMILY AND FRIENDS AVOIDED
11
WORK AND MONEY TROUBLES
12
UNREASONABLE RESENTMENTS
13
NEGLECT OF FOOD
14
MORAL DETERIORATION
15
IMPAIRED THINKING
16
OUT
IN
UNABLE TO INITIATE ACTION
17
VAGUE SPIRITUAL DESIRES
18
COMPLETE DEFEAT ADMITTED
19
OBSESSIVE DRINKING CONTINUES IN VICIOUS CIRCLES
P.K.

Fig. 20.5

earlier in this chapter. Dependence varies between the social drinker for whom companionship is the principal factor, through individuals who take a drink at the end of a working (or indeed any) day, who feel a *need* and who would be reluctant to give it up, to the person who is overcome by need, who cannot resist and whose whole life is ruled by the quest for alcohol. The major factors determining physical dependence are *dose, frequency* of dosing, and *duration* of abuse.

Sudden withdrawal of alcohol from an addict who has developed physical dependence, such as may occur when an ill or injured alcoholic is admitted to hospital, can precipitate an acute psychotic attack (*delirium tremens*) and convulsions as well as agitation, anxiety and excess sympathetic autonomic activity.

Withdrawal is less unpleasant if the patient is sedated, e.g. with a benzodiazepine and a β-adrenoceptor blocker given for the symptoms of sympathetic overactivity. Chlormethiazole (Heminevrin), an anticonvulsant sedative, has a reputation as especially effective, but such a claim is hard to prove one way or the other. General aspects of care, e.g. attention to fluid and electrolyte balance, are important. Psychosocial therapy is more important than drugs, which are only of limited use. 'The surprising beneficial effect of any therapy in the initial period of its trial is explained by the enthusiasm of the therapist combined with insufficient length to follow-up'.*

It is usual to administer vitamins, especially thiamine, in which alcoholics are commonly deficient, and i.v. glucose unaccompanied by thiamine may precipitate Wernicke's encephalopathy.

Alcoholism is a major scourge of the human race and the most dangerous property of alcohol is the readiness with which it produces dependence. Its acute effects and the rapidity of their onset and duration (due to its pharmacokinetic properties) allow users easily to adjust their intake to achieve the desired results, and render alcohol the menace to society that it is, as well as a genial social pleasure.

Daily intake† Knowledge of this is valuable to allow both prediction of disease and prevention, both by users and their medical advisers. Amounts are suggested in relation to risk of hepatic cirrhosis, and not to acute effects. A daily consumption of 10 units (80 g) in *men* and 6 units (48 g) in *women* exposes the drinker to serious liver injury. But such injury may occur with 6 units (*men*) and as little as 2 units (*women*)‡.

If challenged by a patient to advise a safe upper limit (which, in fact, cannot be accurately defined), the doctor might reasonably reply: *men*, 3 units per day: *women*, 2 units per day. Anyone taking more than this should have two alcohol-free days per week.

Alcoholics with established cirrhosis have usually consumed about 23 units (185 g) daily for 10 years. It has long been thought that total consumption accumulated over time was the crucial factor for cirrhosis. It now seems possible that alcohol may cause liver injury by predisposing the individual to its development as well as by direct toxic injury and the relationship to total consumption is less certain. Heavy drinkers may develop hepatic cirrhosis at a rate of about 2% per annum. The type of drink (beer, wine, spirits) is not significantly relevant to the health consequences.

A standard bottle of spirits contains 240 g of alcohol. A standard human cannot metabolise more than about 170 g per day. People whose intake is concentrated at the weekend allow their livers time for repair and have a lower risk of liver injury than do those who consume the same total on an even daily basis.

Indicator of heavy drinking. 50% of men who admit drinking above 450 g (56 units) a week have a raised plasma concentration of the enzyme gamma-glutamyltransferase (GGT; > 50 I.U.). The rise is due to hepatic enzyme induction by alcohol and perhaps also to cellular damage. The finding is not specific for alcohol, indicating only liver injury. Various other enzyme abnormalities have been used as markers, and megaloblastosis, but they are all non-specific.

There is a strong association between road traffic accidents in older car drivers and raised blood GGT concentration, suggesting that older problem drinkers (who often do not have an illegal blood concentration of alcohol at the time of the accident, as is characteristically the case with younger drivers) have an increased accident liability independent of recent alcohol consumption.

Pregnancy and the fetus. Pregnancy is unlikely to occur in severely alcoholic women (who have amenorrhoea secondary to liver injury). Even modest alcohol consumption (2–4 units per week) is associated with miscarriage.

Fetal injury can occur in early pregnancy (fetal alcohol syndrome). It may be due to the metabolite, acetaldehyde, and so acute (binge) consumption is more hazardous than similar total intake on a daily basis. Plainly, disulfiram should not be used in a woman who is or might become pregnant.

The vulnerable period of pregnancy is at 4–10 weeks. Because of this, prevention cannot be re-

* Kalant H. Quarterly Journal of Studies in Alcoholism 1962; 23:52.

† For these and other data on alcohol, see *Alcohol and disease*. Br Med Bull 1982.

‡ Women appear to be more susceptible to liver injury than are men. This is not solely a matter of pharmacokinetics but may be also due to the greater occurrence of autoimmune reactivity that has been shown in women with alcoholic liver disease.

liably achieved after diagnosis of pregnancy (usually 3–8 weeks).

There is no safe level of maternal consumption for fetal safety. But it is plainly unrealistic to leave the matter there and it has been suggested that if the ideal total abstinence is unachievable then two *small* drinks (< 2 units) per day should be the target, or, safer, 5 units per week.

In addition to the fetal alcohol syndrome there is general fetal/embryonic growth retardation (1% for every 10 g alcohol per day).

Fetal alcohol syndrome has the following characteristics: microcephaly, mental deficiency with irritability in infancy, low body weight and length, poor co-ordination, hypotonia, small eyeballs and short palpebral fissures, lack of nasal bridge, etc.*

Children of about 10% of alcohol abusers may show the syndrome, with 13% having some alcohol-related abnormalities. In women consuming 12 units of alcohol per day the occurrence may be as much as 30%.

Disulfiram (Antabuse). In alcoholics who are fairly well *and cooperative*, an attempt may be made to discourage drinking by the use of disulfiram. The drug inhibits the enzyme aldehyde dehydrogenase so that acetaldehyde (toxic metabolite of alcohol) accumulates. This is so unpleasant that the patient does not wish to experience it again: disulfiram thus reinforces the perhaps otherwise ineffectual will power. Such therapy by intimidation, whether self-administered or thrust on the patient, is not to be expected to play an important part in the treatment of alcoholism, a disease that is primarily a manifestation of psychological disorder. When a patient is given disulfiram some have given a test dose of alcohol under supervision, so that he can be taught what to expect and also to induce an aversion from alcohol. That this is not to be lightly undertaken is shown by the fact that, though rare, deaths have occurred following the 'test drink'. Such a test is now considered unwise. A typical reaction of medium severity comes on about 5 min after taking alcohol and consists of generalised vasodilatation and fall in blood pressure, sweating, dyspnoea, headache, chest pain, nausea and vomiting. Severe reactions include convulsions and circulatory collapse. Disulfiram causes a similar reaction with paraldehyde.

It is clear that no patient should be given disulfiram without the fullest previous explanation and the certainty that the possible serious consequences of drinking a lot of alcohol in a few minutes are understood.

The disulfiram-alcohol interaction has long been known to workers in the rubber industry in which the substance is used, but it was not applied to therapeutics until after the chance experience of two Danish pharmacologists.* 'Dr. Hald suggested that disulfiram could be employed as an anthelmintic because it had a very strong fixation to copper ions. It was probable that some enzymes of the oxidation system of intestinal worms were copper-containing, and copper-containing enzymes are known in . . . higher animals, including man.' The drug was tested on rabbits infected with worms and results were sufficiently encouraging to warrant clinical trial.

'According to the custom in this house we never give a new drug to patients before we have taken at least double the recommended dose ourselves. During this routine procedure Dr. Hald and I discovered that we had developed an intolerance to alcohol. We compared symptoms and found them identical. The only thing we have in common was the tablets. A test on a third person in our laboratory confirmed the observation.'† Further investigation disclosed the mechanism of the effect.

Calcium carbimide (Abstem) is similar but is less effective and therefore safer if the patient does drink.

Both disulfiram and calcium carbimide inhibit the metabolism of the *wide range* of drugs subject to oxidative metabolism. They do not affect drug conjugation.

Emetics, administered after drinking, are used in the 'aversion' treatment of alcoholism, to establish a conditioned dislike.

Alcoholic drinks. The pharmacology of alcoholic drinks is not the same as the pharmacology of alcohol. The drinks contain other ingredients that may reduce the rate of absorption of alcohol (carbohydrate in beer), act as a carminative (essen-

* For pictures see Streissguth A P et al. Lancet 1985; 2:85.

† Dr. Erik Jacobsen. Personal communication.

tial oils), or diuretic (juniper oil in gin) or inhibit enzymes that are concerned in some drug metabolism (red wines, but not white, i.e. grape skins are concerned). It is certainly widely believed that the toxicity of all varieties of alcoholic drinks is not solely dependent on their alcoholic content and that ill-effects are likely to be more severe if several varieties are taken within a short time; this is expressed as advice 'not to mix your drinks'. There is no conclusive evidence on this point, but there is reason to believe that the effects of ethanol in some drinks are prolonged by the presence of other substances (propyl to octyl alcohols, ethers, aldehydes, etc.), which delay ethanol metabolism by occupying the same metabolic paths (competition). These other ingredients are themselves hardly more toxic than ethanol. It should be remembered that when enough alcoholic drink has been taken to cause 'hangover', subjects have commonly debauched themselves in other ways too, with tobacco, food, polluted atmosphere and fatigue, and in addition is expecting to feel ill the next day.

Since there are many more important subjects for research, the final elucidation of this point in the near future is unlikely, and indeed very strong evidence would be needed to shake, although not to confirm, the faith of most people that this or that drink or combination is harmless or harmful, for the effects of alcoholic drinks are part of the folklore of society.

Alcohol and other drugs. *All cerebral depressants* (hypnotics, tranquillisers, antiepileptics, antihistamines) can either potentiate or synergise with alcohol, and this can be important at *ordinary* doses in relation to car driving. But, when supplies of hypnotics or tranquillisers are given to patients known to drink heavily, they should be warned to omit the drugs when they have been drinking. Deaths have occurred from this combination.

Alcohol-dependent people with a physical tolerance are relatively tolerant of some other cerebral depressant drugs (hydrocarbon anaesthetics and barbiturates), but of course the synergism with these drugs still occurs. There is no significant acquired cross-tolerance with opioids.

Interaction with *caffeine*, though long believed, appears now to be negligible.

Sulphonylureas (antidiabetics) cause a disulfiram-like reaction, as may *metronidazole*.

Hepatic metabolism. Substantial doses of alcohol depress hepatic hydroxylation and so increase the systemic bioavailability of drugs subject to high hepatic first-pass extraction (e.g. *some* benzodiazepines, [e.g. triazolam]) to an extent that may have clinical importance.

Oral anticoagulants: control may be disturbed by alcohol inhibiting hepatic metabolism directly or enhancing it by enzyme induction: moderate drinking is unlikely to cause trouble.

Anticonvulsants can be metabolised faster due to enzyme induction and this contributes to its well-known adverse effect on epilepsy.

Miscellaneous uses. In addition to those already mentioned, its use in strong solutions as an irritant has given alcohol a reputation as a restorative in fainting. When such stimulation is indicated, a slap in the face is just as irritant, cheaper, always handy and cannot enter the lungs and cause pneumonia. Alcohol precipitates protein and is used to harden the skin in bedridden patients. Local application also reduces sweating and may allay itching. As a skin antiseptic 70% by weight (76% by volume) is most effective. Stronger solutions are less effective. Alcohol injections are sometimes used to destroy nervous tissue in cases of intractable pain (trigeminal neuralgia, carcinoma involving nerves).

METHYL ALCOHOL (METHANOL)

Methyl alcohol is of clinical importance because it is sometimes consumed as a substitute for ethanol. Its acute toxicity is slightly less than ethanol, that is, it makes the subject a little less 'drunk', but it is metabolised at only about one-fifth the rate of ethanol and it is the toxic metabolites produced over a long period that make methanol intoxication so serious (as little as 30 g can kill). As with ethanol, methanol elimination is subject to zero-order kinetics.

Methanol poisoning may appear with or without initial symptoms similar to those of ethanol. There is severe malaise, vomiting, abdominal pain and tachypnoea (due to acidosis). Pancreatitis has been found at autopsy on posioned patients and so morphine should not be used if it is avoidable. Muscle cramps also occur. Coma and circulatory collapse may follow. A prominent symptom is visual disturbance with scotomata and total blindness, which may occur early or late. The mechanism is uncertain (it may be due to formate accumulation) and partial or complete recovery can occur, although permanent blindness with optic atrophy is common. Very small doses can cause blindness and large doses sometimes have failed to do so, which has given rise to the suggestion that the eye changes may be due to an idiosyncracy.

The characteristic symptoms of acute methanol poisoning may be delayed for many hours, or even a day or more if much ethanol has been consumed with it, as is often the case. This is because both alcohols are metabolised by the same enzymes and the rate at which each is metabolised depends on the amount of the other present, i.e. substrate competition. This can be made use of in treatment, the less toxic ethanol being added to delay metabolism of the methanol so that more of the latter is excreted unchanged in urine and breath and the amount of metabolites formed is less.

Methanol is metabolised to formaldehyde and then formate, which produces an intense *acidosis* (which itself enhances pH-dependent hepatic lactate production so that lactic acidosis is added). To combat this is the most urgent need if the most effective treatment, dialysis, is not available.

There is reason to think that the prognosis may depend on the acidosis, which may be reversed by i.v. 5% sodium bicarbonate solution (as much as 2 mol in a few hours may be needed and carries excess sodium in amounts that must be managed). Measurement of the plasma bicarbonate and blood pH are of great value in controlling therapy. In their absence, and in severe cases, it is better to risk overtreatment than undertreatment. Mild cases may be treated by oral administration. As methanol is so slowly metabolised a patient may relapse if sodium bicarbonate administration is stopped too soon.

Experiments in animals and clinical observations suggest that administration of ethanol to delay methanol metabolism is beneficial.

If methanol alone has been taken, a single oral dose of 1 ml/kg ethanol (as 50% soln) should be given, followed by 0.25 ml/kg per h orally or i.v. (a blood ethanol concentration of about 100 mg/100 ml may be about right) and treatment should be continued until the blood methanol concentration is less than 25 mg/100 ml. If unconscious, ethanol can be given i.v.

Many cases of methanol poisoning may be complicated by ingestion of ethanol and other substances and this should be taken into account. If frequent blood concentrations are not available then a combination of clinical judgement and knowledge of the kinetics of both alcohols must guide treatment.

Haemodialysis and peritoneal dialysis can remove both alcohols and dialysis is probably desirable if the blood concentration of methanol exceeds 50 mg/100 ml.

A darkened room is reputed to benefit the eye changes.

The above account is of serious acute intoxication. Chronic intoxication, e.g. by drinking some cleansing fluids, and which is commonly accompanied by ethanol, does not generally require the vigorous measures described, even in the presence of high methanol plasma concentration.*

PSYCHODYSLEPTICS or HALLUCINOGENS

These substances produce mental changes that resemble those of some psychotic states. They are chiefly used by people seeking a new experience or escape.

But psychiatrists also use these drugs in supervised therapeutic sessions to encourage the release and reliving of unconscious material in the hope that, assisted by appropriate psychotherapy, the patient may gain insight and an improved ability to cope with his environment. Such use remains experimental and potentially dangerous (suicide,

* Editorial. Lancet 1983; 1:910.
Heath A. Lancet 1983; 1:339.

prolonged psychosis), and should only be conducted by responsible and sane psychiatrists.

Experiences with these drugs vary greatly with the subject's expectations, existing frame of mind and personality and environment. Subjects can be prepared so that they are more likely to have a good 'trip' than a bad 'trip'. It is impossible to describe the pharmacological effects of psychodysleptics in the fashion that can be adopted for most of the drugs in this book.

The following brief account of **experiences with LSD in normal subjects** will serve as a model. Experiences with *mescaline* and *psilocybin* are similar:

Vision may become blurred and there may be hallucinations; these generally do not occur in the blind and are less if the subject is blind-folded. Objects appear distorted, and trivial things, e.g. a mark on a wall, may change shape and acquire special significance.

Auditory acuity increases, but hallucinations are uncommon. Subjects who do not ordinarily appreciate music may suddenly come to do so.

Foods may feel coarse and gritty in the mouth.

Limbs may be left in uncomfortable positions.

Time may seem to stop or to pass slowly, but usually it gets faster and thousands of years may seem suddenly to go by.

Mental problem-solving becomes difficult.

The subject may feel relaxed and supremely happy, or may become fearful or depressed. Feelings of depersonalisation and dreamy states occur.

The experience lasts a few hours, depending on the dose; intervals of normality then occur and become progressively longer.

Somatic symptoms include nausea, dizziness, paraaesthesia, weakness, drowsiness, tremors, dilated pupils, ataxia. Effects on the cardiovascular system and respiration vary and probably reflect fluctuating anxiety.

So disrupting to the individual are some of these drugs, particularly in respect of thought processes, that special legal control is needed, perhaps especially in view of the possibility of their use in a 'person in a position of high authority when faced with decisions of great importance'.*

There is no shortage of accounts of experience with psychodysleptics, because there has been a vogue amongst intellectuals, begun by Mr. Aldous Huxley,† for publishing their experiences.‡ Subsequent accounts are tedious to most except their authors and to those who would do the same; they have little pharmacological importance and reveal more about the author's egocentricity than about pharmacology. The same applies to published accounts of what it is like to be a drug addict.

Lysergic acid diethylamide (LSD). Lysergic acid provides the nucleus of the ergot alkaloids and it was during a study of derivatives of this in a search for an analeptic that in 1943 a Swiss research worker investigating LSD (which structurally resembles nikethamide) felt queer and had visual hallucinations. This led him to take a dose of the substance and so to discover its remarkable potency, an effective oral dose being about 30 μg. The plasma $t_{\frac{1}{2}}$ is about 3 h.

Tachyphylaxis occurs to LSD. Psychological dependence may occur, physical dependence does not.

Amphetamine potentiates LSD.

LSD has been used in the dying; it induced analgesia and indifference.

Its effect on the brain may partly be due to antagonism of 5-HT and to anticholinesterase effect.

Serious adverse effects include: psychotic reaction (which can be delayed in onset) with suicide; teratogenic and mutagenic effects are speculative and the risk is small at worst.

LSD causes curious effects to occur in animals: green sunfish become aggressive, Siamese fighting fish float nose up, tail down, and goats walk in inaccustomed stereotyped patterns. The elephant exhibits episodically a form of sexual or delinquent behaviour known as 'musth'. LSD 100 μg/kg i.m. was given to an animal (the usual dose for man is up to about 2 μg/kg) to test whether this induced a similar state. The elephant developed laryngospasm and status epilepticus and died.§ Badly planned experiments give useless results.

Mescaline is an alkaloid from a Mexican cactus (peyotl), the top of which is cut off and dried and

* Hoffer A. Clin Pharmacol Ther 1965; 6:183.

† Huxley A. *The doors of preception*. London: Chatto and Windus, 1964.

‡ Published experiences of opium and alcohol are legion and span hundreds of years.

§ Cohen S. Ann Rev Pharmacol 1967; 7:301.

used as 'peyote buttons' in religious ceremonies. Mescaline does not induce serious dependence and the drug has little importance except to members of some North and Central American societies and to psychiatrists and biochemists who are interested in the mechanism of induced psychotic states.

Adrenochrome is an oxidation product of adrenaline. It can produce effects similar to those of mescaline and LSD, a fact that has led to speculation as to the possibility of its playing role in mental disease.

Phencyclidine (angel dust) was made in a search for a better intravenous anaesthetic. It is related to pethidine. It was found to induce analgesia without unconsciousness, but with amnesia, in man. However, the postoperative course was complicated by psychiatric disturbance (agitation, abreactions, hallucinations). As the interest of anaesthetists waned, so that of psychiatrists grew, and the drug has been used in experimental therapy. Ketamine originates from this work.

Psilocybin is derived from varieties of the fungus *Psilocybe* ('magic mushrooms') that grow in many countries. It is related to LSD.

Cannabis is obtained from the annual plant *Cannabis sativa* (hemp) and its varieties *C. indica* and *C. americana*. The preparations that are smoked are called marihuana (grass, pot, weed, etc.) and consist of crushed leaves and flowers. There is a wide variety of regional names, e.g. ganja (India, Caribbean), kif (Morocco), dagga (Africa). The resin scraped off the plant is known as hashish (hash). The term cannabis is used to include all the above preparations. Since most preparations are illegally prepared it is not surprising that they are impure and of variable potency. The plant grows wild in the Americas, Africa and Asia. It can also be grown successfully in the open in the warmer southern areas of Britain.

Prof. Sir William Paton has generously allowed the account that follows to be used here.

Active principles. 'Of the scores of chemical compounds that the resin contains, the most important are the oily cannabinoids, including tetrahydrocannabinol (THC), which is the chief cause of the psychic action. Samples of resin vary greatly in the amounts and proportions of these cannabinoids according to their country of origin; and as the sample ages, its THC content declines. As a result, the THC content of samples can vary from almost zero to eight per cent. Pure THC is unstable unless kept in the dark under nitrogen, but is better preserved in the undamaged plant. One result of these facts is that the dose of THC taken, unless under laboratory control, is far more uncertain than with other drugs.

'In addition to the cannabinoids are certain water-soluble substances, including a small amount of an atropine-like substance (which may contribute to the dry mouth), and some acetylcholine-like substances (which may contribute to the irritant effect of the smoke).

'Little is known about the composition of the smoke from a cannabis cigarette, save that about twenty-five to fifty per cent of the THC content is delivered to the respiratory tract.

'THC and other cannabinoids undergo extensive biotransformation in the body, yielding scores of metabolites, several of which are themselves psychoactive. Study of these requires gas–liquid chromatography combined with mass spectrometry. A radioimmunoassay technique has been developed, however, which, although less specific, recognises THC and some principal metabolites in blood or urine. With this technique a fatal car accident attributable to cannabis was identified, as well as high rates (about 30%) of cannabis use in addiction clinics, and the method makes it possible to establish approximate levels of cannabis use.

'The cannabinoids are extremely fat-soluble, and correspondingly insoluble in water. They and their metabolites therefore persist in the body; thus twenty-four hours after a dose of labelled THC, a rat has eliminated, as metabolites in urine and faeces, about ten per cent of the dose, a rabbit about forty-five per cent, and a man about twenty-five per cent. Metabolism is fairly rapid ($t_{\frac{1}{2}}$, 30 h) and the persistence is due to slow release from THC taken up by the tissues.*

'*Psychopharmacology*. Reactions are very varied, and they are much influenced by the behaviour of the group. Euphoria is common, though not invariable, with giggling or laughter which can

* When a chronic user discontinues, cannabinoids remain detectable in the urine for an average of four weeks and it can be as long as 11 weeks before ten consecutive daily tests are negative (Ellis G M et al. Clin. Pharmacol Ther 1986; 38:572).

seem pointless to an observer. Sensations become more vivid, especially visual, and contrast and intensity of colour can increase, although no change in acuity occurs. Size of objects and distance are distorted. Time as experienced becomes longer than clock time; thus a subject asked to say when sixty seconds has elapsed responds too early, but if asked to say how long some period of time was, overstates it: sense of time can disappear altogether, leaving a sometimes distressing sense of timelessness. Recent memory and selective attention are impaired; the beginning of a sentence may be forgotten before it is finished, and the subject is very suggestible and easily distracted. Psychological tests such as mental arithmetic, digit-symbol substitution and pursuit meter tests show impairment, the effect being greater as the task becomes more complex. The vividness of sensory impressions and distractability gives rise to imagery and fantasy; this can progress with increasing dose from mere fanciful interpretation of actual sensations to hallucination in the sense of vivid sensory impressions lacking an external basis. These effects may be accompanied by feelings of deep insight and truth. They are similar in type, though often more intense, to those experienced in hypnagogic imagery or while recovering from an anaesthetic.

'It seems likely that these effects of cannabis can be explained if it removes a restraining "gate" on the inflow of sensory information. Normally, considerable selection takes place, and familiar stimuli or those judged irrelevant are ignored. A dis-inhibitory action of cannabis, lifting this gate, would allow the "flood of sensation" so often reported. Further, it is believed that time sense depends on the frequency of sensory impressions; and increased flow would therefore give the feeling that more time had elapsed. Finally, it is known that the process of memory involves at least three processes: entry into a sensory "register" and passage into a short-term "store"; rehearsal of information either consciously or unconsciously, leading to consolidation and transfer to a longer-term store; and retrieval. It appears that retrieval is not impaired by cannabis (longstanding memories often form the basis of the imagery), and entry seems normal; but conversion of short-term memory is known to be interfered with by a flow of additional sensory impressions, just as a telephone number is likely to be forgotten if someone speaks to you just after you have heard it. It is likely that the flow of sensory impressions under cannabis interferes with the consolidation of recent information in a similar way. Once memory is impaired, concentration becomes less effective, since the object of attention is less well remembered. With this may go an insensitivity to danger or the consequences of actions.

'A striking phenomenon is the intermittent wave-like nature of these effects — a subject may return towards normal, or bring himself "down" for a period. This intermittence affects mood, visual impressions, time sense, spatial sense, and other functions; it represents, incidentally, one of the many experimental difficulties in analysing cannabis action. The effect of a single dose usually ends with drowsiness or actual sleep.

'The effects can also be unpleasant, especially in inexperienced subjects, particularly timelessness and the feeling of loss of control of mental processes. Feelings of unease, sometimes amounting to anguish, occur, and may well have some physical basis — perhaps associated with the acceleration of the heart rate. There is also, especially in the habitual user, a tendency to paranoid thinking. High or habitual use can be followed by a psychotic state; this is usually reversible, quickly with brief periods of cannabis use, but more slowly after sustained exposures.

'*Other pharmacology*. Cannabis smoked* or taken by mouth produces reddening of the eyeballs (probably the forerunner of the general dilation of blood vessels and fall of blood pressure with higher doses), unsteadiness (particularly for precise movements), and acceleration of heart rate. The latter effect can be substantial, and although the insolubility of the cannabinoids in water makes intravenous abuse difficult, cardiac failure would be a serious risk with such use. The smoke produces the usual smoker's cough, and the tar from reefer cigarettes is as carcinogenic in animal experiments as cigarette tobacco tar. Although increase in appetite is commonly experi-

* The smoke is inhaled and the breath held to allow maximum absorption. Effects usually begin in a few minutes and last 2–3 h.

enced, no explanation for it exists, and cannabis use does not have any striking effect on the blood sugar. In animals, with chronic administration of substantial doses, food intake is reduced and weight loss occurs.

'An important finding in animals is that cannabis prolongs sleeping time after a dose of a barbiturate such as pentobarbitone. This has been shown to be due to an impairment of the ability of the liver to metabolise the barbiturate, as a result of inhibition of the microsomal enzymes. The importance lies in the fact that many drugs used in medicine are also dealt with by these enzymes; and it is to be expected that their function will be impaired in the liver of any recent or habitual cannabis user. The effect is not due to THC itself, but mainly to another constituent of the resin, cannabidiol. One hopes that cannabis users seeking medical treatment would inform their doctors accordingly; the main danger would be of overdosage or of overprolonged action.

'In a number of tests cannabis has been found to produce fetal deformities and fetal resorption in animals (rats, rabbits and hamsters) in doses (per unit weight) ranging down to that used in man. The effect has been shown to be dose-related, and (unlike the teratogenic effect in animals of many drugs, but like thalidomide and other known human teratogens) is exerted at a small fraction of the dose liable to kill the mother. It is not clear what the effect in the human is, and it is to be hoped that it is the human equivalent of fetal resorption (miscarriage) rather than teratogenicity. Tests for chromosome damage in users have sometimes been positive, but there is no evidence for a heritable genetic effect. Similar tests, however, have shown an impairment of cell division by THC, as well as interference with biosynthesis of nucleotides and other cell constituents. This effect has, indeed, been tested for possible use in cancer chemotherapy or immunosuppression. The fetal damage may be due to this, although the evidence from the positive teratogenic tests suggests that these are associated with some other resin constituent.

'**Cannabis and crime**. There has been much debate about the connection between cannabis and criminality. A reasonable view, covering other aspects of behaviour, is that cannabis may accentuate a particular mood or facilitate a train of action and such a process could well explain the cases of violence described. A similar position could hold about the connection with sexual behaviour. But here two other contrasting factors enter: the alteration in time sense would change the apparent duration of sexual intercourse; and the predisposition to fantasy may replace sexual activity with images of it. There is, too, the unexplored possibility that the circulatory effects of cannabis include a mild genital engorgement.

'More important, however, is likely to be the effect of repeated use described as the "amotivational syndrome". This term dignifies a still imprecisely characterised state, ranging from a feeling of unease and sense of not being fully effective, up to a gross lethargy, with social passivity and deterioration. It is difficult to assess, when personal traits and intellectual rejection of technological civilisation are also taken into account. Yet the reversibility of the state, its association with cannabis use, and its recognition by cannabis users make it impossible to ignore.

'*Escalation theory*. Attention has mainly concentrated on progression from cannabis to heroin or other opiates. Although only a very small proportion of casual users progress, it is much commoner with heavy users, and the vast majority of opiate users have prior experience of cannabis. Although it is often said that there is no pharmacological basis for such progression, this in fact exists, since cannabis increases suggestibility and shares with heroin (though in milder form) the ability to produce euphoria and analgesia.

'But the situation is a more general one. It seems probable that amphetamine use also predisposes to heroin use; and the overlap in actions between cannabis and LSD makes intelligible the observed progression to LSD (accepted as significant by the Le Dain Commission).* The role of prior use of "soft" drugs, or use of drugs by "soft" techniques in predisposing to more serious abuse needs much more study, particularly by methods which can establish objectively the actual amount of drug used. Although it can only be one

* Le Dain Report. *Cannabis: a report of the Commission of Inquiry into the Non-medical use of drugs*. Ottawa, Canada: Info. Canada, 1972.

of many factors, it could be important in the prevention of serious abuse.

'*Tolerance and dependence*. Tolerance to the behavioural effects of cannabis and of THC in animals has now been repeatedly demonstrated. As with the fat-soluble barbiturates, the first few doses may cumulate, masking the underlying development of insensitivity to the drug's effects. It is not clear whether the tolerance results from increased destruction of the drug or a resistance at the cellular level.

'In man, tolerance and an abstinence syndrome has now been shown by controlled human experiment.* The tolerance may be partly biochemical, since there is limited evidence that THC disappears somewhat faster from the blood of users as compared with naive subjects; but metabolism is not the rate-limiting step in elimination, and tolerance in animals is not associated with lower levels of cannabinoid in the brain. Withdrawal symptoms of morphine or barbiturate type do not occur: but after heavy use, depression, anxiety, sleep disturbance, tremor and other symptoms develop, and many users find it very difficult to abandon cannabis use. In studies on self-administration by monkeys, spontaneous use did not occur, but once use was initiated, drug-seeking behaviour developed. Subjects who have become tolerant to LSD or opiates as a result of repeated dosage respond normally to cannabis but there appears to be cross-tolerance between cannabis and alcohol. . .

'*Finally*, cannabis occupies a fascinating position in the debate of what society should tolerate, and the outcome of the debate will be important. Despite the damage done in later life by alcoholism, it is possible to draw a line between it and cannabis, since alcohol is taken by mouth, occurs naturally in the body and is disposed of in hours, whereas cannabis is not only smoked, but the smoke must be inhaled and retained, and it and its metabolites persist for weeks. There seems no rational basis for drawing a line between cannabis on the one hand, and LSD, the amphetamines or the low-efficacy opioids on the other, especially now that it is known what high rates of cannabis consumption occur.'

The desired effects of cannabis, as of other psychodysleptics, depend not only on the expectation of the user and the dose, but also on the environmental situation and personality. Thus genial or revelatory experiences cannot be relied on to occur, despite optimistic reports, e.g. 'Haschich Fudge† (which anyone can whip up on a rainy day). This is the food of Paradise . . . euphoria and brilliant storms of laughter, ecstatic reveries and extension of one's personality on several simultaneous planes are to be complacently expected. Almost anything St. Teresa‡ did, you can do better . . .'

Reality is more prosaic. Acute panic can occur as well as 'flashbacks' of previously experienced hallucinations on LSD. Acute overdose causes sleep; it is claimed that death has not occurred.

Cannabis and skilled tasks (e.g. car driving). General performance in both motor and psychological tests deteriorates, more in naive than in experienced subjects. Effects may be similar to alcohol, but experiments in which the subject is unaware that he is being tested (and so does not compensate voluntarily) are difficult to do, as with alcohol. Some scientists claim the effects are negligible but this view has been 'put in proper perspective' by a commentator§ who asked how these scientists 'would feel if told that the pilot of their international jet taking them to a Psychologists' conference, was just having a reefer or two before opening up the controls.'

Legalisation of cannabis: see p. 391.

Medical use: see *nabilone* (Cesamet), an antiemetic.

STIMULANTS

Cocaine

Cocaine (see also local anaesthetics). Cocaine dependence is a widespread and ancient practice

* *Pharmacology of marihuana*: a monography of the National Institute of Drug Abuse. In: Braude M C, et al. eds. New York: Raven Press, 1976.

† From *The Alice B. Toklas Cook Book*. London: Michael Joseph, 1954. The author was companion to Gertrude (a rose is a rose is a rose) Stein (1874–1946).

‡ St. Teresa of Avila (1515–82) was noted for her power of levitation.

§ Dr. G. Milner.

amongst South American peasants who chew the leaves with lime to release the alkaloid. It is claimed to give relief from fatigue, hunger and altitude sickness in the Andes, experienced even by natives when journeying by car or other 'fast' transportation, and also to induce a pleasant introverted mental state. Remarkable feats of endurance attributed to chewing cocaine leaves have been reported, but there is no sound scientific confirmation of them. A United Nations enquiry into coca-leaf chewing reported that there was emotional but no physical dependence. It also reported that its use caused physical exhaustion rather than the reverse, and advocated gradual suppression in the interest of the populations concerned.* But what may have been (or even still may be) an acceptable feature of these ancient stable societies has now developed into a business, not for leaf chewing but for the manufacture and export of pure cocaine to supply an eager and lucrative demand from unhappy but economically richer societies where its use constitutes an intractable social problem. These economically developed societies, which cannot control social demand and importation, seek to eliminate the drug at its source in peasant societies that have come to rely on it for economic subsistence. Great distress results when coca plantations are destroyed, by a combination of economic deprivation and removal of the coca leaf, which, when used in the traditional way, helps to make tolerable lives of deprivation.

Cocaine (snow) is used as snuff (snorting), swallowed, smoked (below) or injected i.v. It is taken occasionally or repeatedly at short intervals (10–45 min) during 'runs' of hours to several days. After the 'run' there follows the 'crash' (dysphoria, irritability, hypersomnia) lasting hours to days. After the 'crash' there may be depression ('cocaine blues') and decreased capacity to experience pleasure for days to weeks.†

Emotional dependence may be severe, but physical dependence is slight or absent, as is tolerance.

The psychotropic effects of cocaine are similar to those of amphetamine (euphoria and excitement) but briefer and are due to blockade of the uptake of noradrenaline into adrenergic nerve endings, thus increasing its concentration at receptors; this information is relevant to treating overdose.

Intranasal use causes mucosal vasoconstriction, anosmia and eventually necrosis and perforation of the nasal septum.

Smoking involves converting the non-volatile HCl into the volatile 'free base' or 'crack' (by extracting the HCl with alkali), then vaporising it by heat (it pops or cracks); inhalation with breath-holding allows pulmonary absorption that is about as rapid as an i.v. injection. It induces an intense euphoric state. The mouth and pharynx become anaesthetized.

Intravenous use gives the expected rapid effect (kick, flash, rush). Cocaine may be mixed with heroin (as 'speedball').

The plasma $t_{\frac{1}{2}}$ of cocaine, is 50 min; it is metabolised by plasma esterases.

Overdose is common amongst users (up to 22% of heavy users report losing consciousness). The desired euphoria and excitement turns to acute fear, and fever, convulsions, hypertension, cardia dysrhythmias and hyperthermia may occur. Treatment is chosen according to the clinical picture (and the known mode of action), from amongst, e.g. chlorpromazine for mental disturbance and hypertension: diazepam for convulsions: labetalol or propranolol for hypertension, and appropriate antidysrhythmic agents.

Traders in illicit cocaine sometimes carry the drug in plastic bags concealed by swallowing or in the rectum ('body packing'). There have been instances of the packages leaking, with the inevitable fatal result.

Amphetamine, p. 362.

Khat

The leaves of the khat shrub (*Catha edulis*) contain an alkaloid (cathinone) structurally similar to amphetamine. They are chewed fresh (for maximum alkaloid content) so that the habit was confined to geographical areas favourable to the shrub (Arabia, E. Africa) until modern transpor-

* Report of commission of enquiry on coca leaf (April 1950). United Nations document E/1666.

† *Medical Letter* (1986) July 18.

tation allowed wider distribution. Khat chewers (mostly male) became euphoric, loquacious, excited, hyperactive and even manic. As with some other drug dependencies subjects may give priority to their drug needs above personal, family and other social and economic responsibilities. Cultivation takes up serious amounts of scarce arable land and irrigation water.*

Other drugs

Barbiturates, etc., see index.

Management of adverse reactions to psychodysleptics ('bad trips')

Mild and sometimes even severe episodes can be managed by reassurance including talk, 'talking the patient down', and physical contact, hand holding, etc. (LSD and mescaline). The objective is to help the patient relate his experience to reality and to appreciate that his mental experiences are drug-induced and will abate. Because short-term memory is disrupted the treatment can be very time-consuming since the therapist cannot absent himself without risking relapse. But with phencyclidine such intervention may have the opposite effect, i.e. overstimulation. It is therefore appropriate to sedate all anxious or excited subjects with diazepam (or chlorpromazine or haloperidol). With sedation the 'premorbid ego' may be rapidly re-established.

If the 'bad trip' is due to overdose of an anticholinergic drug, natural or synthetic, then diazepam is specially preferred, or a neuroleptic with no or minimal anticholinergic effects, e.g. haloperidol. A dose of anticholinesterase that penetrates the central nervous system (physostigmine 2–4 mg i.m.) is effective in severe reaction to an anticholinergic.

Drugs, skilled tasks, car driving

It is convenient to deal with the general topic here. There has already been some discussion on *alcohol* (p. 414) and on *cannabis* (p. 428). But many medicines also affect performance, and not only the obvious examples, *psychotropic drugs of all kinds, but also antihistamines, anticholinergics, analgesics including some NSAIDs (e.g. indomethacin), antiepileptics, antidiabetics (hypoglycaemia), some antihypertensives.*

It is plain that prescribers have a major responsibility here, both to warn patients and, in the case of those who need to drive for their work, to choose medicines having minimal liability to cause impairment. One example must suffice. In a study† of two histamine H_1-receptor blockers, terfenadine did not impair car driving tests (weaving amongst bollards and 'gap acceptance') whereas triprolidine did. Subjects who were aware of drowsiness were yet unable to compensate, so that it is not enough to warn drivers to be more careful if they feel drowsy; they should not drive.

Patients who must drive when taking a drug of known risk (e.g. benzodiazepine) should be specially warned of times of peak impairment.

A patient who has an accident and who was not warned of drug hazard, whether verbally or by labelling, may successfully sue the doctor in law. It is also necessary that patients are advised of the additive effect of alcohol with prescribed medicines.‡

Car driving is a complex multi-function task that includes§:

visual search and recognition
vigilance
information processing under variable demand
decision-making and risk-taking
sensorimotor control

It is evident that drivers may be more accident

* Khan I et al. Trends in Pharmacological Science Aug 1984, p. 326.

† Betts T et al. Br Med J 1984; 288:281.

‡ Nordic countries require that medicines liable to impair ability to drive or to operate machinery be labelled with a red triangle on a white background. The scheme covers antidepressants, benzodiazepines, hypnotics, drugs for motion sickness and allergy, cerebral stimulants, antiepileptics and hypotensive agents.

In the UK there are some standard labels that pharmacists are recommended to apply, e.g. No. 2: 'Warning. May cause drowsiness. If affected to not drive or operate machinery. Avoid alcoholic drink'. They are offered as 'a carefully considered balance between the unintelligibly short and the inconveniently long.' (see Brit. Nat. Formul.)

§ In: Willett R E et al., eds. Drugs, driving and traffic safety. Geneva: WHO, 1983.

prone without any subjective feeling of sedation or dysphoria: the fact that they feel OK does not mean that they are OK.

The criteria for safety in air-crew are necessarily more stringent than with car drivers.

Little is known of impairment and risk in skilled tasks other than driving. Concentration on physical injury should not distract from the possibility that those who live by their intellect and imagination (politicians and even journalists may be included here) may suffer from thoughtless prescribing.

Resumption of car driving or other skilled activity after *anaesthesia* is a special case, and an extremely variable one. The following suggestions may serve. After dentistry under local anaesthesia alone, 2 h. Where a sedative (e.g. i.v. benzodiazepine, opioid or neuroleptic), or any general anaesthetic has been used, 48 h. How the patient *feels* is not a reliable guide to recovery of skills.

GUIDE TO FURTHER READING

On non-medical use; drug dependence

1 Huxley A. The doors of perception. London: Chatto and Windus, 1954
2 De Quincey T. Confessions of an English opium eater. First published in 1821. Many editions since.
3 Final report of the Canadian Government's Commission of Inquiry into non-medical use of Drugs. Ottawa: Queen's Printer, 1973.
4 Schlicht J et al. Medical aspects of large outdoor festivals. Lancet 1972; 1:948.
5 Weiss B et al. Enhancement of human performance by caffeine and amphetamines. Pharmacol Rev 1962; 14:1.
6 Smith G M, et al. Amphetamine, secobarbital, and athletic performance. JAMA 1960; 172: 1502, 1623.
7 Freed D L et al. Anabolic steroids in athletics: crossover double-blind trial on weightlifters. Br Med J 1975; 2:1975.
8 Klein H G. Blood transfusion and athletics, games people play. N Engl J Med 1985; 312:854.
9 Burr A. Increased sales of opiates on the blackmarket in the Piccadilly (London) area. Br Med J 1983; 287:883.
10 Nicholi A M. The nontherapeutic use of psychoactive drugs: a modern epidemic. N Eng J Med 1983; 308:925.
11 Sourindrhin I. Solvent misuse. Br Med J 1985; 290:94.
12 Ghodse A H et al. Deaths of drug addicts in the UK 1967–81. Br Med J 1985; 290:425.
13 Wall M E et al. Metabolism, disposition and kinetics of delta-9-tetrahydrocannabinol in men and women. Clin Pharmacol Ther 1983; 34:352.
14 Bass M. Sudden sniffing death. JAMA 1970; 212:2075.
15 Connell P H et al. Necessary safeguards when prescribing opioid drugs to addicts: experience of drug dependence clinics in London. Br Med J 1984; 288:767.
16 Edwards G. Opium and after. Lancet 1980; 1:351.
17 Musto E F et al. A follow-up study of the new Haven (USA) morphine maintenance clinic of 1920. N Engl J Med 1981; 304:1071.
18 Higgins S T et al. Pupillary response to methadone challenge in heroin users. Clin Pharmacol Ther 1985; 37:460.
19 McCarron M M et al. The cocaine 'body packer' syndrome: diagnosis and treatment. JAMA 1983; 250:1417.

On tobacco

1 Royal College of Physicians, London. Smoking or Health. London: Pitman, 1977; and follow-up Report, Health or Smoking? (1983).
2 Smoking and Health. A report of the Surgeon General. US Dept. Health, Education and Welfare. DHEW Publication No (PHS) 79–50066, 1979.
3 Miller L C et al. Potential hazards of rapid smoking as a technique for modification of smoking behaviour. N Engl J Med 1977; 297:590.
4 Lyon J L et al. Cancer incidence in Mormons and non-Mormons in Utah, 1966–70. N Engl J Med 1976; 294:129.
5 Doll R et al. Mortality among doctors in different occupations. Br Med J 1977; 1:1433.
6 Doll R et al. Mortality in relation to smoking: 22 years' observations on female British doctors. Br Med J 1980; 1:967.
7 Manning F et al. Effect of cigarette smoking on fetal breathing movements in normal pregnancies. Br Med J 1975; 1:552.
8 Benowitz N L et al. Daily intake of nicotine during cigarette smoking. Clin Pharmacol Ther 1984; 35:499.
9 Vahakangas K et al. Cigarette smoking and drug metabolism. Clin Pharmacol Ther 1983; 33:375.
10 Ebert R V et al. Effect of nicotine chewing gum on plasma levels of cigarette smokers. Clin Pharmacol Ther 1984; 35:495.
11 Howe G et al. Effects of age, cigarette smoking, and other factors on fertility: findings in a large prospective study. Br Med J 1985; 290:1697.
12 Deanfield J et al. Cigarette smoking and treatment of angina with propranolol, atenolol and nifedipine. N Engl J Med 1984; 310:951.
13 Gillett R W et al. Deception among smokers. Br Med J 1978; 2:1185.
14 Schottenfeld D. Snuff dipper's cancer. N Engl J Med 1981; 304:778.
15 Wald N J et al. Does breathing other people's tobacco smoke cause cancer? Br Med J 1986; 293:1217.
16 Mulcahy R. Cigar and pipe smoking and the heart. Br Med J 1985; 290:951.
17 Raw M. Does nicotine chewing gum work? Br Med J 1985; 290:1231.
18 Chapman S. Stop-smoking clinics: a case for their abandonment. Lancet 1985; 1:918.
19 Boyd E J S et al. Smoking impairs therapeutic gastric inhibition. Lancet 1983; 1:95.
20 Logan R F A et al. Smoking and ulcerative colitis. Br Med J 1984; 288:751.
21 Daly L E et al. Long-term effect on mortality of stopping

smoking after unstable angina and myocardial infarction. Br Med J 1983; 287:324.
22 Wald N et al. Inhaling and lung cancer: an anomaly explained. Br Med J 1983; 287:1273.
23 Jones R M. Smoking before surgery: the case for stopping. Br Med J 1985; 290:1764.
24 Fielding J E. Smoking: Health effects and control. N Engl J Med 1985; 313:491, 555.
25 Weiss N S. Can *not* smoking be hazardous to your health. N Engl J Med 1985; 313:632.
26 Rosenberg N et al. The risk of myocardial infarction after quitting smoking in men under 55 years of age. N Engl J Med 1985; 313:1511.
27 Connolly G N et al. The re-emergence of smokeless tobacco. N Engl J Med 1986; 314:1020.

On alcohol: drugs and car driving.

1 Auty R M et al. Pharmacokinetics and pharmacodynamics of ethanol, whisky, and ethanol with n-propyl, n-butyl and iso-amyl alcohols. Clin Pharmacol Ther 1977; 22:242.
2 O'Keefe S J D et al. Lunchtime gin and tonic a cause of reactive hypoglycaemia. Lancet 1977; 1:1286.
3 Vestal R E et al. Aging and ethanol metabolism. Clin Pharmacol Ther 1977; 21:343.
4 Havard J D J. Alcohol and the driver. Br Med J 1978; 1:1595.
5 Wilkinson P K et al. Blood ethanol concentrations during constant rate intravenous infusion of alcohol. Clin Pharmacol Ther 1976; 19:213.
6 Vestal R E et al. Antipyrine metabolism in man: influence of age, alcohol, caffeine and smoking. Clin Pharmacol Ther 1975; 18:425.
7 Cohen J et al. The risk taken in driving under the influence of alcohol. Br Med J 1958; 1:1438.
8 Special correspondent. Road accidents: are drugs other than alcohol a hazard? Br Med J 1978; 2:1415.
9 Seppala T. Residual effects and skills related to driving after a single oral administration of diazepam, medazepam or lorazepam. Br J Clin Pharmacol 1976; 3:831.
10 Edwards G. Drinking problems: putting the third world on the map. Lancet 1979; 2:402.
11 Betts T et al. Effects of two antihistamine drugs on actual driving performance. Br Med J 1984; 288:281.
12 Dunbar J A et al. Are problem drinkers dangerous drivers. An investigation of arrest for drinking and driving, serum gamma-glutamyltranspeptidase activities, blood alcohol concentrations, and road accidents. Br Med J 1985; 290:827.
13 Nuotto E et al. Coffee and caffeine and alcohol effects on psychomotor function. Clin Pharmacol Ther 1982; 31:68.
14 Sellers E M et al. Drugs to decrease alcohol consumption. N Engl J Med 1981; 305:1255.
15 Harper C G et al. Brain shrinkage in chronic alcoholics: a pathological study. Br Med J 1985; 290:501.
16 Editorial. Alcohol and the fetus — is zero the only option? Lancet 1983; 1:682.
17 Noranjo C A et al. Nonpharmacologic intervention in acute alcohol withdrawal. Clin Pharmacol Ther 1983; 34:214.
18 Dorian E P et al. Triazolam and ethanol interaction, kinetic and dynamic consequences. Clin Pharmacol Ther 1985; 37:559.
19 Robertson I. Does moderate drinking cause mental impairment? Br Med J 1984; 289:711.
20 Edwards G et al. What happens to alcoholics? Lancet 1983; 2:269.
21 Lloyd G. I am an alcoholic. Br Med J 1982; 285:785.
22 Petersson B et al. Alcohol-related death: a major contributor to mortality in urban middle-aged men. Lancet 1982; 2:1088.
23 Johnson A D et al. Prevention of hazardous drinking: the value of laboratory tests. Br Med J 1985; 290:1849.
24 Lieber C S. To drink (moderately) or not to drink. N Engl J Med 1984; 310:846.
25 Fink R et al. Increased free-radical activity in alcoholics. Lancet 1985; 2:291.
26 Harper C et al. Are we drinking our neurones away? Br Med J 1987; 294: 534.

21

Anaesthesia and neuromuscular block

ANAESTHESIA

Until the mid-19th century such relief of pain as was possible during surgery was achieved with natural substances such as alcohol, opium, hyoscine*, cannabis and occasionally by concussion with a wooden bowl or by partial suffocation. The problem of inducing quick, safe and easily reversible unconsciousness for any desired length of time in man only began to be solved in the 1840s when the long-known substances nitrous oxide, ether and chloroform were introduced in rapid succession.

The details surrounding the first use of surgical anaesthesia make unedifying reading at times for there were bitter disputes on priority of discovery following an attempt to take out a patent for ether.

Sir James Simpson, who was to popularise chloroform, heard of the initial trials of ether in 1846 and wrote,† 'It is a glorious thought, I can think of naught else.' Just before his death in 1870 he summarised the chief events of the introduction of anaesthesia in the USA. 'It appears to me that we might correctly state the whole matter as follows:

'1. That on the 11th December, 1844, Dr. Wells had, at Hartford, by his own desire and suggestion, one of his upper molar teeth extracted without any pain, in consequence of his having deeply breathed nitrous oxide gas for the purpose, as suggested nearly half a century before by Sir Humphrey Davy.

'2. That having with others proved, in a limited series of cases, the anaesthetic powers of nitrous oxide gas, Dr. Wells proceeded to Boston to lay his discovery before the Medical School and Hospital there, but was unsuccessful in the single attempt which he made, in consequence of the gas-bag being removed too soon, and that he was hooted away by his audience, as if the whole matter were an imposition, and was totally discouraged.

'3. That Dr. Wells' former pupil and partner, Dr. Morton of Boston, was present with Dr. Wells when he made his experiments there.

* A Japanese pioneer of about 1800 wished to test the anaesthetic efficacy of a herbal mixture including solanaceous plants (hyoscine-type alkaloids). His elderly mother volunteered as subject since she was anyway expected to die soon. But the pioneer administered it to his wife for, 'as all three agreed, he could find another wife, but could never get another mother'. (JAMA 1966; 197: 10.)

† Comrie J D. *History of Scottish medicine*, 2nd ed. London: Baillière, Tindall and Cox, 1932, for Wellcome History of Medicine Museum.

'4. That on the 30th September, 1846, Dr. Morton extracted a tooth without any pain, whilst the patient was breathing sulphuric ether, this fact and discovery of itself making a NEW ERA in anaesthetics and in surgery.'

5 & 6 That ether was soon used in general surgery* and midwifery.

'7. That on the 15th November, 1847, the anaesthetic effects of chloroform were discovered in Edinburgh. . . .'†

Simpson undertook screening experiments, of a kind that would now only be done on animals, on himself and his colleagues. He tested a variety of substances. 'Late one evening' in 1847 'on returning home after a weary day's labour, Dr Simpson, with his two friends and assistants, Drs Keith and Matthews Duncan, set down to their somewhat hazardous work in Dr Simpson's dining-room. Having inhaled several substances, but without much effect, it occurred to Dr Simpson to try a ponderous material, which he had formerly set aside on a lumber-table, and which, on account of its great weight, he had hitherto regarded as of no likelihood whatever. That happened to be a small bottle of chloroform. It was searched for, and recovered from beneath a heap of waste paper. And, with each tumbler newly charged, the inhalers resumed their vocation. Immediately an unwonted hilarity seized the party; they became bright-eyed, very happy and very loquacious — expatiating on the delicious aroma of the new fluid. The conversation was of unusual intelligence, and quite charmed the listeners — some ladies of the family. . . There was a crash. 'On awaking, Dr Simpson's first perception was mental — "This is far stronger and better than ether" said he to himself.' His second was to note that he was prostrate on the floor and that among the friends about him there was both confusion and alarm.' Dr Duncan was unconscious beneath a chair and Dr Keith was struggling.

* In December 1846 the first operation in England under ether (amputation of the leg of a butler from Harley Street) was conducted at University College Hospital, London. The surgeon, Robert Liston, after removing the leg in 28 sec, a facility necessary to compensate for the previous lack of anaesthetics, turned to the watching students, saying, 'This Yankee dodge, Gentlemen, beats mesmerism hollow'. That night he anaesthetised his House Surgeon 'in the presence of two ladies'. (Merrington W R. *University College Hospital and its Medical School: A History*. London: Heinemann, 1976.)

† Its effects had, however, been discovered by a 17-year-old medical student and used in surgery in London some months earlier (Sykes W S. *Essays on the first hundred years of anaesthesia*. Edinburgh: Livingstone, 1961.)

It was not technical difficulties alone that had to be overcome before surgical anaesthesia could become acceptable.

'Dr Simpson refers, in his pamphlet on the religious objections which have been urged to chloroform, to the first operation ever performed — namely the extraction of the rib of Adam, as having been executed while our primogenitor was in a state of sopor, which the professor learnedly argues was similar to the anaesthesia of chloroform. He further draws a justification of his own proceedings from this history of the creation of man. Putting aside the impiety of making Jehovah an operating surgeon, and the absurdity of suggesting that anaesthesia would be necessary in His hands, Dr. Simpson surely forgets that the deep sleep of Adam took place before the introduction of pain into the world during his state of innocence.'‡

It is significant that the first two effective general anaesthetics, nitrous oxide and ether, are still, when used together, after nearly 150 years, the safest choice for an unpractised doctor who finds himself obliged by circumstances to administer a prolonged anaesthetic.

The next important developments in anaesthesia were in the 20th century when the development of new drugs both as primary general anaesthetics and as adjuvants (muscle relaxants), and new apparatus and clinical expertise in rendering prolonged anaesthesia safe, enabled the surgeon to increase his range. No longer was the duration and kind of surgery determined by patients' capacity to endure pain.

Stages of anaesthesia

Surgical anaesthesia using a single agent, e.g. ether, is classically divided into four *stages*, of

‡ Lancet 1848; 1:292.

which the third stage is subdivided into four *planes* (obviously, each merges with the next).

But the attainment of surgical anaesthesia (sleep, analgesia and muscular relaxation) with a single drug requires high doses that are liable to carry inconveniences and hazards (e.g. slow and unpleasant recovery, depression of cardiovascular function) and modern practice employs different drugs to attain each objective so that the classic stages no longer occur in visible succession.

Nevertheless, since these stages provide a background of understanding and since the conveniences of sophisticated practice are not always available, an account is provided, as follows:

The procession of stages derives from descriptions of ether anaesthesia in unpremedicated patients, a slow, unpleasant process. With modern techniques of i.v. anaesthesia and of premedicated inhalation, stages 1 and 2 may hardly be noticed by patient or anaesthetist, and with analgesics and muscle relaxants it is no longer necessary to give heavy doses of a single drug with its attendant disadvantages (see below). But they are retained here because they assist understanding.

Stage 1. Analgesia. Analgesia is partial until stage 2 is about to be reached. Consciousness and sense of touch are retained and sense of hearing is increased.

Stage 2. Delirium. The patient is unconscious, but automatic movements may occur. He may shout coherently or incoherently, become violent or leap up and run about. The prevention of these unpleasant manifestations lies in a skilful, smooth and quick induction in quiet surroundings. Sudden death, probably due to vagal inhibition of the heart or to sensitisation of the heart to adrenaline by the anaesthetic agent, may occur in a violent second stage.

Stage 3. Surgical anaesthesia. This is divided into four *planes* (See Figure 21.1) and the required depth differs according to the kind of operation to be performed. Depth is determined by noting characteristic changes in respiration, pupils, spontaneous eyeball movements, reflexes and muscle tone.

Stage 4. Medullary paralysis. Arrival at this stage constitutes an anaesthetic accident.

The practice of the anaesthetist

The practice of the anaesthetist has three main parts:

1. **Before surgery**, the assessment of the psychological and physical condition including the relevance of any existing drug therapy, all of which may influence the choice of the *premedication*, which may affect the choice of drugs in 2 below.
2. **During surgery**, the production of:
   a. *unconsciousness*.
   b. *analgesia*.
   c. *muscular relaxation*.

   Whilst all three can be produced by a single drug, e.g. ether, thiopentone, this carries disadvantages of heavy dosage (cardiac and respiratory depression, slow recovery) and it is usual to use a drug for each purpose from the wide range available.
3. **After surgery**, recovery, i.e. reversal of anaesthesia and neuromuscular block, and relief of pain and other aspects of postoperative care.

These three components are interdependent, the choice of drugs to be used at any one point affecting the choice of drugs both before and after; for instance drugs used in premedication may reduce both the amount of general anaesthetic and the postoperative medication required. Safety and comfort for the patient are paramount, and good operating conditions for the surgeon are also in the interest of the patient; but the provision of one may compromise the others. The problem may be approached in many different ways, using different combinations of the wide array of drugs that is available.

Simplicity leads to safety, for it is much easier to reach a clear diagnosis when few drugs have been given than when many drugs have inevitably confused the picture. With drugs, safety does not lie in numbers.

The anaesthetists' job is nowadays complicated by the fact that they are often presented with patients already taking drugs affecting the central nervous and cardiovascular systems.

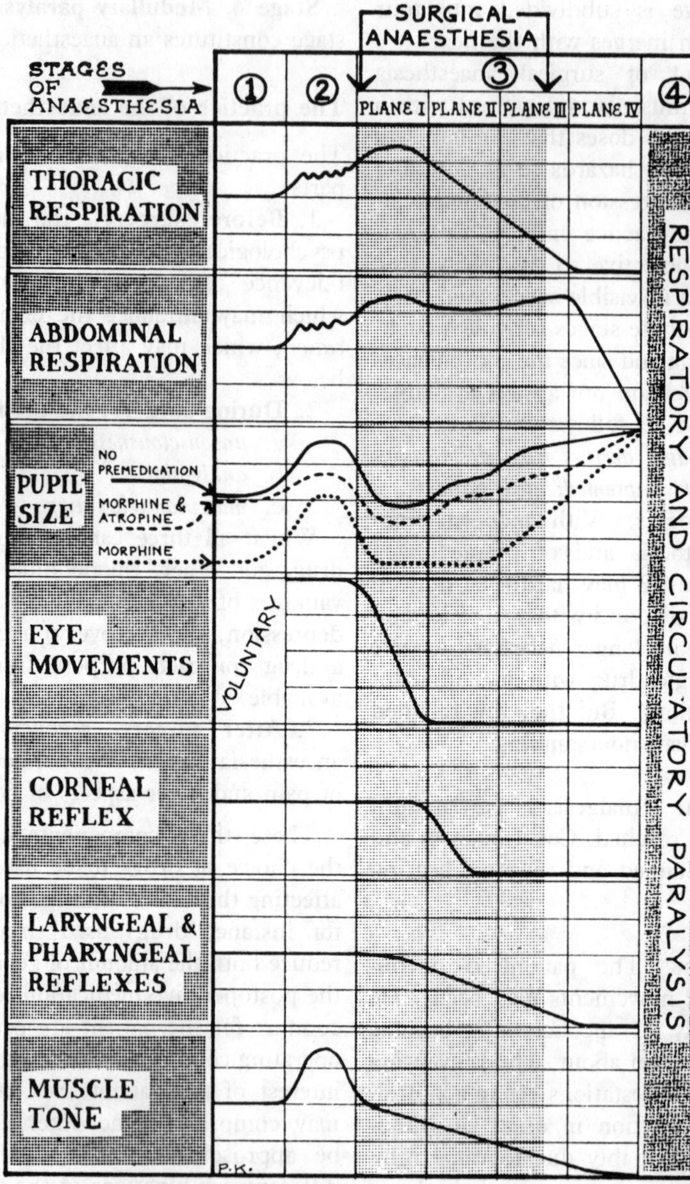

Fig. 21.1

The techniques of administration of anaesthetic drugs and the physical control of respiration are of great importance, but are outside the scope of this book. Premedication is treated relatively extensively as non-anaesthetists are more likely to find themselves concerned with it than with surgical anaesthesia.

Before surgery (premedication). The principal aims are to provide:

1. **Sedation and amnesia**. A patient who is going to have a surgical operation is naturally apprehensive, and it is kind to attempt to reduce this by explanation, reassurance and drugs. In one study a reassuring talk with the anaesthetist was found to have a greater calming effect than a barbiturate.* But it cannot be assumed that all

* Egbert L D et al. JAMA 1963; 185: 553

anaesthetists will be so successful. Preoperative preparation (which may commence on arrival in hospital for planned surgery, e.g. tranquillisers, and not merely 1 h before operation) is not solely humanitarian, for the discharge of adrenaline from the suprarenal medulla and the increased metabolic rate, which are concomitants of anxiety, render the patient both more difficult to anaesthetise and more liable to cardiac dysrhythmias with some anaesthetics (cyclopropane, halothane, trichloroethylene).

Stress-induced increase in plasma cortisol is suppressed by adequate premedication.

Virtually every hypnotic, sedative and tranquillising drug has been applied to premedication and claimed to have special utility, but morphine, morphine derivatives, hyoscine and benzodiazepines can meet most needs.

2. **Analgesia** (an opioid), when there is existing pain or as a supplement to an anaesthetic agent having low analgesic effect (e.g. nitrous oxide, thiopentone). However, if postoperative pain is expected an analgesic may be given both before and at the end of the operation without waiting for the patient to complain of pain. This helps to avoid the postoperative restlessness that occurs if only sedatives were used preoperatively. Subanaesthetic doses of barbiturates actually have an anti-analgesic effect.

3. **Inhibition of the parasympathetic autonomic system (anticholinergic agent)**

a. *the lungs*, to reduce bronchial secretions, which are liable to be profuse if an irritant drug such as ether is used, and to reduce any tendency to bronchospasm.

b. *the salivary glands*, to reduce secretion, for saliva may enter the larynx and cause laryngospasm.

c. *the heart* (vagus), to reduce the likelihood of cardiac dysrhythmias.

Atropine or hyoscine are generally used, s.c. or i.v. Hyoscine can cause confusion in the old. An alternative is *glycopyrronium*; it has low lipid solubility (it is highly ionized) and so it diffuses only slowly across cell membranes (e.g. into the brain, across the gut wall). It is used in anaesthesia because it produces less tachycardia than does atropine but has good mucous membrane antisecretory (drying) action, and because its duration of action is about twice that of atropine it is a better match for the duration of action of neostigmine given to reverse competitive neuromuscular block (see below).

The advent of new sedative and analgesic drugs has naturally led to much experimentation with premedication. In addition, with the increasing knowledge of the physiology and pharmacology of anaesthesia and the development of new anaesthetics, the disadvantages of the classic morphine and atropine routine, which has been in use for over 85 years, have become more obvious.

There is a tendency nowadays to use lighter premedication and to adjust it to the expected needs of the patient and of the procedure to be undertaken. Anaesthetists are no longer content to accept that tranquillity before induction can only be obtained at the cost of slow recovery with vomiting.

The desirability of interfering with parasympathetic responses with atropine has also been questioned. Now that non-irritant gases are available (halothane and allies), there is no need to block salivary and bronchial secretion unless an irritant inhalation (ether) is to be used. In addition, too dry a mucous membrane in the respiratory tract is disadvantageous in that ciliary activity is diminished, and viscous mucus is more likely to obstruct small bronchi. Vagal block is only needed if an anaesthetic that stimulates the vagus (halothane) is used, and then atropine is probably best given i.v. at the time of induction (remembering that it transiently stimulates the vagus before blocking it). Cardiac dysrhythmias due to sympathetic stimulation may be enhanced in the presence of vagal block. The usefulness of atropine and hyoscine as antiemetics, though also disputed, probably remains, especially if morphine has been used in premedication. In one study it was found that when morphine (10 mg) alone was used in premedication 67% of patients vomited after operation. After the addition of atropine (0.6 mg) to the premedication, only 35% of patients vomited, although the incidence of nausea and retching remained high.

Thus, premedication should be chosen in the light of knowledge of patients' temperaments and of the way they react to the approaching ordeal, of their disease, of the nature and likely duration of surgery, of their age and medical history, and of the anaesthetic agents that it is intended to use.

Though it is usual to give premedication 1 h before anaesthetic induction, anxious patients (the majority) will be grateful for sedation (by a benzodiazepine) from the start of the day of surgery or the night before.

Routes of administration. Traditionally, drugs are given s.c., but this is not always essential, and oral premedication can give good results, as well as wasting less of the nurses' time and being pleasanter for the patients, especially children. It is important to restrict the substances taken thus to the minimum amount or the dangers of regurgitation and aspiration are increased. (NB: the stomach is never empty and a tablet or two and a mouthful of water 2 h before surgery are not likely to make a significant addition to the volume of gastric juice already there.) Caution is needed in the case of children who may demand, and receive from too-kindly nurses, jam, sweets and biscuits as the price of co-operation.

Children provide a special opportunity for anaesthetists to demonstrate their skills; whether they and the nurses conspire to keep the children happy and fearless without premedication, and painlessly inject a barbiturate (and perhaps atropine) i.v. in the anaesthetic room, or whether sedation or narcosis* (oral, s.c., i.m.) is used. Rectal administration is acceptable though the dose may be expelled.

The following **suggested choices for premedication** have the sanction of long usage and will serve the unpractised who find themselves obliged to act as anaesthetist. They should only be generally abandoned for the newer techniques when these too have been proved by time. The inexperienced should not readily adopt novel practices in this, or, indeed, in any other complex situation.

Before general anaesthesia where analgesia is or will be needed morphine *plus* atropine (or hyoscine or glycopyrronium).

Before general anaesthesia where analgesia will not be needed benzodiazepine *alone or plus* atropine (or hyoscine or glycopyrronium).

Children: Trimeprazine or promethazine.

Premedication is generally given i.m. 1 h before operation. Hyoscine and promethazine are both sedative and anticholinergic. Many drugs used in anaesthetic premedication, for instance morphine and atropine, alter the pupil size and this will affect the utility of the pupils as a gauge of anaesthetic depth. A single dose of less than 1 mg atropine will not precipitate glaucoma.

A single dose of a gastric antacid may be given before a general anaesthetic as prophylaxis against aspiration of acid gastric contents (acid aspiration syndrome or Mendelson's syndrome); a histamine H_2-receptor blocker (e.g. ranitidine) is an alternative, to reduce gastric secretion volume and acidity.

During surgery.

The modern trend is to induce *sleep, analgesia* and *muscular relaxation* with separate drugs. This triad can be produced with a single drug in large doses but the consequences of the resulting deep anaesthesia are unpleasant and may be dangerous.

A typical general anaesthetic consists of:

1. *Induction*: thiopentone, i.v. (with suxamethonium if intubation is intended).

2. *Maintenance*: (a) with nitrous oxide plus a volatile agent, e.g. halothane or ether, if the patient is to breathe spontaneously.

(b) with nitrous oxide plus i.v. analgesic (e.g. fentanyl, morphine, pethidine) plus a neuromuscular blocking agent (e.g. tubocurarine) if muscle relaxation is needed for abdominal surgery (with tubocurarine, respiration will necessarily have to be provided by the anaesthetist); where neuromuscular block is used there is risk of a paralysed patient regaining consciousness, see under tubocurarine.

If a neuromuscular blocking drug is not used, muscle relaxation can be provided by deep anaesthesia with an inhalation agent (e.g. ether, enflurane, but not halothane; though this is not easy), or by nerve block with a local anaesthetic, according to circumstances.

In addition, special techniques such as the

* Narcosis prior to going to the anaesthetic room is demanding of staff as unconscious patients may not be left alone lest they suffocate.

production of hypotension or hypothermia may be required.

After surgery the anaesthetist ensures that the effects of neuromuscular blocking agents and opioid-induced respiratory depression have either worn off adequately or have been reversed by an antagonist; the patient must never be left alone until conscious, with protective reflexes restored and stable circulation.

'After operation the patient, who has already been submitted to preoperative medication and anaesthesia, may receive antibiotics; analgesics, sedatives and tranquillisers; purgatives and enemas; hypotensive or hypertensive agents; anticoagulants; cardiac stimulants or depressants; steroids, diuretics, and bronchodilators; and parenteral blood-volume expanders. To eliminate unnecessary drugs and reduce the use of others would be an act of clemency besides a welcome economy.'*

Drug elimination may increase in the postoperative period (e.g. increased hepatic metabolism). Reduced gut motility may delay absorption of drugs.

Relief of pain (see Ch. 16) after surgery presents many problems. Morphine and its derivatives are commonly used (usually intermittently, but sometimes by continuous i.v. infusion), but since they constipate, may cause vomiting, and depress cough and respiration, it will be appreciated that they have disadvantages, for instance after operations on the bowel and chest. Pethidine neither constipates nor suppresses spontaneous cough significantly, although it can be useful, given i.v., to reduce cough from an endotracheal tube. There is a wide choice from amongst the opioids and non-steroidal anti-inflammatory drugs. In a substantial study of 14 preparations, the following were found best: levorphanol (2 mg), pethidine (100 mg), oxycodone (10 mg), pentazocine (25 mg), morphine (10, 15 mg) plus cyclizine (50 mg) (Cyclimorph).† Inhalation of nitrous oxide/oxygen mixture (Entonox) is also effective (see nitrous oxide) for brief analgesia, e.g. defaecation after haemorrhoidectomy.

Postoperative **vomiting** is largely preventable by skilled technique including avoidance of drugs that are particularly liable to cause it (ether, cyclopropane). Antiemetics can be effective.

Some special techniques for:

1. *Single-handed operator/anesthetist*: For general anaesthesia this situation is unacceptably dangerous except in emergency.
2. *Repeated small procedures*, e.g. burns dressings.
3. *Minor procedures*, e g cardiac catheterisation, neuroradiology, endoscopy, cardioversion.

These situations require analgesia of varying degrees and sedation, without depression of respiration, so that the operator is not distracted by the need to guard the patient's airway.

Available techniques include:

Dissociative anaesthesia; i.e. a state of analgesia, and a light hypnosis (the eyes may remain open), see *ketamine*.

Neuroleptanalgesia, in which the patient is in a state of analgesia but is cooperative. It is produced by a combination of a neuroleptic (e.g. droperidol) and a high-efficacy opioid analgesic (e.g. fentanyl or alfenatil;) an alternative is use of diazepam (tranquilliser) with pentazocine (analgesic). But it is commonly used as a supplement to general anaesthesia.

Diazepam (i.v.)‡ can be used alone for procedures causing discomfort but not pain, e.g. endoscopy, and with a local anaesthetic where pain is expected, e.g. removal of impacted wisdom teeth. Anterograde amnesia is characteristic, the patient remains cooperative, respiratory depression is not usually important. Dose 10–40 mig i.v. slowly, about 2 mg/min until the patient becomes drowsy, the eyelids droop and speech is slurred; progress of sedation may be monitored by conversation with the patient. Midazolam or lorazepam are alternatives. Thiopentone rectally can be used for similar purposes.

None of the above is completely safe and respiratory depression and apnoea can occur especially in the elderly with cerebral atherosclerosis and patients with respiratory insufficiency. Laryngeal reflexes are not spared and inhalation of oral secretions or dental debris can occur.

* Editorial Lancet 1961; 2:589.
† Morrison J D et al. Br Med J 1971; 3:287.

‡ Diazepam solution is irritant and liable to cause local pain and thrombophlebitis; the complication is reduced by use of an oil-in-water emulsion (Diazemuls).

PHARMACOLOGY OF ANAESTHETIC DRUGS

All the successful general anaesthetics are given i.v. or by inhalation because these routes allow closest control over blood levels and so of brain levels.

Mode of action

How anaesthetics produce complete, controllable, reversible loss of consciousness remains uncertain.

General anaesthetics act on the brain, primarily on the midbrain reticular activating system and the cortex. A primary cellular site of action (of both general and local anaesthetics) seems to be along the axonal lipid bilayer membrane, which is disordered by the drugs so that cation (Na, K) movements through the protein pores, which are associated with action potentials, are obstructed. The fact that increased atmospheric pressure can reverse anaesthesia is held to be compatible with this hypothesis. Other sites of action include neurotransmitter release and effects postsynaptic membranes.

Many anaesthetics are very **fat-soluble** and there is good correlation between this and anaesthetic potency; the more fat-soluble tend to be the more potent anaesthetics, but such a correlation is not invariable. Some anaesthetic agents are not fat-soluble and many fat-soluble substances are not anaesthetic agents. There are no properties common to every agent and it is likely that there are several modes of action.

Pharmacokinetics of inhalation anaesthetics (volatile liquids: gases)

The level of anaesthesia is correlated with the tension (amount) of anaesthetic drug in the brain tissue and this is dependent on the development of a series of tension gradients from the high partial pressure delivered to the alveoli and decreasing through the blood to the brain and other tissues. These gradients are dependent on the physical properties of the anaesthetic and the tissues, as well as on physiological functions (ventilation, blood flow).

'Clinical anaesthetists have administered millions of anaesthetics during more than a century with little precise information of the uptake, distribution and elimination of inhalational and non-volatile anaesthetic agents. Considering how serious is the handicap of not knowing these fundamental and essential facts about the drugs they have used so often, the record of success and safety in clinical anaesthesia is an extraordinary accomplishment indeed. It can in some measure be attributed to the accumulated experience and successful teaching of a highly developed sense of intuition from generation to generation of anaesthetists. It can often be attributed in part to the ability to learn by error observing patients come uncomfortably close to injury and even to death.'*

It is not appropriate to discuss the detailed pharmacokinetics of anaesthetics here as they are chiefly important to professional anaesthetists, but a few points of general interest are mentioned below.

An anaesthetic that is *highly soluble* in blood (ether, methoxyflurane) will, if given at a steady concentration, provide a slow induction. This is because the blood acts as a reservoir for the drug so that it does not enter the brain rapidly until the blood reservoir has been filled. A rapid induction can be obtained by increasing the concentration of drug inhaled initially and by hyperventilating the patient. This is difficult to do with ether because it is so irritant, and dangerous to do with methoxyflurane because it depresses the cardiovascular system.

Agents that are *less soluble* in blood (nitrous oxide, cyclopropane, halothane), on the other hand, provide a rapid induction of anaesthesia because the blood reservoir is small and gas is available to pass into the brain sooner.

During induction of anaesthesia the blood is taking up anaesthetic gas selectively and rapidly and the loss of volume in the alveoli leads to a flow of gas into the lungs that is independent of respiratory activity. When the anaesthetic is withdrawn the reverse occurs and there is a diffusion of gas from the blood into the alveoli, which, in the case of nitrous oxide, can account for as much as 10% of the expired volume and so can significantly lower the alveolar oxygen concentration. Thus

* Papper E M. Br J Anaesth 1964; 36:124.

mild clinical anoxia occurs, and it may last for as long as 10 min, and, though harmless to most, it may be a factor in cardiac arrest in patients with reduced pulmonary and cardiac reserve, especially when administration of the gas has been at high concentration and prolonged, when the outflow is especially vigorous. Oxygen should therefore be given to such patients during the last few minutes of anaesthesia and the early postanaesthetic period.*

This phenomenon, *diffusion anoxia*, occurs with all gaseous anaesthetics, but is most prominent with gases that are relatively insoluble in blood, for they will diffuse out most rapidly when the drug is no longer inhaled, i.e. just as induction is faster, so is elimination. A combination of nitrous oxide and cyclopropane is therefore specially potent in this respect. Highly blood-soluble agents will diffuse out more slowly, so that recovery will be slower just as induction is slower, and with them diffusion anoxia is insignificant.

Pharmacokinetics of intravenous anaesthetics

While intravenous anaesthetics allow an extremely rapid induction because the blood concentration can be raised rapidly, there is no channel of elimination that can compete with the lungs for speed. The metabolic breakdown of many useful agents does not occur fast enough for really quick recovery and so reliance is put on rapid redistribution of the drug (e.g. thiopentone), which can only be satisfactory for brief operations. With prolonged use, recovery from thiopentone must be slower for the body is storing more and more of the drug and with repeated doses recovery depends on the mass of the storage tissues (muscle, fat), the blood flow through them, and the rate of metabolism and excretion of the drug. Attempts to use thiopentone i.v. as a sole anaesthetic agent in war casualties led to its being described as an ideal form of euthanasia†.

Therefore substances rapidly absorbed and rapidly excreted through the lungs still offer the best prospect of precise control (with continuous administration) even in the presence of pulmonary disease, except perhaps severe emphysema. Elimination of inhaled anaesthetics can be hastened by inducing hyperventilation. There is no quick method of eliminating drugs whose action is normally terminated by metabolism or by redistribution. For the present it is usual to approach the ideal by using a combination of drugs in such a way that the disadvantages of each are less prominent.

But the need to reduce atmospheric pollution by inhalation anaesthetics (including nitrous oxide) and the apparently increasing problem of awareness of paralysed patients under nitrous oxide maintenance have been accompanied by a revival of interest in the use of i.v. drugs as sole anaesthetic agents (*total intravenous anaesthesia*). The requirements for prompt and complete termination of anaesthesia are stringent, but they are increasingly being met by the newer agents such as ketamine and by combinations of drugs such as analgesic opioids (fentanyl) and sedatives (etomidate).

Comparisons of anaesthetics under routine clinical conditions are difficult to arrange, but they can be done.

Testing a new general anaesthetic on man presents a specially difficult problem. Now that existing techniques of anaesthesia are so safe it is hard to expect a patient undergoing the anxiety of approaching surgery to consent to an experimental trial of a new drug, and to administer the drug, in however cautious a fashion, without the patient's informed assent is certainly immoral and assuredly illegal. In at least one country (USA) the problem has been approached by paying volunteers to undergo careful administration of graduated doses in a laboratory, with extensive monitoring of cardiovascular, respiratory and central nervous functions.

Comparison of potency of inhalation drugs both for efficacy and adverse effects (e.g. cardiac depression) may be done by measuring the minimum alveolar concentration required to prevent reflex response to a surgical skin incision in 50% of subjects (MAC_{50}), or the MAC that prevents response in 95% of subjects (MAC_{95}),

* Oxygen is important in the post-anaesthetic period for other and often more important reasons, e.g. failure to remove neuromuscular block adequately, central respiratory depression and respiratory obstruction.

† Halford J J. A critique of intravenous anaesthesia in war surgery. Anesthesiology 1943; 4:67.

which is closer to real life clinical practice. A second point on the dose-response curve can be obtained for the MAC that just allows response to a spoken command. For non-volatile i.v. anaesthetics of which a dose can be accurately administered as a bolus or infusion, the equivalent is the anaesthetic dose that prevents movement in response to the noxious stimulus (AD_{95}); or the minimum infusion dose.

INHALATION AGENTS

The preferred inhalation agents are those that are minimally irritant and non-flammable and comprise *nitrous oxide* and the fluorinated hydrocarbons, i.e. *halothane* and its allies, enflurane and isoflurane. But the irritant, explosive ether is cheap and relatively safe in unskilled hands so that it retains a place in some parts of the world.

Nitrous oxide (1844) is a safe anaesthetic gas provided that it is used correctly. Untoward effects are due to anoxia resulting from unskilled use or to megaloblastic bone marrow depression from prolonged use (many hours) in intensive care, e.g. after cardiac operations (inhibition of a vitamin B_{12} coenzyme necessary for folate metabolism). It is an effective analgesic but a comparatively inefficacious anaesthetic and cannot alone maintain surgical anaesthesia. For this reason it is commonly used with other analgesics or as a vehicle for other inhalants such as halothane. It is used alone for very brief operations (e.g. dental). Induction and recovery are rapid. It is not explosive, but supports combustion. Nitrous oxide diffuses into any air- containing space in the body causing an increase in pressure that can be dangerous, e.g. in a pneumothorax.

Nitrous oxide, inhaled as a 50% mixture with oxygen, is used as a self-administered analgesic, in obstetrics, for changing painful dressings, etc., and also in postoperative pain and myocardial infarction; it is also useful to take to the site of accidents. Premixed cylinders (Entonox) are cheaper to produce than are machines that mix the gases from separate cylinders, but they can give trouble in cold climates in one respect; if cooled to −8°C the gases liquefy and practically separate so that at first a high concentration of oxygen is delivered, and pain is not relieved; this is followed by delivery of a dangerously low concentration of oxygen. Apart from avoiding cooling this can be minimised by keeping and using cylinders on their side, not upright; by immersing the cylinder in warm water and inverting it three times before use, or by keeping it at 10°C or more (room temperature) for 2 h before use.

Halothane (Fluothane, 1956) is an extremely convenient anaesthetic, being potent, and only slightly irritant (less coughing and breath-holding). Induction and recovery are quick and it is non-flammable. However it has four important disadvantages; it causes hypotension, respiratory depression, bradycardia and cardiac dysrhythmias; the heart is sensitised to adrenaline and noradrenaline. Despite these and its expense, the good qualities of halothane have gained it a major place in routine anaesthetic practice.

Halothane, especially when administered repeatedly has been incriminated as rarely causing acute hepatocellular damage, *halothane hepatitis*. The mechanisms are uncertain, whether due to idiosyncratic metabolism of halothane, or to an immune reaction in which the drug or its metabolites provoke an altered antigenicity of some hepatic cell components. Controversy continues.

The major difficulties are the rarity of the event (< 1:10 000 and getting rarer as precautions seem to become effective) and that, lacking any clear diagnostic feature, it is difficult to be certain in any one case that the jaundice is not due to another factor, e.g. pre-existing disease, virus infection.

Current practice is to avoid a second administration of halothane within 2 months (ideally 4–6 months), to study the postoperative course of any previous use of halothane for any indication suggestive of minor liver injury, fever (especially unexplained fever lasting more than 5 days) or jaundice, and to avoid halothane in such cases. Additional risk factors appear to be female sex, obesity, middle age, hypoxia and hepatic enzyme induction.

Kinetics. Halothane is a liquid, boiling at 50°C. About 70% is eliminated via the lungs in the 24 h after use, but about 10% is metabolised in the liver and it induces hepatic drug metabolising enzymes; indeed, anaesthetists using it may themselves be in a state of partial enzyme induction.

Enflurane (1966) is similar to halothane but less potent, and it may be safer with adrenaline. It is less metabolised than halothane and may not cause hepatitis. It can cause convulsions.

Isoflurane (1982) is an isomer of enflurane and being somewhat less lipid soluble than either halothane or enflurane it provides quicker induction. It is metabolized to only a small extent (one-tenth that of enflurane and one-hundredth that of halothane), which means that organ toxicity to patients and to personnel is likely to be low*. It is less depressant to the cardiovascular system than its allies, though it causes vasodilatation, which can be useful for deliberate induction of hypotension. It probably sensitizes the heart to catecholamines less than its allies. It can be self-administered for obstetric analgesia. Its use is limited by cost.

Ethyl ether (1842) is relatively non-toxic and is justly reputed to be a safe drug even in unpractised hands. This is because the blood concentration that stops respiration is less than that which stops the heart, so that there is greater opportunity to retrieve an adverse situation. It is easier to provide artificial respiration than it is to start an arrested heart.

But the use of ether is declining because of two big disadvantages. Its vapour is *flammable* in air and explosive in oxygen, and induction of anaesthesia is slow (see pharmacokinetics, above) and therefore unpleasant to patients; though induction can be hastened by adding a little halothane or stimulating respiration with CO_2. The pungent smell is objectionable and irritation of the respiratory tract leads to coughing, laryngeal spasm and increased mucus secretion. Ether also causes vasodilatation, which, in the third plane of the third stage, may be great enough to cause severe fall in blood pressure. It increases capillary bleeding.

A vigorous sympathetic autonomic response normally occurs during ether anaesthesia and counteracts the circulatory effects. If this response fails then circulatory collapse may occur, obviously especially in patients taking a β-adrenoceptor blocker. The hyperglycaemia that occurs is chiefly due to release of adrenaline.

If ether anaesthesia is deep and prolonged, recovery is slow and postoperative vomiting occurs, largely due to swallowing saliva containing ether. Beside these disadvantages must be placed the very practical advantage that, for a given degree of competence, anaesthetic deaths with simple techniques using ether are less common than with more complicated techniques employing other drugs.

Liquid ether boils at 35°C and so may prove inconvenient in hot climates, and as it is heavier than air a dangerous flammable layer may accumulate near the floor of the operating theatre.

When open drop administration is used it is important to avoid getting ether into the eyes or on to the skin because it is irritant.

Convulsions are a rare complication of ether anaesthesia. They are thought to be the result of a combination of circumstances, and are most common in children. They are promoted by deep anesthesia, sepsis, atropine premedication, fever or overheating, and carbon dioxide retention. They are dangerous and can be largely avoided. Treatment is by cooling, and i.v. diazepam or barbiturate for convulsions; oxygen and artificial respiration may be needed after giving the anti-convulsant because convulsions are followed by respiratory depression, which is increased by the treatment.

Ether decomposes, forming toxic aldehydes and peroxides, unless protected from light and heat. Addition of carbon dioxide and copper delay decomposition. Very old ether should be suspected and discarded if possible.

Ethyl chloride (1844) is so highly potent as to be regarded as dangerous even for quick induction, which it provides. It is flammable and explosive; it boils at 12°C and so has to be kept under pressure if it is to be liquid at room temperature. Because of its extreme volatility it may be used for local anaesthesia, for which purpose it is sprayed on the skin, and, in vaporising, paralyses sensory nerve endings by cooling (cryoanalgesia); chlorofluoromethanes are also used.

Chloroform (1847) was the only non-explosive

* Editorial. Isoflurane. Lancet 1985; 2: 537.

potent anaesthetic until the introduction of trichloroethylene in 1934. But now, owing to cardiac depression, hepatic toxicity and the development of alternatives, it is obsolete.

Cyclopropane (1929) is a potent, explosive, non-irritant gas. It is preferable to halothane when a quick induction is desired and it is particularly desired to avoid hypotension. It sensitises the heart to adrenaline and this, together with the carbon dioxide retention that results from respiratory depression, promotes cardiac dysrhythmias. It tends to cause laryngospasm. When cyclopropane is withdrawn there is sometimes a sudden drop in blood pressure, 'cyclopropane shock', which is said to be due to the rapid fall in carbon dioxide in the blood.

Trichloroethylene (1934) is similar to chloroform but less toxic. It is seldom used for surgical anaesthesia because it is both a weak anaesthetic agent and liable to cause tachypnoea and cardiac dysrhythmias. It is an effective analgesic and its use is now almost confined to obstetrics (rarely) where, in special vaporisers that prevent overdose, it can be self-administered. Trichloroethylene should not be used in carbon dioxide absorption systems for it decomposes in contract with soda lime to form toxic products, which may be the cause of cranial nerve damage (especially 5th nerve). It also decomposes if exposed to light and air. It is non-flammable and is non-irritant in anaesthetic concentrations.

Atmospheric pollution of operating theatres by inhalation anaesthetics is suspected of being harmful to theatre personnel. An anaesthetist working with halothane can accumulate in 3–4 h amounts that will not be eliminated completely by the following morning. Epidemiological studies have raised questions relating to excess of fetal malformations and miscarriages, hepatitis and cancer in operating theatre personnel. It seems likely that, at least, the risk of miscarriage is real (due to nitrous oxide). Theatre staff becoming or seeking to become pregnant should not work in a contaminated environment.*

It was reported in 1972† that anaesthetists in the USSR had applied for a 15% salary bonus for working in a hazardous atmosphere. But it would seem a better solution to spend money on eliminating risk than on paying people to accept it. Risk can be reduced by use of circle systems that allow low fresh gas flows, scavenging systems, improved ventilation of theatres (a minor contribution), filters that absorb volatile agents but not nitrous oxide; by using regional anaesthesia or total i.v. anaesthesia (i.e. no other drugs used) in preference to inhalation wherever feasible. The continued dominance of inhalation anaesthesia is a remarkable tribute to the pharmacokinetics of anaesthetic gases.

INTRAVENOUS ANAESTHETICS

Thiopentone sodium is the most widely used i.v. anaesthetic. It is highly effective and quick acting and is especially suited to providing a pleasant induction. Anaesthesia may be induced in a healthy adult by injecting i.v. 4–6 ml of a 2.5% solution (i.e. 100–150 mg) in 30 sec (a 5% solution is prone to cause venous thrombosis) and waiting at least 1 min before injecting more. In those with a slow circulation time (the old, the diseased) injection should be slower. Laryngospasm is said to be comparatively frequent. The great rapidity with which a patient may pass through the stages of anaesthesia (Figure 21.1) means that the first obvious sign of overdose may be apnoea. Great care is therefore necessary when using thiopentone. Anaesthesia may be continued by nitrous oxide, supplemented if necessary by an analgesic i.v. or by another inhalation agent, e.g. halothane, for thiopentone does not prevent reflex response (raised blood pressure and heart rate, muscular contraction) to painful stimuli and it is therefore unsatisfactory by itself for painful operations, struggling and laryngospasm resulting from any attempt to use it thus. Another disadvantage is respiratory depression, which is relatively greater for a given degree of muscular relaxation than is the case with inhalants. It is also dangerous in

* Air in surgical theatres often exceeds the concentrations (nitrous oxide 25 parts per million: halothane 2.0 ppm) recommended by the American National Institute of Occupational Safety and Health.

† Editorial. Anaesthesia 1972; 27: 1.

oligaemic patients because it abolishes compensatory vasoconstriction (as do all anaesthetic agents at high dose) and it may cause dangerous hypotension in the elderly or the arteriosclerotic.

Kinetics. In the early phase of an i.v. injection, the plasma $t_{\frac{1}{2}}$ of thiopentone is 2.5 min and after equilibration the average $t_{\frac{1}{2}}$ is 8 h. Free thiopentone rapidly enters the brain from the blood; consciousness is lost in about 20 sec and equilibration between blood and brain occurs in 30–60 s; it is about 75% bound to plasma proteins and it is this extensive protein uptake that requires the initial i.v. injection to be fairly rapid (see above) to get a high free concentration and so a quick loss of consciousness. Thiopentone is almost completely metabolised.

The comparatively rapid recovery from a single dose is due to *redistribution* of the drug into the well-perfused viscera and lean tissues of the body. Fat is not as important an element in this redistribution as was previously supposed, for, though thiopentone is highly fat soluble, fat has a low blood flow compared with the other tissues. Thus rapid recovery may follow several repeated doses of thiopentone until the time comes when the tissues can store no more drug, i.e. have equilibrated with the blood. A further dose then produces prolonged anaesthesia, as recovery now depends on destruction of the drug and not on redistribution. It is inadvisable to exceed a total of 1.0 g thiopentone in any operation.

Injection other than into the vein is dangerous. If it is given subcutaneously the skin may slough. Given into or around a nerve (usually the median), permanent palsy may follow. To dilute the irritant solution, and to induce local hyperaemia to hasten absorption, 0.5% lignocaine (without adrenaline) may be injected into the site. In the case of nerve injury it may be desirable to incise the area and try to wash out the drug. If thiopentone is accidentally injected into an *artery*, thrombosis occurs and amputation may even become necessary. Treatment of this mishap is to heparinise the patient immediately and perhaps to block the sympathetic supply to the limb, e.g. stellate ganglion block. Vasodilator drugs are probably not helpful. The arm should be kept cold to reduce oxygen requirements. Surgical removal of the clot may be tried after about 6 h if there is no improvement in the physical signs. Heparin may be continued, or oral anticoagulant therapy begun, with allowance for surgery, until it is sure that all is well, which will probably mean about a week. Serious consequences from these mishaps are unlikely if 2.5% solution rather than 5% solution is used, and damage to arteries or nerves is less likely if the lateral border of the forearm and the back of the hand are chosen for injection and the vessel is palpated (without a tourniquet on the arm) before inserting the needle.

Methohexitone is similar, but provides rather quicker recovery and so is suited for use in outpatients.

There are other i.v. agents for general anaesthesia. None has been proved superior in routine use to thiopentone.

Ketamine (Ketalar) is related to phencyclidine (a hallucinogen); it induces 'dissociative anaesthesia', i.e. profound analgesia with light sleep (the eyes may remain open); pharyngeal reflexes are retained, but cannot be relied upon to prevent regurgitation. There is increased muscle tone; the blood pressure commonly rises; respiratory depression can occur. Given i.v. ketamine anaesthetises in about 30 sec and i.m. in about 3 min. Anaesthesia lasts about 5–20 min. The $t_{\frac{1}{2}}$ is 2–4 h. Unpleasant dreams and hallucinations lasting up to 24 h are characteristic and may be accompanied by 'emergence delirium'. These unpleasantnesses can be reduced by concomitant use of an opioid or a benzodiazepine, and provision of tranquil environment during recovery (emergence).

Combinations of a neuroleptic (an antipsychotic drug which also increases muscle tone) **with a potent narcotic analgesic** are used to induce 'neuroleptanalgesia' during which the patient may remain cooperative. Injected slowly i.v. they induce sedation and analgesia in a few minutes. Respiratory depression occurs. Combinations include Thalamonal (droperidol, a butyrophenone; plus fentanyl, related to pethidine); phenoperidine is an alternative to fentanyl.

Diazepam (i.v.) see p. 439.

Etomidate is structurally related to tolazoline (an α-adrenoceptor blocker), it is given i.v. and sleep lasts for 6–10 min. Though asleep, patients are not protected against noxious (painful) stimuli and analgesic premedication is needed for painful operations. Cardiovascular depression is slight. Metabolism is rapid. Prolonged infusion (sedation in intensive care) causes an inhibition of adrenocortical steroidogenesis that is unresponsive to corticotrophin, and etomidate should be confined to induction and brief procedures.

Propofol. An i.v. induction dose produces unconsciousness in about 30 seconds. It is metabolised with a $t_{\frac{1}{2}}$ of 40 min. Recovery occurs about 4 min after the last bolus dose, i.e. there is no clinically important accumulation in tissues.

NEUROMUSCULAR BLOCKING DRUGS

These substances first attracted scientific notice because of their use as arrow poisons by the natives of South America, who use the most famous of all, curare. Specimens of crude curare had been reaching Europe before 1811 when Sir Benjamin Brodie smeared 'woorara paste' on wounds of guinea-pigs and noted that death could be delayed by inflating the lungs through a tube introduced into the trachea. Though he did not continue until complete recovery, he did suggest that the drug might be of use in tetanus. A year later the traveller Charles Waterton visited South America to seek 'the deadly wourali poison'.* He obtained a specimen and tried it on a sloth, 'from the time the poison began to operate, you would have conjectured that sleep was over-powering it and you would have exclaimed, "Pressitque jacentem, dulcis et alta quies, placidæque simillima morti".' He also used it on an ox 'whose flesh was very sweet and savoury at dinner'. Having noted that 'it totally destroys all tension in the muscles' Waterton turned to experiment on a fowl with reputed antidotes. He held the bird up to its mouth in water, poured sugar-cane juice and rum down its throat and filled its mouth with salt, but despite, or perhaps because of, this treatment, the bird died. He discussed the most promising antidote but did not then try it: 'It is supposed by some, that wind introduced into the lungs by means of a small pair of bellows, would revive the poisoned patient, provided the operation be continued for a sufficient length of time. It may be so; but this is a difficult and a tedious mode of cure.'

On his return to England he experimented on a donkey which 'died apparently' in 10 min. He incised the windpipe and inflated the lungs with bellows for 2 h which 'saved the ass from final dissolution'. She recovered, was named Wouralia, and was kept in idleness by a sentimental peer for the remaining 25 years of her life.

Despite attempts to use curare for a variety of diseases including epilepsy, chorea and rabies, the lack of pure and accurately standardised preparations as well as the absence of convenient routine techniques of artifical respiration if overdose occurred, prevented it from gaining any firm place in medical practice until 1942, when these difficulties were removed.

Drugs acting at the myoneural junction produce complete paralysis of all voluntary muscle so that movement is impossible and artificial respiration is needed. Attempts to achieve selective relaxation, sparing respiration, in the treatment of convulsions and disorders of muscle tone, have been unsuccessful.

The necessity for artificial respiration no longer deters anaesthetists, who are now quite accustomed to taking over respiration from the patient as a routine. It is plainly important that a paralysed patient should be in a state of full analgesia and unconscious during surgery (see below).

Neuromuscular transmission and its modification by drugs

When an impulse passes down a motor nerve to voluntary muscle it causes release of acetylcholine at the nerve endings. This modifies the condition of the membrane of the motor end-plate, a specialised area on the muscle fibre. In its resting state the inside of the membrane is electrically negative with respect to the outside and is said to be polarised. The acetylcholine causes an increase in the permeability of this membrane to some ions so that depolarisation occurs, and this triggers the

* Waterton C. *Wanderings in South America*. Revised edition 1828. Reprinted by Hutchinson, London, 1906. Numerous other editions.

action potential that is associated with contraction of the muscle.

Neuromuscular blocking agents used in clinical practice interfere with the process described above. However, substances that prevent the release of acetylcholine at nerve endings exist, e.g. Cl. botulinum toxin A (Dysport), used in blepharospasm, some venoms and analogues of choline.

There are *two principal mechanisms* by which drugs used clinically interfere with neuromuscular transmission:

By competition (tubocurarine, gallamine, pancuronium, alcuronium, vecuronium, atracurim). These drugs compete with acetylcholine for the cholinergic receptors. They do not cause depolarisation themselves but they protect the end-plate from depolarisation by acetylcholine. The result is a flaccid paralysis.

Reversal of this type of neuromuscular block can be achieved with anticholinesterase drugs, such as neostigmine, which prevent the destruction by cholinesterase of acetylcholine released at nerve endings, allow the concentration to build up and so reduce the competitive effect of a given concentration of blocking agent.

By depolarisation (suxamethonium). Such drugs imitate the action of acetylcholine at the motor end-plate and at their first application voluntary muscle contracts, but, as they are not destroyed immediately like acetylcholine, the depolarisation persists. It might be expected that this prolonged depolarisation would result in muscles remaining contracted, but this is not so (except in chickens), probably because the drug also causes a decrease in excitability of the area around the end-plate; although a standing depolarisation of the end-plate persists, it is not strong enough to maintain the muscle in contraction. The cause of neuromuscular block by these drugs may therefore be the reduction in excitability of the muscle rather than the depolarisation, although these two effects may be interdependent.

Anticholinesterase drugs in big doses can produce neuromuscular block by depolarisation but cannot be used clinically for this purpose because of their effect on the central and autonomic nervous systems (but they have been developed for chemical warfare and as selective insecticides). Anticholinesterases are thus not only useless as antidotes to depolarising drugs but may even increase the paralysis. However, with prolonged administration a depolarisation block changes to a competitive block (dual block). Because of the uncertainty of this situation a competitive blocking agent is preferred for anything other than short procedures.

Neuromuscular blocking agents acting by competition (non-depolarising)

Tubocurarine* is an alkaloid that produces neuromuscular block by competition with acetylcholine. The peripheral site of action of curare was demonstrated by Claude Bernard in 1850 in a famous series of simple experiments on frogs. Its chief use is to provide muscle relaxation during surgery without incurring the disadvantages of deep anaesthesia. Its introduction into surgery made it desirable to decide once and for all whether the drug altered consciousness. Doubts were resolved in a single experiment.† A normal subject was slowly curarised after arranging a detailed and complicated system of communication. Twelve minutes after beginning the slow infusion of curare, the subject, having artificial respiration, could move only his head. He indicated that the experience was not unpleasant, that he was mentally clear and did not want an endotracheal tube inserted. After 22 min, communication was possible only by slight movement of the left eyebrow and after 35 min paralysis was complete and direct communication lost. An airway was inserted. The subject's eyelids were then lifted for him and the resulting inhibition of alpha rhythm of the electroencephalogram suggested that vision and consciousness were normal. After recovery, aided by neostigmine, the subject reported that he had been mentally 'clear as a bell' throughout, and confirmed this by recalling what he had heard and seen. The insertion of the endotracheal airway had caused only minor

* Curare is the crude plant preparation. The word is often used loosely when one of the pure alkaloids is, in fact, intended.
† Smith S M et al. Anesthesiology 1947; 8: 1.

discomfort, perhaps because of the prevention of reflex muscle spasm. During artificial respiration he had 'felt that (he) would give anything to be able to take one deep breath' despite adequate oxygenation. In another study curare was excluded from one arm by an inflated cuff so that the subject could make finger signals,* and this isolated forearm technique can be used to detect wakefulness in clinical anaesthesia.†

It is plainly essential to ensure that paralysed patients do not regain awareness unnoticed during surgery. That this is not merely a theoretical risk is shown by the occasion when an anaesthetist, visiting his patient the day after the operation, was horrified when she sympathetically remarked, 'I had no idea you doctors were so badly paid'. He had discussed the inadequacy of his salary with a colleague during the operation. The patient had felt her bowels being manipulated but no pain. However, pain can occur on such occasions, and both anaestheists and patients will wish to avoid them. Awareness is most likely when nitrous oxide and oxygen are being used with neuromuscular block, and reflex signs suggestive of pain include bronchospasm, sweating and response of the pupil to light, as well as movement; but awareness can occur without these accompaniments.

In addition to its neuromuscular blocking effect tubocurarine blocks autonomic ganglia and causes tissue *histamine release*. Both these effects may cause a transient drop in blood pressure (which can be made use of), and the latter may induce bronchospasm.

Curare is *insignificantly absorbed from the alimentary tract*, a fact known to the South American Indians, who use it to procure food, as well as in war.

After an i.v. *injection* the action is maximal in 4 min and lasts usefully for 30 min (the $t_{\frac{1}{2}}$ for *effect* is about 50 min).

Tubocurarine is partly *excreted* unchanged in the urine and partly metabolised. But the brief action of single doses is partly due to redistribution of the drug in the body rather than to its elimination. It follows therefore that repeated use over a few days may result in prolongation of action of the later doses.

Tubocurarine is well tolerated at all ages, except perhaps in neonates, though there is enough individual variation for some anaesthesists to advise a small initial test dose routinely.

Potentiation occurs with ether and with chlorpromazine, and some *antibiotics* (aminoglycosides) can cause neuromuscular block and synergise with competitive blocking agents. But this is only clinically important if they are used in situations where overdose is easy, e.g. when they are tipped into the pleural or peritoneal cavities at operation, e.g. neomycin.

Apart from occasional prolongation of action for unknown reasons, after-effects of tubocurarine are slight, although diplopia may rarely persist for a few days. It is preferred for Caesarian section as it enters the fetus less than do others.

The action of tubocurarine is *antagonised* by anticholinesterase drugs. Neostigmine (2–3 mg of the methylsulphate) is usually given intravenously, preceded by atropine (1.2 mg) or glycopyrronium to prevent the parasympathetic autonomic effects of the neostigmine (especially the vagal bradycardia). The patient may rarely relapse into paralysis again and so must be carefully watched. Too much neostigmine can cause neuromuscular block by depolarisation, which will cause confusion unless there have been some signs of recovery before neostigmine is given. Progress can be monitored with a nerve stimulator.

It is theoretically undesirable to give atropine and neostigmine in full doses i.v. simultaneously, for atropine, before blocking the vagus nerve, causes, by a central action, transient vagal stimulation (except in blacks). If this is added to the effect of neostigmine, excessive cardiac slowing may result. Atropine is therefore best given a few minutes before the neostigmine.

Dose: Tubocurarine: initially 10–15 mg, i.v. (or i.m.); then supplements according to response.

Whenever tubocurarine is used mechanical ventilation is essential.

A variety of alternatives to tubocurarine provide properties that often render them preferable.

Pancuronium and **gallamine** differ from tubocurarine in that they act a little sooner, and do not

* Campbell E J M et al. Clin Sci 1969; 36: 323.
† Wilson M E. Br J Anaesth 1981; 53: 1234.

release histamine, both desirable properties. They cause tachycardia (especially gallamine).

Alcuronium is similar to tubocurarine. **Vecuronium** is shorter acting, does not cause tachycardia and is excreted via the bile.

Atracurium is unique in that it is altered spontaneously in the body to an inactive form by a passive chemical process (Hofman elimination). Duration of action (15–35 min) is thus uninfluenced by the state of the circulation, the liver or the kidneys, a real advantage in patients with hepatic or renal disease and in the aged. It is suitable for Caesarian section. Like tubocurarine it causes histamine release.

Neuromuscular blocking agents acting by depolarisation

Suxamethonium (succinylcholine, Scoline) paralysis is usually preceded by muscular fasciculation, and this may be the cause of the muscle pain lasting 1–3 days that is a common sequence of its use and which can rarely simulate meningeal irritation. The pain can be largely prevented by preceding the suxamethonium with a small dose of a competitive blocking agent. Suxamethonium total paralysis (1–2 mg/kg) lasts up to 4 min with 50% recovery ($t_{\frac{1}{2}}$ for *effect*) of about 10 min. It is particularly useful for brief procedures such as tracheal intubation or electric convulsion therapy. Suxamethonium is destroyed by plasma pseudocholinesterase and so its persistence in the body is increased by neostigmine, which inactivates that enzyme, and in patients with hepatic disease or severe malnurition whose plasma enzyme levels may be lower than normal. Procaine and amethocaine also are destroyed by plasma pseudocholinesterase and so, by competing with suxamethonium for the enzyme, may prolong its action and vice versa (lignocaine and prilocaine are metabolised differently). In addition there are individuals (about 1 in 2500 of the population) with hereditary defects in amount or kind of enzyme, who cannot destroy the drug as rapidly as normals.* Paralysis then lasts for hours; there is no effective way of restoring the enzyme or of eliminating the drug. Treatment consists in ventilating until recovery.

Repeated injections of suxamethonium can cause bradycardia, extrasystoles, other cardiac irregularities and even ventricular arrest. These are probably due to activation of cholinergic receptors in the heart and are prevented by 1.0 mg atropine i.v. High doses stimulate the pregnant uterus. The i.v. dose is 20–100 mg. Continuous i.v. infusions (2–3 mg/min) or intermittent doses can be used for more prolonged and readily variable relaxation, but dual block (see above) may occur.

* When cases are discovered the family should be investigated (plasma cholinesterase) and abnormal individuals warned.

Uses of neuromuscular blocking agents

Drugs acting by competition may antagonise those acting by depolarisation and it would seem better not to use them simultaneously (except as above to prevent initial muscle contraction with suxamethonium). Full doses used concurrently make intubation more difficult because of the difficulty in knowing when the partly antagonized suxamethonuim has taken effect. A dose of suxamethonium for tracheal intubation followed by tubocurarine some minutes later, after its action has worn off, would not, of course, be objectionable.

Neuromuscular blocking agents should only be employed by those who can intubate and ventilate.

In surgery and in **intensive therapy units** they are used to provide muscular relaxation.

In convulsions (e.g. electric convulsion therapy) they are used to prevent injury due to the violence of the fit. In status epilepticus or convulsant drug poisoning, neuromuscular blocking agents with mechanical respiration have been used; they are also used in tetanus.

Intrauterine use in the fetus. Bold and skilled clinicians have used tubocurarine by i.m. injection (fetus) to immobilize the fetus in order to permit intrauterine treatment (blood transfusion of severely rhesus iso-immunized fetuses)†

† de Crespigny L C et al Lancet 1985; 1:1164

Other muscle relaxants

Drugs that provide muscle relaxation by an action on the central nervous system or on the muscle itself are not useful for this purpose for surgery; they are insufficiently selective and full relaxation, even if achievable, is accompanied by general cerebral depression.

But there is a place for drugs that reduce spasm of the voluntary muscles without impairing voluntary movement. Such drugs can be useful in *neurological spastic states, low back syndrome* and *rheumatism* with muscle spasm.

Baclofen (Lioresal) is a derivative of gamma-aminobutyric acid (GABA), an inhibitory central nervous system transmitter. It reduces spasticity and flexor spasms, but as it has no effect on voluntary muscle power, function is commonly not improved. Ambulant patients may need their leg spasticity to provide support and reduction of spasticity may expose the weakness of the limb. It benefits some cases of trigeminal neuralgia. Baclofen is given orally and has a $t_{\frac{1}{2}}$ of 3 h.

Dantrolene (Dantrium) acts directly on muscle and prevents the release of calcium from sarcoplasm stores, see malignant hyperthermia.

Alternatives include orphenadrine (Disipal), diazepam (Valium), carisoprodol (Carisoma), chlormezanone (Trancopal) and methocarbamol (Robaxin). Most are prone to cause objectionable sedation.

LOCAL ANAESTHETICS

Cocaine was the first local anaesthetic discovered. It was isolated in 1860 and suggested as a local anaesthetic for clinical use in 1879. Nothing however was done until 1884 when Dr. Sigmund Freud in Vienna was reinvestigating the alkaloid, and invited Dr. Carl Koller to join him. The latter had long been interested in the problem of local anaesthesia in the eye, for general anaesthesia has disadvantages in ophthalmology. On observing the numbness of the mouth caused by taking cocaine orally he realised that this was a local anaesthetic effect. He tried cocaine on animals' eyes and introduced it into clinical ophthalmological practice,* whilst Freud was on holiday. Freud had already thought of this use and discussed it, but, appreciating that sex was of greater importance than surgery, he had gone off to see his fiancée. The use of cocaine spread rapidly and it was soon being used to block nerve trunks. Chemists then began to search for less toxic substitutes, with the result that procaine was introduced in 1905.

Desired properties. Innumerable compounds have local anaesthetic properties, but comparatively few are suitable for clinical use. Useful substances must be water-soluble, sterilisable by heat, non-irritant, have a rapid onset of effect, a duration of action appropriate to the operation to be performed, be non-toxic when absorbed into the circulation, and leave no local after-effects.

Mode of action. Local anaesthetics act on all nervous tissue to prevent the nerve impulse from arising and from propagating. They do this by combining with a receptor in membrane sodium ion channels and blocking the passage of sodium. They paralyse afferent nerve endings, sensory and motor nerve trunks and the central nervous system, although they may excite the latter first.

The fibres in nerve trunks are affected in order of size, the smallest (autonomic, sensory) first, probably because they have a proportionately high surface area, and then the larger (motor) fibres.

Kinetics: Absorption from mucous membranes varies according to the compound. Those that are well absorbed are used as surface anaesthetics (cocaine, lignocaine, prilocaine). Absorption of topically applied local anaesthetic can be extremely rapid and give plasma concentrations comparable to those obtained by injection. This had led to deaths from overdosage, especially via the urethra.

Prolongation of action by vasoconstrictors. The effect of a local anaesthetic is terminated by its removal from the site of application. Thus anything that delays its absorption into the circulation will prolong its local action and can reduce its systemic toxicity where large volumes are used. Adrenaline or noradrenaline generally (1: 200 000–400 000) are commonly used (dentists use 1:80 000) and they double the duration of effect (e.g. from 1 to 2 h). A vasoconstrictor should not be used for nerve block of an extremity

* Koller C. JAMA 1928; 90: 1742.

(finger, toe, nose, penis). For obvious anatomical reasons, the whole blood supply may be cut off by intense vasoconstriction so that the organ may be damaged or even lost. In dentistry particularly it is sometimes useful to terminate local anaesthesia promptly when the operative job is done. This can be achieved by reversal of adrenaline vasoconstriction by injecting an α-adrenoceptor blocker (phentolamine) into the site.

Enough adrenaline or noradrenaline can be absorbed to affect the heart and circulation and reduce the plasma K. This can be dangerous in cardiovascular disease, with general anaesthetics that sensitise the heart to catecholamines (halothane) and with tricyclic antidepressants and potassium losing diuretics. An alternative vasoconstrictor is felypressin (synthetic vasopressin), which, *in the concentrations used*, does not affect the heart rate or blood pressure and may be preferable in patients with cardiovascular disease. There is no significant added hazard to the use of catecholamines in patients taking an MAOI, except perhaps where there is cardiovascular disease, and felypressin is preferable in these patients in any case.

Administration and fate. Local anaesthetics are usually effective within 5 min of application and have a useful duration of effect of 1–2 h, which may be doubled by adding a vasoconstrictor (above). Obviously, *half* time of *effect* is of less interest to patients undergoing painful procedures than is the duration of *full* effect.

Most local anaesthetics are used in the form of the acid salts, as these are both soluble and stable. This acid salt (usually HCl) must dissociate in the tissues to liberate the free base, which is biologically active. This dissociation is delayed in abnormally acid, e.g. inflamed, tissues. The risk of spreading infection also makes local anaesthesia undesirable in infected areas.

Ester compounds (cocaine, procaine, amethocaine, benzocaine) are hydrolysed by liver and plasma esterases (and their effects may be prolonged where there is genetic deficiency).

Amide compounds (lignocaine, prilocaine, cinchocaine, bupivacaine) are dealkylated in the liver.

It is evident that defective liver function, whether due to primary cellular insufficency, or to low liver blood flow in cardiac failure or due to propranolol, may both prolong the $t_{\frac{1}{2}}$ and allow higher peak plasma concentrations of both types of local anaesthetic. But this is likely only to be important with large or repeated doses or infusions.

The *distribution* plasma $t_{\frac{1}{2}}$ of a *single* dose of a local anaesthetic is a few minutes, determined by distribution into tissues with concentrations approximately in relation to blood flow. But when an i.v. infusion is used an equilibration with all body tissues has been achieved (steady state) then the $t_{\frac{1}{2}}$ is determined solely by elimination (above) and is longer, e.g. lignocaine 1.5 h. These considerations are plainly important in the management of cardiac dysrhythmias.

Antagonists. Procaine and amethocaine, which are derivatives of p-aminobenzoic acid, inhibit sulphonamide antibacterial activity. This probably has no significant effect in antagonising suphonamides throughout the body, but with wounds, or when local anaesthesia is being used for lumbar puncture or other exploration in sulphonamide-treated patients, local sulphonamide antagonism followed by infection is a theoretical risk. Lignocaine and prilocaine do not antagonise sulphonamides.

Other effects. Local anaesthetics also have the following clinically important effects in varying degree:

1. Excitation of parts of the central nervous system, which may show itself by anxiety, restlessness, tremors and even convulsions, which are followed by depression.
2. Quinidine-like actions on the heart.

Uses. Local anaesthesia is generally used for trivial operations, when loss of consciousness is neither necessary nor desirable and also as an adjunct to major surgery to avoid high dose general anaesthesia. It is also used for major surgery, plus sedation, though many patients prefer unconsciousness. It is invaluable when the operator must also be the anaesthetist. Local anaesthetics can also be used topically for short periods to give relief from local pain or itching (but skin allergy is common).

For any but the most trivial operation premedication with a benzodiazepine is theoretically desirable to counteract the central excitant action of local anaesthetics, especially cocaine, but the doses used may in fact provide little or no protection.

Local anaesthetics may be used in several ways to provide:

1. *Surface anaesthesia*; as solution, jelly or lozenge. Chronic use is liable to cause allergy.

2. *Infiltration anaesthesia*, to paralyse the sensory nerve endings and small cutaneous nerves.

3. *Regional anaesthesia*.

a. *Intravenous*; a cuff is applied to the arm, inflated above arterial pressure after elevating the limb to drain the venous system, and the veins filled with local anaesthetic (e.g. 0.5% prilocaine) *without* adrenaline. The arm is anaesthetised in 6–8 min, and the effect lasts for up to 40 min if the cuff remains inflated. The cuff cannot safely be deflated until 20 min have passed. The technique is useful in providing anaesthesia for the treatment of injuries speedily and conveniently, and many patients can leave hospital as soon as 15 min after the cuff has been let down (during which time sensation and power return). The technique must be meticulously conducted for if the *full* dose of local anaesthetic is accidentally suddenly released into the general circulation severe toxicity and even death may result. Even if correctly performed, drug enters the general circulation through vessels in the bone that are not obstructed by the tourniquet. If toxicity occurs, convulsions and cardiac arrest may have to be treated. Patients should be fasted and someone (in addition to the surgeon) who is fully able to resuscitate should be present.

b. *Nerve block*, to anaesthetise a region, which may be small or large, by injecting the drug around, not into, the appropriate nerves, usually either a peripheral nerve or a plexus. Nerve block provides its own muscular relaxation as motor fibres are blocked as well as sensory fibres, although with care differential block can be achieved. Areas of selective sensory, but not motor nerve block, are found at the edges of some regional nerve blocks. Even when motor fibres are intact, provided there is sensory block, muscular relaxation will occur if the patient's consciousness is blunted with a hypnotic drug. There are various specialised forms: paravertebral, paracervical, pudendal block. Sympathetic nerve blocks may be used in vascular disease to induce vasodilatation.

Epidural (extradural) anaesthesia can be used in thoracic, lumbar and sacral (caudal) regions: it is widely used in obstetrics. As the term implies, the drug is injected into the extradural space where it acts on the nerve roots. This technique avoids the potentially serious hazards of putting foreign substances into the CSF; the risk of headache and hypotension is less than with spinal anaesthesia.

c. *Spinal anaesthesia and analgesia* in which the anaesthetic is put into the subarachnoid space. By using a solution of appropriate specific gravity and tilting the patient the drug can be kept at an appropriate level. Hypotension due to block of the sympathetic nervous system outflow occurs.

Serious local neurological complications have occurred rarely, both from the drug and from accidentally introduced bacteria.

Opioid analgesics may also be used intrathecally.

Regional anaesthesia requires considerable knowledge of anatomy and attention to detail for both success and safety.

Adverse reactions. Excessive absorption results in nervousness, tremors and even convulsions. These latter are very dangerous and are followed by respiratory depression. Diazepam or thiopentone, or even suxamethonium, may be necessary to control the convulsions as in status epilepticus. Respiratory stimulants are useless and dangerous as the patient has already passed through a phase of overstimulation. Nausea, vomiting and abdominal pain may occur, and also sudden cardiovascular collapse and respiratory failure for which there is no specific treatment other than respiratory and cardiac resuscitation. When systemic toxicity follows injection of a local anaesthetic into an extremity, a tourniquet may be used to delay entry of what remains into the general circulation, but resuscitation is the first priority. Hypertension can occur with cocaine (see below).

Allergic reactions such as rashes, asthma and anaphylactic shock rarely occur*, and the subject may be allergic to more than one drug. Regular

* Most 'reactions' occurring in the dental chair are the result of fear, posture, dose, and not of allergy.

users are wise if they take care to keep them off their own skin when filling syringes. Reactions are rarer with lignocaine than with procaine.

Routine tests for allergy or intolerance have been advocated before injecting local anaesthetics. Their value is doubtful and they are very time-consuming. A ship's cook aged 62 was to have a bronchogram performed because of suspected bronchial carcinoma. 'He was given an amethocaine lozenge to suck, to indicate whether or not he was allergic to amethocaine. As he showed no reaction, half an hour later his throat was sprayed with 0.5 to 1 ml of amethocaine solution. During this proceduce he suddenly collapsed, had a convulsive fit, and died within three minutes.'*

Local inflammatory or necrotic effects may occur, for these drugs can damage all cells.

Cocaine (an alkaloid and ester) is used medicinally solely as a surface anaesthetic (for *abuse* see p. 428) usually as a 4% solution, (because adverse effects are both common and dangerous when it is injected. Even as a surface anaesthetic sufficient absorption may take place to cause serious adverse effects. Ear, nose and throat surgeons sometimes apply a little pure solid or 10% solution to small areas and do not consider the practice unduly dangerous. Cocaine stimulates the CNS and in overdose causes first, restlessness and tremors, then excitement and convulsions.

Cocaine prevents the uptake of catecholamines (adrenaline, noradrenaline) into sympathetic nerve endings, thus increasing their concentration at receptor sites, so that cocaine has a built-in vasoconstrictor action, which is why it retains popularity as a surface anaesthetic for surgery involving mucous membranes, e.g. nose. Other local anaesthetics do not have this action.

The same mechanism explains the mydriasis that occurs when cocaine is applied to the eye and also the occurrence of general sympathomimetic effects. Adrenaline should never be added to cocaine solution. Injected catecholamines are also potentiated due to the block of nerve uptake (as above), for it is uptake into nerve endings that normally determines the duration and intensity of both naturally released and injected catecholamines. *Overdose* of cocaine causes cardiovascular collapse and sometimes hypertension. Treatment of overdose involves considerations of sedation and anticonvulsant therapy (diazepam) and adrenoceptor block (e.g. by labetalol, chlorpromazine). The $t_{\frac{1}{2}}$ is 50 min, but see pharmacokinetics above.

* Brit Med J 1955; 1:610.

Individual local anaesthetics (Table 21.1)

Lignocaine (Xylocaine, lidocaine; amide) is a successful drug for surface use as well as for injection, combining efficacy with comparative lack of toxicity. It is also useful in cardiac dysrhythmias (see index). Overdose of lignocaine, however, can cause convulsions although this is often preceded by somnolence rather than by excitement. Structurally, lignocaine differs from most other local anaesthetics and so is especially suitable for trial in cases of known allergy to other drugs. For kinetics see above.

Prilocaine (Citanest; amide) is used similarly to lignocaine, but it is less toxic. This was shown in a double-blind experiment in which 20 volunteers received each drug i.v. It can cause methaemoglobinaemia (due to a metabolite) at highest doses and this is only clinically important in patients in whom slight decrease of oxygen-carrying capacity is harmful, e.g. severe heart failure. It is available with adrenaline or felypressin as vasoconstrictors.

Bupivacaine (Marcain; amide) is particularly long acting (see table 21.2) and is used for nerve blocks in general, including obstetric epidural anaesthesia and for post-surgical and chronic pain relief. Whilst onset of effect is comparable to the above, peak effect is at about 30 min.

Procaine (Novocain; ester) is not absorbed through mucous membranes and is useless as a surface anaesthetic. It is rapidly hydrolysed in the blood, which is an advantage when an overdose has been given ($t_{\frac{1}{2}}$, 0.7 min).

Amethocaine (Anethaine; ester) resembles cocaine more than procaine and is effective on surfaces as well as by injection. It is dangerous, being absorbed fast through mucous membranes so that systemic toxic effects may occur.

Proxymetacaine (Ophthaine; amide) is used in the eye if it is important not to dilate the pupil, e.g. for tonometry.

Table 21.1 Approximate data on three widely used local anaesthetics (amide class). Other strengths are used, especially in dentistry.

Drug	*Surface anaesthesia*			*Infiltration*		*Nerve block*		Onset of	Duration:*	Max dose
	Soln. strength (%)	Effective in (min)	Duration (h)	Soln. strength (%)	Max. vol. (ml)	Soln. strength (%)	Max. vol. (ml)	effect: infilt. and nerve block (min)	infilt. and nerve block (h)	mg, (adult) with vasocon (without vasocon)
Prilocaine (Citanest)	4	5	1–2	1.0	40	3	20*	3–6	1½–3	600 (400)
Lignocaine (Xylocaine)	2,4	5	1–2	0.5	40	1.5	25*	5–10	2–4	500 (200)
Bupivacaine† (Marcain)	–	–	–	–	–	0.25 0.5	60 30	4	8 (nerve) 2–3 (epidural)	150 (150)

* With adrenaline or felypressin (but see text): if these are not used to delay absorption the doses in the table are toxic (except bupivacaine) and so *substantially* less should be given (see final col. above). If weaker solutions are used, larger volumes may be injected. Lozenges, lollipops for children, creams, ointments, jellies and suppositories are available for appropriate local use. As anaesthesia develops there is a danger of aspirating a lozenge into the trachea; captive preparations such as the lollipop are safer. All dosage figures apply to the hydrochlorides and are only approximate, larger amounts can often be given safely, but deaths have occurred with smaller amounts, so the minimum amount that will do the job should be used. Widely different solution strengths are used in some cases.

† Specialist use for prolonged anaesthesia

There are numerous other local anaesthetics (e.g. amylocaine, cinchocaine, benzocaine, oxybuprocaine, butacaine, orthocaine), and their omission here is not meant to imply that good results are not obtainable with them.

Choice of local anaesthetic. The many agents available are proof that all have disadvantages and that no agent is unchallengeably the best for all occasions. This is particularly the case for *surface* anaesthesia, although a claim that lignocaine is safest and best could not easily be dismissed, prilocaine is a contender when dosage must be heavy. For *injection* by the occasional user *lignocaine* or *prilocaine* are satisfactory.

There have been many deaths due to confusion of the names, all ending in 'caine' and to the use of wrong concentrations of unfamiliar drugs.

OBSTETRIC ANALGESIA AND ANAESTHESIA

Although this soon ceased to be considered immoral, it has been a technically controversial topic since 1853 when it was announced that Queen Victoria had inhaled chloroform during the birth of her eighth child. The *Lancet* recorded 'intense astonishment . . . throughout the profession' at this use of chloroform, 'an agent which has unquestionably caused instantaneous death in a considerable number of cases'. But the Queen took a different view, writing in her private Journal of 'that blessed chloroform' and adding that 'the effect was soothing, quieting and delightful beyond measure'.

Pain-free labour sometimes occurs spontaneously but, rightly or wrongly, most women in Western civilisations anticipate pain and demand relief. The reason for lack of general agreement on which drugs are best is that requirements are stringent, and much depends on the skill with which they are used. *The ideal drug* must relieve pain without making the patient confused or uncooperative. It must not interfere with uterine activity nor must it influence the fetus (respiratory depression is the chief disadvantage and may occur by a direct action of the drug on the fetus, by prolonging labour or by reducing uterine blood supply). It should also be suitable for use by a midwife without supervision.

Innumerable schemes have been proposed and good results can be obtained with many, by those who take the trouble to familiarise themselves with them. Generally, strong analgesic drugs should not be started before uterine contractions are well advanced as they can arrest labour if started sooner. The following may be taken as a general guide:

Onset of labour, up to three-quarter dilatation of cervix: non-inhalational tranquillisers and analgesics, e.g. pethidine.

From three-quarter dilatation of cervix till birth: inhalation drugs, e.g. nitrous oxide/oxygen, trichloroethylene: this is to avoid respiratory depression of the fetus, which occurs with effective doses of narcotic analgesics.

Pethidine is widely used. It seldom causes serious respiratory depression but has been shown to reduce respiratory minute volume in the baby. The mother may experience drowsiness and nausea. Morphine depresses fetal respiration more than pethidine. Opioids may impair infant feeding for 48 h. Naloxone administered to the mother before birth or to the child after birth will reverse opioid effect. Opioids delay gastric emptying, which can carry hazard of vomiting if general anaesthesia is then needed. The effect is not antagonised by metoclopramide.

Diazepam, as tranquilliser, not analgesic during labour and as anticonvulsant in preeclampsia and eclampsia, has a serious effect on the newborn if the maternal dose exceeds 30 mg in the 15 h before delivery (apnoeic spells, failure to feed, hypothermia), and these effects can last several days.

In general the baby will be about as depressed as the mother at the time of birth, and respiratory depressant should be withheld if birth is imminent. The intervals between doses are judged on clinical progress.

Sympathomimetic amines and other vasoconstrictors may cause fetal distress by reducing placental blood supply. They do not enter the fetus. Extreme hypotension from any cause also results in fetal anoxia.

Nitrous oxide and oxygen (50% of each, Entonox) may be administered for each pain from a machine the patient works herself or supervised by a midwife (about 10 good breaths are needed for maximal analgesia). Nitrous oxide and air mixtures are obsolete because hypoxia is unavoidable at effective concentrations of nitrous oxide. Trichloroethylene in a special vaporiser for self-administration can be used, but onset of analgesia is slower than with nitrous oxide and the patient is liable to become drowsy and so to be less co-operative.

Special techniques, e.g. epidural and pudendal nerve block, are also used by specialists.

General anaesthesia presents a special problem in that the safety of the fetus must also be considered, and the anaesthetist must consider the patient to have a full stomach, so that regurgitation is a particular risk.* All anaesthetics and analgesics in general use cross the placenta in varying amounts and, apart from respiratory depression, produce no important effects except that high doses interfere with uterine retraction and may be followed by uterine haemorrhage. All neuromuscular blocking agents can be used safely, although gallamine crosses the placenta and suxamethonium stimulates the uterus; none interferes with uterine retraction.

ANAESTHESIA IN PATIENTS ALREADY TAKING DRUGS

Anaesthetists are in an unenviable position. They are expected to provide safe service to patients in any condition, taking any drugs. Sometimes there is opportunity to modify drug therapy before surgery but often there is not. Anaesthetists require a particularly complete drug history of the patient.

The most important groups of drugs that affect anaesthesia are adrenal steroids, tranquillisers, antidepressants and antihypertensives. There is a paucity of useful data.

Adrenal steroids, see index.

Antibiotics. Aminoglycosides (e.g. neomycin, gentamicin) are themselves neuromuscular blocking

* Aspiration into the lung of gastric contents containing a high volume of acid juice is specially injurious if pH is < 2.5 (acid aspiration syndrome, Mendelson's syndrome). It should be prevented by giving women in labour a dose of gastric antacid 2-hourly (magnesium trisilicate plus sodium bicarbonate; the bicarbonate is important), or a histamine H_2-receptor blocker (cimetidine, ranitidine). Meloctopramide may be used to promote gastric emptying where time allows; it also increases tone of the lower oesophageal sphincter. So important is this that if an anaesthetic must be given to a patient with a full stomach, 'crash induction' (thiopentone plus suxamethonium) with intubation with a cuffed tube before the patient has time to vomit, is used. Prior to intubation the oesophagus may be occluded by backward pressure on the cricoid cartilage. Thus by combining drugs with other measures the safety of the patients may be attained.

agents in high dose and are additive with non-depolarising neuromuscular blocking drugs.

Anticholinesterases can potentiate suxamethonium.

Anticoagulants, see index. NSAIDs interfere with blood platelet function and may cause oozing at the operation site.

Antiepileptics. Continued medication is essential to avoid status epilepticus. Drugs must be given parenterally until the patient can swallow. Valproate can impair coagulation.

Antihypertensives of all kinds. Hypotension may complicate anaesthesia, but it is best to continue therapy. Hypertensive patients are particularly liable to excessive rise in blood pressure and heart rate during intubation, which can be dangerous if there is ischaemic heart disease. Postoperatively, parenteral therapy may be needed for a time. Abrupt withdrawal of antihypertensive drugs can lead to rebound hypertension, especially with clonidine.

Calcium channel blocking drugs. Patients taking verapamil may develop heart block with halothane.

Digitalis. Cardiac dysrhythmias are more likely with general anaesthesia.

β-adrenoceptor blocking drugs can prevent the homeostatic sympathetic cardiac response to cardiac depressant anaesthetics and to blood loss; bronchospasm may occur.

Diuretics. If hypokalaemia occurs, this will potentiate neuromuscular blocking agents and perhaps general anaesthetics.

Oral contraceptives and postmenopausal hormone replacement therapy predispose to thromboembolism, see index.

Psychotropic drugs. *Neuroleptics* potentiate or synergise with opioids, hypnotics and general anaesthetics. Those with antihypertensive properties, chlorpromazine, reserpine, may cause severe hypotension during anaesthesia.

Antidepressants. Monoamine oxidase inhibitors can potentiate opioids (especially pethidine), and, rarely, general anaesthetics as well as some sympathominetics. Tricyclics potentiate catecholamines and some other adrenergic drugs. For full discussion see Ch. 18.

Lithium may be continued unless there is serious risk of electrolyte disturbance or renal insufficientcy, when it should be stopped a week before surgery.

Opioid analgesics, hypnotics and alcohol. If enough of these has been habitually taken for tolerance to result, there will be some cross-tolerance with general anaesthetics.

ANAESTHESIA IN THE DISEASED, THE OLD AND THE YOUNG

The normal response to anaesthesia may be greatly modified by disease. The possibilities are vast and only some of the more important aspects will be mentioned here.

Respiratory disease and smoking predispose the patient to postanaesthetic pulmonary complications such as collapse and pneumonia. The site of operation and the incidence of pain are also relevant when they cause defective ventilation due to pain and fear of coughing.

Pneumonia due to a drug-sensitive organism is preferable to pneumonia due to a drug-resistant organism. Therefore prophylaxis should be begun immediately before or after operation, not days before, for this would allow colonisation of the lungs by resistant organisms. Routine use of antimicrobials does not prevent postanaesthetic pneumonia in healthy people.

Cardiac disease. The aim is to avoid the circulatory stress (with increased cardiac work which can compromise the myocardial oxygen supply), caused by struggling, coughing, laryngospasm and breath holding. Drugs given i.v. should be injected slowly to avoid hypotension, which may occur with very many substances if they are given too fast.

Patients with fixed cardiac output, e.g. mitral stenosis or constrictive pericarditis, are specially liable to a drop in cardiac output, for which they cannot compensate, with drugs that depress the myocardium and vasomotor centre. Thiopentone induction is liable to do this and inhalation induction may be preferable. Anoxia is obviously harmful. It will be seen that skilled technique rather than choice of drugs on pharmacological grounds is the important factor. If heart failure or dysrhythmias are anticipated from the condition of the patient or the nature of the operation, digoxin or antidysrhythmic drugs may be begun pre-operatively.

Hepatic and renal disease. Very many drugs are metabolised by the liver or excreted by the kidney so that disease of these organs is liable to lead to increased drug effects. This should be taken into account when selecting drugs and their doses. General anaesthetics can also impair hepatic function.

Malignant hyperthermia occurs in from 1: 15 000 (children) to 1: 40 000 of unselected subjects of general anaesthesia. It is a result of an inherited muscle disorder (autosomal dominant). The condition occurs during or within several hours of anaesthesia. It is precipitated by almost any drug, but especially by potent inhalation agents (especially halogenated), and by suxamethonium; but it is possible that it may also result from stress alone. The patient may previously have safely experienced a general anaesthetic. The mechanism involves a sudden rise in release of bound (stored) calcium of the sarcoplasm, stimulating contraction and a hypermetabolic state.

Malignant hyperthermia is a life-threatening medical emergency. Oxygen consumption increases by up to three times normal, and body temperature may rise as fast as 1°C every 5 min, reaching as high as 43°C. Rigidity of voluntary muscles may not be evident at the outset or in mild cases.

Administration of *dantrolene* i.v., 1 mg/kg, is urgently required; further doses are given if there is not a quick response; the average total effective dose is 2.5 mg/kg, but as much as 10 mg/kg may be needed. Dantrolene probably acts by preventing the release of calcium from the sarcoplasm store that ordinarily follows depolarization of the muscle membrane.

Non-specific treatment is needed for the hyperthermia. Cardiac dysrhythmias occur (due to potassium release from contracted muscle).

Any future anaesthesia in patients who have experienced the syndrome can be achieved with minimal risk by using opioids, barbiturates, diazepam, neuroleptics, nitrous oxide or ester-class local anaesthetics.

It is recommended that i.v. formulation of dantrolene should be available in every surgical theatre. Where it is not available (it is extraordinarily expensive) an ester-class local anaesthetic (e.g. procaine) given cautiously i.v. may be better than nothing.

The relation of malignant hyperthermia syndrome with neuroleptic malignant syndrome is uncertain.

Diabetes mellitus. The chief danger is hypoglycaemia caused by giving insulin to a fasted patient. The response to anaesthesia and surgery is hyperglycaemia due to activation of the sympathetic autonomic system (it is particularly marked with ether), but the effect is ordinarily clinically insignificant.

Thyroid disease. Nowadays patients are not operated on for hyperthyroidism until the metabolic rate has been controlled by drugs. If by some mischance an operation must be done whilst the metabolic rate is high and a thyroid 'crisis' follows, it may be treated by methods used in anaesthetic hypothermia; β-adrenoceptor block is used to protect the heart, which is sensitised to catecholamines. Hypothyroid patients are liable to be intolerant of many drugs. Hypothyroidism may be corrected rapidly with liothyronine, but if it is of long standing this must be reversed slowly because of risk of cardiovascular collapse. See Ch. 36.

Porphyria. Barbiturates should never be used as they may precipitate a severe attack. Chlorpromazine is safe for premedication. See index.

Muscle diseases. Patients with myasthenia gravis are very sensitive (intolerant) to competitive but not to depolarising neuromuscular blocking drugs. Those with dystrophia myotonica may recover less rapidly than normal from central respiratory depression and neuromuscular block; they may fail to relax with suxamethonium. All patients with generalised muscular weakness or disease should be treated with special attentiveness.

Genetics. 1. *Sickle-cell disease*: hypoxia can precipitate a crisis.

2. *Atypical pseudocholinesterase (or deficiency)* delays metabolism of suxamethonium seriously: any effect on ester class local anaesthetics is probably unimportant clinically.

Raised intracranial pressure will be made worse by inhalation agents (e.g. halothane, nitrous oxide) by hypoxia or hypercapnia and in response to intubation, it depresses the respiratory centre and these patients are liable to respiratory failure with central nervous depressants, especially opioids. Therefore, premedication may consist of atropine alone.

Sedation in intensive therapy units. Patients who are not too sick are likely to feel frightened. Charity requires that they be relieved (by sympathetic care and, if necessary, by drugs). Benzodiazepines are an obvious choice, e.g. midazolam.

But there are other reasons for sedation. Some patients will 'fight' the mechanical ventilator they require, and endotracheal tubes are extremely uncomfortable and even painful. Opioids are an obvious choice, e.g. phenoperidine (where short $t_{\frac{1}{2}}$, 30 min, is desired). These not only relieve pain and discomfort, but tranquillise and depress respiration so that the patient fights the ventilator less. A competitive neuromuscular blocking agent may have to be added to reduce the need for high doses of opioids, especially where there is reduced renal and hepatic function. But its use adds the risk of death due to accidental disconnection of the ventilator. Neuromuscular blockers do *not* impair consciousness and an aware and paralysed patient is in great distress, and is unable to communicate this to attendants. Everyone will wish to avoid this and it can be done by skilled use of sedative and opioids.

Old age (see p. 140). Old people are liable to become confused by cerebral depressants, especially by hyoscine, and atropine is usually substituted. Apart from this there are no special problems for anaesthesia, but mistakes and overdose are less easily retrieved in the old and frail than in the young and healthy. In general, elderly patients require smaller doses than the young. Hypotension should be especially avoided as it readily causes cerebral hypoxia.

Childhood (see p. 140). Here again the problems are more technical, physiological and psychological than pharmacological. Premedication is often by sedatives, e.g. benzodiazepine, orally or by rectum, rather than by injected morphine or papaveretum with hyoscine, although children in fact tolerate these well. Neonates are said to be intolerant of competitive, and tolerant of depolarising, neuromuscular blocking agents, and also to need little anaesthesia.

GUIDE TO FURTHER READING

1 Epstein R M et al. Influence of the concentration effect on the uptake of anesthetic mixtures: the second gas effect. Anesthesiology 1964; 25:364.

2 Committee on nitrous oxide and oxygen analgesia in midwifery: report to Medical Research Council. Clinical trials of different concentrations of oxygen and nitrous oxide for obstetric analgesia. Br Med J 1970; 1:709.

3 Evans J M et al. Reversal of narcotic depression in the neonate by naloxone. Br Med J 1976; 2:1098.

4 Nimmo W S et al. Narcotic analgesics and delayed gastric emptying during labour. Lancet 1975; 1:890.

5 Cree J E et al. Diazepam in labour: its metabolism and effect on the clinical condition and thermogenesis of the newborn. Br Med J 1973; 4:251.

6 Editorial. Analgesia for endoscopy. Lancet 1976; 2:1125.

7 Editorial. Premedication tradition. Lancet 1977; 2:1066.

8 Leigh J M et al Effect of preoperative anaesthetic visit on anxicty. Br Med J 1977; 2:987.

9 Armstrong R F et al. Anaesthetic waste gas scavenging systems. Br Med J 1977; 1:941.

10 Price H L et al. The uptake of thiopental by body tissues and its relation to the duration of narcosis. Clin Pharmacol Ther 1960; 1:16.

11 Saidman L J et al. Effects of nitrous oxide and of narcotic premedication on the alveolar concentration of halothane required for anesthesia. Anesthesiology 1964; 25:302.

12 Morrison J D et al Controlled comparison of the efficacy of fourteen preparations in the relief of postoperative pain. Br Med J 1971; 3:287.

13 Edwards G et al. Deaths associated with anaesthesia. A report of 1,000 cases. Anaesthesia 1956; 11:194.

14 Editorial. Antanalgesia. Br Med J 1963; 2:129.

15 Editorial. Deaths in the dental chair. Br Med J 1975; 1:293.

16 Editorial. Drug reactions during anaesthesia. Lancet 1985; 1:1195.

17 Nelson T E et al. The malignant hyperthermia syndrome. N Engl J Med 1983; 309:416.

18 Morgan B M et al. Analgesia and satisfaction in childbirth (The Queen Charlotte's 1,000 mother survey). Lancet 1982; 2:808.

19 Keenan D J M et al. Comparative trial of rectal indomethacin and cryoanalgesia for control of early post thoractomy pain. Br Med J 1983; 287:1335.

20 Ngai S H. Effects of anaesthetics on various organs. N Engl J Med 1982; 302:564.

21 Ogg T W. Use of anaesthesia: implications of day-care surgery and anaesthesia. Br Med J 1980; 2:212.

22 Fineberg H V et al. The case for abandonment of explosive anaesthetic agents. N Engl J Med 1980; 303:613.

23 Neuberger J et al. Halothane anaesthesia and liver damage. Br Med J 1984; 289:1136.

24 Vessey M P et al. Occupational hazards of anaesthesia. Br Med J 1980; 281:696.

25 Herbert M et al. Profile of recovery after general anaesthesia. Br Med J 1983; 286:1539.
26 Editorial. Sedation in the intensive care unit. Lancet 1984 1:1388.
27 Amos R J et al. Incidence and pathogensis of acute megaloblastic bone-marrow charge on patients receiving intensive care. Lancet 1982; 2:835.
28 Editorial. Analgesia and the metabolic response to surgery. Lancet 1985; 1:1018.
29 Jones J G, et al. Hearing and memory in anaesthetised patients. Br Med J 1986; 292:1291.
30 Levis B. Deaths and dental anaesthetics. Br Med J 1983; 286:3.
31 Edwards R. Anaesthesia and alcohol(ics). Br Med J 1985; 291:423.
32 Sweeney B et al. Toxicity of bone marrow in dentists exposed to nitrous oxide. Br Med J 1985; 291:567.

22

Cholinergic and anticholinergic drugs

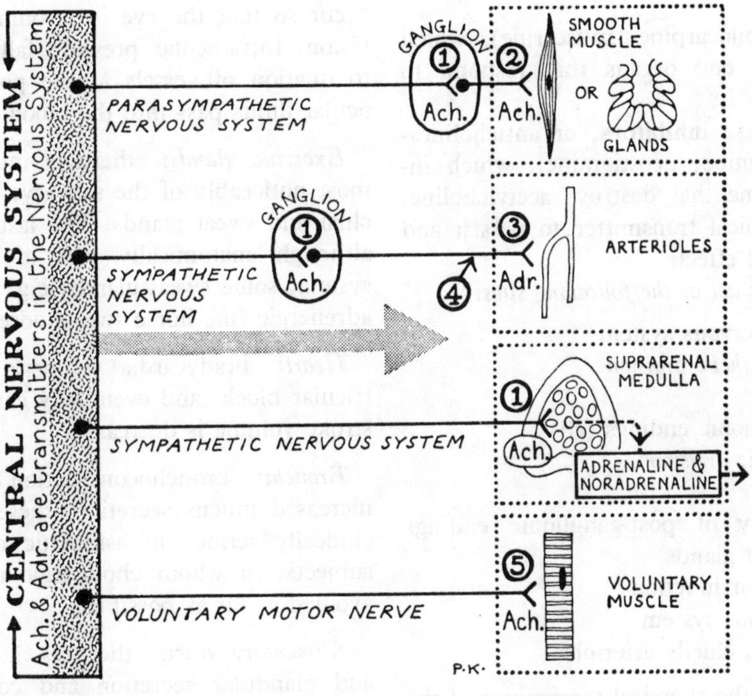

Fig. 22.1 Diagram showing sites of chemical transmitters of nerve impulse. (This is the classic oversimplification that is sufficient for this account.)

Ach. = acetylcholine
Adr. = noradrenaline or adrenaline

Site 1 is blocked by ganglion-blocking agents and stimulated by nicotine and big doses of some choline esters and anticholinesterases.

Site 2 is blocked by atropine and stimulated by some choline esters, anticholinesterases and pilocarpine.

Site 3 is blocked by adrenoceptor blocking agents and function is interfered with by drugs that deplete noradrenaline stores in nerve-endings and end-organs (reserpine).
Sympathomimetic amines stimulate here.

Site 4 is blocked by adrenergic neurone-blocking agents (bethanidine).

Site 5 is blocked by neuromuscular blocking agents and stimulated by choline esters and anticholinesterases.

CHOLINERGIC DRUGS

These substances act on receptors at all the sites in the body where acetylcholine is the transmitter of the nerve impulse. They stimulate and, at higher concentrations, paralyse. In addition, like acetylcholine, they act directly on peripheral blood vessels to dilate them.

Cholinergic drugs may be:

A. **Choline esters** (carbachol, bethanechol), which act at all sites like acetylcholine. Muscarinic effects are more prominent than nicotinic (see below).

B. **Alkaloids** (pilocarpine, muscarine), which act selectively on end organs that respond to acetylcholine.

C. **Cholinesterase inhibitors**, or anticholinesterases (physostigmine, neostigmine), which inactivate the enzyme that destroys acetylcholine, allowing the chemical transmitter to persist and produce intensified effects.

Cholinergic drugs act at the following sites:

1. Autonomic nervous system
   a. *Parasympathetic division*
      ganglia
      post-ganglionic endings (all)
   b. *Sympathetic division*
      ganglia
      a minority of post-ganglionic endings (e.g. sweat glands).
2. Neuromuscular junction
3. Central nervous system
4. Blood vessels, chiefly arterioles.

Acetylcholine is the chemical transmitter of the nerve impulse at all these sites acting on a post-synaptic receptor, except on most blood vessels in which the cholinergic receptor is unrelated to nerve endings. It is also produced in tissues unrelated to nerve endings, e.g. placenta and ciliated epithelial cells, where it acts as a local hormone (autacoid) on local receptors.

A list of principal effects is given below. Not all occur with every drug and not all are noticeable at therapeutic doses, e.g. central nervous system effects of cholinergic drugs are best seen in cases of anticholinesterase agent poisoning. *Atropine antagonises all the effects of cholinergic drugs except those at autonomic ganglia and the neuromuscular junction*, i.e. it does not act at receptors served by neurones arising in the central nervous system.

Autonomic nervous system: actions

Parasympathetic division. Stimulation of cholinergic receptors in autonomic ganglia and at the post-ganglionic endings affects chiefly the following organs:

Eye: miosis and spasm of the ciliary muscle occur so that the eye is accommodated for near vision. Intra-ocular pressure falls, due, perhaps, to dilation of vessels at the point where intra-ocular fluids pass into the blood.

Exocrine glands: there is increased secretion most noticeably of the salivary, lachrymal, bronchial and sweat glands. The last are cholinergic, although anatomically part of the sympathetic system; some sweat glands, e.g. axillary, may be adrenergic (the horse sweats adrenergically).

Heart: bradycardia occurs, with atrioventricular block, and eventually cardiac arrest. The stroke volume is decreased.

Bronchi: bronchoconstriction occurs, also increased mucus secretion, these effects may be clinically serious in asthmatic or other allergic subjects, in whom cholinergic drugs should be avoided as far as possible.

Alimentary tract: there is increased motility and glandular secretion and colicky pain may occur. Sphincter tone is reduced and the patient may defaecate embarrassingly. Lowering of oesophageal sphincter tone creates a risk of regurgitation and inhalation, e.g. in anaesthesia.

Bladder and ureters contract and the drugs promote micturition.

Sympathetic division. *The ganglia* only are stimulated, also the cholinergic nerves to the adrenal medulla. These effects are overshadowed by effects of the drugs on the parasympathetic system and are commonly evident only if atropine has been given to block the latter, when tachycardia, vasoconstriction and hypertension occur.

Neuromuscular junction

The neuromuscular junction has a cholinergic nerve ending, and so is stimulated, causing muscle fasciculation, followed, if excess is given, by a depolarisation neuromuscular block.

Central nervous system

There is usually stimulation followed by depression, but variation between drugs is great, possibly due to differences in penetration into the nervous system. Mental excitement occurs, with confusion and restlessness, insomnia (with nightmares when sleep does come), tremors and dysarthria, and sometimes even convulsions and coma.

Blood vessels

There is stimulation of cholinergic post-synaptic receptors (vasodilator) in addition to the more important dilating action on arterioles and capillaries mediated through non-innervated receptors. Anticholinesterases potentiate acetylcholine, which occurs in the vessel walls independently of nerves.

Nicotinic and muscarinic effects

The actions of acetylcholine and substances acting like it at autonomic ganglia and the neuromuscular junction (i.e. at the end of cholinergic nerve fibres, which arise in the central nervous system) are described as *nicotinic* because they are like the stimulant effects of nicotine. The actions at post-ganglionic cholinergic endings (parasympathetic endings plus the cholinergic sympathetic nerves to the sweat glands) and those uninnervated on blood vessels are described as *muscarinic* because they resemble those of the alkaloid muscarine. The central nervous system actions are not included in this curious categorisation. The terms are useful because it is more concise to say that atropine blocks the muscarinic but not the nicotinic effects of neostigmine than it is to describe this antagonism in any other way. But these terms seem to be unacceptable to clinicians who, although they were nearly all brought up on them, decline to apply them when discussing the clinical use of drugs, perhaps because they find them unnecessary as well as confusing, despite the fact that they were introduced to avoid confusion.

Choline esters

Acetylcholine

Since acetylcholine has such great importance in the body it is not surprising that attempts have been made to use it in therapeutics. But a substance with such a huge variety of effects and so rapidly destroyed in the body is unlikely to be useful when given systemically.

The use of acetylcholine in psychiatry illustrates some facets of the introduction of new remedies as well as providing interesting clinical pharmacological data. It was first injected i.v. as a therapeutic convulsant in 1939, in the justified expectation that the fits would be less liable to cause fractures than those following therapeutic leptazol convulsions. Recovery rates of up to 80% were claimed in various psychotic conditions. Enthusiasm began to wane, however, when it was shown that the fits were due to anoxia resulting from cardiac arrest and not to pharmacological effects on the brain.*

The following composite description of the effects of i.v. injection on many patients shows a mixture of receptor effects of acetylcholine and of anoxia due to acetylcholine-induced cardiac arrest: A few seconds after the injection (which was given as rapidly as possible, to avoid total destruction in the blood) the patient sat up 'with knees drawn up to the chest, the arms flexed and the head bent forward. There were repeated violet coughs, sometimes with flushing. Forced swallowing and loud peristaltic rumblings could be heard.' Respiration was laboured and irregular. 'The coughing abated as the patient sank back in the bed. Forty seconds after the injection the radial and apical pulse were zero and the patient became comatose.' The pupils dilated, and deep reflexes were hyperactive. In 45 sec the patient went into opisthotonos with brief apnoea. Lachrymation, sweating

* Harris M et al. Archives of Neurology and Psychiatry 1943; 50:304.

and borborygmi were prominent. The deep reflexes became diminished. The patient then relaxed and 'lay quietly in bed — cold moist and gray. In about 90 seconds, flushing of the face marked the return of the pulse.' The respiratory rate rose and consciousness returned in about 125 sec. The patients sometimes micturated but did not defaecate. They 'tended to lie quietly in bed after the treatment.' 'Most of the patients were reluctant to be treated.'*

The investigators who conducted this series obtained bad therapeutic results except in one schizophrenic patient who nearly died. In this patient, the pulse first disappeared for 50 sec, returned for 20 sec and disappeared again for 140 sec. It then reappeared for 5 and disappeared for 50 sec, after which the patient 'recovered'. The authors considered that the brain had suffered such extensive anoxic damage 'that obvious schizophrenic symptoms, at least for the time being, (were) impossible.'

These and other results were sufficiently intimidating for therapy to be modified to non-convulsant doses for neurotics. After several favourable reports, a careful study was done in which it was shown that acetylcholine was not a therapeutic agent because the same rate of improvement occurred in control groups, the use of control groups having been neglected by those who popularised the treatment. The authors of this series commented on the necessity for a placebo or dummy in controlled therapeutic trials as being 'nowhere more true than where psychiatric practice is concerned, because a substantial proportion of emotionally disturbed patients show favourable responses to any therapeutic effort which combines enthusiasm, impressiveness and benevolence.'†

As it would clearly be useful to the physician to be able to produce some of the effects of acetylcholine without all others, related substances have been investigated and there is now a variety of drugs available with longer action and varying degrees of selectivity; but none confine their efforts to one organ alone. The principal drugs are described below.

* Cohen L H et al. Archives of Neurology and Psychiatry 1944; 51:171.

† Hawkins J R et al. Journal of Mental Science 1956; 102:60.

Other choline esters

Carbachol is a choline ester that is not destroyed by cholinesterase; its actions are most pronounced on the bladder and bowels, so that the drug is used to stimulate these organs, e.g. after surgery. Carbachol is stable in the alimentary tract (oral dose 1–4 mg). It is extremely dangerous if given i.v. but may be administered s.c. (0.2–0.5 mg).

Bethanechol (Myotonine) (5, 10 mg) is not destroyed by cholinesterase. It acts chiefly on the bowel and bladder and may be more selective than carbachol. The dose is 2–5 mg s.c. or 5–30 mg p.o.

Alkaloids with cholinergic effects

Pilocarpine is an alkaloid from a genus of American plant (*Pilocarpus* spp.). It acts directly on end-organs innervated by post-ganglionic nerves (parasympathetic system plus sweat glands); it also stimulates and then depresses the central nervous system. Its action at the neuromuscular junction and autonomic ganglia is very slight. Its chief clinical use is in the eye as a miotic (1% solution or as sustained-release Pilocarpine Ocuserts). It has an undeserved reputation as a hair restorer but has occasionally found a use as a sialogogue in parkinsonian patients taking large doses of an anticholinergic drug. Objectionable effects, such as sweating, generally outweigh the benefits. Overdose is liable to cause respiratory symptoms due to bronchospasm and profuse bronchial secretion.

Arecoline is an alkaloid in the betel nut, which is chewed in the East. It produces a mild dependence, for like other parasympathomimetic drugs, it stimulates the brain. It has no place in therapeutics.

Muscarine is of no therapeutic use but it has pharmacological interest. It is present in small amounts in the fungus *Amanita muscaria* (fly agaric). This fungus is named after its capacity to kill the domestic fly (*Musca domestica*) and muscarine was so named because it was thought to be the insecticidal principle, but it is relatively non-toxic to flies (by the oral route). The fungus may also contain anticholinergic substances and GABA-receptor agonists in amounts sufficient to be psychoactive in man.

Poisoning with these fungi may present with anticholinergic, with cholinergic or with GABA-ergic effects. All have CNS actions. It is evident that careful clinical observation will be needed to distinguish the state of the patient. But in any case the cerebral excitation will be best treated by sedation (diazepam) rather than by too-clever exercises in clinical pharmacological analysis, which may result in treatment that makes the patient worse. Happily, poisoning by *Amanita muscaria* is seldom serious. Species of *Inocybe* contain larger amounts of muscarine (see index: Fungus poisoning).

The lengths to which man is prepared to go in taking 'chemical vacations' from life when conditions are hard are shown by the inhabitants of Eastern Siberia, who used *Amanita muscaria* recreationally, for its cerebral stimulant effects. They were apparently prepared to put up with the autonomic actions to escape briefly from reality. The fungus was scarce in winter when, no doubt, the greatest need for it was felt, and the frugal devotees discovered that by drinking their own urine they could prolong the intoxication. Sometimes, in generous mood, the intoxicated person would offer his urine to others as a treat. The ancient Vikings reputedly used the fungus to assist them to become berserk*. Unfortunately cheap alcohol has supplanted most such interesting practices.

Anticholinesterases

In the region of cholinergic nerve endings and in erythrocytes there is an enzyme that specifically destroys acetylcholine, 'true' cholinesterase or acetylcholinesterase. In various tissues, especially blood plasma, there are other esterases that are not specific for acetylcholine but that also destroy other esters, e.g. suxamethonium and procaine. These are called non-specific or pseudo-cholinesterases. Chemicals that inactivate these esterases (i.e. anticholinesterases) are used in medicine, and in agriculture as insecticides. They act by allowing naturally formed acetylcholine to accumulate instead of being destroyed and their effects are almost entirely due to this accumulation in the central nervous system, at the neuromuscular junction, autonomic ganglia, post-ganglionic cholinergic nerve endings (which are principally in the parasympathetic nervous system) and in the walls of blood vessels, where acetylcholine is a local hormone not necessarily associated with nerve endings. Some of these effects oppose each other, for instance the effect of an anticholinesterase on the heart will be the resultant of stimulation at sympathetic ganglia and the opposing effect of stimulation at parasympathetic (vagal) ganglia and post-ganglionic nerve endings as well as vasodilatation. Therefore the clinical effects of anticholinesterases are not entirely predictable.

Physostigmine (eserine) is an alkaloid obtained from the seeds of a West African plant, which has long been used both as a weapon and as an ordeal† poison. It acts for a few hours. It is used in the eye to cause miosis, spasm of the ciliary muscle and reduce intra-ocular pressure. The drug crosses the blood–brain barrier and is effective at counteracting the toxic central effects of anticholinergic substances, e.g. tricyclic antidepressants taken in overdose.

Neostigmine (tab 15 mg; inj 0.5, 2.5 mg/ml) is a synthetic anticholinesterase whose actions are more prominent on the neuromuscular junction and the alimentary tract than on the cardiovascular system and eye. It is therefore principally used in myasthenia gravis and to stimulate the bowels and bladder after surgery, and as an antidote to competitive neuromuscular blocking agents. In addition it has a direct stimulant action of its own, unrelated to inhibition of cholinesterase, which may be of importance in myasthenia gravis. Neostigmine is effective orally (15–30 mg, three or four times a day), and by injection (usually s.c.) 0.5–2.0 mg. But higher doses may be used, often combined with atropine (to block unwanted actions), in myasthenia gravis. Anaesthetists use 2.5–5 mg i.v. with atropine to reverse neuromuscular block.

Pyridostigmine (Mestinon) (60 mg) is similar to neostigmine but has a slower onset and slightly longer duration and perhaps fewer visceral effects. It is often used in myasthenia gravis, 4 mg of the

* 'Frenzied fury', highly valued on the battlefield.

† To determine guilt or innocence according to whether the accused died or lived after the judicial dose. The practice had the advantage that the demonstration of guilt provided simultaneous punishment.

bromide being equivalent to 1 mg of neostigmine. Distigmine (Ubretid) is a variant of pyridostigmine (two linked molecules as the name implies). Ambenonium (Mytelase) is similar but has a slightly longer duration of action than pyridostigmine.

Edrophonium (Tensilon; 10 mg/ml) is related to neostigmine. Its duration of action is only minutes and autonomic effects are minimal except at high doses. The drug is used in the diagnosis of myasthenia gravis and in differentiating a myasthenic crisis (when weakness is due to inadequate anticholinesterase treatment or severe disease) from a cholinergic crisis (when weakness is caused by overtreatment with an anticholinesterase). Myasthenic weakness is substantially improved by edrophonium whereas cholinergic weakness is aggravated (dangerously) but the effect is transient — the action of 3 mg i.v. is over in 5 min.

Ecothiopate (Phospholine) and *demecarium* (Tosmilen) are used as long-lasting miotics. Enough can be absorbed to potientiate cholinergic drugs and suxamethonium given systemically, for weeks after cessation of use. Spasm of the ciliary muscle may be intense and cause headache.

Anticholinesterase poisoning. The anticholinesterases used in therapeutics are generally those which reversibly inactivate cholinesterase for a few hours. Insecticides of the carmabate type act by reversible inhibition of cholinesterase but organophosphorus insecticides inhibit the enzyme almost or completely irreversibly so that recovery depends on formation of fresh enzyme. This process may take weeks although clinical recovery is usually evident in days. Cases of poisoning are usually met outside therapeutic practice, for example, after agricultural, industrial or transport accidents. Substances of this type have also been studied for use in war (nerve gas). Diagnosis depends on observing a substantial part of the list of actions below. The prominence of individual effects varies with different agents, e.g. sweating and salivation are not usual in dyflos poisoning.

A typical case of poisoning by cutaneous absorption will, perhaps after a delay, develop headache, confusion, anorexia and a sense of unreality. The patient is often giddy, apprehensive and restless. Conspicuous salivation, rhinorrhoea and sweating follow, with respiratory wheeze and dyspnoea indicating the onset of bronchoconstriction and excessive bronchial secretion. Miosis may occur and cause the headache, but it is not invariable; nor is it an index of severity, for it may be due to a local effect of the poison entering via the conjunctiva. Vomiting and cramping abdominal pains may lead to diarrhoea and tenesmus, and there may also be urinary incontinence. Muscle twitching typically begins in the eyelids, tongue and face, then extends to the neck and limbs and is accompanied by severe weakness. Progressive respiratory difficulty leads to convulsions and coma. Death is due to a combination of the actions in the central nervous system, to paralysis of the respiratory muscles by peripheral neuromuscular block, and to excessive bronchial secretions causing respiratory failure. At autopsy, ileal intussusceptions are commonly found.

Treatment. Since the most common circumstance of accidental poisoning is exposure to insecticide spray or spillage, contaminated clothing should be removed and the skin cleaned. Gastric lavage is needed if any of the substance has been ingested. Attendants should take care to ensure that they do not become contaminated.

Atropine 2 mg is given i.m. or i.v. as soon as possible and repeated every 15–60 min until dryness of the mouth and a heart rate in excess of 70 beats per minute indicate that its effect is adequate. A poisoned patient may require 100 mg or more for a single episode.

Atropine antagonises only anticholinesterase effects that are central and those due to stimulation at post-ganglionic nerve endings (excessive secretion) and vasodilation; i.e. the muscarinic actions. Neuromuscular block is not relieved, for atropine does not antagonise acetylcholine at the endings of nerve fibres that arise in the central nervous system (nicotinic effects). Hence artificial ventilation may be needed to assist the respiratory muscles. Attention to the airway is vital because of bronchoconstriction and excessive secretion and this may require endotracheal intubation and ventilation. Diazepam may be needed for convulsions. Atropine eye-drops may relieve the headache caused by miosis.

Poisoning with reversible anticholinesterases is appropriately treated by atropine and the necessary general support but *irreversible* cholinesterases call for additional measures. The organophosphorus insecticides inactivate cholinesterase by phosphorylating the active centre of the enzyme. *Reactivating substances* are either phosphorylated very easily, so that they compete for the poison in the body, diverting it from cholinesterase, or they may dephosphorylate the enzyme. The principal agents, *pralidoxime* and *obidoxime* (Toxigonin), are held in specially designated centres. They should be administered within 12 hours of poisoning and are probably valueless after 24 hours, for by then insecticide and enzyme are irreversibly bound. Pralidoxime 30 mg/kg should be given 4-hourly i.v. as indicated by the patient's condition. Obidoxime 3–6 mg/kg i.v. may also be administered with advantage at these intervals, for it crosses the blood–brain barrier and may potentiate the action of pralidoxime. Repeated dosing may be particularly important in poisoning with parathion, which is slowly converted into an active form after it enters the body. These reactivators are not effective for all types of organophosphorous or carbomate insecticide.

Erythrocyte or plasma cholinesterase content should be measured if possible, both for diagnosis and to determine when a poisoned worker may return to his task in the event of his being willing to do so. This should not be allowed until the cholinesterase exceeds 70% of normal, which may take several weeks.

Disorders of neuromuscular transmission

Myasthenia gravis

Myasthenia gravis is characterised by weakness or undue fatiguability of extra-ocular, bulbar, neck, limb girdle, distal limb and trunk muscles, usually in that order of onset. Synaptic transmission at the neuromuscular junction is impaired; most cases appear to have an autoimmune basis (85% of patients have autoantibodies to the acetylcholine receptor) but the remaining 15% may have other causes.

Neostigmine was introduced in 1931 for its stimulant effects on intestinal activity. In 1934 it occurred to Dr. Mary Walker that since the paralysis of myasthenia had been attributed to a curare-like substance in the blood, physostigmine (eserine), an anticholinesterase drug known to antagonise curare, might be beneficial. It was and she reported this important observation in a short letter.* Soon after this she used neostigmine by mouth with greater benefit.

The sudden appearance of an effective treatment for a hitherto untreatable chronic disease must always be a dramatic event for its victims. The impact of the discovery of the action of neostigmine has been described by one patient.

'My myasthenia started in 1925, when I was 18. For several months it consisted of double vision and fatigue . . . An ophthalmic surgeon . . . prescribed glasses with a prism. However, soon more alarming symptoms began.' Her limbs became weak and she 'was sent to an eminent neurologist. This was a horrible experience. He . . . could find no physical signs . . . declared me to be suffering from hysteria and asked me what was on my mind. When I answered truthfully, that nothing except anxiety over my symptoms, he replied "My dear child, I am not a perfect fool . . .", and showed me out.' She became worse and at times she was unable to turn over in bed. Eating and even speaking were difficult.

Eventually, her fiance, a medical student, read about myasthenia gravis and she was correctly diagnosed in 1927. '*There was at that time no known treatment and therefore many things to try.*' She had gold injections, thyroid, suprarenal extract, lecithin, glycine, and ephedrine (which enhances neuromuscular transmission). The last had a slight effect. 'Then in February 1935, came the day that I shall always remember. I was living alone with a nurse . . . It was one of my better days, and I was lying on the sofa after tea . . . My fiance came in rather late saying that he had something new for me to try. My first thought was "Oh bother! Another injection, and another false hope." I submitted to the injection with complete indifference and within a few minutes began to feel very strange . . . when I lifted my arms, exerting the effort to which I had become accustomed, they shot into the air, every movement I attempted was grotesquely magnified until I learnt to make less effort . . . it was strange, wonderful

* Walker M B. Lancet 1934; 1: 1200.

and at first, very frightening . . . we danced twice round the carpet. That was my first meeting with neostigmine, and we have never since been separated.'*

Pathogenesis†. Mounting evidence indicates that most cases of myasthenia gravis are caused by specific antibodies that either block or cause complement-mediated lysis of the acetylcholine receptor. In common with all body tissues, this receptor is constantly being broken down and re-synthesised. It persists for about 7 days in normal individuals but its life is only one day in myasthenic patients. The thymus gland is in some way involved in the process and three-quarters of patients have either thymitis or a thymoma.

Diagnosis may be made by anticholinesterase drugs, which dramatically relieve muscular weakness and fatiguability. Neostigmine 1–3 mg may be injected s.c. It is best to give atropine 0.5 mg for each 1 mg of neostigmine to avoid unpleasant visceral effects, e.g. colic, vomiting, defaecation, due to stimulation of the parasympathetic autonomic system. The atropine does not interfere with the effect of neostigmine at the neuromuscular junction, i.e. it antagonises the muscarinic but not the nicotinic effect of acetylcholine.

Edrophonium has fewer autonomic side-effects and is usually preferred for its much briefer action than neostigmine. A syringe is loaded with edrophonium 10 mg; 2 mg are given i.v. and if there is no improvement in weakness in 30 sec the remaining 8 mg are injected. An hour later 15 or 20 mg can be given if there was no response to the first injection.

Treatment is: (a) symptomatic and (b) immunosuppressive.

a. *Symptomatic* treatment aims to increase the concentration of acetylcholine at the neuromuscular junction with anticholinesterase drugs. The mainstay is usually pyridostigmine, starting with 60 mg by mouth 6-hourly and increasing if necessary to 1200 mg per day in 3 or 4 divided doses. The effects of pyridostigmine by mouth begin in about 20 min and are maximal after 2 hours. Pyridostigmine is preferred because its action is smoother than that of neostigmine but the latter is more rapid in onset and can with advantage be given in the mornings to get the patient mobile. Either drug can be given parenterally if bulbar paralysis makes swallowing difficult. Individual variation in response and care in adjusting doses and intervals is rewarding. Too high a dose of anticholinesterase drugs may make the weakness worse by causing excess build-up of acetylcholine (*cholinergic crisis*) and it is important to distinguish this from an exacerbation of the disease (*myasthenic crisis*). There is no simple clinical means of making this distinction, but if the total daily dose of anticholinesterase drug is less than 15 tablets and the pupil diameter exceeds 3 mm the weakness is unlikely to be cholinergic. The pattern of relief of weakness may also help; if it increases more than 2 hours after a dose, and is relieved by the next dose, this suggests myasthenic weakness; if it is marked 1 hour after a dose and is not significantly improved by the next dose, it is likely to be cholinergic. A consideration of the mechanism of action and of the time-course of drug effect shows why this should be so. A dose of edrophonium will make the diagnosis; a myasthenic crisis gets better and cholinergic crisis gets worse — dangerously so if the vital bulbar and respiratory muscles are involved — so this test is best left to those with special experience and mechanical ventilation facilities should be at hand.

The habitual use of atropine to abolish parasympathetic effects is undesirable because it may mask excessive therapy, and so make the differentiation between myasthenic and cholinergic crisis more difficult, for parasympathomimetic effects (miosis, salivation, abdominal cramps, bradycardia) act as a warning that overdose is being approached.

The patient should learn to recognise the symptoms of both overdosage and underdosage. At high doses accumulation may occur over several weeks and culminate in a cholinergic crisis. Eye muscles are relatively resistant to therapy so that forcing the dose to correct diplopia may cause a cholinergic crisis. A cholinergic crisis should be treated by withdrawing all anticholinesterase medication, mechanical respiration if required, and atropine i.v. for muscarinic effects of the overdosage. The neuromuscular block is a nicotinic effect and will be unchanged by atropine.

* Disabilities and how to live with them. London: Lancet, 1952.

† Havard C W H, Scadding G K. Drugs 1983; 26: 174–184.

Pralidoxime may be tried (500 mg by slow i.v. infusion repeated as necessary) though it may be ineffective.

A resistant myasthenic crisis may be treated by withdrawal of drugs and artificial respiration for a few days. Plasma exchange has been tried (to remove antibodies).

b. *Immunosuppressive* treatment is directed at eliminating the acetylcholine receptor antibody, thus correcting the underlying immunological abnormality at least temporarily.

Thymectomy causes remission in 80% of patients under 40 years who do not have a thymoma, although it may take 3–5 years for the full effect to become apparent. Why thymectomy should be effective is not clear, for the thymus is not a major site of anti-receptor antibody, although the gland does contain acetylcholine receptors; it is suggested that thymocytes influence the patient's own lymphocytes to produce specific antibody.

Thymectomy should also be undertaken in myasthenic patients who have a thymoma, but the reason is to prevent local tumour extension for the procedure usually does not improve the muscle weakness.

Prednisolone induces improvement or remission in over 80% of cases. The dose should be increased slowly using an alternate-day regimen until the minimum effective amount is attained and improvement may take several weeks. Some patients initially get worse on corticosteroid therapy, possibly because anticholinesterases are rendered more effective, and a cholinergic crisis is provoked. The risk of such an occurrence is lessened if the initial dose of corticosteroid is low and is increased gradually but it should always be undertaken in a hospital with intensive care facilities.

Corticosteroid treatment is indicated for the seriously ill patient about to undergo surgery, for those who are unsuitable for thymectomy and for patients who have not benefitted from the procedure. In addition, prednisolone may be particularly effective for ocular myasthenia, which is fortunate, for this variant of the disease responds poorly to thymectomy or anticholinesterase drugs.

Azathioprine is also effective but maximum improvement may not be seen for 6–15 months. Patients who are male, over 35 years and who have had the disease for less than 10 years seem to respond best. Prednisolone, together with azathioprine as a corticosteroid-sparing agent, is probably the best combination for the severely affected myasthenic patient.

In summary, treatment of myasthenic gravis comprises:

a. anticholinesterases for symptomatic relief;

b. prenisolone when thymectomy is inappropriate or ineffective;

c. azathioprine as a corticosteroid-sparing agent;

d. thymectomy for patients under 40 years who do not have a thymoma.

Drug-induced disorders of neuromuscular transmission

Quite apart from the neuromuscular blocking agents used in anaesthesia, a number of drugs possess actions that impair neuromuscular transmission and in appropriate circumstances, give rise to:

a. postoperative respiratory depression in persons whose neuromuscular transmission is otherwise normal;

b. aggravation or unmasking of myasthenia gravis or

c. a drug-induced myasthenic syndrome.

These drugs include:

Antibiotics: Aminoglycosides (neomycin, streptomycin, kanamycin, gentamicin) and polypeptides (colistin, polymyxin B) may cause postoperative breathing difficulty if they are instilled into the peritoneal or pleural cavities. It appears that the antibiotics both interfere with the release of acetylcholine and have a curare-like effect on the postsynaptic membrane.

Cardiovascular drugs: Those that possess local anaesthetic effect properties (quinidine, procainamide, lignocaine) and certain β-adrenoceptor blockers (propranolol, oxprenolol, practolol) act by interfering with neurotransmitter release and may aggravate or reveal myasthenia gravis.

Other drugs:

Penicillamine causes some patients, especially

those with rheumatoid arthritis, to form antibodies to the acetylcholine receptor and a syndrome indistinguishable from myasthenia gravis results. Spontaneous recovery occurs in about two-thirds of cases when penicillamine is withdrawn.

Phenytoin may rarely induce or aggravate myasthenia gravis, or induce a myasthenic syndrome, possibly by depressing acetylcholine release.

Lithium may impair presynaptic neurotransmission by substituting for sodium ions in the nerve terminal.

DRUGS WHICH OPPOSE ACETYLCHOLINE

These drugs may be divided into three groups:

A. **Anticholinergic (or anti-acetylcholine)** drugs, which act principally at post-ganglionic cholinergic (parasympathetic) nerve endings, i.e. atropine-like drugs (Figure 22.1, p. 461, site 2).

B. **Ganglion-blocking** agents (Figure 22.1, site 1).

C. **Neuromuscular blocking** agents (Figure 22.1, site 5).

It is not known why drugs oppose acetylcholine more effectively at some sites than at others. The above groups are not perfectly separate, for both curare and atropine have weak ganglion-blocking effects.

Atropine and related drugs block the effect of acetylcholine, at the post-ganglionic cholinergic (parasympathetic) endings, site 2 on the diagram; and also at the non-innervated receptors on the blood vessels (i.e. antimuscarinic) and in the central nervous system. Some drugs of this group have a blocking effect at autonomic ganglia also, but none blocks the neuromuscular junction except in heavy overdose (propantheline).

The actions of atropine will first be described. Other drugs will be dealt with chiefly in how they differ from atropine. Some anticholinergic drugs have a variety of other actions, e.g. histamine-receptor block, but find a place in therapeutics as anticholinergic agents.

Atropine

Atropine is an alkaloid from the plant *Atropa belladonna*, the first name of which commemorates its success as a homicidal poison, for it is derived from the senior of three legendary Fates, Atropos, who cuts with shears the web of life spun and woven by her sisters Clotho and Lachesis (there is a minor synthetic atropine-like drug named lachesine). The term belladonna refers to the once fashionable female practice of using an extract of the plant to dilate the pupils (incidentally blocking ocular accommodation) as part of the process of 'making myself attractive'.

Atropine acts by competing for the same receptors as acetylcholine, occupying them and thus rendering the acetylcholine ineffectual, i.e. it has the same affinity as acetylcholine for the receptors but different intrinsic activity (it is an acetylcholine receptor blocker).

In general, the peripheral effects of atropine are inhibitory but commonly a transient phase of stimulation (partial agonist effect, perhaps in the central nervous system) occurs before the inhibition and in the case of the heart (Vagus nerve) this can have clinical importance. Atropine also blocks the effects of injected cholinergic drugs both peripherally and on the central nervous system. The clinically important actions of atropine are listed below; they are mostly the opposite of the activating effects on the parasympathetic system produced by cholinergic drugs.

Actions at parasympathetic post-ganglionic nerve endings

Exocrine glands. All secretions except milk are diminished. Dry mouth is common and lachrymation is suppressed. Gastric acid secretion is reduced but so also is the total volume of gastric secretion so that H^+ concentration (pH) may be little altered. In doses acceptable to man, atropine does not have enough effect on acid secretion to be of use in peptic ulcer (i.e. it lacks selectivity for the stomach).

Sweating (sympathetic nerve supply, but largely cholinergic) is inhibited. Bronchial secretions are reduced and may become viscid, which can be a disadvantage, as removal of secretion by cough and ciliary action is rendered less effective.

Smooth muscle is relaxed. In the gastrointestinal tract there is reduction of tone and peristalsis. Muscle spasm of the intestinal tract induced by morphine is reduced, but such spasm in the biliary tract is not. Atropine relaxes bronchial muscle, an effect which is useful in some asthmatics. Micturition is slowed and urinary retention may be induced, especially when there is pre-existing prostatic enlargement.

Ocular effects. Mydriasis occurs with a rise in intra-ocular pressure in an eye predisposed to narrow-angle glaucoma (but only rarely in chronic open-angle glaucoma). This is due to the dilated iris blocking drainage of the intra-ocular fluids from the angle of the anterior chamber. An attack of glaucoma may be induced. There is no significant effect on pressure in normal eyes. The ciliary muscle is relaxed and so the eye is accommodated for distant vision. After atropinisation, normal pupillary reflexes may not be regained for two weeks. Atropine is a cause of unequal sized and unresponsive pupils.

Cardiosvascular system. Atropine reduces vagal tone thus increasing the heart rate, and enhancing conduction in the bundle of His, effects that are less marked in the elderly, in whom vagal tone is low. Full atropinisation may increase rate by 30 beats/min in the young, but has little effect in the old.

Transient initial vagal stimulation, probably in the central nervous system, may be of clinical importance when atropine is given with neostigmine, as when the latter is used to antagonise curare-like drugs. This does not occur in blacks, a genetic difference. It is generally advised that atropine be given a few minutes before neostigmine to avoid the transient summation of the two drugs on the vagus.

Atropine has no significant effect on peripheral blood vesels in therapeutic doses, but in poisoning, there is marked vasodilatation.

Central nervous system is stimulated by atropine. Restlessness and mental excitement occur with large doses, and even mania, delirium and hallucinations. Hyperthermia occurs, made worse by the concurrent prevention of sweating.

Atropine is effective against both tremor and rigidity of parkinsonism (see index). It prevents or abates motion sickness.

Antagonism to cholinergic drugs. Atropine opposes the effects of all cholinergic drugs on the central nervous system, at post-ganglionic cholinergic synapses and on the peripheral blood vessels. It does not oppose cholinergic effects at the neuromuscular junction or significantly at the autonomic ganglia (i.e. atropine opposes the muscarine-like but not the nicotine-like effects of acetylcholine).

Pharmacokinetics. Atropine is readily absorbed from the alimentary tract and may also be injected by the usual routes. The occasional cases of atropine poisoning following use of eye drops are due to the solution running down the lacrimal ducts into the nose and being swallowed. The $t_{\frac{1}{2}}$ is 15–40 hours. Atropine is in part destroyed in the liver and in part excreted unchanged by the kidney. Some tolerance occurs.

The usual dose is 0.25–2.0 mg by mouth or 0.4–1.0 mg by i.v. injection; for chronic use it has largely been replaced by other drugs.

Atropine (and other anticholinergic drug) *poisoning* presents with the more obvious peripheral effects — dry mouth (with dysphagia), mydriasis, blurred vision, hot dry skin, and, in addition, hyperexia, restlessness, anxiety, excitement, hallucinations, delirium, mania and later, cerebral depression and coma — or as it has been described with characteristic American verbal felicity 'hot as a hare, blind as a bat, dry as a bone, red as a beet and mad as a hen.'* It may occur in children who have eaten berries of solanaceous plants, e.g. deadly nightshade and henbane. When the diagnosis is doubtful, it is said to be worth putting a drop of the patient's urine in *one* eye of a cat (the rabbit is less sensitive; the test does not seem to have been used in man). Mydriasis, if it results, confirms the diagnosis, but absence of effect proves nothing.

* Cohen H L et al. Archives of Neurology and Psychiatry 1944; 51:171.

The treatment of atropine (and other anticholinergic drug) poisoning is on general lines, e.g. a sedative (diazepam) for excitement. There is evidence that an anticholinesterase drug that enters the central nervous system may be useful in reversing both the central and peripheral effects. Physostigmine (eserine) 1–4 mg i.v. or i.m. is effective, though it may need repeating, as its action (1–2 hours) is shorter than that of atropine; high dose may cause convulsions.

Other anticholinergic drugs

In the accounts that follow, the principal peripheral atropine-like effects of the drugs may be assumed. The points in which they differ from atropine are the main topics.

Hyoscyamine is less active in the central nervous system. Atropine is racemic hyoscyamine, 'hyoscyamine' is the laevo form; the dextro form is only feebly active. Atropine is more stable chemically and so is preferred.

Hyoscine (scopolamine) is structurally related to atropine. It differs chiefly in being a central nervous system depressant, although it may sometimes cause excitment. The old are often confused by hyoscine and so it is avoided in their anaesthetic premedication. Mydriasis is briefer than with atropine. The dose is 0.3–0.6 mg s.c. *Genoscopolamine* is similar to hyoscine.

Atropine methonitrate (Eumydrin) blocks autonomic ganglia as well as having strong peripheral effects, especially on the intestinal tract and salivary secretion. It has been used in the conservative treatment of congenital hypertrophic pyloric stenosis, combined with dietary control, but this tedious treatment has been superseded by surgery.

Hyoscyamus, stramonium and *belladonna* are crude plant preparations containing hyoscyamine, hyoscine and atropine in varying proportions. At one time Bulgarian belladonna had a high reputation as a remedy for parkinsonism. It was taken in white wine 'after the first sleep' and was part of a system of 'cure' which included bathing in water warmed by the sun and sleeping only on the right side. This routine naturally had a marked, though only temporary success. Bulgarian belladonna was soon shown not to be superior to other forms.

Hyoscine butylbromide (Buscopan) also blocks autonomic ganglia. It is effective orally, i.m. or i.v. It is an effective relaxant of smooth muscle, including the cardia in achalasia, the pyloric antral region and the colon. Radiologists and endoscopists use it for this. It may sometimes be useful for colic.

Homatropine is used for its ocular effects (2% solution as eye drops). Its action is shorter than atropine and therefore less likely to cause serious rise of intra-ocular pressure. Its effects wear off in a day or two. Complete cycloplegia cannot always be obtained unless repeated instillations are made every 15 min for 1–2 h. It is especially unreliable in children, in whom atropine is preferred. The pupillary dilation may be reversed by physostigmine eyedrops. Derivatives are available for systemic use but offer no important advantages.

Tropicamide (Mydriacyl) and cyclopentolate (Mydrilate) are useful (as 0.5 or 1% solutions) for mydriasis and cycloplegia. They are quicker and shorter acting than homatropine. The differences between them are trivial. Mydriasis occurs in 10–20 min and cycloplegia shortly after. The duration of action is 6–12 h.

Ipratropium (Atrovent) is used by inhalation as a bronchodilator; it has little effect on mucus viscosity.

Propantheline (Pro-Banthine) is perhaps the best known of a large number of synthetic anticholinergic drugs that have achieved a largely undeserved popularity, especially in the treatment of peptic ulcer. The drug may also be used for irritable bowel syndrome, as a muscle relaxant in diagnostic procedures, and for nocturnal enuresis. It has marked peripheral atropine-like and weak ganglion-blocking actions, so that, although it can interfere with all autonomic functions, its effects are most marked on the parasympathetic division. In overdose it has a curare-like effect at the neuromuscular junction, so it is capable of antagonising acetylcholine at all peripheral cholinergic nerve endings. The unwanted effects are what might be expected: dry mouth, blurred vision, constipation and difficult micturition. Postural hypotension and sexual impotence may occur.

Emepronium (Cetiprin) is similar to propantheline. It has been found useful in reducing bladder motility and increasing bladder capacity in cases of urinary frequency, tenesmus and urgency incontinence. It is noted for causing oesophageal ulceration especially in the elderly (when the tablets are held up).

Flavoxate (Urispas) is similar.

Dicyclomine (Merbentyl) is preferred for infantile pyloric stenosis and infantile colic.

Glycopyrronium (Robinul) is used by anaesthetists (see index).

Many drugs similar to propantheline have been marketed because any really effective and selective parasympathetic-blocking agent might theoretically have some use in treatment of peptic ulcer, but in general they are ineffective under conditions of clinical use. It would be profitless as well as tedious to describe each drug and to enumerate the claims made for it, and so only some of the names will be given here for identification of the type of drug: penthienate (Monodral), tricyclamol, poldine (Nacton), orphenadrine (Benadryl), promethazine (Phenergan).

Other drugs with anticholinergic effects are described under the drug therapy of parkinsonism. For poisoning see under atropine.

Uses of anticholinergic drugs

The clinical uses of anticholinergic drugs are legion.

a. *For their actions in the central nervous system* some (benzhexol, orphenadrine) are used against the rigidity and tremor of *parkinsonism* in which disease doses higher than the usual therapeutic amounts are often needed and tolerated.

They are used as *anti-emetics* (hyoscine, promethazine).

Their *sedative* action is used in anaesthetic premedication (hyoscine).

b. *For their peripheral actions* they (atropine, homatropine, cyclopentolate) are used in *ophthalmology* to *dilate the pupil and to paralyse ocular accommodation*. If it is desired to dilate the pupil and to spare accomodation, a sympathomimetic (e.g. phenylephrine) is useful.

In *anaesthesia* (atropine, glycopyrronium, hyoscine) to block the vagus and reduce secretion.

In the *respiratory tract* ipratopium is an effective bronchodilator, sparing mucus viscosity.

For their actions on the *alimentary tract* they are used against muscle spasm and hypermotility. They are used in ulcerative colitis, and against colic (pain due to spasm of smooth muscle) and to prevent morphine-induced muscle spasm when that analgesic is used against colic.

In the *urinary tract*, emepronium and flavoxate are used to relieve muscle spasm accompanying infection in cystitis and against colic.

In disorders of the *cardiovascular system*, anticholinergic drugs may be useful in attacks of cardiac arrest due to hyperactivity of the carotid sinus reflex and occasionally in heart-block and in bradycardia following myocardial infarction (atropine), but the initial vagal stimulation may be a disadvantage.

In *cholinergic poisoning*, atropine is an important antagonist of both central nervous, parasympathomimetic and vasodilator effects though it has no effect at the neuromuscular junction and will not prevent voluntary muscle paralysis. It is also used to block autonomic effects when cholinergic drugs, such as neostigmine, are used for their effect on the neuromuscular junction in myasthenia gravis and to reverse neuromuscular block in anaesthesia.

Disadvantages of the anticholinergics include their capacity to precipitate narrow-angle glaucoma or urinary retention in the presence of prostatic hypertrophy. In organic pyloric stenosis these drugs may prevent gastric emptying by reducing peristalsis and they may also make oesophageal achalasia worse.

GUIDE TO FURTHER READING

1 Harris et al. Convulsant shock treatment of patients with mental disease by intravenous injection of acetylcholine. Archives in Neurology and Psychiatry 1943; 50:304.
2 Cohen H L et al. Acetlycholine treatment of schizophrenia. Archives in Neurology and Psychiatry 1944; 51:171.
3 Hawkins J R et al. Journal of Mental Science 1956; 102. Intravenous acetlycholine therapy in neurosis. A controlled trial, p 43. Carbon dioxide inhalation therapy in neurosis. A controlled clinical trial, p 52. The placebo response, p 60.
4 Cullumbine H et al. The effects of atropine sulphate

upon healthy male subjects. Quart J Exp Physiol 1955; 40: 309–319.
5 Morton H G et al. Atropine intoxication. J Pediatr 1939; 14:755.
6 Randall W C et al. The pharmacology of sweating. Pharmacol Rev 1955; 7:365.
7 Williams E M V. The mode of action of drugs upon intestinal motility. Pharmacol Rev 1954; 6:159.
8 Grant W M. Physiological and pharmacological influences upon intraocular pressure. Pharmacol Rev 1955; 7:143.
9 Lambert D. Personal paper; Myasthenia gravis. Lancet 1981; 1:937.
10 Editorial. Management of myasthenia gravis. Lancet 1982; 2:135.
11 Scadding G K, Havard C W H. Pathogenesis and treatment of myasthenia gravis. Br Med J 1981; 183: 1008–1012.

23

Cardiovascular system I: Adrenergic mechanisms: Sympathomimetic agents

ADRENERGIC MECHANISMS

Some History

Sir Henry Dale has told of the discovery in 1895 of the hypertensive effect of adrenaline: 'Dr. Oliver . . . was a physician in practice. . . . he appears to have used his family in his experiments, and a young son was the subject of a series, in which Dr. Oliver measured the diameter of the radial artery and observed the effect upon it of injecting extracts of various animal glands under the skin. We may picture Professor Schafer . . . finishing an experiment . . . in which he was recording the arterial pressure of an anaesthetised dog. To him enters Dr. Oliver, with the story of the experiments, and, in particular, with the statement that injection under the skin of a glycerine extract from the calf's suprarenal gland was followed by a definite narrowing of the radial artery. Professor Schafer is said to have been entirely sceptical, and to have attributed the observation to self-delusion. . . . Dr. Oliver, however, is persistent . . . so Professor Schafer makes the injection, expecting a triumphant demonstration of nothing, and finds himself standing 'like some watcher of the skies, when a new planet swims into his ken', watching the mercury rise in the manometer with amazing rapidity and to an astounding height. . . .'*

This discovery led eventually to the isolation and synthesis of adrenaline in the early 1900s. Many related compounds were examined and, in 1910, Barger and Dale invented the word *sympathomimetic*† and also pointed out that noradrenaline mimicked the action of the sympathetic nervous system more closely than did adrenaline. Nevertheless adrenaline was generally thought to be the sympathetic mediator for the next 35 years, partly because noradrenaline was not known to be present in the body, and partly because many of the available preparations of 'adrenaline' did in fact contain a substantial amount of noradrenaline. Clarification of the situation had to wait until accurate methods both of identifying adrenaline and noradrenaline and of estimating them separately were found.

* Dale H. Edinburgh Medical Journal 1938; 45:461

† Compounds which . . . simulate the effects of sympathetic nerves not only with varying intensity but with varying precision . . . a term . . . seems needed to indicate the type of action common to these bases. We propose to call it 'sympathomimetic'. A term which indicates the relation of the action to innervation by the sympathetic system, without involving any theoretical preconception as to the meaning of that relation or the precise mechanism of the action'. (Barger G, Dale, H H. J Physiol 1910; XLI: 19–59.)

CLASSIFICATION OF SYMPATHOMIMETICS BY SITE OF ACTION

Noradrenaline is synthesised and stored at adrenergic nerve terminals and can be released from these stores by stimulating the nerve or by drugs (reserpine, guanethidine, ephedrine, amphetamine). These noradrenaline stores may be replenished by i.v. infusion of noradrenaline, and abolished by cutting the nerve.

Sympathomimetics may be classified thus: those that act:

a. **directly** on the adrenoceptor (adrenaline, noradrenaline, isoprenaline, methoxamine, xylometazoline, oxymetazoline, metaraminol, oxedrine, entirely; and dopamine and phenylephrine mainly).

b. **indirectly**, by causing a release of noradrenaline from stores at nerve endings (amphetamines, tyramine; ephedrine, largely).

c. *by both mechanisms* (a) *and* (b), though often with a preponderance of one or other: other synthetic agents, but also dopamine and ephedrine.

It is evident that *tachyphylaxis* (diminishing response to frequent or continuous administration) is particularly to be expected with drugs in group (b), and that they are less suitable for use in maintaining blood pressure than drugs of group (a). Tachyphylaxis to group (a) may be due to receptor changes.

The *interactions* of sympathomimetics with other drugs affecting the vascular system are complex. Some drugs prevent the uptake of noradrenaline from the circulation into stores (this may account for the potentiation of the pressor effect of noradrenaline by guanethidine and tricyclic antidepressants) and some drugs actively deplete the stores (reserpine) and thus block the action of sympathomimetics that act by releasing noradrenaline from stores. It is now evident that the sympathetic system is a lot more complicated than many had previously supposed, and that some drugs will act differently after acute and after chronic administration, according to whether the noradrenaline stores are depleted or not, and receptors may change in number and activity; and there are subclasses of receptors.

Actions of sympathomimetics: definition of adrenoceptors

Many sympathomimetics are racemic compounds and one form is commonly much more active: for instance levo-noradrenaline is at least 50 times as active as the dextro form.

For 46 years (up to 1958) it was known that the peripheral motor (vasoconstriction) effects of adrenaline were preventable and that the peripheral inhibitory (vasodilatation) and the cardiac stimulant actions were not preventable by the then available antagonists (ergot alkaloids, phenoxybenzamine).

In 1948, Ahlquist introduced a hypothesis to account for this. He proposed **two different sorts of adrenoceptors** (α and β). For a further 10 years, only antagonists of α-receptor effects (α-adrenoceptor block) were known, but in 1958 the first substance to selectively and competitively prevent β-receptor effects (β-adrenoceptor blocker), dichloroisoprenaline, was discovered. However, it was unsuitable for clinical use (it also had strong agonist activity, i.e. it was a partial agonist or agonist/antagonist) and it was not until 1962 that the first reasonably satisfactory β-adrenoceptor blocker (pronethalol) was introduced to medicine. Unfortunately it proved to be carcinogenic in some mice (but not in rats) and was soon replaced by propranolol (Inderal).

It is evident that the site of action has an important role in selectivity, e.g. drugs that act on receptors *directly* and stereospecifically may be highly selective, whereas drugs that act *indirectly* by discharging noradrenaline indiscriminately from nerve endings, e.g. amphetamine, will have less selective effects.

Consequences of activating the adrenoceptor

Catecholamines (adrenaline, noradrenaline, dopamine) act as *first messenger* transmitters, combining with post-synaptic receptors on the outside of the cell membrane, thus activating the enzyme adenylate cyclase on the inside of the cell membrane, which causes an increase in intracellular cyclic AMP, the *second messenger* (destroyed by intracellular phosphodiesterase*). This second messenger initiates a sequence (cascade) of enzymic and ionic changes that mediate the characteristic effect of that receptor, whether this be contraction of arteriolar smooth muscle or release of glucose or potassium from liver cells.

Many hormones act via cyclic AMP. Specificity is provided by the receptor, not by the messengers.

The complexity of adrenergic mechanisms is shown by the following:

Drugs may mimic or impair adrenergic mechanisms:

1. *directly*, binding on adrenoceptors: *agonist* (adrenaline) or *antagonist* (propranolol).
2. *indirectly*, by discharging noradrenaline stored in nerve endings† (amphetamine).
3. by *preventing re-uptake* into the adrenergic nerve ending of released noradrenaline (cocaine, tricyclic antidepressants)
4. by *preventing the destruction* of noradrenaline (and dopamine) in the nerve ending (monoamine oxidase inhibitors).
5. by *depleting the stores* of noradrenaline in nerve endings (reserpine).
6. by *preventing the release* of noradrenaline from nerve endings in response to a nerve impulse (guanethidine).
7. by causing the nerve ending to synthesise a *false transmitter* instead of noradrenaline (methyldopa).

All the above mechanisms operate in both the *central* and *peripheral* nervous systems. This discussion is chiefly concerned with agents that influence peripheral adrenergic mechanisms.

* Aminophylline (in high dose only) inhibits phosphodiesterase and so enhances cyclic AMP concentrations. In the treatment of asthma with a β-receptor agonist plus aminophylline there is thus a desired interaction on the bronchi, but an undesired interaction on the heart.

† Fatal hypertension can occur when this class of agent is taken by a patient treated with a monoamine oxidase inhibitor.

Table 23.1 Clinically relevant aspects of adrenoceptor functions

α-adrenoceptor effects*	β-adrenoceptor effects
Eye†: mydriasis	**Heart** (β_1) increased *rate* (SA node) increased *automaticity* (AV node and muscle) increased *velocity* in conducting tissue increased *contractility* of myocardium decreased *refractory period* of all tissues
Arterioles: *constriction* (only slight in coronary and cerebral)	**Arterioles:** *dilatation* (β_2)
	Bronchi (β_2): relaxation
	Uterus (β_2): relaxation of pregnant uterus.
	Skeletal muscle: tremor (β_2)
Skin: sweat, pilomotor	**Mast cells**: inhibition of release of autacoids (histamine, leukotrienes) in Type I allergy
Male ejaculation	
Metabolic effect: hyperkalaemia	**Metabolic effects:** hypokalaemia (β_2) hepatic glycogenolysis (β_2) lipolysis (β_1)
Bladder sphincter: contraction	**Bladder detrusor**: relaxation
Intestinal smooth muscle relaxation is mediated by α- and β-adrenoceptors.	

* For the role of subtypes (α_1 and α_2) see prazosin.
† Effects on intra-ocular pressure involve both α- and β-adrenoceptor as well as cholinoceptors.

Numerous sympathomimetics are available, they include those that occur in the body, in plants (ephedrine) and a range of synthetic analogues. Agents that act unselectively on α- and β-adrenoceptors, not surprisingly, have only restricted utility (e.g. for local or topical application). The development of selective analogues has provided important therapeutic advances.

Ergot alkaloids act via adrenoceptors and are described in Chapter 37.

CLASSIFICATION OF SYMPATHOMIMETICS BY SELECTIVITY FOR RECEPTORS

The following classification of sympathomimetics and antagonists is based on selectivity for receptors and on use. But *selectivity is relative, not absolute*; if enough is administered, agents will act on a wider range of receptors; the same applies to selective antagonists (receptor blockers); e.g. an agent used to arrest premature labour (β_2-receptor) will also cause tachycardia (β_1) as the dose increases; a β_1-(cardio)selective adrenoceptor blocker can cause severe exacerbation of asthma (β_2) even at low dose. It is important to remember this because patients have died in the hands of doctors who have forgotten or been ignorant of it.

Agonists

α + **β-effects: unselective: adrenaline** — now used as vasoconstrictor (α) with local anaesthetics, as a mydriatic and in the emergency treatment of anaphylactic shock, for which condition it has the right mix of effects (bronchodilator, positive cardiac inotropic, vasoconstriction at high dose): it has been superseded for asthma by more selective (β_2) agents.

α-effects: noradrenaline (with slight β_1 effect on heart) is best left to its essential role in physiology: it is selectively released where it is wanted: as a therapeutic agent it has been almost entirely superseded for hypotensive states by dopamine and dobutamine: also having predominantly α-effects are methoxamine and imidazolines (xylometazoline, oxymetazoline), metaraminol, oxedrine, phenylephrine, phenylpropanolamine, ephedrine, pseudoephedrine: some are used solely for topical vasoconstriction (nasal decongestants).

α-effects in the central nervous system: clonidine.

β-effects: unselective (i.e. β_1 + β_2): **isoprenaline:** its uses as bronchodilator (β_2), for positive cardiac inotropic effect and to enhance conduction in heart block (β_1) have been largely superseded by agents with a more appropriately selective profile of effects. Other agents with unselective β-effects: ephedrine, methoxyphenamine, orciprenaline are also obsolescent for asthma.

β_1-effects, with some α-effects: dopamine: used in vascular shock.

β_1-effects: dobutamine, prenalterol: used for cardiac inotropic effect.

β_2-adrenoceptor agonists, used in *asthma*, include: salbutamol, terbutaline, fenoterol, isoetharine, pirbuterol, reproterol, rimiterol, orciprenaline (partially selective): used to relax the *uterus*: isoxsuprine, orciprenaline, ritodrine, salbutamol, terbutaline.

Antagonists

α-adrenoceptor: prazosin*, indoramin, phentolamine, phenoxybenzamine, thymoxamine, yohimbine†

β-adrenoceptor: propranolol, alprenolol, sotalol, acebutolol, pindolol, metoprolol, timolol, atenolol, oxprenolol, betaxolol, nadolol, penbutolol, practolol (for subclassification of β-adrenoceptor blockers see p. 500).

α- + β-adrenoceptor: labetalol.

The overall effect of a sympathomimetic depends on the *site* of action (direct or indirect acting), on *receptor specificity* and on *dose*; for instance adrenaline ordinarily dilates muscle blood vessels (β_2; mainly arterioles, but veins also) but in very large doses constricts them (α). The actions described in the Table are those of doses used in therapeutics or of amounts ordinarily liberated in the body. The end results are often complex and unpredictable, partly because of the variability of homeostatic reflex responses and partly because what is observed (e.g. a change in blood pressure) is the result of many factors (e.g. vasodilatation [β] in some areas, vasoconstriction [α] in others, and cardiac stimulation [β]).

To block all the effects of adrenaline and noradrenaline, both kinds of antagonist must be

* Prazosin (p. 496) is selective for α_1-adrenoceptors on the effector organ (post-junctional, post-synaptic) and spares presynaptic α_2-adrenoceptors on the nerve ending (the role of which is to mediate negative feedback control and so to reduce noradrenaline release from nerve endings).

† *Yohimbine* blocks α_2 (presynaptic) adrenoceptors, i.e. it blocks the negative feedback effects of released noradrenaline thus preventing the suppression of noradrenaline release, i.e. it indirectly enhances activity of adrenergic endings; it has not found a definitive clinical use although it has had a reputation for restoring enfeebled male sexual function.

Table 23.2 Comparison of noradrenaline, adrenaline and isoprenaline

Effect	Noradrenaline	Adrenaline	Isoprenaline
Heart:			
a. rate	*slowed* (reflexly due to BP rise)	*increased* (direct action)	*increased* (direct action)
b. force of myocardial contraction	little effect	increased (direct action) 'palpitations' due to *a* + *b*	increased (direct action) 'palpitations' due to *a* + *b*
c. cardiac output (stroke)	insignificant or reduced	increased	increased
d. excitability, conductivity	increased	much increased	much increased
Blood pressure:			
a. systolic	rises	rises(due to *b* and *c* above)	little change, or may fall
b. diastolic	rises	falls (due to *a* below)	falls
Vascular beds in:			
a. muscle	usually constricted	dilated	dilated
b. skin & viscera	constricted	constricted	dilated
c. heart	? dilated	dilated	dilated
Total peripheral resistance	*increased*	*decreased*	*decreased*
Metabolism:			
O_2 consumption, liberation of glucose from glycogen	insignificant	increased	insignificant
Central nervous system	insignificant	stimulation: feelings of fear and anxiety, respiration increased, tremor	stimulation
Smooth muscle:			
a. bronchi	little effect	relaxed	relaxed
b. intestine and bladder	relaxed	relaxed	relaxed
c. sphincters	constricted	constricted	constricted
d. uterus (pregnant)	stimulated	usually inhibited	inhibited
Capillary permeabilty	little effect	reduced	?

used. This can be a matter of practical importance, e.g. in phaeochromocytoma.

Adverse effects

Adverse effects of sympathomimetics may be deduced from their actions. Tissue necrosis due to intense vasoconstriction (α) around injection sites is particularly prone to occur as a result of leakage from i.v. infusions. The effects on the heart (β_1) are the commonest cause of deaths due to these drugs (ventricular dysrhythmias), and sympathomimetic drugs should be used with great caution in patients with heart disease.

Sympathomimetics are particularly likely to cause cardiac dysrhythmias (β_1) in patients under trichloroethylene or halothane anaesthesia. The effect of the sympathomimetic drugs on the pregnant uterus is variable and difficult to predict, but serious fetal distress can occur, due to reduced placental blood flow as a result both of contraction of the uterine muscle (α) and arterial constriction (α). β_2-agonists are used to relax the uterus in premature labour, but unwanted cardiovascular actions can be troublesome.

Only about 2% of circulating adrenaline or noradrenaline is excreted unchanged in the urine, but this is enough to be useful in the diagnosis of

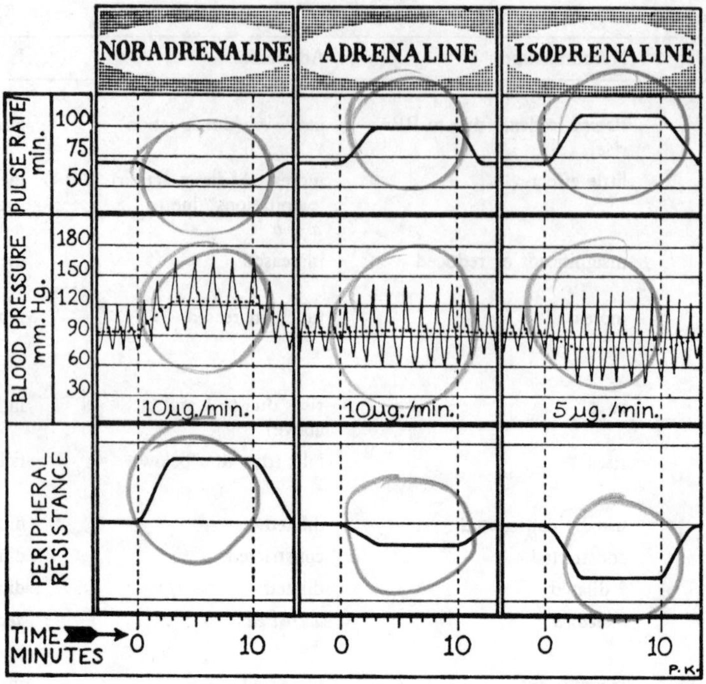

Fig. 23.1 Cardiovascular effects of noradrenaline, adrenaline and isoprenaline; pulse rate/min, blood pressure in mmHg (dotted line is mean pressure), peripheral resistance in arbitrary units. By permission after Ginsburg J. Cobbold A F, In: Vane J R et al., ed. Adrenergic mechanism. London: Churchill, 1960.

phaechromocytoma. The estimation of the breakdown products, metanephrines, and vanilyl mandelic acid (VMA) in the urine is also useful.

Sympathomimetics and plasma potassium

Adrenergic mechanisms have a role in the physiological control of plasma potassium concentration. The biochemical pump that shifts K into cells is activated by β_2-adrenoceptor agonists (adrenaline, salbutamol, isoxsurpine) and can cause *hypo*kalaemia. The effect is blocked by β_2-adrenoceptor antagonists.

The α-adrenoceptor has a suppressive effect on the pump and activation tends to cause *hyper*kalaemia.

The effects of administered (β_2) sympathomimetics may be clinically important in patients having pre-existing hypokalaemia, e.g. due to intense adrenergic activity such as occurs in myocardial infarction*, in fright (admission to hospital is accompanied by transient hypokalaemia), or with previous diuretic therapy, and taking digoxin. In such subjects use of a sympathomimetic infusion or of an adrenaline-containing local anaesthetic may increase the hypokalaemia and precipitate cardia dysrhythmia.

β-adrenoceptor blockers, as expected, enhance the hyperkalaemia of muscular exercise; and one of their benefits in preventing cardiac dysrhythmias after myocardial infarction may be due to block of β_2-receptor-induced hypokalaemia.

Pharmacokinetics

Catecholamines (adrenaline, noradrenaline, dopamine, dobutamine) are metabolised by two enzymes, monoamine oxidase (MAO) and catechol-O-methyltransferase (COMT). These enzymes are present in large amounts in the liver and kidney and account for most of the metabolism of injected catecholamines. MAO is also present in the intestinal mucosa (and in nerve endings, peripheral and central). Because of these enzymes catecholamines are ineffective when swallowed (though isoprenaline in enormous dose can be used by this route

* Normal subjects, infused i.v. with adrenaline in amounts that approximate to those found in the plasma after severe myocardial infarction show a fall in plasma K of about 0.8 mmol/l. Brown M J N Engl. J. Med 1983; 309:1414

to treat heart block); non-catecholamines (e.g. salbutamol, amphetamine) are effective orally.

A physiological note. The *termination of action of noradrenaline* released at nerve endings is by (a) re-uptake into nerve endings where it is stored and also subject to MAO degradation, (b) diffusion away from the area of the nerve ending and the receptor (junctional cleft), and (c) metabolism (by MAO and COMT). These processes are slower than the extraordinarily swift destruction of acetylcholine at the neuromuscular junction by acetylcholinesterase situated outside the cells alongside the receptors. The difference reflects a different physiological requirement, almost instantaneous (millisecond) responses required of voluntary muscle are not required (indeed might be disastrous) of arteriolar muscle.

The *plasma $t_{\frac{1}{2}}$ of catecholamines is 1–2 min.*

Synthetic non-catecholamines in clinical use have $t_{\frac{1}{2}}$ of hours, e.g. salbutamol (albuterol) 4 h, because they are more resistant to enzymic degradation and conjugation. They penetrate the central nervous system and may have prominent effects (e.g. amphetamine). Substantial amounts appear in the urine, where they are subject to pH-dependent kinetics (see index; acid urine enhances urinary elimination and alkaline urine reduces it); this is of little importance in treating overdose since the drugs are relatively short acting and sedation (for CNS effects) by chlorpromazine, which also has useful α-adrenoceptor blocking action, plus a β-adrenoceptor blocker for cardiac dysrhythmia if it occurs, is convenient.

Individual sympathomimetics

The classic type-substances will be described first despite their limited role in therapeutics, and then the more selective analogues that have largely replaced them. See the table on p. 477 for list of receptor actions, which will not be repeated in detail here.

For *pharmacokinetics*, see above.

Adrenaline (**epinephrine**; both α- and β-receptor effects) is used as a vasoconstrictor with local anaesthetics (1 : 80 000 or weaker) to prolong their effects (about × 2); as a topical mydriatic (sparing accommodation; it also lowers intra-ocular pressure); and for allergic reactions, s.c., i.m. (or i.v.). The route must be chosen with care. Given s.c. there is intense vasoconstriction, which slows absorption and so prolongs and smooths effects, if there is circulatory collapse (as in anaphylactic shock) absorption will be too delayed and the i.m. route is preferred; use i.v. requires dilution of the standard solution (1 : 1000, i.e. 1 mg/ml) and careful, frequent monitoring of heart rate and blood pressure. Intracardiac injection is used in cardiac arrest; even though ventricular fibrillation may be provoked, normal rhythm can be restored by electric cardioversion.

Adrenaline is used in anaphylactic shock (i.m.) because its mix of actions, cardiovascular and bronchial, provide the best compromise for speed and simplicity of use in an emergency; it may also stabilise mast cell membranes and reduce release of vasoactive autacoids. The dose for this indication is 0.5–1 mg (0.5–1 ml of 1 : 1000 solution: 1 mg/ml): it is repeated as necessary and generally 2 mg in 5 min should be regarded as maximal. It may be exceeded, but palpitations, cardiac dysrhythmia and hypertension are likely to occur. Lower doses s.c., e.g. 200–500 μg are used for less urgent situations.

Adrenaline (topical) decreases intra-ocular pressure in chronic open-angle glaucoma, as does *dipivefrine*, an adrenaline ester prodrug.

Minor uses that are obsolescent include: hypoglycaemia (to mobilise hepatic glycogen as glucose) and to contract the splenic capsule to discharge malaria parasites into the general circulation for diagnosis.

Thyrotoxic patients are intolerant of adrenaline.

Accidental *overdose* with adrenaline occurs occasionally. It is rationally treated by propranolol to block the cardiac β-effects (cardiac dysrhythmia) and phentolamine to control the α-effects on the peripheral circulation that will be prominent when the β-effects are abolished; labetalol would be an alternative. β-adrenoceptor block alone is hazardous as the then unopposed α-receptor vasoconstriction causes (severe) hypertension; see phaeochromocytoma. Antihypertensives of other kinds are plainly irrational and some may also potentiate the adrenaline.

Noradrenaline (**norepinephrine**; chiefly α-effects). The main effect of administered noradrenaline is to raise the blood pressure by constricting the arterioles and so raising the total peripheral resistance, with reduced blood flow, (except in coronary arteries which have few α-receptors), though it does have slight cardiac stimulant (β_1) effect. Noradrenaline is given by i.v. infusion to obtain a gradual sustained response; the effect of a single i.v. injection would last only a minute or so. It is obsolete except where strong peripheral vasoconstriction is specifically desired, e.g. septic shock. It is available in ampoules of solution containing 1 mg/ml of base and these are diluted (usually 4 ml/litre) in glucose 5%, or NaCl plus glucose: pH < 6; the usual dose is 4–6 μg/min of noradenaline base (8–12 μg of salt); approximately 15–30 drops/min) but the rate is always adjusted according to the response and much higher dose may be needed. After a few hours the solution will have significantly lost potency (0.5 g ascorbic acid/litre will delay this). Blood pressure must be taken at 5-min intervals, and more frequently at the beginning of the infusion. Gangrene of the extremities may follow prolonged infusions and necrotic ulceration of large areas round the infusion site can occur, for even if the needle does not slip out of the vein, some will leak out. The risk of gangrene can be minimised by using a large vein and rapid flow of dilute solution for the shortest possible time. If an extravasation is detected, the α-adrenoceptor blocking agent, phentolamine (5 mg diluted), should be injected into the area. If an infusion of noradrenaline is given for many hours some blood vessels may cease to respond, and the blood pressure may fall, so that the dose has to be increased even though some vessels at the periphery may be so constricted that gangrene begins.

Noradrenaline infusions should be stopped gradually because their sudden cessation may be followed by a catastrophic fall in the blood pressure. Many explanations have been put forward both for this and for the development of tachyphylaxis, but none is established. The difficulties and dangers, including cardiac dysrhythmias, of noradrenaline infusions are undoubted, and the benefits obtained from them in, for instance, hypotensive states may be questioned: infusions should be avoided whenever possible. It is uncertain whether the transient rise of serum potassium that occurs at the beginning of an infusion has practical importance. Noradrenaline is used with injected local anaesthetics (1 : 80 000 or weaker).

Isoprenaline (isoproterenol, isopropylnoradrenaline) is a non-selective β-receptor agonist, i.e. it affects both β_1 and β_2-receptors. It relaxes muscle, including that of the blood vessels, has negligible metabolic or vasoconstrictor effects, but has a vigorous stimulant effect on the heart. This latter is its main disadvantage in the treatment of bronchial asthma and virtually precludes injection except in complete heart block. It can be given as tablets, to be dissolve under the tongue or as a sustained-release preparation (Saventrine) to be swallowed. In asthma it has been superseded by selective β_2-agonists. *Adverse effects* to be expected of a β-adrenoceptor agonist include tachycardia, palpitations, dysrhythmias and tremor, and angina pectoris in predisposed patients.

Dopamine is an agonist for specific *dopamine receptors* in the CNS and the renal artery (dilator), as well as for both α- and β-adrenoceptors; it also has some capacity to release noradrenaline from nerve endings. It is given by continuous i.v. infusion because, like all catecholamines, its $t_{\frac{1}{2}}$ is short (2 min). An i.v. infusion (2–5 μg/kg/min) causes increased renal blood flow due to action on vasodilator dopamine receptors in the renal artery. As the dose rises the heart is stimulated, with tachycardia and increased cardiac output. On the peripheral circulation the combination of α- and β-adrenoceptor effects usually causes overall slight reduction in total peripheral resistance, though at high doses the alpha effects predominate (hypertension occurs). This combination of effects renders dopamine a drug of choice in management of shock (provided any intravascular volume deficit has been corrected), but the use of any drug in this condition should not be undertaken lightly. An i.v. infusion should start at about 2 μg/kg/min and may be increased at intervals of 15–30 min until the desired effect or adverse effects occur, e.g. excessive tachycardia or dysrhythmia. Increasingly close monitoring (blood pressure, urine output, etc.) should be conducted as the rate exceeds 5 μg/kg/min; it should rarely be taken above 20 μg/kg/min. The infusion should be withdrawn gradually over hours to avoid hypotension. Dopamine is stable for about 24 h in sodium chloride or dextrose; it is inactivated by alkaline solutions, e.g sodium bicarbonate. Subcutaneous leakage causes vasoconstriction and necrosis and should be treated by local injection of an α-adrenoceptor blocking agent (phentolamine 5 mg, diluted).

For CNS aspects of dopamine, agonists and antagonists, see index.

Dobutamine is primarily a β_1-adrenoceptor agonist with greater inotropic than chronotropic effects on the heart; it has some α-agonist effect, but less than dopamine. It differs from isoprenaline in causing less tachycardia (any significant rise in rate indicates overdose), and perhaps less dysrhythmia; there is also less reduction in peripheral resistance (β_2-receptor). It may be useful in acute heart failure (in the absence of severe hypertension). The plasma $t_{\frac{1}{2}}$ is 2 min. **Prenalterol** is similar.

Salbutamol, *isoetharine, fenoterol, rimiterol, reproterol, pirbuterol and terbutaline* are β-adrenoceptor agonists that are relatively selective for β_2-receptors, so that cardiac (β_1-receptor) effects are less prominent, though these can be serious with high dosage. They are longer acting than isoprenaline probably because they are not substrates for catechol-O-methyltransferase, which methylates catecholamines in the blood.

Salbutamol (Ventolin) (2 mg) is taken orally, 2–4 mg up to 4 times/day. It acts quickly by inhalation and the effect can last as long as 4 h, which makes it suitable for both prevention and treatment of asthma. Of an inhaled dose (100–200 μg, i.e. 0.1–0.2 mg), about 20% is absorbed and can cause cardiovascular effects. The plasma $t_{\frac{1}{2}}$ is 3 h. It can also be given by injection, e.g. in asthma, premature labour (β_2-receptor) and for cardiac inotropic (β_1) effect in heart failure (where the β_2 vasodilator action is also useful). Clinically important hypokalaemia can occur (shift of K into cells). The other drugs above are similar.

Orciprenaline (metaproterenol) is a non-selective β_1- and β_2-adrenoceptor agonist. *Ritodrine* has some selectivity for β_2-receptors. *Isoxsuprine* is a non-selective β-adrenoceptor agonist that also has a direct vasodilator effect.

Ephedrine (30 mg) is similar to adrenaline and has many similar effects, but it has a relatively greater stimulant effect on the central nervous system in adults, producing alertness, anxiety, insomnia, tremor and nausea. Children may be sleepy when taking it. In practice central effects limit its use as a sympathomimetic in asthma.

Ephedrine is well absorbed when given by mouth and unlike most other sympathomimetics is not much destroyed by the liver: it is largely excreted unchanged by the kidney. It is usually given by mouth but can be injected. It differs from adrenaline principally in that its effects come on more slowly and last longer. Tachyphylaxis occurs, probably because it acts by discharging noradrenaline from stores, which it exhausts.

Ephedrine can be used as a bronchodilator, in heart block, as a mydriatic and as a mucosal vasoconstrictor, but it is being displaced by newer drugs, which are often better for these purposes. It sometimes is useful in myasthenia gravis (adrenergic agents enhance cholinergic neuromuscular transmission). *Phenylpopanolamine* (norephedrine) is similar but with less CNS effect.

Amphetamine (Benzedrine) and **dexamphetamine** (Dexedrine; see also index) are seldom used for their peripheral effects, which are similar to those of ephedrine, but usually for their effects on the central nervous system (narcolepsy, hyperkinesia in children) on which they are relatively more active, producing cortical arousal. For *overdose* see pharmacokinetics, above: for other aspects, see index.

Phenylephrine (Neophryn) has actions qualitatively similar to noradrenaline but has a longer duration of action, up to an hour or so. It can be used as a nasal decongestant (0.25–0.5% solution), but sometimes irritates. In the doses usually given, the central nervous effects are minimal, as are the direct effects on the heart. It is also used as a mydriatic and briefly lowers intra-ocular pressure.

Mucosal decongestants

Nasal and bronchial decongestants (vasoconstrictors) are widely used in allergic rhinitis, colds, coughs and sinusitis, and to prevent otitic barotrauma, as nasal drops or as sprays to be sniffed; The latter reach a greater area of the mucous membrane. All the sympathomimetic vasoconstrictors, i.e. with α-effects, have been used for the purpose, with or without an antihistamine (H_1-receptor), and there is little to choose between them. If used more often than 3-hourly and for above 3 weeks the mucous membrane is likely to be damaged. The occurrence of rebound congestion or allergic reaction is liable to lead to overuse. The least objectionable drugs are ephedrine 0.5% and xylometazoline 0.1% (Otrivine). Naphazoline and adrenaline should not be used, and nor should blunderbuss mixtures of vasoconstrictor, antihistamine, adrenal steroid and antibiotics. Oily drops and sprays may enter the lungs and eventually cause lipoid pneumonia.

It may sometimes be better to give the drugs orally rather than up the nose. They interact with antihypertensives and can be a cause of unexplained failure of therapy unless enquiry into patient self-medication is made. Deaths (hypertension) have occurred when such preparations have been taken by patients treated for depression with a monoamine oxidase inhibitor.

HYPOTENSIVE STATES

(*Anaphylactic shock*: see index)

Shock is a state of inadequate capillary perfusion (oxygen deficiency) of vital tissues to an extent that adversely affects cellular metabolism (capillary endothelium and organs) causing malfunction including release of enzymes and vasoactive substances,* i.e. it is a *low flow* or *hypoperfusion state*. The cardiac output and blood pressure are low in fully developed cases. But a maldistribution of blood (due to constriction, dilatation, shunting) can be sufficient to produce tissue injury even in the presence of high cardiac output and arterial blood pressure (warm shock), e.g. some cases of septic shock.

The essential element, hypoperfusion of vital organs, is present whatever the cause, whether pump failure (myocardial infarction), maldistribution of blood (septic shock) or loss of total intravascular volume (bleeding, or increased permeability of vessels damaged by bacterial cell wall substances, by burns or by anoxia). Function of vital organs, brain (consciousness, respiration) and kidney (urine formation) are clinical indicators of adequacy of perfusion of these organs.

Treatment may be summarised:

1. *Treatment of the cause*: pain, wounds, infections, adrenocortical deficiency.
2. *Replacement of any fluid lost* from the circulation; but extra fluid is dangerous when the primary fault is in the heart or pulmonary circulation.
3. *Maintenance of the diastolic blood pressure and perfusion of vital organs* (brain, heart, kidneys).

Blood flow (oxygen delivery) rather than blood pressure is of the greatest immediate importance for the function of vital organs. But a reasonable blood pressure is needed to ensure organ perfusion, e.g. brain and myocardium, and pressure for secretion of urine. Hypotension due to *low peripheral resistance* is of little importance if the patient is horizontal or tilted head down, for venous return to the heart, and so the cardiac output, are then maintained, and blood flow to brain, myocardium and kidneys remains adequate until the diastolic pressure falls below about 40 mm Hg. But low cardiac output is always serious even though compensatory vasoconstriction maintains the arterial pressure, for blood flow is reduced.

The decision how to treat shock depends on assessment in the individual patient of the pathophysiology, whether cardiac output, and so peripheral blood flow, is inadequate (low pulse volume, cold-constricted periphery), or whether cardiac output is normal and peripheral blood flow is adequate (good pulse volume and warm dilated periphery), whether the patient is hypovolaemic or not, or needs a cardiac inotropic agent, a vasoconstrictor or a vasolidator. See also naloxone.

In poisoning by a cerebral depressant the principal cause of hypotension is low peripheral resistance due to sympathetic block. The cardiac output can be restored by tilting the patient head down and by increasing the venous filling pressure by cautiously expanding the blood volume with plasma. This is particularly necessary if the patient is on a respirator, due to the circulatory effects of the intermittent increased intrathoracic

* In fact, a medley of substances (autacoids), kinins, prostaglandins, leukotrienes, histamine, endorphins, serotonin, vasopressin, angiotensin.

pressure (similar to Valsalva's manoeuvre), which reduces cardiac filling. Use of vascular drugs is unnecessary and may be harmful. They do not reproduce the pattern of the missing sympathetic (neurogenic) vasoconstriction.

In **central circulatory failure** (acute cardiac damage, e.g. myocardial infarction) the cardiac output and blood pressure are low due to loss of pumping power; myocardial perfusion is dependent on aortic pressure. Venous return, (central venous pressure) is normal or high. The low blood pressure may trigger the sympathoadrenal mechanisms of peripheral circulatory failure summarised below.

Not surprisingly, the use of drugs in low output failure due to acute myocardial damage is disappointing. Vasoconstriction (by α-adrenoceptor agonist), by increasing peripheral resistance, may raise the blood pressure by increasing afterload, but this can further reduce cardiac output. Cardiac stimulation with a β_1-adrenoceptor agonist may fail, increases myocardial oxygen consumption and may cause a dysrhythmia. Dopamine or dobutamine offer a reasonable choice.

But if there is bradycardia (as there sometimes is in myocardial infarction), minute output can be increased by vagal block with atropine.

Digitalis is not useful in cardiogenic shock, though it may be needed for other reasons. Vasodilators may be needed to treat severe heart *failure*.

In the case of **pulmonary artery embolus** there is theoretical benefit to be derived from a vasoconstrictor. The output of the right ventricle, and so the volume of blood going to the left ventricle, is reduced and as a result the coronary blood flow to both ventricles falls. The right ventricle is therefore doing more work, against the obstructed pulmonary artery, with less oxygen supply to its muscle. If the peripheral resistance is raised by giving vasoconstrictors (e.g. noradrenaline) the diastolic pressure in the aorta will rise and with higher perfusion pressure the coronary flow may improve, and may benefit the overworked right ventricle.

In **mesenteric infarction**, animal experiments suggest that vasoconstrictor drugs may aggravate intestinal ischaemia.

In **septic shock** (caused by endotoxins from gram-negative organisms and other cell products from gram-positive organisms), the cardiac output may be low or high, but vital organs are underperfused; there is sequestration of blood in the abdominal viscera and lungs and fluid loss into the tissues through damaged capillary endothelium. First there is a peripheral vasodilatation with eventual fall in arterial pressure. This initiates a vigorous sympathetic discharge that causes constriction of arterioles and venules. There is then a progressive peripheral anoxia of vital organs and acidosis. The arterioles dilate, but the venules do not, so that blood is sequestrated in the periphery and *effective* circulatory volume falls because of this and fluid loss into the extravascular space.

The immediate aim of treatment is to restore cardiac output by increasing venous return to the heart and to reverse the maldistribution of blood. This can be done by increasing intravascular volume (plasma transfusion), keeping a close watch on central venous pressure to avoid overloading the heart, and by tilting the patient head down. Oxygen is useful as there is often uneven pulmonary perfusion.

In addition a vasodilator drug may allow the release of the sequestered blood, and α-adrenoceptor blockers (e.g. phentolamine) have been used for this. Unfortunately the blood is liable to stay sequestered despite reduction of the obstructive venular constriction. Administration of a vasodilator drug to a patient with a low blood volume is, of course, disastrous.

Drugs that increase peripheral resistance (sympathomimetics with α-effects and *no* β_1-effect) are likely only to make matters worse by further reducing blood flow to vital organs, in the event of the resistance vessels (arterioles) retaining their reactivity and responding to them, which they may not do. Noradrenaline does have some cardiac inotropic (β_1) effect and may be used if substantial vasoconstriction is judged necessary. But *dopamine* provides a 'mix' of actions that is least likely to do harm and even may do good (α + β-effects + renal vasodilatation).

Adrenocortical steroids in enormous (and costly) doses (e.g. dexamethasone 2–6 mg/kg i.v. as single injection, repeated in 2–6 h and after that as clinical judgement counsels for a maximum of 2–3 days) may benefit by reducing the consequences of damage to cellular membranes by toxins or anoxia and so preventing the release of biologically active damaging substances. The effect probably has nothing to do with the ordinary actions of corticosteroids. Proof of clinical efficacy is hard to get and this treatment is not definitively evaluated. It probably has little or no efficacy in endotoxin (septic) shock (see p. 660). Ordinary replacement doses of adrenocortical steroid are useless. Use of these high doses in cardiogenic shock may cause cardiac dysrhythmia (hypokalaemia) and may possibly delay healing of the infarct.

Hypotension in patients with atherosclerosis (occlusive vascular disease) is more serious than in others, for they are specially dependent on pressure to provide the necessary blood flow in vital organs because the vessels are less able to dilate. Dopamine may be considered.

Choice of drug in shock. On present knowledge the best drug would be one that stimulates the myocardium as well as selectively modifying peripheral resistance to increase flow to vital organs.

Dopamine meets these requirements best. Where high doses are being used and vasoconstriction predominates it may sometimes be useful to add a vasodilator, e.g. an α-adrenoceptor blocking drug. As well as reducing peripheral blood flow, prolonged vasoconstriction reduces blood volume due to passage of fluid into the extravascular space. Thus cessation of use may be followed by a drop in cardiac output.

Dobutamine is used when cardiac inotropic effect is the primary requirement.

Noradrenaline is used when vasoconstriction is the first priority, plus some slight cardiac inotropic effect.

Technique of use. Continuous infusion i.v. of dopamine is preferred. Modern monitoring by both invasive and non-invasive techniques has reached such heights of complexity that it can give more information than some doctors know how to put to good use, even if it is indeed the right information. We are liable 'to measure everything at once, losing ourselves in a sea of numbers many of which are derived by arithmetical exercises from other numbers'*.

At least the heart rate and rhythm, blood pressure and urine flow should be closely watched. No attempt should be made to raise the pressure to normal; about 80–90 mm Hg systolic pressure is enough, for the drugs are not restoring normal physiology. Prognostic indices tell us 'whether the patient will live or die, but such studies do not reveal by which parameters we should 'fly' the patient, and so we end up flying the patient by the seat of our pants instead of our other end'*. These words, of an expert, may give some comfort when the complexities of management seem overwhelming.

Warning. The use of drugs in shock is secondary to accurate assessment of cardiovascular state and to other essential management — treatment of infection, maintenance of intravascular volume, etc.

Restoration of intravascular volume. Ideally the transfusion should be similar to that which has been lost — blood for haemorrhage, plasma for burns, saline for gastrointestinal loss. But in an emergency, speed of replacement is more important than its nature. **Note on dextrans** (polysaccharides): Dextran 150, 110 or 70 (these are the molecular weights in thousands; albumin MW is 69 000) can be used as plasma substitutes to restore volume; they are retained in the circulation and largely eliminated by metabolism. Dextran 40 should not be used for this purpose; its small molecule means that it is rapidly (few hours) excreted by renal glomerular filtration; it is concentrated in the urine and, especially if there is oliguria, this results in a highly viscous urine that blocks renal tubules causing acute renal failure. It is also commonly presented in hypertonic form so that its brief effect in increasing plasma volume is by drawing interstitial fluid into the vascular system; it is used to improve peripheral blood flow by decreasing plasma sludging of cells, e.g. peripheral vascular disease and post-surgical thromboembolism. Large volumes of all

* Thompson W L Proceedings of the Royal Society of Medicine 1977; 70:25.

dextrans (above 1.5 l) can interfere with platelet function. They also interfere with blood group cross-matching and clinical biochemical measurements.

Gelatin and polygeline (MW approx. 35 000) are alternatives to dextrans; as is **hetastarch**; and these are replacing dextrans. Anaphylactoid reactions may occur with any of the above.

Orthostatic hypotension, whether idiopathic (Shy–Drager syndrome), or secondary to diabetes mellitus or parkinsonism, is due to degeneration of the autonomic pathways; there is a (compensatory) increase in the number of end-organ adrenoceptors. Initial treatment is by expansion of blood volume by using a sodium-retaining adrenocortical steroid (fludrocortisone) plus elastic support stocking to reduce venous pooling of blood when erect. The possibility that vasodilator prostaglandins in excess could be a factor in some cases had led to trial of an inhibitor of prostaglandin synthesis (indomethacin) with success, particularly when combined with fludrocortisone.

Other measures include α- adrenoceptor agonist with *veno* rather than arterioconstrictor action, e.g. dihydroergotamine, and use of a *partial agonist, non-selective* β-adrenoceptor blockers (pindolol); also metoclopramide (dopamine receptor blocker).

Postprandial fall in blood pressure (probably due to redistribution of blood to the splanchnic area) is characteristic of this condition; it especially occurs after breakfast (blood volume is lower in the morning). Substantial doses of caffeine (two large cups of coffee) can mitigate this, but they need to be taken early in the meal and not right at the end. The action may be due to block of vasodilator adenosine receptors.*

Regimens of indirectly acting sympathomimetic (eg. tyramine) combined with a monoamine oxidase inhibitor have been used successfully but plainly require the utmost caution lest there be a hypertensive crisis.

The discrepant reported results of drug therapy may be due to differences in adrenergic function dependent on whether the degeneration is central, peripheral, preganglionic or postganglionic.

* See Onrott J et al. N Engl J Med 1985; 313:549.

GUIDE TO FURTHER READING

1 Ahlquist R P. A study of adrenotropic receptors. Am J Physiol 1948; 153:586

2 Monroe R R et al. Oral [ab]use of stimulants obtained from inhalers. JAMA 1947; 135:909

3 Barcroft H et al. On the actions of noradrenaline, adrenaline and isopropylnoradrenaline on the arterial blood pressure, heart rate and muscle blood flow in man. J Physiol 1949; 110:194

4 Williams M E et al. Catecholamine modulation of rapid potassium shifts during exercise. N Engl J Med 1985; 312:823

5 Epstein F H et al. Adrenergic control of serum potassium. N Engl J Med 1983; 309:1450

6 Barnes P J. Radioligand binding studies of adrenergic receptors and their clinical relevance. Br Med J 1981; 282:1207

7 Bristow M R et al. Decreased catecholamine sensitivity and β-adrenergic receptor density in failing human hearts. N Engl J Med 1982; 307:205

8 Fowler M B et al. Comparison of haemodynamic responses to dobutamine and salbutamol in cardiogenic shock after acute myocardial infarction. Br Med J 1982; 284:73

9 Cryer P E. Physiology and pathophysiology of the human sympathoadrenal neuroendocrine system. N Engl J Med 1980; 303:436

10 Motulsky H J et al. Adrenergic receptors in man: direct identification, physiologic regulation and clinical alterations. N Engl J Med 1982; 307:18

11 Editorial. Gas gangrene from adrenaline. Br Med J 1968; 1:721

12 Sprung C L et al. The effects of high-dose corticosteroids in patients with septic shock. N Engl J Med 1984; 311:1137. Also Editorial (Kass E H), p. 1178

13 Patrick J M et al. The effect of a weeks [duration] β-adrenoceptor antagonism on daytime heart rates, subjective responses to exercise, and physical activity in normal subjects. Br J Clin Pharmacol 1985; 19:177

24

Cardiovascular system II: Drugs used in arterial hypertension and angina pectoris

Reduction of blood pressure follows on the reduction of *peripheral arteriolar resistance* and/or *cardiac output* by a variety of mechanisms at a variety of sites, as listed below.

The *principal mechanisms* are the following:

1. Dilatation of *arteriolar resistance vessels*, the heart pumps against lower resistance (afterload).

2. Dilatation of *venular capacitance vessels*, reduced venous return to the heart (preload) leads to reduced cardiac output, especially in the upright position

3. Reduction of *sympathetic drive to the heart* leads to lower cardiac output, especially in response to stress, e.g. vertical posture, exercise, emotion.

The drugs preferred in therapy are those that lower blood pressure with minimal interference with homeostatic control, i.e. posture, exercise. Postural and exercise hypotension may be particularly limiting with antihypertensives that block the sympathetic neurone (that are more effective at high rates of impulse transmission, i.e. standing, than at low rates, i.e. lying), that block both α_1- and α_2-adrenoceptors (i.e. negative-feedback control is lost) and that dilate capacitance vessels (venules). If α-adrenoceptor block is sufficient, on standing upright the reduced arterial constriction allows a fall in blood pressure and gravitational venous pooling, with a consequent brisk drop in cardiac output).

The β-adrenoceptor blockers are particularly free from these inconveniences.

SITES OF ACTION OF ANTIHYPERTENSIVE AND VASOLIDATOR DRUGS

There is a variety of mechanisms of action and some drugs appear under more than one heading.

1. **Blood**
   a. *volume: diuretics*
   b. *plasma enzyme: angiotensin converting enzyme inhibitors*: captopril, enalapril.

2. **Blood vessel (arteriole, venule, capillary) wall**

a. *nitrates* (muscle of vessels): glyceryl trinitrate, isosorbide dinitrate/mononitrate, etc.
b. *calcium channel blockers* (muscle of vessels): verapamil, nifedipine, diltiazem, lidoflazine.
c. *angiotensin converting enzyme (ACE) inhibitors* (capillary endothelium): captopril, enalapril.
d. *miscellaneous: diuretics; sodium nitroprusside; diazoxide; minoxidil; hydralazine; dipyridamole; xanthines.*

3. **The adrenoceptors on blood vessels and myocardium**
a. *α-adrenoceptor block*: prazosin, phentolamine, indoramin, ergot alkaloids, etc.
b. *β-adrenoceptor block*: propranolol, alprenolol, acebutolol, etc.
c. *α + β-adrenoceptor block*: labetalol.
d. *serotonin (5-HT) receptor + α-adrenoceptor block*: ketanserin.

[For adrenoceptors in the central nervous system, see below]

4. **The peripheral sympathetic adrenergic nerve terminal**:
a. *adrenergic neurone blockers*: bethanidine, debrisoquine, guanethidine.
b. *depletion of stored transmitter* (noradrenaline): reserpine.
c. (*formation of false transmitter*: methyldopa), see central nervous system below.

5. **Inhibition of synthesis of noradrenaline and adrenaline (adrenal medulla and adrenergic nerve endings)**: metirosine.

6. **Autonomic ganglion block**: trimetaphan, pentolinium.

7. **Central nervous system**:
a. *α_2-adrenoceptor agonist*: clonidine.
b. *false adrenergic transmitter*: methyldopa

8. **Afferent nerve endings**: veratrum

There follows *an account of antihypertensive and vasodilator (anti-anginal) drugs* according to the above classification.

1. Drugs acting on blood

a. **Diuretics**, particularly the thiazides, are useful antihypertensives. They cause sodium loss with reduced volume of blood and extracellular fluid (up to 10% with chronic treatment).

b. **Angiotensin converting enzyme (ACE) inhibitors**. A small proportion of this enzyme is present in plasma; the major proportion being associated with capillary endothelium cell membrane, below.

2. Drugs acting on blood vessel walls (arteriole, venule, capillary)

a. Organic nitrates

Both nitrites and organic nitrates were introduced into medicine in the 19th century; they relax smooth muscle. Their chief use is in angina pectoris. Principal effects are:

The vascular system. There is a generalised dilatation of *venules* (capacitance vessels) and to a less extent of *arterioles* (resistance vessels) resulting in a fall of blood pressure that is postural at first; they dilate the larger *coronary arteries* especially. The drugs are used to relieve angina pectoris, and the mechanisms of this are discussed below. A severe drop in blood pressure will reduce coronary flow as well as cause fainting due to reduced cerebral blood flow, and so it is vital to ensure that an overdose is not taken. Patients should be instructed on the signs of overdose: palpitations, dizziness, blurred vision, headache and flushing followed by pallor, and that if these occur they should lie down and spit out or swallow any remains of a sublingual tablet. The optimum dose is probably that which causes slight tachycardia and a feeling of fullness in the head.

The urinary, biliary and alimentary tracts. Transient relief of pain due to spasm of smooth muscle (colic), can sometimes be obtained.

Preparations of nitrates (and nitrites)

Glyceryl trinitrate (1879) (trinitrin, nitroglycerin; 300, 500, 600 μg) is an oily, non-flammable liquid that explodes on concussion with a force greater than that of gunpowder. However, physicians meet it mixed with inert substances and made into a tablet, in which form it is both innocuous and fairly stable. Tablets more than 8 weeks old or exposed to heat or air will have lost potency by evaporation and should be discarded.

Glyceryl trinitrate is the drug of choice in the treatment of an attack of angina pectoris. The tablets should be bitten up and dissolved under the tongue, where absorption is rapid and reliable. Time spent ensuring that patients understand the way to take the tablets and that the feeling of fullness in the head is harmless is time well spent. The $t_{\frac{1}{2}}$ is 3 min. The action begins in 2 min and lasts up to 30 min. The initial dose is 300 or 500 μg, but the amount required for each patient must be found by trial, up to 6 mg a day total. It is taken at the onset of pain, when stopping exercise to find and take the tablet no doubt contributes to the relief, and as a prophylactic immediately before any exertion that experience has taught usually brings on the pain. The drug is occasionally given as a diagnostic test for angina pectoris, but it is unwise to use it if myocardial infarction is seriously suspected. Absorption from the intestine is good, but there is such extensive hepatic first-pass metabolism that the sublingual route is preferred; an oral mucosal spray (Nitrolingual Spray) is an alternative. For *prophylaxis*, glyceryl trinitrate can be given via the skin (ointment under an occlusive dressing; Transiderm-Nitro) or from a special tube (the dose is measured by length: Percutol); this can be useful for victims of nocturnal angina.

An i.v. formulation is available for use in congestive *heart failure* and severe angina.

Amyl nitrite (1867) is a flammable volatile liquid. It is inhaled through the open mouth. The social disadvantage of having to break (pop) a glass capsule and the distinctive smell, with no compensatory advantage, has rendered it obsolete for angina pectoris.

'Poppers' (amyl nitrite and allies) have acquired a spurious reputation as an aphrodisiac and indeed may seem so to those individuals who cannot distinguish between genital vasodilatation and true sexual pleasure. No sympathy need be expended on individuals who suffer severe hypotension by such misuse. Nor on its use to relax the anal sphincter to accommodate sexual procedures. More sinister adverse effects associated with heavy use for sexual recreation (e.g. immunosuppression) are suggested but unproved.

Isosorbide dinitrate (Cedocard; $t_{\frac{1}{2}}$, 30 min) is used for prophylaxis of angina pectoris and for congestive heart failure (tabs, sublingual and to swallow). It is subject to extensive hepatic first-pass metabolism.

Isosorbide mononitrate (Elantan; $t_{\frac{1}{2}}$, 5 h) is used for prophylaxis of angina (tabs to swallow). Hepatic first-pass metabolism is much less than for the dinitrate.

Pentaerythritol tetranitrate (Peritrate; $t_{\frac{1}{2}}$, 8 h) is less efficacious than its metabolite *pentaerythritol trinitrate* ($t_{\frac{1}{2}}$, 11 h).

Pharmacokinetics

The nitrates are generally well absorbed through oral and intestinal mucosae and the skin and are used by these routes. They are subject to extensive and rapid metabolism in the liver at first pass after absorption from the gut, as is shown by the substantially larger doses required by that route over sublingual (this is why it is acceptable to swallow a sublingual tablet to terminate excess effect should it be socially embarrassing to spit it out). They are first denitrated to mononitrates (and to glycerol) and then conjugated with glucuronic acid. The $t_{\frac{1}{2}}$ periods vary, see above. The *systemic* bioavailability and $t_{\frac{1}{2}}$ increase when there is hepatic insufficiency.

Mode of action on smooth muscle appears to be to calcium entry in to the cells but with substantial difference from calcium channel blockers.

Tolerance to nitrates

Tolerance to the characteristic vasodilator headache comes and goes quickly. Explosives factory workers exposed to a nitrate-contaminated environment lost it over a weekend and some chose to maintain their intake by using nitrate impregnated headbands (transdermal absorption) rather than have to accept the headaches and reacquire tolerance so frequently. However, this obtains only with doses higher than those used clinically, and with ordinary use in angina pectoris tolerance is not a problem.

Adverse effects of nitrates

Collapse due to fall in blood pressure resulting from overdose or allergy may occur. The patient should remain supine, and his legs should be raised above his head to restore venous return to the heart.

These drugs are obviously contraindicated for the pain of myocardial infarction and in angina due to anemia.

Nitrate headache, which may be severe, is probably due to the stretching of pain-sensitive tissues around the meningeal arteries resulting from the increased pulsation that accompanies the cerebral vasodilatation. If headache is severe the dose should be halved.

Methemoglobinemia occurs with heavy dosage; sodium nitrite is preferred in cyanide poisoning (see index).

b. Calcium channel blockers

Calcium channel blockers (antagonists) are effective in angina pectoris and hypertension. They block the passage of calcium through special ion channels in the cell membrane. Calcium is necessary for the contraction of muscle. The effect of these drugs is to relax vascular smooth muscle (peripheral resistance arterioles and coronary arteries; but not veins) and to reduce myocardial contractility. These actions reduce the oxygen consumption of the heart and benefit angina pectoris. The drugs are structurally heterogeneous and are not therapeutically equivalent.

Calcium antagonists (below) are metabolised in the liver and half-lives are about 4 h.

Nifedipine (Adalat) (5, 10 mg) is useful especially where there is active coronary vasoconstriction; it may usefully be combined with a β-adrenoceptor blocker. Dose: 10 mg up to ×3/day with food, increased to 20 mg if necessary: start with half dose for the elderly: for immediate effect in angina or acute hypertension the capsule is bitten and the liquid contents held in the mouth. A sustained-release tablet (20 mg) allows once-daily administration.

Diltiazem (Tildiem) is similar but it may cause bradycardia, which is additive with a β-adrenoceptor blocker.

Verapamil (Cordilox) has cardiac antidysrhythmic actions in addition; depression of conduction can be additive with β-adrenoceptor blockers.

Lidoflazine (Clinium) and *prenylamine* (Synadrine) are similar.

Adverse effects of the group include hypotension, heart failure, bradycardia, heart block, oedema. A rebound of disease may occur with abrupt withdrawal.

A *further account* will be found under cardiac dysrhythmias.

c. Angiotensin converting enzyme (ACE) inhibitors

Renin is an enzyme produced by the kidney in response to adrenergic activity (diminished adrenergic activity reduces renin production), and to sodium depletion. Renin converts a circulating globulin (angiotensinogen) into the biologically inert angiotensin I, which is then changed by *angiotensin converting enzyme* (ACE: kininase II) into the highly potent *vasoconstrictor* angiotensin II (ACE is located chiefly on the luminal surface of capillary endothelial cells, particularly in the lungs; there is also some in plasma and inside cells). Angiotensin II also stimulates production of aldosterone (sodium-retaining hormone) by the adrenal cortex. It is evident that angiotensin II can have an important effect on blood pressure.

Bradykinin (an endogenous vasodilator occurring in blood vessel walls) is also a substrate for ACE; it is uncertain whether this has general clinical importance, although inhibition of its breakdown by ACE inhibition may be at least partly responsible for the blood pressure lowering effect in patients with low plasma renin concentrations.

The antihypertensive effect of ACE inhibitors results primarily from vasodilatation (reduction of peripheral resistance) with little change in cardiac output or rate; renal blood flow may increase (desirable): a fall in aldosterone production may also contribute.

ACE inhibitors are particularly efficacious when

the raised blood pressure results from excess renin production (renovascular hypertension). An effect (sometimes excessive, particularly if the patient is taking a diuretic) is seen after the first dose, and it may increase progressively over weeks with continued administration (as with other antihypertensives). They combine well with a diuretic.

ACE inhibitors can be useful in refractory heart failure.

Pharmacokinetics

Captopril has a $t_{\frac{1}{2}}$ of 2 h and is partly metabolised and partly excreted unchanged; in renal failure elimination is reduced and adverse effects are more common.

Adverse effects include loss of taste (which may recover though therapy is continued), stomatosis (like aphthous ulcers), abdominal pain, liver injury, raised plasma K (see effect on aldosterone above), deterioration of renal function, proteinuria and blood disorders, occasionally with high doses.

Captopril (Capoten) and *enalapril* (Innovace) are available. Enalapril is a prodrug: it inhibits ACE maximally for 10 h and still has useful effect at 24 h, thus allowing once-daily administration: it may cause fewer adverse effects.

d. Miscellaneous

Diuretics reduce plasma volume but they also reduce arteriolar peripheral resistance and vasoconstriction response to noradrenaline, perhaps by altering sodium balance in the arteriolar wall (see diazoxide below).

Diazoxide (Eudemine) is a thiazide but without diuretic effect; indeed it causes salt and water retention. It is a potent antihypertensive by reducing *arteriolar* peripheral resistance with little effect on veins. Sympathetic homeostatic reflexes can still act so that there is generally little postural hypotension except shortly after an i.v. injection.

It is chiefly used to obtain immediate control of *severe hypertension* and heart failure. 150–300 mg is given i.v. *rapidly* (30 s; the patient must be lying down). The reason for speed is that diazoxide is so extensively bound to plasma protein that a sufficiently high free plasma concentration may not be attained if the dose is given slowly.* The maximum effect occurs within 5 min and lasts for at least 4 h. It is strongly alkaline and extravasation should be avoided. The dose may be repeated according to response; i.v. use will rarely need to be prolonged beyond 24 h. *Slower* infusion over 30 min is safer but less effective. The $t_{\frac{1}{2}}$ is 30 h.

In life-threatening situations 600 mg may be needed. Alternative therapy should be instituted at the same time, either oral diazoxide or other therapy suitable for long-term use.

Diazoxide causes excessive sodium retention, which can be opposed, if necessary, by a (non-thiazide) diuretic. It relaxes the uterus and may stop labour, which may be restarted with oxytocin.

Diazoxide causes hyperglycaemia by inhibiting release of *stored* (but not of newly synthesised) insulin from β-islet cells; the hyperglycemia can be antagonised by a sulphonylurea. This action renders it unsuitable for long-term oral use in hypertension.

Diazoxide is also used to treat *tumours of pancreatic β islet cells*. It does not cause permanent diabetes. *Oral* long-term use is practicable but is rarely needed.

Hydralazine (25, 50 mg) has a place in combined drug therapy of hypertension. It reduces peripheral resistance by directly relaxing *arterioles*, but has negligible effect on veins. For this reason postural hypotension is not generally a problem. The compensatory baroreceptor-mediated sympathetic discharge induced by the hypotension causes tachycardia and increased cardiac output, even causing angina pectoris in predisposed subjects, and there is transiently increased renal blood flow. This sympathetic discharge, and the usual compensatory increase in blood volume that occurs with all drugs that increase the intravascular capacity, lead to loss of effect (tolerance). But the compensating mechanisms can be eliminated by a β-adrenoceptor blocker (or other drug interfering with sympathetic activity) and a diuretic (to prevent increased

* This matter is controversial and some would prefer to inject i.v. at gradually increasing rate.

blood volume), and such combined therapy is usual practice. Some of the adverse effects of hydralazine can be accounted for by the hyperkinetic circulatory changes — headache, flushing, nasal and conjunctival congestion, lacrimation, palpitations and vomiting. With prolonged use of doses above 200 mg total/day, a reversible syndrome of myalgia and arthralgia proceeding to disseminated lupus erythematosus is liable to occur.

Hydralazine is metabolised by acetylation with the same genetic variation as isoniazid. The $t_{\frac{1}{2}}$ in fast acetylators is 4 h and in slow acetylators 5 h. This difference is clinically insignificant, particularly as there is substantial hepatic first-pass metabolism and the duration of antihypertensive action is much longer than is to be expected from the $t_{\frac{1}{2}}$, as is also the case with β-adrenoceptor blockers. Twice-daily dosing is usual, starting with 25 mg each dose and increased every 2–3 days to the maximum of 100 mg total per day.

In hypertensive emergency hydralazine 20–40 mg i.v. may be given; the maximum effect will be seen in 10–80 min; it can be repeated according to need and the patient transferred to oral therapy within 1–2 days.

Minoxidil is a vasodilator selective for *arterioles* rather than for veins similar to diazoxide and hydralazine; it is highly effective in severe hypertension, but can cause hirsutism (see baldness) and oedema.

Sodium nitroprusside is a highly effective hypotensive agent when given i.v. Its effect is almost immediate and lasts for 1–5 min. Therefore it must be given by infusion and its action is accurately controllable by altering the infusion rate. It dilates both *arterioles and veins*, which would be disastrous if the patient stood up. But no patient who needs this drug is likely to want to stand up. Nitroprusside action is terminated by metabolism. It penetrates erythrocytes, where electron transfer from haemoglobin iron to nitroprusside yields methaemoglobin and an unstable nitroprusside radical. This breaks down, liberating cyanide radicals. Most of the cyanide remains in the erythrocytes and is firmly bound, it is the free cyanide that passes into the plasma that is toxic, diffusing throughout the body and inhibiting cellular respiration (cytochrome oxidase). The cyanide is converted to thiocyanate and so accumulates over days as the infusion is prolonged (3 days should generally not be exceeded).

Measurement of plasma thiocyanate may be useful in determining whether the patient is suffering from toxicity from prolonged (days) infusion. Poisoning can cause delirium and psychotic symptoms. Metabolic acidosis may occur as a result of cell metabolism becoming anaerobic.

Animals and man poisoned by nitroprusside are reputed to manifest the characteristic cyanide smell.

Prolonged infusions of nitroprusside may be made safer by concurrent administration of hydroxocobalamin by i.v. infusion, to take up cyanide and become cyanocobalamin, and of sodium thiosulphate intermittently. These should not be mixed before administration (see also *cyanide poisoning*).

It is plain that use of this drug requires unusual knowledge and care.* It is particularly dangerous in patients with renal or hepatic insufficiency.

Sodium nitroprusside is used in *hypertensive emergencies, refractory heart failure and for controlled hypotension in surgery*. An infusion may be begun at 0.5 to 1.5 μg/kg/min and control of blood pressure is likely to be established at 0.5 to 8 μg/kg/min; close monitoring of blood pressure is mandatory; rate changes of infusion may be made every 5–10 min.

Dipyridamole (Persantin) relaxes smooth muscle but also may have metabolic effects on the myocardium. Its value in angina is controversial. It reduces platelet aggregation.

Cholinergic drugs reduce blood pressure but produce too many other effects to be used for this purpose.

Other vasodilators include nicotinic acid derivatives (inositol nicotinate [Hexopal], nicofuranose [Bradilan], nicotinyl alcohol [Ronicol]); naftidrofuryl (Praxilene); bamethan (Vasculit), which has

* Light causes sodium nitroprusside in solution to decompose; when made, a solution should be immediately protected by an opaque cover, e.g. metal foil, and used fresh; the fresh solution has a faint brown colour; if the colour is strong it should not be used.

complex metabolic effects; and cinnarizine (Stugeron). They are used in peripheral vascular disease.

Vasodilators in heart failure (see also p. 538). The capacity of these drugs to relieve both cardiac 'preload' (by dilating the veins) and cardiac 'afterload' (by dilating arterioles) has led to their use in heart failure, whether or not hypertension is present. In such cases the cardiac output is low and the heart cannot respond to the high filling pressure, and is working against a high resistance. Reduction of both filling pressure and peripheral resistance can, by taking excessive loads off the heart, lead to improved function (see *heart failure*). The drugs most suitable for this purpose are those that act strongly on veins as well as on arterioles (organic nitrates, sodium nitroprusside) rather than those that are relatively selective for arterioles (hydralazine).

Drugs in peripheral vascular disease

The aim has been to produce peripheral arteriolar vasodilatation without a concurrent significant drop in blood pressure, so that an increased blood flow in the limbs will result. Drugs are naturally more useful in patients in whom the decreased flow of blood is due to *spasm* of the vessels (Raynaud's phenomenon) than where it is due to *organic obstructive* changes that may make dilatation in response to drugs impossible (arteriosclerosis, Buerger's disease).

α-adrenoceptor blocking agents are used in peripheral vascular disease, but they increase blood flow to skin rather than muscle. They have been successfully used in the treatment of superficial ulcers (varicose and traumatic).

Drugs do not remove the cause of the disease, but may delay the onset of gangrene or limit its spread and relieve some of the symptoms. That treatment is unsatisfactory is shown by the wide range of drugs used. More recently it has been realised that cellular metabolic changes may be primary actions of the drugs. Benefit, when it occurs, may thus be from a mixture of effects on cell metabolism and increased blood flow. They are worth trying in troublesome cases but conclusive clinical evidence to allow firm recommendations is lacking. Unsubstantiated claims are rife. If a drug does not benefit in a few weeks it should be withdrawn. A choice may be made from amongst those listed above (*other vasodilators*). *Night cramps* occur in the disease and quinine has a somewhat controversial reputation in their management.

Raynaud's phenomenon may be helped by nifedipine, reserpine, prazosin or phenoxybenzamine, also by topical glyceryl trinitrate and, curiously, griseofulvin, which has a vasodilator effect.

β-adrenocedptor blockers exacerbate peripheral vascular disease by leaving α-receptor vasoconstriction unopposed.

Senile cerebral insufficiency: see co-dergocrine below; also *intellectual function*. For *induced vascular spasm*, e.g. with surgery, phenoxybenzamine and papaverine may be used intravascularly.

Blood viscosity and blood flow. Viscosity of blood in the microcirculation depends on plasma viscosity (e.g. fibrinogen concentration) and erythrocyte deformability (the smallest vessels are half the diameter of a red cell). *Oxpentifylline* (Trental), a methylxanthine, increases the flexibility of erythrocytes by activating cyclic AMP; it also reduces aggregation of exythrocytes and platelets and the fibrinogen content of blood; it appears to have less efficacy in peripheral vascular disease than does regular exercise.

Dextran 40 reduces blood viscosity briefly.

3. Drugs acting on the adrenoceptors on blood vessels and myocardium

Adrenoceptor blocking drugs prevent the response of effector organs to adrenaline and noradrenaline (and other sympathomimetic amines) whether released in the body or injected; circulating adrenaline and noradrenaline are antagonised more readily than the effects of adrenergic nerve stimulation.

The drugs act by competition with adrenaline and noradrenaline for the α or β receptors on the effector organs (they neither alter the agonists themselves nor affect their synthesis).

Some adrenoceptor blocking drugs have to be altered in the body before they become effective (i.e. they are pro-drugs), and this explains the slow onset of action of phenoxybenzamine.

For details of *receptor effects* see Table 23.1.

a. α-adrenoceptor blocking drugs

There are two sub-types of α-adrenoceptor: the α_1-*adrenoceptor*, on the effector organ (postsynaptic), mediates vasoconstriction. The α_2-adrenoceptor, on the nerve ending (presynaptic), mediates a reduction of release of chemotransmitter (noradrenaline), i.e. it mediates negative feedback control of transmitter release.

Most α-adrenoceptor blockers are unselective, blocking both α_1 and α_2-receptors. When subjects taking such a drug rise from supine to erect posture or take exercise the sympathetic system is physiologically activated. The normal vasoconstrictive (α_1) effect (to maintain blood pressure) is blocked by the drug and the failure of this response causes the sympathetic system to be further activated and to release more and more transmitter. This increase in transmitter would normally be reduced by negative feedback via the α_2-receptors; but these are blocked too.

The β-adrenoceptors however are not blocked and the excess transmitter released at adrenergic endings is free to act on them, causing a tachycardia that may be unpleasant. It is for this reason that unselective α-adrenoceptor blockers are not used alone in hypertension.

An α_1-adrenoceptor blocker that spared the α_2-receptor so that negative feedback inhibition of noradrenaline release was maintained, could be useful in hypertension (less tachycardia and postural and exercise hypotension); *prasozin* is such a drug.

Adverse effects of α-adrenoceptor block are postural hypotension, nasal stuffiness, red sclerae and in the male, failure of ejaculation. Effects peculiar to each drug are mentioned below.

Prazosin (Hypovase) acts as just described. It has a curious transient disadvantage, the 'first-dose effect'; within 2 h of the first (rarely after another) dose there may be a brisk hypotension sufficient to cause loss of consciousness. It is prudent to initiate treatment with a low dose, with food, at home and on going to bed, since to experience this effect would not be a reassuring introduction to what is likely to be life-long therapy. Lower doses of prazosin may be used if it is combined with a diuretic or β-adrenoceptor blocker. The $t_{\frac{1}{2}}$ is 2 h.

Phentolamine (Rogitine) is given i.v. for brief effect in adrenergic hypertensive crises, e.g. phaeochromocytoma or MAOI-sympathomimetic interaction. It can be used to terminate dental anaesthesia when adrenaline has been used to provide vasoconstriction (for convenience or to reduce self-injury by cheek and tongue chewing as is liable to occur in mentally retarded subjects). In addition to α-receptor block it has direct vasodilator and cardiac inotropic actions. Dose for hypertensive crisis 5–10 mg i.v. or i.m. repeated as necessary (minutes to hours). The use of phentolamine as a diagnostic test for phaeochromocytoma is only appropriate when biochemical measurements are impracticable, since it is less reliable.

Phenoxybenzamine (Dibenyline, Dibenzyline) (10 mg) is a powerful α-adrenoceptor blocking drug whose effects may last 2 days or longer. Accumulation may therefore occur at the beginning of treatment and the dose must be increased slowly. It is impossible to reverse the circulatory effects of an overdose by noradrenaline or other sympathomimetic drugs, because, although the amount of receptor binding at the outset is competitive, once the drug is on the receptor it binds irreversibly and is not displaced by administering increased amounts of agonist, i.e. its effects are unsurmountable, which may be a useful property for treating phaeochromocytoma, and this is why its action is so prolonged. The full effect of an i.v. dose may take up to an hour to develop, since it is a pro-drug (see above).

It is wise to observe the effects of a single test dose closely before starting regular administration. Phenoxybenzamine is used in bladder neck dysfunction, e.g. in prostatism.

Indigestion and nausea are common with oral therapy. The oral dose is 10–80 mg three or four times a day. By i.v. infusion, 10–70 mg, according to the response, may be given over 20 min.

Thymoxamine (Opilon) and **indoramin** (Baratol) are alternatives.

Labetalol has *both* α- and β-receptor blocking activities, see under β-adrenoceptor block, below.

Ergot alkaloids (see index). The naturally occurring alkaloids with effective α-adrenoceptor blocking actions are also powerful α-adrenoceptor agonists (i.e. partial agonists); the latter action obscures the vasodilatation that is characteristic α-adrenoceptor blocking drugs.

Chemical reduction of the natural alkaloids largely eliminates α-adrenoceptor smooth muscle agonist effect but spares α-adrenoceptor block. The alkaloids are also thought to reduce sympathetic tone by a depressant action on the central nervous system. The principal preparation is co-dergocrine (Hydergine; a mixture of three dihydrogenated alkaloids). It is liable to cause malaise, nausea and vomiting at effective doses. Co-dergocrine may increase cerebral blood flow without lowering the blood pressure and its use has been associated with improvement in senile cerebral insufficiency, but the mechanism of any benefit is more likely to be enzyme changes secondary to effects on receptors than to changes in flow.

Chlorpromazine has many actions of which α-adrenoceptor block is a minor one, but sufficient to cause hypotension.

Yohimbine is an alkaloid from a West African tree. It is a weak α_2-adrenoceptor blocking agent (i.e. it blocks the negative feedback receptor so that sympathetic activity is enhanced). It also stimulates the central nervous system, causing a release of antidiuretic hormone. When given with a barbiturate it causes seminal ejaculation in mice, but despite this it is no longer regarded as an effective aphrodisiac in man, even when mixed with strychnine, pemoline and methyltestosterone (Potensan forte).

An **aphrodisiac** would be a drug that would provide a reliable, selective dose-related increase in sexual desire and performance, lasting, ideally, we suppose, a few hours. There is no such drug. If there were, its social disadvantages might well be found to outweigh any benefits to an occasional individual.

Uses of α-adrenoceptor blocking drugs

These include:

1. **Hypertension**
   a. phaeochromocytoma
   b. essential: prazosin
2. **Heart failure** as vasodilator
3. **Peripheral vascular disease**
4. **Miscellaneous**: in *chilblains*, with dubious benefit; in *causalgia* the mechanism of relief, if any, is obscure, but anything (also i.v. regional guanethidine block) is worth trying in this diabolical condition.

b. β-adrenoceptor blocking drugs

Pharmacodynamics. These drugs block only the β-effects of adrenaline and will *convert the characteristic adrenaline effect on blood pressure to that of noradrenaline* (i.e. rise in blood pressure, see also phaeochromocytoma).

The cardiovascular effects of β-adrenoceptor block depend on the amount of sympathetic tone present. The chief *cardiac effects* result from reduction of sympathetic drive. They are *reduced heart rate* (automaticity) and *reduced myocardial contractility* (rate of rise of pressure in the ventricle). With reduced rate the cardiac output/min is reduced and the overall oxygen consumption falls. These effects are more evident on the response to exercise than at rest. With acute administration of a β-adrenoceptor blocker without partial agonist activity *peripheral vascular resistance* tends to rise, probably chiefly a reflex response to the reduced cardiac output, but also because the α-adrenoceptor (vasoconstrictor) effects are no longer partially opposed by β-adrenoceptor (dilator) effects. With chronic use peripheral resistance returns to about pre-treatment levels or a little below, varying according to presence of partial agonist activity. *Hepatic blood flow* may be reduced by as much as 30% and this is enough to prolong the $t_{\frac{1}{2}}$ of the lipid-soluble members whose metabolism is much dependent on hepatic flow, i.e. those with extensive hepatic first-pass metabolism, including propranolol itself; also lignocaine, which is liable to be used concomitantly for cardiac dysrhythmias. The *cold extremities* that are characteristic of chronic therapy are probably due chiefly to reduced cardiac output with reduced peripheral blood flow, rather than to the blocking of (β_2) dilator receptors, for the effect occurs, though less commonly, with cardioselective (β_1 selective) blocking members of the group.

At first sight the *cardiac effects* might seem likely to be disadvantageous rather than advantageous. Fortunately the heart has substantial functional reserves so that use may be made of the desired properties in the diseases listed below, without inducing heart failure. But heart failure due to the drug does occur in patients with seriously diminished cardiac reserve (but see *uses*).

The *resting blood pressure* is little affected by a single dose, but long-term administration generally results in a fall in pressure that may not reach its maximum for 4 weeks or more. This may seem odd since the β-adrenoceptors are blocked at once. But the elimination of peaks and rate of rise of blood pressure during the day (due to exercise and anxiety) may secondarily allow a slow reversal of arteriolar hypertrophy; but this is speculative, and the precise mechanism(s) for efficacy of β-adrenoceptor blocking drugs in hypertension remain unelucidated.

A substantial advantage of β-block in hypertension is that physiological stresses such as *exercise, upright posture and high environmental temperature* are not accompanied by hypotension as they are with agents that interfere with α-adrenoceptor mediated homeostatic mechanisms. With β-block these necessary adaptive α-receptor constrictor mechanisms remain intact.

Effect on *plasma potassium concentration*, see p. 480.

β-adrenoceptor selectivity: *cardioselectivity* (see table of receptor effects p. 500). Cardioselective β-adrenoceptor blockers have a higher affinity for β_1- (cardiac) receptors than for β_2- (vasodilator, bronchodilator) receptors.

The question is whether the differences constitute clinical advantages.

Potential advantages include less likelihood of causing bronchoconstriction and of provoking or prolonging hypoglycaemia in diabetics.

Some β-blockers (antagonists) also have agonist action, i.e. they are *partial agonists*. This is sometimes described as having intrinsic sympathomimetic activity. These agents cause somewhat less fall in heart rate, resting and with exercise, than do the pure antagonists (blockers) and may be less effective in severe angina pectoris in which reduction of heart rate is particularly important. There is also less fall in cardiac output and possibly fewer patients experience unpleasantly cold extremities, though intermittent claudication may be worsened by β-block whether or not there is partial agonist effect. Both classes of drug can precipitate heart failure and indeed no important difference is to be expected since patients with heart failure have existing high sympathetic drive.

Abrupt withdrawal may be less likely to lead to a rebound effect if there is some partial agonist action, since proliferation of receptors such as occurs with prolonged block may not occur (see p. 501).

Some β-blockers have *membrane stabilising* (quinidine-like or local anaesthetic) effect, but this, with currently available drugs, is probably clinically insignificant except that members having this effect will anaesthetise the eye if applied topically for glaucoma (timolol is used in the eye and does not have this action). Membrane stabilising action inhibits sperm motility, and the *d*-isomer of propranolol (lacking β-blocking activity) has potential efficacy as a vaginal contraceptive.

The justification for mentioning these differences, which are not great enough to warrant firm general recommendations for drug selection, is that in individual cases they may be important.

Intrinsic heart rate. If the sympathetic (β) and the parasympathetic (vagus) drives to the heart are simultaneously adequately blocked by a β-adrenoceptor blocker plus atropine, the heart will be its own master and will beat at its 'intrinsic' rate. The intrinsic rate at rest is usually about 100/min (i.e. normally there is parasympathetic vagal dominance, which decreases with age).

The *ankle jerk relaxation time* is prolonged by β_2-adrenoceptor block, which may be misleading if the reflex is being relied on in diagnosis and management of hypothyroidism.

Duration of action. First-order kinetics applies to elimination, but receptor block follows a zero-order decline*. The reasons for this are complex but the practical application is important, e.g. within 4 h of 20 mg propranolol i.v. the plasma concentration falls by 50%, but the receptor block (as measured by exercise tachycardia) falls by only 36%*. The duration of effect will also depend on

* McDevitt D G et al. Clin Pharmacol Ther 1975; 18:708. Levy G. Clin Pharmacol Ther 1966; 7:362.

the dose. With a high dose the extent of receptor block will be greater than with a low dose, but the decline in block will proceed at the same rate, so that it will take longer for the block following a high dose to fall to clinically insignificant levels. With a high dose giving a high plasma concentration it also, of course, takes longer for the concentration to fall to a subeffective level, though the $t_{\frac{1}{2}}$ is unchanged (see half life).

Most β-adrenoceptor blockers can be given once daily in either ordinary or sustained-release formulations because the $t_{\frac{1}{2}}$ of pharmacodynamic effect exceeds the elimination $t_{\frac{1}{2}}$ of the substance in the blood.

Esmolol is an ultra-short-acting β-adrenoceptor selective agent; it is given by i.v. infusion, reaches a steady state in 5 min and its effects wear off substantially in 2 min and entirely in 18 min; it may find a role in acute control of hypertension and cardiac dysrhythmias.

Pharmacokinetics

β-adrenoceptor blockers can be considered according to their relative solubility in lipids and in water.

Lipid-soluble agents are more rapidly absorbed (across lipoprotein membranes) and are extensively metabolised (hydroxylated, conjugated) to water-soluble substances (some of which are active) that can be eliminated by the kidney. In particular they are subject to extensive hepatic first-pass metabolism after oral administration (e.g. 70% propranolol). Being lipid soluble they readily cross cell membranes and so have a high apparent volume of distribution; they readily enter the central nervous system (e.g. the liposoluble propranolol reaches concentrations in the brain ×20 those of the water-soluble atenolol); they have shorter $t_{\frac{1}{2}}$ than do water soluble members. Plasma concentrations of drugs subject to extensive hepatic first-pass metabolism vary greatly between subjects (up to ×20) because the process is so much affected by two highly variable factors, speed of absorption and hepatic blood flow, which latter is the rate-limiting factor (when hepatic processes become saturated, as does occur, a further increase in dose results in a dramatic rise in plasma concentration); β-blockers reduce hepatic blood flow (30%) and so, with chronic use, reduce their own metabolism, e.g. the $t_{\frac{1}{2}}$ of propranolol may increase ×3; but this effect is less with partial agonists with which blood flow is maintained.

Water soluble agents show more predictable plasma concentrations because they are less subject to liver metabolism, being excreted unchanged by the kidney; thus their half lives are much prolonged in renal failure (e.g. atenolol $t_{\frac{1}{2}}$ increased from 7 to 20 h). Patients with renal disease are best not given drugs (of any kind) having a long $t_{\frac{1}{2}}$ and whose action is terminated by renal elimination. Water-soluble agents may also have a lower incidence of some effects attributed to penetration of the central nervous system, e.g. nightmares.

Lipid soluble agents (with $t_{\frac{1}{2}}$ in hours): propranolol (3), alprenolol (3), oxprenolol (3), metoprolol (4), timolol (5), labetalol (4). *Intermediate*: pindolol (4), acebutolol (3). *Water soluble*: atenolol (7), practolol (9), sotalol (10), nadolol (11).

Considerations of pharmacokinetics are of particular importance not only because β-adrenoceptor blockers are widely used but also because a high proportion of patients is elderly.

Classification of β-adrenoceptor blocking drugs (Table 24.1)

1. *Pharmacokinetic*: lipid soluble, water soluble: see above.

2. *Pharmacodynamic*. The associated properties (partial agonist action and membrane stabilising action) certainly have only minor clinical importance with current drugs at doses ordinarily used and may be quite insignificant in most cases. But it is desirable that they be known, for they probably can sometimes matter and they may foreshadow future developments. For example, drugs having partial β-adrenoceptor agonist effect cause less reduction of cardiac output at rest, as is to be expected.

Other *β-adrenoceptor blockers** include: *non-selective*: penbutolol, betaxolol, bunolol, bufetolol,

* More than 30 are available worldwide.

Table 24.1 β-adrenoceptor blocking drugs

	Drug	Partial agonist effect (intrinsic sympathomimetic effect)	Membrane stabilising effect (quinidine-like effect)
Division I: non-selective ($\beta_1 + \beta_2$) block			
Group I	oxprenolol }	+	+
	alprenolol }		
Group II	propranolol	−	+
Group III	pindolol	+	−
Group IV	sotalol }		
	timolol }	−	−
	nadolol }		
Division II: β_1 (cardio) selective block*			
Group I	acebutolol	+	+
Group III	practolol	+	−
Group IV	atenolol }	−	−
	metoprolol }		
	bisoprolol	−	±
Division III: non-selective β-block + α-block			
Group II	labetalol	−	+
Division IV: β_1 (cardio) selective block + α-block no example yet available.			

* β_1 (cardio) selective drugs are 50–100 times as effective against β_1-receptors as are non-selective drugs. But as the dose (concentration at receptors) rises this selectivity is gradually lost.

bufuralol, bunitrolol. β_1-*receptor selective*: bevantolol, pafenolol, tolamolol.

Uses

β-adrenoceptor blocking drugs are likely to be of use in any condition where reduction of adrenergic activity involving β-adrenoceptors can be beneficial, whether peripheral sympathetic autonomic, adrenal medullary secretion, or CNS adrenergic activity. Such conditions are various.

A. **Cardiovascular**

1 *Angina pectoris* (β-block reduces cardiac work and oxygen consumption).

2. *Hypertension* (β-block reduces cardiac output and rate): there is little interference with homeostatic reflexes.

3. *Cardiac tachydysrhythmias*: (β-block reduces drive to cardiac pacemakers: subsidiary properties, see table, may also be relevant).

4. *Myocardial infarction and reinfarction*, prevention (mechanisms uncertain): 'cardioprotective' effect; possible effect on platelet aggregation.

5. *Aortic dissection and after subarachnoid haemorrhage* (by reducing force and speed of systolic ejection [contractility] and blood pressure).

6. *Obstruction of ventricular outflow* where sympathetic activity occurs in the presence of anatomical abnormalities, e.g. Fallot's tetralogy (R. ventricle: cyanotic attacks): hypertrophic subaortic stenosis (L. ventricle: angina).

7. Prevention and treatment of gastro-intestinal bleeding in hepatic cirrhosis (reduction in portal pressure, see p. 696).

8. Some cases of heart failure due to cardiomyopathy, and a few selected cases of other myocardial disease, are associated with high sympathetic activity (usually, but not invariably, with tachycardia) that renders the cardiac contractility process uneconomic in terms of oxygen consumption. There is evidence that β-adrenoceptor block can be beneficial. Obviously the correct selection of cases is critical as these drugs can also cause heart failure, see above.

B. **Endocrine**

9. *Hyperthyroidism* (which see) β-block reduces unpleasant symptoms of sympathetic overactivity: there may also be an effect on metabolism of thyroxine).

10. *Phaeochromocytoma* (block of β-agonist effects of circulating catecholamines).

C. Central nervous system

11. *Anxiety* with somatic symptoms (see *anxiety*).

12. *Migraine* prophylaxis.

13. Essential *tremor*, some cases.

14. Alcohol and opioid acute *withdrawal symptoms*.

D. Eye

15. *Glaucoma* (timolol or carteolol eye drops) may act by altering production and out-flow of aqueous tumour.

Adverse reactions

1. **Due to β-adrenoceptor block**

Bronchoconstriction (β_2-receptor). As expected, which is more likely in asthmatics (in whom even eye drops can be fatal)* and bronchitics and with the non-selective blockers. But β_1-receptor (cardio) selective members are not totally selective and these drugs may precipitate asthma; however, non-β-receptor mechanisms may also operate.

Cardiac failure. Patients near to cardiac failure need sympathetic drive to give adequate cardiac output/min: a drop in rate may be enough to induce cardiac failure.

Heart block may be made dangerously worse.

Incapacity for vigorous exercise due to failure of the cardiovascular system to respond to sympathetic drive.

Hypertension may occur whenever block of β-receptors allows pre-existing α- effects to be unopposed, e.g. phaeochromocytoma. But it occasionally occurs with acute administration without obvious cause.

Reduced peripheral blood flow, especially with non-selective members, leading to cold extremities, which, rarely, can be severe enough to cause necrosis; intermittent claudication may be worsened.

Reduced blood flow to liver and kidneys, reducing metabolism and elimination of drugs, and liable to be important if there is hepatic or renal disease.

Hypoglycaemia, especially with non-selective members, which block β_2-receptors, and especially in diabetes, due to impairment of the normal sympathetic-mediated homeostatic mechanism for maintaining the blood sugar, i.e. recovery from iatrogenic hypoglycaemia is delayed. But since α-adrenoceptors are not blocked, hypertension may occur as the sympathetic system discharges in an 'attempt' to reverse the hypoglycaemia. In addition, the symptoms of hypoglycaemia, insofar as they are mediated by the sympathetic (anxiety, palpitations), will not occur (though sweating will) and the patient may miss the warning symptoms of hypoglycaemia and slip into coma. Cardioselective (β_1) drugs are preferred in diabetes.

Sexual function: interference is unusual.

* A 36-year-old woman asthmatic collected from a pharmacy, chlorpheniramine for herself and oxprenolol for a friend. She took a tablet of oxprenolol by mistake. Wheezing began in one hour and worsened rapidly; she experienced a convulsion, respiratory arrest and ventricular fibrillation. She was treated with positive-pressure ventilation (for 11 h) and i.v. salbutamol, aminophylline and hydrocortisone. She survived. (Williams I P et al Thorax 1980; 35:160.)

2. **Not certainly due to β-adrenoceptor block**

Effects include loss of general well-being, tired legs, fatigue, depression, sleep disturbances including insomnia, dreaming, feelings of weakness, gut upsets, rashes.

Oculomucocutaneous syndrome occurred with chronic use of practolol.† Other members either do not cause it, or so rarely do so that they are under suspicion only, and, properly prescribed, the benefits of their use far outweigh such a very low risk. But the mechanism of the syndrome is uncertain and, that being so, prediction from tests in animals is likely to remain elusive; it may have an immunological basis.

The patient's protection, should another drug in fact cause the syndrome, lies in the alertness of his doctor with regard to early reactions involving eyes or skin. Symptoms related to the gut are so common and have so many causes that they are a poor early warning of impending disease. It is also a matter of concern that some manifestations of the syndrome have been recorded as developing after cessation of therapy.

Abrupt cessation of therapy can be dangerous in ischaemic heart disease, and prudence counsels

† *Practolol* was developed to the highest current scientific standards; it was marketed (1970) only after independent review by the UK drug regulatory body. All seemed to go well for about 4 years (though skin rashes were observed) by which time there had accumulated about 200,000 patient years of experience with the drug, and then, wrote the then Research Director of the industrial developer, 'came a bolt from the blue and we learnt that it could produce in a small proportion of patients a most bizarre syndrome, which could embrace the skin, eyes, inner ear, and the peritoneal cavity' and also the lung (oculomucocutaneous syndrome). The cause is likely to be an immunological process to which a small minority of patients are prone, 'with present knowledge we cannot say it will not happen again with another drug.'

That the drug caused this peculiar syndrome was recognised by an alert ophthalmologist who ran a special clinic for external eye diseases. In 1974 he suddenly became aware that he was seeing patients complaining of dry eyes but with unusual features. Instead of the damage (blood vessel changes with metaplasia and keratinisation of the conjunctiva) being on the front of the eye exposed by the open lids it was initially in the areas behind and protected by the lids. He noted that these patients were all taking practolol. Quite soon the whole syndrome was defined, as above. Some patients became blind and some required surgery for the peritoneal disorder and a few died as a consequence.

The drug is now available only for brief use by injection in emergency control of disorders of heart rhythm.

The developer acknowledged moral (though not legal) liability for the harm done and paid compensation to affected patients.

that withdrawal should be gradual. The risk of exacerbation of disease appears to be less with partial agonists. The body responds to any interference by adaptive mechanisms that can include increased drive in the system interfered with and also growth of extra receptors in response to continuous block. It should not be a matter of surprise if sudden withdrawal of β-adrenoceptor block is sometimes followed by sympathetic overactivity (overshoot) and that this could be harmful to a diseased cardiovascular system, e.g. worsening of angina, dysrhythmias, hypertension.

Second, patients may have responded to freedom from angina by increasing their habitual exercise, so that when the drug is withdrawn they continue with the higher level of physical activity.

Overdose, including self-poisoning, causes bradycardia, heart block, hypotension and low output cardiac failure that can proceed to shock; bronchoconstriction can be severe, even fatal, in patients subject to any bronchospastic disease; loss of consciousness may occur with lipid-soluble agents that penetrate the central nervous system. β-Adrenoceptor block will outlast the persistence of the drug in the plasma that might be expected from the plasma $t_{\frac{1}{2}}$. Rational treatment includes; atropine (0.5–3 mg i.v. as one or two bolus doses) to eliminate the unopposed vagal activity that contributes to bradycardia; i.v. injection or infusion of a β-adrenoceptor agoinst, e.g. isoprenaline (4 μg/min, increasing at 1–3 min intervals until the heart rate is 50–70 beats/min); in severe poisoning the dose may need to be high and prolonged to overcome the competitive block*; other sympathomimetics may be used as judgement counsels, according to the desired receptor agonist actions (β_1, β_2, α) required by the clinical condition, e.g. dobutamine, dopamine, noradrenaline, adrenaline.

But this approach is not always successful and glucagon, which has cardiac inotropic and chronotropic actions independent of the β-adrenoceptor (dose 10 mg i.v. followed by infusion of 2–3 mg/min) has been thought useful (controlled trials, obviously, are lacking).

Aminophylline has non-adrenergic cardiac inotropic and bronchodilator actions.

* The present published record seems to be 115 mg isoprenaline i.v. over 65 h, held by Lagerfelt J et al. Acta Med Scand 1976; 199:517.

Interactions

Pharmacokinetic. Lipid soluble agents metabolised in the liver provide higher plasma concentrations when another drug that inhibits hepatic metabolism (e.g. cimetidine) is added. Enzyme inducers enhance the metabolism of this class of β-blockers. β-adrenoceptor blockers themselves reduce hepatic blood flow (fall in cardiac output) and reduce the metabolism of other β-blockers, of lignocaine and of chlorpromazine.

Pharmacodynamic. The effect on the blood pressure of sympathomimetics having both α- and β-receptor agonist actions is increased by block of β-receptors leaving the α-receptor vasoconstriction unopposed; the pressor effect of abrupt clonidine withdrawal is enhanced, probably by this action. Other cardiac antidysrhythmic drugs are potentiated (hypotension, bradycardia, heart block etc). Combination with a calcium channel blocker (notably verapamil, but nifedipine seems safe) may be particularly adverse when cardiac function is already impaired.

Most non-steroidal anti-inflammatory drugs attenuate the antihypertensive effect of β-blockers (but not perhaps of atenolol), presumably due to inhibition of formation of vasodilator prostaglandins.

β-adrenoceptor blockers potentiate the effect of other antihypertensives particularly when an increase in heart rate is part of the homeostatic response (α-adrenoceptor blockers).

Non-selective ($\beta_1 + \beta_2$) receptor blockers potentiate hypoglycaemia of insulin and sulphonylureas.

Pregnancy

β-adrenoceptor blocking agents are used in hypertension of pregnancy, including pre-eclampsia. Both lipid- and water-sòluble members enter the fetus and may cause neonatal bradycardia and hypoglycaemia. In early pregnancy they appear not to be teratogenic.

Individual β-adrenoceptor blockers

Propranolol (Inderal) (10, 40, 80, 160 mg) standard and sustained-release (160 mg) formulations. Once or twice a day oral administration of 80 mg is effective in *hypertension*; the dose may be increased weekly. Maintenance dose is likely to be

160–320 mg total/day. For *angina pectoris* the maintenance dose will be 120–240 mg total/day. For *prophylaxis of myocardial infarction* 160 mg total/day. When given i.v. (1 mg/min up to 10 mg) for *cardiac dysrhythmia* or *thyrotoxicosis* it should be preceded by atropine (1–2 mg i.v.) to prevent excessive bradycardia.

Atenolol (Tenormin) (50, 100 mg) is used for angina pectoris and hypertension, 50–100 mg orally once a day.

Oxprenolol is used similarly.

Practolol is used only by injection for short-term control of cardiac dysrhythmias.

c. α + β-adrenoceptor blocking drug

Labetalol (Trandate) (100, 200, 400 mg) is a β-adrenoceptor blocker (non-selective) that also blocks α-adrenoceptors; its dual effect on blood vessels minimises the vasoconstriction characteristic of unselective β-block so that for practical purposes the outcome is similar to using a cardioselective β-blocker. See the Table 24.1.

The approximate ratio between α- and β-adrenoceptor block is 1:3 with oral administration and 1:7 after i.v. administration.

Ordinary β-adrenoceptor blockers are unsuitable for quick antihypertensive effect because a quick drop in blood pressure triggers a compensatory sympathetic discharge that increases peripheral vascular resistance (via α-adrenoceptors). Block of β-adrenoceptors alone cannot prevent this compensatory response. But the addition of α-receptor block can. It is this latter action that renders labetalol suitable for gaining quick control of blood pressure (orally or i.v.) In phaeochromocytoma the additional α-receptor block has been found sufficient to prevent the characteristic rise in blood pressure that occurs with β-receptor block alone.

Chronic use of labetalol is accompanied by normal cardiac output with reduced peripheral resistance, whereas chronic pure β-receptor block is accompanied by low cardiac output and about normal peripheral resistance.

Postural hypotension (characteristic of α-receptor block) is liable to occur at the outset of therapy and if the dose is increased too rapidly. But with chronic therapy when the β-receptor component is largely responsible for the antihypertensive effect it is not a problem.

The plasma $t_{\frac{1}{2}}$ of labetalol is 4 h; it is extensively metabolised.

The initial oral dose is 200 mg total/day in two doses with food; it may be doubled after 2 weeks. The more severe cases may need a total daily dose of up to 2400 mg/day.

For emergency control of severe hypertension 50 mg i.v. may be given over 1 min with the patient supine, and repeated at 5 min intervals up to a maximum of 200 mg. Slow i.v. infusion is an alternative. After i.v. labetalol patients are highly responsive to posture for about 3 h.

d. Serotonin (5 HT) receptor + α-adrenoceptor blocking drug

Ketanserin (Sufrexal) appears to act principally to block serotonin vasoconstrictor (subtype S_2 or 5-HT_2) receptors and also has some α-adrenoceptor blocking effect (its affinity ratio of serotonin block to adrenoceptor block is 1:5). It is an effective antihypertensive (alone and in combination) and it remains to be seen whether it has a role in other cardiovascular diseases.

Serotonin (synthesised in enterochromaffin cells, largely in the gut, and also extensively taken up into blood platelets from which it is released to have vascular effect) has complex effects on the cardiovascular system, varying with the vascular bed and its physiological state; it generally constricts arterioles and veins and induces blood platelet aggregation; it also modulates (enhances/inhibits) noradrenergic transmission.

4. The peripheral sympathetic adrenergic nerve terminal

a. Adrenergic neurone blocking drugs

Adrenergic neurone blocking drugs are selectively taken up into adrenergic nerve endings by the active, energy-requiring, saturable amine (noradrenaline) pump mechanism. They accumulate in the noradrenaline storage vesicles from which they are released in response to nerve impulses. The consequences of this uptake are, in importance:

First. Sympathetic nerve impulses release less noradrenaline than normal. The mechanism is uncertain; it is not simply a consequence of the reduction of noradrenaline stores.

Second. Noradrenaline uptake into nerve endings is inhibited.

Noradrenaline stores in nerve endings are depleted; but a single initial large dose of some members (guanethidine, debrisoquine) causes transient release of noradrenaline with the expected result, transient hypertension.

Damage to noradrenaline storage mechanisms occurs with prolonged use.

'Denervation' supersensitivity occurs, i.e. an enhanced sensitivity of the end organ to noradrenaline, probably a compensatory response to prolonged exposure to reduced amounts of transmitter (which results in the formation of more receptors).

There is also an immediate sensitisation of end organs.

A rise in blood pressure occurs in hypertension due to phaeochromocytoma (probably due both to inhibition of neurone uptake of catecholamines and simultaneous end-organ sensitisation).

In addition there is membrane stabilising (local anaesthetic) effect that renders the drugs effective in cardiac dysrhythmias and may contribute to the principal action (above) by stabilising the neuronal membrane from inside.

That this group of drugs is occupying selectively a physiological process is illustrated by the fact that stimulation of the sympathetic nerves causes release of guanethidine from the nerve ending. Thus guanethidine can be said to form a false transmitter, though this does not seem to be the mechanism of its antihypertensive effect.

General consequences of administration are an indiscriminate reduction of sympathetic activity of veins (preload), arterioles (afterload), with reduction of cardiac rate and output. The result is that supine blood pressure is not well controlled and troublesome postural and exercise hypertension occur; also failure of ejaculation.

Interactions. Competition for the amine pump, depletion of noradrenaline stores and denervation supersensitivity all contribute to clinically important interactions, e.g. injected adrenaline or noradrenaline is potentiated (blocked uptake into nerve endings, and end-organ supersensitivity): but indirectly acting sympathomimetics (which see) are less effective since their action is dependent on the release of stored noradrenaline in the nerve endings. There is antagonism of hypotensive effect by other substances that compete for the amine pump, tricyclic antidepressants, phenothiazine and butyrophenone neuroleptics, amphetamines (including related appetite suppressants, but not fenfluramine) and ephedrine and other vasoconstrictors (decongestants) found in common cold and cough remedies available for self-medication and therefore only known to the physician if he questions the patient whose blood pressure control is unaccountably lost: MAO inhibitors may cause hypertension.

For the above reasons adrenergic neurone blockers have been superseded as drugs of first choice in hypertension.

The principal members are *guanethidine, bethanidine* and *debrisoquine* (the latter drug is known particularly because the population is separable into slow [10%] and fast hydroxylators of this and of other drugs by inheritance [autosomal recessive], see *pharmacogenetics*).

b. Depletion of stored transmitter (noradrenaline)

Reserpine (Serpasil) is an alkaloid from plants of the genus *Rauwolfia*, used in medicine since ancient times in southern Asia, particularly for insanity. In 1931 the hypotensive effect of plant extracts was reported, but it was largely ignored until 1949. Reserpine was isolated in 1952. About 50 *Rauwolfia* alkaloids are known. Reserpine has had extensive use in psychiatry but is now obsolete, though it retains a minor place in hypertension.

Reserpine depletes adrenergic nerves of noradrenaline primarily by blocking the storage mechanism within the nerve ending, so that there is less transmitter available for release. It does not block the amine pump by which extraneuronal noradrenaline is taken up into nerve endings. Its antihypertensive action is due chiefly to peripheral action, but it enters the CNS, where it causes adverse effects, see below.

Reserpine is generally used in combination, e.g. with a thiazide diuretic or hydralazine in hypertension. Numerous fixed-dose formulations are available, e.g. reserpine plus hydrochlorothiazide.

It is extremely important to restrict the dose to avoid mental depression and it should not be used in patients liable to endogenous depression.

Adverse effects are fairly common, but at doses recommended are seldom serious. The following occur: lethargy and apathy, nasal stuffiness, gain in weight and diarrhoaea. Dyspnoea, not associated with cardiac failure, occurs, and onset of cardiac failure has also been reported. Anaesthesia in patients taking reserpine, or within two weeks of ceasing, may cause severe hypotension.

Older domestic male turkeys are liable to fatal hypertensive dissecting aneurism of the aorta. This can cause serious economic loss. The addition of reserpine to their drinking water reduces their blood pressure and preserves their lives without noticeably moderating their natural rage,* as may β-adrenoceptor blockers.

Other alkaloids, *deserpidine* (Harmonyl) and *methoserpidine* (Decaserpyl) are alternatives.

c. Formation of false transmitter

See adrenergic neurone blocking drugs and methyldopa.

5. Inhibition of synthesis of noradrenaline and adrenaline (adrenal medulla and adrenergic nerve endings

Metyrosine (α-methyltyrosine) is an inhibitor of the enzyme tyrosine hydroxylase, which converts tyrosine to dopa; lack of dopa means lack of dopamine and therefore of noradrenaline and adrenaline, which are made from it by further enzyme processes. It is used orally to treat phaeochromocytomas that cannot be removed surgically. Catecholamine synthesis is reduced by up to 80% over 3 days.

6. Autonomic ganglion blocking drugs

Because they are not selective and block sympathetic and parasympathetic systems alike, the ganglion-blockers are obsolete in routine therapy of hypertension. *Trimetaphan* (Arfonad), a short-acting agent (given by i.v. infusion) also has direct vasodilator effect; it is used for producing hypotension to provide a blood free field during surgery, and can be used for emergency control of hypertension; it provides 'minute-to-minute' control.

The principal unwanted effects of ganglion block can be predicted from a knowledge of autonomic physiology (students may care to make the attempt). When used for long-term control of hypertension (mecamylamine, pentolinium, pempidine, hexamethonium) the most troublesome effects were postural and exercise hypotension (inevitable from the site of action), severe constipation (parasympathetic ganglia) and male sexual impotence (parasympathetic plus sympathetic ganglia), but these latter are not significant with brief use during surgery.

7. Central nervous system

a. α-adrenoceptor agonist

Clonidine is an agonist to α_2-adrenoceptors (postsynaptic) in the brain, suppressing sympathetic outflow and reducing blood pressure. At high doses it also acts on the peripheral α_2-adrenoceptors (presynaptic) on the adrenergic nerve ending; these mediate negative feedback supression of noradrenaline release. (In overdose clonidine can stimulate α_1-adrenoceptors [postsynaptic] and thus cause hypertension), i.e. there is a therapeutic window. It is evident that, as is so often the case, receptor selectivity is not an absolute property, but is relative and dose related, i.e. as with the locks on 'cheap' cars, one key may open the whole range, though this is not intended by the manufacturer. Clonidine was discovered to be hypotensive, not by the pharmacologists who tested it in the laboratory but by a physician who used it on himself as nose drops for a cold.†

Clonidine reduces blood pressure with little postural or exercise drop and would be a drug of first choice were it not for a serious handicap. Abrupt or even gradual withdrawal, e.g. forgetfulness, intercurrent illness, need for surgery, often causes a rebound hypertension (in up to 50% of cases) (with high plasma catecholamine concen-

* Conference on use of tranquilising agent Serpasil in animal and poultry production. College Agriculture, Rutgers State University, USA, 1959. Wild turkeys have a blood pressure of 120/60 mm Hg, but domestic turkeys are hypertensive (204/144 mm Hg). Digoxin increases the incidence of aneurysm. It seems that it is the *rate* of rise of pressure in the aorta that is important in this disease (probably in man also) and that reserpine and β-adrenoceptor blockers benefit by attenuating this.

† Page L H N Engl J Med 1981; 304:1371.

tration) akin to the hypertensive attacks of phaeochromocytoma. The onset may be rapid (a few hours) or delayed for as long as two days; it subsides over 2 to 3 days. Treatment is either to reinstitute clonidine, i.m. if necessary ($t_{\frac{1}{2}}$ 9 h), or to treat as for phaeochromocytoma*. Although it does not occur invariably on withdrawal the disadvantage is potentially serious and therefore, since there are plenty of alternative drugs for hypertension, clonidine cannot be regarded as a drug of first choice, though its use is justified in resistant cases. Patients taking clonidine will need to be assessed for reliability of compliance as well as given careful instructions. Common adverse effects include sedation and dry mouth.

Clonidine provides effective prophylaxis in some cases of *migraine* and allied vascular headaches and in some cases of *menopausal flushing*. A special low-dose oral formulation (Dixarit, 0.025 mg) is used, tablets of which contain one-quarter the dose of the smaller of the tablets used for hypertension (Catapres; 0.1, 0.3 mg). The dose for migraine prophylaxis is free from serious withdrawal hypertension (see above). Initially 50 μg (2 tablets Dixarit) is given twice a day, increased to a maximum of 75 μg (3 tablets Dixarit) one or twice daily, after not less than 2 weeks or in accordance with the frequency of the headaches if they occur at longer intervals. This use is an instance when, conscious of human frailty in remembering and writing doses, and placing decimal points, it may be thought prudent to use the proprietary name to ensure that amounts carrying the hazard described above are not inadvertently prescribed. It is unusual for different size tablets of the same drug to have different clinical uses. (*Note*: the naive hope that clonidine would be a useful shaving soap adjuvant, causing α-adrenoceptor mediated piloerection, has not been realised.)

Guanabenz (Wytensin) is similar to clonidine.

b. False transmitter

Since chemotransmitters and receptors in the CNS and in the periphery are similar, the drugs in this section also have peripheral actions, as is to be expected.

Methyldopa (Aldomet) (125, 250, 500 mg) probably acts primarily in the brain stem vasomotor centres. It is a substrate for othe enzymes that synthesise noradrenaline (dopa → dopamine → noradrenaline), but it follows the path (α-methyldopa → α-methyldopamine → α-methylnoradrenaline). Nervous activity then releases a mixture of true transmitter (noradrenaline) and false transmitter (α-methylnoradrenaline). The false transmitter is more persistent than the true transmitter and this enhances the agonist effect on CNS α_2-adrenoceptors that mediate inhibition of sympathetic outflow with the result that there is reduction in peripheral vascular resistance and sometimes a slight reduction in cardiac output, and blood pressure falls. See clonidine.

The false transmitter is also produced at peripheral adrenergic endings, but as it is there about as effective an agonist as the true transmitter, peripheral action is clinically insignificant.

The chief clinically important advantage of methyldopa is that it interferes with homeostatic reflexes less than do adrenergic neurone blockers, i.e. the blood pressure is controlled equally whether the patient is supine, standing or exercising.

Methyldopa is reliably absorbed from the gut and readily enters the CNS. It has a plasma $t_{\frac{1}{2}}$ of about 1.5 h. It can be given i.v. Its metabolites, as might be expected, are capable of interfering with plasma and urinary catecholamine determinations for the diagnosis of phaeochromocytoma.

Adverse effects are largely those expected of its mode of action, and also allergy; they include sedation (frequent), headache, nightmares, depression, involuntary movements, nausea, flatulence, constipation, sore or black tongue, positive Coombs test with, occasionally, haemolytic anaemia, leucopenia, thrombocytopenia, hepatitis.

Gynaecomastia and lactation occur due to interference with dopaminergic suppression of prolactin secretion. Any failure of male sexual function is probably secondary to sedation. Because of its adverse effects methyldopa is no longer a drug of first choice in routine management of hypertension.

* Though prazosin (selective α_1-adrenoceptor block) may be preferred to an unselective agent (α_1 + α_2 block) because it is undesirable, at least theoretically, to block α_2-receptors, which are the site of agonist action of clonidine.

Dose: 250 mg two or three times a day for 2 days increased by 250 mg (total) every 2 days; a single dose at bedtime is adequate for some patients. The usual total daily dose range is 500 mg to 3.0 g. It can be given slowly i.v. (not i.m.), 250–500 mg, 6-hourly.

8. Afferent nerve endings

Veratrum plant alkaloids sensitise baroreceptors so that they respond more intensely to pressure and so enhance the physiological vasodepressor activity, including the vagus nerve causing a characteristic bradycardia. Vomiting is common. Veratrum is now obsolete.

TREATMENT OF ANGINA PECTORIS*

An attack of angina pectoris[†] *occurs when the need of the myocardium for oxygen exceeds the amount delivered to it by the coronary circulation*. The principal forms relative to choice of drug therapy are *angina of exercise* (more common), and *angina at rest* (variant angina) in which coronary artery spasm is of major significance (less common).

The *objective of treatment is to unload the heart or to prevent/suppress spasm of the coronary arteries* so that oxygen need is adequately met.

Myocardial oxygen consumption is chiefly determined by *preload*, i.e. the venous filling and stretching of the heart and its muscle fibles, which evokes the *contractility* (extent and velocity of fibre shortening during systole); the *afterload*, i.e. the peripheral arteriolar resistance against which the heart must eject blood, and including the peak systolic pressure that must be reached; and the heart *rate*, which determines the duration of diastole during which intramyocardial pressure is low enough to allow myocardial perfusion to occur via the coronary arteries.

All these determinants of oxygen consumption are influenced by the activity of the *sympathetic nervous system* and it is no surprise that continuous use of a β-*adrenoceptor blocking drug* benefits angina pectoris, reducing the frequency of attacks. This is achieved by diminishing sympathetic cardiac stimulation due to exercise, anxiety or excitement.

The heart can be unloaded, i.e. its oxygen needs diminished, by:

a. halting the *provocative exercise* (physical or emotional).
b. reducing the *preload* (venous return).
c. reducing the *afterload* (arteriolar resistance).
d. reducing the *rate*.
e. *dilating* the coronary arteries (even though diseased, the larger arteries may double their diameter).

Antianginal drugs provide benefit as follows:

1. *Organic nitrates* reduce *preload* and *afterload* and *dilate* the main coronary arteries (rather than the arterioles).
2. β-*adrenoceptor blocking drugs* reduce myocardial *contractility* and slow the heart *rate*.
3. *Calcium channel blocking drugs* reduce cardiac *contractility*, *dilate* the coronary arteries and reduce *afterload* (dilate peripheral arterioles).
4. Aspirin reduces the incidence of non-fatal myocardial infarction and sudden cardiac death in patients with unstable (crescendo) angina, presumably by an antiplatelet effect (see Ch 28).

These classes of drug complement each other and can be used together.

Summary of treatment of angina pectoris

1. The *cause* is treated when possible, e.g. anaemia.
2. *Arrangement of life* so as to reduce the number of attacks. Weight reduction can be very helpful.
3. For *immediate pre-exertional prophylaxis*: glyceryl trinitrate sublingually; nifedipine is an alternative.
4. For *an acute attack*: glyceryl trinitrate.
5. For *long-term prophylaxis*

a. β-*adrenoceptor block*, e.g. proparanolol, or a cardioselective member to avoid blocking the dilator (β_2) receptors in the coronary vessels, given continuously (not merely when an attack is

* For a personal account by a physician of his experiences of angina pectoris, coronary by-pass surgery, ventricular fibrillation and recovery, see Swyer G I M. Br Med J 1986 292:337. Compelling and essential reading.

† *Angina pectoris: angina*, a strangling; *pectoris*, of the chest.

expected). Dosage is adjusted by results. Some put an arbitrary upper limit to dose, but others recommend that if complete relief is not obtained the dose should be raised to the maximum tolerated, provided the resting heart rate is not reduced below 55/min; or raising the dose to a level at which an increase causes no further inhibition of exercise tachycardia. In severe angina a pure antagonist, i.e. an agent lacking partial agonist activity, is preferred, since the latter may not slow the heart sufficiently.

b. a *calcium channel blocking drug*: nifedipine: an alternative to a β-adrenoceptor blocker, especially if coronary spasm is suspected or if the patient has myocardial insufficiency or any bronchospastic disease. It can also be used with a β-blocker, *or*

c. a *long-acting nitrate*: isosorbide dinitrate or mononitrate.

6. Drug therapy may be adapted to the *time of attacks*, e.g. nocturnal (percutaneous glyceryl trinitrate or isosorbide mononitrate orally at night).

7. *Smoking* should be discouraged.

8. *Antiplatelet therapy* (aspirin) reduces the incidence of fatal and of non-fatal myocardial infarction in patients with unstable angina (i.e. intermediate between stable angina and acute myocardial infarct)*.

9. *Surgery* in selected cases.

Warning. Therapy, especially with short $t_{\frac{1}{2}}$ β-adrenoceptor blocker, should not be withdrawn suddenly (see p. 501).

Drug evaluation

Organic nitrates have been found to prevent the ECG changes induced by measured exercise. Ethyl alcohol taken as whisky reduced the pain induced by exercise but did not modify the ECG changes (which finally dismissed the belief that alcohol is a useful coronary vasodilator).

Therapeutic trials of the efficacy of drugs in preventing or relieving angina must be designed and conducted meticulously. The disease is very variable and the pain, having particularly sinister associations, is liable to be much influenced by emotion. Cessation of attacks may be due to patients changing their physical habits rather than to the drug, e.g. development of angina is related to heart rate and blood pressure rather than to amount of effort; regular exercise can reduce cardiac effects of a given amount of work.

The principal criteria of efficacy are relief and prevention of attacks in daily life, and the amount of measured exercise that precipitates an attack; in addition may be measured the ECG changes associated with myocardial ischaemia (depression of ST segment), and, in the background, on-demand consumption of glyceryl trinitrate tablets.

* Cairns J A et al. N Engl J Med 1985; 313:1369.

TREATMENT OF ARTERIAL HYPERTENSION

Evaluation of antihypertensives

Evaluation falls into two classes:

1. Whether long-term reduction of blood pressure benefits the patient by preventing complications and prolonging life; these studies take years.

2. Whether a drug is capable of effective, safe and comfortable control of blood pressure; these studies last weeks or months. They commonly are conducted double-blind, which can involve complicated arrangements when accurate titration of the dose/effect of drugs is involved. Careful design and conduct are essential because of the very great natural variations in the disease. Emotion may result in changes of up to 100 mm Hg systolic and 40 mm Hg diastolic over a few minutes. In addition, these changes may persist for weeks. In therapeutic trials the short period of control observation on new patients that often precedes a few weeks treatment can be valueless for comparative purposes. 'A period of treatment is a period of reassurance to a hypertensive patient, and reassurance will obviously lead to greater emotional calmness and a lowering of blood pressure. . . . I have seen many patients whose blood pressure at the first visit may be, for example, 260 systolic and 120 diastolic, and at a second visit, a few weeks later, may be 118 systolic and 80 diastolic after only mild sedation and great assurance. I have given placebos to hypertensive patients and obtained 80% sympto-

matic improvement.' The author of those words* has also shown that merely increasing the frequency of a patient's visits to the physician can result in a drop in blood pressure, presumably due to the reassuring effect of such a frequent contact. 'Yet this scheme of increased frequency of visits is commonly applied by clinical investigators of new drugs . . .' It is also known that the appearance of a doctor to measure the blood pressure has itself a pressor effect (peaks within 4 min, largely over by 10 min).

In another study it was found that regular placebo injections i.m. were accompanied by a reduced blood pressure for over a year, whereas an oral placebo had insignificant effect.

It is clear that double-blind carefully controlled studies are essential when evaluating the response to treatment in hypertension, especially over short periods†, for effective hypotensive drugs are capable of causing serious harm and it is important that only those who will actually benefit from their pharmacological effects should take them.

The aim of treatment is to reduce the blood pressure as near to normal as possible in the erect posture, and to keep it there whether the patient is lying, standing or exercising and whether the environment is hot or cold. This is expecting a lot, but it often can be achieved though there may be a price to pay in well-being. When this aim is achieved in *severe cases* there is usually great symptomatic improvement, retinopathy clears and vision improves; headaches are often abolished. However, a variable amount of irreversible damage has often been done by the high blood pressure before treatment is started; renal failure may progress despite treatment; arterial damage leads to cardiac or cerebral catastrophes. It is obviously desirable to start treatment before irreversible changes occur, and in mild and moderately severe cases this often means advising treatment to symptom-free people discovered by screening.

It is also obvious that to recommend what may be life-long drug treatment to youngish people who are symptom-free and who may find they feel less well taking treatment than they did before demands exact knowledge of the natural history of the disease, and of the effects of careful long-term drug use, as well as considerable knowledge of the drugs themselves and of human nature.

Which patient to treat. The prognosis in untreated **malignant (accelerated) hypertension** is so bad that it was ethically impossible to withhold treatment from any patients when ganglion-blocking drugs became available (1951). Thus in the therapeutic trials of hexamethonium (the first ganglion blocker to be used in therapy) the controls had to be similar patients observed in previous years (historical controls). In a series of 82 patients suffering from malignant hypertension treated with ganglion-blocking drugs the expectation of life was six to eight times that of patients not so treated.‡ All such patients require treatment to save their lives.

There is substantial evidence that effective treatment of patients with a diastolic pressure consistently above 110 mm Hg reduces the risk of strokes, renal failure and heart failure, though not of myocardial infarction (except perhaps with β-adrenoceptor blockers).

Treatment requires as much care and attention as the use of insulin in diabetes. Treatment will be life-long.

Women are more resistant to the effects of hypertension than are men (some risk of strokes: lower risk of myocardial infarction) and some would only treat them routinely if the diastolic pressure exceeds 115 mm Hg.

Patients over 65 years require special consideration. Benefits are likely to be less and therapeutic misadventures are more common. Nor do old people have the resilience (psychological or physical) to endure even the milder adverse effects, e.g. loss of energy, depression; and postural hypotension is particularly dangerous in the old. The old may be adequately treated by

* Ayman D. JAMA 1949; 141:974.

† The biggest trial ever done in hypertension was *single* blind for logistic, not for scientific, reasons. It was deemed to be impracticable to manage a study involving treatment adjustments in 17 354 patients and lasting 5½ years if the double blind technique was used. The study cost £4.5 million (US$5.85 million). (Medical Research Council Working Party. Br Med J 1985; 291:97.)

‡ Harington M et al Br Med J 1959; 2:969.

very low doses very well spaced out. The *minimum* effective dose should be consciously sought. The evidence suggests that treatment of the elderly reduces cardiac deaths significantly but has little or no benefit on cerebrovascular deaths.*

Considerations of *quality of daily life* weigh specially heavily, and therapy, when it is used, should be less aggressive than in younger people who have so much more to gain, e.g. a slight reduction in pressure may be acceptable in the old, rather than aiming at 'normal' levels.

The World Health Organization classifies blood pressure thus:

Normal: equal to or below 140/90 mm Hg.

Hypertensive (adults): 160/95 mg Hg or above.

Borderline or intermittent: 140–159/90–94 mm Hg (using fifth Korotkoff phase for diastolic pressure).

Patients having a diastolic pressure consistently *in excess of 115 mm Hg* deserve treatment unless there are definable reasons for not undertaking it (these can be heterogeneous, e.g. advanced age, certainty of non-compliance).

Mild hypertension defined by the UK Medical Research Council as diastolic pressure above 90 mm Hg and below 110 mm Hg (for the trials results of which are summarised below) presents a difficult problem of balancing potential benefit against risk, and clinicians will make a decision based on their knowledge of their patients, the disease, the drugs and the results of large therapeutic trials.

An enormous study has been done†, lasting 5½ years:

17 354 patients were recruited.

85 572 patient years of observation were accrued.

Patients were randomly allocated to treatment with a *thiazide diuretic* (bendrofluazide) or with a *β-adrenoceptor blocker* (propranolol) or with *placebo*.

Stroke rate was reduced on active treatment (bendrofluazide was effective in smokers and in non-smokers whereas propranolol was effective in non-smokers only).

Coronary event rate was not reduced overall (but non-smokers taking propranolol shared a lower rate).

All cardiovascular event rate was uninfluenced overall except that it was lower in non-smokers taking propranolol.

Mortality from 'all causes' was not significantly influenced except that it was lower in non-smokers taking propranolol (but there was a slight decrease in men and increase in women).

It is not possible to define precisely the *individuals* who will benefit from drug treatment.

Non-smoking may provide more benefit than drug treatment.

Women may not benefit from drug treatment.

Overview. 'If 850 mildly hypertensive patients are given active antihypertensive drugs for one year about one stroke will be prevented. This is an *important but infrequent* benefit. Its achievement subjected a substantial percentage of the patients to chronic side effects, mostly but not all minor. Treatment did not appear to save lives or substantially alter the overall risk of coronary heart disease. More than 95% of the control patients remained free of any cardiovascular event during the trial.

'Neither of the two drug regimens had any clear overall advantage over the other. The diuretic was perhaps better than the β-blocker in preventing stroke, but the β-blocker may have prevented coronary events in non-smokers.

'For all categories of events, and in both treated and placebo groups, rates were lower in non-smokers than in smokers.'

It is obvious that *adverse effects of therapy are important in that very large numbers of patients must be treated in order that very small numbers may gain*; this is a salient feature of the use of drugs to *prevent* disease.

In this trial about 40% of patients stopped the treatment to which they were initially randomized for one reason or another, e.g. rise of blood pressure, suspected adverse drug reaction. Of those whose blood pressure rose above the mild range, 76 were taking active treatment and 1011 were taking placebo.

Adverse reactions were as follows:

Diuretic: impaired glucose tolerance; gout;

* See ref (3) at the end of this chapter.

† Medical Research Council Working Party. Br Med J 1985; 291:97. The trial began in 1977 and the choice of drugs and dose inevitably follow the then current opinion.

sexual impotence; lethargy; nausea; dizziness, headache.

β-*adrenoceptor blocker*: Raynaud's phenomenon, skin disorder; dyspnoea; lethargy; nausea; dizziness; headache; sexual impotence (rarely).

It may be that these adverse effects would be diminished by use of a lower dose of diuretic (e.g. bendrofluazide 2.5 mg/day rather than the 10 mg used in this study and which is more in accord with current opinion), by combination therapy, or by use of other agents, e.g. calcium channel blockers (introduced since the trial began), although these might introduce their own novel problems. Enormous trials such as this take so long that they are partially outdated by the time they are concluded and reported.

Principles of antihypertensive therapy

Blood pressure is determined by:

1. *blood volume*,
2. *cardiac* contractility and output,
3. *peripheral resistance* (arterioles),

and the blood pressure may be reduced by interfering with any one or more of these. But drugs are selective and when this is done with one drug alone the factors that are uninfluenced are liable to adapt (homeostatic mechanism), to oppose the useful efect and to restore the previous state. There are two principal mechanisms of such adaptation:

a. *Increase in blood volume.* This occurs with any drug that reduces peripheral resistance or cardiac output due to activation of the *renin–angiotensin–aldosterone* system. Glomerular flow falls and in response to this plasma volume increases and cardiac output and blood pressure rise. This compensatory effect can be prevented by using a diuretic in combination with the other drug, and this is commonly done. Indeed a diuretic should be regarded as a usual constituent of any *multi*-drug regimen both for its primary antihypertensive effect and because it prevents adaptation to the effects of other drugs.

b. *Baroreceptor reflexes.* A fall in blood pressure evokes reflex activity of the sympathetic system, causing increased peripheral resistance and cardiac activity (rate and contractility).

'Therefore, whenever high blood pressure is proving difficult to control and whenever a number of hypotensive drugs are used in combination, the drugs chosen should between them act on all three main determinants of blood pressure — blood volume, peripheral resistance and the heart. Such combinations will achieve three objectives:

(i) maximise antihypertensive efficacy by adding actions exerted at three different points in the cardiovascular system;

(ii) minimise the opposing homeostatic effects by blocking the compensatory changes in blood volume, vascular tone and cardiac function;

(iii) minimise side effects by permitting smaller doses of each drug each acting at a different site and having different side effects.'*

A gradual regimen for treating hypertension where there is no haste can be proposed

1. Start with a single morning dose of either a *diuretic* (bendrofluazide) or a β-*adrenoceptor blocker* (atenolol). Efficacy will begin to be seen within 2–3 days and most of it will have developed within 14 days (dose of β-blocker can be monitored by heart rate response to standard exercise).

2. If the pressure is not controlled in 2–3 weeks, *add the second drug*, above. The dose of diuretic will be fixed, but that of the β-adrenoceptor blocker will be in the small-to-moderate range.†

3. If this is insufficient add a *vasodilator* e.g. hydralazine, prazosin or nifedipine. At this point efficacy can be increased by moving from the convenient once-daily administration to twice-daily administration.

4. If this fails either *raise the dose of the* β-*adrenoceptor blocker* until pressure is controlled or the pulse rate on standing has fallen to 55/min, or for a β-blocker with partial agonist activity, inhibits exercise tachycardia, *or*,

* Chalmers J P Australian Prescriber 1977; 2:6.

† Drugs having a *short steep dose-response curve* for efficacy (that quickly reach a plateau) are given in fixed dose (e.g. to increase the diuretic does not add to efficacy though it does add to toxicity). Drugs having *long sloping dose-response curves* can be titrated for efficacy as well as being used as fixed-dose components of multi-drug regimens.

5. Add a drug of another class, e.g. a calcium channel blocker (nifedipine) if this has not already been instituted, or a centrally acting drug (methyldopa), an ACE inhibitor (enalapril), an adrenergic neurone blocker (bethanidine), or spironolactone.

High-efficacy drugs with quick onset of action should be given after food to avoid high peak-plasma concentrations and consequent postural hypotension; food may enhance the total amount of some drugs reaching the systemic circulation (guanethidine) probably due to food-induced changes in splanchnic blood flow and gut activity.

In a few patients with severe hypertension, lowering the blood pressure may make the patient worse, for instance if there is severe renal impairment (blood urea above 17 mmol/l), or advanced cerebral or coronary arteriosclerosis. In these cases blood flow in vital organs may depend upon a high perfusion pressure; but when such patients have severe hypertensive symptoms a very cautious trial of hypotensive drugs is worthwhile. Weight reduction in an obese hypertensive patient often relieves breathlessness on exertion and sometimes lowers the blood pressure, although this may be more apparent than real, since arm thickness affects sphygmomanometer readings, fat arms providing higher readings than thin arms. Sympathomimetic appetite suppressants (but not fenfluramine) will antagonise the effects of many antihypertensive drugs.

Treatment and severity

Mild hypertension will commonly be adequately treated by a *single drug*, stage 1 above.

Moderately severe hypertension may be treated from the start as in stage 2 above (*two drug* regimen).

Severe hypertension may be treated from the start as in stages 3 to 5 above (*three drug* regimen).

Alternatives. It is obvious that there are numerous alternative regimens, and the fact that they are not all mentioned does not mean that good results are not obtainable; but some aspects deserve special mention.

1. *Diet*. Milder cases (diastolic pressure < 105) can often be controlled by *low salt diet*, without need for drugs. But such is human nature that many patients may find a daily tablet of diuretic preferable to the inconveniences of constant concern about diet. In either case, obesity should be reduced.

2. *Initial therapy*. Many would now begin with a β-adrenoceptor blocker rather than a diuretic. The metabolic effects of diuretics (diabetes, hyperuricaemia, hypokalaemia) are avoided and this may be thought of special importance in the young who may be going to take the drugs for decades, and in the old who are more liable to adverse effects and who are more likely to be taking digoxin (risk with hypokalaemia). It is also possible that β-adrenoceptor block confers some protection against myocardial infarction (cardioprotection) which is not the case with other antihypertensives.

3. *Where there is haste*, then labetalol will provide quicker control than do other β-adrenoceptor blocking drugs because of its added α-adrenoceptor blocking property; alternatively, use an adrenergic neurone blocker, which is later exchanged for less unpleasant drugs.

4. *Centrally acting drugs*, e.g. methyldopa, are alternatives to β-adrenoceptor block, e.g. in asthmatics.

5. *Where there is renal failure*, a loop diuretic, e.g. frusemide, is more effective than a thiazide.

Monitoring

Obviously the blood pressure will be monitored by doctor and also sometimes by the patient.

Diuretics and potassium.* The potassium losing (kaliuretic) diuretics used in hypertension deplete body K by 10–15%. Routine potassium chloride supplements are not required, but occasional cases of hypokalaemia will occur. Uncomplicated patients should be monitored for K loss at 3 months and thereafter 6–12 months†, but special cases will need more frequent tests.

* The case for potassium as an actual antihypertensive agent and deserving of use for that reason has not been validated. The risks of hyperkalaemia are undoubted in patients with renal insufficiency, the elderly, diabetics and patients taking β-adrenoceptor blockers, etc.

† WHO/ISH meeting. Lancet 1983; 1:457.

Since K is mostly intracellular, plasma concentrations are not always a reliable guide. Control of K balance is particularly important if the patient is also taking digoxin.

Fixed-dose diuretic/potassium formulations contain only a little K and provide only marginal protection.

The addition of a K-retaining diuretic to a K-losing diuretic is feasible in troublesome cases of K loss but great care is needed if renal function is inadequate as serious hyperkalaemia may occur.

Citrus fruits have a reputation as a source of K. The flesh of an average-size orange provides 7–8 mmol (mEq) of K; tomatoes and bananas provide similar amounts. A tablet of Navidrex-K contains 8.1 mmol of K plus cyclopenthiazide, and of Slow-K (sustained-release formulation) 8 mmol of K and of chloride. The normal daily requirement of K is 60–120 mmol. Non-chloride K (e.g. bicarbonate, citrate) as is found in fruits only provides effective replacement if the patient is not chloride deficient (alkalotic). See also p. 553.

Compliance. It is obvious that multidrug therapy will pose a substantial problem of compliance. Since treatment will be life-long it is well worthwhile taking trouble to find the most convenient regimen for each individual.

A single daily dose would be ideal and to achieve this slow-release formulations and fixed-dose combinations are used.

Perhaps the best course is to gain control of the blood pressure with separate tablets of each drug and, when the patient is stabilised, to seek to adapt the therapy to its most convenient form.

Fixed-dose formulations are useful as above, but routine *initial* use is undesirable in mild cases as a patient may well be indefinitely condemned to taking one drug he does not need and to suffer its adverse effects.

It is reasonable to employ these formulations initially in moderately severe cases. But in severe cases it is particularly important to be able to adjust doses of each drug separately and to determine the patient's need accurately, before giving priority to the convenience provided by fixed-dose formulations.

Examples include: Co-betaloc (metoprolol + hydrochlorothiazide), Inderex (propranolol + bendrofluazide), Tenoretic (atenolol + chlorthalidone), Trasidrex (oxprenolol + cyclopenthiazide), and Spiroprop (propranolol + spironolactone).

Accelerated (malignant) hypertension

Usually prompt oral treatment with the objective of reducing the blood pressure over at least 12 hours will suffice, e.g. labetalol (α + β-adrenoceptor block; but see phaeochromocytoma below). Alternatives are nifedipine, hydralazine or methyldopa.

Abrupt drops in blood pressure are dangerous because cerebral blood flow may fall so low as to cause serious ischaemia (stroke, blindness). Cerebral blood flow is substantially reduced when *mean* pressure falls by 25%. The blood pressure should not be acutely reduced below 160/100 mm Hg and this level should be attained over hours. A drop of 25% in pressure is about the maximum that can be tolerated over minutes. Blood pressure should be lowered slowly (24 h) in the elderly, but may be reduced more rapidly (say, 12 h) in younger patients.

When there is encephalopathy, *parenteral* therapy is essential, not only for speed but for certainty that the drug is in the blood.

Sodium nitroprusside is a drug of first choice but its action is so fast that it needs extremely careful (1 min) monitoring. Alternatives for parenteral use are diazoxide or labetalol.

Lower-than-usual doses should be used if antihypertensive drugs have recently been taken or if renal function is impaired.

Blood pressure monitoring is plainly essential and doses and intervals are judged by response. It is obvious that a drug acting quickly and briefly (sodium nitroprusside) needs closer supervision than a drug with slower onset of a smoother action, and availability of monitoring is a factor in choice of drug.

Posture may be made use of to potentiate the drug and to diminish the effects of inadvertent overdose.

Severe tachycardia consequent on pressure reduction may be controlled by propranolol i.v.

Oral maintenance treatment for severe hypertension should be started at once if possible; parenteral therapy is seldom necessary for more than 48 h.

Pregnancy hypertension

Effective treatment of hypertension improves fetal and perinatal survival. Controlled trials are difficult to do and present considerable ethical problems. Methyldopa has long been a favoured agent for oral therapy* and parenteral hydralazine for emergency reduction of blood pressure. Because of possible consequence to the fetus choice of drug is conservative. But β-adrenoceptor blockers (labetalol, oxprenolol) are increasingly regarded as effective and safe for both mother and fetus. Severe hypotension in the mother must be avoided since it jeopardises the fetus.

Thiazide diuretics should not be used in prevention or treatment of pre-eclampsia as there is no evidence of efficacy and their metabolic effects may increase risk to both mother and fetus; they cause hyperuricaemia, which is itself a useful predictor of the disease; reduction of vascular volume may lead to fetal hypoperfusion.

Unwanted interactions (see also individual drugs)

Sympathomimetics, including appetite suppressants (but excluding fenfluramine) and tricyclic antidepressants can, even in small doses, reverse the effects of antihypertensives, especially of adrenergic neurone blockers. Phenothiazine and butyrophenone *neuroleptics* exert a similar antagonism. The mechanism is interference with the noradrenaline pump and therefore with both noradrenaline and drug uptake into nerve endings.

Methyldopa plus an *MAO inhibitor* may cause excitement and hallucinations.

Non-steroidal antiinflammatory drugs (NSAIDs), e.g. indomethacin, attenuate the antihypertensive effect of β-adrenoceptor blockers and of diuretics, perhaps by inhibiting the synthesis of vasodilator prostaglandins. This can also be important when a diuretic is used for severe left *ventricular failure*.

Cimetidine inhibits hepatic metabolism of lipid-soluble β-adrenoceptor blockers.

Surgical anaesthesia may lead to a brisk fall in blood pressure in patients taking antihypertensives. Antihypertensive therapy should not ordinarily be altered before surgery, although it obviously can complicate care both during and after the operation.

Sexual function and cardiovascular drugs

All drugs that interfere with sympathetic autonomic activity, including diuretics, can interfere with sexual function. In men they cause failure of ejaculation and difficulty with erection. Substitution of a drug having a different site of action (e.g. vasodilator or ACE inhibitor; or even changing the drug within a group) may solve this problem, in which pharmacological effects may be potentiated by psychology. Centrally acting drugs (methyldopa, clonidine) cause sedation as well as reducing sympathetic drive, and this is an additive factor. Also, hypertensive patients are commonly of an age when non-drug causes of decline in sexual activity are increasingly common and patients may be influenced by fear of ill-health and of the consequences of their disease in general and the likelihood that sexual activity may be hazardous, as indeed it sometimes may be.

Sexual intercourse and the cardiovascular system. Normal sexual intercourse with orgasm is accompanied by transient but brisk physiological changes, e.g. tachycardia of up to 180 beats/min, with increases of 100 beats/min over less than one min, can occur. Systolic blood pressure may rise by 120 mm Hg and diastolic by 50 mm Hg. Orgasm may be accompanied by transient pressure of 230/130 mm Hg in normotensive individuals. Electrocardiographic abnormalities may occur in healthy men and women. Respiratory rate may rise to 60/min.

Such changes in the healthy may reasonably be thought to bode ill for the unhealthy (hypertension, angina pectoris, post-myocardial infarction), and 'sudden deaths do occur during or shortly after sexual intercourse, but usually in clandestine circumstances such as the bordello or the mistress's boudoir, or when the relationship is

* Follow-up studies show no intellectual impairment in children up to age 7½ years.

between an older man and a younger woman — or are these the ones that make the news? In one series, 0.6% of all sudden deaths were attributable to sexual intercourse and in about half of these cardiac disease was present . . . Clearly it is undesirable that the patient with coronary heart disease should achieve the haemodynamic heights attainable in youth . . .'*

If symptoms attributable to haemodynamic stress do occur during sexual intercourse a modest dose of β-adrenoceptor blocker about 2 h before the estimated time of achievement may well be justified; it is unlikely significantly to affect performance. That which helps the tremulous violinist or ski-jumper or examinee (see *anxiety*) should surely not be denied for this allied purpose when the theoretic basis (reduction of excessive sympathetic autonomic activity) is similar. Patients taking a β-blocker long term for angina prophylaxis have showed reductions in peak heart rate during coitus from 122 to 82 beats/min.

Patients suffering from angina pectoris will use glyceryl trinitrate or isosorbide dinitrate as usual for pre-exertional prophylaxis 10 min before intercourse.

Phaeochromocytoma

This tumour of the adrenal medulla secretes principally noradrenaline, but also variable amounts of adrenaline. Symptoms are related to this. Hypertension may be sustained or intermittent.

Diagnostic tests include measurement of catecholamine concentrations in blood and urine or concentrations of metabolites in urine. Some chemical determinations can be interfered with by methyldopa, levodopa, phenothiazine neuroleptics, labetalol, MAO inhibitors, tetracyclines and by large amounts of caffeine-containing drinks, chocolate, bananas, ice-cream, vitamins, etc, but with modern techniques such interference is less troublesome than formerly.

Antihypertensive drugs may alter catecholamine concentrations (particularly those that induce a reflex increase in sympathetic activity, e.g. vasodilators).

* Editorial Br Med J 1976; 1:414.

False-positive results in tests are common and patients have undergone unnecessary operations because the tests have been regarded as more reliable than they are.†

A variety of *pharmacological tests* is also used; they too can give erroneous results and must be carried out meticulously:

a. *Phentolamine test.* An i.v. dose of this α-adrenoceptor blocker causes a subsantial drop of blood pressure in cases with sustained hypertension.

b. *Clonidine suppression test.* By its action on α-adrenoceptors in the central nervous system, clonidine reduces sympathetic outflow and so the release of catecholamines at nerve endings; it does not supress the catecholamine output by a phaeochromocytoma, which is not under neural control.

c. *Pentolinium suppression test.* This works on the same principle as clonidine though it reduces sympathetic activity at a different site (the sympathetic ganglion).

d. *Provocative tests. Glucagon* (and tyramine and histamine) cause the tumour to release catecholamines and the blood pressure to rise; provocative tests are dangerous and an α-adrenoceptor blocking drug (phentolamine) must be ready for instant use.

A phaeochromocytoma may also be stimulated to secrete and cause a hypertensive attack by metoclopramide and by any drug that releases histamine (opioids, curare). The pressor effect of circulating catecholamines is potentiated by adrenergic neurone blocking drugs and by β-adrenoceptor blockers used alone (below).

Control of blood pressure and heart rate when the tumour cannot be located or removed is

† On the other hand, a positive test must not be ignored. In 1954, a hospital clinical chemistry laboratory was asked to set up a biological assay for catecholamines in the urine. The head of the laboratory tested urine from the lab staff to obtain a reference range for the assay. All were negative except his own which was strongly positive. He felt well and regarded the result as showing insufficient specificity of the test. Two years later a fluorimetric assay became available. The urines of the lab staff were tested again with the same result. The head of the laboratory still felt well, but this time he decided to consult a physician colleague. A few days later, before the consultation, he was quietly reading a newspaper at home in the evening when he had a fatal cerebral infarction. Autopsy revealed a phaeochromocytoma. (Robinson R. Tumours that secrete catecholamines. Chicheste: Wiley, 1980).

achieved best by a combination α- and β-adrenoceptor block (see preparation for surgery, below).

The α-block chiefly controls the blood pressure by abolishing peripheral vasoconstriction, and the β-block controls the tachycardia. A β-receptor blocker should not be given alone, for although it blocks the cardiac stimulation, it also abolishes the peripheral vasodilator effects of adrenaline, leaving the powerful α-effects unopposed, so that there is a rise in peripheral resistance and a further rise of blood pressure. At present, no β-blocker is sufficiently selective for the heart to avoid this effect; but the combined β- and α-receptor blocker (labetalol) can be used successfully (though cases of hypertension have been reported).

For *surgical removal*, where the site of the phaeochromocytoma is known, the patient may be spared the effects of liberation of dangerous amounts of catecholamines due to anaesthesia and handling of the tumour, by preparation for 2 to 3 days with an α- and a β-blocker (phenoxybenzamine* or prazosin *plus* propranolol or atenolol), so that operation is conducted under complete or partial receptor blockade. This prolonged preparation allows the reduced blood volume (due to vasoconstriction) to be restored to normal before surgery. The patient must, of course, be kept supine if large doses of α-blocker are used. Maintenance of blood volume during and after surgery is essential, for the blood pressure depends on it, though the vessels retain their responsiveness to angiotensin, which could be used in a postsurgical hypotensive emergency.

* Phenoxybenzamine may be preferred because it combines irreversibly with receptors and consequently its action is not surmountable by a sudden surge of catecholamine released from the tumour.

When the site of the tumour is unknown, blood pressure changes can provide a useful guide to indicate when the surgeon has found it; complete adrenoceptor block would prevent this. A quick-acting α-blocker (phentolamine), plus a β-blocker should be kept at hand to control the blood pressure and heart rate and rhythm; sodium nitroprusside i.v. is used for short-term control of hypertension. After the adrenal veins have been clamped, a pressor infusion may be needed to maintain the blood pressure (but it may be preferable to expand plasma volume because patients can become dependent on sympathomimetic pressor infusions).

Metirosine (*α-methyltyrosine*) has been used successfully to block catecholamine synthesis. It inhibits tyrosine hydroxylase, which converts tyrosine to dopa, a precursor of dopamine and noradrenaline; it is used to control hypertension when the phaeochromocytoma cannot be removed.

Metaiodobenzylguanidine (mIBG; an analogue of guanethidine) is an adrenergic neurone blocker. It is actively taken up by adrenergic tissue and is concentrated in phaeochromocytomas. Radioactive forms allow localization of tumours and detection of metastases; also selective therapeutic irradiation of functioning metastases. It is subject to the interactions of adrenergic neurone blockers, e.g. tricyclic antidepressants. It may also be similarly useful in other tumours of chromaffin tissue (e.g. carcinoid).

GUIDE TO FURTHER READING

1 Page I H. Antihypertensive drugs: our debts to industrial chemists. N Engl J Med 1981; 304:615.

2 Medical Research Council Working Party, MRC Trial of treatment of mild hypertension. Br Med J 1985; 291:97. Also Editorial. Breckenridge A, p. 89.

3 European Working Party. Mortality and morbidity results from the European Working Party on High Blood Pressure in the elderly trial. Lancet 1985; 1: 1349. Also Editorial, p. 1369.

4 Editorial. Calcium antagonists and blood pressure. Lancet 1983; 2:22.

5 McAreavey D et al. 'Third drug' trial comparative study of antihypertensive agents added to treatment when blood pressure remains uncontrolled by a beta-blocker plus thiazide diuretic. Br Med J 1984; 288:106: also Editorial, Breckenridge A. Br Med J 1984; 289:859.

6 WHO/International Society for Hypertension. Mild Hypertension Liasion Committee. Trials of the treatment of mild hypertension Lancet 1982; 1:149.

7 Bayliss J et al. Clinical importance of the renin-angiotension system in chronic heart failure: double-blind comparison of captopril and prazosin. Br Med J 1985; 290:1861.

8 Watkins J et al. Attenuation of hypotensive effect of propranolol and thiazide diuretics by indomethacin. Br Med J 1980; 281:702.

9 Gould B A et al. Does placebo lower blood pressure? Lancet 1981; 2:1377.

10 Gill J S et al. Hypertension and well-being. Br Med J 1983; 287:1490.

11 Mancia G et al. Effects of blood pressure measurement by the doctor on patients' blood pressure and heart rate. Lancet 1983; 2:695.

12 Anonymous. I had a phaeochromocytoma. Lancet 1982; 1:922.
13 Bravo D L et al. Phaeochromocytoma: diagnosis, localization and management. N Engl J Med 1984; 311:1298.
14 Editorial. Lowering blood pressure without drugs. Lancet 1980; 2:459.
15 Ball S G et al. A need for new converting enzyme inhibitors. Br Med J 1985; 290:180.
16 Benson H et al. Angina pectoris and the placebo effect. N Engl J Med 1979; 300:1424.
17 Abrams J. Nitroglycerin and long-acting nitrates. N Engl J Med 1980; 302:1234.
18 Silverman K J. Angina pectoris: natural history and strategies for evaluation and management. N Engl J Med 1984; 310:1712.
19 Fox K et al. Interaction between cigarettes and propranolol in treatment of angina pectoris. Br Med J 1980; 281:191.
20 Hiatt W R et al. Beta-2 adrenergic blockade evaluated with epinephrine after placebo, atenolol, and nadolol. Clin Pharmacol Ther 1985; 37:2.
21 Stokes G S et al. On the combination of alpha and beta-adrenoceptor blockade in hypertension. Clin Pharmacol Ther 1983; 34:576.
22 Leenen F H H et al. Antihypertensive effect and degree of beta-adrenoceptor blockade after short-term and semi-chronic propranolol therapy. Br J Clin Pharmacol 1984; 17:745.
23 Breckenridge A M et al, eds. Beta-adrenoceptor blocker/drug interactions: a symposium. Br J Clin Pharmacol 1984; 17: 1S–114S.
24 Wilcox R G et al. The effects of acute or chronic ingestion of propranolol on the physiological response to prolonged submaximal exercise in hypertensive men. Br J Clin Pharmacol 1984; 17:273.
25 Quyyumi A A et al. Effect of partial agonist activity in beta-blockers in severe angina pectoris, a double-blind comparison of pindolol and atenolol. Br Med J 1984; 289:951.
26 Asplund J et al. Patients' compliance in hypertension. Br J Clin Pharmacol 1984; 17:547.
27 Bulpitt C J et al. Side effects of hypotensive agents evaluated by a self-administered questionnaire. Br Med J 1973; 3:485, and subsequent correspondence.
28 Harington M et al. Results of treatment in malignant hypertension. Br Med J 1959; 2:969. A historic study.
29 Personal paper. Trials and tribulations of a symptom-free hypertensive physician receiving the best of care. Lancet 1977; 2:291.
30 Skegg D et al. Frequency of eye complaints and rashes among patients receiving practolol and propranolol. Lancet 1977; 2:475.
31 Gersh B J et al. Comparison of coronary artery bypass surgery and medical therapy in patients 65 years of age or older: a nonrandomized study from the Coronary Artery Surgery Study (CASS) Regulations. N Engl J Med 1985; 313:217.
32 Gould S H et al. The effects of antihypertensive therapy on the quality of life. N Engl J Med 1986, 314:1657.

25

Cardiovascular system III: Cardiac dysrhythmia and cardiac failure

The pathophysiology of cardiac dysrhythmias is complex and the actions of drugs that are useful in stopping or controlling them may seem equally so. Nevertheless many patients with dysrhythmias respond well to therapy with drugs and a working knowledge of their effects and indications pays dividends, for irregularity of the heart-beat may be at least inconvenient and at worst fatal.

SOME PHYSIOLOGY AND PATHOPHYSIOLOGY

There are two types of heart cell from the electrophysiological point of view.

The first type is the *conducting* cell and is found in the sino-atrial (SA) node, the atrioventricular (AV) node and in the His–Purkinje system of the ventricles; this cell is distinguished by being able to discharge automatically (i.e. it exhibits *automaticity*). When it does so, an action potential (electrical impulse) is formed and spreads to adjacent cells. The rate of automatic discharge is normally fastest in the most proximal conducting tissue; thus the SA node (70 discharges per min) controls the contraction rate of the heart, making the cells more distal in the conducting system fire more rapidly than they would do spontaneously. If the SA node fails to function, the next fastest part takes over. This is often the AV node (45 discharges per min) or a site in the His–Purkinje system (25 discharges per min). *Altered rate of automatic discharge* or *abnormality of the mechanism by which an impulse is generated* from a centre in the conducting tissue is one cause for cardiac dysrhythmia; circulating catecholamines, for example, increase the rate of automatic discharge.

The second type of cardiac cell is the *contracting* or myocardial muscle cell. This differs from the first cell type in lacking the capacity to discharge spontaneously, but when an impulse reaches it through the conducting system, discharge occurs and the cell contracts.

In the resting state the interior of the cell is electrically negative with respect to the exterior and during discharge there is a rapid change in potential to positive within the cell (depolarisation). After discharging, both the conducting cells and the muscle cells gradually repolarise to the resting potential again. In the process of depolarisation and repolarisation various phases are recognised and each is characterised by movement of particular ions into and out of cells. *Antidysrhythmic drugs* act on different points of this cycle and hence a simplified account of the *phases of polarisation* follows:

Phase 0: is the rapid depolarisation of the cell membrane and it is associated with a fast inflow of *sodium ions* through channels that are selectively permeable to these ions (the transmembrane electrical potential within the cell alters from about −60 to +30 millivolts (mV) relative to the extracellular fluid).

Phase 1: is a short initial period of rapid repolarisation brought about mainly by an outflow of *potassium ions* (the transmembrane electrical potential alters from +30 to +10 mV).

Phase 2: is a period when there is a delay in repolarisation caused mainly by a slow movement of *calcium ions* from exterior into the cell through channels that are selectively permeable to these ions (the transmembrane electrical potential alters from +10 to −10 mV).

Phase 3: is a second period of rapid repolarisation during which *potassium ions* move out of the cell (the transmembrane electrical potential alters from −10 to −70 mV).

Phase 4: is the fully repolarised state (transmembrane electrical potential −70 mV) during which *potassium ions* move back into and *sodium and calcium ions* move out of the cell again to enable the next cycle to begin.

The automaticity of the pacemaker cell is due to its electrical instability in this phase, for it allows sodium to leak back *into* the cell. The result is a slow discharge to a critical threshold (transmembrane electrical potential −60 mV) when there is rapid depolarisation and the cycle is repeated. Cardiac muscle cells do not leak sodium during this phase and remain in the repolarised state; they thus have no inherent automaticity and only discharge when stimulated.

In phases 1 and 2 the cell is in an *absolutely refractory* state and is incapable of responding further to any stimulus, but during phase 3, the *relative refractory* period, the cell will depolarise again if a stimulus is unusually strong. In the conducting system the orderly sequence of depolarisation and transmission of an action potential may not proceed uniformly. Ischaemia, for example, can retard conduction in a part of the system. An impulse conducted down a normal Purkinje fibre may spread to an adjacent fibre that has transiently failed to transmit, and pass up it in the reverse direction. If this retrograde impulse should in turn re-excite the cells that provided the original impulse, a repetitively firing *re-entrant* circuit is established. Re-entrant tachycardia can also occur within the AV node if a premature atrial impulse reaches it when some of the cells are in the relative refractory period; it can develop within minor branches of the Purkinje system, indeed many ectopic foci may be micro re-entry circuits in aggregates of cells.

In summary, most cardiac dysrhythmias are probably due to either

1. *altered rate of spontaneous discharge* in conducting tissue or
2. *impaired conduction* in part of the system leading to the formation of re-entry circuits.

CLASSIFICATION OF DRUGS

It would seem reasonable, therefore, that drugs used to treat cardiac dysrhythmias ought to influence automatic discharge or to affect conduction in re-entry circuits. In practice, the antidysrhythmic drugs do not fall naturally into such a classification. Many facts about their electropharmacology are known but it is not always possible to use these satisfactorily to explain why a drug will stop one type of dysrhythmia and not another. Nevertheless, in the preclinical stage of development, the antidysrhythmic drugs are classified according to their electropharmacological actions* and this provides a widely used system for grouping clinically useful drugs of similar properties. It is presented below together with an indication of why the actions by which drugs are classified may be useful in dysrhythmias.

The system does not encompass all drugs that are used to treat dysrhythmias and others are described in a subsequent section.

Class 1: Sodium channel blockade

These drugs restrict the rapid inflow of sodium during Phase 0 and thus slow the maximum rate of depolarisation. Local anaesthetics act in this way. The general term for this property is *membrane stabilising activity*; it may contribute to

* Vaughan Williams E M. J Clin Pharmacol 1984; 24: 129–147

stopping dysrhythmias by limiting the *responsiveness to excitation* of cardiac cells in general. The drugs may be sub-classified according to their effect on the refractoriness of conducting cells after rapid depolarisation, as follows:

A. *Drugs that prolong refractoriness*
   e.g. quinidine, procainamide, disopyramide
B. *Drugs that shorten refractoriness*
   e.g. lignocaine, mexiletine, phenytoin, tocainide
C. *Drug that has little effect on refractoriness*
   e.g. flecainide

Class II: Sympathetic blockade

These drugs reduce the activity of the sympathetic nervous system in the myocardium. Their antidysrhythmic effects are probably related to reduction in background sympathetic tone, reduction of automatic discharge and protection against adrenergically induced ectopic pacemakers, e.g. propranolol and other β-adrenoceptor antagonists and bretylium (peripheral adrenergic neurone blockade).

Class III: Prolongation of refractoriness without alteration of the rate of depolarisation

Prolongation of cellular refractoriness beyond a critical point may prevent a re-entry circuit being completed and may thereby abolish a re-entrant tachycardia (see above), e.g. amiodarone.

Class IV: Calcium channel blockade

By blocking the slow calcium channels these drugs depress the rate of discharge of the SA node and prolong conduction and refractoriness in the AV node, which may explain their effectiveness in terminating paroxysmal supraventricular tachycardia, e.g. verapamil, diltiazem.

Although the antidysrhythmics have been entered into this classification according to a characteristic major action, most have other effects as well. For example, quinidine (class I) also has class III effects; propranolol (class II) also has class I effects; and sotalol (class II) also has class III effects. Paradoxically, antidysrhythmic drugs may actually be the cause of dysrhythmia, e.g. if used in too high a dose. These effects are described in more detail in the accounts of individual drugs which follow.

CLASS IA

Quinidine (200 mg) is described first as it is the prototype class I drug, although not now the most frequently used. It is the optical isomer of quinine; both substances have cardiac and antimalarial effects but their relative potencies differ. The cardiac effect of quinine was observed in 1749 when it was used against 'rebellious palpitation' but this was not followed up. In 1912, Wenckebach* was visited by a Dutch merchant who wished to get rid of his attacks of atrial fibrillation, which, although they did not unduly inconvenience him, offended his notions of good order in life's affairs. On receiving a guarded prognosis, the merchant enquired why there were heart specialists if they could not accomplish what he himself had already achieved. In the face of Wenckebach's incredulity, he promised to return the next day with a regular pulse, which he did, at the same time revealing that he had done it with quinine. At that time quinine had a reputation as a general remedy rather like that of aspirin today, and taking it empirically the merchant had found that a gram of quinine would abolish his attacks in about 25 minutes.† Examination of quinine derivatives led to the introduction of quinidine in 1918.

Quinidine has a number of *cardiac actions*.

1. The capacity for and rate of automatic firing of pacemaker cells (automaticity) are reduced (class I); this effect serves to suppress premature beats or an ectopic pacemaker.

2. The responsiveness of atrial, ventricular and Purkinje cells to excitation, and the conduction velocity of impulses, are reduced (class I); both effects help to limit the spread of an abnormal impulse.

* Karel Frederick Wenckebach (1864–1940). Dutch physician; he described a disorder of cardiac conduction, 'Wenckebach block'.
† Wenckebach K F. JAMA 1923; 81:472.

3. The refractory period of atrial, ventricular and Purkinje cells is prolonged; this is due to a class III action and may extend the refractoriness of cells beyond a critical point, prevent the completion of a re-entry circuit and thus terminate a re-entrant tachycardia.

4. The contractility of the myocardium is depressed (negative intropic effect); this is only slight at ordinary doses with a normal myocardium but may be important with the diseased heart.

5. The vagus nerve activity on the heart is reduced (an atropine-like effect).

Electrocardiographic changes occur with therapeutic doses. The most characteristic effect is prolongation of the Q–T interval due to lengthening of ventricular systole. In addition, there may be prolongation of the P–R interval (atrioventricular conduction block) and inversion and prolongation of the T wave.

Absorption of quinidine from the gut is rapid. It is 80% bound to plasma proteins. About 75% of the drug is metabolised and the remainder is eliminated unchanged in the urine. Its $t_{\frac{1}{2}}$ is 6 h. There is wide individual variation in plasma concentration following standard doses, and maximum benefit with minimum risk can be got by controlling therapy with measurements of plasma concentration (effective range, 2–5 mg/l).

Quinidine can suppress and prevent supraventricular, nodal and ventricular ectopic beats and tachycardias, for example after myocardial infarction or following DC shock. It may also be used to restore or maintain sinus rhythm in patients who have had atrial fibrillation or flutter but it should never be used alone for these conditions as its anticholinergic action enhances AV conduction (see later, atrial fibrillation and flutter).

The dose is 200–400 mg orally 3–4 times daily; it is often administered as a slow-release preparation (Kinidin Durules 500 mg twice daily).

Adverse effects include anorexia, nausea, vomiting and diarrhoea. Cinchonism occurs, as with quinine, and generalised muscle weakness. Cardiac effects include the induction of dysrhythmias, notably of ventricular origin, causing syncope. The negative inotropic action (above) may result in hypotension and cardiac failure. Allergic reactions of various types occur. Quinidine should be stopped if adverse effects more serious than nausea, tinnitus or mild diarrhoea occur, if the QRS complex on the electrocardiogram exceeds the control value by more than 25%, or if there are frequent (one every 6 sec) ectopic beats. Plasma digoxin concentration is raised by quinidine and the dose of digoxin should be decreased when the drugs are used together.

Procainamide (250 mg) has effects on the heart that are essentially the same as those of quinidine, namely

1. membrane stablisation (reduced automaticity, reduced responsiveness to excitation, reduced conduction velocity; class I)

2. prolongation of the cardiac refractory period (classes I and III)

3. anticholinergic effects (milder than those of quinidine).

Procainamide is well absorbed from the alimenary tract and gives a maximum effect in one hour. Less than 20% is bound to plasma proteins and the $t_{\frac{1}{2}}$ is 3 h. The drug is acetylated in the liver and there are genetically fast- and slow-acetylator phenotypes; most of a dose is eliminated either unchanged or as the acetylated metabolite in the urine. The therapeutic plasma concentration of procainamide alone is 4–10 mg/l; when N-acetylprocainamide is measured as well, the range is 10–30 mg/l.

Procainamide is used to suppress and prevent supraventricular, nodal and ventricular dysrhythmias, especially those that follow myocardial infarction.

The dose is as follows: by mouth 250 mg every 4–6 h; by *slow* i.v. injection 25–50 mg/min with ECG monitoring until the dysrhythmia is controlled (max. 1 g); maintenance treatment by mouth is as above and by i.m. injection 100–250 mg every 4–6 h.

Adverse effects of procainamide include hypotension due to its negative inotropic effect and induction of dysrhythmias. In long-term use up to 80% of patients taking procainamide develop abnormal titres of antinuclear factor in the blood and 30% proceed to a systemic lupus-like syndrome. The effect is dose-related, is more common in slow acetylators and usually regresses when the drug is withdrawn. Allergic reactions of various types occur and there is cross-allergy with procaine.

Disopyramide (100 mg) possesses membrane-stabilising properties (class I), prolongs the cardiac refractory period (classes I and III) and has anticholinergic activity.

Absorption of disopyramide from the gut is rapid and almost complete. Plasma protein binding is 27%. About 50% of a dose is eliminated in the urine by glomerular filtration and the remainder is metabolised. The $t_{½}$ is 6 h, but is prolonged after myocardial infarction, probably because diminished cardiac output reduces renal clearance and $t_{½}$ may be 25 h when impairment is severe. The therapeutic plasma concentration is 3–6 mg/l.

Disopyramide is effective in both supraventricular and ventricular dysrhythmias, especially after myocardial infarction. It may also be used for paroxysmal supraventricular tachycardias of the Wolff–Parkinson–White (WPW) syndrome.

The dose is: by mouth 300–800 mg daily in divided doses according to response; by slow i.v. injection 2 mg/kg body weight over 5 min with ECG monitoring (not more than 150 mg in total) and maintained at 0.4 mg/kg hourly by i.v. infusion, the total daily dose not to exceed 800 mg.

Adverse effects on the cardiovascular system include hypotension and cardiac failure due to its negative inotropic effect, and induction of cardiac dysrhythmia. Anticholinergic activity is a significant problem and may lead to dry mouth, blurred vision, glaucoma and urinary hesitancy and retention.

CLASS IB

Lignocaine (inj. 100 mg, 1 mg/ml, 2 mg/ml; see also *local anaesthetics*), like quinidine possesses membrane-stabilising (class I) effects but unlike quinidine it *reduces* the cardiac refractory period. It is probably because of this difference that lignocaine can sometimes terminate a dysrhythmia when quinidine and procainamide fail, and vice versa.

Lignocaine is used by the i.v. or occasionally by the i.m. route; dosing by mouth is unsatisfactory because the $t_{½}$ (90 min) is too short to maintain a constant plasma concentration by repeated administration and because the drug, although well absorbed from the gastrointestinal tract, undergoes extensive pre-systemic (first-pass) elimination in the liver and plasma concentrations are variable. The i.v. route is safe to use and the short $t_{½}$ makes for greater ease in dose adjustment than with most antidysrhythmics. Lignocaine is almost entirely metabolised in the liver and the rate at which it is cleared from the blood depends on liver blood flow. Patients in cardiac failure have higher blood concentrations of lignocaine on a standard dosing regimen because liver blood flow is reduced. The therapeutic blood concentration is 2–5 mg/l.

Lignocaine is used for ventricular dysrhythmias, especially those complicating myocardial infarction.

A satisfactory regimen is a loading dose of 1–2 mg/kg as an i.v. bolus injection, followed by a continuous i.v. infusion of 4 mg/min for 30 min, 2 mg/min for 2 h, then 1 mg/min. In an emergency outside hospital, 4–5 mg/kg may be given by i.m. injection.

Adverse effects are not common unless infusion is rapid or there is significant cardiac failure; they include hypotension, dizziness, blurred sight, sleepiness, subjective difficulty in talking or swallowing, numbness, sweating, confusion, twitching and fits.

Mexiletine (50, 200, 360 mg; inj. 25 mg/ml) is similar to lignocaine in that it possesses membrane-stabilising properties (Class 1) and reduces the cardiac refractory period.

Absorption of mexiletine from the gut is normally almost complete but delayed or incomplete absorption may occur if narcotic analgesics have been used, as may be the case after myocardial infarction. Mexiletine is eliminated mainly by metabolism, only about 10% being excreted unchanged in the urine. The $t_{½}$ is 10 h in healthy subjects but may be longer in cardiac patients. The therapeutic plasma concentration lies between 0.7 and 1.5 mg/l.

Mexiletine is used for ventricular dysrhythmias, especially those complicating myocardial infarction and those induced by cardiac glycosides.

The dose is as follows: by mouth 400–600 mg as a loading dose, followed after 2 h by 200–250 mg three or four times daily for maintenance; i.v. 100–250 mg should be administered at 25 mg per minute and the plasma concentration is maintained by infusing 250 mg in one hour followed by 250 mg in two hours followed by 0.5 mg/min for as long as is necessary.

Adverse effects are related to dose and include nausea, vomiting, hiccough, tremor, drowsinesss, confusion, dyasrthria, diplopia, ataxia, cardiac dysrhythmia and hypotension.

Tocainide (400, 600 mg; inj. 50 mg/ml; inf. 10 mg/ml) is structurally related to lignocaine, has membrane-stabilising (class I) properties and shortens the cardiac refractory period. It is however suitable for repeated administration by mouth, being well absorbed from the gastrointestinal tract and having a $t_{\frac{1}{2}}$ of 11 h. Elimination unchanged by the kidney accounts for half of the dose and metabolism for the remainder. Tocainide is effective in the control of ventricular dysrythmias especially following myocardial infarction; it may be used to continue antidysrhythmic treatment in place of an infusion of lignocaine.

Adverse effects are dose related and include hypotension, bradycardia and other dysrhythmias, and aggravation of cardiac failure; central nervous system effects similar to those experienced with lignocaine may also occur.

Phenytoin (see also under *antiepileptics*; 25, 50, 100 mg; inj. 50 mg/ml) is used as an antidysrhythmic drug because of its membrane-stabilising properties (class I). Like lignocaine, phenytoin shortens the cardiac refractory period.

Phenytoin is given mainly for ventricular and supraventricular dysrhythmias associated with digoxin overdose. The therapeutic plasma concentration is 10–25 mg/l. Care must be taken in dosing because the elimination processes for phenytoin are saturable and progressive increments in dose results in a disproportionate rise in plasma concentration. Individual variation in plasma concentration may also arise from enzyme induction.

CLASS IC

Flecainide has membrane-stabilising properties (class I) and slows conduction in all cardiac tissues including the anomalous pathways responsible for the Wolff–Parkinson–White (WPW) syndrome; it has little effect on the cardiac refractory period. The drug is well absorbed from the gastrointestinal tract. Plasma protein binding is 30–60%. Its action is terminated both by metabolism in the liver and by elimination in the urine. The $t_{\frac{1}{2}}$ is 14 h in healthy adults but may be over 20 h in patients with cardiac disease, in the elderly and in those with poor renal function.

Flecainide is effective mainly for ventricular but also for supraventricular dysrhythmias including those of the WPW syndrome. It should be reserved for cases resistant to other drugs and treatment should be initiated under specialist supervision.

Adverse effects involving the nervous system include nausea, dizziness, blurred vision, tremor, abnormal taste sensations and paraesthesia. Dysrhythmia may be precipitated in patients with cardiac disease and its negative inotropic effect may induce cardiac failure.

CLASS II

β-adrenoceptor antagonists (see index) are effective probably because they counteract the dysrhythmogenic effect of catecholamines. The following actions appear to be relevant.

1. The rate of automatic firing of the SA node is accelerated by β-adrenergic stimulation and this effect is abolished by β-blockers. Some ectopic pacemakers appear to be dependent on adrenergic drive.

2. β-blockers prolong the refractoriness of the AV node, which may prevent re-entrant tachycardia at this site.

3. Many β-blocking drugs (propranolol, oxprenolol, alprenolol, acebutolol) also possess membrane-stabilising (class I) properties, particularly when there is myocardial ischaemia or acidosis. Sotalol prolongs cardiac refractoriness (class III) but has no class I effects; it is often preferred when a β-blocker is needed.

β-adrenoceptor antagonists can be used for a range of supraventricular dysrhythmias, in particular those associated with exercise, emotion or thyrotoxicosis. They are useful in WPW syndrome and in digoxin-induced dysrhythmias. Sotalol may be given to suppress ventricular ectopic beats and ventricular tachycardia.

For long-term use, any of the oral preparations

is suitable. In emergencies, practolol 5 mg may be given by slow i.v. injection and repeated if necessary. There is no danger of inducing the oculomucocutaneous syndrome in such short-term use. Alternatively, propranolol may be given i.v. at a rate of 1 mg per min to a maximum of 10 mg, preceded by atropine 1–2 mg for vagal block.

Adverse effects from overdosage include heart block or even cardiac arrest. Heart failure may be precipitated when a patient is dependent on sympathetic drive to maintain output. Concomitant administration of verapamil (and probably diltiazem) is contraindicated because cardiac contractility is further reduced and AV block is increased. The relatively cardioselective antagonists metoprolol, atenolol and practolol are less likely to provoke acute airways obstruction in asthmatic or bronchitic patients but are not free from the risk.

Bretylium blocks the release of noradrenaline from sympathetic nerves. In the heart it prolongs the refractory period (class III) without affecting the rate of propagation of the cardiac impulse. Formerly used for hypertension, it is now obsolete, as tolerance soon develops and absorption from the gut is variable. The $t_{\frac{1}{2}}$ is 9 h and 80% of a dose is excreted in the urine unchanged. It may be used for resistant ventricular tachyrhythmias, especially those complicating myocardial infarction or cardiac surgery. The main adverse effects are hypotension, bradycardia and parotid pain.

CLASS III

Amiodarone (100, 200 mg; inj. 50 mg/ml) prolongs the effective refractory period of myocardial cells, the AV node and anomalous pathways by a class III action. Extension of the refractory period beyond a critical point may be sufficient to prevent a re-entry circuit being completed and so terminate a re-entrant tachycardia. The drug may also antagonise α-and β-adrenoceptors non-competitively.

Amiodarone is absorbed from the gastrointestinal tract and its enormous apparent distribution volume (5000 litres/70 kg) indicates that little remains in the blood; it is lipid soluble and is stored in fat and many other tissues. The drug is metabolised in the liver and eliminated via the biliary and intestinal tracts. It is slowly released from its storage sites and the $t_{\frac{1}{2}}$ is about 30 days, but may be as long as 100 days.

Amiodarone is effective for chronic ventricular dysrhythmias. In atrial fibrillation it slows the ventricular response and may restore sinus rhythm; it may be used to maintain sinus rhythm after cardioversion for atrial fibrillation or flutter. It is also effective for the management of resistant re-entry supraventricular tachycardias associated with the WPW syndrome.

The very long $t_{\frac{1}{2}}$ indicates that amiodarone accumulates slowly to steady state on daily dosing. A loading dose is therefore necessary to achieve an early effect. Usually 0.6 g daily for one week will suffice; thereafter therapy may be maintained with 0.2 g daily. It may also be given i.v. 5 mg/kg over 20–120 min, then 15 mg/kg for 24 h, by a central line to avoid phlebitis.

Adverse cardiovascular effects are uncommon apart from prolongation of the Q–T interval, which predisposes to dysrhythmias. Almost all patients develop corneal microdeposits that cause visual haloes and photophobia. These are dose-related, resolve when the drug is discontinued and are not a long-term threat to vision. Each 200 mg tablet of amiodarone contains about 75 mg of iodine, which is enough to interfere with thyroid function, and both hyperthyroidism and hypothyroidism are reported. Peripheral conversion of thyroxine (T_4) to tri-iodothyronine (T_3) is inhibited, so that patients on long-term therapy generally have increased T_4 and decreased T_3 plasma concentrations; thyroid function should be checked before a patient begins treatment. Photosensitivity reactions are common and amiodarone may cause a bluish discolouration on exposed areas of the skin. Less commonly, pulmonary fibrosis and hepatitis occur.

Interaction with digoxin (by displacement from tissue binding sites and interference with its elimination) and with warfarin (by inhibiting its metabolism) results in increased effect of both these drugs, which may commonly be administered with amiodarone. β-blockers and calcium channel antagonists augment the depressant effect of amiodarone on SA and AV node function and patients with disorders of the cardiac conducting system should be carefully supervised when these drugs are used in combination.

CLASS IV

The calcium channel blockers

Calcium is involved in the function of cardiac conducting and contracting cells and of arterial smooth-muscle cells. It is appropriate to discuss here its action at both these sites.

Cardiac cells

1. After the initial *fast* transmembrane influx of sodium that depolarises the cell (phase 0) and the partial repolarisation by outflow of potassium (phase 1) there is a secondary *slow* inward current through channels that are selective for calcium ions (phase 2). This inflow through *slow calcium channels* delays repolarisation and causes a plateau in the action potential; during this plateau the cell is absolutely refractory, i.e. it cannot respond to any stimulus, however great.

2. Contraction of cardiac muscle cells requires an influx of calcium ions, which trigger the release of calcium from intracellular stores. This calcium is delivered during phase 2 to the immediate vicinity of the myofibrils. Intracellular calcium is necessary for contraction

(i) through the supply of chemical energy released when the high-energy phosphate bond of adenosine triphosphate (ATP) is broken down by calcium-dependent ATPase and

(ii) through its binding to a protein complex named troponin, which regulates the formation of cross-bridges between the contractile proteins actin and myosin, which thus draw closer and produce the shortening of the muscle.

Arterial smooth muscle cells

Contraction of smooth muscle in coronary and systemic arteries and in arterioles is also dependent on calcium ions, which enter through channels equivalent to those in cardiac cells when an appropriate stimulus is received. The mechanism is similar to that in the myocardium but differs in that the calcium binds to a molecular complex known as calmodulin, which activates the enzyme that phosphorylates the light chains of myosin; these in turn activate the actin–myosin cross-bridges that generate the contraction.

Calcium channel blocking drugs

A large number of drugs interfere with the availability of calcium for its physiological functions and may be described as having a calcium antagonist action. They include local anaesthetics, β-adrenoceptor antagonists, neomycin, phenytoin and barbiturates. Their action agaisnt calcium is usually non-specific, unrelated to the main effect and must be regarded as separate from the specific effect that some drugs have on the slow calcium channels.

The calcium-channel blockers prevent the influx of calcium through the slow ion channels. They are active at low concentrations of calcium and have negligible effect on the sodium influx that generates the action potential. The drugs may also interfere with the functions of calcium within the cell. It is convenient to think of them further as:

1. Specific, potent blockers such as verapamil, diltiazem and nifedipine. These drugs are structurally unrelated but they all block the movement of calcium into cardiac and arterial smooth muscle cells and so cause them to relax. The resulting dilatation of coronary arteries relieves angina (verapamil, nifedipine, diltiazem) and of arteriolar resistance vessels benefits hypertension (nifedipine). Cardiac muscle contractility is reduced (verapamil, diltiazem). Verapamil also blocks slow calcium channels in the SA and AV nodes and is effective against supraventricular dysrhythmias.

2. Less specific, less potent drugs, e.g. lidoflazine and prenylamine, which also relax arteriolar smooth muscle and are used to prevent angina.

It is convenient to discuss here verapamil, nifedipine and diltiazem, although only the former is used for dysrhythmias.

Verapamil (40, 80, 120 mg; inj. 2.5 mg/ml) prolongs conduction and refractoriness in the AV node and depresses the rate of discharge of the SA node. It also reduces cardiac contractility, dilates coronary arteries, especially those that are in spasm, and dilates peripheral arterioles. Verapamil is well absorbed from the gastrointestinal tract and undergoes extensive first-pass extraction in the liver such that only about 20% of the oral dose reaches the systemic circulation (50% in patients with diseased livers). A metabolite, norverapamil, accumulates in plasma and has some effects that are similar to those of the parent compound. Verapamil has large distribution volume, about 90% of the drug in the blood is bound to plasma proteins and the $t_{\frac{1}{2}}$ is 4 h.

The particular place of verapamil as an antidysrhythmic drug is to terminate paroxysmal supraventricular tachycardia when given i.v.; it may be less effective by mouth to prevent this dysrhythmia because of variable first-pass extraction by the liver (above). Verapamil benefits both stable and unstable angina, especially when there is associated coronary artery spasm, e.g. in Prinzmetal's variant form. It may also be used to treat hypertension (see Chapter 24).

The dose by mouth is as follows: for dysrhythmias 40–120 mg × 3/day; for angina 80–120 mg × 3/day; for hypertension 120–240 mg × 2/day. The i.v. dose for dysrhythmias is, by slow injection, 5 mg, repeated in 5–10 min if necessary, or by infusion, 5–10 mg over 1 h, maximum dose 100 mg in 24 h.

Mild adverse effects are fairly common and include constipation, headache, flushing, peripheral oedema and giddiness, all of which may improve with continued use. Verapamil should not be given to patients with sick sinus syndrome, second- or third-degree AV block, bradycardia or heart failure. Patients who are taking a β-blocker should only be given verapamil by mouth if they show no tendency to cardiac failure and they should not receive the drug i.v. Verapamil reduces the renal clearance of digoxin by about 50% and the dose of digoxin should be decreased when the drugs are used together.

Diltiazem (60 mg) dilates coronary arteries and arterioles, which increases myocardial perfusion and decreases peripheral resistance; it also weakens cardiac contractility but because there is reduced afterload the tendency to cardiac failure is limited. The drug prolongs AV conduction but to a lesser extent than does verapamil. Diltiazem is rapidly and completely absorbed from the gastrointestinal tract and about 50% of an oral dose is extracted in the first pass through the liver; a metabolite, desacetyldiltiazem, possesses about half the pharmacological activity of the parent drug. Diltiazem in the blood is more than 80% bound to plasma proteins and the $t_{\frac{1}{2}}$ is 5 h. The drug is used to prevent both stable and unstable angina. The dose is 60 mg × 3/day (or × 2/day for elderly patients) to a maximum of 360 mg per day.

Adverse effects include ankle oedema, headache and nausea. Diltiazem should not be used in patients with sick sinus syndrome, second- or third-degree AV block or severe bradycardia.

Nifedipine (5, 10, 20 mg) dilates resistant arterioles and coronary arteries at plasma concentrations that have relatively little effect on myocardial contractility. Any direct effects on the cardiac conducting system are negligible. The drug is well absorbed from the gastrointestinal tract but only about 55% of an oral dose reaches the systemic circulation because it is extracted in first pass through the liver; it is 95% bound to plasma proteins and the $t_{\frac{1}{2}}$ is 1.5 h. Nifedipine is effective for the prevention of stable and unstable angina, especially when there is coronary artery spasm, for hypertension and for Raynaud's phenomenon (see Chapter 24). The dose is 10–20 mg × 3/day but it may be preferred to start with 5 mg × 3/day in the elderly. Adverse effects are related to vasodilatation and include headache, flushing and dizziness; these are improved if the dose is lowered or if drug is used with a β-blocker.

OTHER DRUGS USED TO TREAT CARDIAC DYSRHYTHMIAS

Some of the drugs used in dysrhythmias exert their actions through the autonomic nervous system by mimicking or antagonising the effects of the parasympathetic or sympathetic nerves that supply the heart.

The vagus nerve (cholinergic, parasympathetic), when stimulated, has the following effects on the heart:

1. bradycardia due to decreased automaticity of the SA node
2. slowing of conduction through and increased refractoriness of the AV conducting tissue

3. reduced force of contraction (contractility) of the heart
4. shortening of the refractory period of atrial muscle
5. decreased myocardial excitability

Effects 1, 2, 4 and 5 are used in the therapy of dysrhythmias.

The vagus nerve may be stimulated reflexly by various physical manoeuvres. Vagal stimulation may slow or terminate supraventricular dysrhythmias and should if possible be carried out under ECG control.

Carotid sinus massage activates stretch receptors and is the method most commonly used: external pressure is applied gently to one side at a time but *never* to both sides at once. Some individuals are very sensitive to the procedure and develop severe bradycardia and hypotension.

Other methods include the Valsalva manoeuvre (deep inspiration followed by expiration against a closed glottis, which stimulates stretch receptors in the lung and also reduces venous return to the heart); the Muller procedure (deep expiration followed by inspiration against a closed glottis); production of nausea and retching by inviting patients to put their *own* fingers down their throat. Eyeball pressure, although effective, is not recommended as it is painful when undertaken properly and may damage the retina.

Cardiac glycosides (see below) increase vagal nerve action.

The vagus nerve is blocked by atropine, an action that is used to accelerate the heart during episodes of sinus bradycardia as may occur after myocardial infarction. The dose is 0.6 mg i.v. and repeated as necessary to a maximum of 3 mg per day. Adverse effects are those of cholinergic blockade, namely dry mouth, blurred vision, urinary retention, confusion and hallucination.

Other antidysrhythmia drugs that have a vagal blocking (anticholinergic) action include quinidine, procainamide and disopyramide.

The sympathetic division (adrenergic component of the autonomic nervous system), when stimulated, has the following effects on the heart (receptor effects):

1. tachycardia due to increased rate of discharge of the SA node
2. increased automaticity in the AV node and His–Purkinje system
3. increase in conductivity in the His–Purkinje system
4. increased force of contraction
5. shortening of the refractory period

(It may be noted that the effects of the two lists above are not all opposites).

Isoprenaline, a β-adrenoceptor agonist, may be used to accelerate the heart and to raise cardiac output when there is extreme bradycardia due to heart block (e.g. after myocardial infarction) before the insertion of an electrical pacemaker.

The dose is as follows: i.v. 0.5–10 μg per minute; by mouth 30 mg every 8 h to a maximum of 840 mg per day (note the enormous difference).

Adverse effects are those of β-adrenergic stimulation and include tremor, flushing, sweating, palpitation, headache and diarrhoea.

Digoxin and cardiac glycosides

> 'We think the Public under great obligations to Dr. Withering. . .'
> (From a 1785 review of *An Account of the Foxglove*, by William Withering)

In 1775, Dr William Withering was making a routine journey from Birmingham (England), his home, to see patients at the Stafford Infirmary. Whilst the carriage horses were being changed half way, he was asked to see an old dropsical woman. He thought she would die and so some weeks later, when he heard of her recovery, was interested enough to enquire into the cause.*

Recovery was attributed to a herb tea containing some twenty ingredients, amongst which Withering, already the author of a botanical textbook, found it 'not very difficult . . . to perceive that the active herb could be no other than the foxglove'. He began to investigate its properties, trying it on the poor of Birmingham, whom he used to see without fee each day. The results were inconclusive and his interest flagged until one day he heard that the principal of an Oxford College had been

*Peck T W, Wilkinson K D. William Withering. Bristol: Wright, 1950.

cured by foxglove after 'some of the first physicians of the age had declared that they could do no more for him'. This put a new complexion on the matter, and pursuing his investigation, Withering found that foxglove extracts caused diuresis in some oedematous patients. He defined the type of patient who might benefit from it, and equally important, he standardised his foxglove leaf preparations and was able to lay down accurate dosage schedules. His advice, with little amplification, would serve today. Crude foxglove preparations are called 'digitalis'.

Considerable skill and practice were needed to get the best results from digitalis and Withering knew this when, after ten years study, he wrote: 'it is better the world should derive some instruction, however imperfect, from my experience, than that the lives of men should be hazarded by its unguarded exhibition, or that a medicine of so much efficacy should be condemned and rejected as dangerous and unmanageable.'* In other words, digitalis, like most effective therapeutic agents, can be an effective poison if misused. What Withering feared might happen did happen; physicians ignored his instructions based on careful observation and long experience, poisoned their patients and blamed him. After seeing how other physicians used digitalis, Withering remarked: 'Shall we wonder then that patients refuse to repeat such a medicine, and that practitioners tremble to prescribe it?'

The result was that digitalis fell into disrepute, although it continued to be used for various diseases, including tuberculosis. One hundred and fifty years were to pass before it finally became accepted as the asset that it is, and the details of its use in heart failure and cardiac dysrythmias were worked out.

Digitalis contains a number of active glycosides (digoxin, digitoxin, lanatosides) the actions of which are qualitatively similar, differing principally in rapidity of onset and duration. The following account refers to all the cardiac glycosides; the crude preparation of dried leaf (Prepared Digitalis) that had to be standardised biologically is no longer used since the pure individual glycosides are available.

* Withering W. An Acount of the Foxglove. London: Robinson, 1785.

Mode of action. Cardiac glycosides affect the heart both directly and indirectly in complex interactions, some of which oppose each other.

In summary, *the clinically important effects* are:

On the myocardium	—	*increased excitability and increased contractility*
On SA and AV nodes and conducting tissue	—	*decreased generation and propagation*

These effects are now described in greater detail.

1. **The direct effect** of cardiac glycosides is to inhibit the membrane-bound (ATPase) that, by hydrolysing ATP, supplies energy for the system that pumps sodium out of, and transports potassium into cardiac cells. The resulting rise in intracellular sodium and fall in potassium affect the activity of the heart as follows:

(a) *Electrical activity*. The transmembrane electrical potential and the duration of the cardiac refractory period decrease whilst the rate of spontaneous depolarisation of pacemaker cells increases. In consequence the myocardial effects are:

(i) *increased excitability* (capacity to respond to a stimulus) and

(ii) *increased automaticity* (capacity to initiate beats), leading to cardiac *dysrhythmias*.

(b) *Mechanical activity*. Changes in the distribution of sodium raise the free intracellular calcium concentration, which *enhances myocardial contraction*. In consequence: this *increased contractility* (force and velocity of contraction, or positive inotropic effect) reduces the size of the failing, dilated heart (overstretched muscle is less efficient) and increases cardiac output.

2. **The indirect effect** of cardiac glycosides is to enhance *vagal* nerve activity. In consequence there is:

(a) *decreased automaticity* of the *SA node*,

(b) *decreased refractory period* of *atrial muscle*, which favours conversion of flutter to fibrillation and

(c) *increased refractory period* and *decreased*

conduction in the *AV* conducting tissue: the ventricles are thus protected from excessive bombardment in atrial dysrhythmias (but high dose may cause bradycardia and sometimes even complete heart-block).

The *electrocardiographic effects* of the cardiac glycosides are as follows: the T wave becomes smaller, disappears or may become inverted; the ST segment sags below the iso-electric line; the PR interval is prolonged (delayed conduction); the QT interval is shortened (increased contractility).

Pharmacokinetics. Digoxin is described since it is most widely used. Other glycosides are referred to as appropriate. Digoxin may be administered by mouth (see pharmaceutical bioavailability, below) or i.v. and distributes widely throughout the body (e.g. serum:cardiac tissue ratio, 1:67) and the apparent distribution volume is about 500 litres/70 kg. Plasma protein binding is 30%. Digoxin is elimated 80–85% unchanged by the kidney and the remainder is metabolised by the liver. The $t_{\frac{1}{2}}$ is 36 h. By contrast *digitoxin* depends very largely on hepatic metabolism for elimination and little is excreted unchanged; the plasma $t_{\frac{1}{2}}$ is also much longer, 150 h. It follows that in renal failure the elimination of digitoxin is little changed, whereas that of digoxin is markedly impaired and the $t_{\frac{1}{2}}$ approaches that of digitoxin. For this reason, digitoxin may be preferred in progressive renal failure.

The principal uses of cardiac glycosides are in:

1. *Atrial fibrillation*, benefiting chiefly by the vagal effects on the AV conducting tissue thus slowing the ventricular rate.

2. *Paroxysmal supraventricular tachycardia*, benefiting chiefly by the vagal effects on the SA node, slowing its rate of discharge, and on the AV tissue, as in 1, above.

3. *Atrial flutter*. Cardioversion is preferred but digoxin may be effective, chiefly by the vagus nerve action of shortening the refractory period of the atrial muscle, to convert flutter to fibrillation, in which the ventricular rate is more readily controlled.

4. *Cardiac failure*, benefitting the patient chiefly by the direct action to increase myocardial contractility. Digoxin is used in left ventricular or congestive cardiac failure due to ischaemic, hypertensive or valvular heart disease, especially in the short term. It is of little value in heart failure due to chronic cor pulmonale and should be used only with close supervision in hypertrophic obstructive cardiomyopathy with atrial fibrillation and rapid ventricular response, when the positive inotropic effect may increase outflow tract obstruction but the effect of slowing heart rate is beneficial.

Dosing. That of *digoxin* (62.5, 125, 250 μg) is described here; doses of other glycosides appear below. Oral administration is normally satisfactory because digoxin is absorbed quickly and will begin to have an effect on the heart within 1–2 hours, becoming maximal within 3 hours. If the oral route is unsuitable and a quicker onset of action is desired, digoxin 0.25 mg may be injected i.v. slowly; this will start to affect the heart rate within 30 min.

The loading dose: Therapeutic concentrations of plasma digoxin are achieved following the oral administration of 0.75–1.5 mg in a 70 kg person. This total amount may be given in three or four divided doses at 6-hour intervals. Since pharmaceutical bioavailability of the tablet is 67%, the i.v. loading dose should be two-thirds of the oral loading dose.

The maintenance dose is the dose that will replace the amount eliminated from the body in any given time. In a patient with normal renal function, about one-third of the total body content of digoxin is removed in any 24-hour period: thus, if the patient is watched carefully during the loading period and found not to show adverse effects, administration of about one-third of the loading dose once very day will maintain a therapeutic concentration. This is usually 0.125–0.5 mg (but the range may be as wide as 0.0625 mg to 1.0 mg).

If there is no great urgency to achieve an early effect, the loading dose may be omitted altogether, but the above principle can be used to decide what daily dose should be given, i.e. on the basis of the patient's weight an estimate is made of the loading dose that would have been required and one-third of this amount is administered daily. The patient can be assumed for practical purposes to have attained a steady-state plasma concentration on this dose 7–8 days (5 × $t_{\frac{1}{2}}$) later, if renal function is normal. Adjustments in the daily maintenance dose may be required according to clinical response and '*Many lives have probably been saved by the simple rule that a dose should be omitted if the heart rate falls below 60 beats/min*'.*

Reduced dosing of digoxin is called for in certain clinical situations, as follows:

1. *Renal impairment*. Both the distribution volume and rate of elimination of digoxin are reduced. Correspondingly, less digoxin is required for loading and for maintenance doses. Although there is not general agreement, it has been suggested that as little as half the normal loading dose should be used and further increments made according to clinical response. Calculation of the maintenance dose is based on the fact that with progressive renal impairment, the clearance of digoxin falls in relation to the fall in creatinine clearance (see: dosing regimens for patients with renal impairment, Chapter 27). As a general rule, for patients with creatinine clearances in excess of 60 ml/min, the principles for administration of digoxin to individuals with normal renal function will suffice, i.e. careful observation while loading doses are given, followed by the administration of one-third of the loading dose as the maintenance dose.

2. *The elderly* in general experience adverse effects of digoxin more readily than do younger individuals. This results largely from a decline in renal clearance with age.

3. *Hypothyroid* patients are intolerant of digoxin and should be given lower than normal doses (and hyperthyroid patients are resistant to digoxin).

4. *Electrolyte disturbances*. Hypokalaemia accentuates the effects of digoxin, as may be anticipated from its mode of action, which is to inhibit the membrane-bound sodium-potassium ATPase and lower intracellular potassium. This can be a hazard because patients on digoxin are also likely to be taking potassium-depleting diuretics. Hypomagnesaemia may also accentuate digoxin toxicity.

Therapeutic plasma concentrations are difficult to define precisely but concentrations below 0.7 μg/l† are usually ineffective and concentrations in excess of 1.7 μg/l are associated with increasing risk of toxicity. The difficulty in defining the safe upper level merely reflects the number of other influences that affect the response of the heart to digoxin: electrolyte imbalance, age, thyroid status and renal function. These factors have to be taken into account in interpreting the significance of a plasma digoxin measurement.

* Hamer J. Br J Clin Pharmacol 1979; 8:109.
† 1 μ/l = 1ng/ml = 1.3 nmol/l.

The **principal preparations** are:

Digoxin (Lanoxin) is available as a tablet (0.25, 0.125, 0.0625 mg), as an oral paediatric/geriatric elixir, and as an injection; see above for dose.

Digitoxin is available as a tablet (0.1 mg) and as an oral solution. The loading dose is 1–1.5 mg and the maintenance dose 0.05–0.2 mg daily.

Lanatoside C is available as a tablet (0.25 mg); the loading dose is 1.5–2 mg daily for 3–5 days and the maintenance dose 0.25–1 mg daily.

Medigoxin (Lanitop) is a methylated form of digoxin that is more completely absorbed and more rapidly effective. The $t_{\frac{1}{2}}$ is 60 h.

Ouabain Inj. acts on the heart within 5–10 min of an i.v. injection, the full effect being obtained within 1–2 h. Up to 1 mg may be given by slow i.v. injection.

The choice of preparation is easy. *Digoxin* is generally satisfactory for all purposes. Digitoxin may be preferred when there is progressive renal impairment or in those rare patients who vomit when given low doses of digoxin.

Pharmaceutical bioavailability of digoxin in different formulations (i.e. the amount of drug released from a tablet and so available for absorption) has in the past varied substantially and has given rise to adverse effects if a patient's drug was changed from one brand to another. These differences were closely related to variation in the rates of tablet dissolution. The introduction of standardised dissolution rate tests has resulted in much greater uniformity between brands; on average the pharmaceutical bioavailability of tablets is now 67% and of the solution (elixir) 80%.

Adverse effects of cardiac glycosides

Adverse effects of digitalis are well described by Withering, who wrote: 'The Foxglove, when given in very large and quickly-repeated doses, occasions sickness, vomiting, purging, dizziness, confused vision, objects appearing green or yellow . . . slow pulse, even as slow as 35 in a minute, cold sweats, convulsions, syncope, death.'

Modern experience confirms his observations.

Symptoms of intoxication have been reported in 7–20% of patients receiving routine treatment.

Abnormal cardiac rhythms are the most serious adverse effects and usually take the form of ectopic dysrhythmias (ventricular ectopic beats, ventricular tachydysrhythmias, paroxysmal supraventricular tachycardia) and heart block. The concurrence of an ectopic dysrhythmia (due to the direct effect of cardiac glycosides of increasing cardiac excitability) with heart block (due to the indirect, vagal, effect on the AV node) is a characteristic of cardiac glycoside overdosage. Any other type of dysrhythmia may also occur.

Gastrointestinal effects are common. Anorexia usually precedes vomiting and is a warning that dosage is excessive. Vomiting is principally central, due to stimulation of the chemoreceptor trigger-zone connected to the vomiting centre in the medulla, but is to some extent a local effect on the alimentary tract. Diarrhoea may also occur.

Visual effects commonly include disturbances of colour vision, e.g. yellow (xanthopsia) but also red or green vision, photophobia and blurring.

Gynaecomastia may occur in men and breast enlargement in women with long-term use. The structures of the cardiac glycosides have similarities with those of the oestrogens.

Mental effects include confusion, restlessness, agitation, nightmares and acute psychoses.

Self-poisoning with digoxin is associated with nausea and vomiting; in addition there is hyperkalaemia because inhibition of the sodium-potassium ATPase pump prevents intracellular accumulation of potassium. The classic electrocardiographic changes associated with the prolonged use of digoxin may be absent. There may be exaggerated sinus dysrhythmia, bradycardia and ectopic rhythms with or without heart block.

Interactions. Adverse reactions may develop in stabilised patients due to depletion of body potassium from therapy with diuretics or with adrenal steroids. Quinidine displaces digoxin from its tissue-binding sites and interferes with its elimination by the kidney. The result is a substantial rise in plasma digoxin concentration when quinidine is given to a patient who is already taking digoxin; when both drugs are given together the dose of digoxin should be reduced by half. Verapamil, nifedipine and amiodarone also raise steady-state plasma digoxin concentrations and the digoxin dose should be lowered when any of these is added. AV block caused by digoxin is increased by verapamil and β-adrenoceptor blockers.

Treatment of adverse effects should first involve stopping the drug and for milder manifestations this need be only for a day or two. Dangerous cardiac dysrhythmias demand admission to hospital. Hypokalaemia (serum potassium < 3.5 mmol/l) can be corrected by infusion of potassium (0.3–0.5 mmol/min) provided the electrocardiogram is monitored continuously. Too-rapid injection is liable to stop the heart. Potassium itself prolongs the myocardial refractory period and slows conduction, and these effects may be as important as replacement of myocardial cellular potassium. When there is increased ventricular excitability due to cardiac glycosides, potassium should be given even if there is no hypokalaemia. Phenytoin 100 mg i.v. is useful in the management of digoxin-induced dysrhythmias. This dose can be repeated every 5 min until there is adverse effect or the dysrhythmia is brought under control. If there is bradycardia, atropine can be used to accelerate the heart by blocking the vagus. Dialysis is not useful as less than 1% of the drug in the body is in the blood. Electrical pacing may be needed; but direct current shock may lead to ventricular fibrillation.

The use of *antibodies* to digoxin to treat digoxin poisoning has been tried experimentally in animals but failed because the whole antibody molecule (raised in another species) was itself antigenic. The problem has been overcome by the synthesis of the digoxin-specific binding (Fab) fragment of the antibody (*Digibind*), infusion of which inactivates digoxin in the plasma and is an effective treatment for severe digoxin overdose. Because it lacks the Fc segment, this fragment is non-immunogenic and it is sufficiently small to be eliminated as the digoxin–antibody complex in the urine. Its use complicates subsequent assay of plasma digoxin.

THE CHOICE BETWEEN DRUGS AND ELECTRIC SHOCK THERAPY TO TERMINATE DYSRHYTHMIAS

Direct current (DC) electric shock applied externally is often the best way to convert cardiac dysrhythmias to sinus rhythm. Many atrial or ventricular dysrhythmias start as a result of transiently operating factors, but once they have begun, the abnormal mechanisms are self-sustaining. When an electric shock is given, the heart is depolarised, the ectopic focus is extinguished and the SA node, the part of the heart with the highest automaticity, resumes as the dominant pacemaker.

Electric conversion has the advantage that it is immediate, unlike drugs, which may take days or longer to act; also, the effective doses and adverse effects of drugs are largely unpredictable and can be serious.

Electric conversion is used in supraventricular and ventricular tachycardia, in ventricular fibrillation, and in atrial fibrillation and flutter. Drugs can be useful to prevent a relapse.

DRUG TREATMENT OF CARDIAC DYSRHYTHMIAS

The anatomical site of a dysrhythmia is often identifiable accurately and rapidly with an electrocardiogram. Notwithstanding the previously described eletrophysiological classification, it is therefore useful to categorise drugs according to their principal site of antidysrhythmic action, as follows:

Sites of drug action; direct and indirect

On SA node and atrium
β-blockers
Digoxin
Verapamil
Amiodarone
Disopyramide
Quinidine
Flecainide
Atropine
Isoprenaline

On AV node
Verapamil
Digoxin
β-blockers
Flecainide
Atropine
Isoprenaline

On anomalous pathways
Amiodarone
Disopyramide
Procainamide
Quinidine
Flecainide

On ventricle
Lignocaine
Tocainamide
Mexiletine
Disopyramide
Procainamide
Quinidine
Phenytoin
Amiodarone
Flecainide

Sinus bradycardia

Sinus bradycardia requires treatment if there is hypotension with reduced blood flow to brain, heart or kidneys or escape rhythms. It may be caused by drugs, e.g. β-adrenoceptor blockers, opioid analgesics (which stimulate the vagal centre) or digoxin. It may complicate acute (especially inferior) myocardial infarction and extreme bradycardia may allow a ventricular focus to take over and lead to ventricular tachycardia. The foot of the bed should be raised to assist venous return and atropine 0.6 mg should be given i.v. and repeated if necessary after 10 min and after 30 min (but the total dose in 24 h should not exceed 3 mg).

Atrial ectopic beats

Atrial ectopic beats are not due to organic heart disease and seldom demand drug treatment. Reduction in the intake of tea, coffee and other xanthine-containing drinks, and use of tobacco may suffice. When action is needed, reassurance and sedation are best tried first, but a small dose of a β-adrenoceptor blocker may be used. Atrial ectopic beats after myocardial infarction may precipitate atrial tachycardia and, if frequent (> 6/min) and persistent, should be prevented by a β-adrenoceptor blocker or quinidine.

Paroxysmal atrial and nodal tachycardia

Many attacks are self-limited. The mainstays of therapy are *vagal stimulation* by physical manoeuvres (see above) and *drugs*.

Prevention. Recurrent attacks may be prevented by a β-adrenoceptor blocker (e.g. sotalol) or by digoxin; the lowest effective dose should be used. Causes such as thyrotoxicosis, excessive tea or coffee drinking or smoking should be eliminated.

Treatment. If vagal stimulation is unsuccessful, verapamil i.v. is highly effective, failing which a DC shock may be administered, for this has an immediate effect. If there is any heart block, digoxin should be suspected as the cause of the dysrhythmia. Phenytoin or potassium may then be used, but verapamil is *contraindicated* because of the AV block.

Atrial fibrillation

The heart is less efficient in atrial fibrillation because cardiac output is reduced, e.g. some ventricular beats fail to open the aortic valves and so are completely wasted. Patients feel and perform better when sinus rhythm is restored.

Control. The patient needs rate control to allow adequate diastolic time for the ventricle to be filled. Digoxin is the drug of choice. When heart disease is severe, a rapid ventricular rate should be reduced as quickly as possible with digoxin i.v. If digoxin does not achieve this, e.g. in thyrotoxicosis, propranolol may be added, rather than increasing the dose of digoxin. With long-standing rheumatic mitral valvular disease, it is generally better to control the heart rate with digoxin than to attempt to convert it to sinus rhythm.

Conversion to sinus rhythm. Electrical conversion has supplanted drugs. The chief indications are uncontrollable ventricular rate and atrial fibrillation persisting after treatment of its cause, e.g. myocardial infarction, pneumonia, hyperthyroidism. Electric conversion should be avoided if digoxin toxicity is suspected but may proceed if the patient's dose of digoxin, serum potassium and renal function are normal. Quinidine will be required, at least for a time, to prevent relapse, and may be started 24 hours before the DC shock. In atrial fibrillation, quinidine alone may, paradoxically, lead to an abrupt increase in ventricular rate because it can reduce a high rate of atrial contraction with a considerable degree of heart-block, to a lower rate without heart-block; the result can be disastrous. Thus, if 500 impulses per minute come from the atrium and the AV conducting tissue transmits one out of four, the ventricular rate will be 125/minute. When quinidine slows the atrial rate to 200/minute and exerts an anticholinergic (facilitating) effect on AV conduction, all impulses may be transmitted so that the ventricular rate rises suddenly from 125 to 200/minute.

When atrial fibrillation has been present for less than six months it is usually possible to stop it but there is a risk of arterial thromboembolism. This is the result of the resumed coordinated atrial contraction detaching recent, rather than old, organised, thrombus from the atrial wall. It occurs whether fibrillation is of recent onset or of long duration. *All patients* should therefore be given anticoagulants for two weeks before conversion.

Atrial flutter

Treatment is urgent if a fast ventricular rate is causing cardiac failure or threatens extension of an area of myocardial infarction. Cardioversion is usually preferred. Should it prove unsuccessful the heart rate may be reduced with digoxin either alone or incombination with verapamil of a β-adrenoceptor blocker or amiodarone or quinidine; this may in addition convert the patient to sinus rhythm or at least to atrial fibrillation in which the ventricular rate is more easily controlled. Quinidine should *never* be used alone as it may facilitate 1:1 conduction as in atrial fibrillation (above).

Heart block

The use of artificial pacemakers is beyond the scope of this book. In an emergency, AV conduction may be improved by atropine (vagal block; 0.6 mg i.v.) or by isoprenaline (sympathetic stimulation; 0.5–10 μg/min, i.v.).

For prolonged therapy, if a pacing facility is not available, isoprenaline orally (sustained-release formulation, Saventrine) may be used.

Pre-excitation (Wolff–Parkinson–White) syndrome

This occurs in otherwise healthy young adults, who experience attacks of dysrhythmia, mainly supraventricular tachycardia or atrial fibrillation. They possess an anomalous (accessory) pathway through which a sinus impulse may pass from the atria and activate the ventricles sooner than would have been the case had the impulse travelled in the normal path. Episodes of re-entrant dysrhythmia result. Drugs that delay conduction through the AV node are used to prevent it, i.e. a β-adrenoceptor blocker (sotalol), amiodarone or flecainide. Verapamil and digoxin may increase conduction through the anomalous pathway and should be avoided. Treatment of an attack with a very rapid ventricular rate may demand a DC shock to restore sinus rhythm.

Ventricular premature beats

These may occur in apparently healthy persons and are precipitated by tea, coffee or tobacco; no drug treatment is then required. They may be caused by overdosage with digoxin or diuretic drugs (hypokalaemia). Ventricular premature contractions are common after myocardial infarction. The particular significance is that during the early or peak phases of the T-wave, the heart is especially vulnerable to abnormal stimuli and an ectopic beat developing at this time may precipitate ventricular tachycardia or fibrillation (the R-on-T phenomenon). About 80% of patients with myocardial infarction who proceed to ventricular fibrillation have preceding ventricular premature beats. Lignocaine is effective in suppressing ectopic ventricular beats; in the absence of clear evidence that routine prophylaxis reduces mortality, many specialists in coronary care give lignocaine if there are more than six ventricular ectopics per minute, if they occur near to the peak of the T-wave, if there are runs of two or more in succession or if they are multifocal. Tocainide, mexiletine, disopyramide or sotalol are alternative drugs.

Ventricular tachycardia

Ventricular tachycardia demands urgent treatment since it frequently leads to ventricular fibrillation and circulatory arrest. A powerful thump of the fist on the mid-sternum or precordium may stop a tachycardia. If the patient is in good condition i.v. treatment may begin with lignocaine or, should that fail, amiodarone i.v. For recurrent ventricular tachycardia amiodarone is often preferred but the choice is wide and includes mexiletine, tocainide, disopyramide, procainamide, quinidine or sotalol by mouth. The selection of a particular drug may be influenced by anticipated adverse effects, e.g. disopyramide and quinidine have anticholinergic effects that would be undesirable in a patient with glaucoma or prostatism.

Electrical conversion is the treatment of choice if there is rapid haemodynamic deterioration. It should be followed by lignocaine 100 mg i.v. and continued with an i.v. infusion of 2–4 mg/min for as long as experience and wisdom counsel.

Ventricular fibrillation (see Cardiac arrest, below)

Ventricular fibrillation is usually due to severe organic heart disease, e.g. it may follow acute myocardial infarction or episodes of ischaemia in patients with coronary heart disease. It may also be caused by excessive dosage of digoxin, procainamide, quinidine, adrenaline, cyclopropane, tricholoroethylene or chloroform. In the case of the three anaesthetics, the dysrythmia is probably due to the interaction of the drugs and naturally secreted adrenaline on the heart; it therefore follows that adrenaline should not be given to patients anaesthetised with these drugs. Dopamine is less dangerous in this respect.

CARDIAC ARREST

Anyone who uses drugs may find him or herself faced with, and indeed sometimes the cause of, this emergency.*

'Cardiac arrest is a term used to describe sudden failure of the heart to maintain an adequate cerebral circulation. It may be due to a marked weakening or slowing of the normal heart beat, to asystole or to ventricular fibrillation. The circulatory stasis that results leads to tissue hypoxia, cellular damage, and ultimately, death. The organ most sensitive to hypoxia is the brain: at normal body temperatures irreversible changes may occur if the circulation fails for more than 2 or 3 min. If, however, the circulation is restored within this time, complete recovery is possible. Indeed, effective treatment by artificial ventilation and external cardiac compression sometimes produces a complete return of consciousness, even though the heart is in asystole or ventricular fibrillation.

'Successful treatment depends on speed. Diagnosis must be rapid and an effective artificial ventilation and circulation must be produced without delay. Once this has been achieved the immediate danger is over and specific treatment designed to restart the heart may be delayed until an electrocardiogram has been obtained.

* We are grateful to Professor M. K. Sykes for the following account. DRL, PNB.

'The diagnosis of cardiac arrest is based on four signs: *unconsciousness, absent pulses, absent respirations, and, usually, widely dilated pupils*. These signs indicate that the cerebral circulation is inadequate and that external aid is required.

'All other attempts to establish a diagnosis are valueless and only waste time. For example, normal ECG complexes can persist for up to a minute after cessation of effective cardiac contractions.

'Treatment of cardiac arrest

'1. Move the patient to the firm edge of the bed or place a board under the mattress. Raise the legs to improve venous return.

'2. Clear the airway by removing the pillow and extending the neck fully. If foreign material in the pharynx is suspected, turn the head to one side and scoop it out with the forefinger before extending the neck.

'3. Perform mouth-to-mouth or mouth-to-nose artificial ventilation. Check that the chest expands well with each breath. If expansion is poor, extend the neck further, pull the chin forward and try again.

'4. After 2 or 3 breaths, commence external cardiac compression. Place the left hand over the lower end of the sternum and press the right hand sharply on the back of the left so that the chest is compressed (60 to 80 times a minute). The sternum should be depressed 3 to 5 cm. Check that a pulse is produced in the femoral or carotid arteries. Since chest compression does not produce effective pulmonary ventilation, intersperse one breath of mouth-to-mouth ventilation between each group of 6 to 8 cardiac compressions. Continue this sequence until normal ventilation and circulation are re-established.

'Effective treatment should produce a good pulse, and the pupils should constrict. If treatment has been initiated rapidly, spontaneous ventilation may return at this stage. Return of consciousness during cardiac compression is unpleasant, in different ways, for both patient and operator. For this reason the resuscitation trolley should contain anaesthetic drugs, and pre-mixed 50% nitrous oxide/oxygen cylinders.

'5. Pass an endotracheal tube and ventilate with oxygen.

'6. Take an electrocardiograph:

'(a) if normal complexes are present, give (i.v.) a vasopressor or inotropic drug (for hypotension), atropine (for sinus bradycardia) or isoprenaline (for heart block).

'(b) If ventricular fibrillation is present, defibrillate with a DC defibrillator. Cover the electrodes with conductive jelly and place one over the sternum and another over the cardiac apex region. Give a shock of 100–400 joules. Start at the lower figure and if this fails increase the setting. Ensure an adequate coronary blood flow by effective external compression between shocks. If a defibrillator is not available, it is worth giving lignocaine 1 mg/kg i.v. as a bolus (not by slow infusion).

'(c) If asystole is present, inject 5 ml of 10% calcium chloride i.v. Continue cardiac compression and defibrillate when rapid fibrillation appears. If asystole persists, inject 5 ml of 1 in 10,000 adrenaline (i.e. one in ten dilution of Adrenaline Inj. BP, which is 1:1,000 or 1 mg/ml) into the heart through the fourth left intercostal space, 2 cm lateral to the left border of the sternum. If asystole still persists, consider exposing the heart by a left thoracotomy through the fifth interspace; compression then being performed directly. The above drugs may be repeated at 10-min intervals. A transvenous pacemaker may be inserted if heart block persists.

'7. Give 120–240 mmol of sodium bicarbonate i.v. to correct the metabolic acidosis resulting from tissue hypoxia.

'8. If consciousness is slow to return, consider the use of dehydrating agents, dexamethasone or induced hypothermia.'

[*Note*: When i.v. injection is impracticable, double doses of adrenaline, atropine and lignocaine may be given via an endotracheal tube. Administration via an oropharyngeal airway is unlikely to be useful.]

CARDIAC FAILURE

The essential function of the heart is to maintain a circulation of blood sufficient to meet the metabolic needs of the body. The heart may fail from disease of the myocardium itself, mainly ischaemic, or from an excessive workload imposed on it by arterial hypertension, valvular disease or an arteriovenous shunt. The management of cardiac failure requires both the relief of any treatable underlying or aggravating cause, e.g. hypertension, and therapy directed at the failure itself.

Some physiology and pathophysiology

Cardiac output (CO) depends on the heart rate (HR) and the volume of blood that is ejected with each beat, i.e. the stroke volume (SV). It is expressed by the equation:

$$CO = HR \times SV$$

There are three factors that regulate the stroke volume, namely preload, afterload and contractility.

Preload refers to the load on the heart created by the volume of blood that occupies the left ventricle at the end of diastole and that it must eject with each contraction. It can also be viewed as the amount of stretch that the left ventricle is subject to as a result of the volume of blood that it contains; as the preload rises so also does the degree of stretch and the length of cardiac muscle fibres. Preload is thus a *volume* load and can be excessive, for example, when there is valvular incompetence or an arteriovenous shunt.

Afterload refers to the load created by the resistance to blood flow in the arterial system, i.e. the total peripheral resistance. Afterload is thus a *pressure* load and is excessive, for example, in arterial hypertension.

Contractility refers to the capacity of the myocardium to generate the force necessary to overcome preload and afterload.

When the circulation fails to meet the metabolic demands of the body, various mechanisms are recruited to help maintain the cardiac output.

(a) *The heart dilates*, especially in response to excessive preload. The greater the length of individual cardiac fibres the greater the tension the myocardium cab develop (the Frank–Starling relationship). Thus for a time, dilatation of the heart helps to sustain cardiac output.

(b) *The sympathetic drive to the heart increases*. There is greater rate and force of cardiac contraction (*increased contractility*), constriction of peripheral venous capacitance vessels (*increased preload*) and arteriolar resistance vessels with raised peripheral resistance (*increased afterload*). These circulatory changes divert blood from the liver, kidneys and skin to maintain flow to the heart and brain.

(c) *The renin–angiotensin–aldosterone system is activated*; aldosterone causes sodium to be retained, thus increasing blood volume (*increased preload*) and angiotensin causes peripheral vasoconstriction (*increased afterload*).

In the early stages of cardiac failure these physiological adjustments serve to maintain the blood supply to the tissues but as failure progresses they outlive their usefulness and actually impair the effectiveness of the circulation. Elevated peripheral resistance, apart from adding directly to cardiac work, increases the tension of the left ventricular wall, which raises the myocardial consumption of oxygen. Thus a cycle is set up that further impairs cardiac performance, and with reduced cardiac output the patient experiences fatigue. Excessive retention of salt and water together with heightened venous tone, raise the ventricular filling pressure beyond the capacity of the myocardium to cope, the lungs become congested and the patient is dyspnoeic.

The distinction between the capacity of the myocardium to pump blood and the load against which the heart must work is useful in therapy. For years the approach to treating cardiac failure was to cause the myocardium to contract more effectively and the mainstay of therapy was digoxin for its inotropic (contractility) effect. Yet the failing heart is already being strongly stimulated to contract by increased sympathetic drive. The logical alternative is to alleviate the load imposed on the failing heart by the physiological adjustments to cardiac failure and indeed drugs that reduce preload or afterload have been found to be very effective, especially when the left ventricular volume is raised (less predictably so for failure of the right ventricle). The main hazard of their use is a drastic fall in cardiac output in those occasional patients whose output is dependent on a high left ventricular filling pressure, e.g. those that are volume depleted by diuretic use or those with severe mitral stenosis.

Drugs used to treat cardiac failure may therefore be classified as follows:

1. Reduction of preload

Diuretics increase salt and water loss, reduce blood volume and lower excessive venous filling pressure. Their use is described in Chapter 27.

Nitrates (see also Chapter 24) dilate the smooth muscle in venous capacitance vessels, increase the volume of the venous vascular bed (which normally may comprise 80% of the whole vascular system), and reduce ventricular filling pressure, thus decreasing heart wall tension and reducing myocardial oxygen requirements. The drugs have an arteriolar dilating action but it is relatively mild. Glyceryl trinitrate may relieve angina more by its venodilating than by its arteriolar dilating action. It may be given sublingually 0.3–1 mg for acute left ventricular failure and repeated as often as necessary or by i.v. infusion, 10–200 μg/min. For chronic left ventricular failure, isosorbide dinitrate 40–160 mg per day may be given by mouth in divided doses or pentaerythritol tetranitrate 20–60 mg × 3–4/day by mouth. Exercise capacity is improved but tolerance to this effect may develop with chronic use. Headache, which tends to limit the dose of nitrate used for angina, is less of a problem in cardiac failure perhaps because the patients are more vasoconstricted.

The immediate beneficial effect of frusemide and morphine in acute left ventricular failure is probably due to the venodilating action of these drugs rather than to diuresis and relief of pain and anxiety respectively.

2. Reduction of afterload

Hydralazine (see also Chapter 24) relaxes vascular smooth muscle and reduces peripheral vascular resistance. The dose is 100 mg/day by mouth but up to 200 mg/day may be needed and the beneficial effect may diminish with repeated use. Reflex tachycardia occurs and lupus erythematosus may be induced when the dose exceeds 200 mg per day.

Salbutamol stimulates β_2-adrenoceptors to cause peripheral vasodilatation and reduce systemic vascular resistance. It may, however, increase heart rate (β_1-receptor) which is a disadvantage.

3. Reduction of preload and afterload

Angiotensin-converting enzyme (ACE) inhibitors (see also Chapter 24) act as follows:

(a) by reduction of afterload, preventing the conversion of angiotensin I to the active form angiotensin II, which is a powerful vasoconstrictor and is present in the plasma in high concentration in cardiac failure.

(b) by reduction of preload, because the formation of aldosterone, and thus retention of salt and water, is prevented.

Captopril or *enalapril* are effective at improving exercise capacity. A test dose should *always* be given to patients who are in cardiac failure or are already taking a diuretic; maintenance of blood pressure in such individuals may depend greatly on the activated renin–angiotensin–aldosterone system and a standard dose of an ACE inhibitor can cause a catastrophic fall in blood pressure. With captopril the first dose should be 6.25 mg by mouth increasing to 25 mg × 3/day; for enalapril 2.5 or 5 mg by mouth initially increasing to 20–40 mg once daily. Tolerance to the beneficial effect is less likely to develop than with other vasodilators. Once therapy with an ACE inhibitor is established a diuretic may usefully be added.

Prazosin (see also Chapter 24), a selective α_1-adrenoceptor antagonist, dilates smooth muscle in arterioles and in veins, so relieving both preload and afterload. To avoid hypotension the first dose should be 0.5 mg by mouth, then 1 mg × 3–4/day, increasing to 4–20 mg/day total. The beneficial effect may diminish with repeated use and if prazosin is withdrawn abruptly the cardiac failure may worsen markedly.

Phentolamine and *sodium nitroprusside* may also be used; both must be given by i.v. infusion.

4. Stimulation of the myocardium

Digoxin improves myocardial contraction most effectively in the dilated, failing heart but also in the longer term, once an episode of cardiac failure has been brought under control (inotropic effect). This effect occurs in patients in sinus rhythm and is separate from its (chronotropic) action of reducing ventricular rate and improving ventricular filling in atrial fibrillation (see before for details of dose).

Dopamine (Intropin), a precursor of noradrenaline, has a positive cardiac inotropic effect by its agonist action on myocardial β_1-adrenoceptors; these effects are enhanced by its capacity to release noradrenaline from nerve endings. It has a lesser accelerating effect on heart rate than does isoprenaline for an equivalent degree of inotropism. A further action of dopamine is to cause renal cortical vasodilatation by stimulating dopamine receptors in renal arteries, so increasing renal blood flow, glomerular filtration and sodium excretion. The combination of cardiac inotropism with renal vasodilatation makes dopamine a useful agent in hypotensive states, e.g. cardiogenic shock, especially if there is associated fluid overload. Dopamine is given by i.v. infusion and the rate must be carefully monitored against the amount of urine produced (see Chapter 23 for details of dose). The $t_{\frac{1}{2}}$ of dopamine in blood is only 2 min, which is an advantage when infusion rates require to be changed repeatedly (recalling that plateau blood concentrations are attained in $5 \times t_{\frac{1}{2}}$).

Adverse effects are due to excessive sympathetic stimulation and include nausea, vomiting, vasoconstriction, cardiac dysrhythmias and angina; phentolamine, a short-acting α-adrenoceptor antagonist, may be needed to reverse unwanted effects. Extravasation of dopamine during infusion may cause ischaemic necrosis.

Dobutamine (Dobutrex) is a β_1-adrenoceptor agonist that has relatively more powerful cardiac inotropic than chronotropic activity. Unlike dopamine (above) it does not cause renal vasodilation but renal blood flow may be improved as cardiac output rises. Dobutamine is used to provide inotropic support after cardiac surgery and in shock, e.g. cardiogenic or septic. Its $t_{\frac{1}{2}}$ is 2 min. The dose is 2.5–10 μg/kg/min, according to the response.

Adverse effects are similar to those of dopamine.

Prenalterol (Hyprenan) is a selective β_1-adrenoceptor agonist that increases cardiac output but its effect on heart rate is negligible. It is used to provide inotropic support in heart failure after myocardial infarction, cardiac surgery or shock. Prenalterol may also be given to counteract adverse effects of β-blockade, e.g. after overdosage. The $t_{\frac{1}{2}}$ is 2 h.

The drug management of cardiac failure may be summarised thus:

(a) Mild cardiac failure should be treated with a loop diuretic in low dose, say frusemide 40 mg, to which amiloride 5 mg may be added to help conserve potassium; if necessary this combination may be increased two-or three-fold.

(b) If failure is not adequately controlled by diuretics, as above, a vasodilator may be added. An ACE inhibitor may be preferred if hypotension is not a problem, or alternatively isosorbide dinitrate with which hydralazine may later be combined.

(c) Digoxin may be added if failure persists and the diuretic regimen may be intensified, e.g. by increasing the amount of loop diuretic and by replacing amiloride with spironolactone.

(d) Other inotropic agents should be reserved for urgent situations such as cardiogenic or septic shock. Dobutamine produces a predictable inotropic effect and is less likely than dopamine to cause peripheral vasoconstriction.

GUIDE TO FURTHER READING

1 Hillis W S, Whiting B. Antiarrhythmic drugs. Br Med J 1983; 286: 1332–6.
2 Aronson J K. Cardiac arrhythmias: theory and practice. Br Med J 1985; 290: 487–8.
3 Forfar J C, et al. Thyrotoxic atrial fibrillation: an underdiagnosed condition? Br Med J 1982; 285: 909–10.
4 Shaw D B. Ventricular premature beats — stormy petrels? Br Med J 1982; 284: 367–8.
5 Ward D E, et al. Recurrent ventricular tachycardia. Br Med J 1985; 290: 1926–7.
6 Ruskin J N. Ventricular extrasystoles in healthy subjects. N Engl J Med 1985; 312: 238–9.
7 Cobb L A. Cardiac arrest during sleep. N Engl J Med 1984; 311: 1044–5.
8 Graboys T B. The treatment of supraventricular tachycardias. N Engl J Med 1985; 312: 43–4.
9 Orme M L'E. Antidepressants and heart disease. Br Med J 1984; 289: 1–2.

10 Graboys T B, et al. Coffee, arrhythmias and common sense. N Engl J Med 1983; 308: 835–6.
11 Horgan J H. Cardiac pacing. Br Med J 1984; 288: 1942–4.
12 Editorial. Flecainide acetate. Lancet 1984; 1: 85–6.
13 McKenna W J, et al. Amiodarone: the experience of the past decade. Br Med J 1983; 287: 1654–6.
14 Lipkin D P, et al. Treatment of chronic heart failure: a review of recent drug trials. Br Med J 1985; 291: 993–6.
15 Bristow M R. The adrenergic nervous system in heart failure. N Engl J Med 1984; 311: 850–1.
16 LeJemtel T H, et al. Should the failing heart be stimulated? N Engl J Med 1984; 310: 1384–5.
17 Braunwald E, et al. Vasodilator therapy of heart failure. Has the promissory note been paid? N Engl J Med 1984; 310: 459–61.
18 Editorial. Angiotensin-converting-enzyme inhibitors in treatment of heart failure. Lancet 1985; 2: 811–2.
19 Wilkins M R, et al. William Withering and digitalis, 1785 to 1985. Br Med J 1985; 290: 7–8.
20 Editorial. Endogenous foxglove. Lancet 1983; 2: 1463–4.
21 George C F. Interactions with digoxin: more problems. Br Med J 1982; 284: 291–2.
22 George C F. Digitalis intoxication: a new approach to a old problem. Br Med J 1983; 286: 1533–4.
23 Johnston G D. Alternatives to digitalis glycosides for heart failure. Br Med J 1985; 290: 803–4.
24 Editorial. Beta-agonists and heart failure. Lancet 1983; 2: 1063–4.
25 Colucci W S, et al. New positive inotropic agents in the treatment of congestive heart failure. N Engl J Med 1986; 314: 290–9 and 349–58.
26 Opie L H. Drugs and the heart. Lancet 1980; 1: 693–8: 750–5: 806–9: 861–8 : 912–8: 966–72: 1011–7.
27 Opie L H. Drugs and the heart four years on. Lancet 1984; 1: 496–501.

26

Cardiovascular system IV: Hyperlipidaemias

Physiology
Classification
Drugs
Management of hyperlipidaemias

Some physiology

Dietary triglyceride is carried in the bloodstream on chylomicrons, which become progressively smaller as lipolysis takes place. This is accomplished by the enzyme lipoprotein lipase, which is attached to the capillary endothelium of certain tissues including adipose tissue, skeletal and cardic muscle. Fatty acids released during lipolysis are taken up by the tissues and the chylomicron remnants are cleared by the liver.

Endogenous triglyceride, synthesised by the liver and carried bound to very low density lipoproteins (VLDL) is progressively removed from the circulation by the same lipolytic mechanism as above. The low density lipoproteins (LDL) that are formed as a result of this process constitute the major system for delivering cholesterol to the tissues in man. LDL are small enough to pass through the vascular endothelium, bind to specific high-affinity LDL apoprotein receptors on cell membranes and enter cells by pinocytosis. Cholesterol within the cell is needed for membrane growth and repair and to form steroids.

High density lipoproteins (HDL), the other cholesterol-rich particles, appear to act as a *reverse* transport mediator, mobilising peripheral cholesterol, e.g. in arterial walls, and taking it to the liver for elimination; they are thus protective in ischaemic vascular disease.

Management of hyperlipidaemias should be viewed against the background of the following facts.

1. Hyperlipidaemias are common; about 25% of the adult population have a plasma cholesterol concentration in excess of the level associated with cardiovascular risk (5 mmol/l).

2. Investigation of hyperlipidaemia must be directed initially at excluding secondary causes, which include liver and biliary disease, obesity, hypothyroidism, diabetes, diet and alcohol excess.

3. Most hyperlipidaemias that are not explained by a secondary cause are multifactorial in origin (i.e. environmental plus genetic).

4. Some are primarily genetic, and the classification of hyperlipidaemias is based on these types.

5. When hyperlipidaemia is proven, all members of the patient's family must also be investigated.

6. The vast majority of cases of hyperlipidaemia seen in general medical practice and perhaps half those who attend special lipid clinics can be managed by *diet* alone. Much of the work of lipid clinics is taken up with attending to patients' other risk factors, including hypertension, diabetes, thyroid disease and smoking, as well as to the lipid abnormality.

7. The justification for using drugs that lower blood lipid is most easily made in the relatively small number of patients who have major abnormalities of their lipid profiles as this reduces their risk of ischaemic heart disease.

The biochemical diagnosis should be made on a blood sample taken after a 14-h fast; if lifelong treatment is to be contemplated, two or three such samples should be taken at weekly intervals. In those who have sustained myocardial infarction or other serious illness, plasma triglyceride concentrations rise and cholesterol falls and these lipids are not stable till 3 months have elapsed, but an estimation in the first 24 h after the event (i.e. before metabolic changes have had time to occur) gives an acceptable result.

Classification

Hyperlipidaemias are classified as follows*:

Type I is rare, characterised by high concentrations of chylomicrons and triglycerides in the blood due to deficiency of lipoprotein lipase, and is associated with abdominal pain, pancreatitis and eruptive xanthomata.

Type IIa is common, characterised by high concentrations of LDL and cholesterol in the blood, and is associated with ischaemic heart disease. A proportion of these patients (0.2% of the general population) have heterozygous monogenic familial hypercholesterolaemia, which is associated with severe premature heart disease and tendon xanthomata.

Type IIb is common, characterised by high concentrations of LDL and VLDL, cholesterol and triglycerides in the blood, and is associated with ischaemic heart disease.

Type III is uncommon, characterised by high concentrations of 'broad-β' lipoprotein, cholesterol and triglyceride in the blood due to an inherited abnormal apolipoprotein, and is associated with palmar xanthomata and ischaemic heart and peripheral vascular disease.

Type IV is common, characterised by high concentrations of VLDL and triglyceride in the blood, may be associated with obesity, diabetes and high alcohol intake and gives rise to ischaemic heart and peripheral vascular disease.

Type V is uncommon, characterised by high concentrations of chylomicrons, VLDL and triglyceride in the blood of some patients, in part due to excessive alcohol intake or diabetes. These patients are liable to develop pancreatitis.

Drugs used to treat hyperlipidaemias

Cholestyramine (Questran) (sachets, 4 g) is an anion-exchange resin that binds bile acids in the intestine. Bile acids are formed from cholesterol in the liver, pass into the gut in the bile and are reabsorbed at the terminal ileum. The total bile acid pool is only 3–5 g but because such enterohepatic recycling takes place 5–10 times a day, on average 20–30 g of bile acid are delivered into the intestine every 24 h. Bile acids bound to cholestyramine are lost in the faeces and the depletion of the bile acid pool stimulates conversion of cholesterol to bile acid: the result is that plasma LDL cholesterol falls by 20–25%. In some patients there is a compensatory increase in hepatic cholesterol synthesis. The dose is 16–24 g per day but up to 36 g may be needed for resistant cases. This is uncomfortably large and patients do not like it. About half the patients who take cholestyramine experience constipation and some complain of anorexia, abdominal fullness and occasionally of diarrhoea. Because the drug binds anions, impaired absorption of warfarin, digoxin, thiazide diuretics, phenobarbitone and thyroid hormones may occur when these drugs are given with cholestyramine. Drugs should be given one hour before cholestyramine.

Colestipol (Colestid) is similar to cholestyramine.

Nicotinic acid (100 mg) lowers plasma triglyceride and cholesterol concentrations. It probably acts as an antilipolytic agent in adipose tissue, reducing the supply of non-esterified free fatty acids and hence the availability of substrate for hepatic lipoprotein synthesis. Treatment of hyperlipidaemias requires 1–2 g three times daily (the normal human nutritional needs are less than 30 mg/day). Flushing of the skin and gastrointestinal upset commonly occur; the unpleasantness may be diminished by gradually building up the dose over 6 weeks and in time tolerance to the adverse effects develops.

Nicofuranose (tetranicotinoylfructose; Bradilan) is a fructose ester of nicotinic acid that may be better tolerated.

Clofibrate (500 mg) (Atromid) inhibits hepatic lipid synthesis, causing plasma cholesterol to decline by 10–15% and triglyceride by 25% in unselected patients, but patients with Type III hyperlipidaemia respond by twice this amount or more. Clofibrate is reliably absorbed from the gastrointestinal tract and is extensively bound to plasma proteins; its action is terminated by metabolism in the liver or by excretion unchanged in the

* Beaumont J L et al. Bull WHO 1970; 43: 891.

urine. The dose is 500 mg twice or thrice daily after meals. Adverse effects are generally mild but an acute myalgia may rarely develop, especially in hypoproteinaemic states such as the nephrotic syndrome, in which the concentration of unbound drug is unusually high. A placebo-controlled trial* of clofibrate in the primary prevention of myocardial infarction involving 15 745 men showed that the incidence of non-fatal myocardial infarctions was 25% less in those who received the active drug. Surprisingly, the study also revealed that deaths unrelated to ischaemic vascular disease were *increased* in those who received clofibrate; this finding has not been explained. The clofibrate group also showed a much higher incidence of gallstone requiring surgery in this and other studies.

Interactions with oral anticoagulants, frusemide and sulphonylureas may occur because competition with clofibrate for binding sites on plasma albumin increases free concentration and thus the effect of these drugs at standard doses.

Bezafibrate (Bezalip) has similar effects to clofibrate and lowers plasma triglyceride and cholesterol concentrations.

Probucol (Lurselle) increases the excretion of bile acids and reduces cholesterol biosynthesis; the resulting fall in plasma lipid concentration affects both LDL and the 'protective' HDL. The drug is well tolerated but some patients experience gastrointestinal upset and abdominal pain.

Management of hyperlipidaemias

Management may proceed as follow:

1. *Any medical disorder* that may be causing hyperlipidaemia, e.g. diabetes or hypothyroidism, should be treated first.

* Report of Committee of Principal Investigators. Br Heart J 1978; 40: 1069. Lancet 1984; 2: 600.

2. *Dietary adjustment*. The following applies to all patients.

a. Those who are overweight should reduce their total caloric intake until they have returned to the weight that is appropriate for their height; this automatically assumes reduced intake of alcohol and animal fat. Elevated triglyceride concentrations may respond particularly well to alcohol withdrawal.

b. Those who fail to achieve adequate weight reduction or are already at their ideal weight should reduce their total fat intake; polyunsaturated fats or oils may partially substitute for the reduction in animal fats. There is seldom need for a specific low cholesterol diet (e.g. by excluding egg yolks, sweetbreads) as reducing fat intake largely achieves this effect.

3. *Specific types of hyperlipidaemia* are treated thus:

a. *Types I (and some Type V)*. Reduce dietary fat to 10% of total caloric intake; this may be assisted by partial substitution of fat by medium chain triglycerides, which are not carried to the systemic circulation on chylomicrons but enter the liver directly by the portal circulation.

b. *Type IIa* usually respond to diet but those with familial hypercholesterolaemia almost always need an anion-exchange resin (cholestyramine or colestipol) and often another agent.

c. *Type IIb and IV* are usually related to being overweight, to diabetes, food and alcohol, and respond to the measures indicated above; nicotinic acid, clofibrate or bezafibrate may be added in resistant cases.

d. *Type III* are usually diet-sensitive, failing which clofibrate or bezafibrate are the drugs of choice and are very effective.

e. *Poorly responsive patients* with familial hypercholesterolaemia (IIa) and those with severe (Types III, IV and V) hyperlipidaemia should preferably be referred to a specialist.

GUIDE TO FURTHER READING

1 Oliver M F. Does control of risk factors prevent coronary heart disease? Br Med J 1982; 285: 1065–1066.
2 Lewis B. The lipoproteins: predictors, protectors, and pathogens. Br Med J 1983; 287: 1161–1164.
3 Goldstein J L et al. Defective lipoprotein receptors and atherosclerosis. N Engl J Med 1983; 309: 288–296.
4 Oliver M F. Why measure cholesterol after myocardial infarction, and when? Br Med J 1984; 289: 1641–1642.
5 Oliver M F. Hypercholesterolaemia and coronary heart disease: an answer. Br Med J 1984; 288: 423–424.
6 Murchison L E. Hyperlipidaemia. Br Med J 1985; 290: 535–538.
7 Schaefer E J, Levy R I. Pathogenesis and management of lipoprotein disorders. N Engl J Med 1985; 312: 1300–1310.

27

Kidney and urinary tract

A diuretic is any substance which increases urine and solute production, but this wide definition includes substances not commonly thought of as such. For instance, everyone has personal experience of the diuretic properties of water. *To be therapeutically useful a diuretic should increase the output of sodium as well as of water*, since diuretics are normally used to remove oedema fluid, which is composed of water and solutes, of which sodium is the most important.

SOME PHYSIOLOGY

Each day the body produces 200 l of glomerular filtrate, which is modified in its passage down the renal tubules and appears as 1.5 l of urine. Thus *a 1% reduction in reabsorption of water will double urine output*. Clearly drugs that act on the tubule have considerable scope to alter body fluid and electrolyte balance and a brief account of tubular function with particular reference to sodium will help to explain how diuretic drugs act.

Sodium is filtered at the glomerulus and is reabsorbed at the proximal tubule both actively and passively. Active sodium transport is linked to that of filtered glucose, of amino acids and of bicarbonate. About 85% of filtered bicarbonate is reabsorbed in the proximal tubule, which is one reason why the urine is slightly acid. Carbonic anhydrase in proximal tubular epithelial cells catalyses the generation of $H_2CO_3^-$, which dissociates to H^+ and HCO_3. H^+ is actively secreted into tubular fluid in exchange for Na^+, which passively enters the cells to form $NaHCO_3$. Overall, 65% of the filtered sodium is reabsorbed and isotonically takes with it back into the blood the same fraction of the glomerular filtrate. The epithelium of the proximal tubule is described as 'leaky' because of its free permeability to water and a number of solutes and it is the principal site of action of the *osmotic diuretics* (see Figure 27.1, Site 1).

The fluid now passes into the loop of Henle, where 25% of the filtered sodium is reabsorbed. The physiological changes are best understood by considering first the ascending limb; in the *thick* segment (Site 2), chloride is transported actively from the tubular fluid into the interstitial fluid, taking with it sodium but not water, to which this part of the tubule is impermeable. Thus, the interstitium becomes hypertonic and fluid in the descending limb, which is permeable to water, becomes concentrated as it approaches the tip of the loop, because the hypertonic interstitial fluid sucks it out. The system thus has the characteristics of a *countercurrent multiplier*, which by active transport of ions converts a small change in osmolarity into a steep osmotic gradient. The high osmotic pressure in the medullary interstitium is sustained by the straight blood vessels (vasa rectae) that lie close to the loops of Henle and, making a 'hairpin' turn, act as *countercurrent exchangers*, for the incoming blood receives sodium from the outgoing blood*. As the tubule re-enters the renal cortex, sodium and chloride continue to be actively extruded into the interstitial tissue (Site 3) but are rapidly removed because cortical blood flow is high and there are no vasa rectae present. The significant fact is that interstitial fluid tonicity ranges from *low* in the cortex to *high* in the medulla; the powerful *loop diuretics* act by reducing this osmotic gradient.

In the distal tubule, sodium is reabsorbed in exchange for potassium and hydrogen under the influence of aldosterone. This site (Site 4) accounts for only 5% of the total sodium reabsorbed. Diuretics that act proximal to this site cause potassium depletion because more sodium is made available to exchange with potassium, which is lost in the urine.

The collecting tubule then travels back down into the medulla to reach the papilla; in doing so it passes through strata of successively higher osmotic pressure, which tend to draw water out of tubular fluid. This final concentration of urine is under the influence of antidiuretic hormone, the action of which is to prevent water from leaving the tubular fluid.

DIURETIC DRUGS

That organic mercurials have some diuretic effect has been known since the 16th century, but the first potent diuretic for clinical use was introduced in Vienna in 1920, when a mercury compound, merbaphen (Novasurol) was tried as an anti-syphilitic in a hospital ward where measurement of urine output was part of the nursing routine. Merbaphen, though unsatisfactory as an anti-syphilitic, was then given to many oedematous patients, in whom it proved to be an effective diuretic, though toxic. It was soon replaced by mersalyl, which is now obsolete.

The next important development arose from the observation that acidosis occurred in patients taking sulphanilamide (this does not occur with currently used sulphonamides). The acidosis was found to be due to inhibition of the enzyme carbonic anhydrase in the kidney. Further research resulted in the introduction in 1951, as a diuretic, of a potent carbonic anhydrase inhibitor, acetazolamide. In 1957, chlorothiazide was introduced following studies of compounds related to acetazolamide, but chlorothiazide is only a weak carbonic anhydrase inhibitor and does not owe its diuretic effect to this property. Both acetazolamide and the thiazides are structurally related to sulphanilamide.

Further modification of molecular structures has led to the introduction of diuretics with greater efficacy (frusemide, ethacrynic acid, bumetanide) or potassium-sparing actions (triamterene, amiloride).

Diuresis may be initiated by *renal* or by *extra-renal* mechanisms.

1. *Outside the kidney*:

a. by inhibiting the release of antidiuretic hormone, e.g. water, hypotonic solutions, ethanol.

b. by raising the cardiac output and increasing renal blood flow, e.g. dobutamine and dopamine.

2. *On the kidney*. Diuretics act within the tubular cells and tubular lumen where they attain high concentration. Most are organic anions and are secreted into tubular fluid by the nephron. The principal sites of action of clinically useful diuretics are conventionally numbered as follows (Fig. 27.1):

Site 1. Proximal renal tubule: an *isotonic* movement of water follows the active reabsorption of sodium from the tubular lumen: *osmotic* diuretics here act by raising the osmolarity of tubular fluid and preventing water reabsorption.

* The most easily comprehended countercurrent exchange mechanism (in this case for heat) is that in wading birds in cold climates whereby the veins carrying cold blood from the feet pass closely alongside the arteries carrying warm blood from the body and heat exchange takes place. The result is that the feet receive blood below body temperature (which birds do not mind) and the blood from the feet, which is often very cold, is warmed before it enters the body so that the internal body temperature is more easily maintained. The principle is the same for maintaining medullary hypertonicity.

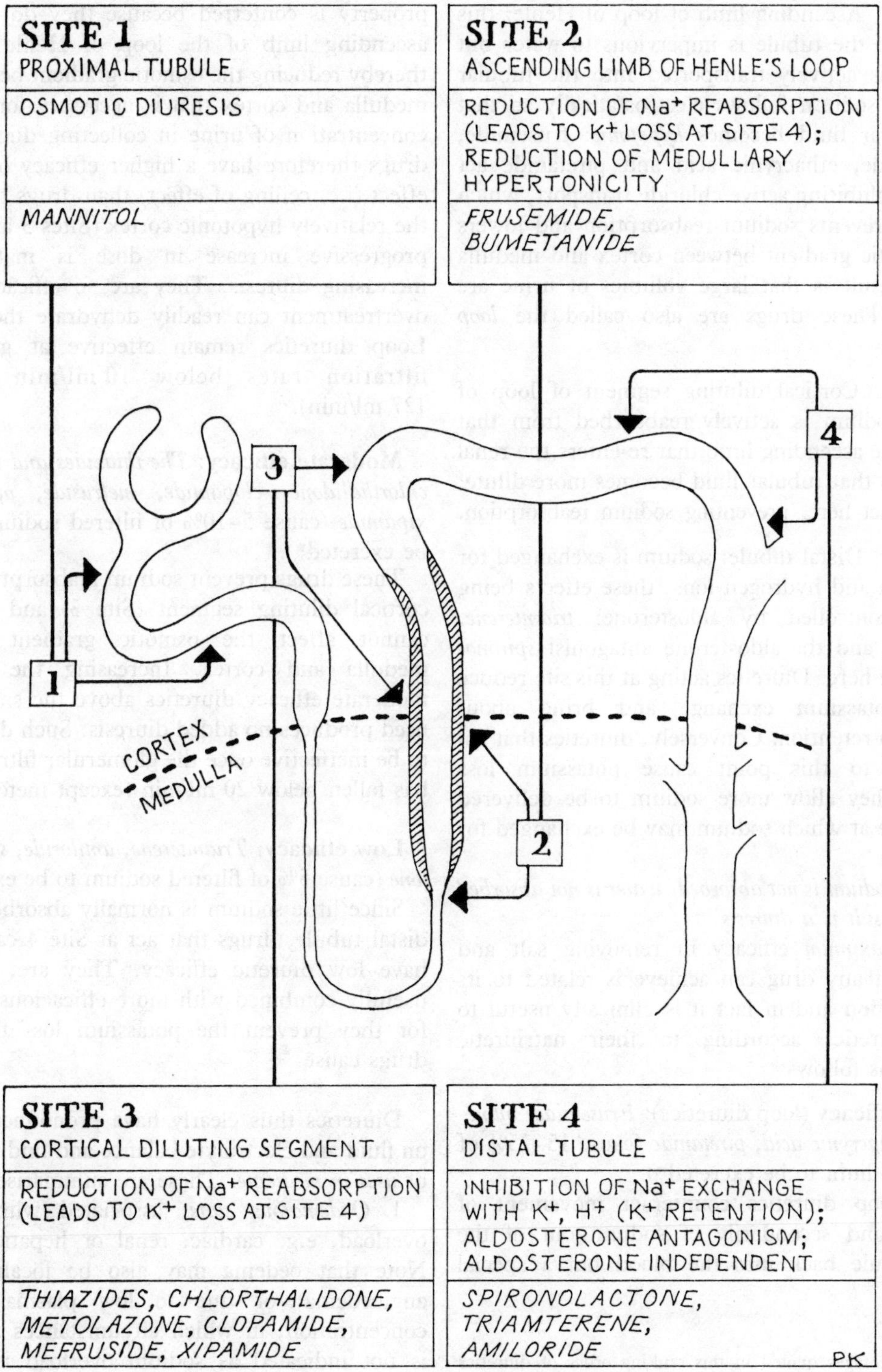
SITE 1
PROXIMAL TUBULE
OSMOTIC DIURESIS
MANNITOL
SITE 2
ASCENDING LIMB OF HENLE'S LOOP
REDUCTION OF Na+ REABSORPTION (LEADS TO K+ LOSS AT SITE 4); REDUCTION OF MEDULLARY HYPERTONICITY
FRUSEMIDE, BUMETANIDE
3
4
1
2
CORTEX
MEDULLA
SITE 3
CORTICAL DILUTING SEGMENT
REDUCTION OF Na+ REABSORPTION (LEADS TO K+ LOSS AT SITE 4)
THIAZIDES, CHLORTHALIDONE, METOLAZONE, CLOPAMIDE, MEFRUSIDE, XIPAMIDE
SITE 4
DISTAL TUBULE
INHIBITION OF Na+ EXCHANGE WITH K+, H+ (K+ RETENTION); ALDOSTERONE ANTAGONISM; ALDOSTERONE INDEPENDENT
SPIRONOLACTONE, TRIAMTERENE, AMILORIDE
PK

Fig. 27.1 Sites of action of diuretic drugs

Site 2. Ascending limb of loop of Henle: this portion of the tubule is impervious to water but chloride is actively transported into the tubular cells and sodium follows electrostatically so that the tubular fluid becomes *hypotonic*: frusemide, bumetanide, ethacrynic acid and piretanide act here by inhibiting active chloride transport, which in turn prevents sodium reabsorption and lowers the osmotic gradient between cortex and medulla — the result is that large volumes of urine are formed. These drugs are also called the *loop diuretics*.

Site 3. Cortical diluting segment of loop of Henle: sodium is actively reabsorbed from that part of the ascending limb that re-enters the renal cortex, so that tubular fluid becomes more dilute: *thiazides* act here, preventing sodium reabsorption.

Site 4. Distal tubule: sodium is exchanged for potassium and hydrogen ions, these effects being mainly controlled by aldosterone: *triamterene*, *amiloride*, and the aldosterone antagonist *spironolactone* act here. Diuretics acting at this site reduce sodium/potassium exchange and bring about potassium retention. Conversely, diuretics that act proximal to this point cause potassium loss because they allow more sodium to be delivered to the site at which sodium may be exchanged for potassium.

When sodium is not absorbed, water is not absorbed and the result is a diuresis.

The *maximum* efficacy in removing salt and water that any drug can achieve is related to its site of action and in fact it is clinically useful to rank diuretics according to their natriuretic capacity as follows:

High efficacy (loop diuretics): *Frusemide, bumetanide, ethacrynic acid, piretanide* (cause 15–25% of filtered sodium to be excreted*).

The loop diuretics counteract movement of chloride and secondarily of sodium out of the renal tubule back into the blood but a special property is conferred because they do so in the ascending limb of the loop of Henle (Site 2), thereby reducing the osmotic gradient between the medulla and cortex that is necessary for the final concentration of urine in collecting ducts. These drugs therefore have a higher efficacy of diuretic effect (i.e. ceiling of effect) than drugs that act in the relatively hypotonic cortex (Sites 3 and 4) and progressive increase in dose is matched by increasing diuresis. They are so efficacious that overtreatment can readily dehydrate the patient. Loop diuretics remain effective at glomerular filtration rates below 10 ml/min (normal 127 ml/min).

Moderate efficacy: *The thiazides and the related chlorthalidone, clopamide, mefruside, metolazone, xipamide* (cause 5–10% of filtered sodium load to be excreted*).

These drugs prevent sodium reabsorption in the cortical diluting segment (Site 3) and therefore cannot affect the osmotic gradient between medulla and cortex. Increasing the dose of moderate efficacy diuretics above the small range used produces no added diuresis. Such drugs tend to be ineffective once the glomerular filtration rate has fallen below 20 ml/min (except metolazone).

Low efficacy: *Triamterene, amiloride, spironolactone* (cause 5% of filtered sodium to be excreted*).

Since little sodium is normally absorbed by the distal tubule, drugs that act at Site 4 can at best have low diuretic efficacy. They are, however, usefully combined with more efficacious diuretics for they prevent the potassium loss that these drugs cause.

Diuretics thus clearly have pronounced effects on fluid and electrolyte balance and find a number of *uses in medicine*. These are summarised below:

1. *Oedematous states* associated with sodium overload, e.g. cardiac, renal or hepatic disease. Note that oedema may also be localised, e.g. angioedema, or due to low plasma albumin concentration, in which circumstances a diuretic is not indicated as sodium overload is not the underlying problem.

2. *Hypertension*, by reducing intravascular volume and probably by other mechanisms too,

* The percentages quoted in this ranking order of diuretics refer to the highest fractional excretion of filtered sodium under carefully controlled conditions and should not be taken to represent the average fractional sodium loss during clinical use of the diuretics.

e.g. reduction of sensitivity to noradrenergic vasoconstriction.

3. *Hypercalcaemia*. Frusemide reduces calcium absorption in the ascending limb of the loop of Henle and this action may be utilised in the emergency reduction of elevated plasma calcium in addition to rehydration and other measures (see index).

4. *Idiopathic hypercalciuria*, a cause of renal stone disease, may be treated with thiazide diuretics; reduction of intravascular volume favours proximal renal tubular resorption of calcium.

5. *The syndrome of inappropriate secretion of antidiuretic hormone secretion (SIADH)* may be treated with frusemide if there is a dangerous degree of volume overload. Other measures will also be required; these include withdrawal of a drug if is the cause (e.g. chlorpropamide), water restriction, demeclocycline (see index), and salt replacement.

6. *Nephrogenic diabetes insipidus*, paradoxically, responds to diuretics which, by contracting vascular volume, increase salt and water reabsorption in the proximal tubule, and thus reduce urine volume.

The high efficacy or loop diuretics

Frusemide (furosemide, Lasix) (20, 40, 500 mg; inj. 10 mg/ml) is structurally related to the thiazides but its principal site of action is in the thick portion of the ascending limb of the loop of Henle (Site 2) where it interferes with chloride and sodium reabsorption (see foregoing discussion on loop diuretics). Because more sodium is delivered to the aldosterone-sensitive portion (Site 3), *exchange for potassium leads to urinary potassium loss and hypokalaemia* (see 'Some physiology', above). Chloride loss results in hypochloraemia. Since almost all the filtered bicarbonate has already been absorbed in the proximal tubule, continued use of frusemide causes hypochloraemic and hypokalaemic alkalosis. However, the drug has a mild carbonic anhydrase inhibiting effect in the proximal tubule and in high doses, the resulting bicarbonate loss counteracts the tendency to metabolic alkalosis. Magnesium and calcium loss are increased by frusemide to about the same extent as that of sodium; the effect on calcium is utilised in the emergency management of hypercalcaemia (see index).

Pharmacokinetics. Frusemide is well absorbed from the gastrointestinal tract, is highly bound to plasma proteins and is mostly excreted unchanged or as a glucuronide in the urine. The plasma $t_{\frac{1}{2}}$ is 2 h but this rises to over 10 h in renal failure. It crosses the placenta.

Uses. Frusemide is highly successful for the relief of oedema. Progressive increase of dose is matched by increase in urine production. Taken orally it acts within an hour and diuresis lasts about 6 h. Enormous volumes of urine (e.g. 10 l in 24 h) can result and such overtreatment can cause hypovolaemia and circulatory collapse. Given i.v. it acts within 30 min and can relieve acute pulmonary oedema, perhaps due partly to a vasodilator action that precedes the diuresis. An important feature of frusemide is its efficacy in the presence of glomerular filtration rates of 10 ml/min or less as in severe heart and renal failure where other diuretics fail.

The *dose* is 20–120 mg by mouth per day; i.m. or i.v. 20–50 mg is given initially. For use in renal failure, special high-dose tablets of frusemide (500 mg) are available, and a solution of 250 mg in 25 ml, which should be infused i.v. at a rate not greater than 4 mg/min. A low-dose continuous i.v. infusion of 4–16 mg/h may be successful in some cases of refractory oedema.

Adverse effects in addition to electrolyte disturbance and hypotension (low plasma volume) and those mentioned in the general account (below) are uncommon. They include nausea, pancreatitis and, rarely, deafness, which is usually transient and associated with rapid i.v. injection in renal failure. Non-steroidal anti-inflammatory drugs, notably indomethacin, reduce frusemide-induced diuresis.

Bumetanide (Burinex) (1, 5 mg; inj. 0.5 mg/ml) is similar in action to frusemide, i.e. it acts on the ascending limb of the loop of Henle.

The drug is rapidly and completely absorbed from the gut, about two-thirds of a dose is quickly eliminated unchanged in the urine, and the remainder is metabolised. The $t_{\frac{1}{2}}$ is 1.5 h. The diuretic action begins within half an hour of an oral dose and is complete within 4–6 h.

Bumetanide is used in the same clinical circumstances as frusemide.

The dose is 1–5 mg by mouth. In acute pulmonary oedema 2 mg may be given i.v.

It may induce metabolic disturbances less readily than frusemide. Apart from the adverse effects listed in the general account, bumetanide may cause muscle pains in high dosage; ototoxicity occurs but is infrequent.

Ethacrynic acid (Edecrin) (50 mg: inj. 50 mg) is structurally different from the other loop diuretics, but its action on the nephron is similar to that of frusemide. It is eliminated partly by metabolism in the liver and partly unchanged in the urine; the $t_{\frac{1}{2}}$ is 40 min.

It is indicated in the same clinical conditions as is frusemide but has tended to be less widely used possibly because of gut upset and gut haemorrhage. As with frusemide, the diuretic response may be torrential, so that acute saline depletion and hypotension due to serious reduction in plasma volume may occur. The oral dose is 50–150 mg for 1 or 2 doses but more (up to 400 mg/day) may be given in refractory cases. It is too iritant to be given s.c. or i.m.

Ethacrynic acid may cause hearing loss with oral use as well as i.v.; deafness may be transient or permanent.

Piretanide (Arelix) (6 mg) in common with the other loop diuretics inhibits chloride transport in the ascending limb of the loop of Henle. After an oral dose most of the drug is eliminated unchanged in the urine and the $t_{\frac{1}{2}}$ is 2 h. Piretanide relaxes vascular smooth muscle and is used for mild-to-moderate hypertension.

Thiazides and related drugs

Thiazides are widely used because they are reliably effective when taken orally and produce few adverse effects except potassium depletion in short-term or intermittent use. In long-term use (hypertension) the metabolic effects (diabetes, hyperuricaemia) are more important.

Actions. Thiazides depress sodium transport in the cortical diluting segment (Site 3) of the nephron just proximal to the point of sodium–potassium exchange. They have an additional though lesser action on the proximal tubule (Site 1). This group of drugs also raises *potassium excretion* to an important extent. Thiazides are *hypotensive*, chiefly due to reduction in intravascular volume but probably also to reduction of peripheral vascular resistance (thiazides diminish the responsiveness of vascular smooth muscle to noradrenaline). Other diuretics, e.g. the loop type, also reduce blood pressure, but for the same degree of natriuresis the effect is greater with the thiazides.

Pharmacokinetics. Thiazides are generally well absorbed from the gut and most have diuretic effect within an hour of being taken by mouth. There are numerous thiazide derivatives and their differences lie principally in duration of action. The relatively water soluble (*cyclopenthiazide, chlorothiazide, hydrochlorothiazide*) are most rapidly eliminated, their main effect occurring within 4–6 h and being complete by 10–12 h. They are excreted unchanged in the urine and active secretion of thiazides by the proximal renal tubule contributes to high renal clearance ($t_{\frac{1}{2}}$ usually less than 4 h). The relatively lipid-soluble members of the group (*polythiazide, methyclothiazide, hydroflumethiazide*) distribute more widely into body tissues and act for over 24 h, which can be objectionable if the drug is used for diuresis, though useful for hypertension.

Adverse effects. Some are discussed below. Rashes (sometimes photosensitive), thrombocytopenia and agranulocytosis occur.

Bendrofluazide (2.5, 5 mg) is a satisfactory member of this group for routine use. The oral dose is 5–10 mg and diuresis usually lasts less than 12 h so that it should be given in the morning. Bendrofluazide, *used primarily for a diuresis* may be given daily for the first few days, then, say, three days a week. Potassium supplements are best retained if not given on the same day or if on the same day, not at the same time.

As an antihypertensive bendrofluazide is given daily; in the absence of a diuresis clinically important potassium depletion is uncommon, but plasma potassium concentration should be checked in potentially vulnerable groups such as the elderly.

Cyclopenthiazide (0.5 mg) is a satisfactory alternative. The oral dose is 0.25–1 mg daily.

Other members of the group include: *chlorothiazide, hydrochlorothiazide, hydroflumethiazide, methyclothiazide and polythiazide.*

Diuretics related to the thiazides

There are several compounds that, although strictly not thiazides, do have structural similarities with them and probably act at the same site on the nephron; they are therefore of moderate efficacy. They have, on the whole, a greater duration of action, like the thiazides are indicated for oedema and hypertension, and have a similar profile of adverse effects. These drugs include:

Chlorthalidone acts for 48–72 h after a single oral dose.

Xipamide is structurally related to chlorthalidone and to frusemide. Elderly patients may be troubled by its brisk and prolonged diuresis.

Clopamide also acts for about 24 h.

Metolazone is effective when renal function is impaired. This drug potentiates the diuresis produced by frusemide and the combination can be effective in resistant oedema provided the patient's fluid and electrolyte loss is carefully monitored.

Mefruside is structurally related to frusemide but closer to the thiazides in its site of action. The main effect occurs 6–12 h after administration and may last for 24 h.

Indapamide is structurally related to chlorthalidone but lowers blood pressure at subdiuretic doses, perhaps by altering calcium flux in vascular smooth muscle. The drug is thus indicated for hypertension and not oedema and it has little apparent effect on potassium, glucose or uric acid excretion.

Potassium-sparing diuretics

Spironolactone (Aldactone) (25, 50, 100 mg). Certain synthetic steroid lactones that are structurally similar to aldosterone competitively inhibit the renal tubular action of this hormone. One of these, *spironolactone*, is useful in the therapy of refractory oedema. Aldosterone promotes sodium reabsorption and potassium loss in the distal tubule. Excessive secretion of aldosterone contributes, at least in part, to fluid retention in hepatic cirrhosis and nephrotic syndrome, and it is in such cases that spironolactone is most useful. It may also benefit congestive heart failure.

Pharmacokinetics. After oral administration, spironolactone is largely converted in the gut and liver to the active metabolite *canrenone* (i.e. it is a prodrug) which has a $t_{\frac{1}{2}}$ of about 9 h. Most of the diuretic effect of spironolactone is probably due to this metabolite, which is available as a drug in its own right, potassium canrenoate. Canrenone has been shown to improve myocardial contraction, an additional action that may prove beneficial for patients in cardiac failure.

Uses. In common with other diuretics that act on the distal tubule, spironolactone is relatively ineffective when used alone, causing less than 5% of the filtered sodium load to be excreted, but it may with advantage be combined with a drug that reduces sodium reabsorption proximally in the tubule, e.g. a loop diuretic. Addition of spironolactone can relieve oedema resistant to a loop diuretic used on its own. Spironolactone is also effective in hypertension, used alone, but since the drug is carcinogenic in rats, it might be prudent not to prescribe it long-term in young patients who have a good prognosis.

Spironolactone will reduce the potassium loss that occurs with thiazide and other diuretics, though it may not abolish the need for potassium supplements (use of K supplement with a K-sparing diuretic requires great care to avoid hyperkalaemia). It should not be used in combination with other potassium-retaining diuretics as this will lead to hyperkalaemia. A dangerous degree of potassium retention may also develop if spironolactone is prescribed for patients with impaired renal function.

Dose. Spironolactone is given orally, 50–100 mg/day total, in one or more doses. The maximum diuresis is delayed for up to 4 days but if after 5 days the response is inadequate, 200 mg/day may be administered.

Adverse effects are uncommon but include gynaecomastia (which reverses when the drug is withdrawn), mental confusion, drowsiness, rashes, abdominal pain and menstrual irregularities. It causes slight urate retention. Spironolactone induces hepatic microsomal enzymes. The therapeutic effect of carbenoxolone in peptic ulcer is abolished by spironolactone.

Potassium canrenoate (Spiroctan-M) (inj. 200 mg in 10 ml) is metabolised in the body to canrenone, the active metabolite of spironoclactone (see above). Indications for use are essentially those of spironolactone and the same precautions should apply. Normally, up to 800 mg i.v. is given each day either as a single injection or in divided doses. Local venous irritation or pain may occur unless the injection is given slowly.

Amiloride (Midamor) (5 mg) a pteridine derivative, is structurally related to triamterene. It increases sodium loss and *reduces* potassium loss by a direct action on ion transport in the distal tubule, i.e. it does not antagonise the action of aldosterone and, in contrast to spironolactone, it is effective when there is no aldosterone excess. Its action is therefore complementary to that of the thiazides and, used with them, sodium loss is increased and potassium loss is reduced. One such combination, Moduretic (amiloride 5 mg plus hydrochlorothiazide 50 mg) is used for mild hypertension or oedema. The maximum effect of amiloride occurs about 6 h after an oral dose and the action may last 24 h; the $t_{\frac{1}{2}}$ is 6 h. The oral dose is 5–20 mg daily.

Triamterene (Dytac) (50 mg) is a potassium-sparing diuretic that has an action and use similar to that of the structurally related amiloride. Triamterene is quite extensively metabolised but some is excreted unchanged in the urine and the $t_{\frac{1}{2}}$ is less than 2 h. The diuretic effect extends over 10 h. Hyperkalaemia can occur especially if potassium supplements, already in use with a thiazide, are inadvertently continued when triamterene is added. Gastrointestinal upsets occur. The oral dose is 50–300 mg.

Adverse effects of diuretics in general

Potassium depletion. Diuretics which act at Sites 1, 2 and 3, proximal to the aldosterone-sensitive site in the distal tubule (Site 4), increase potassium excretion. This subject warrants some discussion since hypokalaemia, amongst other adverse effects, may cause cardiac dysrhythmia especially in patients at risk, e.g. after myocardial infarction, in those taking digoxin and in those with a history of dysrhythmia.

More than 98% of the body's potassium is intracellular and the plasma potassium is not a reliable indicator of body stores. The significance of hypokalaemia is that adverse effects of potassium depletion probably depend on the *ratio* between extracellular and intracellular potassium rather than the total body stores and it is the circulating potassium that is the more subject to fluctuation and much the more easily monitored. The safe lower limit for serum potassium concentration is normally quoted as 3.5 mmol/l. Whether or not diuretic therapy causes significant lowering of serum potassium depends both on the drug and on the circumstances in which it is used.

a. The *loop diuretics* cause a smaller fall in serum potassium than the thiazides, for equivalent diuretic effect, but have a greater capacity for diuresis (i.e. higher efficacy), especially in large dose and so are associated with greater decline in potassium.

b. *Low dietary intake* of potassium predisposes to hypokalaemia; the risk is particularly notable in the elderly, many of whom ingest less than 50 mmol per day (dietary normal 60–120 mmol).

c. Ingestion of certain *other substances* aggravates potassium loss. These include: adrenocortical steroids, ACTH, carbenoxolone and liquorice, which is sometimes used to flavour medicines or may be taken in substantial amounts as confectionery, unknown to the doctor.

d. Hypokalaemia during diuretic therapy is also more likely in the *hyperaldosteronism* whether primary or, more commonly, secondary to severe liver disease, congestive heart failure or nephrotic syndrome.

e. Potassium loss occurs with *diarrhoea*, *vomiting* or *small bowel fistula*, which may develop during diuretic therapy.

f. If a patient has *oedema* and diuresis is brisk and continuous, potassium depletion is likely to occur.

g. When a thiazide diuretic is used for *hyper-*

tension, there is no case for automatic prescription of a potassium supplement in the absence of predisposing factors. If hypokalaemia does develop, it is usually evident within three months of starting therapy and the serum potassium should be measured at that time and thereafter 6-monthly or annually.

Symptoms and signs of hypokalaemia include muscle weakness, constipation and anorexia. ECG changes commonly take the form of S–T depression, low amplitude or inversion of the T wave, which, merging with the U wave, gives the impression of prolongation of the Q–T interval. Cardiac dysrythmias may follow. Renal tubular damage and paralytic ileus are unusual unless there is an additional cause of potassium loss such as diarrhoea.

Potassium depletion can be *minimised* or *corrected* by:

1. maintaining a good dietary intake
2. intermittent use of potassium losing drugs (drug holidays)
3. potassium supplements
4. combining a potassium losing with a potassium retaining drug.

Regular estimation of serum potassium is the most satisfactory way to monitor the adequacy of potassium replacement.

Potassium *chloride* is preferred because chloride is the principal anion excreted along with sodium when high efficacy diuretics are used, i.e. they cause hypochloraemic alkalosis. Where there is chloride lack the exchange of potassium for sodium in the distal tubule is enhanced and potassium depletion proceeds further. Unfortunately, solid KCl is unpleasant to take (gastric irritation) and enteric-coated tablets are liable to disintegrate at one site in the small bowel, causing ulceration, or may not disintegrate at all.

Satisfactory formulations include:

Potassium chloride effervescent tabs (Sando-K tabs) containing 12 mmol K and Cl: the dose is 2–6 tabs daily or alternate days.

Potassium chloride slow-release tabs (Slow-K tabs) containing 8 mmol each of K and Cl: the dose is 2–6 tabs daily or alternate days.

If a supplement is required at least 24 mmol of potassium should be given daily if diet and renal function are normal. Even with slow-release forms of the oesophagus may occur; it appears that this may result from poor oesophageal motility or from obstruction to the passage of the tablet by an enlarged left atrium compressing the oesophagus. Patients, particularly the elderly, should be warned never to take such tablets dry but always with several large mouthfuls of liquid and sitting upright or standing. Combined tablets of diuretics and KCl may not provide enough KCl. Also potassium supplement is better retained if it is not given on the same day, or if on the same day, not at the same time as the diuretic.

Potassium conserving diuretics can be combined with the potent potassium depleting drugs; amiloride is satisfactory.

Hyperkalaemia may occur and regular measurement of serum potassium concentration is necessary when potassium conserving diuretics are used or if potassium supplements are given to patients with impaired renal function.

Symptoms and signs of hyperkalaemia include abdominal discomfort, muscle weakness, metallic taste and stiffness and paraesthesiae in the hands and feet. ECG changes are: tall T wave, low P wave, spreading of the QRS complex. But symptoms may be absent until cardiac arrest occurs.

Treatment of hyperkalaemia

a. In a severe case, the initial objective is to shift potassium rapidly from plasma into cells. This can be done most quickly by giving (1) sodium bicarbonate i.v. (40–160 mmol) and repeating it in a few minutes if ECG changes persist, (2) dextrose 20%, 300–500 ml plus insulin 1 unit/3 g dextrose by i.v. infusion.

b. If ECG changes are marked, calcium may be given to oppose the myocardial effect of potassium (calcium gluconate 10% solution, 10 ml i.v. and repeat if necessary in a few minutes). Calcium may potentiate digoxin and should be used cautiously, if at all, in a patient taking this drug. Sodium bicarbonate and calcium salt must not be mixed because calcium precipitates.

c. Subsequently, a cation-exchange resin (polystyrene sulphonate resin, see later) can be used orally or rectally to remove body potassium via the gut.

d. Dialysis is, of course, highly effective.

Magnesium deficiency. Thiazide and loop diuretics cause significant urinary loss of magnesium; potassium-retaining diuretics probably also cause magnesium retention. Magnesium deficiency brought about by diuretics seems rarely to be severe enough to induce the classical picture of neuromuscular irritability and tetany but cardiac dysrhythmias, mainly of ventricular origin, do occur and respond to repletion of magnesium (using chloride, citrate or gluconate). Other reported features include depression, muscle weakness, refractory hypokalaemia and atrial fibrillation resistant to digoxin.

Hypovolaemia can result from overtreatment. Acute loss of excessive fluid leads to postural hypotension and dizziness. A more insidious state of *chronic hypovolaemia* can develop especially in the elderly. After initial improvement, the patient becomes sleepy and lethargic. Blood urea concentration rises but sodium and chloride concentrations are usually normal. Clearly, hypovolaemia responds to adjustment of the dose of diuretic and transiently increased fluid intake.

Urinary retention. Sudden vigorous diuresis can cause acute retention of urine in the presence of bladder neck dysfunction, e.g. due to prostate enlargement.

Sexual impotence may occur with prolonged use.

Hyponatraemia. Diuretics can bring about hyponatraemia by causing sodium loss in patients who continue to ingest adequate water. Additional mechanisms are probably also involved including enhancement of antidiuretic hormone (ADH) release. Such patients have reduced total body sodium and extracellular fluid and are oedema-free. The treatment is to discontinue the diuretic and perhaps to administer isotonic saline i.v. This condition should be distinguished from hyponatraemia *with* oedema, a state that develops in some patients with congestive cardiac failure, cirrhosis or nephrotic syndrome. Here salt and water intake should be restricted because the extracellular fluid is expanded. Hyponatraemia with a normal extra-cellular fluid volume occurs in the syndrome of inappropriate ADH secretion, which responds to water restriction and other measures (p. 549).

Urate retention with hyperuricaemia and sometimes clinical gout occurs with the *high efficacy diuretics* — frusemide, bumetanide (possibly to a lesser extent) and ethacrynic acid. All *moderate efficacy diuretics*, i.e. thiazide and similar drugs, cause hyperuricaemia.

Two mechanisms appear to be responsible. First, diuretics cause volume depletion that induces increased absorption of almost all solutes in the proximal tubule including urate. Second, diuretics and uric acid are organic acids and compete for the transport mechanism that carries such substances from the blood into the urine. Diuretic-induced hyperuricaemia can be antagonised by allopurinol or probenecid.

Carbohydrate intolerance. Carbohydrate tolerance is impaired by those diuretics that produce prolonged hypokalaemia, i.e. the thiazide and loop type. It appears that intracellular potassium is necessary for the formation of insulin and the glucose intolerance is probably due to insulin deficiency. The result is an increase in insulin requirement of diabetic patients or manifest disease in latent diabetics. The effect is generally reversible over several months. It is a serious consideration in selecting therapy for young hypertensives who will require treatment for decades.

Alkalosis. The thiazides and the loop diuretics (notably ethacrynic acid) cause sodium, potassium and chloride excretion, which leads to a metabolic alkalosis.

Calcium homeostasis. *Loop diuretics* increase renal calcium loss; in the short term this is not a serious disadvantage and indeed frusemide may be used in the management of hypercalcaemia after rehydration has been achieved. In the long term this effect may be undesirable especially in elderly patients who tend in any case to be in negative calcium balance. By contrast the *thiazides* decrease renal excretion of calcium and this property may influence the choice of diuretic in a potentially calcium-deficient individual. The hypocalciuric effect of the thiazides has been used effectively to reduce episodes of renal colic in patients with idiopathic hypercalciuria.

Interactions. Loop diuretics potentiate ototoxicity of aminoglycosides and nephrotoxicity of some cephalosporins. Indomethacin and other non-steroidal anti-inflammatory drugs reduce the diuresis induced by frusemide and possibly other diuretics, perhaps by inhibiting synthesis of vasodilator prostaglandins.

Abuse of diuretics. Psychological abnormality sometimes takes the form of abuse of diuretics and/or purgatives. The subject usually desires to 'slim' to become 'attractive' or 'healthy' or may have anorexia nervosa. There can be severe depletion of sodium and potassium, with renal tubular damage (due to chronic hypokalaemia).

Osmotic diuretics

Any substance that filters through the glomerular membrane* and is not completely reabsorbed in the renal tubules necessarily has some diuretic effect as it is excreted with its isosmotic equivalent of water. Non-electrolytes of small molecular weight are used.

Osmotic diuretics act mainly in the proximal tubule, where they prevent reabsorption of water. The sodium in the tubular fluid thus becomes diluted and a steep concentration gradient develops between tubular and interstitial fluid. Less sodium is thus absorbed at the proximal tubule and at the ascending limb of the loop of Henle, so disturbing the osmotic gradient between medulla and cortex. Some of the sodium delivered to the distal tubule exchanges with potassium. The result is that urine volume increases according to the load of osmotic diuretic and sodium and potassium loss increase.

Glucose (MW 198) excess in diabetes mellitus provides an example of a pathological osmotic diuresis. In diabetic ketoacidosis it is responsible for much of the sodium and water loss that leads to hypovolaemia, hypoperfusion and acidosis.

Uses

1. For rapid reduction of *intracranial or intraocular pressure* by osmotic effect in the blood, drawing fluid out of tissues (*not* primarily by diuresis).

2. Rarely, to maintain urine flow, e.g. preoperatively in jaundiced patients with a high risk of acute tubular necrosis. A major disadvantage of the osmotic diuretics arises if the kidneys are too impaired to form urine even after an osmotic load; a patient could inadvertently be given a hypertonic solution that his body is not capable of eliminating and the ensuing expansion of intravascular volume may cause heart failure and pulmonary oedema.

The following are used:

Mannitol (MW 182) is a polyhydric alcohol that is filtered across the glomeruli but not reabsorbed to any significant extent in the tubules. It is given i.v. (or orally, when it induces osmotic diarrhoea).

Urea (MW 60). If urea is given to the patient, the amount filtered will increase. The blood urea is necessarily raised, but this is not in itself of any clinical importance. Urea (30% solution) i.v. is an effective agent for transient *reduction of intracranial pressure* but careful attention to detail is necessary. Obviously, it is pointless to use urea in a patient with renal failure.

Xanthine diuretics

The general properties of the xanthines (theophylline, theobromine, caffeine) are discussed elsewhere. These compounds are weak diuretics and are useless for this purpose in therapeutics. They act by inhibiting absorption of sodium, chloride and water in the renal tubules to produce a small diuresis. Theophylline (as aminophylline) can be used to increase glomerular filtration by its cardiac action, which increases renal blood flow.

Carbonic anhydrase inhibitors

Carbonic anhydrase facilitates the reaction between carbon dioxide and water to form carbonic acid:

$$CO_2 + H_2O \overset{\text{Carbonic anhydrase}}{\rightleftharpoons} H_2CO_3 \rightleftharpoons H^+ + HCO_3^-$$

the rate being slow in the absence of the enzyme. This reaction is fundamental to the production of either acid or alkaline secretions, and a high concentration of carbonic anhydrase is present in the gastric mucosa, pancreas, eye and kidney. Within the proximal tubule cells of the kidney, carbonic anhydrase provides a supply of hydrogen ions that are exchanged for sodium in the tubular fluid so that body sodium is conserved. The

* All molecules having MW < 10 000 (all drugs) and some substances up to MW 50 000.

hydrogen ions in the tubular fluid then combine with bicarbonate to form carbonic acid, which is metabolised to CO_2 and H_2O by carbonic anhydrase on the luminal surface of the tubule cells. Hence inhibition of carbonic anhydrase reduces the supply of hydrogen ions so that sodium and bicarbonate remain in the tubular fluid. An alkaline urine with high sodium bicarbonate content results. The increase in sodium excretion leads to a diuresis. Furthermore, increased delivery of sodium to the distal tubule, where there is exchange with potassium, causes potassium loss. *Tolerance* quickly develops because continued loss of bicarbonate leads to a metabolic acidosis that eventually provides an adequate supply of hydrogen ions in the tubular fluid without the action of carbonic anhydrase. At this stage diuresis ceases. Carbonic anhydrase inhibition is therefore effective for diuresis only when it is used intermittently, and as a means of treating sodium overload it is obsolete.

But *inhibitors of carbonic anhydrase have uses in medicine*.

1. They have been found to *reduce intra-ocular pressure*. This action is due not to diuresis (thiazides actually raise intra-ocular pressure slightly). The formation of aqueous humour is an active process that requires a supply of bicarbonate ions that is dependent on the presence of carbonic anhydrase. Inhibition of carbonic anhydrase reduces formation of aqueous humour and lowers intra-ocular pressure. This is a local action and is not affected by the development of acid–base changes elsewhere in the body, i.e. tolerance does not develop.

2. Carbonic anhydrase inhibition also appears to be useful for *prophylaxis of acute mountain sickness*. This condition affects unacclimatised people at altitudes in excess of 3000 metres, especially if ascent has been rapid and exertion great; symptoms range from nausea, lassitude and headache to pulmonary and cerebral oedema. The explanation may be that at high altitude, hyperventilation in response to falling oxygen tension is inhibited because alkalosis is also induced. The rationale for using a carbonic anhydrase inhibitor is that the induced metabolic acidosis increases respiratory drive and helps maintain arterial oxygen tension. In double-blind trials, climbers who took acetazolamide experienced fewer symptoms and performed better than those who took placebo.*

Acetazolamide (Diamox) (250 mg; inj. 500 mg) is most widely used. It is well absorbed from the gut and is elminated only by the kidney. The $t_{\frac{1}{2}}$ is 3 h. The drug accumulates in erythrocytes.

In acute congestive glaucoma 250–1000 mg are given by mouth each day, in divided doses for amounts over 250 mg. A single daily dose of 500 mg in a sustained-release preparation is taken at night for prophylaxis of acute mountain sickness. Acetazolamide is also used in the treatment of epilepsy and periodic paralysis. Adverse effects are not common; paraesthesiae, drowsiness, fever, rashes occur; and blood disorders are rare. It should not be used in liver failure, as it has occasionally precipitated hepatic coma. Renal calculi may occur, perhaps because the urine calcium is in less soluble form owing to low citrate content of the urine.

Inhibition of carbonic anhydrase in sites other than the kidney produces few significant effects. Acid secretion in the stomach is reduced, but not enough to be useful.

Dichlorphenamide (Daranide) is similar to acetazolamide.

Cation-exchange resins

The discovery of the phenomenon of ion exchange occurred in the mid-19th century when an English landowner became interested in the possible loss of ammonia from his manure heaps. He consulted a chemist who began an experimental study, in the course of which he found that if an ammonium sulphate solution percolated down a soil column, calcium sulphate came out at the bottom. This was a surprise for him, not least because the phenomenon of electrolytic dissociation of salts was then unknown.† Cation- exchange resins may be used to remove cations (e.g. sodium, potassium) from the intestinal contents. Though not themselves diuretics, they found their initial

* Birmingham Medical Research Expeditionary Society Mountain Sickness Study Group. Lancet 1981; 1:180. Green M K et al. Br Med J 1981; 283:811.

† Kitchener J A. Ion Exchange Resins. London: Methuen, 1957.

clinical use as part of long-term diuretic and oedema prevention regimens until modern effective diuretics abolished the need for them. The chief use now is in *hyperkalaemia*.

The resins consist of aggregations of big insoluble molecules carrying a fixed negative charge, which therefore loosely bind positively charged ions (cations). The cations are exchangeable with the cations in the fluid environment and the order of natural affinity for cations runs from large divalent to small monovalent ions, thus Ca > Mg > K > NH_4 > Na > H.

One of the principal difficulties in the use of cation-exchange resins is to ensure as nearly as possible that only the desired ion is removed from the body.

In hyperkalaemia, oral administration or retention enemas of *polystyrene sulphonate resin* may be used. The resin does not merely prevent absorption of ingested potassium when given orally, but takes up the potassium normally secreted into the intestine and ordinarily reabsorbed. A *sodium*-phase resin (Resonium A) should not be used in patients with renal or cardiac failure as sodium overload may result. A *calcium*-phase resin (Calcium Resonium) may cause hypercalaemia and should be avoided in patients with multiple myeloma, metastatic carcinoma, hyperparathyroidism and sarcoidosis. The usual dose is 15 g by mouth ×3 or ×4/day or 30 g rectally. Enemas should ideally be retained for at least 9 h but this is usually impossible.

Use of diuretic drugs

Choice of diuretic

Oral administration is obviously preferable and a thiazide is satisfactory, but the shorter duration of action of loop diuretics is an advantage. If a quick and vigorous response is needed, frusemide and bumetanide orally, or i.v. or i.m. in very urgent cases, are preferred. Spironolactone should be given only in combination with other diuretics when these fail to be effective. Other considerations such as the presence of a high serum urate concentration may influence the selection of particular diuretics (see adverse effects of diuretics).

Combinations of diuretics

There is no advantage in combining two diuretics that are very similar to each other structurally. In general, dissimilar diuretics summate with or potentiate each other. However, the most effective diuretics (frusemide, bumetanide or ethacrynic acid) do not generally need the assistance of a second drug, though they may be combined with triamterene, amiloride or spironolactone in order to reduce potassium loss (as well as to enhance natriuresis) when prolonged use is contemplated. Where there is hyperaldosteronism, spironolactone may usefully be added.

Therapeutic efficacy

The most effective (loop) diuretics have such a vigorous effect that they are useful in acute pulmonary oedema but they can cause collapse due to serious acute loss of extracellular volume.

Because oral agents are easily given repeatedly, lack of supervision can result in insidious overdose. *Early signs of overdose are postural dizziness* (hypotension) due to reduced blood volume, and a *rising blood urea* concentration due to falling glomerular blood flow (filtration); electrolyte imbalance follows.

Measurement of weight changes is the simplest guide to the success or failure of diuretic regimens. Fluid intake and output charts are more demanding of time and often less accurate.

Salt restriction

When abnormal retention of sodium occurs, retention of water follows; thus one obvious way of removing oedema is to reduce sodium intake. Clinically useful diuretics increase the excretion of sodium, but this will only lead to mobilisation of oedema fluid if its replacement by sodium from the diet is prevented. Dietary sodium restriction was an important part of treatment until the introduction of effective oral diuretics. A normal diet contains about 10 g of sodium chloride per day (1 g of sodium chloride contains about 17 mmol sodium). If no salt is added in cooking or at mealtimes this may fall to about 2–5 g a day, which is often low enough, but special low-salt diets (about 1 g daily) may be needed. Really extreme salt restriction is usually intolerable and unnecessary. It is unnecessary to restrict water intake unless hyponatraemia is present.

Treatment of oedema

The removal of oedema involves more than simply giving diuretic drugs. It is also important to ensure that there is adequate glomerular filtration, in the absence of which diuretics acting on the renal tubule are less effective.

Cardiac oedema occurs when the cardiac output is not sufficient to perfuse the kidneys adequately. The extracellular fluid then increases as a result of altered renal haemodynamics. It can be lowered by increasing sodium output (diuretics) or by reducing intake (low sodium diet). Dopamine infusion (see index) can be used to improve renal blood flow and thereby to increase urine production. Therapy can also be directed both to reducing the demands of the body for blood flow and to increasing the efficiency of the heart. The body's demands can be reduced by rest and sometimes by treating disease, as when hyperthyroidism is reduced (drugs, surgery), anaemia is corrected (drugs, transfusion), an arteriovenous shunt is abolished (surgery) or peripheral resistance is reduced (vasodilators).

Renal oedema. By the time chronic renal disease causes oedema, reversal of the disease process in the kidney is seldom practicable. The oedema of *nephrotic syndrome* arises as follows: loss of albumin causes a fall in plasma oncotic (colloid osmotic) pressure and the resulting diversion of intravascular volume into the interstitium stimulates the renin–angiotensin–aldosterone system, which causes sodium avidly to be retained.

The chief therapeutic aims are the reduction of dietary sodium intake and the prevention of excessive sodium retention using diuretic drugs. Reduction of sodium reabsorption in the renal tubule by diuretics is most effective when glomerular filtration has not been too much reduced by disease. But the high-efficacy drugs, frusemide, bumetanide or ethacrynic acid, can be effective even when it is very low. The combination of frusemide plus metolazone is particularly effective at low glomerular filtration rates but the resulting diuresis should be carefully monitored for safety.

Spironolactone may be added usefully to potentiate the loop diuretic, antagonise the secondary hyperaldosteronism and conserve potassium, loss of which can be severe.

An adrenal steroid or immunosuppresive drug may be needed.

In *acute renal failure* use of diuretics is controversial once the condition is established, but they may be effective in preventing it. In this case the potent loop diuretics are used but not osmotic diuretics for if the kidneys are not capable of producing urine the patient would be left with a hypertonic solution in the circulation.

Diuretics are not usually needed in acute nephritis as most cases recover spontaneously, but they may be necessary if pulmonary oedema develops (frusemide).

Hepatic ascites and oedema is due to portal venous hypertension together with decreased plasma colloid osmotic (oncotic) pressure and hypoproteinaemia causing hyperaldosteronism as is the case with nephrotic oedema (above). Furthermore, in the kidney, diversion of blood flow from the cortex to the medulla favours sodium retention. The aim of treatment is therefore to reduce dietary sodium intake and to limit sodium reabsorption by use of diuretics. This may be achieved with a loop diuretic plus an aldosterone antagonist used to produce a slow or gradual diuresis. If it is vigorous, depletion of sodium and potassium and hypochloraemic alkalosis occur, which may result in hepatic coma.

Large accumulations of ascites are sometimes removed by abdominal paracentesis partly for the sake of speed. Ascitic fluid contains large amounts of protein and repeated paracenteses will aggravate hypoproteinaemia, so this approach should be avoided if at all possible. Every effort should be made to control cirrhotic ascites by diuretics and salt restriction alone.

Refractory oedema

Oedema sometimes persists despite a vigorous diuretic regimen. This is most common in the terminal phase of an illness, when homeostasis is grossly deranged, but certain points are worth remembering.

1. Bed rest by improving renal circulation can itself restore drug responsiveness.

2. Strict adherence to low-sodium diet may bring about improvement.

3. Fluid restriction may be necessary if the plasma sodium concentration falls.

4. Frusemide in a dose of 2–3 g daily may be required, and spironolactone up to 300 mg daily in divided doses. Alternatively frusemide may be combined with metolazone.

5. Failure of response may be due to poor absorption of diuretic from an oedematous gut mucosa or because of injection into oedematous tissue from which it is too slowly absorbed. The i.v. route is then preferred; in addition, frusemide may be given by continuous *infusion* at doses sufficient to ensure a diuresis without risking deafness.

6. Some patients in severe cardiac failure may respond to an i.v. infusion of dopamine.

ALTERATION OF URINE pH

It is sometimes useful to alter urine pH by drugs and the indications for such therapeutic manoeuvres are summarised below.

Alkalinisation of urine

a. Increases the elimination of aspirin/salicylate, phenobarbitone and phenoxyacetate herbicides (e.g. 2, 4-D; MCPA). (See pH partition hypothesis, p. 115.)

b. Prevents urate and cystine stone formation and reduces the risk of crystalluria with sulphonamides.

c. Reduces irritation in an inflamed urinary tract.

d. discourages the growth of certain organisms, e.g. *Esch. coli*.

The urine can be made alkaline by sodium bicarbonate i.v. or by sodium bicarbonate or potassium citrate by mouth; the latter is oxidised and the cation combines with bicarbonate in the renal tubular fluid. To be effective, potassium citrate at least 3–6 g by mouth 6-hourly is needed (Potassium Citrate Mixture) or sodium bicarbonate powder, 5–10 g daily.

The cation can be dangerous in heart failure (sodium overload) or renal failure (sodium or potassium overload).

The use of sodium bicarbonate by i.v. infusion to treat salicylate or phenobarbitone overdose is described in Chapter 10.

Acidification of urine

a. Is used as a test for renal tubular acidosis.

b. Increases elimination of phencyclidine, fenfluramine and amphetamine although it is very rarely needed and then only in severe and acute poisoning with these drugs. For further discussion see Chapter 10.

The urine may be made acid by ammonium chloride or arginine hydrochloride (equivalent to drinking HCl); by a sulphur-containing amino acid (methionine; equivalent to drinking H_2SO_4), or by ascorbic acid.

Ammonium choride is converted by the liver into urea and hydrogen ions leading to a hyperchloraemic metabolic acidosis. High doses cause gastric irritation, abdominal pain, nausea and vomiting, but any dose may be dangerous in a patient with poor renal function. Neither should patients with hepatic failure be given ammonium chloride because they cannot convert the ammonium into urea and may therefore go into coma.

DRUGS AND THE KIDNEY

The kidneys comprise only 0.5% of body weight, yet they receive 25% of the cardiac output. Thus, it is hardly surprising that *drugs can damage the kidney* and that *disease of the kidney affects responses to drugs*.

Drug-induced renal disease

Drugs and chemicals damage the kidney by:

1. **Direct biochemical effect.**

Substances that cause direct toxicity include:
Heavy metals (mercury, gold, iron, lead)
Antimicrobials (aminoglycosides, amphotericin, sulphonamides, cephalosporins)

X-ray contrast media (chiefly biliary agents)
Analgesics (aspirin)
Solvents (carbon tetrachloride, ethylene glycol)
2. **Indirect biochemical effect.**
Uricosurics may cause urate to be precipitated in the tubule.
Calciferol may cause renal calcification.
Diuretic and laxative abuse can cause tubular damage through potassium and sodium depletion.
Sulphonamides can crystallise in the kidney and urinary tract.
Anticoagulants may cause haemorrhage into the kidney.
Worcestershire sauce (acetic acid, spices, salt) has caused renal stones when consumed in enormous quantities by people with perverted taste for this excellent condiment.
3. **Immunological effect.**
A wide range of drugs produce a wide range of injuries.

Drugs: phenytoin, gold, penicillins, sulphonamides, hydralazine, isoniazid, rifampicin, procainamide, penicillamine and others.

Injuries: arteritis, glomerulitis, interstitial nephritis, systemic lupus erythematosus.

A drug may cause damage by more than one of the above three mechanisms (e.g. sulphonamides).

The *sites and pathological types of injury* are as follows:

Glomerular damage. The large surface area of the glomerular capillaries renders them susceptible to damage from circulating immune complexes; glomerulonephritis, proteinuria and nephrotic syndrome may result, e.g. following treatment with penicillamine, when the patient has made an immune response to the drug. The degree of renal impairment is best reflected in the *creatinine clearance*, which provides a measure of the glomerular filtration rate because creatinine is filtered and not reabsorbed.

Tubular damage. By concentrating 200 l of glomerular filtrate into 1.5 l of urine each day, renal tubular cells expose themselves to much greater amounts of solutes and environmental toxins than do other cells in the body. The proximal tubule, through which most water is reabsorbed, experiences the greatest concentration and so suffers most drug induced injury. Specialised transport processes concentrate acids (salicylate, cephalosporins) and bases (aminoglycosides) in renal tubular cells. Heavy metals and radiographic contrast media also cause damage at this site. Proximal tubular toxicity is best shown by leakage of *glucose, phosphate,* HCO_3 and *amino acids* into the urine.

The counter-current multiplier and exchange systems of urine concentration (see p. 545) cause some drugs to accumulate in the renal medulla. Analgesic nephropathy is often first evident in this site partly because of high tissue concentration, and partly, it is believed, because of ischaemia through inhibition of locally produced vasodilator prostaglandins. The distal tubule is also the site of lithium-induced nephrotoxicity. Damage to the medulla and distal nephron is manifested by failure to *concentrate* the urine after fluid deprivation and by failure to *acidify* urine after ingestion of ammonium chloride.

Tubular obstruction. Given certain physicochemical conditions, crystals can deposit within the tubular lumen. Methotrexate is relatively insoluble at low pH and can precipitate in the distal nephron when the urine is acid.

Successful treatment of a leukaemia may be followed by the development of fatal urate nephropathy if breakdown of nucleic acids released by destruction of leukaemic cells delivers large amounts of insoluble urate to tubular fluid. This outcome can be prevented by starting the patient on allopurinol before the leukaemia is treated, for allopurinol inhibits xanthine oxidase and the more soluble precursor, hypoxanthine, is excreted.

Other drug-induced lesions of the kidney include:
Vasculitis: caused by sulphonamides, allopurinol, isoniazid.

Allergic interstitial nephritis: caused by penicillins sulphonamides, thiazides, allopurinol, phenytoin.
Systemic lupus erythematosus: caused by hydralazine, procainamide.

Drugs may thus induce any of the common clinical syndromes of renal injury, namely:
acute renal failure (aminoglycosides, cisplatin)

nephrotic syndrome (penicillamine, gold, captopril)
chronic renal failure (non-steroidal anti-inflammatory drugs, amphotericin B)
functional impairment (reduced ability to dilute and concentrate urine, potassium loss in urine and acid base imbalance, as above)

Prescribing for patients with renal impairment

Drugs may:

1. *Exacerbate* renal disease;
2. *Accumulate* due to failure of renal excretion or by changes in protein binding.
3. Be *ineffective* (e.g. thiazide diuretics in moderate or severe renal failure; uricosurics).

Problems of safety arise especially in patients with renal failure, who must be treated with drugs that are potentially toxic and are wholly or largely eliminated by the kidney. A knowledge of, or at least access to sources of, pharmacokinetic data is essential for safe therapy for such patients.

Drugs may be classified in terms of their dependence on renal elimination as the following examples show:

1. *Drugs that are eliminated almost exclusively by the kidney*

	Plasma $t_{\frac{1}{2}}$ *(h)*	
	Normal	*Severe renal impairment**
Benzylpenicillin	0.5	8
Ampicillin	1	14
Acyclovir	2.5	20
Gentamicin	2.5	50
Sotalol	5	41
Atenolol	6	100
Tetracycline	8	75

The prolongation of $t_{\frac{1}{2}}$ indicates that special care must be exercised if these drugs are used in patients with impaired renal function.

2. *Drugs that are almost entirely metabolised*:

	Plasma $t_{\frac{1}{2}}$ *(h)*	
	Normal	*Severe renal impairment**
Paracetamol	2	2
Clindamycin	2	3
Propranolol	3	3
Rifampicin	3	3
Lorazepam	15	15
Doxycycline	18	18
Nortriptyline	30	30
Warfarin	40	40

The normal $t_{\frac{1}{2}}$, despite severe uraemia, indicates that such drugs can generally be used in normal dose when renal function is impaired. However, this advice must be tempered by the realisation that many drugs produce pharmacologically active metabolites that tend to be more water-soluble than the parent drug, are dependent on the kidney for their elimination, and accumulate in renal failure.

Drugs that produce pharmacologically active metabolites include: acebutolol, allopurinol, carbamazepine, chlordiazepoxide, clobazam, clorazepate, diazepam, 5-fluorouracil, flurazepam, hydralazine, iproniazid, isosorbide dinitrate, metronidazole, nicoumalone.

3. *Drugs that are partly metabolised and partly eliminated by the kidney*.

	Plasma $t_{\frac{1}{2}}$ *(h)*	
	Normal	*Severe renal impairment**
Lincomycin	5	12
Trimethoprim	10	25
Amphetamine	12	24
Chlorpropamide	36	200
Digoxin	36	120
Digitoxin	150	240

Doses of some drugs in this class must be modified when renal function is impaired, notably digoxin.

Dosing regimens for patients with renal impairment

1. **Initial dose**. When the problem is one of elimination it might be expected that the initial (or where necessary the priming or loading) dose (see Drug Dosage, p. 132) would be the same in the uraemic as in the healthy subject, for the volume in which the drug has to distribute should

* Glomerular filtration rate < 5 ml/min: normal 127 ml/min

not be different. However, binding of drug to plasma proteins may be reduced because of hypoproteinaemia or because of competition for binding sites with metabolic byproducts that accumulate in renal failure. Therefore it may be prudent to initiate drug therapy with a dose that is lower than would normally be used until its effect can be observed, especially with an extensively protein-bound drug or in a patient who is hypoproteinaemic or in advanced renal disease.

2. **Maintenance dose**. The dose that is required to maintain an effective concentration in the tissues depends on the rate of drug elimination and the physician requires some estimate of the extent to which elimination is reduced in the individual patient. The most convenient and useful guide is the *creatinine clearance*. This is best illustrated by drugs that are wholly excreted by the kidney (penicillins, many cephalosporins, aminoglycosides) since for these the rate of drug elimination declines in proportion to the creatinine clearance. Put another way, drug $t_{\frac{1}{2}}$ is inversely proportional to creatinine clearance and if the *creatinine clearance is halved, then the drug* $t_{\frac{1}{2}}$ *is doubled*; if the creatinine clearance is one-quarter of normal, the drug $t_{\frac{1}{2}}$ is quadrupled and so on. Once an estimate of drug $t_{\frac{1}{2}}$ can be made in an individual patient, there are two main approaches to calculating the maintenance dose.

a. The normal maintenance dose is given but the interval between doses is lengthened. Using the principle that each maintenance dose replenishes the fall in plasma concentration in the previous $t_{\frac{1}{2}}$ (see Drug Dosage, p. 133), this approach involves giving a normal maintenance dose at intervals equal to the (prolonged) $t_{\frac{1}{2}}$ in the patient. This, however, may call for an inconvenient frequency of dosing — a drug that has a $t_{\frac{1}{2}}$ of 8 h in persons with normal renal function, given to a patient whose creatinine clearance is 25% of normal, would have to be administered every 32 h.

b. A reduced maintenance dose is given but the interval between doses is unchanged. The reduction in maintenance dose may be related directly to the creatinine clearance, i.e. a patient with a creatinine clearance 50% of normal would receive half the normal maintenance dose.

The purpose of the present discussion is to illustrate *principles* of dosing for patients with impaired renal function by taking the simplest case, i.e. drugs that are eliminated wholly by the kidney. The issue becomes more complicated for drugs that are partly excreted by the kidney and partly metabolised by the liver for then the simple relation between creatinine clearance and rate of drug elimination must be modified*. *In practice it is often the case that the only knowledge the doctor has is (a) the class of drug that is to be prescribed and (b) the approximate degree of renal impairment. The following general rules are then appropriate:*

1. *Drugs that are wholly or largely excreted by the kidney or drugs that produce active, renally eliminated metabolites* — give a normal or slightly reduced initial dose and reduce the maintenance dose *or* increase the dose interval in proportion to the degree of renal impairment (which is indicated by the creatinine clearance).

2. *Drugs that are wholly or largely metabolised to inactive products* — give normal doses (except when renal failure is advanced, or there is hypoproteinaemia, or the drug is extensively plasma protein bound, in which case a smaller initial dose may still be desirable because more free drug may be available to fill a reduced distribution volume).

3. *Drugs that are partly eliminated by the kidney and partly metabolised* — give a normal initial dose and modify the maintenance dose or dose interval in the light of what is known about the patient's renal function and the drug, its dependence on renal elimination and its inherent toxicity; the latter is a matter of individual judgement. The proviso in 2 (above) also applies.

Time to reach steady-state blood concentration

It is important to remember that the *time* to reach steady-state plasma concentration is dependent *only* on drug $t_{\frac{1}{2}}$ and that a drug reaches 97% of its ultimate steady-state concentration in five $t_{\frac{1}{2}}$ periods. If $t_{\frac{1}{2}}$ is prolonged by renal impairment, so also will be the time to reach steady state. An individual with normal renal function receiving a constant dose of digoxin ($t_{\frac{1}{2}}$, 36 h) can be expected to be at plateau concentration in about 7 days, but

* Dettli L. Clin Pharmacokinet 1976; 1: 126–134.

when kidney function is severely depressed the process may take two weeks or more.

Schemes for modifying drug dosage for patients with renal disease do not abolish their increased risk of adverse effects; *such patients should be observed particularly carefully during a course of drug therapy*. Ideally, dosing should be monitored by drug plasma concentration measurements, but this service is not available to most of the world population.

Selection of drugs for patients with renal disease

The following general guides apply:

Analgesics

Opioids that are inactivated by metabolism may yet present particular problems for the uraemic patient.

Morphine has increased hazard because reduced plasma protein binding may accentuate the free plasma concentration and so its respiratory depressant effect.

Pethidine should be avoided as it forms an active metabolite (norpethidine) that can accumulate in renal failure to cause seizures.

Codeine, dihydrocodeine and dextropropoxyphene should also be avoided.

Methadone is transformed into inactive metabolites and is to be preferred.

Naloxone, the competitive opioid antagonist, requires no dose modification.

Non-steroidal anti-inflammatory drugs

These should in general be avoided as they may cause fluid retention and deterioration in renal function. Some specific comments are relevant.

Diflunisal, azapropazone and sulindac are eliminated by the kidney; alternatives should be used.

Aspirin is best avoided because it may aggravate a pre-existing bleeding tendency and because salicylate metabolism is readily saturated, whereupon further elimination depends on renal function.

Paracetamol is acceptable as it is metabolised.

Anticonvulsants

Phenytoin, sodium valproate and carbamazepine may be used in normal dose as they are metabolised.

Antidiabetic drugs

Chlorpropamide should not be used because its normally long duration of action ($t_{\frac{1}{2}}$, 36 h) is even longer in renal failure.

Glipizide ($t_{\frac{1}{2}}$, 7 h) is acceptable because it is metabolised but active metabolites can produce hypoglycaemia and blood sugar should be monitored with extra frequency.

Metformin should be avoided because of the risk of serious lactic acidosis.

Insulin requirements diminish.

Antimicrobial drugs

Aminoglycosides (gentamicin, tobramycin, amikacin, streptomycin) should be given in reduced dose when there is any degree of renal impairment. These drugs are almost wholly dependent on elimination by the kidney and have a relatively narrow therapeutic ratio. The effectiveness and safety of the dosing regimen should be checked by monitoring plasma concentrations (peak and trough).

Cephalosporins vary in the extent to which they are dependent on renal elimination (see p. 219) and the dose may need to be lowered.

Penicillins are relatively non-toxic and can be tolerated in normal doses even when renal function is moderately reduced. In severe renal impairment penicillins should be given in reduced dose. *Carbenicillin and ticarcillin* are presented as sodium salts and can cause fluid overload in patients with reduced renal function.

Sulphonamides should be avoided as there is increased risk of crystalluria and other adverse effects.

Tetracyclines should be avoided not only because they are eliminated by the kidney but they also aggravate pre-existing uraemia by interfering with protein synthesis (anti-anabolic effect), so that the kidneys have to excrete an extra load from amino acid metabolism. There are two exceptions; *doxycycline* and *minocycline* are not eliminated by the renal route and may be used when a tetracycline is essential for a patient with impaired renal function: but they retain antianabolic effect.

Urinary antimicrobials. Nitrofurantoin, a metabolite of which accumulates and may cause polyneuritis, and nalidixic acid, which is more likely to cause adverse effects, should be avoided.

Other drugs that should be avoided or used in reduced dose include: acyclovir, amphotericin B, chloramphenicol, ethambutol, isoniazid, trimethoprim, vancomycin.

Anti-parkinsonism drugs

Amantadine should be avoided.
Levodopa and bromocriptine may be used in normal dose.

Cardiovascular drugs

Digoxin should be given in reduced dose, the plasma concentration should be monitored; the risk of toxicity is increased by electrolyte disturbance.

β-adrenoceptor blocking drugs. Propranolol, labetalol, oxprenolol, timolol and metoprolol are metabolised and should be preferred to acebutolol, nadolol, sotalol, pindolol and atenolol, which are excreted by the kidney. Most experience has been gained with propranolol, which is effective for hypertension, angina and cardiac dysrhythmia, in patients with renal impairment.

Other antihypertensives are given in doses that relate to their response.

Hydralazine, prazosin, nifedipine, minoxidil, diazoxide and methyldopa can be used in normal maintenance doses but it is advisable to start with a smaller dose than usual.

Sodium nitroprusside will reduce blood pressure rapidly but should not be infused for longer than 48 h because it is metabolised to thiocyanate, which accumulates and is toxic (cyanide poisoning).

Captopril and enalapril should be used in reduced dose.

Bethanidine, debrisoquine and guanethidine should be avoided.

Cardiac antidysrhythmics

Lignocaine and quinidine can be used in normal doses.

Procainamide and disopyramide form active metabolites and their dose interval should be increased in severe renal impairment.

Diuretics

Thiazides are ineffective when the glomerular filtration rate falls below 20 ml/min.

Frusemide, bumetanide and metolazone continue to be active at glomerular filtration rates of 10 ml/min and below, but should be used with special care because they may induce volume depletion, which is indicated by a rising plasma creatinine or blood urea concentration.

Amiloride, triamterene and spironolactone are contraindicated in advanced renal disease because they cause dangerous hyperkalaemia.

Ethacrynic acid should be avoided because its ototoxicity is increased.

Gastrointestinal drugs

Gastric antacids and other drugs that contain substantial amounts of sodium (e.g. salts of antimicrobials) and potassium (e.g. potassium citrate) should be avoided, because these cations accumulate and the composition of all antacids and particularly of effervescent preparations should be examined before prescribing them.
Aluminium hydroxide, see p. 615.
Carbenoxolone causes fluid retention and should be avoided.
Cimetidine and ranitidine should be used in reduced dose.

Psychoactive drugs

Lithium should be avoided as it is difficult to avoid toxicity even when plasma concentrations can be measured.

Diazepam and chlordiazepoxide are satisfactory anxiolytics in normal doses but the patient should be watched for over-sedation.

Temazepam ($t_{\frac{1}{2}}$, 6–8 h) and *triazolam* ($t_{\frac{1}{2}}$, 2–4 h) are short-acting and satisfactory for night sedation.

Diphenhydramine, an antihistamine (H_1- receptor), provides both sedation and relief from uraemic pruritis but the dose should not exceed 25–50 mg twice daily.

Tricyclic antidepressants and the *phenothiazine antipsychotics* are metabolised and patients with impaired renal function should respond normally to conventional doses of these drugs.

Uricosuric agents

Probenecid and sulphinpyrazone are ineffective in renal failure.

Allopurinol, because it blocks uric acid synthesis, is an effective alternative in gout prophylaxis, especially if the gout is the cause of the renal impairment, but the dose should be lowered.

NEPHROLITHIASIS

Calcareous stones result from hypercalciuria, hyperuricosuria, hyperoxaluria and hypocitraturia. Hypercalciuria and hyperoxaluria render urine supersaturated in respect of calcium salts; citrate lowers the urinary saturation of calcium oxalate and inhibits its precipitation from solution.

Non-calcareous stones occur most commonly in the presence of urea-splitting organisms, which increase the ammonium ion content and alkalinity of the urine and favour formation of magnesium ammonium phosphate (struvite) stones. Urate stones form in conditions of unusual acidity of urine (pH < 5.5). Patients with cystinuria form cystine stones.

Management. Passage of a single calcium-containing stone by a patient who does not have renal calcification probably needs no treatment as the risk of recurrence is small, especially in those over 50 years of age. If there is recurrence, some may benefit from continued observation and advice to maintain a daily urine output exceeding 2.5 litres. There appears to be little case for restricting dietary calcium but it may be worthwhile reducing the intake of oxalate-rich foods (rhubarb, spinach, tea, chocolate, peanuts).

Thiazide diuretics reduce the excretion of calcium and oxalate in the urine without affecting calcium absorption from the gastrointestinal tract and probably halve the rate of stone formation. *Cellulose phosphate* (Calcisorb) binds calcium in the gut, reduces urinary calcium excretion and may benefit calcium stone-formers. *Allopurinol* is effective in those who have normal excretion of calcium but high excretion of urate in the urine. *Potassium citrate*, which alkalinises the urine, should be given to prevent formation of pure uric acid stones.

PHARMACOLOGICAL ASPECTS OF MICTURITION

Some physiology

The smooth muscle fibres of the detrusor comprise the body of the bladder and are continued into the urethral wall. The base of the bladder is formed by the trigone and its muscle fibres extend both into the ureters and into the urethra. The internal sphincter is a concentration of smooth muscle at the bladder neck; it is only well developed in the male and its principal function is to prevent retrograde flow of semen during ejaculation. Distal to this lies the external sphincter, which is composed of striated muscle; its innervation is uncertain but it is capable of sustained contraction. It is separate from the striated musculature of the pelvic floor.

The detrusor is innervated mainly by *cholinergic* fibres, which are excitatory and cause the muscle to contract and urine to be voided. The smooth muscle of the internal sphincter and the urethra is rich in α_1 *adrenoceptors*, activation of which causes contraction. There is an abundant supply of *oestrogen* receptors in the distal two-thirds of the female urethral epithelium, which degenerates after the menopause causing loss of urinary control.

When the detrusor relaxes and the sphincters close, urine is stored; this is achieved by central inhibition of cholinergic tone accompanied by a reflex increase in α-adrenergic activity. Voiding requires contraction of the detrusor accompanied by relaxation of the sphincters. These acts are coordinated by a micturition centre probably in the pons.

Functional abnormalities

The main abnormalities that require treatment are:

Increased bladder activity characterised by uninhibited, unstable contractions of the detrusor, which may be of unknown aetiology or secondary to an upper motor neurone lesion or bladder neck obstruction.

Decreased bladder activity or hypotonicity due to a lower motor neurone lesion or overdistension of the bladder or to both.

Urethral sphincter dysfunction, which is due to various causes including weakness of the muscles and ligaments around the bladder neck, descent of the urethrovesical junction and periurethral fibrosis; the result is stress incontinence.

Atrophic change effects the distal urethra in females.

A number of drugs are used to alleviate abnormal micturition as is now discussed.

Anticholinergics act by blocking the parasympathetic supply to the bladder and are effective for incontinence due to uninhibited contractions of the detrusor. Emepronium bromide or propantheline are used and give considerable benefit to some sufferers but often at the cost of the adverse effects that accompany cholinergic blockade (see p. 470).

Smooth muscle relaxants include flavoxate, which has a papaverine-like action, and dicyclomine, which in addition to having a direct effect on smooth muscle is a cholinergic antagonist.

Tricyclic antidepressants. Imipramine is effective especially for nocturnal but also for daytime incontinence. Its parasympathetic blocking action is probably in part responsible but imipramine may also benefit by altering the patient's sleep profile.

α-adrenoceptor antagonist. Phenoxybenzamine may alleviate obstructive symptoms in about three-quarters of patients with benign hypertrophy of the prostate by relaxing the proximal urethra. It appears to be most useful in patients who are awaiting prostatectomy and are at risk of urinary retention.

Oestrogens either applied locally to the vagina or taken by mouth may benefit urinary incontinence due to atrophy of the urethral epithelium in menopausal women.

Cholinergic drugs may be used to stimulate the detrusor when the bladder is hypotonic. Distigmine is preferred but as its effect is not sustained, intermittent catheterisation is also needed when the hypotonia is chronic.

GUIDE TO FURTHER READING

1 Maclean D, Tudhope G R. Modern diuretic treatment. Br Med J 1983; 286: 1419–1422.
2 Editorial. Carbonic anhydrase. N Engl J Med 1985; 313: 179–181.
3 Editorial. Fending off the potassium pushers. N Engl J Med 1985; 312: 785–787.
4 Editorial. Magnesium deficiency and diuretics. Br Med J 1982; 285: 1377–1378.
5 Editorial. Magnesium, the mimic/antagonist of calcium. N Engl J Med 1984; 310: 1253–1254.
6 Wasnich R D et al. Thiazide effect on the mineral content of bone. N Engl J Med 1983; 309: 344–347.
7 Editorial. Treatment of hypercalciuria. N Engl J Med 1984; 311:116.
8 Murphy M B et al. Glucose intolerance in hypertensive patients treated with diuretics; a fourteen year follow-up. Lancet 1982; 2: 1293–1295.
9 Editorial. Kidney function and drug action. N Engl J Med 1985; 313: 816–817.
10 Editorial. Analgesic nephropathy. Br Med J 1981; 282: 339–340.
11 Resnick N M, Yalla S V. Management of urinary incontinence in the elderly. N Engl J Med 1985; 313: 800–804.
12 Malone-Lee J. The pharmacology of urinary incontinence. In: Barbagallo-Sangiorgi G, Exton-Smith A N, eds. Aging and drug therapy. New York and London: Plenum Press, 1984: 419–440.

28

Blood I: Drugs and haemostasis

The haemostatic system permits blood to remain liquid within vessels, yet to form a solid plug when a vessel is breached. The system is complex but can be separated into three major components, namely:

1. *the formation of fibrin (coagulation)*
2. *the degradation of fibrin (fibrinolysis)*
3. *the platelets*

Drugs which interfere with the haemostatic system are valuable in the management of pathological thrombus formation within blood vessels, or of pathological bleeding. They may be classified according to the components of the system they affect.

THE COAGULATION SYSTEM

In simplified form **the blood coagulation system** is as shown in Figure 28.1.

The *prothrombin time* monitors the *extrinsic system*. The *kaolin cephalin clotting time (KCCT)* monitors the *intrinsic system*.

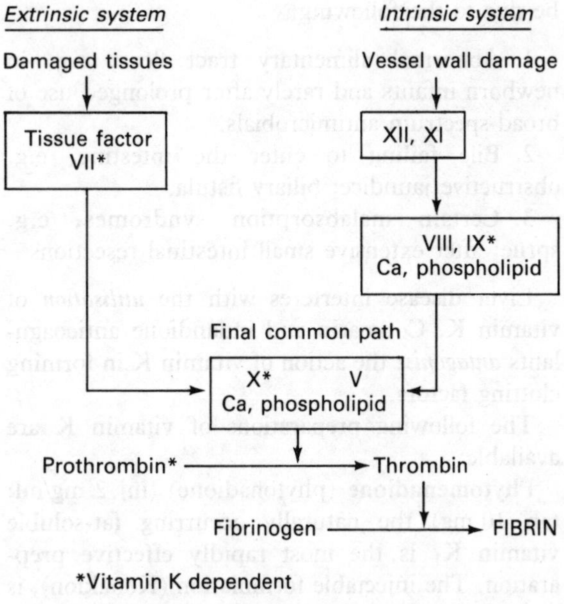

Fig. 28.1 The blood coagulation system

Promotion of coagulation

Vitamin K

Vitamin K (Koagulation vitamin) is necessary for the formation of prothrombin and factors VII, IX and X in the liver. It was discovered during feeding experiments on chicks in which it was found that deficiency of an ether-soluble substance caused a bleeding disease. At about the same time the bleeding tendency in obstructive jaundice was found to be due to prothrombin deficiency and that vitamin K was effective treatment. There are two naturally occurring vitamins K. K_1 is widely distributed in plants and K_2 is synthesised in the alimentary tract by bacteria. Bile is required for the absorption of natural vitamin K, which is fat-soluble.

Metabolism and utilisation take place in the liver. Therefore vitamin K is less effective against hypoprothrombinaemia due to hepatic insufficiency. Indeed the response to vitamin K may be used to assess liver function, since failure of a prolonged prothrombin time to shorten after parenteral administration of vitamin K indicates considerable liver damage. A bleeding tendency due to dietary deficiency of vitamin K probably does not occur in man. However deficiency may be due to the following:

1. Abnormal alimentary tract flora, e.g. in newborn infants and rarely after prolonged use of broad-spectrum antimicrobials.
2. Bile failing to enter the intestine, e.g. obstructive jaundice; biliary fistula.
3. Certain malabsorption syndromes, e.g. sprue; after extensive small intestinal resections.

Liver disease interferes with the *utilisation* of vitamin K. Coumarin and indandione anticoagulants *antagonise* the action of vitamin K in forming clotting factors.

The following preparations of vitamin K are available:

Phytomenadione (phytonadione) (inj 2 mg/ml; tab 10 mg) the naturally occurring fat-soluble vitamin K_1 is the most rapidly effective preparation. The injectable formulation (Konakion), is used in emergency and must be administered slowly as flushing, sweating, chest tightness and peripheral vascular collapse may occur, probably due to the castor oil it contains to make it water miscible. Otherwise phytomenadione may be given i.m. (with care to cause minimum trauma because of the bleeding disorder), s.c. or orally.

Dose. For a bleeding emergency due to prothrombin deficiency induced by a coumarin, phytomenadione 20 mg (by slow i.v. injection) will render the patient refractory to oral anticoagulant (not to heparin) for about 2 weeks. A dose of 10–15 mg for less severe bleeding (orally or i.m.) will allow anticoagulant therapy to continue comparatively smoothly. A dose of 5–10 mg by mouth may be given if there has been no bleeding but the prothrombin time is so prolonged as to cause alarm; otherwise it is sufficient to omit one or two doses of anticoagulant as is judged appropriate.

A substantial dose of vitamin K_1 will reduce prothrombin time in 6–12 h, occasionally 24 h, and more quickly by injection than by mouth; in severe cases doses may need to be repeated (in, say, 24 h).

Menadiol sodium phosphate (Synkavit) (tabs 10 mg; inj. 19 mg/ml) is a synthetic analogue of vitamin K. It is water-soluble and is therefore preferred in malabsorption or in states in which bile flow (necessary for absorption of fat-soluble vitamins) is deficient. The main disadvantage is that it takes 24 h to act but its duration of action is several days.

The dose is 5–40 mg daily; it may be given orally, i.v. or i.m.

Menadiol sodium phosphate cause haemolytic anaemia in moderate doses. The drug should not be given to neonates, especially those that are deficient in glucose-6-phosphate dehydrogenase; their immature livers are unable to cope with the heavy bilirubin load caused by haemolysis and there is danger of kernicterus.

Fat-soluble analogues of vitamin K, which are available in some countries, include acetomenaphthone and menaphthone.

Indications for vitamin K or its analogues are:
1. Bleeding or threatened bleeding due to the coumarin or indandione anticoagulants. Phytomenadione is preferred for its rapid action. Dosage regimens vary according to the degree of urgency, as described above.
2. Hypoprothrombinaemia of the newborn and prematurity. The prothrombin concentration of newborn infants' blood is low, and can be corrected by prophylactic administration of phytomenadione to the mother (1–5 mg) 4–24 h before delivery, or, for greater reliability, to the baby (0.3 mg/kg).
3. Hypoprothrombinaemia due to intestinal malabsorption syndromes. Menadiol sodium phosphate should be used as it is water-soluble.
4. Hypoprothrombinaemia due to salicylates in overdose.

Prevention of coagulation

There are two sorts of anticoagulants:

Indirect acting: coumarin and indandione

drugs. These take about 72 h to become fully effective, act for several days, are given orally and can be antagonised, albeit comparatively slowly, by vitamin K. They are only effective *in vivo*.

Direct acting: heparin, ancrod. These are rapidly effective, only act for a few hours and must be given parenterally. They are effective *in vitro* as well as *in vivo*.

Indirect acting anticoagulants: coumarin and indandione drugs

History. In the early 1920s, in North America, a new and mysterious cattle disease began to trouble farmers. There was haemorrhage, often copious, which was sometimes spontaneous but more often followed trauma; for example, 21 out of 22 cows died following dehorning; 12 out of 25 young bulls died after castration. All had bled to death. Schofield, a veterinary pathologist who first described the disease, quotes a farmer who, 'following the traditions of his elders, cut a slice of skin and cartilage from the ears of all his yearling cattle and then retired for the night. This was to have had the mysterious effect of a blood tonic. The application of ligatures the following morning saved his cattle from immediate death, but due to a continuation of the feed they all succumbed' to haemorrhage within a few weeks. It was found that bleeding only occurred in cattle which had eaten sweet clover, a new fodder crop.* Schofield, observed that it was only mouldy sweet clover that was toxic and performed a simple experiment: 'Good clover stalks and damaged clover stalks were picked from the same hay mow. The good were fed to one rabbit and the damaged to another. The rabbit which ate the good remained well, while the rabbit which ate the bad, died, showing typical (haemorrhagic) lesions. This experiment was duplicated, using a different sample of clover hay. The results were the same.'

This report, and the economic importance of the disease, led to a lot of research, which after 20 years culminated in the isolation of the toxic agent, dicoumarol, which subsequently became widely used in medicine.

Coumarins are present in many plants and are important in the perfume industry; the smell of new mown hay and grass is due to coumarin.

Coumarins include: warfarin (Marevan) (1, 3, 5 mg) and nicoumalone (acenocumarin, Sinthrome) (4 mg).

Indandiones (phenindione) are obsolescent because of allergic adverse reactions unrelated to coagulation, but phenindione (Dindevan) is still available.

The principal differences between these drugs are pharmacokinetic rather than pharmacodynamic so they will be described together.

Mode of action. During the formation of clotting factors II, VII, IX and X in the liver, vitamin K is converted to a biologically inactive metabolite that is then reduced back to the active vitamin by the enzyme epoxide reductase. Coumarins, which are structurally similar to vitamin K, are believed to act as competitive inhibitors of this enzyme and thus limit the availability of the active form of the vitamin to form clotting factors. The great *advantage* over heparin is that they can be given orally: their chief *disadvantage* is the time-lag before they exert their effect due to their *indirect mode of action*, i.e. although synthesis of these clotting factors is quickly prevented, anticoagulation is delayed until the clotting factors already present in the circulation have been cleared. The individual factors are eliminated at different rates (i.e. their $t_{\frac{1}{2}}$ periods differ) and the net result is that anticoagulant protection is not effective until about 72 h after the first dose.

Pharmacokinetics. Warfarin and nicoumalone are readily absorbed from the alimentary tract. All the oral anticoagulants are more than 90% bound to plasma proteins and their action is terminated by metabolism in the liver, except for nicoumalone, which is eliminated in the urine mainly in the unchanged form. The $t_{\frac{1}{2}}$ of warfarin is usually quoted as 44 h but the drug is a racemic mixture, i.e. it is in effect two drugs, namely, the enantiomorphs S(−) ($t_{\frac{1}{2}}$, 32 h) and R(+) ($t_{\frac{1}{2}}$, 54 h). S(−) warfarin is four times more potent than R(+) warfarin. Drugs that interact with warfarin affect these components differently. The $t_{\frac{1}{2}}$ of nicoumalone is 24 h and that of phenindione 5 h.

Management of oral anticoagulants. *Warfarin* is the most generally satisfactory and widely used oral anticoagulant. The following discussion there-

* Schofield F W. J Am Vet Med Assoc 1924; 64:553.

fore refers to it although the principles apply to all drugs of this type.

Monitoring of therapy is by the *prothrombin time*. In the UK a standardised reagent is used and the results are expressed by the laboratory as the British Comparative Ratio (BCR), which is the ratio of the prothrombin time in the patient to that in a normal, un-anticoagulated person (approx 12 sec). Alternatively, the commercially available Thrombotest reagent may be used, in which case the results are expressed as the percentage of normal prothrombin activity.

Oral anticoagulation is often undertaken in patients who are already receiving heparin. The BCR and Thrombotest reliably reflect the degree of prothrombin activity provided that the kaolin cephalin clotting time (KCCT; which measures the anticoagulant effect of heparin, see later) is within the therapeutic ratio range of 1.5–2.5. The BCR may be significantly affected if heparin is administered by repeated i.v. injection, which inevitably induces peaks and troughs in anticoagulant activity but a normal KCCT ratio is usually obtainable if heparin is given by constant i.v. infusion as is now usual. The transfer of a patient from heparin to warfarin can then be accomplished as is described in the following section.

Dosage. There is much inter-individual variation in dose requirements and modification may be required for susceptible persons, for example, those with cardiac failure in whom liver congestion reduces requirements. A detailed scheme relating initial doses of warfarin to BCR that should bring the ratio smoothly into the theraputic range, is reproduced below (Table 28.1), with the permission of the authors and the Editor of the *British Medical Journal*.[*]

Table 28.1 Loading dose schedule for warfarin administration

Day	BCR[†]	Warfarin dose (mg)
1	<1.4	10.0
2 (16 h after 1st dose)	<1.8	10.0
	1.8	1.0
	>1.8	0.5
3 (16 h after 2nd dose)	<2.0	10.0
	2.0–2.1	5.0
	2.2–2.3	4.5
	2.4–2.5	4.0
	2.6–2.7	3.5
	2.8–2.9	3.0
	3.0–3.1	2.5
	3.2–3.3	2.0
	3.4	1.5
	3.5	1.0
	3.6–4.0	0.5
	>4.0	nil
		Predicted maintenance dose
4 (16 h after 3rd dose)	<1.4	>8.0
	1.4	8.0
	1.5	7.5
	1.6–1.7	7.0
	1.8	6.5
	1.9	6.0
	2.0–2.1	5.5
	2.2–2.3	5.0
	2.4–2.6	4.5
	2.7–3.0	4.0
	3.1–3.5	3.5
	3.6–4.0	3.0
	4.1–4.5	Miss next days dose, then give 2 mg.
	>4.5	Miss next 2 days doses, then give 1 mg

Formerly a single priming dose of warfarin 30 mg was used but this is undesirable since the risk of bleeding is increased and the change in the BCR during the first 1–2 days reflects mainly the disappearance of the short-lived factor VII, absence of which confers only doubtful antithrombotic effect.

Maintenance therapy should aim to keep the BCR in the range 2.0–4.5. Warfarin 3–9 mg/day should normally achieve this. When the prothrombin control is stable the BCR need only be measured fortnightly or less often.

The level of anticoagulation is usually adjusted according to the clinical condition and the following guidelines:[‡]

BCR 2.0–2.5 for prophylaxis of deep vein thrombosis including high-risk surgery.

BCR 2.0–3.0 for treatment of active deep vein thrombosis, pulmonary embolism, transient ischaemic attacks, and prophylaxis after hip surgery and surgery for fractured femur.

* Fennerty A et al. Br Med J 1984; 288:1268.

† British Comparative Ratio (see text)

‡ British Society for Haematology guidelines on oral anticoagulants, 1984. Quoted by Poller L. Br Med J 1985; 290:1683.

BCR 3.0–4.5 for recurrent deep vein thrombosis, pulmonary embolism, arterial disease including myocardial infarction, arterial grafts, and prosthetic heart valves and grafts.

Adverse effects. Bleeding is the commonest. A review of 167 studies found that the risk was highest in those with ischaemic cerebrovascular disease (29%), venous thromboembolism (23%) and ischaemic heart disease (19%).* An identifiable risk factor was often present when bleeding was major; in venous thromboembolism these were cancer, recent surgery and paraplegia which are also predisposing factors for thrombosis. Bleeding may occur at any site, but especially the alimentary and renal tracts and brain in those with cerebrovascular disease. Patients with liver disease or vitamin K deficiency are exceptionally intolerant of these compounds.

Warfarin should be avoided in early pregnancy because, apart from the danger of bleeding, it can cause a characteristic abnormality known as the 'fetal warfarin syndrome'.† The drug should also be discontinued near term as it crosses the placental barrier and exacerbates neonatal hypoprothrombinaemia; heparin may be substituted at this stage for it can be discontinued before labour and the anticoagulant effect passes off in about 6 h.

Management of bleeding. Haemorrhage threatening life or major organs should be treated with fresh frozen plasma or concentrates of vitamin K-dependent factors for immediate repair despite the infective and thrombotic risks so created. For lesser bleeding, vitamin K_1 10–20 mg by slow i.v. injection will reduce the BCR to normal in 3–5 h, or orally in up to 12 h, although response may be delayed for up to 24 h. Mild episodes such as bruising, melaena or haematuria call only for the temporary cessation of oral anticoagulant, although if the physician is alarmed, vitamin K_1 5 mg by mouth will reduce the BCR without wholly eliminating the anticoagulant effect.

* Levine M N. Drugs 1985; 30:444.

† Bossed forehead, sunken nose, upper airways obstruction due to underdeveloped cartilage; foci of calcification in the epiphyses giving rise to a stippled appearence on radiographs; the incidence is believed to be 5% in infants exposed to vitamin K antagonists especially in the 6–9th weeks of pregnancy.

Withdrawal of oral anticoagulant. There is evidence that a higher incidence of thrombotic episodes occurs after withdrawal of anticoagulant therapy. The most likely explanation seems to be that this is a 'catching up' phenomenon, i.e. the patients now develop thromboses they would have had earlier but for anticoagulant therapy.

At one time it was thought that *abrupt* withdrawal might be associated with a higher incidence of thromboembolism than gradual withdrawal due to a rebound hypercoagulable state. Withdrawal over several weeks was advocated. However the prolonged effect of warfarin means that sudden cessation of administration amounts to withdrawal of effect over several days. The balance of evidence is that abrupt, as opposed to gradual cessation of therapy does not, of itself, add to the risk of thromboembolism.

Interactions. Oral anticoagulant control requires to be precise both for safety and efficacy. Thus interference by other factors has only to be slight to have clinical importance. Addition of *any* new agent to the treatment of a patient receiving an oral anticoagulant should be undertaken in the knowledge that it may alter the degree of anticoagulation. If a drug that alters the action of warfarin must be used, the BCR should be monitored frequently and the dose of warfarin adjusted during the period of institution *and* withdrawal of the new drug.

The following list, although not comprehensive, identifies medicines that should be avoided and those that may safely be used with warfarin.‡

Analgesics. Avoid aspirin and other NSAIDs because gastric erosions may bleed (they also have antiplatelet effect) and dextropropoxyphene (which inhibits warfarin metabolism, exaggerating its effect) but use paracetamol, ibuprofen, or naproxen. Dextromoramide, methadone and morphine and pethidine may also be used.

Cardiac antidysrhythmics. Avoid amiodarone (which potentiates the effect of warfarin) but atropine, disopyramide and lignocaine may be used.

Antimicrobials. Avoid chloramphenicol, co-trimoxazole, metronidazole, miconazole, lata-

‡ Scott A, Orme M L'E. Adverse Drug Reaction Bulletin 1983; No 103:380. Report. Br Med J 1982; 285: 274.

moxef, long-acting sulphonamides, nalidixic acid and tetracyclines, which inhibit warfarin metabolism, and neomycin (oral) and kanamycin (oral), which impair vitamin K absorption — these all potentiate anticoagulant effect. Rifampicin stimulates warfarin metabolism by enzyme induction and reduces its effect. Penicillins, sodium fusidate and most cephalosporins appear to be safe.

Anticonvulsants. Avoid carbamazepine, Phenytoin and phenobarbitone, enzyme inducers that increase warfarin metabolism, but ethosuximide and sodium valproate are safe.

Antidepressants. Avoid MAOIs, which inhibit warfarin metabolism, but tricyclics may be used.

Antihypertensives. Hydralazine, methyldopa, nifedipine and prazosin may be used.

β-Adrenoceptor blockers. Lipid-soluble drugs (propranolol, metoprolol) may impair warfarin metabolism and a water-soluble agent (atenolol) should be preferred.

Bronchodilators. Aminophylline, salbutamol and terbutaline may be used.

Diuretics. Avoid ethacrynic acid but frusemide and the thiazides may be used.

Gastrointestinal drugs. Avoid cimetidine, which inhibits warfarin metabolism, and preparations containing liquid paraffin, which impairs vitamin K absorption, but ranitidine and most antacids and laxatives may be used.

Hypoglycaemics. Sulphonylureas and biguanides may be used.

Sedatives and anxiolytics. Benzodiazepines may be used.

Oral contraceptives. Avoid, except for progestogen-only.

Others. Careful monitoring of anticoagulation is needed with cholestyramine and clofibrate for these potentiate warfarin.

Direct-acting anticoagulants: *heparin*

Heparin was discovered by a medical student, J. McLean, working at Johns Hopkins Medical School in 1916. Seeking to devote one year to physiological research he was set to 'determine the value of the thromboplastic (clotting) substance in the body'. He found that extracts of various tissues (brain, heart, liver) accelerated clotting but that activity deteriorated during storage. To his surprise, the extract of liver that he had kept longest not only failed to accelerate but actually retarded clotting. His personal account proceeds:

'After more tests and the preparation of other batches of heparphosphatide, I went one morning to the door of Dr. Howell's office, and standing there (he was seated at his desk), I said "Dr. Howell, I have discovered antithrombin." He smiled and said, "Antithrombin is a protein, and you are working with phosphatides. Are you sure that salt is not contaminating your substance?"

'I told him that I was not sure, but that it was a powerful anticoagulant. He was most skeptical. So I had the Deiner, John Schweinhant bleed a cat. Into a small beaker full of its blood, I stirred all of a proven batch of heparphosphatides, and I placed this on Dr. Howell's laboratory table and asked him to call me when it clotted. It never did clot.'* It was heparin.

* Jay McLean expands the tale. 'The discovery of heparin came as a result of my determination to accomplish something by my own ability. . . I was reared without a father, and a child knows when there is no breadwinner to rely upon.' His stepfather was unsympathetic to McLean's plans for a medical education. 'The earthquake and fire in San Francisco in 1906 stripped us of all accumulated assets, our house burned, my stepfather's place of employment burned'. He entered the University of California but had to leave after his second year to work for 15 months to earn money to support his third university year. He joined friends going to the Mojave Desert gold mine and worked as a 'mucker', 'chuck-tender', apprentice miner and mill-hand, 'where we processed ore into beautiful gold bricks'. He returned to University, continuing spare-time jobs (office, blood-counts and urinalysis, museum, book-stores, deck-scrubbing on the San Francisco Bay ferry-boats, lumberyards, railway mail-clerk). He then applied to Johns Hopkins University because he knew that there was a good physiology laboratory there and already he had his mind set on becoming a surgeon trained in physiology rather than the conventional anatomy. But 'my Dean at the University of California had written to the Dean at Johns Hopkins that "I was not the kind of man Hopkins sought"', though McLean did not then know this. After earning enough money to pay for his transcontinental journey (drilling oil-wells for another 15 months) he travelled to Johns Hopkins University. The Registrar 'was surprised to see me and asked if I had not received a letter denying me admission. I told him I had but figured on working a year; and I started to look for a job. The next day word was sent to me to see the Dean. I was informed

Heparin is a mucopolysaccharide, occurs in tissues in mast cells and is prepared commercially from ox lung or bovine or porcine intestinal mucosa.

Mode of action. Heparin is the strongest organic acid in the body and in solution carries an electronegative charge. It depends for its action on the presence in plasma of a substance, antithrombin III, which is a naturally occurring inhibitor of several clotting factors, in particular of activated factor X (Xa) and thrombin. In the presence of small quantities of heparin, antithrombin becomes vastly more active. Inhibition of factor Xa is patricularly important since this factor has a role in both the intrinsic and extrinsic coagulation systems. Furthermore, inhibition of coagulation at the factor Xa stage requires much less heparin that does inhibition at the later thrombin stage. This is the rationale for the use of low doses of subcutaneous heparin in *preventing* thrombus formation as opposed to the high doses that are required to *treat* established thrombosis (see below).

Heparin also reduces the lipaemia that follows a fatty meal by liberating lipoprotein lipase, which hydrolyses triglycerides to free fatty acids that pass into the tissues.

It is suggested that heparin is beneficial in arterial embolus, not only on account of its anticoagulant properties, but also by virtue of its slight vasodilator effect, which may promote collateral circulation.

that there was an unexpected vacancy and I had been admitted to the school. I promptly paid the fees. . . I immediately called on Dr. Howell (professor of physiology) and told him of my desire to prepare for an academic career in surgery and that I wished to devote one whole year to physiological research now. . . I felt I could never do it after graduation. I wanted to determine if I could solve a problem by myself. I told him my savings would just last one year and after that I would have to work for a year before returning to the School. . . I was assigned a sink and attached 'table-drainboard' with a shelf over the sink.' The professor of physiology and other staff 'lunched together, but I was not invited to join them. I was not a colleague. This may have been in part because my drying tissues produced an all-pervading insufferable odour. . .' He also undertook study of organic chemsitry (to remedy an entrance deficiency) and German language in order to read the German chemistry literature. He 'worked nights, Saturdays and Sundays'. After the initial demonstration (above) Dr. Howell 'still did not believe me,' but after further demonstrations he 'became associated with my research problem' (on anticoagulation substance) and they gave heparin to a dog i.v. Dr. Jay McLean was writing this account of the discovery of heparin in 1957 when he died, leaving it uncompleted. See, McLean J. Circulation 1959; XIX:75.

Pharmacokinetics. Heparin is mainly metabolised by the liver but it is partly taken up by the reticuloendothelial system and some is excreted unchanged by the kidney. Delayed elimination occurs in patients with impaired renal function. Differing values are often quoted for the $t_{\frac{1}{2}}$ of heparin because $t_{\frac{1}{2}}$ *increases with the dose given* and also because it may be expressed either as the $t_{\frac{1}{2}}$ of heparin assayed in the plasma or as the $t_{\frac{1}{2}}$ of its anticoagulant effect on the clotting time. With average doses the $t_{\frac{1}{2}}$ of heparin in the plasma is about 80 min and the $t_{\frac{1}{2}}$ of its effect on the clotting time is about 100 min (but with high doses as long as 5 h). Heparin is ineffective by mouth because it is precipitated by acid. Given i.v. the maximum effect is immediate.

Control of heparin therapy. The kaolin cephalin clotting time (KCCT) is the method of choice for measuring the effect of heparin in the UK. The optimum therapeutic range is 1.5–2.5 times the control.

Dose. a. *Treatment of established thrombosis*. The usual regimen is a bolus injection of 5000 units, followed by a constant rate i.v. infusion that delivers 30 000–40 000 units in 24 h. There is very striking variation between individuals in their response to standard doses of heparin. The KCCT should therefore be measured 4–6 h after starting therapy and the infusion rate should be adjusted to keep it in the optimum therapeutic range; this usually requires daily measurements of KCCT.

b. *Prevention of thrombosis*. Heparin is used in *lower doses* for prophylaxis of venous thrombosis in high-risk cases, e.g. postoperatively, or after myocardial infarction. It is usual to give 5000 units s.c. 8 or 12 hourly*. Preparations containing this amount of heparin either as its sodium or calcium salts in 0.2 ml of water are available.

Adverse effects. Bleeding is the only serious acute complication of heparin therapy. It is

* Adjusted, as opposed to fixed-dose, s.c. heparin may be even more effective. Leyvraz P F, et al. N Engl J Med 1983; 309:954.

uncommon, except after surgery. Subfractions of different molecular weights prepared from crude heparin are currently under study to determine whether some retain useful antithrombotic effect with less risk of haemorrhage. Thrombocytopenia occurs in about 2–3% of patients. Osteoporosis tends to develop in patients who have received therapeutic doses of heparin for more than 4 months and may lead to spontaneous bone, including vertebral, fracture. Allergic reactions and skin necrosis occur but are rare. Transient alopecia has been ascribed to heparin.

Heparin antagonism. Heparin effects wear off so rapidly that an antagonist is seldom required except after perfusion for open-heart surgery. When antagonism is needed:

Protamine, a protein obtained from fish sperm, may be used to reverse the anticoagulant action of heparin. It is as strongly basic as heparin is acidic, which explains its immediate antagonism. It is given by slow i.v. injection as protamine sulphate and 1 mg neutralises about 100 units of heparin derived from mucosa (mucous) or 80 units of heparin from lung; but if the heparin was given more than 30 min previously, the dose must be scaled down. Protamine itself has some anticoagulant effect and overdosage must be avoided. The maximum dose must not exceed 50 mg.

Ancrod (Arvin) is an enzyme preparation from the venom of the Malayan pit viper. Its anticoagulant effect is due to a direct proteolytic action on fibrinogen which forms an unstable form of fibrin that is removed from the blood not by fibrinolysis but by the reticuloendothelial system. Ancrod (i.v.) thus depletes fibrinogen and offers an alternative to heparin. Spontaneous haemorrhage with ancrod is rare and although it is weakly antigenic, resistance does not commonly develop. It is contraindicated in pregnancy, in septicaemia and concomitantly with dextran plasma expanders. A specific antidote of highly purified globulins will rapidly reverse the effect of ancrod.

Uses of anticoagulants

The thrombus that forms in leg veins characteristically has a white 'head' consisting principally of platelets adherent to the vessel wall and a red 'tail' which may be only loosely attached to the vessel wall and is comprised of a framework of fibrin in which are caught up the various formed elements of the blood; it is the red part of the thrombus that may threaten life by breaking loose and embolising in the lungs. A thrombus in an artery has a different structure; the swifter flow of blood washes out many of the looser elements such as red cells, and the thrombus consists to a much greater extent of masses of platelets and leucocytes moulded to the shape of the vessel wall. It is therefore not surprising that, in general: *anticoagulant drugs*, which stop formation of fibrin thrombus, are more effective in venous than in arterial thrombosis and *antiplatelet* drugs (see later) are used in arterial but not venous thrombosis.

Anticoagulant drugs are used for the following conditions:

1. **Venous disease.**

a. **Established venous thromboembolism.** The rationale for the use of anticoagulants in the management of deep vein thrombosis and pulmonary embolism is clear — extension of an existing thrombus must be avoided because fresh thrombus is more likely to detach and embolise, and is particularly dangerous if it is in large proximal veins. Effective anticoagulation also helps recanalisation of veins and is believed to clear vein valves of thrombus; it should thus prevent long-term consequences such as swelling of the leg and stasis ulceration. Management is related to the site of thrombosis; for a thrombus in a large proximal vein either surgery or thrombolysis (by urokinase or streptokinase) is often preferred therapy, and an anticoagulant is used to prevent recurrence of thrombosis; small distal thrombi require only elevation and binding of the limb (to increase flow in deep veins) and no anticoagulant; thrombosis in tibial veins should be treated with anticoagulant. Ideally the site of thrombosis should first be established by venography but this is not always feasible. Heparin should be used initially because of its rapid onset of effect. It should be continued until the signs of thrombosis (heat, swelling of the limb) have settled, which may take 5–7 days. Also there is evidence that it takes this long for a thrombus to become firmly adherent to the vessel wall. Usually oral anticoagulant is started on the 3rd to the 5th day in the knowledge that at least 2 days must elapse before the prothrombin time (as BCR) is in the therapeutic range. The risk of recurrence reduces with passage of time after the initial event. In cases of deep vein thrombosis uncomplicated by pulmonary embolus, 3 months of anticoagulant therapy appears adequate.* When there is evidence of pulmonary embolus it is common practice to continue therapy for 6 months.

Clearly these guidelines may have to be modified in the light of individual circumstances.

Anticoagulant therapy may be lifesaving in *thrombo-embolic pulmonary hypertension*.

b. **Prevention of venous thrombosis**. It has been clear for a number of years that oral anticoagulants reduce the risk of thromboembolism in conditions in which there is special hazard, e.g. after surgery. Partly because of the danger of bleeding and partly because of the effort of maintaining control, oral anticoagulants have not been widely adopted in this role but effective use has been made of mechanical methods such as intermittent calf compression during surgery. However numerous trials have shown the protective effect of low doses of heparin (5000 units 8- or 12-hourly s.c.) against deep leg vein thrombosis. The significant fact is that it takes a lot less heparin to *prevent* venous thrombosis than it does to *treat* established thrombosis. This is possibly because heparin acts at an early stage in the cascade of coagulation factors, that leads to fibrin formation (see before). *Dihydroergotamine* is also effective in preventing post-operative deep vein thrombosis, especially in combination with low-dose heparin. The α-adrenergic action of dihydroergotamine increases venous tone and discourages venous pooling.

Apart from its use after surgery, low-dose heparin can be used to prevent venous thromboembolism in other high-risk patients, e.g. those hospitalised and immobilised with strokes, cardiac failure or malignant disease. Spontaneous bleeding has not been a problem with this form of anticoagulant treatment.

Low molecular weight *dextrans* can reduce postoperative thromboembolism if infused i.v. at the time of operation. Dextran 70 (molecular weight 70 000) is used; it may act by reducing platelet adhesiveness.

2. **Cardiac disease.**

Indications for *long-term* oral anticoagulation include:

a. **Atrial fibrillation**, especially when it accompanies mitral stenosis and the danger of systemic embolus is high. Patients with atrial fibrillation from other causes (thyrotoxicosis, chronic sinoatrial disease) probably also benefit particularly when cardiac enlargement indicates a sluggish circulation.

b. **Mitral stenosis with sinus rhythm.** There is a hazard of systemic embolus with stenosis that is more than minimal.

c. **Cardioversion**, to restore sinus rhythm in patients with atrial fibrillation carries some risk of embolism especially in those with rheumatic valve disease and a history of previous embolism. Oral anticoagulant may be started one month before cardioversion and continued for one month after sinus rhythm has been restored.

d. **Acute myocardial infarction**. Anticoagulants were formerly widely used but are now given much less often, although pooling of the data from 32 clinical trials†, some of which gave negative results, indicated that anticoagulation was beneficial. There is certainly a case for anticoagulating patients who have had large infarcts and are in particular danger of forming arterial emboli from *mural thrombus*. Another benefit from anticoagulant therapy may be the prevention of *venous thrombo-embolism* due to immobility and sluggish circulation such as occurs in bad-risk patients (with shock, cardiac dysrhythmias, heart failure). Low-dose subcutaneous heparin will also prevent venous thrombosis in these patients but it is less certain that it will protect against mural thromboemboli.

e. **Crescendo (unstable) angina.** It is usual to

* Lagerstedt C I et al. Lancet 1985; 2:515.

† Chalmers T C et al. N Engl J Med 1977; 297:1091.

hospitalise and anticoagulate the patient and at the same time attempt to control the angina with a nitrate, a β-adrenoceptor blocker and a calcium channel blocker. Clear evidence of the value of anticoagulant therapy in this disorder is lacking. Aspirin, however, appears to protect against myocardial infarction and cardiac death in patients with unstable angina (see index).

f. **Cardiomyopathy**. Mural thrombus may form in both the dilated and hypertrophic types.

g. **Cardiac surgery**. There is a high incidence of embolism from *artificial* aortic and mitral valves although *tissue* valves are less prone to this complication.

3. **Arterial disease**.

a. Heparin may prevent extension of a *thrombus* and hasten its recanalisation; it is commonly used in the acute phase following thrombosis or embolism.

b. Oral anticoagulant therapy may be used to prevent *recurrence* in patients who have suffered a stroke due to thromboembolism but 3 weeks should elapse before starting therapy as there is a danger of precipitating cerebral haemorrhage. In *transient ischaemic attacks* there is no good evidence that anticoagulation reduces the risk of recurrence or of subsequent cerebral infarction. Low-dose aspirin is increasingly used for its antiplatelet effect.

There is no case for treating *peripheral vascular disease*, e.g. intermittent claudication, with an oral anticoagulant.

Long-term anticoagulant therapy

The decision to use long-term therapy in a patient must take into account non-drug factors. The patient should be told of the risk of haemorrhage including those introduced by taking other drugs, and of the signs of bleeding into the alimentary or urinary tracts. All patients should carry a card stating that they are receiving an oral anticoagulant. Anticoagulant therapy should be withheld from a patient who is considered to be unlikely or unable to comply with the requirements of regular medication and blood testing because the danger of the treatment is too great.

The experience of haemorrhagic events is directly related to the level of anticoagulation; safety and good results can only be obtained by close attention to detail. When anticoagulation therapy is well conducted the risk of fatal cerebral haemorrhage is about 1 per 300 years at risk and that for fatal gastrointestinal bleeding is 1 per 1000 to 1 per 2000 years at risk.*

Contraindications to Anticoagulant Therapy

These are mostly conditions in which there is a tendency to bleed and the contraindication is relative rather than absolute, the dangers being balanced against the possible benefits. It is convenient to think of contraindications in the following categories:

1. *Haematological*: a pre-existing bleeding disorder.
2. *Neurological*: recent stroke or surgery to the brain or eye.
3. *Cardiovascular*: severe uncontrolled hypertension.
4. *Alimentary*: active peptic ulcer, inflammatory bowel disease, oesophageal varices, cirrhosis.
5. *Renal*: if function is severely impaired.
6. *Behavioural*: inability or unwillingness to cooperate, dependence on alcohol.
7. *Pregnancy*: in early pregnancy the fetal warfarin syndrome is a hazard and bleeding may cause fetal death in late pregnancy.

Surgery in patients taking anticoagulants

Capillary bleeding stops normally in the presence of coumarin anticoagulants if the prothrombin time (BCR) is at the lower limit of the therapeutic range, for immediate cessation of bleeding depends on platelet activity and vessel retraction. Therefore operations in which good control of larger vessels is assured may safely be performed if the prothrombin concentration is not unduly low. Neurosurgery and ophthalmic and prostatic surgery are particularly hazardous; drainage tubes left in the body and blind needling procedures are

* Loelinger E A, Broekmans A W. In: Dukes M N G, ed. Meyler's Side Effects of Drugs, 10th Ed. Amsterdam: Elsevier 1984:651.

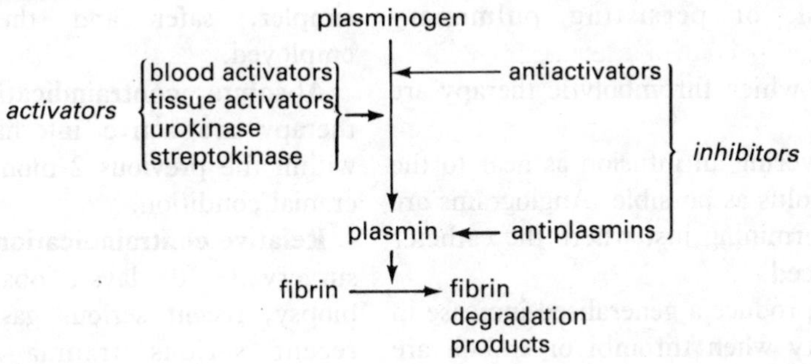

Fig. 28.2 The fibrinolytic enzyme system

liable to provoke bleeding by damaging small arteries.

For elective surgery the oral anticoagulant may be withdrawn about 5 days before the operation and resumed about 3 days after if conditions seem appropriate; low-dose heparin may be used in the intervening period. For dental extractions, omission of the drug for 1–2 days to adjust control to the lower limit of the therapeutic range is adequate; it can be resumed the day after surgery.

For emergency surgery it may be necessary to antagonise the warfarin by vitamin K, and to use heparin as judged appropriate.

DRUGS THAT ACT ON THE FIBRINOLYTIC SYSTEM

The preservation of an intact vascular system requires not only that blood be capable of coagulating but also that there should be a mechanism for removing the products of coagulation when they have served their purpose of stopping a vascular leak. This is the function of **the fibrinolytic system,** the essential features of which are summarised in Figure 28.2.

Since fibrin is the framework of a thrombus, its dissolution clears the clot away. The coagulation and fibrinolytic systems can be seen as being in a state of dynamic equilibrium.

The therapeutic potentialities of fibrinolytic substances are obvious. *Anticoagulants* may *prevent* thrombosis, *fibrinolytics* can *remove* formed thrombi and emboli. Inhibitors of the fibrinolytic system

Inhibitors of the fibrinolytic system can be of value in certain bleeding states characterised by excessive fibrinolysis.

Promotion of fibrinolysis

The approach is to infuse a **plasminogen activator.** There are two preparations:

Streptokinase is extracted from β-haemolytic streptococci. It is antigenic and since most people have circulating antibodies to streptococci, therapy must start with a loading dose large enough to neutralise or inhibit antibodies in the bloodstream.

Urokinase is derived from cultured human renal tubular cells or normal urine; it appears to be non-antigenic.

Both have a $t_{\frac{1}{2}}$ of less than 20 min and must be given by continuous i.v. infusion.

When standard doses are used laboratory control of therapy is probably not needed but the patient must be watched carefully to detect signs of bleeding.

The **objectives** of thrombolytic therapy are*:

a. to restore the circulation to normal by removing obstructing thrombi.

b. to prevent venous valve damage because it is believed that many thrombi originate here and are cleared by effective thrombolysis; damaged venous valves probably cause the post-phlebitic syndrome — the chronically swollen limb that tends later to develop stasis ulceration.

c. to prevent permanent damage due to thromboemboli in lung blood vessels and to

* Report. Br Med J 1980; 280:1585.

reduce the risk of persisting pulmonary hypertension.

The **modes** by which thrombolytic therapy are given are:

Locally by delivering an infusion as near to the thrombus or embolus as possible. Angiograms are invaluable in determining just where the catheter tip should be placed.

Systemically to produce a generalised increase in fibrinolytic activity when thrombi or emboli are multiple.

Uses. Therapy is most useful when thrombosis is of recent origin (<7 days). Thrombolysis is undertaken for extensive occlusion of pelvic and proximal leg veins and for massive pulmonary embolism with shock; in the latter case embolectomy may be avoided.

Thrombi susceptible to thrombolytic therapy disappear dramatically within hours. In arterial thrombosis, thrombolysis is likely to be most effective in those situations in which tissue death distal to the block is slowest, giving time to institute therapy before permanent damage is done, for example in occlusion of limb vessels.

Despite demonstrated value, thrombolytic therapy has never been widely abdopted for the management of thromboembolic disease. Streptokinase and urokinase have the disadvantage that neither is well absorbed *by fibrin thrombi*. Thus they generate plasmin *in the circulation* where it is wasted, or is actually harmful as it also destroys *fibrinogen* and bleeding may result.

Interest has therefore been created by another fibrinolytic agent, namely the plasminogen activator produced by *human tissues*, which is avidly absorbed onto fibrin. This material has been cloned and expressed in bacteria as *recombinant tissue-type plasminogen activator*. Studies in which tissue-type plasminogen activator was administered i.v. in patients with acute myocardial infarction have indicated that it digests thrombi in coronary arteries at least as well or better than streptokinase without depleting plasma fibrinogen to a major degree.* If this material fulfils its promise, thrombolytic therapy should become simpler, safer and therefore more widely employed.

* Verstraete M et al. Lancet 1985; 1: 842 and 2: 965–969.

Absolute contraindications to thrombolytic therapy are active internal bleeding, a stroke within the previous 2 months or an active intracranial condition.

Relative contraindications include recent major surgery (<10 days), obstetric surgery, organ biopsy, recent serious gastrointestinal bleeding, recent serious trauma and severe arterial hypertension.

Adverse effects. The commonest complication is **bleeding** (treated with tranexamic acid) and this occurs more often than in patients treated with heparin. Streptokinase causes allergic reactions, which should be treated with hydrocortisone.

Stanozolol has fibrinolytic activity and is used to treat lipodermatosclerosis, which may complicate deep vein thrombosis.

Prevention of fibrinolysis

Drugs that inhibit fibrinolysis are useful in a number of bleeding disorders.

Tranexamic acid (500 mg) binds to the sites on fibrin that normally accept plasminogen (to be converted to plasmin that dissolves fibrin); fibrinolysis is thus retarded. The $t_{\frac{1}{2}}$ of the drug is about 80 min after an i.v. bolus injection and it is excreted almost entirely in the urine.

Uses. When tissues rich in plasminogen activator are damaged, a hyperplasminaemic bleeding state may occasionally result. The principal proposed indication for tranexamic acid is to prevent excessive bleeding after prostatic surgery, tonsillectomy, uterine cervical conisation and menorrhagia, whether primary or induced by an intra-uterine contraceptive device. Direct evidence of benefit to individual patients is often difficult to define and quantify but there is probably less blood loss and a reduced requirement for blood transfusion. Tranexamic acid may also reduce bleeding after ocular trauma and in haemophiliacs after dental extraction. Claims that the drug prevents rebleeding after subarachnoid haemorrhage have not been substantiated. The drug benefits some patients with *hereditary angioneurotic oedema* presumably by preventing the plasmin-induced uncontrolled activation of the complement system that characterises that condition.

Dose is 1.0–1.5 g, 2–4 times daily by mouth or 1.0 g thrice daily by slow i.v. injection.

Adverse effects are rare; nausea and diarrhoea occur and sometimes hypotension.

Aminocaproic acid is similar to but less effective than tranexamic acid.

Aprotinin (Trasylol) is a naturally occurring inhibitor of proteolytic enzymes that has been used for the treatment of pancreatitis and disseminated intravascular coagulation. Obviously, controlled therapeutic trials in these serious conditions are difficult and the value of aprotinin remains uncertain (it is very costly).

DRUGS THAT AFFECT PLATELET ACTIVITY

Some physiology

Platelets do not stick to healthy endothelium but if a vessel wall is breached they react at the site in the following sequence:

1. Platelets *adhere* to the exposed tissues, especially collagen, and release materials including adenosine diphosphate (ADP) and thromboxane, in response to which,

2. platelets *aggregate* on the original deposition releasing further ADP and thromboxane, whereupon,

3. platelets *transform* into a solid plug and simultaneously *release* their granule contents, including proteins, enzymes, enzyme inhibitors, vasoactive and other peptides and agents that participate in the coagulation process. The system that enables platelets to distinguish between healthy and damaged endothelium involves prostaglandins as shown in Figure 28.3.

The figure summarises the sequences of events through which platelet prostaglandin activity is mediated as a basis to understanding how drugs alter these processes. It may best understood if it is followed thus:

a. As in so many biological systems, *cyclic AMP* plays a key role. *High* concentrations of intra-platelet cyclic AMP inhibit adhesion, aggregation and the release reaction and *low* concentrations have the opposite effect.

b. The quantity of cyclic AMP within platelets is under enzymic control for it is formed by the action of *adenylate cyclase* and degraded by *phosphodiesterase*.

c. Platelet adenylate cyclase in turn is stimulated by *prostacyclin* (from the endothelium) and inhibited by *thromboxane* (from within platelets). Hence the action of thromboxane lowers cyclic AMP concentration and promotes platelet adhesion; prostacyclin raises cyclic AMP concentration and prevents platelet adhesion.

d. Both prostacyclin and thromboxane are derived from arachidonic acid, which is a constituent of cell walls, both platelet and endothelial. *Cyclooxygenase*, an enzyme present in both sites, converts arachidonic acid to endoperoxides, which are further metabolised by *prostacyclin synthase* to prostacyclin in the endothelium and by *thromboxane synthase* to thromboxane in platelets. Thus prostacyclin is principally formed in the endothelium, whereas thromboxane is mainly generated in platelets.

e. The selective activity in prostaglandin synthesis between endothelium and platelets is important; the intact vascular endothelium does not attract platelets because of the high concentration of prostacyclin in the intima. However sub-intimal tissues contain little prostacyclin and immediately they are exposed to the circulation by a breach in the intima, platelets, under the influence of thromboxane, adhere and aggregate. Atheromatous plaques do not generate prostacyclin, which could explain platelet adhesion at these sites.

Inhibitors or activators of aggregation act directly or indirectly by altering the rate of formation or degradation of platelet cyclic AMP.

Drugs that affect platelet activity

Aspirin (75, 300 mg) ($t_{\frac{1}{2}}$ 15 min) inhibits cyclo-oxygenase by acetylation of the enzyme; the salicylate part of the molecule ($t_{\frac{1}{2}}$, 3 h upwards, i.e. saturation kinetics) is irrelevant to this action. The acetylation is irreversible and hence lasts the lifetime of the platelet (7–9 days). It follows from what has been written above that aspirin is capable of preventing formation of *both* thromboxane and prostacyclin and therapeutic interest in its anti-

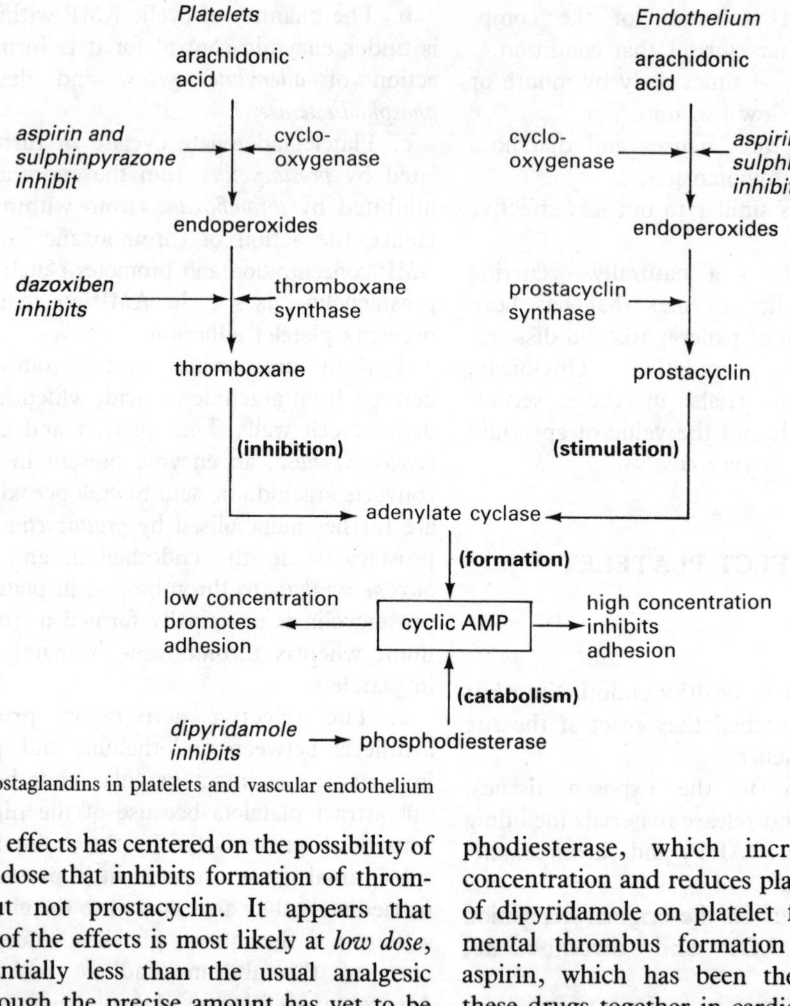

Fig. 28.3 Prostaglandins in platelets and vascular endothelium

thrombotic effects has centered on the possibility of defining a dose that inhibits formation of thromboxane but not prostacyclin. It appears that separation of the effects is most likely at *low dose*, i.e. substantially less than the usual analgesic doses, although the precise amount has yet to be established. Perhaps it is not surprising that large scale (and costly) trials of aspirin for preventing arterial occlusion in the substantial doses of 1.0 g per day and more have shown marginal or no benefit from the drug.

Sulphinpyrazone inhibits several platelet functions possibly by competitive antagonism of platelet cyclo-oxygenase; its effects are dose dependent and reversible. Some days must elapse before the full effect of sulphinpyrazone appears and disappears, probably because active metabolites are formed. The drug is active by mouth and has a $t_{\frac{1}{2}}$ of about 4 h; it is partly metabolised in the liver and partly excreted unchanged. Sulphinpyrazone is a uricosuric and its primary use is in hyperuricaemia and gout.

Dipyridamole reversibly inhibits platelet phosphodiesterase, which increases cyclic AMP concentration and reduces platelet activity. Effects of dipyridamole on platelet function and experimental thrombus formation are potentiated by aspirin, which has been the reason for testing these drugs together in cardiovascular disease.

Dextrans, particularly of molecular weight 70 000 (dextran 70), reduce platelet activity and prolong the bleeding time. These substances differ from the other antiplatelet drugs, which are used for arterial thrombosis; dextran 70 reduces the incidence of postoperative *venous* thrombo-embolism if it is given during or just after surgery.

Dazoxiben was produced as a consequence of an understandably intensive search for drugs that inhibit synthesis of thromboxane but not prostacyclin synthesis. The drug inhibits plasma thromboxane production in a dose-dependent manner and it has negligible activity against prostacyclin synthesis. Its role in cardiovascular disease is being evaluated.

See also: *epoprostenol* (prostacyclin; Flolan), *misoprostol*.

Uses of antiplatelet drugs

Cerebrovascular disease. Patients who suffer *transient ischaemic attacks* are at particular risk of stroke. One multicentre study* compared aspirin 1300 mg/day, sulphinpyrazone 800 mg or both with placebo in 585 patients with threatened stroke. When the effect of sulphinpyrazone and aspirin were calculated separately, sulphinpyrazone was not associated with benefit, but men taking aspirin had a 48% reduction in stroke or death; women taking aspirin experienced no benefit in this study. Until the position is clarified by further trials it seems reasonable to treat patients with transient cerebral or retinal ischaemia with aspirin provided there are no obvious contraindications to its use; in the absence of a reliable guide to dose, 75–150 mg/day is commonly given.

Ischaemic heart disease. Several secondary-prevention trials (i.e. in survivors of myocardial infarction) have shown either no benefit or slight benefit from aspirin, dipyridamole or sulphinpyrazone. The reduction in mortality was similar to that achieved by anticoagulation with warfarin in the past. Until some consensus emerges there seems to be no case routinely to treat patients with ischaemic heart disease with these drugs.

Aspirin does, however, appear to exert a protective effect against myocardial infarction and sudden cardiac death in patients with unstable (crescendo) angina.†

Cardiac surgery. Addition of dipyridamole to conventional anticoagulation with warfarin appears to reduce the risk of thromboembolism in patients with prosthetic (artificial) heart valves. Dipyridamole and aspirin may improve vein-graft patency in patients who have undergone coronary bypass surgery. These reports are encouraging and indicate a possible role for antiplatelet agents in occlusive vascular disease.

Attention is also turning towards the possibilities of modifying platelet function advantageously by manipulating *dietary factors*. For many years it has been known that the Inuit (Eskimos) have a low incidence of acute myocardial infarction and a prolonged bleeding time, but this has been regarded as a matter of interest rather than of emulation. It now seems that these characteristics are due to the nature of the polyunsaturated fatty acids in the Inuit diet (cold-water marine animals), notably eicosapentaenoic acid. This difference in animal fats appears to be related to the necessity for survival of cold water animals that their fats should not solidify at low temperatures. The usual fatty acid acid prostaglandin precursor in fats of other animals is arachidonic acid, consumption of which gives rise to the balanced prostacyclin/thromboxane state described above. A diet rich in fish-oil fatty acid increases the content of eicosapentaenoic acid in platelet and endothelial cell membranes at the expense of arachidonic acid, the metabolism of which is also inhibited because both substances compete for cyclo-oxygenase. It is believed that eicosapentaenoic acid is converted in the platelet into an inactive form of thromboxane, but in the endothelium into a prostacyclin, which is an effective platelet anti-aggregating substance; the haemostatic balance is thereby favourably altered. This view is supported by the results of a 20-year dietary study that showed an inverse relation between fish consumption and coronary heart disease.‡

Local and systemic haemostatics

Many local haemostatic preparations are available; most act by providing a network of fibres that promotes coagulation. They are particularly effective on oozing surfaces, e.g. in tooth sockets.

Human or bovine thrombin is prepared as a powder; if a solution is used it must be freshly made; thrombin is useful in haemophilia and, together with fibrin, in neurosurgery and also when fixing skin grafts. It must never be injected.

Fibrin foam is available as a dry mass of fibrils; it is usually used with thrombin and is absorbed in the body.

Oxidised cellulose (Oxycel) is not well absorbed; it is not used with thrombin on account of its acidity. It is suitable for surface haemostasis,

* The Canadian Cooperative Study Group. N Engl J Med 1978; 299:53.

† Lewis H D et al. N Engl J Med 1983; 309: 396. Cairns J A et al. N Engl J Med 1985; 313:1369.

‡ Kromhout D et al. N Engl J Med 1985; 312: 1205.

but should not be left on as a dressing as it interferes with repair of the epithelium.

Adrenaline may be useful in epistaxis, stopping haemorrhage by inducing local vasoconstriction when applied by packing the nostril with ribbon gauze soaked in adrenaline solution.

Ethamsylate (Dicynene) is given systemically to reduce capillary bleeding, e.g. in menorrhagia.

Sclerosing agents. A variety of chemicals is used to cause inflammation and thrombosis in varicose veins and so induce permanent obliteration. They include injections of ethanolamine oleate and sodium tetradecyl sulphate (given i.v. for varicose veins) and phenol in oil (given submucously for haemorrhoids). Local reactions and embolus can occur.

Haemophilia

Management is a matter for those with special expertise but the following points are of general interest. Bleeding in haemophilia can sometimes be stopped by pressure: edges of superficial wounds should be strapped, not stitched. Tranexamic acid (p. 578) may be used to reduce bleeding after dental extraction. Antihaemophilic globulin (factor VIII) concentrate should be used for bleeding that is more than minor. Desmopressin (DDAVP) increases plasma concentration of factor VIII and its administration may on occasion render transfusion unnecessary, so avoiding the risk of transmitted infection.

GUIDE TO FURTHER READING

1 Gallop P M et al. Carboxylated calcium-binding proteins and vitamin K. N Engl J Med 1980; 302: 1460–1466.
2 Wessler S, Gitel S N. Warfarin. From bedside to bench. N Engl J Med 1984; 311: 1645–1652.
3 Shinton N K (editorial). Standardisation of oral anticoagulant treatment. Br Med J 1983; 287: 1000–1001.
4 Poller L. Editorial. Oral anticoagulants reassessed. Br Med J 1982; 284: 1425–1426.
5 Report. Drug interactions with coumarin derivative anticoagulants. Br Med J 1982; 285: 274–275.
6 Poller L. Therapeutic ranges in oral anticoagulant administration. Br Med J 1985; 290: 1683–1686.
7 Fennerty A G et al. Audit of control of heparin treatment. Br Med J 1985; 290: 27–28.
8 Saltzman E W. Editorial. Treatment of venous thrombosis with subcutaneous heparin. N Engl J Med 1982; 306: 232–233.
9 Editorial. Familial antithrombin III deficiency. Lancet 1983; 1: 1021–1022.
10 Swan H J C, Editorial. Thrombolysis in acute evolving myocardial infarction. N Engl J Med 1983; 308: 1345–1355.
11 Relman A S. Editorial. Intravenous thrombolysis in acute myocardial infarction. A progress report. N Engl J Med 1985; 312: 915–916.
12 Laffel G L, Braunwald E. Thrombolytic therapy. A new strategy for the treatment of acute myocardial infarction. N Engl J Med 1984; 311: 710–717, 770–776.
13 Report. Thrombolytic therapy in treatment. Summary of an NIH consensus conference. Br Med J 1980; 280: 1585–1587.
14 Sharma GVRK et al. Thrombolytic therapy. N Engl J Med 1982; 306: 1268–1276.
15 The Anturane Reinfarction Trial Research Group. Sulphinpyrazone in the prevention of sudden death after myocardial infarction. N Engl J Med 1980; 302: 250–256.
16 Editorial. The Anturane reinfarction trial: reevaluation of outcome. N Engl J Med 1982; 306: 1005–1008.
17 Saltzman E W. Editorial. Aspirin to prevent arterial thrombosis. N Engl J Med 1982; 307: 113–115.
18 de Gaetano G et al. Pharmacology of antiplatelet drugs and clinical trials on thrombosis prevention: a difficult link. Lancet 1982; 2: 974–977.
19 Hampton J R. Editorial. Platelets and coronary disease, round three. Br Med J 1985; 290: 414–415.
20 Glomset J A. Editorial. Fish, fatty acids and human health. Br Med J 1985; 312: 1253–1254.
21 Editorial. DDAVP in haemophilia and von Willebrand's disease. Lancet 1983; 2: 774–775.
22 Editorial. Factor VIII inhibitors in haemophilia. Lancet 1983; 1: 742–743.
23 Buckler P, Douglas A S. Antithrombosis treatment. Br Med J 1983; 287: 196–198.
24 Chalmers T C et al. Evidence favoring the use of anticoagulants in the hospital phase of acute myocardial infarction. N Engl J Med 1977; 297: 1091–1096.
25 Ruckley C V. Editorial. Management of pulmonary embolism. Br Med J 1982; 285: 831–833.
26 Saltzman E W. Editorial. Progress in preventing venous thromboembolism. N Engl J Med 1983; 309: 980–982.

29

Blood II: Iron, vitamin B_{12} (cobalamin) and folic acid

IRON

Iron, which was the metal symbolising strength in magical systems, used to be given to people suffering from weakness, and no doubt many were benefitted, some psychologically (placebo reactors) and others because they had anaemia. The rational use of iron could not begin until both the presence of iron in the 'colouring matter' of the blood and the 'defective nature of the colouring matter' in anaemia were recognised. Early in the 19th century Dr. Pierre Blaud recognised many of the important principles of iron therapy. He said that iron should be given in inorganic form, that small doses should be given at first and increased gradually. He introduced his Pills, containing ferrous carbonate and sulphate. Unfortunately a number of eminent physicians towards the end of the last century considered, for purely theoretical reasons, that inorganic iron could not be absorbed, so that many expensive and relatively ineffective organic iron preparations were developed. Modern research has shown that Dr. Blaud was right.

Some facts and figures

- total body iron 2–6 g (male 50 mg/kg: female 35 mg/kg).
- haemoglobin contains about two-thirds of total iron
- stores comprise about one-third (ferritin and haemosiderin) in marrow, spleen and muscles.
- most of the iron released from the 3 × 10^6 erythrocytes destroyed every sec is reconverted to haemoglobin.
- 6.3 g of haemoglobin (21 mg iron) is cycled/24 h.
- diet (average Western) contains 10–15 mg iron/day.
- normal man absorbs up to 10% dietary iron (i.e. 1–4 mg/day), which is adequate.
- anaemic man absorbs about 30% of dietary iron.
- iron is lost from the body mainly by desquamation from the gut and skin.
- total iron loss/day 0.5–1 mg.
- menstrual loss is about 30 mg/period; menstruating woman are therefore liable to be in negative balance.
- a pregnant woman needs 2.5 mg iron/day extra for the fetus, placenta and normal blood loss at delivery.

Iron absorption takes place chiefly in the upper part of the small intestine where the acid medium enhances solubility, but also throughout the gut, allowing sustained-release preparations to be used. Most iron in food is ferric. Ferrous iron is more readily absorbed than ferric and a reducing agent, such as ascorbic acid, greatly increases the amount of ferrous form; however, substantial doses (200 mg 8-hourly with the iron) are needed to produce a useful clinical effect and combined formulations often do not contain enough. Succinic acid also enhances absorption.

The *process of absorption* after oral administration involves transport of iron into the mucosal cell. Inside the cell there is a protein, apoferritin, which binds iron to form ferritin. The amount of apoferritin in the cell varies in accordance with the state of the body's iron stores, i.e. its need for iron. Iron that is not bound to apoferritin or that dissociates from it, i.e. iron in the so-called labile iron pool, passes on into the plasma where it is bound to the protein, transferrin, and is transported to the bone marrow normoblasts (which incorporate it into haem), the placenta, and iron stores in the liver cells as ferritin) as well as to other cells for the synthesis of myoglobin and iron-containing enzymes. The small amount of *ferritin* in the blood comes from breakdown of iron-storage (ferritin-containing) cells. Its measurement gives a good indication of the state of the body's iron stores.

Iron-deficient subjects absorb up to 20 times as much administered iron as those not in need. When iron is given in large doses the control mechanism fails, resulting in excess absorption and eventually haemosiderosis.

Abnormalities of the small intestine may interfere with either the absorption of iron, as in the malabsorption syndromes and coeliac disease, or possibly with the conversion of iron into a soluble and reduced form. Partial gastrectomy often leads to reduced iron absorption.

The formation of insoluble iron salts (such as phosphate and phytate) in the alkaline medium of most of the small intestine probably explains why much of the iron taken by mouth is not absorbed, even in severe iron deficiency.

It used to be thought that many forms of iron could not be utilised. However, using a radioactive isotope of iron (^{59}Fe) it has not been shown that a varying proportion of the iron in almost all iron compounds, ranging from steel filings to haemoglobin, can be converted into a soluble ferrous form and absorbed.

Interactions. Iron and *tetracycline* bind together in the gut and impairment of absorption of both occurs to a clinically important extent. Doses should be separated by 3 h.

Ascorbic acid increases absorption (above) and *desferrioxamine* binds iron and reduces absorption (below); in *pica* (compulsive eating of non-foods) ingestion of clay (which acts as an ion-exchange resin) reduces iron absorption enough to cause anaemia.

Iron deficiency. The symptoms and signs of iron deficiency are mostly due to anaemia, which is usually microcytic and hypochromic, and is characterised by a low mean corpuscular volume (MCV), low mean corpuscular haemoglobin (MCH), low mean corpuscular haemoglobin concentration (MCHC), low plasma iron concentration, high total iron binding capacity (TIBC, represented by transferrin) and low plasma ferritin (representing iron stores). The sore tongue, atrophic skin and nail changes found in iron deficiency anaemia are due to a reduction in the amount of iron-containing enzymes, which are necessary for renewal of epithelial cells.

Iron therapy

Iron therapy is only indicated for the prevention or cure of iron deficiency. 25 mg of iron per day must be available to the bone marrow if an iron deficiency anaemia is to respond with a rise of 1% of haemoglobin (0.15 g Hb) per day.

(In anaemia of chronic inflammatory disease, e.g. rheumatoid arthritis, the plasma ferritin is normal [or raised], indicating that there is a failure to utilise stored iron, and not lack of iron; iron therapy is not indicated.)

When oral therapy is used it is reasonable to assume that about 30% of the iron will be absorbed and to give about 180 mg of elemental iron daily. However, calculations are not necessary except when iron is given by injection.

Total i.v. iron required (mg) 3 × body wt in kg × Hb deficit* in g/100 ml blood. This formula allows about 0.5 g to replenish stores.

With iron dextran *i.v.* all the iron is biologically available. But with *i.m.* iron dextran about 30% of iron remains bound to muscle, and with iron sorbitol i.m. about 30% is lost by renal excretion. This is taken into account when calculating an i.m. course of iron: 40 mg i.m. = 30 mg i.v.; in pregnancy it is usual to add 0.5 g for needs of placenta, fetus and blood loss at delivery.

Injectable preparations, Iron Dextran and Iron Sorbitol contain 50 mg/ml.

Iron stores are less easily replenished by oral therapy than by injection, and oral therapy should be continued for 2 months after the haemoglobin concentration has returned to normal.

It is illogical to give iron in haemolytic anaemias unless there is also haemoglobinuria, for the iron from the lysed cells remains in the body, and haemosiderosis may ultimately occur.

Iron therapy is needed:

1. *In iron deficiency due to chronic blood loss.*

* i.e. normal Hb (14–16) g/100 ml − patient's Hb/100 ml. Manufacturers provide tables so that doctors do not have to perform arithmetic, which they are liable to get wrong.

2. *In pregnancy*. The fetus takes up to 600 mg of iron from the mother even if she is iron deficient, but the iron stores of a baby born to an iron deficient mother may be abnormally low. Dietary iron is seldom adequate and iron should be given from the fourth month to pregnant women who should be particularly *warned not to let children get at the tablets*, which are often attractively coloured and needlessly sugar-coated.

3. *In various abnormalities of the gastrointestinal tract* in which the proportion of dietary iron absorbed may be reduced (e.g. in malabsorption syndromes generally).

4. *In premature babies*, since they are born with low iron stores, and in babies weaned late. There is very little iron in human milk and even less in cow's milk.

5. *During the treatment of severe pernicious anaemia* with hydroxocobalamin, as the iron stores occasionally become exhausted by the sudden increase in blood formation.

Oral iron preparations

There is an enormous variety of official and proprietary iron preparations. For each milligram of elemental iron taken by mouth, ferrous sulphate is as effective and no more toxic than more expensive preparations. Solutions of iron salts are seldom used as they stain the teeth. It is particularly important to avoid initial overdosage with iron as the resulting symptoms may cause the patient to abandon therapy. A small dose is given at first and increased after a few days. The objective is to give 100–200 mg of elemental iron per day. If given on a full stomach iron causes less gastrointestinal upset but less is absorbed than if it is given between meals. Commonly used preparations, given in divided doses, include:

Ferrous Sulphate Tabs, 200–600 mg daily. Each 200 mg tablet contains 60 mg of elemental iron.

Ferrous Gluconate Tabs, 300–1200 mg daily. Each 300 mg tablet contains 35 mg of elemental iron.

Ferrous Fumarate Tabs, 200–600 mg daily. Each 200 mg tablet contains 65 mg of elemental iron. *Ferrous succinate* and *ferrous glycine sulphate* are alternatives.

Choice of oral iron preparation. Oral iron is widely used, both for therapy and for prophylaxis (pregnancy) of anaemia in people who are feeling little, if at all, ill. Because of this, the occurrence of gastrointestinal upset is particularly important as it is liable to cause the patient to give up taking iron; in one study 32% of pregnant women were not taking the iron prescribed*.

Gastrointestinal upset is minimal if the dose does not exceed 180 mg elemental iron/day.

The evidence as to which preparation provides best iron absorption with least adverse effects is conflicting. Unfortunately, many of the studies on which claims for rival preparations are made, are found, on close inspection, to be inadequate. There is little doubt that valid comparisons can only be made with doses of preparations containing equal amounts of elemental iron *and* under strict double-blind conditions. It has been shown that gastrointestinal upsets can be greatly influenced by expectation.

All the available iron preparations are not listed here, partly because the effort to find and classify them is just not worth making; there are more than 30 marketed in Britain; many contain unnecessary added vitamins (but see ascorbic acid above).

The following course is suggested: Start a patient on ferrous sulphate.† If this seems to cause gastrointestinal upset, try ferrous gluconate, succinate or fumarate. Addition of adequate amounts of ascorbic or succinic acid increases the amount of iron absorbed and so may allow smaller amounts of iron to be given with a lower incidence of gastrointestinal upset. If simple preparations are unsuccessful, and this is unlikely, then the pharmaceutically sophisticated, and expensive preparations may be tried, e.g. formulations that release iron slowly and only after passing the pylorus, from resins, chelates (sodium iron edetate) or plastic matrices (Slow-Fe, Sytron, Feospan etc.) so that iron is released in the lower rather than the upper small intestine. It is often said that the lesser incidence of symptoms is due to less iron being released and absorbed. But this is not invariably so and patients who cannot

* Bonnar J et al Lancet 1969; 1:457.

† Ferrous sulphate is the most toxic form in acute overdose and it may be thought best not to prescribe it to members of households where there are small children.

tolerate standard forms even when taken with food may get as much iron with fewer unpleasant symptoms if they use a sustained-release formulation.

Liquid formulations are available for adults who prefer them and for small children, e.g. *Ferrous Sulphate Mixture, Paediatric*: 5 ml contains 12 mg of elemental iron. *Polysaccharide–iron complex* (Niferex): 5 ml contains 100 mg of elemental iron (it is diluted before use).

There are numerous other iron preparations which can give satisfactory results.

Sustained-release and **chelated** forms of iron (see above) have the advantage that poisoning is less serious if a young mother's supply is consumed by children, a real hazard.

Iron therapy blackens the faeces but does not generally interfere with tests for occult blood (commonly needed in investigation of anaemia), though it may give a false positive with some occult blood tests (e.g. guaiac test).

Duration of therapy: in general a full dose (see above) should be given until the Hb level is normal and then continued at reduced dose for 2 months to replenish stores. Prolonged heavy dose can cause haemosiderosis.

Parenteral iron administration

Parenteral iron administration may be required if iron cannot be absorbed from the intestine, if a sure response is essential in a severe iron deficiency anaemia, as in late pregnancy (though here a blood transfusion may be preferred); if, as sometimes happens for no known reason, oral iron therapy fails or the patient cannot be relied on to take it.

The *speed of response is not quicker* than that with full doses of oral iron reliably taken and normally absorbed, for both provide as much iron as an active marrow can use.

The approximate *total requirement* can be calculated from the haemoglobin level (see above).

The ionised salts of iron are extremely powerful protein precipitants that cannot be used parenterally and un-ionised iron complexes have been developed.

Management is best left to a haematologist if one is available.

Oral iron therapy should be stopped 2 days before injections begin; not only is it unnecessary, but it may promote adverse reactions to the injections by saturating the plasma protein (transferrin) binding sites so that the injection gives higher unbound iron plasma concentration than is safe. This occurs with iron sorbitol; the large molecule of iron dextran does not bind to transferrin.

Intravenous iron. Iron Dextran is used (see below). There is no reason to give intermittent i.v. injections, so it is given by **total dose infusion** (enough iron to correct anaemia and to replenish stores on a single occasion). The technique has obvious advantages: it avoids the inconvenience and unpleasantness of repeated i.m. injections and of incomplete treatment due to non-compliance. The disadvantages are that the patient must arrange to attend hospital for a day, that close supervision is necessary and that ill-effects, sometimes serious (collapse) and death, rarely, can occur. It should only be used where it is essential to do so. A history of any allergy is a contraindication. Resuscitation equipment should be at hand. Technique must be studied and compliance by the doctor must be meticulous.

Intramuscular iron. Iron Sorbitol Inj (Jectofer; 1 ml = 50 mg Fe) is an iron–sorbitol–citric-acid complex of low molecular weight that is rapidly absorbed into the blood from the site of injection (unlike iron dextran). About 30% of a dose is excreted by the kidney in 24 h and the urine may turn black transiently at the time of peak iron excretion. It may also, though normal when passed, turn black on standing for some hours, probably due to formation of iron sulphide by bacterial action.

Iron sorbitol has been found to increase the urinary leucocyte excretion rate in patients with urinary tract infections or non-infective renal disease, and it should probably be avoided in such patients, in whom iron dextran i.m. may be preferred.

Iron sorbitol is bound to the plasma globulin, transferrin, and is stored in the marrow and liver. It is not substantially taken up in the reticulo-endothelial system. Excess unbound iron is excreted in the urine. Iron sorbitol is unsuitable for total dose infusion, probably because, after rapid saturation of transferrin, there would be very high free (toxic) iron levels in the blood (compare with iron dextran below).

Iron sorbitol is given by deep i.m. injection, which can be painful. It stains the skin, but this can be minimised by inserting the needle through the skin and then moving the skin and subcutaneous tissue laterally before entering the muscle so that the needle track becomes angulated when the needle is withdrawn. The dose is up to 1.5 mg/kg/day until the total amount of iron required has been given. The injections are usually painful and general reactions (headache, dizziness, disorientation, nausea, vomiting) occur and sometimes a metallic taste, up to 2 h after injection.

Iron Dextran Inj. (Imferon; 1 ml = 50 mg Fe) given i.m., has been widely used as the least toxic preparation of iron for parenteral use. After iron dextran had been in use for some years it was found that huge doses repeatedly injected into the same site in rats caused local sarcoma but there is no evidence that this constitutes a hazard to man.

Iron dextran has a high molecular weight and is absorbed slowly from the injection site into the lymphatics. It is possible that the prolonged local residual concentration (25% remains after 3 weeks) is relevant to carcinogenesis. Iron sorbitol injection, however, has a low molecular weight and is rapidly absorbed into the blood, and is not carcinogenic in animals, so that, for i.m. use, it may be preferable. However, iron sorbitol probably causes more immediate adverse reactions than iron dextran. The immediate ill-effects of both preparations i.m. are similar in kind. The dose is 2 to 5 ml of the solution i.m. daily in active patients, or once or twice a week in inactive patients.

Iron dextran is not bound to transferrin and is stored in the reticulo-endothelial system (unlike iron sorbitol, see above) and this may be why the total requirements to correct anaemia and to replenish stores can be given in a single slow infusion (see above).

Folic acid deficiency may be unmasked by effective iron therapy. Where there is a deficiency of both iron and folic acid, the deficiency of the latter may not be obvious because haemopoiesis is held back by lack of iron. If iron is supplied there will be an increased formation of red cells and the folic acid deficiency will be disclosed. This is liable to happen in pregnancy and so folic acid is commonly given to all pregnant patients with anaemia (see below); it also ocurs in malabsorption syndromes.

Adverse effects

Some adverse effects of therapeutic doses have been mentioned above.

Ordinary doses of iron preparations sometimes, and slight overdoses very frequently, cause mild gastrointestinal disturbances. These are minimised if the initial dose is small and then slowly increased. Nausea, abdominal pain, and either constipation or diarrhoea, may occur. Gossip in clinics leads expectant mothers to anticipate being upset by iron tablets, and one blind controlled trial has shown that nausea, heartburn, flushes, constipation and diarrhoea were just as common in the control group receiving dummy tablets as in the group taking adequate amounts of iron.

High doses of iron salts by mouth can cause severe gastrointestinal irritation and even necrosis of the mucous membrane. Large amounts are absorbed and cardiovascular collapse occurs. Autopsy has shown severe damage to brain and liver. Tablets of most iron preparations are attractive to children because they are senselessly coloured and sugar-coated. Death may occur if an infant swallows a quantity of these 'sweets' whose danger is not sufficiently recognised. Sustained-release forms are safer in homes where heedless parents live with small children.

Cautionary tale. '. . . a girl aged 19 months was found vomiting after taking 15 or 16 ferrous sulphate tablets. She was taken to hospital and there given salt and water and she vomited again. The mother was told that there were no bed available and she was sent to another hospital. Here she was told that the tablets were not poisonous and would do the child no harm. The child was retching now but not vomiting and the mother was told to take her home and give her plenty of milk to drink. The mother was not satisfied and took the child to another doctor on the way home. He told her to give the child orange juice to drink and she would be all right. The mother then took the child home, put her in her cot, and went to make some orange juice. When she returned the child was dead . . . about four hours after the child had taken the tablets.'* Patients such as this can be saved by prompt chelation therapy.

The clinical course of a typical case of acute iron poisoning has four phases.†.

First, ½–1 h after ingestion: abdominal pain, vomiting, bloody diarrhoea, acidosis and cardiovascular collapse, with coma and death in 4–6 h in 20% of cases.

Second, in 80% of cases, a period of improvement lasting 8–16 h, which may be permanent or which may pass into —

Third, cardiovascular collapse, convulsions, coma and sometimes death about 24 h after ingestion.

Fourth, 1–2 months later, gastrointestinal obstruction from scarring.

Treatment of acute iron poisoning is urgent and immediate efforts to chelate iron in the blood and in the intestine must be made. Raw egg and milk help to bind iron until a chelating agent is available.

The first step should be to give *desferrioxamine* 1–2 g i.m. (repeated 3- to 12-hourly in severe cases) or i.v. (see below); same dose in adults and children.

Only after this should gastric lavage or emesis (see index) be performed. If lavage is used, the water should contain 2 g desferrioxamine/litre. After emptying the stomach, 10 g desferrioxamine in 50 ml water should be left in the stomach.

After this, an i.v. infusion should be set up to correct abnormalities of electrolyte and water balance. Desferrioxamine may also be given i.v. in saline or dextrose, up to 15 mg/kg/h with a maximum dose of 80 mg/kg in 24 h (or 2 g i.m. 12-hourly).

Poisoning is severe if the plasma iron concentration exceeds 90 μmol/l (500 μg/100 ml) or plasma becomes pink (vin rosé) due to the large formation of ferrioxamine (below); i.v. rather than i.m. administration of desferrioxamine is then indicated.

* Spencer I O B Br Med J 1951; 2:1112.

† Aldrich R A In: Wallerstein R O, Metier S R, etd. Iron in Clinical Medicine. University of California Press, 1958.

Chelating capacity. 5 g desferrioxamine chelates iron contained in about 10 tabs ferrous sulphate or gluconate (100 mg desferrioxamine chelates about 8.5 mg iron); this does not apply under the different conditions of iron overload, below.

Where anuria occurs, exchange transfusion should be considered, for the toxicity of large amounts of the iron chelate (ferrioxamine) is unknown.

Desferrioxamine (Desferal) is an iron-chelating agent (see *chelating agents*). During a systematic investigation of Actinomycete metabolites iron-containing substances (sideramines) were discovered; they probably play a part in iron absorption. One of these substances was ferrioxamine. The iron in this can be removed chemically, leaving desferrioxamine. This provides an example of the pharmaceutical industry at its best.

When desferrioxamine comes into contact with ferric iron, its straight-chain molecule twines around it and forms a non-toxic complex of great stability (ferrioxamine), which is excreted in the urine giving it a reddish colour. It has a negligible affinity for other metals in the presence of iron excess and serious adverse effects (retina) are rare.

Desferrioxamine has been shown to be effective in the therapy of acute iron poisoning and in the treatment and perhaps the diagnosis of diseases associated with chronic iron accumulation. A topical formulation is available for ocular siderosis.

Desferrioxamine reduces aluminium accumulation in renal dialysis.

Chronic iron overload The body is unable to excrete any excess of iron so that, if there is uncontrolled iron intake, it accumulates in the body. Grossly excess parenteral iron therapy or a hundred or more blood transfusions (as in treatment of thalassaemia‡) can lead to haemosiderosis. Oral iron therapy has also been reported to cause it over many years.

The treatment of chronic iron overload (e.g. haemochromatosis, haemolytic anaemias and thal-

‡ A 26-year-old subject with β-thalassaemia major had been transfused 404 units of blood over his lifetime. His iron stores were so high (estimated at above 100 g) that he triggered a metal detector at an airport security checkpoint. (Jim R T S Lancet 1979; 2:1028.)

assaemia with transfusional iron overload). Iron may be removed by repeated venesection when there is not anaemia (haemochromatosis) or by chelation (transfusional overload).

The amount of iron bound by desferrioxamine and eliminated in the urine varies with age and route of administration, intermittent i.m., or continous s.c. infusion from a pump carried on a belt.

The most effective way of administration is by 12-hourly nocturnal daily s.c. infusion of desferrioxamine together with ascorbic acid to increase the availability of free iron for chelation. This regimen can put a patient living a life dependent on red-cell transfusions into the desired negative iron balance. High doses of desferrioxamine can damage the retina. The expense of doing this over a long period is currently enormous and raises serious ethical problems in relation to the large numbers of patients with thalassaemia major. There is need for a cheap orally effective alternative.

A single venesection of 500 ml blood, in the absence of anaemia, removes 200 mg iron and can be repeated weekly.

A large intake of tea binds non-haem iron (as in iron-reinforced bread) and may play a modest but useful part in iron overload states; the tannins in tea are probably responsible.

Deficiencies of other metals

Copper, cobalt, molybdenum and manganese deficiencies have all been postulated as rare causes of otherwise unexplained anaemias. The evidence is seldom convincing and they have no place in therapeutics at present. Goitre and nephritis have occasionally followed the use of cobalt in anaemia.

EXTRINSIC AND INTRINSIC FACTORS IN PERNICIOUS ANAEMIA

In 1925, Castle performed classic experiments demonstrating that two factors were required to cure pernicious anaemia. He showed that beef muscle and normal human gastric juice were ineffective when given separately by mouth, but that when they were given *together* a good reticulocyte response was obtained. 'Consequently it was assumed that some unknown but essential interaction between beef muscle as an extrinsic (food) factor and normal human gastric juice as an intrinsic factor appeared to be required for the restoration of normal hematopoiesis in the patient with pernicious anaemia.'* During the succeeding 20 years many successful attempts were made to isolate both the extrinsic and intrinsic factors from various sources. Soon after crystalline cyanocobalamin (vitamin B_{12}) was isolated in 1948 it was generally accepted to be the extrinsic factor. Intrinsic factor (secreted by the gastric mucosa) is a glycoprotein and relatively crude preparations from animal stomachs have been used in the oral therapy of pernicious anaemia. Intrinsic factor acts solely as a vehicle for carrying the important extrinsic factor into the body, but if large oral doses of cobalamins are given they are absorbed independently of intrinsic factor.

Vitamin B_{12} (the cobalamins)

The cellular coenzyme B_{12} is formed in the body from cobalamins (different forms of vitamin B_{12}). *Hydroxocobalamin* is preferred for clinical use.

Pure crystalline cyanocobalamin was prepared from liver simultaneously and independently in the USA and in England in 1948, 22 years after Minot and Murphy first demonstrated the effectiveness of oral liver therapy in pernicious anaemia. The delay was mainly due to the great difficulties of assay of the vitamin. Assay of different fractions is obviously essential during any purification procedure, and for many years the production of a reticulocyte response in patients with pernicious anaemia was the only method. Research has been greatly helped by the discovery that some micro-organisms (*Lactobacillus casei, Euglena gracilis*) require vitamin B_{12} as a growth factor, and this has been used to develop a relatively simple microbiological assay, which is interfered with if the patient is taking antimicrobials; radioimmunoassay now eliminates this inconvenience. Vitamin B_{12}, as prepared, was soon shown

* Castle W B N Engl J Med 1953; 249:603.

to contain cobalt and a cyanide radicle and so was given the chemical name cyanocobalamin, which is now the official name. Its structural formula has been elucidated by crystallographic analysis. Cyanocobalamin is made from cultures of streptomyces.

Function. A deficiency of vitamin B_{12} in the body leads to:

1. A megaloblastic anaemia (Addisonian or pernicious anaemia).
2. Degeneration of the brain, spinal cord and peripheral nerves (subacute combined degeneration): symptoms may be psychiatric or physical.
3. Abnormalities of epithelial tissue, particularly of the alimentary tract (e.g. sore tongue and malabsorption).

The exact **mechanism of action** of vitamin B_{12} in megaloblastosis remains uncertain, but it is known to be a coenzyme for an essential stage in folate metabolism and may affect folate transport into cells.

Requirements of cobalamins are about 1–5 μg daily. Absorption takes place mainly in the ileum. After absorption it is carried in plasma bound to proteins (transcobalamins). It is not significantly metabolised, and excretion is via the bile (there is enterohepatic circulation) and via the kidney. Several years' supply (2–5 mg) is normally stored throughout the body (with about 1 mg in the liver). Most animals cannot synthesise cobalamin and so are directly or indirectly dependent upon micro-organisms for it. Man gets most of his cobalamin from meat; organisms in the human colon synthesise it but it is not absorbed from this part of the intestine, and if rabbits in the wild did not eat their own faeces they would suffer from pernicious anaemia.

Cobalamin does not occur in plants (except in legumes in which it is made by bacteria in root nodules) and **dietary deficiency** occurs amongst people who have not enough money to buy meat, as well as amongst the Vegans, who are a sect of particularly uncompromising vegetarians.* A rare form of dietary deficiency is due to Scandinavian fish tapeworms which live in the gut and take up all the cobalamin before the host has a chance to absorb it.

* Smith A D M. Br Med J 1962; 1:1655.

The fate of cobalamin has been studied by labelling it with radioactive cobalt.

Indications for vitamin B_{12}

Indications for administration are the prevention and cure of conditions due to its deficiency, which commonly presents as megaloblastic anaemia, though neurological or mental disorder (with anaemia) can occur.

In pernicious (Addisonian) anaemia the gastric mucosa is unable to produce intrinsic factor and so vitamin B_{12} deficiency occurs. A pentagastrin-fast achlorhydria is invariably present. Despite its name, the prognosis of a patient with uncomplicated pernicious anaemia, properly treated, is little different from that of the rest of the population. The neurological complications, particularly spasticity, are often permanent, although there may be considerable improvement under treatment. Total removal of the stomach or atrophy of the mucous membrane in a post-gastrectomy remnant may, after several years, lead to a similar anaemia.

Malabsorption syndromes. In coeliac disease and idiopathic steatorrhoea vitamin B_{12} and folic acid deficiency is common although megaloblastic anaemia occurs only relatively late.

A variety of drugs can cause malabsorption including neomycin, colchicine, metformin, slow-release KCl and antiepileptics.

Deprivation of vitamin B_{12} by abnormal bowel flora occurs in tropical sprue, multiple jejunal diverticular, bowel fistulae and blind-loop syndrome. This can be remedied by a broad-spectrum antibiotic, e.g. tetracycline.

Cyanocobalamin has been tried **empirically**, sometimes in enormous doses, without striking success, in a variety of neurological conditions. In some types of peripheral neuritis, especially the diabetic, it has been thought to give benefit, but controlled trials are lacking. Hydroxocobalamin is worth giving in **tobacco amblyopia** where it is possible there is an element of cyanide intoxication from the tobacco, and cyanocobalamin may be formed.

Diagnostic use. Large doses of hydroxocobalamin may induce an incomplete response in pure folic acid deficiency, but response to a tiny dose (2–4 μg) is diagnostic of cobalamin deficiency.

In addition the *Schilling test* of vitamin B_{12} absorption may be used. *First*: the patient is given a small dose of radioactive vitamin B_{12} *orally*, followed shortly by a large dose of non-radioactive vitamin B_{12} *i.m.* The large injected dose saturates binding sites in the body so that if any of the oral radioactive dose is absorbed it will not find any binding sites available and will be eliminated in the urine where it can easily be measured. In pernicious anaemia gut absorption and therefore urinary elimination of radioactivity is negligible. *Second*: the test is then repeated with intrinsic factor added to the oral dose. The radioactive vitamin B_{12} is now absorbed and is detected in the urine. Both stages of the test are needed to maximise reliability of diagnosis of pernicious anaemia.

Contraindications: *undiagnosed anaemia*; Therapy of pernicious anaemia must be both adequate and life-long, so that accurate diagnosis is essential. Even a single dose interferes with diagnosis by blood picture for weeks, although the Schilling test remains abnormal. Inclusion of small amounts of cyanocobalamin in oral tonics is probably harmless but implies an irresponsible attitude in both promoter and prescriber. It is a bad thing that a patient's health should ever depend on not absorbing the physician's inadequate therapy.

Preparations and dosage

Hydroxocobalamin is bound to plasma protein to a greater extent that is *cyanocobalamin*, with the result that there is less free to be excreted in the urine after an injection so that rather lower doses at longer intervals are adequate. This is why it is preferred to cyanocobalamin, though the latter can give satisfactory results (except in tobacco amblyopia).

The initial dose in cobalamin deficiency anaemias, including uncomplicated pernicious anaemia, is hydroxocobalamin 1 mg i.m. every 2–3 days for 5 doses to induce remission and to replenish stores. Maintenance may be 1 mg 3-monthly; higher doses will not find binding sites and will be eliminated in the urine. But higher doses should probably be used in renal and hepatic disease (due to defects in conversion to the active coenzyme and excretion).

The initial stimulation of haemoglobin synthesis often depletes the *iron* and *folate* stores and supplements of these may be needed.

Hypokalaemia may occur at the height of the erythrocyte response in severe cases. It is attributed to uptake of K by the rapidly increasing erythrocyte mass. Oral K should be given.

Failure to respond implies inaccurate diagnosis or the presence of other disease such as carcinoma, hypothyroidism or chronic infection. If neurological complications have occurred the dosage can be doubled, though this probably does no good, but some would give all cases milligram doses initially as hydroxocobalamin is non-toxic.

Because of increased urinary excretion when high blood levels are achieved, inadequate response should be treated by increased frequency of injections as well as increased amount.

Haemoglobin estimations are necessary at least every 6 months to check adequacy of therapy and for early detection of iron deficiency anaemia due to carcinoma of the stomach, which occurs in about 5% of patients with pernicious anaemia.

When injections are refused or are impracticable (rare allergy), administration as snuff or aerosol has been effective, but these routes are potentially less reliable. Large daily oral doses (300 μg) are probably preferable. Monitoring of the blood must be close.

Adverse reactions virtually do not occur, but its use as a 'tonic' is an abuse of a powerful remedy for it may obscure the diagnosis of pernicious anaemia, which is a matter of great importance in a disease requiring life-long therapy and prone to serious neurological complications.

Liver extracts contain folic acid and cyanocobalamin. They were the mainstay of therapy for pernicious anaemia for about 20 years, but the introduction of pure cobalamins has made them obsolete.

In pernicious anaemia, folic acid should not be used. Although it will improve the anaemia, it allows progression of subacute combined degeneration of the nervous system. A patient with pernicious anaemia who has been given folic acid is in a dangerous situation.

There are oral preparations containing a miscellany of substances necessary for blood formation, including iron, folic acid, cyanocobalamin and other vitamins, liver, stomach extracts, etc, generally in doses insufficient to cure anaemias, but often sufficient to interfere with diagnosis. They are promoted to preserve the aged in health, for anaemia and as tonics.

Both their indiscriminate promotion by commercial interests and their use by physicians in undiagnosed cases shows a disregard for patients' interests that is inconsiderate at best and callous at worst. Regulatory authorities are in a position to eliminate the preparations.

FOLIC ACID (PTEROYLGLUTAMIC ACID)

Folic acid was so named because it was discovered as a bacterial growth factor present in spinach leaves (folium = a leaf). It is one of the B group of vitamins and was soon shown to be the same substance as that present in yeast and liver which cured a nutritional macrocytic anaemia in Indian women, a similar experimental anaemia in monkeys, an anaemia and growth failure in chicks, and to be a growth factor for a variety of micro-organisms.

Functions. Folic acid is itself inactive. It is converted into the biologically active coenzyme tetrahydrofolic acid, which is important in the biosynthesis of amino and nucleic acids, and therefore in cell division. The formyl derivative of tetrahydrofolic acid is folinic acid or citrovorum factor (leucovorin) and this can be used where the body fails to effect the conversion of folic acid (see folic acid antagonists).

Ascorbic acid protects the active tetrahydrofolic acid from oxidation, and the anaemia of scurvy, although usually normoblastic, may be megaloblastic due to deficiency of tetrahydrofolic acid.

Deficiency of folic acid leads to a megaloblastic anaemia probably because it is necessary for the production of the purines and pyrimidines, which are essential precursors of deoxyribonucleic acid (DNA). The megaloblastic marrow of cobalamin deficiency is due to interference with folic acid utilisation since the morphological changes of such deficiency can be reversed by folic acid. However, it is vital to realise that folic acid does not provide adequate treatment for pernicious anaemia. Folic acid antagonists (which see) are sometimes used in treatment for acute leukaemias.

Occurrence and requirements. Folic acid is widely distributed, especially in green vegetables, yeast and liver. It is present in food mostly in conjugated forms (polyglutamates). Many body tissues contain an enzyme that releases the folic acid from the conjugates. Daily requirement of pure folic acid is about 50 μg and a diet containing 400 μg of polyglutamates will provide this. It is synthesised by bacteria in the large intestine, but as the sole site of absorption is the jejunum, this is irrelevant. Body stores are adequate for several months only.

Indications are the prevention and cure of the megaloblastic anaemia due to deficiency of folic acid:

Dietary deficiency. There is enough folic acid in an ordinary Western diet for normal people, but its deficiency plays some part in the complex nutritional macrocytic anaemias that are common in the economically underdeveloped areas of the world. A megaloblastic anaemia of infancy has been caused by dietary deficiency of folic acid, which was absent from certain brands of dried milk. **Body stores** are smaller than of vitamin B_{12}, there being only several months supply.

In malabsorption syndromes, particularly steatorrhoea, gluten enteropathy and sprue, poor absorption of folic acid from the small intestine often leads to a megaloblastic anaemia.

In pregnancy, folate requirement is increased from 400 μg to 800 μg/day and mild deficiency is common, with a minority of cases developing severe megaloblastic anaemia. For this reason routine folic acid administration is added to routine iron administration. The dose needed is about 300 μg folic acid a day, which is insufficient to alter the blood picture of pernicious anaemia and so there is no risk of masking that disease, which is also very rare in women of reproductive age and is probably incompatible with a successful pregnancy. A large number of preparations of iron with folic acid is available, e.g. *Iron and Folic Acid Tabs*: ferrous fumarate 304 mg (100 mg iron) plus folic acid 350 μg. They are only suitable for prevention. Larger doses may be used in therapy of the anaemia (below); it will remit spontaneously some weeks after delivery. Vigorous iron therapy in pregnancy may unmask a folic acid deficiency.

In chronic haemolytic states folic acid requirement is increased.

Anticonvulsant drugs, particularly phenytoin, primidone and phenobarbitone, occasionally cause a macrocytic anaemia that responds to folic acid. This may be due to enzyme induction by the anticonvulsants increasing need for folate to perform hydroxylations (see under *epilepsy*) but other factors may be involved. Some **antimalarials** (e.g. pyrimethamine) may interfere with conversion of folates to the active tetrahydrofolic acid, causing macrocytic anaemia, as may nitrofurantoin.

Diagnostic use is similar to that of cyanocobalamin.

Preparations and dosage. Synthetic folic acid (5 mg) is taken orally; 5 mg daily is usually given for 4 months, or indefinitely if the cause of deficiency cannot be removed. The sodium salt is available for injection and it is reasonable to start treatment of a severe deficiency with it. After the first few doses oral supplements are adequate even in the malabsorption syndromes. There is no advantage in giving folinic instead of folic acid, except in the treatment of the toxic effects of folic acid antagonists in order to by-pass the site of metabolic block.

For dose in pregnancy, see above.

Adverse reactions: allergy occurs rarely.

GUIDE TO FURTHER READING

1 Crosby W H. Who needs iron? N Engl J Med 1977; 297:543.
2 Weinbren K et al. Intramuscular injections of iron compounds and oncogenesis in man. Br Med J 1978; 1:683.
3 Bonnar J et al. Do pregnant women take their iron? Lancet 1969; 1:457.
4 Callender S. Quick- and slow-release iron: a double-blind trial with a single daily dose regimen. Br Med J 1969; 4:531.
5 De Alarcon P A et al. Iron absorption in thalassaemia syndromes and its inhibition by tea. N Engl J Med 1979; 300:5.
6 Neuvonen P J et al. Interference of iron with absorption of tetracyclines in man. Br Med J 1970; 4:532.
7 Castle W B. Development of knowledge concerning the gastric intrinsic factor and its relation to pernicious anaemia. N Engl J Med 1953; 249:603.
8 Smith E L. Crystalline anti-pernicious-anaemia factor. Br Med J 1949; 2:1367.
9 Chalmers J N M. Comparison of hydroxocobalamin and cyanocobalamin in the treatment of pernicious anaemia. Lancet 1965; 2:1305.
10 Castle W B. Treatment of pernicious anaemia: historical aspects. Clin Pharmacol Ther 1966; 7:147.
11 Rosenberg I H. Folate absorption and malabsorption. N Engl J Med 1975; 293:1303.
12 Editorial. Folate and aplasia of the bone marrow. N Engl J Med 1978; 298:506.
13 Reizenstein P et al. Overprescribing iron tablets to elderly people in Sweden. Br Med J 1979; 2:962.
14 Bjorn-Reemusen E. Iron absorption: present knowledge and controversies. Lancet 1983; 1:914.
15 Finch C A et al. Perspectives in iron metabolism. N Engl J Med 1982; 306:1520.
16 Wolfe L et al. Prevention of cardiac disease by subcutaneous deferoxamine in patients with thalassemia major. N Engl J Med 1985; 312:1600.
17 Nienhuis A W. Vitamin C and iron. N Engl J Med 1981; 304:170.
18 Lewes G J. Do women with menorrhagia need iron? Br Med J 1982; 284:1158.

30

Respiratory system

COUGH

There are two sorts of cough, the useful and the useless. Cough is useful when it effectively expels secretions, exudates, transudates or extraneous material from the respiratory tract, i.e. when it is *productive*; it is useless when it is *unproductive*. Useful cough should be allowed to serve its purpose and be suppressed only when it is exhausting the patient or is dangerous, e.g. after eye surgery. Useless cough should be stopped, or, if it is due to thick secretions that cannot be expelled, made useful if possible.

Clinical assessment of the frequency and intensity of cough of disease by objective recording by way of a microphone allows assessment of antitussives despite the great spontaneous fluctuations. Such recording has shown patients' own reports of their cough to be too unreliable to provide valid drug comparisons.

Experimental cough, induced by inhalation of an irritant, e.g. citric acid, does not correlate well with cough of disease, so that it is unreliable for detecting antitussive effect, but it can be used to delineate the time course of action of drugs.

Placebo effects in cough are great.

Sites of action

Sites of action of useful antitussives are:

1. Periperal sites

(a) On the *afferent side of the cough reflex* by reducing input of stimuli from throat, larynx, trachea, e.g. a warm moist atmosphere, demulcents* in the pharynx.

(b) On the *efferent side of the cough reflex*: measures to render secretions more easily removable (mucolytics, postural drainage) will reduce the amount of coughing needed, by increasing its efficiency.

The best antitussive is removal of the cause of the cough by, for example, chemotherapy or surgery.

2. Central nervous system

Agents may act on the medullary paths of the cough reflex (opioids), on the cerebral cortex and on the sub-cortical paths (opioids and sedatives in general).

If it is true that cough can result from summation of sub-threshold stimuli from mechano- and chemoreceptors from many parts of the respiratory tract and outside it, e.g. diaphragm and

* From Latin, *demulcere*, to carress soothingly.

pleura, it is not surprising that it may be reduced by drugs apparently acting at sites far removed from the site of the disease, e.g. demulcents in bronchitis, though it has not been conclusively shown that any such relief is other than a placebo effect. Also, there is no doubt that a cough can be induced by psychogenic factors such as by anxiety not to cough, when it is socially disadvantageous to do so, e.g. when in hiding or during the quiet parts of a musical concert, and can be reduced by a placebo.

Cough is also under substantial voluntary control, as witness the increase during the louder passages of a London winter orchestral concert. A good woman with a cough may sleep better alone and free from fear of depriving her exhausted spouse of sleep, whilst a child may cough less if in reassuring company in his or her parents' room. Considerations such as these are relevant to practical therapeutics.

COUGH SUPPRESSION

Antitussives that act peripherally

The patient should stop smoking.

When the cough arises *above the larynx* then syrups and lozenges that glutinously and soothingly coat the pharynx (*demulcents*) may be used, e.g. Simple Linctus (mainly syrup; sugar). Small children are prone to swallow lozenges and so a confection on a stick may be preferred.

Linctuses are demulcent preparations that can be used alone and as vehicles of other antitussives. That their exact constitution is not critical was known and taught to medical students in 1896*. 'Many of you know that this (simple) linctus used to be very much thicker than it is now, and very likely the thicker linctus was more efficacious. The reason why it was made thinner was this. It was discovered that a large number of children came to the surgery complaining of cough, and they were given the linctus, but instead of their using it as a medicine, they took it to an old woman out in Smithfield, who gave them each a penny, took their linctus, and made jam tarts with it.'*

* Brunton L (1897). Lectures on the action of medicines. London: Macmillan.

When cough arises *below the larynx*, water aerosol inhalations and a warm environment often give relief. If it is wished to make the inhalation smell therapeutic, Benzoin Tincture Cpd† may be added to the hot water. Benzoin inhalation may also promote secretion of dilute mucus and so help to give a protective coating to the inflamed mucous membrane but its effects are more probably solely psychological. Menthol and eucalyptus provide similar therapeutic smell.

Intractable cough can be a severe problem in patients with bronchial carcinoma. Lignocaine administered by a nebuliser appears to control this type of cough effectively and delays the need to use potent opioids such as diamorphine.

Antitussives that act on the central nervous system

In general, when it is desired to suppress cough, drugs that act on the pathways of the cough reflex in the medulla are used. When these drugs are opioids then part of the effect may result from their actions on higher nervous centres as tranquillisers. The morphine-related antitussives principally used are relatively non-addicting and have little depressant effect on the respiratory centre, though they may dry the mucosa and thicken the sputum. They include codeine, pholcodine, noscapine (narcotine) and dextromethorphan. It is possible that as good results can be obtained with these as with more addicting substances, e.g. morphine, diamorphine and methadone, which are powerful respiratory depressants. Linctuses of codeine, pholcodine and methadone are often used. Codeine needs to be given in high doses, say 60 mg, and a tablet is satisfactory. In bronchogenic carcinoma Strong Pholcodeine Linctus or even Diamorphine Linctus may be required.

Sedation reduces cough. Antihistamines (H_1-receptor) with sedative and anticholinergic actions (e.g. diphenhydramine) can also suppress cough by these (but not by antihistamine) actions; they may need to be given in doses that also cause drowsiness and thus they are usually combined with other drugs. A great many synthetic,

† Friar's Balsam.

centrally acting non-opioid antitussives have come and gone; patients will not suffer if the physician ignores these.

MUCOLYTICS AND EXPECTORANTS

Normally about 100 ml of fluid is produced from the respiratory tract each day and most of it is probably swallowed. Respiratory mucus consists largely of water and its slimy character is due to glycoproteins linked together by disulphide bonds to form polymers. In pathological states much more mucus may be produced and proteins exude from bronchial cells, bond with glycoproteins and form larger polymers with the result that the mucus becomes more viscous. Patients with chest disease can have difficulty in clearing their chests of viscous sputum by cough because the bronchial cilia are rendered ineffective. They can be assisted by drugs that liquify mucus.

Mucolytics

Bromhexine (Bisolvon) (8 mg) is a synthetic derivative of a plant alkaloid (vasicine) that has been used as an expectorant in the East for many years. Taken orally, it can reduce viscosity of bronchial secretion. Larger volumes of sputum are thus expectorated, but ventilatory function is not necessarily improved. Bromhexine may be worth trying in bronchitics with slight-to-moderate airway obstruction. The oral dose is 8–16 mg 6- to 8-hourly. It may cause gastrointestinal irritation.

Acetylcysteine (Airbron) and methylcysteine (Visclair) have free sulphydryl groups that open disulphide bonds in mucus and reduce its viscosity. They are given by inhalation (or instillation) and may be useful chiefly when particularly viscous secretion is a problem (cystic fibrosis, care of tracheostomies). *Carbocisteine* (Mucodyne) is an alternative. Acetylcysteine may also be taken by mouth and achieves high concentration in the lung. It may cause gastrointestinal irritation and allergic reactions.

Detergents given as aerosols, e.g. tyloxapol (Alevaire) are probably not significantly superior to the above.

Iodide stimulates the production of thin bronchial secretion by a direct action on secretory cells. It is generally necessary to give it to the limits of tolerance and so it is not popular. Iodide has an unpleasant metallic taste and may cause painful swelling of the salivary and lachrymal glands after a few doses. With long-term treatment gastric intolerance or hypothyroidism may occur but these are largely avoided if treatment is intermittent.

Water inhalation as an aerosol, though cheap, is not to be despised. The visible vapour from a boiling kettle is an aerosol of water, it is not steam, which is invisible. Simply hydrating a dehydrated patient can have a beneficial effect in lowering sputum viscosity.

Expectorants

Expectorants are held to encourage productive cough by increasing the volume of bronchial secretion; they may have little more than placebo value. The group includes iodide, chlorides, bicarbonates, acetates, squill, ipecacuanha, creosotes, volatile oils and guaiacols.

Cough mixtures

There are innumerable combinations of antitussives, expectorants, mucolytics, bronchodilators and sedatives. Sedative antihistamines are included in some mixtures. Every formularly is replete with cough mixtures. A selection is mentioned below. Choice is not critical.

CHOICE OF DRUG THERAPY IN COUGH

Choice of drug therapy in cough depends on numerous factors. For example, cough due to invasion of a bronchus by a neoplasm requires different treatment to that due to chronic bronchitis with broncospasm. As always, it is necessary to have a clear idea of what it is intended to achieve before starting to use drugs.

The following are general recommendations only; there is usually a wide choice of agents of approximately equal efficacy for any one case.

1. *For simple suppression of useless cough.* Codeine, pholcodine, methadone linctuses (in

increasing order of efficacy) may be used in large, infrequent doses. In children, cough is nearly always useful and sedation at night is more effective to give rest than is codeine. Pertussis is an exception and sedation, codeine and atropine methonitrate may be tried; salbutamol 0.3 mg/kg/day orally has been claimed to be effective.

2. *To increase bronchial secretion slightly and to liquefy what is there*. Water inhalations with or without Menthol and Benzoin Inhalation, or Menthol and Eucalyptus Inhalation may provide comfort harmlessly.

Bromhexine or acetylcysteine orally may be useful.

If a brisk increase in secretion is desired potassium iodide is effective but adverse effects may be unavoidable.

3. *For cough originating in the pharyngeal region*. Glutinous sweets or lozenges (demulcents), incorporating a cough suppressant or not, as appropriate, are used.

All drug formularies include numerous remedies for cough, some of which contain both an expectorant and a suppressive, e.g. Opiate Squill Linctus (Gee's Linctus). The rationale of this apparent therapeutic incompatability is to make coughing more effective whilst also controlling it. Such mixtures have not been evaluated scientifically.

4. *For bronchoconstriction complicating cough*. Bronchodilator drugs can be used, e.g. orciprenaline, perhaps with bromhexine (Alupent Expectorant). Atropine is undesirable as it thickens bronchial secretion. Oxygen inhalation thickens secretions and patients having oxygen may need expectorants. The oxygen must be bubbled through water to avoid drying the secretions and so rendering them even more viscous.

RESPIRATORY STIMULANTS (ANALEPTICS)

The drugs used are central nervous system stimulants and the therapeutic dose is close to that which causes convulsions. Their use must therefore be carefully monitored.

Nikethamide causes an increase in the rate and depth of respiration by stimulating the medullary respiratory centres both directly and reflexly through the carotid body. Its effect is transient and it is given by slow i.v. injection, repeated at 15–30 min intervals as necessary. Adverse effects include restlessness and twitching (at first round the mouth), itching, vomiting, flushing and cardiac dysrhythmias.

Doxapram (Dopram) acts like nikethamide but produces a greater effect on the depth than on the rate of respiration. Although the benefit from a single i.v. injection is only about 5 min, doxapram has a larger margin between therapeutic and toxic doses than other respiratory stimulants and is suitable for maintenance treatment. It is given by i.v. infusion, 0.5–4 mg per minute according to the response of the patient. Coughing and laryngospasm that develop after its use may represent a return of normal protective responses. The adverse effects are as described for nikethamide and in addition it causes patients to experience a feeling of perineal warmth; in high doses the blood pressure is elevated.

Ethamivan (Clairvan) is similar to nikethamide.

Aminophylline is a respiratory stimulant and may be infused slowly i.v. (500 mg in 6 h).

Acetazolamide (see also Chapter 27) promotes bicarbonate diuresis and metabolic acidosis, which may be a useful stimulus to respiration during exacerbation of chronic obstructive lung disease or weaning from mechanical ventilation.

Uses. Respiratory stimulants have some place in some cases of acute ventilatory failure due to the following:

(a) acute exacerbations of chronic lung disease with hypercapnia, drowsiness and inability to cough. As a short-term measure, stimulation of respiration with supervised sputum clearance may obviate tracheal intubation and mechanical ventilation and 'buy time' for chemotherapy to control infection.

(b) removal of the hypoxic drive to respiration by giving oxygen at too high a concentration to patients with chronic lung disease.

(c) apnoea in premature infants; aminophylline may benefit some cases.

Avoid respiratory stimulants if possible in patients with epilepsy (risk of convulsions), ischaemic heart disease or hypertension.

Contraindications. Respiratory stimulants should not be used unless hypoxaemia is accompanied by hypercapnia, i.e. not in acute asthma, neurological or muscular disease or drug overdose. In chronic ventilatory failure with hypercapnia, although alveolar ventilation may increase so does the muscular work of breathing. Thus, increased CO_2 production offsets the CO_2 eliminated by increased ventilation.

A number of other agents have been favoured on rather dubious grounds as respiratory stimulants but are now obsolete. They include *picrotoxin* (a powerful convulsant from an Asian plant that was also used as a bitter in beer until its effect was defined), *strychnine, lobeline* and *menthol* (occasionally, cases of poisoning occur from menthol included in proprietary inhalations and 'cold' remedies to make them smell therapeutic). *Thujone* is a convulsant that used to be an ingredient of absinthe (a potent alcoholic drink flavoured with the plant *Artemisia*, which contains thujone).

Irritant vapours, to be inhaled, have an analeptic effect in fainting, e.g. Aromatic Solution of Ammonia (sal volatile). No doubt they sometimes 'recall the exorbitant and deserting spirits to their proper stations' (Thomas Sydenham, 1624–1689).

OXYGEN THERAPY

Oxygen as used in therapy should be presented with the same care as any other drug: it should be used for a well-defined purpose and its effects should be monitored objectively. Air contains 21% oxygen.

The absolute indication to supplement air is inadequate tissue oxygenation. As clinical signs may be imprecise, arterial blood gases should be measured whenever suspicion arises. Tissue hypoxia can be assumed when the partial pressure of arterial oxygen (PaO_2) falls below 6.7 kPa (50 mm Hg) in a previously normal acutely ill patient, e.g. with myocardial infarction, acute pulmonary disorder, drug overdose, musculoskeletal or head trauma. Chronically hypoxic patients may maintain adequate tissue with PaO_2 below 6.7 kPa by compensating through raised red cell mass and cerebral vasodilatation. Oxygen therapy is used as follows:

1. *High concentration oxygen therapy* is used where a low PaO_2 is associated with a normal or low $PaCO_2$, as in pulmonary embolism, pneumonia or pulmonary oedema. Here concentrations up to 60% may be used for short periods for there is little risk of inducing hypoventilation and CO_2 retention.

2. *Low concentration oxygen therapy* is reserved for patients with low PaO_2 and raised $PaCO_2$, notably those with chronic obstructive lung disease during an infective exacerbation. The normal stimulus to respiration is elevation of the $PaCO_2$ but this control is blunted in chronically hypercapnic patients whose respiratory drive comes from hypoxia. Elevating the PaO_2 in such patients by giving them high concentrations of oxygen removes their stimulus to ventilate, exaggerates CO_2 retention and may cause fatal respiratory acidosis. The objective of therapy in such patients is to provide just enough oxygen to alleviate hypoxia without exaggerating the hypercapnia and respiratory acidosis; normally the administered oxygen concentration should not exceed 28% and in some 24% may be sufficient.

3. *Continuous long-term (domiciliary) oxygen therapy* is given to patients with severe persistent hypoxaemia and cor pulmonale due to chronic bronchitis and emphysema. Clinical trial evidence indicates that taking oxygen for more than 15 h per day improves survival.

HISTAMINE, ANTIHISTAMINES AND ALLERGIES

Histamine is a naturally occurring amine that fascinates pharmacologists and physicians. It is found in most body tissues in an inactive bound form, often in mast cells, and pharmacologically active free histamine is released from cells in response to stimuli such as physical trauma or antigen–antibody reactions. Various chemicals can also cause release of histamine. The more powerful of these (proteolytic enzymes and snake venoms) have no place in therapeutics, but a number of useful drugs, such as tubocurarine, morphine and even some antihistamines cause histamine release, although not usually enough to do more than transiently lower blood pressure or cause a local reaction.

The *physiological functions* of histamine are suggested by its distribution in the body. In body surface membranes — the alimentary canal, the respiratory tract and in the skin — its role is to react against foreign substances. In glands — gastric, intestinal, lachrymal or salivary — it mediates part of the secretory process. In most cells near blood vessels it plays a role in regulating the microcirculation.

Histamine acts as a local hormone (autacoid) similarly to serotonin or prostaglandins, i.e. it is a local chemical transmitter between the cell from which it is released and cells in the immediate vicinity. In the context of gastric secretion, for example, stimulation of receptors on the histamine-containing cell causes release of histamine, which in turn acts on receptors on parietal cells, which then secrete hydrogen ions (see gastric secretion, Chapter 31).

The **actions of histamine** that are clinically important are those on:

Smooth muscle. In general, histamine causes smooth muscle throughout the body to contract (excepting arterioles but including the larger arteries). Stimulation of the pregnant human uterus is insignificant. A brisk attack of bronchospasm may be induced in subjects who have any allergy, particularly asthma, when it may occur even in the presence of an antihistamine.

Arteries are dilated, with a consequent fall in blood pressure. The characteristic throbbing headache that occurs after histamine injections is due to stretching pain-sensitive structures in the dura mater by alterations in pressures in blood vessels and cerebrospinal fluid.

Capillaries dilate and their permeability to plasma increases, which responses comprise two parts (the flush and the wheal) of the 'triple response' described by Thomas Lewis.* The third part, the flare, is arteriolar dilatation due to an axon reflex.

Itch. Histamine release in the skin can cause itch.

Gastric secretion. Histamine increases the acid and pepsin content of gastric juices. This effect is antagonised only trivially by atropine and not at all by H_1-receptor antihistamines. H_2-receptor antihistamines are highly effective. Histamine has been used to test the capacity of the gastric mucosa to secrete acid, but it has been replaced by *pentagastrin* (a hormone analogue), which is selective for the stomach, unlike histamine.

The suprarenal medulla is stimulated to release adrenaline and noradrenaline in amounts that are insignificant in normal subjects but that are sufficient to raise the blood pressure in patients with phaeochromocytoma, in whom i.v. injection of histamine has been used as a diagnostic test.

As may be anticipated from the above actions, *anaphylactic shock*, which is largely due to histamine release, is characterised by circulatory collapse and bronchoconstriction. The most rapidly effective antidote is adrenaline (see index) and an antihistamine (H_1-receptor) may be given as well.

Metabolism and fate. Histamine is formed from the amino acid histidine and is inactivated by metabolism, largely by deamination and by methylation. In common with other local hormones, the process of inactivation of histamine is extremely rapid and it is not normally detectable in the blood, although a little appears in the urine.

* Lewis T, et al. Heart 1924; 11:209.

Histamine antagonists

When it became clear that release of histamine by tissue injury had unpleasant and even harmful effects, it was evident that histamine antagonists might have therapeutic importance, especially in allergic conditions.

The effects of histamine can be opposed in three ways:

1. By using a drug with opposite effects, e.g. histamine constricts bronchi, causes vasodilatation and increased capillary permeability. Adrenaline opposes these effects. This is physiological antagonism.
2. By preventing histamine from reaching its site of action (receptors), e.g. by competition, the H_1- and H_2-receptor antagonists.
3. By preventing the release of histamine; adrenal steroids and sodium cromoglycate can suppress the effects on the tissues of antigen–antibody reactions.

The first drugs to competitively block histamine receptors were introduced in 1947. They compromise what are conventionally called the 'antihistamines' and they effectively inhibit the increased *capillary permeability, flare and itch* responses of histamine; they also partially prevent the vascular smooth muscle (blood-pressure lowering) action but they have *no* effect on histamine-induced gastric secretion. Indeed, the standard method of testing a patient's capacity to secrete gastric acid used to be to inject histamine after first giving a large dose of a conventional antihistamine to block the other undesired effects of the infusion. Thus, if a group of drugs blocked certain actions of histamine but had no effect on other actions, it was reasoned that there must be more than one kind of histamine receptor. This was the basis for the search for drugs that block histamine-induced gastric secretion (see Chapter 31) and its success established that there are at least two types of *histamine receptor*:

H_1-receptor: mediates vascular effects (oedema, vasodilatation).

H_2-receptor: mediates the effect on gastric secretion and some vascular effects.

Thus, *histamine antagonists* may now be classified:

H_1-receptor antagonists: see account below.

H_2-receptor antagonists: cimetidine, ranitidine (see Chapter 31).

The term 'antihistamine' is still often applied to H_1-receptor antagonists alone since for many years they were the only antagonists available, but the use of this term is now confusing.

H_1-RECEPTOR ANTAGONISTS

Since their introduction, the number of H_1-antihistamines available has increased rapidly. This is both because they are relatively easy to make and because they control some allergic conditions without curing them, so that they are in constant demand. A substantial proportion of the population, perhaps as much as 10–15%, suffer allergic reactions at some time in their life, so that an effective antihistamine can be very profitable commercially.

The term antihistamine is unsatisfactory, for the drugs have numerous other actions. This partly derives from the fact that there is a considerable similarity of structure amongst such local hormones as histamine, adrenaline, serotonin and acetylcholine. A compound that may block the action of one substance may also be capable of blocking the action of another. Thus, the H_1-antihistamines may also have anticholinergic or sometimes α-adrenoceptor antagonist effects, and anticholinergic drugs may exhibit some antihistaminic actions. Thus H_1-antihistamines are used as hypnotics, antiparkinsonians, antitussives and expectorants, all actions that are not obviously related to antihistaminic effect. These unwanted features are a disadvantage when H_1-antihistamines are used specifically to counteract the effects of histamine, e.g. for allergies, but the introduction of H_1-antihistamines largely free of anticholinergic and sedative effects (terfenadine, astemizole) has been a useful advance.

Although the drugs differ in various ways, these are not of very great importance, except to an occasional individual patient, and they can be conveniently discussed together.

Actions. H_1-antihistamines oppose, to varying degrees, all the effects of liberated histamine except those on gastric secretion (which are H_2-receptor: see above), i.e. the oedema-producing and vascular effects. They are of negligible use in asthma, in which numerous mediators other than histamine are involved. Conventional H_1-antihistamines are *competitive* inhibitors of the action of histamine except for astemizole (at therapeutic doses) and terfenadine (at very high doses), which dissociate very slowly from the receptor and exhibit unsurmountable antagonism (see Chapter 8). H_1-antihistamines are therefore more effective if used *before* histamine has been liberated. Reversal of effects of histamine after it has been released is more readily achieved by *physiological* antagonism by adrenaline, which should first be used in life-threatening allergic reactions.

H_1-antihistamines also affect the central nervous system, usually to depress but sometimes to stimulate, and these actions are not related to histamine receptors. They can occasionally make petit mal worse. They can be beneficial in parkinsonism and motion sickness, and this may be attributable to their anticholinergic effects.

Pharmacokinetics. H_1-antihistamines taken orally are readily absorbed. They are mainly metabolised in the liver. Enough may be excreted in the milk to cause sedation in infants. They are generally administered orally and can also be given i.m. or i.v.

Uses. The H_1-antihistamines are used for symptomatic relief of allergies such as hay faver and urticaria (see below). They are of broadly similar therapeutic efficacy.

Notes on individual H_1-antihistamines

Astemizole (Hismanal) (10 mg) is largely free from sedative and anticholinergic effects; it rarely causes psychomotor impairment and does not potentiate the effects of alcohol or benzodiazepines. It may cause weight gain. The $t_{\frac{1}{2}}$ is 5 days and that of an active metabolite is 10 days, so steady state may not be reached for weeks. A loading dose of 30 mg daily by mouth for up to 7 days is appropriate, then 10 mg daily.

Terfenadine (Triludan) (60 mg) is similar to astemizole. The $t_{\frac{1}{2}}$ is 20 h. The dose is 60 mg × 2/day by mouth.

Mequitazine (Primalan) (5 mg) is less sedative than most other H_1-antihistamines but more so than astemizole. The dose is 5 mg × 2/day by mouth.

Chlorpheniramine (Piriton) (4 mg) is effective when urticaria is prominent and its sedative effect is then useful. The $t_{\frac{1}{2}}$ is 23 h. The oral dose is 4 mg × 3–4/day.

Diphenhydramine (Benadryl) (25 mg) causes marked sedation and anticholinergic effects; it is also used in parkinsonism and motion sickness. The $t_{\frac{1}{2}}$ is 7 h. The dose is 25 mg × 3/day by mouth.

Promethazine (Phenergan) (10, 25 mg) causes marked sedation and acts for 20 h. The $t_{\frac{1}{2}}$ is 12 h. It is used as a hypnotic in adults and children. The dose is as follows: by mouth 20–75 mg in divided doses or as a single dose at night; i.m. or i.v. 25–50 mg, maximum 100 mg.

Cyproheptadine (Periactin), *azatadine* (Optimine), *brompheniramine* (Dimotane), *clemastine* (Tavegil), *dimethindine* (Fenostil), *mebhydrolin* (Fabahistin), *mepyramine* (Anthisan), *oxatomide* (Tinset), *phenindamine* (Thephorin), *pheniramine* (Daneral), *trimeprazine* (Vallergan) and *triprolidine* (Actidil, Pro-Actidil) are similar.

Adverse effects are common with H_1-antihistamines and can be very troublesome although persistence is worthwhile if a good therapeutic effect has been obtained, as tolerance sometimes develops. Apart from sedation, these include dizziness, fatigue, insomnia, nervousness, tremors, gastroinstetinal disturbance and dry mouth. Dermatitis and agranulocytosis can occur. Severe poisoning due to overdose results in coma and sometimes in convulsions.

DRUG MANAGEMENT OF ALLERGIC STATES

The association between hay fever and the air pollen count was first described in 1873 by Charles Blackley*, a general practitioner from Manchester (UK). A sufferer from seasonal hay fever, he experienced an unexpected attack in winter when he entered an unused room to move a vase of dried grasses. Looking down a microscope, he identified the pollen grains and showed their effect on his body by scratching pollen onto the skin of his arm where it raised a weal. He devised a pollen trap attached to a kite and proved that there were pollen grains in the air at 1000 feet. Then, calculating that the symptoms of hay fever could be produced by very small amounts of pollen, his interest turned to homoeopathy (see Chapter 1), which he practised for the remainder of his career.

Histamine is released in many allergic states, but it is not the sole cause of symptoms, other chemical mediators, e.g. leukotrienes and prostaglandins, also being involved. Hence the usefulness of H_1-antihistamines in allergic states is variable, depending on the extent to which histamine rather than other mediators is the cause of the clinical, manifestations.

Hay fever

If symptoms are limited to rhinitis, a *corticosteroid* (beclomethasone, budesonide, flunisolide) or *sodium cromoglycate* applied topically as a spray or

* Blackley C H. Experimental researches on the causes and nature of catarrhus aestivus (hay fever or hay asthma). London: Ballière Tindall and Cox, 1873.

insufflation is often all that is required. Ocular symptoms alone respond well to *sodium cromoglycate* drops. When both nasal and ocular symptoms occur, or there is itching of the palate and ears as well, a systemic *H_1-antihistamine* is indicated. Astemizole or terfenadine are preferred if sedation is a problem with H_1-antihistamines. *Sympathomimetic vasoconstrictors*, e.g. ephedrine, are immediately effective if applied topically, but rebound swelling of the nasal mucous membrane occurs when medication is stopped. Rarely, a *systemic corticosteroid*, e.g. prednisolone, is justified for a severely affected patient to provide relief for a short period, e.g. during academic examinations.

Urticaria

Acute urticaria (named after its similarity to the sting of a nettle, *Urtica*) and *angioneurotic oedema* usually respond well to H_1-antihistamines, although severe cases are relieved more quickly by adrenaline (Adrenaline Inj., 1 mg/ml: 0.1–0.3 ml, s.c.).

Cold urticaria is due to release of autacoids on exposure to cold. It may respond to combined H_1- and H_2-receptor antagonists; the combination is needed fully to block the vascular effects of histamine, which cause flush and hypotension. Cyproheptadine is usually preferred as the H_1-antihistamine.

Chronic urticaria may respond to an H_1-antihistamine plus ephedrine or terbutaline, or to a H_1- plus a H_2-antihistamine.

Hereditary angiooedema, with deficiency of C_1 esterase (a complement inhibitor), does not respond to antihistamines or corticosteroid but only to *fresh frozen plasma*. Delay in initiating treatment may lead to death from laryngeal oedema.

Non-urticarial drug eruptions are not helped and may be made worse by H_1-antihistamines.

Anaphylactic shock, see p. 167.

BRONCHIAL ASTHMA

Asthma is characterised by episodes of wheeze and breathlessness due to variable obstruction of large and small airways. These reverse either spontaneously or as a result of treatment. The condition affects 2–5% of the UK population.

Some pathophysiology

In asthma the bronchi are hyper-reactive to a number of stimuli, which include immunological and psychological factors, infection, physical irritation and exercise. Inflammatory mediators are liberated, principally from mast cells. Some of these are pre-formed and are present as cytoplasmic granules, e.g. histamine, eosinophil and neutrophil chemotactic factors; others are formed after activation of the mast cells, e.g. bradykinin and products of arachidonic acid metabolism either by the lipoxygenase pathway (leukotrienes) or by the cyclooxygenase pathway (prostaglandins, thromboxanes or prostacyclin). The relative importance of the many individual mediators is not yet defined but they interact to produce the bronchial changes of asthma.

In an attack, the bronchial muscle contracts, the mucosa may become oedematous, further reducing the airway, and the bronchial secretion is sticky and hard to dislodge. This results in bronchial plugging, which is an important factor in the ventilatory insufficiency and prevents access of inhaled drug to the periphery. It is a reason why inhaled bronchodilators can fail to give full relief.

Early in an attack there is hyperventilation so that PaO_2 is maintained and $PaCO_2$ is lowered but with increasing airways obstruction the PaO_2 declines and $PaCO_2$ rises; hypoxia with hypercapnia signify a serious asthmatic episode.

Types of asthma

The following are recognised:

1. Asthma associated with specific allergic reactions

This 'extrinsic' type is the commonest and occurs in patients who develop allergy to antigenic substances in the inspired air. In some individuals who have a special liability to develop allergy (atopic), the resulting reaction is of the immediate (type 1) type involving antibodies of immunoglobulin class IgE; in other (non-atopic) persons the reaction is delayed for some hours (type 3) and is associated with the production of precipitating antibodies. Avoidance of exposure to allergens and, possibly, hyposensitisation are particularly relevant to this type of asthma, in addition to the other drug therapies described below.

2. Asthma not associated with known allergy

Some patients exhibit wheeze and breathlessness that is not attributable to any allergic reaction; they may be referred to as having 'intrinsic' asthma. There being no known allergen, it follows that avoidance and hyposensitisation have no place in the therapy of this type of asthma.

3. Exercise-induced asthma

Some patients develop wheeze that regularly follows within a few minutes of exercise; they should take a β-adrenoceptor agonist or sodium cromoglycate (see below) prior to the activity that provokes the asthma.

4. Asthma associated with chronic obstructive lung disease

A number of patients who have persistent airflow obstruction also exhibit considerable variation in airways resistance and are benefitted by drugs used for asthma. It is important to recognise the association and to test their responses to bronchodilators or corticosteroids.

Approaches to treatment

The following are recognised:

1. Prevention of exposure to an antigen

This approach assumes that there is a known antigen and is therefore appropriate for 'extrinsic' asthmatics. Identifying an antigen may be aided by the patient's history (wheezing in response to contact with grasses, pollens, animals), by skin prick or by intradermal injection of selected antigens (Bencard Skin Testing Solutions) or by demonstrating antibodies in the patient's serum. Avoiding an allergen may be practicable when it is related to some special situation, e.g. occupation, but is not feasible if it is widespread, as with house-dust mite. Some clinicians favour giving a course of injections of the antigen in increasing dose to stimulate the production of blocking (IgG and IgA) antibodies, which neutralise the antigen and prevent its reaction with IgE (hyposensitisation). This has been been effective for asthma due to grass pollens.

2. Reduction of the bronchial response

(a) *Corticosteroids* enter cells passively and induce the formation of lipocortin. This protein has a key role in the inflammatory process for it inhibits phospholipase A_2, the enzyme that is responsible for generating arachidonic acid, which in turn gives rise to a host of inflammatory mediators (e.g. prostaglandins and leukotrienes). The corticosteroids used in asthma include *prednisolone* (*or corticotrophin or tetracosactrin*), *beclomethasone, betamethasone and budesonide* (see Chapter 34).

(b) *Other drugs* that reduce the bronchial response include *sodium cromoglycate and ketotifen* (see below).

Specific antagonism of substances liberated in the bronchial reaction has not proved an effective approach; antihistamines, for example, have been tried but they are ineffective in asthma.

3. Dilatation of narrowed bronchi

This is, in effect, an example of physiological antagonism of bronchial muscle contraction and may be achieved as follows:

(a) **β_2-adrenoceptor agonists**. These are regarded as drugs of choice because the adrenoceptors in bronchi are mainly β_2 in type and their stimulation causes bronchial muscle to relax. The drugs include *salbutamol, terbutaline, fenoterol, pirbuterol, reproterol, rimiterol and isoetharine* (see Chapter 23).

Less selective adrenoceptor agonists such as adrenaline, ephedrine, isoprenaline, methoxyphenamine, orciprenaline are regarded as much less safe, being more likely to cause cardiac dysrhythmias. α-adrenoceptor activity contributes to bonchoconstriction but α-adrenoceptor antagonists have not proved effective. Similarly, production of bronchial mucosal vasoconstriction by oral sprays of α-adrenoceptor agonist (adrenaline) is not useful.

(b) **Xanthines.** These are described below and include *aminophylline, choline theophyllinate, theophylline, acepifylline, diprophylline and proxyphylline*.

(c) **Anticholinergic (antimuscarinic) bronchodilators.** Antimuscarinic drugs inhibit the action of acetylocholine at vagal nerve endings to constrict bronchial smooth muscle and may benefit some, notably older, patients with intrinsic asthma. Atropine has been used thus but has largely been replaced for asthma by *ipratropium* (see Chapter 22).

Several of the **drugs used to treat asthma** are described elsewhere. Accounts of those that are not follow below.

Sodium cromoglycate (Intal) stabilises the sensitised mast cell membrane probably by preventing the intracellular movement of calcium; this prevents the cell from releasing bronchoconstrictor substances that ordinarily result from the combination of antigen with antibody on its surface. Thus sodium cromoglycate does not interfere with the actual union of antigen with antibody, but only with the tissue consequences of the combination. It is ineffective unless present before the antigen challenge occurs. Hyposensitisation procedures are not blocked by sodium cromoglycate. Since it does not antagonise the bronchoconstrictor effect of the active substances after they have been released it is not effective in terminating an existing attack, i.e. it prevents bronchoconstriction as opposed to inducing bronchodilatation; it is thus used to *prevent* asthmatic attacks.

Sodium cromoglycate is poorly absorbed from the gastrointestinal tract but it is well absorbed from the lung, which is fortunate so that it can be given by inhalation; it is eliminated unchanged in the urine and bile.

Sodium cromoglycate is chiefly of value in *extrinsic* (allergic) asthma including asthma in children and those whose asthma is made worse by exercise. The effect may be delayed by several weeks. It may reduce the necessity to use oral adrenocortical steroid in some patients, but asthmatics who are truly steroid-dependent do not benefit from it.

The drug is given as a powder by inhalation (Intal Spincap). Inhalation of any powder may, non-specifically, induce bronchospasm. When this happens, one or two puffs of a β_2-adrenoceptor agonist bronchodilator (salbutamol) may be used before inhalation of powder. This is preferable to the fixed-dose formulation of cromoglycate + isoprenaline (Intal Compound) since intelligent use of the drugs separately avoids confounding the benefit of the bronchodilator with the benefit, or lack of benefit, from sodium cromoglycate. A special inhaler (Spinhaler) is required and the dose is one 20-mg capsule (of which only 1–2 mg reach the small bronchi) every 3–6 h. It may also be given by aerosol inhalation, 2 mg (2 puffs) 4–8 times daily, or by inhalation of a nebulised solution, 20 mg 4–6 times daily.

Special formulations are used for *allergic rhintis* (Rynacrom) and *allergic conjunctivitis* (Opticrom). Sodium cromoglycate (Nalcrom) may be used by mouth for food allergy, in association with avoidance of known allergens; the dose is 200 mg 4 times daily. Sodium cromoglycate is remarkably non-toxic. Apart from cough and bronchospasm induced by the powder (above) it may rarely cause allergic reactions. Application to the eye may produce a local stinging sensation and the oral form may cause nausea.

Nedocromil may be effective in a wider range of patients than sodium cromoglycate.

Ketotifen has histamine H_1-receptor blocking and antianaphylactic actions in animals; it may prevent asthmatic attacks but the results of clinical studies are variable. It is taken by mouth and may have to be continued for several weeks to achieve its maximum benefit. In common with other antihistamines it causes drowsiness.

Theophylline is a *xanthine*, a group of substances with numerous pharmacological activities (see Chapter 18). What makes theophylline of relevance to asthma is its ability to relax bronchial smooth muscle. It inhibits phosphodiesterase, the enzyme that metabolises cyclic-AMP; high intracellular concentration of cyclic-AMP maintains smooth muscle in the relaxed state, although there is doubt about the relevance of this action at therapeutic doses. Theophylline also increases the rate and force of cardiac contraction and it raises the rate of urine production. More recently, and of relevance to their role in respiratory disease, xanthines have been found to improve diaphragmatic contraction.

Absorption of theophylline from the gastrointestinal tract is usually rapid and complete. It is widely distributed in the body, 60% is bound to plasma proteins and 90% is metabolised in the liver. The $t_{\frac{1}{2}}$ is 8 h but there is wide variation and it is prolonged in patients with severe cardiopulmonary disease and liver cirrhosis. Smoking enhances theophylline clearance by causing hepatic enzyme induction.

Attention to these factors may explain lack of responsiveness or adverse reactions to theophylline when plasma concentration measurements are not available. Increasing bronchodilator effects with minimal toxicity are achieved between plasma concentrations of 5 and 20 mg/l, although at the upper level, nausea, vomiting, headache or nervousness can occur. Between plasma concentrations of 20 and 40 mg/l there is a danger of cardiac dysrhythmias and when the concentration exceeds 40 mg/l, convulsions or cardiac arrest may occur.

Theophylline is relatively insoluble and it is commercially available as various derivatives that increase its solubility and duration of action (see xanthines, above). It is used for both chronic asthma (by mouth) and status asthmaticus (i.v.); a suppository at night may be effective for those whose asthma is especially worse in the early morning ('morning dippers'). Theophylline is also used in the emergency treatment of left ventricular failure.

Aminophylline Injection contains 250 mg in 10 ml. An adult may receive up to 20 ml (500 mg; or 5–6 mg/kg) i.v. at a rate not in excess of 2 ml (50 mg) per minute, provided the patient has received no aminophylline in the previous 24 hours (patients should be *asked* about oral theophylline consumption), in which case dosage must be reduced. Suggested i.v. maintenance doses are 0.7 mg/kg/hr in patients under 50 years or 0.4 mg/kg/hr for those over 50 years. Lower rates are required for patients with impaired elimination (see above). The dose by mouth is 100–300 mg, 3–4 times daily, and by rectum 360 mg once or twice daily; formulations are numerous.

Adverse effects are related to plasma concentration as is described above.

Assessment of therapy in asthma

The effectiveness of changes in dose and of alterations to the therapeutic regimen should be monitored by serial use of the simpler respiratory function tests such as forced vital capacity and peak expiratory flow rate. These measurements can be easily performed on outpatients, should be routine in hospital wards, and, indeed, should be as customary as blood pressure recording in hypertensive patients. Neither the patients' feelings nor ordinary physical examination are sufficient to determine whether there is still room for useful improvement with drugs. When an asthmatic attack is severe, arterial blood gases should be monitored.

'The effort that has to be made to force air through small tubes decreases in proportion to the fourth power of their radius. This explains why even a very slight increase in the bore of the bronchioles gives such welcome relief to a distressed patient.'*

Inhalation of drugs for asthma

The inhalational route has been developed to advantage because the undesirable effects of systemic administration are reduced by the smaller doses that are needed. Routes of drug administration are discussed generally in Chapter 8 but some further matters are relevant to inhaled drugs for asthma.

Drugs intended to be inhaled must first be converted into particulate form and the optimum *particle size* to reach the small bronchi is 2 μm. An *aerosol* consists of particles dispersed in a gas and may be produced as follows.

Pressurised aerosol. Drug is dissolved in a low-boiling-point liquid (usually one or more fluorocarbons) in a canister under pressure; when the valve is opened, a metered dose of liquid is ejected, forms an aerosol and is inhaled. Coordinating the act of opening the valve with that of

* Wade O L. Prescribers Journal 1964; 4:48

inhalation may be difficult, especially for the young and the elderly; this problem can be overcome by interposing between the aerosol source and the patient's mouth an extension tube (*spacer*) that prevents dispersion of the aerosol before the patient inhales.

Nebulisers convert a solution or suspension of drug into an aerosol. *Jet* nebulisers require a driving gas, usually air from a compressor unit for home use, or oxygen in hospital; the solution in the nebulising chamber is broken into droplets by the jet and the larger droplets are filtered off leaving the smaller ones to be inhaled. *Ultrasonic* nebulisers convert a solution into particles of uniform size by vibrations created by a piezo-electric crystal*. With either method the nebulised solution is delivered to the patient by a mouthpiece or facemask, so no coordination is needed, and the dose can be altered by changing the strength of the solution. Much larger doses can be administered by nebuliser than by pressurised aerosol.

Dry powder inhalers. The drug is formulated as a micronised powder and placed in a device (e.g. Spinhaler) from which it is inhaled. Some patients can use these when they fail with metered-dose aerosols (see sodium cromoglycate, above).

DRUG TREATMENT OF ASTHMA

This naturally varies with the severity and type of asthma, but the following is a summary.

For constant and intermittent asthma

A β-*adrenoceptor* agonist should be given by metered dose aerosol and dosing adjusted to the patients' symptoms. Suitable drugs include salbutamol, terbutaline and the other β_2-adrenoceptor agonists referred to above. The usual dose is 1–2 puffs 4–8 hourly. The patient should be carefully instructed how to use the inhaler when treatment is begun, since failure to benefit is often due to improper use; time spent doing this is never wasted. An oral β-adrenoceptor agonist can be used, e.g. salbutamol 4 mg, 3–4 times daily, but is more likely to give rise to tremor and headache.

If attacks persist, *sodium cromoglycate* should be added and continued for about 4 weeks properly to assess its benefit. It is most likely to prevent attacks in extrinsic and asthmatics but may be helpful in other forms.

Ipratropium by metered-dose aerosol, 1–2 puffs 3–4 times daily may benefit some asthmatics, especially elderly intrinsic asthmatics who may also have chronic bronchitis.

For the patient whose condition fails to improve on sodium cromoglycate, *inhalation of a corticosteroid* by metered-dose aerosol may control symptoms. Since the drug is delivered directly to the site of action, only a fraction of the oral dose is used (50–250 μg per puff). Furthermore, 90% of the inhaled dose is either exhaled or is swallowed and then both poorly absorbed from the gut and rapidly metabolised by the liver. Although reduced hypothalamic–pituitary–adrenal responsiveness has been demonstrated with inhaled steroid, it is not ordinarily a clinical problem. Candidiasis of the mouth and throat can develop in a minority of cases but is readily treated with nystatin mouthwashes or amphotericin B lozenges without interrupting therapy. Washing out the mouth with water after each inhalation reduces the chance of recurrence. Beclomethasone diproprionate (Becotide, 50 μg per dose, 100 μg 3 or 4 times a day) and betamethasone valerate (Bextasol, 100 μg per dose, 200 μg 4 times a day) are used and adjusted to the minimum effective dose. They are about as effective as oral prednisolone 5–10 mg.

To abort exacerbations, a β-receptor agonist aerosol, e.g. salbutamol, may be sufficient.

For more severe relapses, short courses of oral adrenal steroid may be used, thus: days 1 and 2, prednisolone 20 mg per day; days 3 and 4, 15 mg per day; days 5 and 6, 10 mg per day; day 7, 5 mg.

Chest infections increase reversible airways resistance and should be treated vigorously. The requirement of β_2-receptor agonist may increase.

Long-term *oral* therapy with *adrenal steroid* is used only when all else has failed in patients who relapse repeatedly into status asthmaticus or who

* Converts electricity into mechanical vibration

are too disabled to lead a reasonably normal working life. This is more often the case in intrinsic asthma. Because of the dangers of prolonged corticosteroid treatment, objective evidence of benefit should, if possible, be obtained by spirometry. Therapy may begin with prednisolone, say 40 mg per day total, reducing it as soon as feasible to a maintenance dose of 10 mg per day, at which dose the complications of steroid therapy are uncommon. If relapses occur, as they may, the dose may be increased to 30 mg for one day, after which it is reduced by 5 mg per day until the maintenance dose is regained. Adrenal suppression is minimised by giving the corticosteroid as a single dose in the early morning, when endogenous cortisol peaks, for there is then less negative feedback effect on the hypothalamic-pituitary-adrenal system. Although the $t_{\frac{1}{2}}$ of prednisolone is 3 h, once-daily administration is reasonable as the $t_{\frac{1}{2}}$ *of effect* is 18–36 h.

Patients taking long-term systemic (oral) adrenal steroid therapy should also use an inhaled steroid. The reason for this is that the inhaled steroid may allow the dose of oral steroid to be lower than it otherwise would be, and so contribute to reducing the incidence of adverse effects of long-term systemic therapy.

If systemic adrenal steroid therapy has lasted more than 6 months, great caution is required during withdrawal because of a risk of catastrophic relapse. Enzyme induction, e.g. by an antiepileptic drug, can reduce the effect of a corticosteroid by increasing its metabolism.

Sometimes corticotrophin is effective when oral and inhaled corticosteroid fails; it is preferred in children to avoid growth suppression but there is less flexibility in dose adjustment.

In **status asthmaticus**, a serious medical emergency, early vigorous treatment is important, for the bronchi may become refractory to β-receptor agonists (refractory to one means refractory to all) after 36 hours, perhaps the result of respiratory acidosis. In addition, drugs given by metered dose aerosol may fail to reach the narrowed bronchi.

(a) In such cases *salbutamol* should be given by nebuliser (as effective as an intermittent positive pressure ventilator); the dose is salbutamol 2.5–5 mg (as 0.1–0.2% solution) over about 3 min, repeated in 15 min. Alternatively, salbutamol may be injected i.m. in a dose of 8 μg/kg body weight or i.v. slowly 4 μg/kg continuing, if necessary, with an i.v. infusion of 10 μg/min. Nebulised salbutamol is usually preferred.

If this fails, *ipratropium* by nebuliser may usefully be added and/or *aminophylline* i.v. (see above). Infusions of aminophylline or salbutamol may continue for 1–2 days.

(b) There should be no hesitation in using an adrenal steroid. *Hydrocortisone* 200 mg is given i.v. initially, and repeated 4-hourly or according to response. It does not act instantly and response may not be maximal for several hours. Hydrocortisone acts slightly quicker than prednisolone and the parenteral route is preferred at the outset because delayed gastric emptying may render oral administration unreliable. Once there is a response, prednisolone 15 mg 6-hourly by mouth may be used instead; this high dose may be needed for 24–48 h, after which it can be reduced rapidly.

(c) Whilst waiting for the steroid to act, attention may be given to ensuring that the patient is well oxygenated (*humidified* O_2), which will often reduce some of the distress of dyspnoea. CO_2 narcosis is rare in asthma but it is generally preferable to start with O_2 28% and to check that the $PaCO_2$ has not risen before delivering O_2 35%. Excessive secretion of bronchial mucus adds significantly to the degree of respiratory obstruction; dehydration, which is common, thickens mucus and should be remedied by i.v. fluid. Anticholinergics reduce, but thicken, secretion. Infection does not usually play an important part in an exacerbation but should be treated with a broad-spectrum antimicrobial such as amoxycillin if suspected. Severe cases may need assisted respiration or bronchial lavage, but these special techniques are beyond the scope of this book.

Sedation in severe asthma

These patients are hypoxic whilst exerting maximum respiratory effort so that any diminution of respiratory drive due to depression of the respiratory centre may lead to serious underventilation. Opioids (morphine) are obviously contraindicated; even a small dose may stop the patient breathing altogether.

The least dangerous sedatives and hypnotics are probably diazepam, chloral derivatives, chlorpromazine and promethazine. But any sedation that will ensure sleep in a severe asthmatic may adversely effect the respiratory drive and useful cough.

Asthma may be precipitated by β-adrenoceptor block. Since this is competitive, it may be overcome with a sufficient dose of a β-receptor agonist but *the only safe course is* to *avoid the use of β-adrenoceptor antagonists* altogether in patients with a history of asthma; fatal asthma has been precipitated by β-blocker eye-drops.

Interactions. A patient in a severe attack who has been taking large amounts of β-adrenoceptor agonist in an effort to stop it may have absorbed enough to cause substantial cardiac stimulation. Further drugs with cardiac effects (adrenaline or aminophylline) may summate dangerously if given in full doses or rapidly i.v.

Deaths from asthma in the young

In the mid-1960s, there was an epidemic of sudden deaths in young asthmatics outside hospital. It was associated with the introduction of high-dose, unselective ($\beta_1 + \beta_2$) adrenoceptor agonist (e.g. isoprenaline) metered aerosols and did not occur in countries where these high concentrations were not marketed.* The epidemic declined in Britain when the profession was warned and the aerosols were restricted to prescription only. Though the relation between the use of β-receptor agonists and death is inescapable, the actual mechanism of death is uncertain; overdose causing cardiac dysrhythmia is not the sole factor. The subsequent development of selective β_2-receptor agonists is a contribution to safety.

* Stolley P D. Am Rev Resp Dis 1972; 105:883

GUIDE TO FURTHER READING

1 Editorial. Acute oxygen therapy. Lancet 1981; 1: 980–1.
2 Editorial. Long term oxygen and advanced chronic bronchitis. Lancet 1981; 1: 701–2.
3 Editorial. Oxygen in the home. Br Med J 1981; 282: 1909–10.
4 Howard P. (Editorial). Drugs or oxygen for hypoxic cor pulmonale? Br Med J 1983; 287: 1159–60.
5 Rees J. (Editorial). Treatment of pulmonary hypertension in chronic bronchitis and emphysema. Br Med J 1984; 289: 1398–9.
6 Cochrane G M. (Editorial). Slow release theophyllines and chronic bronchitis. Br Med J 1984; 289: 1643–4.
7 Holgate S T, et al. What's new about hay fever? Br Med J 1985; 291: 1–2.
8 Lessof M H. Allergy and its mechanisms. Br Med J 1986; 292: 385–7.
9 Editorial. Inflammatory mediators in asthma. Lancet 1983; 2: 829–31.
10 Weisssmann G. (Editorial). The eicosanoids of asthma. N Engl J Med 1983; 308: 454–5.
11 Goetzl E J. (Editorial). Asthma: new mediators and old problems. N Engl J Med 1984; 311: 252–3.
12 Editorial. Aspirin sensitivity in asthmatics. Br Med J 1980; 281: 958–9.
13 Editorial. Asthma at night. Lancet 1983; 1: 220–2.
14 Barnes, P J. (Editorial). Nocturnal asthma: mechanisms and treatment. Br Med J 1984; 288: 1397–8.
15 McFadden E R, et al. Exercise-induced asthma. N Engl J Med 1979; 301: 763–9.
16 Holgate S T. Changing attitudes to exercise induced asthma. Br Med J 1983; 287: 1650–1.
17 Editorial. Theophylline benefits and difficulties. Lancet 1983; 2: 607–8.
18 Rees J. (Editorial). Clinical trials in asthma. Br Med J 1983; 287: 376–7.
19 Editorial. The nebuliser epidemic. Lancet 1984; 2: 789–90.
20 Editorial. The proper use of aerosol bronchodilators. Lancet 1981; 1: 23–4.
21 Benatar S R. Fatal asthma. N Engl J Med 1986; 314: 423–8.
22 Editorial. Autonomic abnormalities in asthma. Lancet 1982; 1: 1224–5.
23 Editorial. Acute asthma. Lancet 1986; 1: 131–3.
24 Rudd R. (Editorial). Corticosteroids in chronic bronchitis. Br Med J 1984; 288: 1553–4.

31

Gastrointestinal system I: Control of gastric secretion and mucosal resistance: Peptic ulcer

Peptic ulcer kills few patients but troubles many. About 10% of adult males show evidence of past or present ulcer, although the incidence is declining in many Western countries. Ulcers may be transient, recurrent or chronic, and drug therapy is valuable for the relief of symptoms and to aid healing.

SOME PATHOPHYSIOLOGY

The concept of a balance between the agressive capacities of acid plus pepsin and the defensive mechanisms of the mucosa is useful. An ulcer is thought to develop when the equilibrium is disturbed either by enhanced agressiveness or by lessened mucosal resistance.

The relation between peptic ulcer and acid plus pepsin secretion is not simple. On average, patients with duodenal ulcer produce about twice as much HCl as normal subjects, but there is much overlap and about half the patients with duodenal ulcer have acid outputs on the normal range. Patients with gastric ulcer produce normal or reduced amounts of acid. Duodenal ulcer does not occur at very low rates of acid formation but gastric ulcer does. When there is anacidity no peptic ulcers form, i.e. the maxim 'no acid — no ulcer' holds.

The factors that protect the mucosa comprise its impermeability to H^+ ion (the mucosal 'barrier' to H^+), its ability to secrete mucus and bicarbonate ion, its blood flow and its capacity rapidly to replace damaged epithelial cells; endogenous prostaglandins are probably involved in all these mechanisms. Use of non-steroidal anti-inflammatory drugs, cigarette smoking and heredity (male sex, possession of blood group O) influence the equilibrium unfavourably and are associated with increased incidence of peptic ulcer.

In general terms, duodenal ulcer is thought to relate to excessive secretion of acid plus pepsin while defective mucosal resistance probably plays a more important part in the genesis of gastric ulcer.

Drugs can alter the balance towards prevention or healing of ulcer in the following ways:

1. **Reduction of acid secretion by** ***histamine*** H_2-*receptor antagonists*, e.g. cimetidine or ranitidine and *anticholinergic drugs*, e.g. pirenzepine.
2. **Neutralisation of secreted acid by** ***antacids***, e.g. magnesium trisilicate, aluminium hydroxide.
3. **Enhanced mucosal resistance by various mechanisms**, e.g. carbenoxolone, deglycyrrhizinized liquorice, bismuth compounds, sucralfate or prostaglandins.

DRUGS USED FOR PEPTIC ULCER

Fibreoptic endoscopy has made reliable the assessment of these medicines in therapeutic trials and it is clear that certain drugs do have a healing effect. This should be seen against the background that many ulcers heal spontaneously, or in the case of gastric ulcer, respond to measures such as bedrest (uneconomic and boring) or cessation of smoking (requires self-discipline). The use of medicines is justified because they *accelerate* healing with reduced risk of complications and quicker relief of symptoms.

Drugs that reduce gastric acid secretion

Histamine H_2-receptor antagonists

An account of the pharmacology of histamine appears in Chapter 30. Clinically, the most important histamine H_2-receptors are those on the gastric parietal cells. H_2-receptors are also present in vascular smooth muscle and activation of these is partly responsible for the blood-pressure-lowering (vasodilator) effect of histamine; they are also found in lymphocytes, heart, uterus, brain and skin, but antagonising these has not yet been shown to have any important clinical effects. Numerous factors increase acid secretion by the stomach, including food, caffeine, psychological conditioning and drugs. The effects of these are mediated at the parietal cells by three substances, namely, histamine, gastrin and acetylcholine. A significant fact is that H_2-receptor antagonists inhibit not only the acid secretion provoked by histamine, they also prevent acid production by gastrin and acetylcholine. Thus the various influences on gastric acid secretion appear to mediate their effects finally via histamine, and it is no surprise that histamine H_2-receptor blockade has become clinically important.

Cimetidine (Tagamet) (200, 400, 800 mg) was the first clinically important histamine H_2-receptor antagonist. It inhibits gastric secretion stimulated by injected histamine, by insulin, caffeine, protein-rich meals and by cholinergic drugs. All phases of gastric secretion are reduced namely, fasting, nocturnal and food-stimulated. Both the volume and the hydrogen ion concentration of gastric juice are reduced. Although the concentration of pepsin is not reduced, the total amount secreted falls because the volume of gastric juice is less. Parietal cells secrete intrinsic factor as well as hydrogen ions but in normal doses cimetidine does not have a sufficient effect on vitamin B_{12} turnover to lead to haematological or neurological complications. Cimetidine does not affect gastric emptying, unlike anticholinergic drugs, which delay it.

Pharmacokinetics. Cimetidine is readily absorbed from the upper small gut. The $t_{\frac{1}{2}}$ is 2 h and 60% of an oral dose is recovered as unchanged drug in the urine, the remainder appearing as metabolites. Total absorption of cimetidine is unimpaired if it is taken with food, although peak blood concentrations are lower.

Uses. Cimetidine is used for conditions in which reduction of gastric secretion is beneficial. These are principally *duodenal ulcer, benign gastric ulcer, stomal ulcer and reflux oesophagitis.* Before treating gastric ulcer, particular care must be taken to confirm by endoscopy and biopsy that it is benign since the symptoms of *gastric carcinoma* can be relieved by cimetidine so that apparently successful treatment may fatally delay the correct diagnosis.

Its use for *gastrointestinal bleeding* is controversial but when this is due to gastric erosions complicating the stress of such serious disease as fulminant heptic failure, trauma or renal failure, there are reasonable grounds for giving cimetidine by i.v. infusion. Renal transplant patients are also prone to gastric haemorrhage, the incidence of which can be reduced by cimetidine. This success contrasts with bleeding in patients with peptic ulcer, oesophagitis and Mallory–Weiss syndrome (laceration of oesophagogastric junction) in which there may be erosion or trauma to larger blood vessels, and in which clinical trials have failed consistently to show benefit.

Other uses. Cimetidine is also used to prevent and treat *stress ulcers* in gravely ill or burned patients. It is given *before anaesthesia for emergency surgery* and *before labour* to lessen the risk of aspirating gastric acid. In the *Zollinger–Ellison syndrome*, cimetidine controls the excessive acid secretion that is the cause of diarrhoea, weight loss and peptic ulcers; it can be used to improve a patient's condition prior to gastrectomy or as a permanent alternative to surgery in the infirm. In *chronic pancreatic insufficiency* oral enzyme supplements may fail to reach the duodenum in sufficient amount since they are destroyed by acid in the stomach; steatorrhoea and weight loss may be prevented if cimetidine is taken with the enzyme preparations. Cimetidine is also used in the malabsorption and fluid loss that occurs in patients who have had *massive small gut resection* (short bowel syndrome) and develop hypergastrinaemia and gastric hypersecretion.

Dose. Cimetidine 400 mg × 2/day with breakfast and at bedtime is usually satisfactory for peptic ulcer. Alternatively, patients with duodenal ulcer, who usually have a high nocturnal acid secretion, may receive 800 mg as a single dose at bedtime. Most patients become symptom-free in about 8 days but treatment should continue for at least 4 weeks, and for 6 weeks in the case of gastric ulcer. Response rates vary, but after 8 weeks treatment, 85–90% of duodenal and 60% of gastric ulcers can be expected to heal, i.e. the spontaneous healing rate is about doubled. After ulcer healing has been achieved, many patients experience periodic dyspeptic symptoms for a few days at a time. It is reasonable to treat these with short (a few days), intermittent courses of cimetidine. When cimetidine is withdrawn, acid secretion returns to its original level and in some patients, particularly high acid secretors, the tendency to relapse is strong; cimetidine 400 mg as a single daily dose at bedtime may then be given as maintenance therapy. A patient with a long history of recurrence of ulcer should probably be treated surgically but recurrent courses or long-term treatment with cimetidine are acceptable for those who are unfit for surgery.

Higher doses are needed for reflux oesophagitis (400 mg × 4/day), the Zollinger–Ellison syndrome (400 mg × 4/day or more) and to prevent haemorrhage from stress ulcers (up to 2.4 g/day by i.v. injection or infusion).

In patients with severe renal impairment (creatinine clearance 2 ml/min) excretion is delayed. Cimetidine is removed from blood by dialysis and a dose of 200 mg × 2/day in patients undergoing regular haemodialysis will suffice.

Adverse effects and drug interactions are few in short-term use. Minor complaints include headache, dizziness, diarrhoea, tiredness, muscular pain and constipation. Bradycardia and cardiac conduction defects may also occur. Cimetidine is a weak antiandrogen and may cause gynaecomastia and sexual dysfunction in men. In the elderly, particularly, it may cause CNS disturbances including lethargy, confusion and hallucinations. Cimetidine is an inhibitor of hepatic drug oxidising enzymes and raised plasma concentrations or enhanced activity of warfarin, phenytoin, lignocaine, propranolol, theophylline, some benzodiazepines and imipramine result when these drugs are administered with it. Indeed when cimetidine is given there is a potential for increased effect with any drug that is inactivated by oxidation in the liver.

Concern has been expressed that long-term use of highly effective antisecretory drugs may increase the risk of gastric cancer either by a direct action on the mucosa or through the effects of hypochlorhydria favouring the growth in the stomach of bacteria that convert ingested nitrates into carcinogenic nitrosamines. Surveillance studies to date have not provided evidence that this is a real hazard of histamine H_2-receptor antagonists, and it is certainly unlikely with short-term use. Cimetidine may retard diagnosis of existing gastric cancer by relieving symptoms.

Ranitidine (150, 300 mg) is a histamine H_2-receptor antagonist and its actions, uses and therapeutic efficacy are essentially those of cimetidine (above). Its differences from cimetidine lie chiefly in its dose and profile of unwanted effects.

Ranitidine is rapidly absorbed from the upper gastrointestinal tract and excreted mainly unchanged by the kidney; the $t_{\frac{1}{2}}$ is 2 h.

Dose. Ranitidine 150 mg × 2/day taken in the morning and in the evening will usually suffice; a single dose of 300 mg at night may be used as an alternative for duodenal ulceration. A course of treatment should last at least 4 weeks and ulcers that have not healed at this stage are normally healed by a further 4 weeks of therapy. Those with a history of recurrent ulcer may benefit from a maintenance dose of 150 mg nightly. Patients with Zollinger–Ellison syndrome should receive 150 mg × 3/day or more as is necessary.

Adverse effects are few but include headache, rash, dizziness, nausea, constipation and diarrhoea. Ranitidine does not block androgen receptors and it does not cause gynaecomastia or impotence, as does cimetidine. It does not inhibit drug metabolism in the liver and accordingly the drug interactions reported with cimetidine are not to be anticipated with ranitidine.

Pentagastrin, an analogue of gastrin, is used to test the capacity of the stomach to secrete acid (see p. 600).

Anticholinergic drugs

A general account of these is given in Chapter 22. Despite expectations, on the basis of theoretical considerations of the importance of the parasympathetic autonomic system in gastric secretion, these drugs have not proved to have great importance in the therapy of peptic ulcer, largely because of the unwanted effects of anticholinergic blockade.

Pirenzepine (50 mg) inhibits gastric secretion at doses lower than are required to affect gastrointestinal motility, ocular, salivary, urinary and central nervous function. It owes this relative selectivity to its high affinity for and blockade of M_1-muscarine receptors, which are present in autonomic ganglia; it has low affinity for the M_2-receptors of the smooth muscle on the ileum and urinary bladder. In the stomach pirenzepine appears to inhibit transmission in parasympathetic enteric ganglia.

Pirenzepine is poorly absorbed from the gastrointestinal tract and it is excreted mainly unchanged in the urine and bile. It is 16% bound to plasma proteins and the $t_{\frac{1}{2}}$ is 11 h.

It is used for duodenal and gastric ulcer. The dose is 50 mg × 2/day increasing to × 3/day. Treatment should continue for 4–6 weeks but up to 3 months may be needed for resistant cases.

Adverse effects include dry mouth, difficulty in visual accomodation, constipation, diarrhoea and headache, but it is generally well tolerated.

Proton pump inhibitors

Drugs of this new class reduce gastric acid secretion not by blocking cholinergic or histamine H_2-receptors, but rather by inhibiting the action of the H^+, K^+-ATPase in the parietal cell. This enzyme catalyses the exchange of protons (H^+) for potassium ions at the cell membrane, i.e. the final step in the acid secretory process, sometimes called the proton pump. An example is *omeprazole*, which produces a profound, dose-related and long-lasting inhibition of both basal and stimulated acid secretion. It is undergoing clinical evaluation; patients with excessive gastric acid production, e.g. those with Zollinger–Ellison syndrome, may derive special benefit.

Neutralisation of secreted acid: antacids

Antacids are basic substances that reduce gastric acidity by neutralising HCl. The *hydroxide* is the base most commonly employed but *trisilicate*, *carbonate* and *bicarbonate* ions are also used. The therapeutic efficacy and adverse effects depend as well on the metallic ion with which the base is combined, and this is usually *aluminium*, *magnesium* or *sodium*. Calcium and bismuth have largely been abandoned for this purpose because they caused systemic toxicity, and calcium carbonate causes rebound acid secretion, which is not a problem with the above.

The benefit of antacids probably depends on protecting the ulcer from acid (by neutralisation) and from pepsin (which is inactive above pH 5 and which in addition is inactivated (adsorbed) by aluminium hydroxide and magnesium trisilicate. For 90% of peptic ulcer patients 50 mmol neutralising capacity *per hour* (male, duodenal ulcer) and 26 mmol *per hour* (female, duodenal ulcer; male, gastric ulcer) is adequate. Dosage of antacids to achieve this are given below:

Amounts of antacids required to raise pH of 50 mmol HCl to 4.5

Sodium bicarbonate	4.4 g*
Magnesium oxide or hydroxide	5.9 g
Magnesium trisilicate	50 g
Magnesium carbonate	63 g
Aluminium hydroxide gel	715 ml
(as Aludrox)	(294 ml)

Many patients find these large doses unendurable. It is obvious from the above that the first two are much the most efficient. Also, they react quickly, which is important, because half a single dose of antacid will generally have left the stomach in 30 min, i.e. the half-time of gastric emptying. Magnesium trisilicate and aluminium hydroxide are relatively slow acting.

* A level teaspoon of the solid is 3.5–4 g.

The amount of antacid needed depends on the rate of acid secretion, on the presence or absence of food in the stomach and on the rate of gastric emptying. The dose, therefore, cannot be accurately calculated for any one case.

The rate of gastric emptying is the most important limiting factor in achieving continuous elevation of pH by intermittent administration. The significant fact is that however large or small the gastric contents, if it is liquid, half will have left in about 30 min. Thus, relatively more of a total dose spends time in the stomach if small amounts are taken frequently. Conventional doses of antacids act for only 20–40 min in the fasting state but continuous sucking of antacid tables is an effective method of prolonging the effect. Aluminium compounds delay gastric emptying by a direct effect on gastric motility, though combination with magnesium may lessen this action.

Antacids are generally used to relieve symptoms of ulcer and non-ulcer dyspepsia and they are therefore taken when symptoms arise, i.e. intermittently. Evidence indicates that there is a considerable placebo effect. *Large* amounts of a liquid magnesium-aluminium hydroxide mixture (equivalent to 1,008 mmol of neutralising capacity per day) can accelerate duodenal ulcer healing with minimal adverse effects but compliance with the regimen, which requires taking 30 ml × 7/day, overtaxes the diligence of most patients. While a dose of antacid lower than this may also be effective, histamine H_2-receptor antagonists are normally preferred as ulcer-healing agents but an antacid may be taken for occasional symptomatic relief during a course of cimetidine or ranitidine, especially during the first few days.

Alginic acid may be combined with an antacid to encourage adherence of the mixture to the mucosa, e.g. for reflux oesophagitis.

Dimethicone is sometimes included in antacid mixtures as an antifoaming agent to reduce flatulence. It is a silicone polymer that lowers surface tension and allows the small bubbles of froth to coalesce into large bubbles that can more easily be passed up from the stomach or down from the colon. The substance is biologically inactive and is not absorbed from the gastrointestinal tract. Dimethicone on its own probably relieves mild post-operative or post-prandial gastrointestinal symptoms; claims that it protectively coats mucous membranes require supporting evidence. It may help aviators to belch at high altitudes.

Antacids may be classified as:

1. *Systemic*: absorbed, and can cause metabolic alkalosis, e.g. sodium bicarbonate.
2. *Non-systemic*: not significantly absorbed and so will not disturb acid–base balance of the body, e.g. magnesium and aluminium salts.

Individual antacids

Sodium bicarbonate reacts with acid and relieves pain within minutes. It is absorbed and causes alkalosis, which in short-term use may not cause symptoms but can be a serious matter in patients with renal insufficiency. Alkalosis can also cause confusion in diagnosis for it may develop in peptic ulcer patients due to loss of chloride in vomit; this is accompanied by dehydration and renal ischaemia and gives rise to severe symptoms. Both kinds of alkalosis may be present simultaneously.

Sodium bicarbonate can release enough CO_2 in the stomach to cause discomfort and belching, which may have a psychotherapeutic effect or not, according to the circumstances. Excess sodium intake may cause oedema and heart failure in patients with cardiac or renal disease.

Magnesium oxide and **hydroxide** react quickly but cause diarrhoea, as do all magnesium salts, which are also used as purgatives.

Magnesium carbonate is rather less effective.

Magnesium trisilicate reacts slowly, to form magnesium chloride, which reacts with intestinal secretions to form the carbonate, the chloride being released and reabsorbed. Acid–base balance is thus not significantly altered. It adsorbs pepsin. Magnesium salts are trivially absorbed, but retention in renal insufficiency can cause bradycardia.

Aluminium hydroxide reacts with HCl to form aluminium chloride, which reacts with intestinal secretions to produce insoluble salts, especially phosphate, the chloride being released and reabsorbed. It does not alter acid–base balance. In addition to neutralising acid, aluminium hydroxide adsorbs pepsin. It tends to constipate. Sufficient aluminium may be absorbed from the intestine to create a risk of encephalopathy in patients with chronic renal failure. Aluminium hydroxide causes hypophosphataemia and hypophosphaturia by binding phosphate so that it is not absorbed from the gut. The use of aluminium hydroxide to reduce hyperphosphataemia in uraemic patients is inappropriate as antacids that contain aluminium also increase urinary and faecal loss of calcium and reduce the absorption of fluoride, which in the long term results in skeletal demineralisation. Prolonged phosphorus depletion causes anorexia, muscle weakness and osteomalacia.

Magaldrate (Dynese) is a complex of magnesium and aluminium hydroxides that dissociates in gastric acid; it is not just a mixture. Other readily dissociating antacid complexes include alexitol, almasilate and hydrotalcite.

Calcium- and bismuth-containing antacids should generally be avoided. Calcium ion stimulates the release of gastrin to cause rebound hypersecretion. Furthermore, excessive doses, especially combined with heavy milk drinking, which was often advised in peptic ulcer, can cause the hypercalcaemic (milk–alkali) syndrome characterised by headache, weakness, anorexia, nausea, vomiting, abdominal pain, constipation, thirst, polyuria with temporary, or rarely permanent, renal damage. Bismuth may also be absorbed and causes encephalopathy and arthropathy.

Adverse effects of antacid mixtures

Those that apply to individual antacids are described above. Some further general points are relevant.

(a) Many antacid **mixtures** contain *sodium*, which may not be readily apparent from the name and for this reason may be dangerous for patients with cardiac or renal disease. For example, a 10-ml dose of Magnesium Carbonate Mixture contains 9.8 mmol of sodium and of Magnesium Trisilicate Mixture contains 6.3 mmol, whereas the same dose of Magnesium Hydroxide Mixture contains less than 0.1 mmol of sodium. The risk may be known to the physician but we 'do not always remember as we scribble our prescriptions.'*

(b) *Aluminium*- and *magnesium*-containing antacids may interfere with the absorption of other drugs by binding with them or by altering gastrointestinal pH or transit time. Reduced biological availability of iron, digoxin, warfarin and some non-steroidal anti-inflammatory drugs has been ascribed to this type of interaction. It is probably advisable to avoid using antacids concurrently with drugs that are intended for systemic effect by the oral route.

* Editorial. Lancet 1960; 2:695.

Choice of antacid and administration. It is plain that no single antacid is satisfactory; mixtures are often used. They often consist of sodium bicarbonate for quickest effect, supplemented by magnesium hydroxide or carbonate. Sometimes magnesium trisilicate or aluminium hydroxide is added, but these are often used alone, though they are relative slow-acting. All formularies contain numerous antacid preparations; the choice is not critical.

Disturbed bowel habit can be corrected by altering the proportions of magnesium salts that tend to cause diarrhoea and aluminium salts that tend to constipate, sometimes severely.

Tablets are more convenient for the patient at work but, swallowed whole, they act more slowly as they have first to disintegrate; they may be chewed or sucked for speedier effect. A liquid may be more acceptable for frequent use. An antacid taken when the stomach is empty may be effective for only 20–40 min (see above) but if it is taken an hour after a meal, when the buffering action of food has ceased, the effect may last 2–3 h. Patients will find their own optimal pattern of use.

Enhancement of mucosal resistance

Drugs can enhance or augment mucosal resistance by different mechanisms, which are described in the accounts of the various agents.

(a) **Liquorice derivatives**: crude liquorice contains two sources of anti-ulcer activity, one related to glycyrrhizin (a glycoside) and one that remains after glycyrrhizin is removed.

Carbenoxolone (Biogastrone) is derived from glycyrrhetinic acid, which is made from the glycoside in liquorice root. It was discovered as a result of investigations of the casual observation that patients who took an indigestion mixture containing liquorice (for flavour) got better unexpectedly soon. It accelerates healing of gastric ulcer by various related actions that augment mucosal resistance. Carbenoxolone (i) increases the amount and quality of mucus so that the ulcer is protected, (ii) reduces diffusion of H^+ ion from the lumen into the mucosa, especially in the presence of agents such as bile, which promote such back-diffusion, and (iii) reduces the rate of shedding of gastric mucosal cells (i.e. prolongs their life). The ulcer-healing effect depends on direct contact of the drug with the mucosa.

Carbenoxolone is well absorbed from the stomach and is excreted mainly unchanged in the bile. The $t_{\frac{1}{2}}$ is 16 h. The drug is 99% protein-bound in plasma.

Carbenoxolone is used to treat gastric ulcer, 40–70% of which heal after 6 weeks of treatment. This benefit is approximately equivalent to that of bed rest, though the two measures are not additive. It is also effective for duodenal ulcer. Because the drug is absorbed in the stomach and its therapeutic effect is topical (as opposed to systemic), special position-release capsules (Duogastrone) have been devised to lodge in the pylorus and discharge the carbenoxolone into the duodenum. Carbenoxolone combined with alginic acid (to encourage adherence to the mucosa) and antacids (Pyrogastrone) is used for oesophageal inflammation and ulcer caused by gastric reflux. Because of its adverse effects (below), carbenoxolone takes second place to histamine H_2-receptor antagonists in treatment of the above conditions.

Adverse effects. Carbenoxolone has a steroid chemical structure and aldosterone-like activity. It induces sodium retention, which may lead to oedema, hypertension and heart failure. Carbenoxolone should therefore not be used in the elderly. Hypokalaemia also occurs. Spironolactone can correct this but only at the cost of abolishing the therapeutic effect.

Deglycyrrhinized liquorice preparations do not cause fluid retention but retain some ulcer-healing effect. Preparations include Caved-S, a mixture that includes antacids, and Rabro, which in addition to antacids contains frangula bark (a mild bulk purgative).

(b) **Bismuth chelate** (tripotassium dicitratobismuthate, colloidal bismuth, bismuth subcitrate, De-Nol; 120 mg, 120 mg/5 ml), acts by selectively chelating with protein material in the ulcer base, so forming a coating that protects it from the adverse influences of acid, pepsin and bile. The drug also has anti-peptic activity. It is used for both gastric and duodenal ulcer and has a therapeutic efficacy approximately equivalent to histamine H_2-receptor antagonists. There is evidence that peptic ulcers are less likely to relapse after being healed with bismuth chelate than with cimetidine.

The dose is 5 ml of the elixir with 15 ml of water or one tablet chewed × 4/day. As bismuth chelate may adhere to food rather than to the ulcer, these should be taken 30 min before the three main meals of the day, and 2 h after the last meal. A course should last 4 weeks.

Bismuth chelate, particularly as the elixir, darkens the tongue, teeth and stool; the tablet is less likely to do so and is thus more acceptable. Systemic absorption of bismuth from the chelated preparation appears to be well below the levels at which encephalopathy occurs, but as bismuth is eliminated by the kidney it is prudent to avoid giving the drug to patients with impaired renal function.

(c) **Sucralfate** (Antepsin) (1 g) is a basic aluminium salt of sucrose octasulphate (sucrose substituted with eight sulphate groups). In the acid environment of the stomach, the aluminium moiety dissociates and the negatively charged sucrose octasulphate binds electrostatically to positively charged protein molecules that transude from damaged mucosa. The result is that sucralfate forms a viscous paste that adheres selectively to the ulcer base. Its efficacy also appears to derive from binding to and inactivation of pepsin and bile acids; it has negligible acid-neutralising capacity but may prevent damaging back-diffusion of H^+ from the lumen to the mucosa.

Sucralfate is used for gastric and duodenal ulcer and for gastritis; it has a therapeutic efficacy approximately equal to the histamine H_2-receptor antagonists but may be better at prolonging remission after healing has occurred. Maintenance treatment is effective at preventing relapse.

The dose is 1 g × 4/day, one hour *before* meals and at night (to avoid binding to food proteins), but up to 8 g/day may be used. A course normally lasts 4–6 weeks but 12 weeks may be needed for resistant ulcers.

Sucralfate may cause constipation but is otherwise well tolerated. The aluminium moiety is absorbed from the gastrointestinal tract; the concentration of aluminium in the plasma may be elevated in uraemic patients, but not if renal function is normal. As the drug is effective only in acid conditions, an antacid should not be taken 30 min before or after a dose of sucralfate. The aluminium content of sucralfate may cause it to interfere with absorption of other drugs (see *antacids*, above).

(d) **Prostaglandin analogues** are being developed for the treatment of peptic ulcer. Interest in their use in this role stems from the observation that endogenous prostaglandins are important contributors to the integrity of the gastrointestinal mucosa. This mucosal protective (cytoprotective) effect derives from a number of related mechanisms, for prostaglandins:

(i) stimulate secretion of mucus and bicarbonate by the mucosa,

(ii) increase mucosal blood flow; maintenance of an adequate flow not only ensures a supply of oxygen and nutrients but also helps to remove H^+, which readily diffuses from the lumen into damaged or ischaemic tissues,

(iii) prevent luminal H^+ from diffusing into the mucosa, e.g. in response to aspirin, ethanol and bile acids,

(iv) enhance the rate of cell replication in the mucosa, to hasten the repair of damaged epithelium,

(v) can reduce gastric acid secretion.

Prostaglandin analogues, e.g. *misoprostol*, are being developed in the belief that they will mimic the effects of their endogenous counterparts to improve mucosal resistance. They may provide a means of curing those peptic ulcers that fail to heal with histamine H_2-receptor antagonists or of benefitting those conditions in which these drugs have achieved more limited success, e.g. gastritis, duodenitis and oesophagitis.

PEPTIC ULCER THERAPY

A complete account of the medical management of this disease involves a lot more than the mere use of drugs and is outside the scope of this book but it may be summarised thus:

1. *General advice* should be given to stop smoking and to avoid non-steroidal anti-inflammatory drugs (NSAIDs) and alcohol. Healing of ulcers with histamine H_2-receptor drugs is retarded by smoking and ingestion of NSAIDs.

2. *Healing* of peptic ulcer can be accelerated by a number of types of drug. Care must be taken to establish by biopsy that a gastric ulcer is benign for a malignant gastric ulcer may respond temporarily (both symptoms and apparent healing) to drug therapy. A *histamine H_2-receptor antagonist* is generally preferred and ranitidine has fewer adverse effects than cimetidine. If healing has not taken place after 4 weeks, treatment should continue for 8 weeks; the dose may be increased for resistant ulcers. *Pirenzepine, sucralfate* and *bismuth chelate* are alternatives that are approximately as effective as histamine H_2-receptor antagonists. The need for multiple daily dosing may limit compliance with sucralfate and bismuth chelate but they may be effective for some ulcers that have failed to heal with cimetidine or ranitidine. *Carbenoxolone* is no longer a drug of choice because of its adverse effects. *Antacids* as sole treatment can accelerate ulcer healing but must be taken frequently to achieve this; their use is now generally limited to providing supplementary symptomatic relief, e.g. in the first few days of a course of cimetidine or ranitidine for intermittent subsequent use.

3. *Prevention of relapse*, in those individuals who are prone to it, is best achieved with a *histamine H_2-receptor antagonist* taken as a single dose at night, regularly, long-term. Resort to surgery may be required for patients whose ulcers recur despite all other measures.

GUIDE TO FURTHER READING

1 Editorial. Gastric ulcer or cancer. Lancet 1985; 1: 202–3.
2 McNulty CAM, et al. (Editorial). Gastric microflora. Br Med J 1985; 291: 367–8.
3 Editorial. Acid reduction or mucosal protection for peptic ulcer. Lancet 1982; 2: 473–4.
4 Editorial. Cimetidine-resistant duodenal ulcers. Lancet 1985; 1: 23–4.
5 Wormsley K G. (Editorial). Duodenal ulcers which do not heal rapidly. Br Med J 1984; 289:1095.
6 Editorial. Management of gastro-oesophageal reflux. Lancet 1984; 1: 1054–6.
7 Pounder R E. Model of medical treatment for duodenal ulcer. Lancet 1981; 1: 29–30.

8 Sonnenberg A. Comparison of different strategies for treatment of duodenal ulcer. Br Med J 1985; 290: 1185–7.
9 Colin-Jones D G, et al. Postmarketing surveillance of the safety of cimetidine: mortality during second, third, and fourth years of follow up. Br Med J 1985; 291: 1084–8.
10 Langman M J S. Antisecretory drugs and gastric cancer. Br Med J 1985; 290: 1850–2.
11 Collins R, et al. Treatment with histamine H_2 antagonists in acute upper gastrointestinal haemorrhage. N Engl J Med 1985; 313: 660–6.
12 Langman M J S. (Editorial). Antacids for duodenal ulcer? Br Med J 1982; 285: 1520–2.

32

Gastrointestinal system II: Drugs for vomiting, constipation and diarrhoea

VOMITING

If the cause of vomiting cannot be removed, it may be desirable to attempt to prevent or to suppress it by drugs.

The pharmacology of vomiting was little studied until the second world war, when motion sickness attained military importance because 'when a landing has to be made in the face of resistance, it is easy to see that seasickness might on occasion become a handicap'. The British military authorities and the Medical Research Council therefore organised an investigation that has provided a standard for many subsequent drug trials.*

The aim was to find what drugs in what dose would prevent seasickness without interfering with physical and mental efficiency. The only guide to choice of drugs for the trial was the numerous claims based on uncontrolled observations in the past, which, however, made it clear that anticholinergic drugs (atropine and hyoscine) were likely to be important. Attempts to use swing sickness in the hope of being able to avoid 'the disadvantage which the inconstancy of the sea imposed' were not satisfactory, as those who were sick on a swing were not necessarily sick at sea. Reluctantly, the workers turned to the sea for their experiments, observing that 'dependence on so fickle an element for experimental conditions imposed a considerable strain on the patience of the investigator. Chronic sufferers of seasickness may be astonished to learn that on most days throughout the year, an obstinate and baffling calm haunts the waters around this island.'

Whenever there was a prospect of sufficiently rough weather, about 70 soldiers were sent to sea in small ships, again and again, after being dosed with a drug or a dummy tablet and having had their mouths inspected to detect non-compliance. The ships returned to land when up to 40% of the soldiers had vomited. 'On the whole the men enjoyed their trips'; some of them, however, being soldiers, thought the pills were given in order to make them vomit and some 'believed firmly in the efficacy of the dummy tablets.' It was concluded that, of the remedies tested, hyoscine (0.6 mg or 1.2 mg) was the most effective.

* Holling H E et al. Lancet 1944; 1: 127.

This study has been followed by many others on the physiology and pharmacology of nausea and vomiting due to motion, drugs and disease.

Some physiology

Vomiting is in essence a protective mechanism for eliminating irritant or otherwise harmful substances from the upper gastrointestinal tract. The act of emesis is controlled by the vomiting centre in the medulla, and close to it lie other visceral centres, e.g. for respiration, salivation and vascular control, which give rise to the other prodromal sensations associated with vomiting. The vomiting centre does not initiate, but rather it co-ordinates, the act of emesis on receiving stimuli from various sources, namely (a) the chemoreceptor trigger zone (CTZ), a nearby area that is extremely sensitive to the action of drugs and other chemicals, (b) the vestibular system, (c) the periphery (e.g. distension or irritation of the gut, myocardial infarction, biliary or renal stone) and, (d) cortical centres.

The vomiting centre contains many muscarinic cholinergic and histamine H_1-receptors; the CTZ is rich in dopamine receptors.

Antiemetic drugs

Drugs that are effective for nausea and vomiting are classified as follows:

Drug	**Site of action**
1. *Anticholinergics*	
hyoscine and some drugs classed as histamine H_1-receptor blockers (cyclizine, dimenhydrinate, diphenhydramine, meclozine, mepyramine, promethazine)	vomiting centre
2. *Dopamine antagonists*	
domperidone, metoclopramide	CTZ and gut
haloperidol	CTZ
phenothiazines, e.g. chlorpromazine, prochlorperazine, thiethylperazine	vomiting centre and CTZ

4. *Other agents*
(for vomiting due to cytotoxics)
corticosteroids (dexamethasone, methylprednisolone)
cannabinoids (nabilone)
benzodiazepines (diazepam, lorazepam)

Antiemetics acting on the vomiting centre (hyoscine, meclosine, promethazine) alleviate vomiting from any cause, but drugs acting on the CTZ (haloperidol) are only effective for vomiting mediated by the chemoreceptors (morphine, digoxin, uraemia). The most efficacious drugs act at more than one site (see above); the success of many of the H_1-receptor antihistamines as antiemetics is due to the fact that they also block cholinergic receptors.

Anticholinergic and antihistamine drugs are described elsewhere; an account of those dopamine antagonists that are used principally as antiemetics follows below.

Metoclopramide (Maxolon, Primperan) (10 mg; inj 5 mg/ml) has an antiemetic effect, centrally by blocking dopamine receptors in the CTZ and peripherally by enhancing the action of acetylcholine at muscarine receptors in the gut. It raises the tone of the lower oesophageal sphincter, relaxes the pyloric antrum and duodenal cap and increases peristalsis and emptying of the upper gut. The peripheral actions are also utilised to facilitate intubation procedures, radiological examination of the gut, and to empty the stomach before emergency anaesthesia and in labour. If an opioid analgesic has been given, metoclopramide may fail to overcome the inhibition of gastric emptying that opioids produce and thus the risk of vomiting and inhaling gastric contents remains. The direct effects on the gut are antagonised by atropine and other anticholinergic drugs, and are increased by cholinergic drugs. The peripheral action of metoclopramide on the gut is not prevented by surgical vagotomy and the drug can accelerate gastric emptying when this is delayed after a vagotomy and drainage procedure. Gastric secretion is unaffected.

The action of metoclopramide is terminated by metabolism in the liver; the $t_{\frac{1}{2}}$ is 4 h.

Metoclopramide is *used* for nausea and vomiting associated with gastrointestinal disorders, with postoperative conditions, and with cytotoxic drugs and radiotherapy. It is also an effective antiemetic in migraine. The dose is 10 mg 8-hourly orally, i.m. or i.v.

Adverse reactions are characteristic of dopamine receptor antagonists and include extrapyramidal dystonia (torticollis, facial spasms, trismus, oculogyric crises), which occurs more commonly in children and young adults and in those who are concurrently receiving phenothiazine drugs. The reaction is rapidly abolished by the anticholinergic benztropine, given i.v. Long-term use of metoclopramide may cause tardive dyskinesia in the elderly. Metoclopramide stimulates prolactin release and may cause gynaecomastia and lactation. Motor restlessness and diarrhoea also occur.

Domperidone (Motilium) (10 mg; suppos. 30 mg) is a dopamine receptor antagonist. Its antiemetic actions are both central at the CTZ and peripheral in the upper gut, where it increases the pressure in the lower oesophageal sphincter, enhances contractions of the gastric antrum and relaxes the pyloric sphincter. Domperidone crosses the blood–brain barrier poorly; this does not limit its therapeutic efficacy for the CTZ is functionally outwith the barrier, but there is less risk of adverse effects in the central nervous system. The $t_{\frac{1}{2}}$ is 7 h and is prolonged in patients with impaired renal function.

Domperidone is used for nausea or vomiting associated with gastrointestinal disorders and with cytotoxic and other drug treatment. The dose is 10–20 mg every 4–8 h.

Dystonic reactions are much fewer with domperidone than with metoclopramide. It may cause gynaecomastia and galactorrhoea. Cardiac dysrhythmia may be induced if an i.v. bolus exceeds 50 mg and an infusion avoids this risk.

Nabilone (Cesamet) is a synthetic cannabinoid and has properties similar to tetrahydrocannabinol (the active constituent of marijuana), which has an antiemetic action. It is used to relieve nausea or vomiting caused by cytotoxic drugs. Adverse effects include somnolence, dry mouth, decreased appetite, dizziness, euphoria, dysphoria, postural hypotension, confusion and psychosis. These may be reduced if prochlorperazine is given concomitantly.

The drug treatment of various forms of vomiting is now discussed.

Motion sickness

There was a young lady of Spain
Who was dreadfully sick in a train,
Not once, but again,
And again and again,
And again and again and again*

Motion sickness is more easily prevented than cured. It is due chiefly to overstimulation of the vestibular apparatus; it does not occur if the labyrinth is destroyed. Other factors also contribute; visually, a moving horizon can be most disturbing, as can the sensations induced by the gravitational inertia of a full stomach when the body is in vertical movement. That the environment, whether close and smelly or open and vivifying, is important, is a matter of common experience amongst all who have passed between England and France by sea on a rough day. Psychological factors, including observation of the fate of one's companions are also important. Tolerance to the motion occurs, generally over a period of days.

Some drugs effective against motion sickness

These drugs all have anticholinergic actions and all except hyoscine happen to be antihistamines (H_1-receptor).

Once motion sickness has started, oral administration of drugs may fail, not only because they are vomited but because the pylorus may be closed, so that they cannot reach their site of absorption in the small intestine. Injections or suppositories are then indicated. It is as well to remember that prevention of motion sickness may be possible only at the expense of troublesome unwanted effects — sleepiness, dry mouth or blurred vision. Holidaymakers travelling for one-and-a-half hours or less from Dover to Calais by sea or from London to Paris by air may not be grateful for prophylaxis at any cost, especially if drugs as long-acting as meclozine or promethazine are used; also, if they are going to drive cars, the unwanted effects are dangerous, and they must be warned of this, as well as being told to take no alcohol. The duration of exposure is relevant to the choice of drugs: *hyoscine* may be as good as

* Anonymous limerick.

Non-proprietary name	*Proprietary names (tablet size in mg)*	*Oral dose (no. of doses per day)*	*Remarks*
Meclozine	Bonamine (25) Sea-legs (12.5)	50 mg (1)	Low incidence of side-effects. May cause sleepiness; good for prolonged prophylaxis.
Promethazine	Phenergan (25) Avomine (25)	25 mg (1–3)	Best taken in evening as sleepiness fairly common.
Diphenhydramine	Benadryl (25)	25–50 mg (3–4)	May cause sleepiness
Dimenhydrinate	Dramamine (50)	50–100 mg (2–3)	The theoclate of diphenhydramine to which in equiv. dose it is probably not superior. May cause sleepiness.
Cyclizine	Valoid (50)	50 mg (3)	Low incidence of side-effects. May cause sleepiness. Good for prolonged prophylaxis.
Hyoscine	Kwells, Sereen (0.3)	0.6 mg (3)	Useful in single dose for short journeys. Side effects too troublesome for prolonged use. Atropine is probably equally effective.

Table 32.1 Drugs for motion sickness

other drugs for brief, but not for prolonged exposure.

It is usual to take antimetics prophylactically 30–60 min before exposure to the motion, but longer-acting drugs may be begun 12–24 h before.

Choice of drugs. Many drugs are effective, and details of those most commonly used are given in the table. A suitable choice would be meclozine or cyclizine (repeated) for prolonged or hyoscine or cyclizine for brief prophylaxis.

Protection rates are clearly likely to vary a lot with the conditions under which the drugs are used, but about 70% protection may be expected by the right doses given at the right time. Confident prediction of what will happen to any one subject about to take a drug of this kind for the first time may be unwise but much may be gained by an assured air on the part of the prescriber. A sedative, e.g. diazepam, can be a useful adjunct if the patient is anxious or distressed. Much may be done to prevent motion sickness by simple commonsense behaviour over meals and environment.

Vomiting due to drugs

Emetic drugs may act in the central nervous system on the chemoreceptor trigger zone (e.g. morphine or apomorphine) or in the gastrointestinal tract. Digitalis glycosides and ipecacuanha probably act at both these sites.

The best treatment of drug-induced vomiting is to withdraw or reduce the dose of the drug, but if this cannot be done, an attempt, often unsatisfactory, may be made to oppose it by another drug. In general, chlorpromazine or another phenothiazine or metoclopramide are best. However, in the case of opioid-induced vomiting, diphenhydramine, dimenhydrinate or cyclizine, which are normally used for motion sickness, may be better. Cyclizine and morphine are combined as Cyclimorph. Cerebral depressant effects of morphine and the antiemetics are additive, and chlorpromazine potentiates morphine, so that caution is needed.

A usual dose of chlorpromazine is 25–50 mg orally 8-hourly, but if vomiting has already begun, the first dose at least may be given i.m. Larger doses can be needed.

Vomiting due to cytotoxic drugs is probably due to stimulation of the CTZ but the mechanisms may differ as there is a variable interval between dosing with different agents and symptoms. Not all cytotoxic agents cause vomiting but those that do include cyclophosphamide, doxorubicin and nitrosoureas; cisplatin is notably emetic. A phenothiazine, e.g. prochlorperazine, is effective against moderate emesis but tolerance develops with frequent use. Metoclopramide, up to 10 mg/kg i.v. over 8 hours, domperidone or nabilone may then be preferred. Vomiting with highly emetic drugs may be alleviated by a parenteral corticosteroid, e.g. dexamethasone or methylprednisolone. Addition of a sedative, e.g. lorazepam, may help. A combination of drugs given i.v. is often successful and metoclopramide in high dose plus lorazepam plus a corticosteroid may be an optimal regimen.

Radiation sickness

Radiation sickness is treated with prochlorperazine or metoclopramide.

Postanaesthetic vomiting

Postanaesthetic vomiting can be reduced effectively by metoclopramide, which may be given before or after the operation. Chlorpromazine potentiates anaesthetic agents and analgesics and hypnotics and this must be taken into account when it is used, for waking may be delayed. The sedative effects of meclozine and cyclizine may summate with those of other drugs.

Vomiting in pregnancy

Vomiting in pregnancy reaches a peak at 10–11 weeks and usually resolves by 13–14 weeks of gestation. All drugs should be avoided in early pregnancy as far as possible, and much can be done by reassurance that the problem is transient and a discussion of diet, e.g. taking food before getting up in the morning. When a decision is taken to use a drug, promethazine, meclozine or metoclopramide are often preferred and are apparently free from teratogenic effects. Although pyridoxine deficiency has not been shown to complicate simple pregnancy vomiting, it may occur in hyperemesis gravidarum, which requires i.v. fluids and multivitamin supplement. Pyridoxine has been widely used in pregnancy vomiting, alone and with meclozine. It can be considered as a suitable placebo to support psychotherapy if the prescription of a tablet will itself provide useful reassurance that something definite, i.e. not just talk, is being done.

Vomiting of disease

When removal of the cause is not possible, this may be helped by chlorpromazine, metoclopramide, cyclizine or meclozine.

Vertigo

A great range of drugs has been recommended for vertigo and labyrinthine disorders. All the antiemetic drugs are used, also a hodge-potch of remedies the variety of which indicates the absence of scientific evidence of their value, e.g. vasoconstrictors, central nervous system stimulants and depressants, and inevitably, vitamins. Perhaps sedation and an antiemetic (promethazine, cyclizine) are most likely to help. Betahistine, cinnarazine or thiethylperazine may be useful.

Therapeutic emesis

Except for ingested poisons, therapeutic emesis is rarely required. Of course, no emetic should ever be administered to an unconscious patient or when a corrosive substance has been swallowed. The relative usefulness of emesis and of gastric lavage in acute poisoning is discussed elsewhere (see Chapter 10).

Ipecacuanha is the best *emergency emetic*. It contains emetine and cephaline and acts both peripherally (stomach) and centrally (CTZ). It has the advantage that it can be used safely by non-medical people in emergency.

Apomorphine is a semisynthetic, morphine-like alkaloid with the emetic action of morphine greatly enhanced. It also has the other central actions of morphine and can cause coma, especially if given to a patient whose central nervous system is already depressed. It is now obsolete. It was used in aversion therapy of alcoholism, i.e. the subject took a glass of whisky, was then injected with apomorphine and vomited violently; no doubt some patients were helped and some just made their escape from treatment. Overdose responds to naloxone.

MISCELLANEOUS

Reflux oesophagitis

General measures include, (a) weight reduction in the overweight, (b) avoidance of substances known to aggravate the condition, e.g. fatty or hot foods, or to stimulate gastric secretion, e.g. alcohol, (c) avoidance of smoking, because nicotine relaxes the lower oesophageal sphincter, (d) avoidance of stooping when possible and (e) elevating the head of the bed on blocks to discourage nocturnal reflux.

Drugs readily relieve symptoms, but healing of an inflamed or ulcerated mucosa takes substantially longer. Antacids combined with alginic acid (an insoluble viscous substance obtained from seaweed), e.g. Gaviscon or Gastrocote, provide relief for milder degrees of oesophagitis. They supposedly produce a floating viscous gel that blocks reflux and coats the oesophagus. When the condition is more severe, a histamine H_2-receptor antagonist is better, e.g. cimetidine 400 mg × 4/day for 4–8 weeks continuing with 400 mg at night, or ranitidine 150 mg × 2/day for 4–8 weeks continuing with 150 mg at night should maintenance treatment be necessary. Metoclopramide 10 mg × 3–4/day, the last dose taken at night, may usefully be added to reduce reflux by completing gastric emptying.

Reflux oesophagitis may be aggravated by drugs with anticholinergic activity (e.g. tricyclic antidepressants, H_1-receptor antihistamines or phenothiazines), which impair oesophageal peristalsis and cause the lower oesophageal sphincter to relax. Tablets and capsules taken just before going to bed and without an accompanying drink may remain in the oesophagus and damage its mucosa, e.g. non-steroidal anti-inflammatory drugs, emepronium (Cetiprin), potassium tablets or tetracyclines.

Others

Diffuse oesophageal spasm and achalasia may be helped by isosorbide dinitrate 5 mg sublingually or 10 mg swallowed, or by nifedipine 10 mg sublingually or swallowed.

Hiccup. Numerous remedies have been tried. Success has been claimed with granulated sugar, swallowed dry, but when the condition is troublesomely persistent, chlorpromazine, perphenazine, prochlorperazine or metoclopramide appear to offer most prospect of benefit.

Carminatives are substances that are used to assist in expelling gas from the stomach and intestines*. They have been shown to induce relaxation of the cardiac oesophageal sphincter. Examples are peppermint, dill, anise and other herbs that are commonly included in liqueurs and in non-alcoholic solutions for babies, and may be useful in irritable bowel syndrome.

Charcoal is also used for flatulence (to adsorb gas in the stomach). It may help sometimes but the theory of action is unproved (see also *activated charcoal*).

Bitters are substances taken before meals to improve appetite. They have not been scientifically investigated. They include gentian, nux vomica and quinine. Preparations can be found in the BNF and at wine merchants (Byrrh, Dubonnet, Campari).

Demulcents coat and soothe mucous membranes. They are used in sore throat, gastritis, peptic ulcer and in cases of ingestion of corrosive or irritant poisons. They include starch, tragacanth, acacia, mucin, raw egg-white (albumin) and milk.

* The eccentric Roman Emperor Claudius (AD 10–54) 'planned an edict to legitimise the breaking of wind at table, even noisily, after hearing about a man who was so modest that he endangered his health by an attempt to restrain himself.' (Suetonius, trans R. Graves.)

Chlorophyll. Whether chlorophyll in any form taken orally is an effective general body or breath deodorant remains a subject of dispute.* The comment by one critic of claims on its behalf that:

'The goat that stinks on yonder hill
Has browsed all day on chlorophyll,'

has been stigmatised as irrelevant as well as unfair. Local application of high concentrations in wounds or in the gut may have some deodorant effect.

CONSTIPATION

The terms purgative, cathartic, laxative, aperient and evacuant may be considered synonymous.

Purgatives may be classified as (1) bulk, (2) faecal softeners, and (3) stimulant. The time a purgative takes to act determines whether it should be given in the morning or evening, and will be found in the table below together with the dose.

Bulk purgatives

Bulk purgatives act by *increasing the volume and lowering the viscosity* of intestinal contents, so both encouraging and rendering more effective, normal reflex bowel activity.* If taken repeatedly with too little fluid, they can cause intestinal obstruction, especially if there is any organic obstruction or if peristalsis is weak. They include two different groups of substances:

1. **Hydrophilic colloids and indigestible vegetable fibre**, which promote a large, soft, solid stool by holding water in the gut (lowering viscosity).

Bran is the residue left when flour is made from cereals. It contains between 25% and 50% of *fibre*, which is essentially the cell walls of plants. Fibre consists of a group of carbohydrate compounds including cellulose and hemicelluloses and also a non-carbohydrate polymer, lignin. Medicinally, fibre has two notable properties: *first*, it is not broken down by the enzymes in the gut, so it enters the colon intact, and *second*, it has a vast capacity for retaining water; for example, 1 g of carrot fibre can hold as much as 23 g of water.† Taken with insufficient water bran can cause intestinal obstruction. It has been proposed that as humans have progressively refined the carbohydrates in their diet over the centuries, so they have deprived themselves of fibre, particularly from cereal, and that the resultant underfilling of the colon is an important cause of *constipation*, *irritable bowel syndrome* and *diverticular disease*. Certainly, African rural people who have a daily dietary fibre intake of over 50 g and who pass stools weighing more than 250 g daily have a much greater freedom from colonic disease than urbanised Westerners, whose daily diet may contain less than 20 g and whose stools weigh about 100 g daily. Adding fibre (bran) to the diet results in stools that are softer, bulkier and passed more easily and more often. It is thus a safe and natural way of treating constipation. In patients with diverticular disease, bran appears to reduce intracolonic pressure waves and to relieve symptoms. It may also help a proportion of patients with irritable bowel syndrome. Whether returning bran to the diet alters the natural history of these conditions remains to be seen. Miller's bran is obtained in health food shops; for the management of colonic diverticular disease, about 24 g per day is recommended, but prevention should be the aim, since once the anatomical changes have occurred, they cannot be reversed and the sudden addition of a full regimen of bran to the diet of such a person may exacerbate symptoms. The fibre content of normal diet can be increased by eating wholemeal bread and bran cereals.

Methylcellulose takes up water to swell to a colloid about 25 times its original volume. It can be taken as tablets, granules or in solution (e.g. Celevac, Cologel), in control of colostomies, in diverticular disease of the colon (when the high colonic pressures are lowered) and in irritable bowel syndrome. Its use to fill the stomach and suppress appetite in obesity (see index) is probably irrational. It is also used as a suspending agent in pharmacy, in lubricating jellies, in contact-lens

* JAMA 1953; 153: 728, 749. Br Med J 1953; 1: 832–3.

† McConnell A A, et al. J Sci Food Agric 1974; 25: 1427.

wetting solutions and in artificial tears. Sodium carboxymethylcellulose is similar.

Agar is obtained from seaweed; with water it swells and forms a jelly.

Psyllium seeds (Isogel) contain mucilage that swells with water. Various other mucilaginous plant substances that swell with water, include *slippery elm bark, isphagula, frangula, sterculia** and *plantago*.

Prunes and figs act as bulk purges and also contain mild irritant organic substances. It should be remembered that Compound Figs Elixir BNF, and proprietary preparations in which the word 'fig' is prominent, implying mild and 'physiological' action particularly suited to children, owe most of their efficacy to the substantial doses of cascara or senna that are incorporated. They can be violently effective.

Bulk purgatives are often combined with liquid paraffin and stimulant purges in proprietary preparations.

2. **Osmotic laxatives**, which are but little absorbed and increase the bulk and reduce viscosity of intestinal contents to promote a fluid stool.

Inorganic salts (saline purgatives) retain water in the intestinal lumen, or, if given as hypertonic solution, withdraw it from the body. The principal ions are magnesium, sulphate and tartrate. The main substances used as saline purges are magnesium sulphate (Epsom† salt), sodium sulphate (Glauber's‡ salt) and sodium potassium tatrate (Rochelle salt§); the latter mixed with tartaric acid and sodium bicarbonate as in Compound Effervescent Powder BP (Seidlitz§ powder) makes a not wholly unattractive effervescent drink that is promoted also for its psychological effect when taken on getting up in the morning. If prescribed, it is as well to mention to the patient how to prepare the drink, for it is reported that one young man swallowed the ingredients separately. 'He afterwards declared that his stomach exploded and that he was thrown against a wall.' Fortunately the gastric rupture was successfully repaired.‖

Lactulose (3.35 g/5 ml) is a synthetic disaccharide. Taken orally (Duphalac Syrup) it is unaffected by small intestine disaccharidase, is not absorbed and thus acts as an osmotic laxative. In the colon it is fermented to lactic and acetic acids and this is the basis for its use in treatment of hepatic encephalopathy, which is aggravated when ammonia produced in the colon gains access to the systemic circulation. Lactulose, by lowering pH, inhibits the growth of colonic ammonia-producing organisms and reduces non-ionic diffusion of ammonia from the colon into the blood. The dose is, for constipation 15 ml × 2/day, and for hepatic encephalopathy, 30–50 ml × 3/day.

All saline purges are nauseating if taken in too little water; a cupful is minimal, except with magnesium hydroxide, which is insoluble in water and is also used as a gastric antacid; the soluble magnesium salts formed in the alimentary tract act as a saline purge. It is relatively feeble and much used for children and for counteracting the constipating effects of aluminium and calcium salts in gastric antacid therapy. It is often combined with liquid paraffin in an emulsion.

In patients with renal failure the small amount of magnesium absorbed when the sulphate is frequently used can be enough to cause magnesium poisoning, the central nervous effects of which somewhat resemble those of uraemia. Magnesium poisoning can also occur with hypertonic magnesium sulphate enemas for lowering intracranial pressure. Again, the symptoms of poisoning and those of the disease process may be confused.

Faecal softeners (emollients)

1. *Surface-active agents*, e.g. dioctyl sodium sulphosuccinate (docusate sodium; Dioctyl) and poloxamers, e.g. poloxalkol (poloxamer 188) soften faeces by lowering the surface tension of fluids in the bowel, which allows more water to remain in the faeces. They are often combined in

* Named after Sterculinus, a god of ancient Rome who presided over agricultural muck-spreading.

† Epsom, a town near London, known for its mineral spring water and for horse racing.

‡ J. R. Glauber (1604–1648), German chemist.

§ Rochelle, named after La Rochelle, France. Seidlitz, a village in Bohemia, Czechoslovakia, having mineral springs of water of similar constitution.

‖ Tanner N C. Proceedings of the Royal Society of Medicine 1959; 52:379.

Common Purgatives

Mode of action	*Purgative (formulation size in mg)*	*Dose*	*Conventional time of oral administration (time to act)*
Bulk			
solid stool (small & large intestine)	agar	4–16 g	morning (1–3 h)
	bran	8–24 g	
	ispaghula	3–6 g	
	methylcellulose	1.5–6 g	
	pysllium	5–15 g	
	sterculia*		
Bulk			
semi-liquid stool (small & large intestine)	magnesium carbonate	2–5 g	morning (1–3 h)
	magnesium hydroxide	2–4 g	
	magnesium sulphate	5–15 g	
	sodium sulphate	5–15 g	
	sodium potassium tartrate	8–16 g	
Faecal softener			
	dioctyl sodium sulphosuccinate (20) (docusate)	up to 500 mg daily	divided doses (1–2 days)
	liquid paraffin	10–30 ml	evening or in 2–4 equally spaced doses
Stimulant			
semi-liquid stool (small intestine)	castor oil	5–20 ml	morning on an empty stomach (2–6 h)
Stimulant			
semi-liquid stool (large intestine)	bisacodyl (5) (10, suppos)	5–10 mg	night (6–10 h)
	cascara (20)	20–40 mg	night (8–10 h)
Note: danthron is carcinogenic in animals and is being withdrawn.	danthron (combined formulations)	25–75 mg	night (6–12 h)
	sodium picosulphate	5–15 mg	night (6–10 h)
	senna†		night (6–10 h)

* Sterculia B P 62% in preparations of Normacol; 1–2 heaped 5 ml spoonfuls × 1–2/day after meals.
† A variety of biologically standardised (in rats) proprietaries with differing doses, e.g. Senokot Tabs., dose 2–4.

a capsule with a stimulant purgative, e.g. bisacodyl + docusate (Dulcodos). They should not be used with liquid paraffin because they may increase its absorption.

2. *Liquid paraffin* is a chemically inert mineral oil and is not digested. It is tasteless although some find its oiliness nauseating. It is generally said to act by lubricating the bowel, although only about the last few feet can be in need of this, for elsewhere the contents are fluid. Paraffin has been said to increase the rate of passage of small intestine contents by reducing water absorption and it may be this effect as well as the softening powers of the oil (in the colon) that promotes the passage of softer faeces rather than the naive notion of lubrication.

Some paraffin is absorbed from the intestine and collects in the mesenteric lymph nodes where paraffinomas may form. Absorption of fat-soluble vitamins is reduced, but there is no conclusive proof that harm has resulted from either of these effects, although harm is clearly possible.

Liquid paraffin (or other oils) taken over long periods orally, especially at night, or as nasal drops may cause chronic lipoid pneumonia, especially in the old or very young. An unusual case resulted from successful attempts by a patient to lubricate his larynx with liquid paraffin.

Large doses may leak out of the anus causing both physical and social discomfort.

Liquid paraffin may not be as harmless as its chemical inertness suggests and long continued use has been associated with a slightly increased risk of gastrointestinal cancer. Because of these disadvantages, it should never be used long-term as a laxative. It has been administered in circumstances when straining at stool may be painful, as after anal surgery, although it may retard the healing of anal wounds. It is often presented in emulsions with magnesium hydroxide.

Stimulant purgatives

Bisacodyl (Dulcolax) is a synthetic substance. Few new purgatives are introduced, for with the range of drugs available, research by a commercial organisation would not offer attractive prospects of financial return, and academic institutions, not surprisingly though perhaps mistakenly, see little of interest in the study of purgatives.

Bisacodyl stimulates sensory endings in the colon by direct action from the lumen (oral or suppository). In geriatric patients, bisacodyl suppositories reduce the need for regular enemas. There are no important unwanted effects. *Sodium picosulphate* (Picolax) is similar.

Castor oil acts as a purgative after its hydrolysis (i.e. it is a prodrug) in the small intestine to ricinoleic acid, which stimulates peristalsis and reduces fluid absorption. The liquid contents of the small intestine pass rapidly onwards, resulting in a soft or fluid stool after 2–6 h. Having regard to the fact that it has to be digested, castor oil should obviously be given on an empty stomach. The ricinoleic acid is absorbed and there is insignificant stimulation of the large intestine. Colic (griping) is usually trivial, and so complete is the evacuation of the intestine that there is usually constipation afterwards. Castor oil is therefore used chiefly as a 'once and for all' purgative, as after a dietetic error. Its irritant action is powerful enough for it to be capable of starting labour in pregnant women.

Most patients find castor oil objectionable to taste. It is less offensive if given well cooled and floating in fruit juice, milk or whisky, according to taste.

Castor oil is also used in ointments, hair lotions and eye drops as a simple, non-irritant lubricant and vehicle.

The *anthraquinone group* of purgatives includes *cascara, senna, rhubarb* and *aloes*. In the small intestine soluble anthraquinone derivates are liberated and absorbed. These are excreted into the colon and act there, along with those that have escaped absorption, probably after being structurally changed by bacterial action. They are said to stimulate Auerbach's plexus in the large intestine and so provide 'physiological purgation'. Enough may be excreted in the milk to cause colic in a suckling infant.

Patients taking senna or rhubarb may notice their urine is coloured brown (if acid) or red (if alkaline) due to the presence of chrysophanic acid. Prolonged use of this group can cause melanosis of the rectum.

Erratic results with these purgatives, which are usually crude plant extracts, have in the past been due not only to the marked individual variation that occurs and to the development of tolerance, but also to the absence of methods of biological assay, employment of which has now revealed great variations in potency of official preparations. Biologically standardised (in rats) senna preparations are available.

Cascara is obtained from the Californian buckthorn. It is popular for self-medication.

Senna is obtained from an Arabian shrub. Extracts of the fruit (pod) are said to be less griping than those of the leaf, and these are used in the modern biologically standardised preparations of sennosides, e.g. Senokot. For those who like ritual and are not concerned about precision, the practice of soaking pods in water and drinking the extract may be preferred.

Rhubarb (a Chinese plant, not the familiar garden vegetable) and *aloes* are still supplied in the more old-fashioned mixtures. There is nothing much to be said either for or against them, but they are still popular with the self-medicating public because they work.

The *drastic purgatives* (jalap*, colocynth and podophyllum) are obsolete as they are too drastic and so is croton oil. Sulphur (brimstone), although not drastic, is obsolete because of its offensiveness.

Phenolphthalein. The purgative action of phenolphthalein was discovered in 1900 by von Vamossy who was investigating its properties because the Hungarian government wished to use it to 'denature' artificial wines. He administered it to his pet dog, which was at first indifferent, although later it passed a constipated stool. Unsuspecting, von Vamossy and a colleague took 1.5 and 1 g, respectively (normal adult dose, 0.1–0.2 g) and in a few hours passed three to five watery stools, repeated in the evening and again the following morning. They reported no griping and their work, unspecified, was not hindered. Clinical trials followed and phenolphthalein was introduced into clinical practice in 1902. Stories that phenolphthalein was put in wine and its purgative action discovered by the general population are denied by von Vamossy.†

Solid phenolphthalein stimulates the colon directly. It is dissolved in the small intestine, a little is absorbed and excreted in the urine and bile. The excretion of some in the bile tends to prolong its action, as von Vamossy discovered. If the urine or faeces are alkaline they will become red, which may alarm the patient or parent inspecting babies' nappies.

Uses. In addition to their use for relieving constipation, laxatives are sometimes indicated before radiological examination of the bowel (cascara, senna, bisacodyl or sodium picosulphate), for the removal of ingested poisons (a saline purge or castor oil), in hepatic coma (magnesium sulphate), in megacolon and with some drugs that cause constipation, such as opioids.

There are innumerable preparations of purgatives (see any formulary), many of the proprietary ones being elegant and pleasanter than the official preparations. Both are effective, except some of the official anthraquinone group, but elegance must be paid for.

Suppositories (bisacodyl, glycerin) may be used to obtain a bowel action in about 1 h.

For anal and rectal disease, suppositories that are astringent (hamamelis) or anti-inflammatory (adrenal steroid) or which are imagined to provide an inert coating of the mucous membrane (bismuth subgallate) or local anaesthesia (lignocaine) are used as seems necessary.

Enemas produce defaecation by softening faeces and distending the bowel. They are used in preparation for surgery, radiological examination and endoscopy.

Plain water or preparations with sodium phosphate (poorly absorbed and so retains water in the gut) or dioctyl sodium sulphosuccinate are generally used.

Enemas to be retained may be used to provide topical therapy for ulcerative colitis or Crohn's disease of the colon. They may also be given to reduce intracranial pressure for a few hours; saturated magnesium sulphate solution 150 ml, is slowly run into the rectum where it withdraws water from the body into the bowel. Magnesium poisoning may occur in patients with poor renal function.

Constipation and its management

In general, constipation is better treated by *increasing the bulk and decreasing the viscosity of the faeces* than by increasing the motor activity of the gut. Constipation may arise in the following settings:

1. *Habitual constipation* is best corrected by adjusting the diet to contain more fibre, for example, by including unpeeled fruit and vegetables, wholemeal bread, bran-based cereals,

* In the 19th century 'young men proceeding to Africa' were advised to take pills named Livingstone's Rousers, consisting of rhubarb, jalap, calomel and quinine. Br Med J 1964; 2: 1583.

† Vamossy A von. Is phenolphthalein harmful? Am J Dig Dis 1936–37; 3: 22.

muesli* or simply by adding unprocessed bran. This may be sprinkled on in the morning cereal or made up as a separate drink, the disagreeable nature of which is only partially disguised by mixing with fruit juice or milk.

Faecal softeners may also be tried, and if a stimulant is necessary, senna or danthron are perhaps the least objectionable. In general, choice of purgative is not critical.

2. *Painful anal lesions* frequently lead to constipation because when defaecation hurts it is postponed for as long as possible, with the result that the more water is absorbed and the motion becomes harder and so hurts even more when it is eventually passed. This vicious cycle is best broken by the cure of the anal lesion, but a faecal softener or a saline purgative to make the stool semi-fluid may give relief temporarily.

3. *Pregnancy*. Constipation is best treated by ensuring adequate fibre in the diet and if, despite this, the bowel sluggishness persists, one of the milder stimulant purgatives (e.g. senna) should be used, as vigorous purgation can cause abortion, though this is less reliable than some women hope. The use of vigorous purgation, traditionally castor oil, to promote the onset of labour is unpleasant for the patient but moderately effective and is now obsolete.

4. *Acute illness* may lead to sluggish bowel habit, especially if it involves confinement to bed and is accompanied by loss of appetite. Dependence on others for assistance to the lavatory or, worse, to bring a bedpan, is also a factor. The bedpan is not only objectionable as a cause of constipation, but it has also been shown that its use requires a 50% greater oxygen consumption than does the use of a bedside commode, so that the humiliation of a bedpan should only be inflicted on those for whom it is absolutely necessary. These are fewer than is sometimes imagined.† If severe enough to warrant attention, this kind of constipation can usually be dealt with by bulk purgatives, by faecal softeners with or without danthron or by senna or cascara or by suppositories of glycerine or bisacodyl.

5. *Psychological factors* are important. One study of bran extract found that after the substitution of an 'inert placebo . . . an average of almost one bowel movement a day was reported by patients who claimed to be constipated.' Many physicians would echo the authors' statement that, 'At least, in our clinics, constipated persons are those who think they are not having enough bowel movements.'‡ An explanation that normal bowel habit may vary between three motions per day and two per week, may be of more value to the patient than the prescription of a laxative.

6. *Drugs* may cause constipation. *Opioid* analgesics raise the tone of intestinal circular muscle and reduce the force of peristaltic contraction (i.e. increased segmentation and decreased propulsion). Drugs with *anticholinergic* action reduce intestinal motility by blocking the muscarinic action of acetylcholine on gut smooth muscle; these include antispasmodics (e.g. propantheline), antiparkinsonian drugs (e.g. orphenadrine) and tricyclic antidepressants (e.g. amitriptyline). Benzodiazepines used as minor tranquillisers may constipate some patients. When withdrawal of the drug is not feasible, e.g. when treating intractable pain with an opioid, constipation should be anticipated and a laxative should be prescribed with the analgesic.

Misuse of purgatives

Dependence (abuse) may arise following laxative use during an illness or in pregnancy, or the individual may have the mistaken notion that a daily bowel motion is essential for health, or that the bowels are only incompletely opened by nature and that poisons are being retained, or have more complex psychological problems, and so indulge in regular purgation. This effectively prevents the easy return of normal habits because the more powerful purges empty the whole colon, whereas normal defaecation empties only the descending colon. Cessation of use after a few weeks is thus inevitably followed by a few days' constipation whilst sufficient material collects to restore the

* A Swiss invention, being a delicious mixture of chopped cereals, nuts, dried fruits, honey: from German *Gemüseli*, little vegetable.

† Benton J G, et al. (1950). Energy expended by patients on the bedpan and bedside commode. JAMA 1950; 144:1442.

‡ Greiner T, et al. J Chronic Dis 1957; 6:244.

normal state. This may be claimed by the patient as evidence of the continued necessity for purgatives and such reasoning should be forestalled by proper explanation.

To prevent purgative dependence is easier than to cure it; patients feel they understand their own bowels far better than anyone else possibly could, an opinion they seldom extend to other organs, except perhaps the liver. In Britain, there is a tradition that nurses have an intuitive understanding of the bowels that is denied to doctors.

Laxative dependence, which may be solely emotional at first, may be followed by physical dependence. Excessive use of stimulant purgatives* may, especially in the old, lead to severe water and electrolyte depletion, even to hypokalaemic paralysis; also to malabsorption and protein-losing enteropathy. Atonic colon due to damage to gut nerve plexus may occur (cathartic colon) leading to 'pipestem colon', and there may be melanosis; cognoscenti may make the diagnosis through an endoscope.

Purgatives are dangerous if given to patients with undiagnosed abdominal pain, inflammatory intestinal disease or obstruction. Nor should they be used to get rid of hardened masses of faeces in the rectum, for they will fail and cause pain. Digital removal, generally prescribed by a senior and performed by a junior doctor, is required. A faecal softener helps to prevent recurrence.

Constipation may be part of the syndromes associated with obstruction of the bowel, but other symptoms are then always more prominent; treatment is of the cause, and laxatives are dangerous.

Paralytic ileus: when this condition is due to potassium deficiency, the treatment is clear. In other cases, the mechanism is uncertain. Use of cholinergic drugs has been unsatisfactory, and intestinal suction and attendance to electrolyte balance are the proper approach.

Purgatives should be avoided in patients taking broad-spectrum antimicrobials orally, as they may precipitate severe diarrhoea.

* The Roman Emperor Nero (AD 37–68) murdered his severely constipated aunt by ordering the doctors to give her 'a laxative of fatal strength.' He 'seized her property before she was quite dead, and tore up the will so that nothing should escape him.' (Suetonius, trans R Graves)

All stimulant laxatives can cause colic and this can be combated, if necessary with atropine or other anticholinergic drugs, but generally it is a symptom of overdose.

Routine use of purgatives in children, on the principle that a 'good clear out' is healthful is deplorable and casts doubt on either the intelligence or the mental health of the prescriber.

DIARRHOEA

Diarrhoea ranges from a mild and socially inconvenient illness to a major cause of malnutrition (chronic d.) among children in developing countries, and the cause of 4–5 million deaths (acute d.) throughout the world annually. Drugs have a place in its management but *the first priority of therapy is to preserve or restore fluid and electrolyte balance*. The condition is often assumed to be infectious, but it may be caused by anxiety, food, drugs or microbial or other toxins. Diarrhoea is measured by *volume* and *frequency* of stools.

Some physiology

Absorption and secretion of water and electrolytes occur throughout the intestine, probably as separate processes, for absorption is a function of the cells of the intestinal villi and the surface cells of the colon, while cells in the crypts between villi are responsible for secretion. Water follows the osmotic gradients that result from shifts of electrolytes across the intestinal epithelium, and sodium and chloride transport mechanisms are central to the causation and management of diarrhoea, especially that caused by bacteria and viruses.

Absorption of sodium into the epithelium is effected by:

1. *Sodium-glucose coupled entry*. Glucose stimulates the absorption of sodium and the resulting water flow also sweeps additional sodium and chloride along with it (solvent drag). *This important mechanism remains active in diarrhoea of various aetiologies and improvement of sodium and water absorption by glucose (and amino acids) is the basis of oral rehydrating regimens* (below).

2. *Sodium-ion coupled entry*. Na^+ and Cl^- enter the epithelial cell, either as a pair, or, as seems more likely, there is a double exchange; Na^+ (extracellular) with H^+ (intracellular) and Cl^- (extracellular) with OH^- or HCO_3^- (intracellular). Oral rehydrating solutions (below) contain sodium, chloride and bicarbonate.

Secretion is the opposite process to that of absorption. In response to various stimuli, crypt cells transport chloride into the gut lumen and sodium and water follow. This *stimulus-secretion coupling* is modulated by cyclic nucleotides (cyclic AMP, cyclic GMP), calcium, prostaglandins and leukotrienes.

Motility patterns in the bowel. Segmental contractions of the smooth muscle mix the intestinal contents, and there are well recognised patterns of peristaltic contraction that propel the contents along the gut. Abnormal gut motility can be produced by infecting animals with bacteria and it has been suggested that disordered intestinal motility contributes to infective diarrhoea in man. *Patients with diarrhoea commonly have less spontaneous activity of the sigmoid colon than do people with normal bowel habit, and patients with constipation have more*. An important factor in diarrhoea may be loss of the normal segmenting contractions that delay passage of food, so that an occasional peristaltic wave has greater propulsive effect. Also, liquid faeces can trickle along passively to reach the sensory areas for the defaecation reflex in the rectum (stretch receptors) and anus (touch receptors). Some antidiarrhoel drugs act by altering intestinal motility (*antimotility drugs*).

Therapy for diarrhoea involves *first, the correction of fluid and electrolyte imbalance*, and *second*, the use of drugs (in some cases).

Fluid and electrolyte therapy

Oral rehydration therapy (ORT) with glucose-electrolyte solution is sufficient to treat the vast majority of episodes of watery diarrhoea. As a simple, effective, cheap and readily administered therapy for a potentially lethal condition, *ORT must rank as one of the major recent therapeutic advances in medicine*. It is effective because absorption by glucose-coupled sodium transport continues during diarrhoea and provides a means of replacing water and electrolyte losses in the stool. The composition of different glucose-electrolyte formulations varies in detail but two commonly used solutions have the following content:

Glucose-electrolyte formulations for ORT

(mmol/l)	WHO/UNICEF*	Sodium Chloride and Glucose Oral Powder, Compound BNF
Glucose	111	200
Sodium	90	35
Potassium	20	20
Chloride	80	37
Bicarbonate	30	18

* World Health Organization/United Nations Children's Fund (originally the words *international* and *emergency* were included)

The addition of *glycine* further enhances absorption. The choice of sodium 90 mmol/l in the WHO/UNICEF solution is based on measures of sodium concentrations in diarrhoeal stools, but a low-sodium high-glucose (e.g. BNF) preparation may be preferred for infants whose faecal losses are less. Sodium Chloride and Glucose Oral Powder, Compound BNF may be prepared by a pharmacist or is available as a 8.8 g sachet (Dioralyte), which should be dissolved in water 200 ml. The dose is, for adults 1–2 sachets* and for children 1 sachet, after each loose motion; infants should receive one to one-and-a-half times the usual feed volume. When no approved formulation is immediately available a finger pinch of salt and a teaspoonful of sugar dissolved in of 250 ml water (a large glass), will suffice. Adding fruit squash will also supply potassium. Rehydration therapy with commercial soft drinks alone will fail because their sodium content is too low (usually less than 6 mmol/l).

In children fluid and electrolyte depletion is especially dangerous and hospitalisation and i.v. replacement may be needed but *prompt* use of ORT will almost always obviate this. *Antimotility*

* A *sachet* is a small soft impermeable envelope or bag.

drugs (see below) are inappropriate for severe diarrhoea in young children; any marginal efficacy they may have is liable to be counterbalanced by hazard.

Drug treatment

There are two types of drug that are often used in combination. Both types increase viscosity of faeces.

1. *Drugs that increase the viscosity of gut contents directly*: kaolin, chalk. These *adsorbent powders* have been generally thought to act by providing a coating for the bowel and by adsorbing toxic substances, both unsatisfactory explanations. They probably do not coat the bowel; adsorption is not selective and most of their adsorptive capacity may well be to take up non-toxic substances. But whatever the explanation, their therapeutic efficacy is at best marginal, as is shown by the fact that they are often combined with an opioid antimotility drug. *Preparations include*: Kaolin Mixture BNF; 10–20 ml 4-hourly. Kaolin and Morphine Mixture BNF; 10 ml 4-hourly (contains morphine 916 μg/10 ml).

2. *Drugs that delay passage of gut contents (antimotility drugs)* so that there is time for more water to be absorbed: opioids, smooth muscle depressants or anticholinergics. Their use in small children whose recovery, and indeed whose life depends on fluid and electrolyte replacement as primary therapy, is generally contraindicated.

(i) *The opioid group of drugs* activate receptors on the smooth muscle of the bowel, reducing peristalsis and increasing segmentation contractions so that passage of contents is delayed and there is more time for absorption of water.

Codeine (15, 30 mg) is effective. The dose is 15–60 mg 4–6 hourly (see also Ch. 16).

Diphenoxylate is related to pethidine and affects the bowel like morphine. It is effective in diarrhoea. The drug is offered mixed with a trivial dose of atropine (to discourage abuse by causing dry mouth) as Lomotil; four tablets are taken initially, then two tablets 6-hourly (it is unsuitable for small children). Nausea, vomiting, abdominal pain and depression of the central nervous system may be caused. In overdose with Lomotil, respiratory depression may be serious and can occur up to 16 h after ingestion because gastric emptying is delayed. Its action is antagonised by naloxone.

Loperamide (Imodium) (2 mg) is structurally similar to diphenoxylate. Its precise mode of action remains obscure but it impairs propulsion of gut contents by effect on intestinal circular and longitudinal muscle that are at least partly due to an action on opioid receptors. The $t_{\frac{1}{2}}$ is 15 h. The dose is 4 mg initially, then 2 mg after each loose stool to a maximum of 16 mg/day. It may cause nausea, vomiting and abdominal cramps; its potential for abuse appears to be low; its use in small children is controversial.

Codeine 30 mg, *diphenoxylate* 5 mg and *loperamide* 2 mg are therapeutically equivalent. Adverse effects are few in adults, but are slightly more common with diphenoxylate; loperamide is least likely to depress the central nervous system.

(ii) *Smooth muscle depressant*

Mebeverine (Colofac) (135 mg) is a reserpine derivative that has a direct effect on colonic muscle activity, especially, it appears, on colonic hypermotility. It may be used to relieve spasm of intestinal muscle, e.g. associated with organic disease of the gut, and in irritable bowel syndrome. The dose is 135 mg × 3/day. Not being anticholinergic, it does not demonstrate the troublesome side-effects of that group of drugs.

Alverine is an amine with papaverine-like smooth muscle relaxant effect. *Peppermint oil* (in enteric coated formulation) acts similarly.

(iii) *Anticholinergic drugs* such as atropine, dicyclomine, mepenzolate and propantheline are sometimes helpful in chronic diarrhoeas when it is undesirable to use opioids indefinitely, but intestinal paralysis may be precipitated by large doses of propantheline, which also blocks autonomic ganglia.

Travellers' diarrhoea

So familiar is travellers' diarrhoea that is has acquired a variety of popular names: the Aztec Two-step, Montezuma's Revenge, Delhi Belly, Rangoon Runs, Tokyo Trots, Gyppy Tummy, Hong-Kong Dog, Estomac Anglais and Casablanca Crud, all indicate some of the areas deemed dangerous to visitors. The Mexican name *turista* indicates the principal sufferers. Even international conferences of gastroenterologists have been disrupted by the disorder.

A considerable body of medical folklore has arisen among prospective travellers fearful of the consequences of being stricken during their coach tour of five European capitals in seven days. However it is now clear that suggested explanations such as changed environment, diet and psychological causes must give way before mounting evidence that most cases are infective. While the responsible pathogen(s) must vary with the location, much of the diarrhoea that afflicts visitors to tropical and subtropical countries is associated with enterotoxigenic strains of *Escherichia coli*, which produce toxins that stimulate copious fluid secretion by the gut. Enteroviruses and other bacterial, e.g. staphylococcal, toxins are also implicated.

In prophylaxis trials it had been found that antimicrobial drugs (neomycin, tetracyclines and the less-absorbed sulphonamides) can reduce substantially the incidence of diarrhoea and its severity, but probably not its duration when it occurs. Prophylactic drug therapy also has undesirable effects by altering bowel flora, causing rashes and hindering diagnosis of serious infection, and the temptation to use it routinely is best resisted. A wider issue is the possible development and spread of antibiotic-resistant organisms. Thus, while there can be benefits to the *individual* at present, they must be weighed against the risk to the *community* in the future, which in most instances will require that prophylactic antimicrobials should not be used. Antimicrobial drugs are therefore suitable only for use as prophylactics on very special occasions, and then only for less than three weeks. They are not appropriate for the ordinary summer holiday.

Whether or not prophylaxis is to be used, travellers will often want something to take should they fall victim to this unpleasant disorder, which, even in its mild form, can wreak social havoc in any but the most completely equipped holiday motor coach. A reasonable course for holiday travellers in Europe and the Mediterranean area is to take advice on hygiene, and to carry a symptomatic remedy (see below) to be used at the start of diarrhoea.

Treatment. Travellers' diarrhoea can ordinarily be satisfactorily managed by oral rehydration (see above), and one of the opioids that increase gut tone (segmentation) and reduce gut propulsion provides a socially useful reduction in frequency of stools. Loperamide, codeine phosphate and diphenoxylate plus atropine (Lomotil) have not been superseded for both efficacy and convenience, and the patients can control their own dosage safely and within a wide range. Other opioid and kaolin preparations can be used, but many of these are liquids that are cumbersome to transport. An antimicrobial is seldom necessary for the disease is usually self-limiting.

If these remedies fail, then the diarrhoea is fairly severe and the patient should consult a doctor, for the only alternative is to assume such an attack to be both infective and to need specific treatment. Choice of therapy can then be based on local knowledge allied to an attempt to identify a specific organism. Generally it is undesirable to provide patients who are leaving home with a full therapeutic course of broad-spectrum antimicrobial therapy.

Specific infective diarrhoeas

Accounts of appropriate chemotherapy for episodes of diarrhoea caused by specific organisms, e.g. amoebic dysentery, giardiasis or typhoid fever, are given in Table 11.1 and in the section on infection of the intestines (Chapter 13).

Irritable bowel syndrome

This is the commonest condition seen by gastroenterologists; it is characterised by abnormal bowel activity without obvious organic cause and symptoms include colicky abdominal pain, constipation and diarrhoea. Sometimes areas of gut spasm may be seen on barium enema. Stress, psyche, lack of fibre in the diet and food allergy contribute variably to its pathogenesis. An explanation of the functional nature of the disease and avoidance of foods that obviously precipitate symptoms are important initial measures. The condition is not regularly improved by drugs but benefit may be derived by increased dietary fibre, by loperamide or diphenoxylate for diarrhoea, by metoclopramide for nausea and abdominal distension, by sedation with a benzodiazepine, by use of smooth-mucle relaxants such as mebeverine, an anticholinergic, peppermint oil (Colpermin), or occasionally, by an antidepressant.

Ulcerative colitis

The management of ulcerative colitis involves a lot more than giving drugs. General measures to correct anaemia and fluid and electrolyte losses and to improve the general nutritional state are important. The objectives of management are (a) to terminate an acute attack with drugs, (b) to maintain remission with drugs and (c) to select appropriate patients for radical surgery.

Management and drugs

Mild attacks are associated with less than four motions a day, little blood in the stools and only mild systemic upset. These can be managed outside hospital and a regimen of prednisolone 20 mg by retention enema* at night; oral prednisolone 5 mg × 4/day and sulphasalazine 0.5 g × 4/day (see below) will usually suffice. The prednisolone can be tailed off after a few weeks but the sulphasalazine should be continued.

Moderately severe attacks are characterised by frequent passage of stools consisting of larger amounts of blood but occasionally with some solid faeces, and with constitutional disturbance. Drug therapy should comprise prednisolone by retention enema night and morning, oral prednisolone 10 mg × 4/day, and sulphasalazine 0.5 g × 4/day. It the initial response is good, the patient may be managed at home and the regimen should be maintained for one month, when the corticosteroid should be tailed off but the sulphasalazine should be continued. A course of iron by mouth may be needed. If the response is inadequate, the patient should be admitted to hospital without delay.

Severe attacks are recognised by profuse bloody diarrhoea with more than 12 bowel actions in a day, abdominal pain or tenderness, high fever, weight loss, anaemia and weakness. Hospitalisation is essential and management may proceed as follows:

1. Begin with prednisolone 60 mg per day given in divided doses into an i.v. infusion.
2. Three litres or more of fluid and electrolyte may be required daily and particular attention should be paid to ensuring that the potassium supplement is adequate. Blood transfusion may be needed.
3. Parenteral nutrition may also be indicated.
4. Broad-spectrum antibiotic by mouth is *contraindicated* as it may cause an enterocolitis and make the condition worse.
5. The patient should be reviewed closely since failure to respond to this intensive regimen means that colectomy may be required.
6. As the patient's condition improves, i.v. corticosteroid may be replaced by oral prednisolone 40 mg daily in divided doses.
7. Corticosteroid by enema plays a valuable part in the management of ulcerative colitis in general; but the patient with a severely inflamed colon will be unable to retain the standard enema. Under these circumstances an intrarectal drip of hydrocortisone 100 mg in 120 ml of water twice daily has been found useful. Once the patient can tolerate it, an enema may be given, or alternatively Prednesol tablets (prednisolone sodium phosphate, 5 mg) may be dissolved in water to make up an enema; the advantage of the latter is that as the patient improves, it may be possible to use a larger volume of liquid (150 ml or more) and bring corticosteroid into contact with a greater area of mucosa.
8. Sulphasalazine should be reintroduced once improvement has been maintained, and iron supplements will usually be required.

Prevention of relapse is a major aim of management. Relapse may be precipitated by intercurrent gut infection, by broad-spectrum antimicrobial given orally, or by psychological stress. Sulphasalazine 2 g daily definitely lessens the chance of relapse; in this dose adverse reactions are infrequent and generally mild and the drug may be continued indefinitely or for at least a year.

* Predsol, prednisolone 20 mg as the sodium phosphate salt in 100 ml; or Predenema, prednisolone 20 mg as metasulphobenzoate sodium in 100 ml, which is absorbed less

Corticosteroids do not prevent recurrences of the disease in contrast to their usefulness in the acute attack, although a minority of patients may require prolonged therapy. Azathioprine is effective for maintenance therapy although it should be regarded as a second-choice drug; it may also be used as a steroid-sparing agent in those patients who require long-term corticosteroid. Antidiarrhoeal agents, e.g. opioids and anticholinergics, are generally of limited value in ulcerative colitis and may induce toxic megacolon.

Idiopathic proctitis. If an upper limit to inflammation can be seen with the sigmoidoscope, prednisolone suppositories (5 mg) are appropriate.

Crohn's disease. A corticosteroid is best to induce remission in an acutely ill patient and some benefit from continued corticosteroid therapy with or without azathioprine. Metronidazole is effective for Crohn's disease of the perianal region. Sulphasalazine with a corticosteroid is effective for colonic disease.

Inflammation of the ano-rectal area (e.g. due to haemorrhoids) may be treated with Hydrocortisone Suppositories.

Sulphasalazine (Salazopyrin) (0.5 g) consists of two compounds, sulphapyridine and 5-aminosalicylic acid, joined by a diazo bond. Sulphasalazine is poorly absorbed from the small intestine and bacteria in the colon split the diazo bond to release the component parts. The active moiety is now known to be 5-aminosalicylic acid, which is available as a drug in its own right, *mesalazine* (below). Its precise mode of action is unknown. Sulphapyridine is well absorbed, is acetylated in the liver and excreted in the urine; 5-aminosalicylic acid largely remains in the colon.

Sulphasalazine is used to maintain remission in patients with ulcerative colitis. It is inferior to corticosteroids for treatment of the acute attack. The drug may also be used as a disease-modifying agent in rheumatoid arthritis (see index), the condition for which it was originally introduced in the 1930s.

The dose is 1–3 g/day (in four doses), usually 2 g/day achieves best effect with fewest adverse effects. The latter comprise headache, malaise, anorexia, nausea and vomiting. These are dose-related and are more common in genetically slow acetylators. Allergic reactions also occur and include rash, fever and lymphadenitis; rarely leucopenia and agranulocytosis are induced. Reversible infertility may be caused in men. Several of these adverse effects are probably caused by the sulphapyridine part of sulphasalazine.

Mesalazine (400 mg) is 5-aminosalicylic acid (see above). When it is administered by mouth on its own only 20% is recovered in the urine, most remaining in the intestine. Various sustained-release preparations and prodrugs for mesalazine are being evaluated, the objective being to achieve high colonic concentration. Mesalazine is used to maintain remission in ulcerative colitis. Patients who are intolerant of sulphasalazine usually tolerate mesalazine. The dose is 1.2–2.4 g/day (in three doses). The profile of adverse effects due to mesalazine alone (i.e. without sulphapyridine) includes nausea, abdominal pain and watery diarrhoea. These may be confused with symptoms of the ulcerative colitis but if due to mesalazine, they stop when the drug is withdrawn.

Drug-induced diarrhoea

Antimicrobials are the commonest drugs that cause diarrhoea, probably due to alteration of bowel flora. It may range from a mild inconvenience to life-threatening enterocolitis (see the section on antibiotic-associated colitis, Chapter 11). Magnesium-containing antacids may produce diarrhoea, if they are given in excess, as may neostigmine (for myasthenia gravis) and chenodeoxycholic acid (for gall stones). Antihypertensive drugs (e.g. methyldopa or guanethidine), antirheumatic drugs (e.g. indomethacin, mefenamic acid or flurbiprofen) and various metabolic agents (metformin, fenfluramine or chlorpropamide) may also cause diarrhoea.

GUIDE TO FURTHER READING

1 Trounce J R. (Editorial). Antiemetics and cytotoxic drugs. Br Med J 1983; 286: 327–8.
2 Hey H, et al. Oesophageal transit of six commonly used tablets and capsules. Br Med J 1982; 285: 1717–9.
3 Orme M L'E, et al. (Editorial). Metoclopramide and tardive dyskinesia in the elderly. Br Med J 1984; 289: 397–8.
4 Editorial. Idiopathic constipation. Lancet 1985; 1: 795–6.
5 Editorial. Constipation in young women. Lancet 1986; 1: 778–9.
6 Eastwood M A, et al. Dietary fibre. Lancet 1983; 2: 202–6.
7 Taylor R H. Bran yesterday . . . bran tomorrow? Br Med J 1984; 289: 69–70.
8 Carpenter C C J. (Editorial). Oral rehydration. Is it as good as parenteral therapy? N Engl J Med 1982; 306: 1103–4.
9 Editorial. Traveller's diarrhoea. Lancet 1982; 1: 777–8.
10 Gorbach S L. (Editorial). Traveller's diarrhoea. N Engl J Med 1982; 307: 881–3.
11 Editorial. Management of acute diarrhoea. Lancet 1983; 1: 623–5.
12 Taylor D N, et al. Polymicrobial aetiology of travellers' diarrhoea. Lancet 1985; 1: 381–3.
13 Lennard-Jones J E. Functional gastrointestinal disorders. N Engl J Med 1983; 308: 431–5.
14 Editorial. An irritable mind or an irritable bowel. Lancet 1984; 2: 1249–50.
15 Denman A M. (Editorial). Food allergy. Br Med J 1983; 286: 1164–6.
16 Pearson D J. (Editorial). Pseudo food allergy. Br Med J 1986; 292: 221–2.
17 Kirsner J B, Shorter R G. Recent developments in 'nonspecific' inflammatory bowel disease. N Engl J Med 1982; 306: 775–85 and 837–48.

33

Gastrointestinal system III: Liver and biliary tract

DRUGS AND THE LIVER

The liver is the most important organ in which drugs are structurally altered into metabolites, some of which may be biologically inactive, some active, some toxic. Furthermore, it is exposed to drugs at higher concentrations than are most organs because drugs that are administered orally and are absorbed from the gastrointestinal tract (i.e. most drugs) must pass through the liver to reach the systemic circulation; subsequently, 20% of the cardiac output passes through the liver. It is hardly surprising therefore that:

1. *Drugs can cause direct damage to the liver or otherwise interfere with its function.*
2. *Pharmacokinetic and pharmacodynamic changes are induced by liver disease.*.

These issues are here considered.

Drug-induced injury

1. **Drug-induced liver injury or interference with its function*** may be classified broadly as *predictable* and *unpredictable*.

* See Davis M, Williams R. In: Textbook of Adverse Drug Reactions, ed Davies D M, Oxford University Press, Oxford, 1985; 250–290.

Predictable (dose-dependent) type

(a) *Direct liver cell (hepatocellular) injury* occurs with some drugs as the dose is raised. These include:

Paracetamol: when taken in overdose (see Chapter 15).

Salicylate: acute hepatic injury or chronic active hepatitis may develop in patients with connective tissue disorders who receive more than 2 g/day.

Tetracyclines: fatty changes in liver cells and hepatic failure develop when high doses are used; this is avoided if < 2 g/day is given orally and < 1 g/day i.v.

Methotrexate: hepatic fibrosis or cirrhosis may develop with prolonged use, e.g. for psoriasis; the risk is lessened by giving a large dose weekly rather than a smaller dose daily and by monitoring progress by liver biopsy, after every 1.5–2 g of methotrexate.

Azathioprine and its metabolite *6-mercaptopurine*: cholestasis and hepatic necrosis may occur.

Iron: when taken in overdose.

Non-medicinal chemicals including *carbon tetrachloride*, also cause direct hepatotoxicity.

(b) *Interference with bilirubin metabolism and excretion*. Some drugs interfere selectively with bilirubin kinetics in the liver to cause jaundice with minimal disturbances of other liver function tests. The rise in plasma bilirubin is related to dose, and recovery ordinarily occurs on stopping the drug. Examples are:

C-17-substituted testosterone derivatives impair bilirubin excretion into the hepatic canaliculi; the block is biochemical not mechanical. Drugs in this class include androgens and anabolic steroids (e.g. methyltestosterone, nandrolone, oxymetholone, stanozolol), also oestrogens and progestogens used as oral contraceptives, but jaundice is rare with the low-dose formulations now preferred. All the steroid hormones that are cholestatic are pharmacologically active by mouth. Androgens that are active only by injection, e.g. testosterone propionate and nandrolone esters, are not of this group and do not cause jaundice.

Rifampicin impairs hepatic uptake and excretion of bilirubin and plasma unconjugated and conjugated bilirubin (i.e. both before and after conjugation in liver cell microsomes) may be elevated during the first 2–3 weeks of dosing.

Sodium fusidate interferes with hepatic bilirubin excretion to cause conjugated hyperbilirubinaemia.

Cholecystographic media compete with bilirubin for uptake into the hepatic cell, and serum bilirubin may be transiently raised after an oral cholecystogram.

Unpredictable (dose-independent) type

A large number of drugs can cause hepatic damage that is unrelated to dose; the incidence with any single agent is low (if it was not, the drug would not be used). The reaction may or may not be associated with features of generalized allergy (fever, arthralgia, skin rash, lymphadenopathy) and characteristic patterns of injury are:

(a) *Acute hepatocellular necrosis*. This reaction varies from a transient disturbance of liver function tests to acute hepatitis. It can be induced by several drugs including general anaesthetics (*halothane*), anticonvulsants (*carbamazepine, phenytoin, sodium valproate, and phenobarbitone*), antidepressants (*MAO inhibitors*), anti-inflammatory drugs (*indomethacin and ibuprofen*), antimicrobials (*isoniazid, ethionamide, pyrazinamide, PAS and sulphonamides*) and cardiovascular drugs (*methyldopa and quinidine*).

(b) *Chronic active hepatitis*. This may develop when treatment with certain drugs is prolonged, e.g. *methyldopa, isoniazid, dantrolene, or nitrofurantoin*.

(c) *Cholestatic hepatitis*. The picture is of obstructive jaundice though the block is biochemical rather than mechanical. This type is particularly associated with the phenothiazine tranquillisers, especially *chlorpromazine*. The jaundice generally occurs within the first month of therapy, its onset may be insidious or acute, with abdominal pain, and can be accompanied by features suggesting allergy (fever and rash eosinophilia). Direct cell injury can occur simultaneously. Recovery is usual. *Chlorpropamide* and *thiouracil* also cause this type of reaction.

Other effects of drugs on the liver

Synthetic androgens, usually in high dose, and *oral contraceptives*, after prolonged use (more than 5 years), are associated with the appearance of benign liver tumours; there is also increased risk of developing hepatocellular carcinoma, although the absolute risk of this complication is low. Malignant liver tumours associated with the contraceptive pill are highly vascular and may cause recurrent, acute abdominal pain if they rupture and bleed.

In summary, drugs may cause any of the common, and some of the uncommon, forms of liver disease. The possibility of drug-induced injury should be considered when:

(i) plasma transaminases of hepatic origin are raised
(ii) jaundice is unexplained
(iii) acute hepatitis, chronic active hepatitis or cryptogenic cirrhosis are diagnosed
(iv) primary hepatic tumour is present
(v) there is liver disease of obscure cause.

2. Pharmacokinetic and pharmacodynamic changes induced by liver disease

Pharmacokinetic changes

Liver disease causes pharmacokinetic changes because:

(a) drug metabolising capacity is reduced since liver cells are either sick or, if functioning normally, are reduced in number,

(b) liver cells that metabolise drugs are bypassed when portal–systemic shunts develop in cirrhosis,

(c) drug-binding capacity is reduced when liver disease causes hypoproteinaemia and more unbound and pharmacologically active drug may circulate,

(d) drug may distribute into ascitic and oedema fluid when it is ineffective.

The following discussion refers to stable liver disease such as cirrhosis or chronic active hepatitis; there is less information about altered pharmacokinetics in acute liver disease, e.g. viral hepatitis or toxic liver necrosis. The pattern of change that is induced by disease depends on the manner in which a drug is treated by the healthy liver. Drugs that are metabolised by the liver may be broadly divided into two classes:

(i) *Drugs that are rapidly metabolised and highly extracted in a single pass through the liver.* Such drugs are said to undergo *presystemic* elimination after oral administration, i.e. to exhibit the first-pass effect (see Chapter 8). Poor liver cell function means that less drug is extracted from the blood as it passes through the liver and portal systemic shunts allow a proportion of blood to by-pass the liver altogether. Therefore the predominant change in the kinetics of drugs that are given orally is *increased systemic availability*, i.e. the amount that reaches the systemic circulation is larger than normal, and its effect is correspondingly greater. Accordingly the initial doses of such drugs should be smaller than usual, at least until some assessment of their clinical effect has been obtained. The normally low systemic availability of *labetalol, propranolol, pentazocine, pethidine and chlormethiazole*, for example, is much increased in cirrhotic patients. When liver function is severely impaired, the $t_{\frac{1}{2}}$ of drugs in this class may also be lengthened.

(ii) *Drugs that are slowly metabolised and are poorly extracted in a single pass through the liver*, i.e. those that do not exhibit first-pass effect after oral administration. The major change that is brought about by liver disease is *prolongation of* $t_{\frac{1}{2}}$. Consequently the interval between doses of such drugs may have to be lengthened and the time to reach steady-state concentration in the plasma ($5 \times t_{\frac{1}{2}}$) is increased. *Diazepam, lorazepam, phenobarbitone, theophylline and clindamycin*, for example, have materially increased $t_{\frac{1}{2}}$ values in patients with chronic liver disease.

Pharmacodynamic changes

Liver disease causes pharmacodynamic changes because:

(a) tissue response to drugs may alter (e.g. CNS response to opioids, sedatives and antiepileptic drugs),

(b) fluid and electrolyte balance are altered (sodium retention may be induced; ascites and oedema may be refractory to diuretics),

These issues are now discussed, as they affect the use of drugs.

Prescribing for patients with liver disease

It is especially important that all drugs should be prescribed only if there are clear indications and the physician knows and is prepared to deal with adverse effects.

Central nervous system. The brain receives concentrations of toxic substances (ammonia and amines) to which it is normally not exposed, as a result of failure of liver cells to metabolise naturally occurring substances and also of shunting of blood from the portal to the systemic circulation. Its function becomes impaired (hepatic encephalopathy) and its response to drugs is *qualitatively* abnormal.

Opioids should be avoided as coma may be caused, but if one is essential, pethidine is probably less dangerous than morphine. Lorazepam and oxazepam are preferred as anxiolytics and temazepam as an hypnotic for their $t_{\frac{1}{2}}$ values are short. Anti-epileptics should be used in the lowest effective dose; phenobarbitone may induce coma and sodium valproate should be avoided as there is risk of hepatotoxicity. A tricyclic antidepressant may be used when drug therapy is deemed necessary but MAO inhibitors are hazardous.

Non-steroidal anti-inflammatory drugs may cause sodium retention and there is increased risk of gastrointestinal bleeding because of the haemostatic defects of liver disease; paracetamol or ibuprofen may be used in low dose.

Cardiovascular system. β-adrenoceptor blockers that are metabolised (e.g. propranolol and labetalol) should be used in reduced dose as should cardiac antidysrhythmics (e.g. lignocaine, tocainide and mexiletine). Hypokalaemia may precipitate coma so plasma electrolytes should be monitored carefully during diuretic therapy and a potassium-sparing drug should be included in the regimen.

Gastrointestinal system. Antacids that contain much sodium may cause fluid retention and those that contain aluminium and calcium may constipate, which predisposes such patients to encephalopathy as there is greater opportunity for absorption of toxic substances from the gut.

Carbenoxolone may cause oedema and hypokalaemia, both of which are especially undesirable.

Infection. Many antimicrobials are eliminated by the kidney, so ordinary doses of these are safe. Avoid prodrugs such as esters of ampicillin that must be hydrolysed by the liver to be effective, e.g. pivampicillin, talampicillin. Avoid or use in reduced dose those drugs that are associated with risk of hepatotoxicity, e.g. isoniazid, pyrazinamide, erythromycin estolate, fusidic acid, rifampicin and tetracyclines. The sodium content of some penicillins may be hazardously high.

Endocrine system. Prednisone must be converted in the liver to the active prednisolone, so the latter should be used. Avoid androgens and anabolic steroids that are C-17-substituted testosterone derivatives for they are hepatotoxic (see above). Avoid oral contraceptives especially in cholestatic liver disease. Metformin is normally inactivated by the liver and should be avoided as it may cause lactic acidosis; the same applies to chlorpropamide and tolbutamide, which are more likely to induce hypoglycaemia.

BILE SALTS AND DIGESTIVE ENZYMES

Bile salts and gallstones

Gallstone disease affects about 15% of women and 6% of men of middle age in the UK, and the prevalence increases with age. Stones that lie in the gall bladder are often silent but those that find their way into the bile ducts cause significant complications. Cholesterol is the commonest constituent of stones in countries where gallstone disease is common; some stones consist almost exclusively of cholesterol while others also contain bile pigments, calcium and protein. Stones that are rich in cholesterol are amenable to medical treatment.

Some pathophysiology

Human bile has a capacity for maintaining more cholesterol in solution than, say, an equivalent volume of water. The explanation is that bile contains bile acids (mainly cholic, deoxycholic and chenodeoxycholic acids) and phospholipids (mainly lecithin), which together form molecular aggregates called *mixed micelles* that are capable of keeping cholesterol dissolved within them. It follows that bile can become saturated and that cholesterol can precipitate out of solution (forming gallstones), (a) if the concentration of bile acids is too low or (b) if the concentration of cholesterol in the bile is too high.

Bile acids are synthesised from cholesterol in the liver to the amount of 0.2–0.6 g per day and the total body pool is 3–5 g. This on its own is far too little for the biological needs of absorbing lipids from the gut, but the system functions efficiently because bile acids are actively reabsorbed from the terminal ileum and returned to the liver; in any one day bile acids go round the *enterohepatic cycle* 5–10 times.

Non-obese gallstone patients have a reduced bile acid pool, i.e. their underlying abnormality is *bile acid deficiency*. Patients in whom the ileum is diseased are also prone to form gallstones as bile acid reabsorption does not take place and their bile acid pool is depleted.

Obese gallstone patients have a normal bile acid pool but supersaturate their bile because they secrete excessive amounts of cholesterol into it.

As might be expected, gallstones form slowly. In female Pima Indians of south-west USA, who have an unusually high incidence of the disease, there is a lag-time of about 8 years between the occurrence of the cholesterol-saturated bile and the formation of gallstones.

Enhancing the cholesterol-holding capacity of bile is the basis of medical treatment for gallstone and it is achieved either by increasing the bile acid content or by reducing the cholesterol content of bile.

Chenodeoxycholic acid (CDCA; Chendol) comprises about 40% of the naturally occurring bile acids and when it is taken as a medicine to treat gallstones the proportion in bile rises to 70%. CDCA acts mainly by inhibiting cholesterol synthesis in the liver and to a lesser extent by expanding the bile acid pool. The result is that bile contains less cholesterol and more bile acid; saturated bile is converted into unsaturated bile, which can redissolve cholesterol that has precipitated out as gallstones. The dose is given either as a single amount at bedtime or divided throughout the day. An oral cholecystogram after 6 months will show whether therapy is proving effective. Treatment should continue for up to 24 months depending on the size of the stone(s) and should be maintained for 3 months after dissolution.

Adverse effects Diarrhoea occurs in about 40% of patients but this can be avoided if the dose is decreased and then increased gradually. It occurs when bile acid that is not absorbed by the terminal ileum reaches the colon, where it stimulates the secretion of water. Concentrations of plasma aspartate transaminase may be raised early in treatment but no adverse effect of this has been shown. Chenodeoxycholic acid should not be given to patients at risk of pregnancy or to patients with chronic liver disease or inflammatory bowel disease.

Ursodeoxycholic acid (UDCA) is another naturally occurring bile acid that is effective at dissolving gallstones. It is given as a single dose at night or divided throughout the day. UDCA rarely causes diarrhoea and does not elevate transaminases; it is therefore usually preferred to CDCA.

A *terpene* mixture (Rowachol) also increases cholesterol solubility in bile but less effectively than CDCA or UDCA. It may be used in addition to CDCA and UDCA for stones in the common bile duct but is not so effective for gallbladder stones.

Dehydrocholic acid stimulates the formation of thin, watery bile; it is used after surgery to flush small calculi out of the bile ducts, and in radiology to help visualisation of the gallbladder.

Use of drugs to dissolve gallstones

Certain criteria must be met for treatment to stand a reasonable chance of success. The *gallstone(s)* must be completely radiolucent, for even a thin covering of calcium salts usually prevents dissolution. Pigment stones are also radiolucent but are usually associated with haemolytic disorders. Small stones (5–10 mm diameter) respond better because the surface area for dissolution is relatively large. The *gallbladder* must be shown to be functioning by cholecystography; in many patients with recurrent cholecystitis the gallbladder is shrunken and cannot concentrate bile. The *patients* for whom the treatment is most appropriate are mainly those for whom surgery is inadvisable, i.e. the elderly, the obese and the otherwise unfit. Symptoms should be infrequent, for treatment may take 1–2 years. Patients who have asymptomatic gallbladder stones need not be treated at all for such stones tend to remain silent.

Cholestyramine (Questran) is an anion exchange resin that, taken orally, binds bile acids in the bowel and so prevents their absorption. Its use as an hypolipidaemic agent is described in Chapter 26. Excess of bile acids in the colon causes diarrhoea, e.g. after ileal resection. Cholestyramine can be used to bind the bile acids and stop the diarrhoea, though this may result in some steatorrhoea. It is also used to relieve pruritus due to accumulation of bile acids in biliary obstruction, provided the obstruction is partial, i.e. that there is some escape of bile acids into the intestine where they can be bound.

Digestive enzymes

In pancreatic exocrine insufficiency, the aim of therapy is to prevent weight loss and diarrhoea and to maintain adequate growth in children. The problem of getting enough enzyme to the duodenum concurrently with food is not as simple as it might appear. Gastric emptying varies with the composition of meals, e.g. excessive fat, calories or protein cause delay, and pancreatic enzymes taken by mouth are destroyed by gastric juice. On the other hand, only one-tenth of the normal pancreatic output is sufficient to prevent excess fat (steatorrhoea) or excess nitrogen (azotorrhoea) loss, and it is not essential to eliminate these totally.

Preparations are of variable potency. Pancreatin BNF, *Cotazym* and *Nutrizym* appear to be satisfactory. A reasonable course is to start the patient on the recommended dose of a reliable formulation and to vary this according to the individual's needs and the size and composition of meals. The extract may taken before, during and after food to limit destruction by gastric acid, and antacids, cimetidine or ranitidine taken 30–45 mins before the extract may improve its efficacy. Enteric-coated formulations (Pancreatin Granules, Tablets) are available.

GUIDE TO FURTHER READING

1 Sherlock S. The spectrum of hepatotoxicity due to drugs. Lancet 1986; 2: 440–4.
2 Neuberger J, et al. Oral contraceptives and hepatocellular carcinoma. Br Med J 1986; 292: 1355–7.
3 Forman D, et al. Cancer of the liver and the use of oral contraceptives. Br Med J 1986; 292: 1357–61.
4 Editorial. Halothane-associated liver damage. Lancet 1986; 1: 1251–2.
5 Bouchier A D. Gallstone dissolving agents. Br Med J 1983; 286: 778–80.
6 Bouchier I A D. (Editorial). Brides of quietness: silent gallstones. Br Med J 1983; 286: 415–6.
7 Bateson M C. (Editorial). Progress in gallstone disease. Br Med J 1984; 289: 1163–4.
8 Heaton K W. (Editorial). The sweet road to gallstones. Br Med J 1984; 288: 1103–4.

34

Endocrinology I: Adrenal cortex, corticotrophin, corticosteroids and antagonists

In 1855, Dr. Thomas Addison, assisted in his observations by three colleagues, published his famous monograph '*On the constitutional and local effects of disease of the suprarenal capsules*'. In the following year a physiologist whose principal fame lies elsewhere (neurology) made a contribution to the study of the adrenal glands. Brown-Séquard performed bilateral adrenalectomy in animals and demonstrated that the glands were essential to life, but his work was discounted because, it was said, the animals would die of such surgery whether the glands were removed or not.

Before the end of the 19th century attempts were being made to treat patients with Addison's disease by adrenal gland extracts. By 1896, Osler, using glycerin extracts of fresh hog adrenals given orally, had treated six cases, with improvement in one.

The fact that the secretions of the adrenal cortex differed from that of the medulla was not appreciated in 1901, when adrenaline was first isolated, so that the failure of attempts to maintain life in adrenalectomised animals and to benefit Addison's disease with the newly discovered adrenaline was a great disappointment.

It was not until the 1920s that the vital importance of the adrenal cortex was appreciated and the distinction between the hormones secreted by the two parts of the gland became clear. At this time it was said 'the literature so-called of the physiology and pathology of the adrenal bodies presents a very confused and baffling picture, which only begins to clear somewhat when it is recognised that no mean proportion of the total mass of printed matter, and the portion which contributes most to the haze, can and ought to be stricken from the record on internal evidence alone. . . . Nowhere, perhaps, in experimental work is it more necessary to remember the differences between *post hoc* and *propter hoc*.† Anyone who looks into the literature will see how often this rule has been neglected.'*

By 1929, a year of grave economic upheaval, a reliable adrenal cortical extract was being prepared and its potency determined on cats (biological assay). This involved injecting, over a period, some 500 US dollars' worth of material into each cat. These valuable beasts 'were viewed with some economic misgiving by those of us who, as graduate students in the Princeton laboratories at the time, were not sharing in the alleged prosperity of early 1929.'‡ However, the first clinical trial of this extract reassured any doubters by rapidly reviving a moribund patient suffering from Addison's disease.

By 1936, numerous steroids were being crystallised from cortical extracts, but not enough could be obtained to provide supplies for clinical trial.

* Stewart G N Physiol Rev 1924; 4:163.
† If an event follows another in time (*post hoc*). This does not mean that the first event *caused* the second (*propter hoc*).
‡ Gaunt R et al. Ann NY Acad Sci 1949; 50:511.

The first steroid to be synthesised was deoxycortone (DOCA, DCA) in 1937, and this was done before it had been isolated from cortical extracts, in which only very small amounts occur.

In 1948 cortisone was made from bile acids in quantity sufficient for clinical trial, and the dramatic demonstration of its power to induce remission of rheumatoid arthritis was published in the following year. In 1950 it was realised that cortisone is biologically inert and that the active natural hormone is hydrocortisone (cortisol). Since then an embarrassingly large number of synthetic steroids has been made and offered to the clinician. They are made by a complicated process from natural substances (chiefly plant sterols), the constitutions of which approach most nearly to that of the steroids themselves. A principal aim in research is to produce steroids with more selective action than hydrocortisone, which induces a greater variety of effects than desired in any patient who is not suffering from adrenal insufficiency.

About the same time as cortisone was introduced, corticotrophin became available for clinical use. In 1927 it has been shown that removal of the pituitary gland in animals was followed by atrophy of the adrenal cortex. In 1933 it was found that administration of pituitary gland extracts to animals was followed by hypertrophy of the adrenal cortex. In the 1940s the pure substance in the pituitary, corticotrophin, was isolated, and in the 1960s it was synthesised.

CORTICOTROPHIN (ADRENOCORTICOTROPHIC HORMONE, ACTH)

Natural corticotrophin is a 39-amino-acid polypeptide secreted by the anterior pituitary gland; it is obtained from animal pituitaries.

The biological activity resides in the first 24 amino acids (which are common to many species) and most immunological activity resides in the remaining 15 amino acids.

The pituitary output of corticotrophin responds rapidly to physiological requirements by the familiar negative-feedback homoeostatic mechanism. Since the plasma half-life of corticotrophin is 10 min and the adrenal cortex responds rapidly (within 2 min) it is plain that adjustments of steroid output can be quickly made.

Synthetic corticotrophins have the advantage that they are shorter amino acid chains (devoid of amino acids 25–39) and so are less likely to cause serious allergy, though this can happen. In addition they are not contaminated by animal protein which is a potent allergen.

Tetracosactrin consists of the biologically active first 24 amino acids of natural corticotrophin (from man or animals) and so it has similar properties, e.g. 10 min $t_{\frac{1}{2}}$.

Actions

Corticotrophin binds to receptors on cortical cells and activates adenylate cyclase to form cyclic-AMP, which activates enzymic conversion of cholesterol to pregnenelone (the rate-limiting step in steroid synthesis). It thus stimulates the synthesis of corticosteroids (of which the most important is hydrocortisone) and to a lesser extent of androgens, by the cells of the adrenal cortex. It has only a minor (transient) effect on aldosterone production, which can proceed independently. In the absence of corticotrophin the cells of the inner cortex atrophy.*

The release of natural corticotrophin by the pituitary gland is controlled by the hypothalamus via corticotrophin releasing hormone (CRH or corticoliberin), production of which is influenced by environmental stresses as well as by the level of circulating hydrocortisone. High plasma concentration of any steroid with glucocorticoid effect prevents release of corticotrophin releasing hormone and so of corticotrophin, lack of which in turn results in adrenocortical hypofunction. This is the reason why catastrophe may follow sudden withdrawal of steroid therapy, especially in the chronically treated patient. The steroid must be tailed off gradually to give time for the normal pituitary production of corticotrophin to be resumed and, in the case of prolonged therapy, for the recovery of the atrophied suprarenal gland.

* But not of the outer cortex (zona glomerulosa), which secretes aldosterone and is not under pituitary control.

Corticotrophin is of no use in restoring hypothalamic/pituitary function suppressed by prolonged steroid therapy when this is withdrawn.

In chronic steroid therapy the cortex atrophies because plasma corticotrophin concentration is not high enough throughout the day to stimulate it. It is only in response to a *low* plasma steroid concentration that the natural corticotrophin secretion returns, induces recovery of the cortex, and re-establishes the normal circadian rhythm (maximum plasma concentration in the early morning, irregularly falling during the day and early night). Administered corticosteroid suppresses the capacity of the hypothalamus/pituitary to respond to low plasma hydrocortisone (cortisol) concentration. Therefore after withdrawal of corticosteroid therapy it is necessary to wait until the pituitary recovers its capacity to respond (by secreting corticotrophin) to a low concentration of hydrocortisone in the blood before normal function can be resumed. If exogenous corticotrophin were administered for a prolonged period when the steroid therapy was withdrawn it would certainly stimulate the atrophied adrenal cortex to secrete normal or high levels of steroid, but this would still further delay the recovery of the capacity of the pituitary to respond to low plasma hydrocortisone concentration. Recovery of both may take 6–9 months, and patients are at risk during this period.

If corticotrophin is used as sole therapy, hypothalamic/pituitary/adrenal responsiveness to stress is substantially maintained, and this constitutes a definite advantage. The reasons for this may be that blood corticosteroid levels do not reach the heights that are usual with orally administered steroids, and there is some evidence that smaller amounts of corticotrophin from a recovering pituitary produce adequate output from a hypertrophied adrenal, but have little effect on the atrophied cortex induced by prolonged exogenous steroid therapy.

Corticotrophin suppresses growth less than do exogenous steroids and so it is preferred for long-term therapy in children.

The effects of corticotrophin are those of the steroids (hydrocortisone, androgens) liberated by its action on the adrenal cortex. Prolonged heavy dosage causes the clinical picture of Cushing's syndrome.

Corticotrophin is used both in diagnosis and in treatment. It is inactive if taken orally and this limits its usefulness in therapy.

Diagnostic use: as a test of the function of the adrenal cortex in cases of suspected Addison's disease and hypopituitarism.

A convenient technique for the diagnosis of hypoadrenalism in the Outpatient Department is to inject 0.25 mg of Tetracosactrin Inj. i.m. and to take blood after 30 min and after 60 min. Preferably the test should be carried out about 9 a.m. If the plasma cortisol increases by more than 70 μg/l (200 nmol/l) or reaches a level above 200 μg/l (550 nmol/l) hypoadrenalism can be excluded. This is the 'short' tetracosactrin test. An inadequate response means the adrenals are either diseased (Addison's disease) or atrophic (secondary to either pituitary or hypothalamic disease or to steroid therapy). The distinction between these can be assisted by the 'long' tetracosactrin test, in which the patient is given a depot preparation daily for 3 days, but measurements of plasma concentrations of corticotrophin and aldosterone are now preferred.

It is convenient here to summarise some other tests for integrity of the hypothalamic–pituitary–adrenocortical system that involve administration of hormones or drugs by the physician wishing to establish the site and magnitude of disorder, whether due to natural disease or to therapy (e.g. pituitary irradiation). But first a **reminder of some physiology**: changes in plasma concentration of hydrocortisone (cortisol), stress, etc., cause the *hypothalamus* to modify production of corticotrophin-releasing hormone (CRH): this factor acts on the *pituitary* and the released corticotrophin acts on the *adrenal cortex* to secrete hydrocortisone, which is monitored by the *hypothalamus* by a *negative feedback* mechanism.

Defects in this cycle can be isolated by stimulating or suppressing it at these different sites and measuring the consequences (corticotrophin or cortisol in the blood or cortisol in the urine):

Other tests of hypothalamic/pituitary/adrenocortical function. The following test procedures allow analysis of the site of abnormality in this axis.

a. *Dexamethasone suppression*. Dexamethasone acts on the hypothalamus (like hydrocortisone), to reduce output of corticotrophin releasing hormone (CRH), but it does not interfere with measurement of corticosteroids in blood or urine. Normal suppression of cortisol production indicates that the hypothalamic/pituitary/adrenal axis is intact. Failure of suppression implies pathological hypersecretion of ACTH by the pituitary or of cortisol by the adrenal. Dexamethasone is used because its action is prolonged (24 h). The hypothalamic/pituitary axis is most vulnerable to suppression at night. A simple low-dose test is used to diagnose Cushing's syndrome. One milligram of dexamethasone is given orally at 11 p.m. and blood taken for plasma cortisol at 8 a.m. the following day. If there is suppression, all is well. But if there is not or there are complicating factors, a more stringent test is needed (0.5 mg 6-hourly for 48 h) with 24-hour urine collections. Where it is necessary to distinguish between pituitary ACTH hypersecretion and other causes of Cushing's syndrome, a high-dose test is used (either 8 mg as a single dose of 2 mg 6-hourly for 48 h). The high dose will suppress ACTH production by most pituitary tumours, but it is less effective against ectopic ACTH-producing tumours and is ineffective against adrenal tumours. Enzyme induction of corticosteroid metabolism, by e.g. phenytoin, may cause suppression to fail and so give a false result.

b. *Corticotrophin (ACTH)*, see above.

c. *Corticotrophin releasing hormone* (CRH, corticoliberin), a 41-amino-acid peptide, has obvious diagnostic value in testing pituitary integrity.

d. *Insulin hypoglycaemia* constitutes a stress that stimulates the hypothalamus to produce corticotrophin releasing hormone (CRH). A normal response indicates integrity of the whole axis (since cortisol production is measured). The test is potentially hazardous if there is a defect in response to the stress.

e. *Metyrapone* blocks synthesis of hydrocortisone (cortisol) in the adrenal cortex. A dose is given at night and blood is taken in the morning. If function is normal, plasma cortisol will fall and that of the precursor proximal to the enzyme (11β-hydroxylase) block will rise; it implies integrity of both pituitary and adrenal cortex. Metyrapone is sufficiently short acting for there to be little risk of precipitating acute adrenal insufficiency.

Aminoglutethimide and *trilostane* also inhibit corticosteroid synthesis. See p. 662.

Therapeutic use of corticotrophin

Either (*a*) when adrenocortical hormone effects are desired to treat a disease, or (*b*) when it is desired to stimulate inactive adrenal glands.

a. *The aim is to produce intense adrenocortical stimulation to provide high blood levels of hydrocortisone (and some androgen).* Corticotrophin has the disadvantge that it must be given by injection and the effectiveness of the adrenal response remains uncertain unless blood or urine steroid levels are measured. But, unlike corticosteroids, it does not retard growth in children and adolescents and may be preferred for long-term therapy for this reason.

b. *To stimulate an adrenal cortex that has atrophied as a result of hypopituitarism or suppression of the anterior pituitary gland by steroid therapy.* This is not useful during withdrawal of the steroid, but can be used if these patients have an infection or other severe accidental stress during the succeeding 1–2 years when pituitary responsiveness may still be inadequate.

The effects of exogenous corticotrophin differ from those of exogenous adrenal steroid administration in some important respects:

1. Corticotrophin causes an *increased adrenal secretion of anabolic steroids (androgens) as well as of catabolic steroids (e.g. hydrocortisone)*. Exogenous corticosteroids are catabolic and inhibit the hypothalamus resulting in pituitary adrenal suppression, so that even the normal amount of anabolic steroid is not produced; there is thus an increase in urinary 17-oxogenic steroids (metabolites of hydrocortisone, etc.) and a *decrease* in oxosteroids (metabolites of androgens). Muscle wasting and osteoporosis are thus less likely to occur with corticotrophin than with corticosteroids and this is a consideration in the treatment of muscle wasting diseases,e.g. dermatomyositis, polymyositis.

2. *Adrenocortical atrophy* occurs with exogenous steroid, due to hypothalamic/pituitary inhibition,

but *adrenocortical hypertrophy* occurs with exogenous corticotrophin.

3. Exogenous corticotrophin therapy causes *much less hypothalamic* suppression than corticosteroid therapy so that the patient receiving corticotrophin is less likely to suffer acute adrenal insufficiency as a result of intercurrent illness or other stress, or following withdrawal of treatment, than is the patient on corticosteroid therapy.

4. With corticotrophin, *the amount of adrenal stimulation is limited* by the capacity of the gland to about four times the resting output, whereas with exogenous steroid there is no upper limit. This fact may contribute to the lower incidence and lesser severity of some adverse effects in clinical practice. Overdosage with oral steroid is only too easy, particularly with the newer and more potent preparations.

5. Corticotrophin *cannot provide selective anti-inflammatory effect*, for it principally increases endogenous production of hydrocortisone. Therefore electrolyte disturbances, such as *sodium retention*, are inevitable with vigorous therapy.

6. *Adverse effects*. With long-term exogenous corticotrophin therapy there is a *lesser incidence and severity of* osteoporosis and muscle wasting (see 1 above), bruising, gastric upset, peptic ulcer and growth arrest in children, but a *higher incidence* of acne (because of androgen secretion) and of hypertension due to the large amounts of hydrocortisone (cortisol) secreted.

7. Because *immunological resistance* is liable to develop even to synthetic corticotrophin, it is necessary to monitor therapy by measuring plasma hydrocortisone.

Choice between corticotrophin and an orally active steroid for therapy. There must be strong reasons to justify abandoning the convenience of oral therapy for the inconvenience and unpleasantness of twice-weekly i.m. injections, even if self-administered. The *advantages of corticotrophin* are that hypothalamic/pituitary/adrenal response to stress and some unwanted effects are less common, though some others are more common (see 6 above). The risk of chronic overdose is also less and withdrawal is safer and easier (see 3 above). These considerations may sometimes cause corticotrophin to be preferred in individual patients, particularly growing children. Otherwise the indications and contraindications for corticotrophin are similar to those for exogenous steroid, excepting, of course, in cases where the adrenal cortex itself is diseased.

It is important to use the minimum dose for the required response in order to avoid unwanted effects. General contraindications for corticotrophin therapy are the same as those for adrenal steroids. Dosage of corticotrophin cannot be expressed in equivalence with oral steroid. Adrenal response may be monitored by measuring the metabolites of hydrocortisone (17-oxogenic steroids) in the urine.

Preparations. *Tetracosactrin Injection* is a powder dissolved in water immediately before injection i.v. or s.c., 0.25 mg. It is used for diagnostic tests only as it has such a short half-life (15 min).

Tetracosactrin Zinc Injection (Synacthen Depot) in which the hormone is adsorbed on to zinc phosphate from which it is slowly released. This is the form used in therapy, for it can be given i.m. twice a week (0.5 to 1.0 mg) and the doses then spaced according to response.

Corticotrophin preparations from animals (mixed with carboxymethyl-cellulose or gelatin for prolonged effect) remain available, but pure synthetic preparations are always preferable to inevitably impure biological preparations.

ADRENAL STEROIDS AND THEIR SYNTHETIC ANALOGUES

Hormones normally produced by the adrenal cortex include hydrocortisone (cortisol), corticosterone, aldosterone and some androgens and oestrogens, but not cortisone. Cortisone is a pro-drug, i.e. it is biologically inert and must be converted (largely in the liver) to hydrocortisone for biological activity; its use is obsolete for this reason. Numerous other steroids have been isolated from the gland and many more have been made in the laboratory.

Adrenal steroids are chiefly used in medicine for their anti-inflammatory and immunosuppressive effects (pharmacotherapy). These are only obtained when the drugs are given in doses far above those needed for *physiological* (*replacement*) effect. Their metabolic effects, which are of the greatest importance to the normal functioning of the body, then become adverse reactions or side-effects. Much successful effort has gone into separating *glucocorticoid* from *mineralocorticoid* effects and some steroids (prednisolone, dexamethasone) have virtually no mineralocorticoid activity. It has not yet proved possible to separate the glucocorticoid effects from each other, so that if a steroid is used for its anti-inflammatory action the risks of osteoporosis, diabetes, etc., remain. But one important physiological effect, sodium retention, has been eliminated by the introduction of a double bond that transforms hydrocortisone to prednisolone — a small structural change that has a big biological effect.

In the account that follows, the effects of hydrocortisone will be described and then other steroids insofar as they differ. In the context of this chapter 'adrenal steroid' means a substance with hydrocortisone-like activity. Androgens are described elsewhere.

Mechanism of action

Adrenocortical steroids enter cells where they combine with steroid receptors in the cytoplasm, and the combination then enters the nucleus. This results in the synthesis of protein, including enzymes, that regulate vital cell activities over a wide range of metabolic functions including all aspects of inflammation (there is formation of protein that inhibits the enzyme phospholipase A_2, which is needed to allow the supply of arachidonic acid from which mediators of inflammation are formed. These mediators cause increased vascular permeability and so oedema, leucocyte migration, fibrin deposition, etc. (See mode of action of NSAIDs.)

The actions of hydrocortisone are as below. Naturally there is a distinction between *replacement therapy (physiological effects)* and the higher doses of *pharmacotherapy*.

On inorganic metabolism (**mineralocorticoid** effects): increased retention of sodium by the renal tubule, and increased potassium excretion in the urine.

On organic metabolism (**glucocorticoid** effects):

a. *Carbohydrate metabolism*: gluconeogenesis is increased and peripheral glucose utilisation (transport across cell membranes) may be decreased (insulin antagonism) so that hyperglycaemia and sometimes glycosuria results. Latent diabetes becomes overt, and this effect has been used as a test for the prediabetic state.

b. *Protein metabolism: anabolism* (conversion of amino acids to protein) is decreased but *catabolism* continues unabated or even faster, so that there is a negative nitrogen balance with muscle wasting. Osteoporosis (reduction of bone protein matrix) occurs, growth slows in children, the skin atrophies and this, with increased capillary fragility, causes bruising and striae. Healing, of peptic ulcers or of wounds, is delayed as is fibrosis.

c. *Fat deposition*: this is increased on shoulders, face and abdomen.

Inflammatory response is depressed, regardless of its cause, so that as well as being of great benefit in 'useless' or excessive inflammation, steroids can be a source of danger in infections by limiting useful protective inflammation.

Allergic responses are suppressed. The antigen–antibody interaction is unaffected, but its injurious inflammatory consequences do not follow.

Antibody production is reduced by heavy doses.

Lymphoid tissue is reduced (including leukaemic lymphocytes).

Renal excretion of uric acid is increased.

Blood eosinophils are reduced in number, and this has been used as a test of activity.

Euphoria or psychotic states may occur, perhaps due to CNS electrolyte changes.

Anti-vitamin D action, see calciferol.

Reduction of hypercalcaemia chiefly where this is due to excessive adsorption of Ca from the gut (sarcoidosis, vitamin D intoxication).

Urinary calcium excretion is increased and renal stones may form.

Growth reduction where new cells are being *added* (growth in children), but not where they are *replacing* cells as in adult tissues.

Suppression of hypothalamic/pituitary/adrenocortical system occurs with high doses, so that sudden withdrawal leaves the patient in a state of adrenocortical insufficiency. The normal daily secretion of hydrocortisone is 10–30 mg. Exogenous daily dose of hydrocortisone 40–80 mg or prednisolone 10–20 mg, or its equivalent of other agents is needed daily for complete cortical suppression and for useful anti-inflammatory effect. A steroid-suppressed adrenal continues to secrete aldosterone.

Notes on individual adrenal steroids

All drugs in Table 34.1 except deoxycortone and aldosterone are active when swallowed, being protected from hepatic metabolism by high binding to plasma proteins. Some details of preparations and equivalent doses are given in the table. Injectable and topical forms are available (creams, suppositories, eye drops, etc.).

Hydrocortisone (cortisol) is the principal naturally occuring steroid; it is taken orally; a soluble salt can be given i.v. (as Hydrocortisone Sodium Succinate Inj.) for rapid effect in emergency. A suspension of the insoluble Hydrocortisone Acetate Inj. can be given i.m. for prolonged effect, and also intra-articularly.

Cortisone can also be given orally or i.m. It is a pro-drug, i.e. it is biologically inactive and is converted to hydrocortisone in the liver, so it is unsuitable for topical application. Though satisfactory as replacement therapy in most patients, hepatic insufficiency may result in inadequate conversion to hydrocortisone, so that it is better to use hydrocortisone as routine replacement therapy in Addison's disease.

Choice of parenteral preparation for systemic effect: the soluble Hydrocortisone Sodium Succinate Inj. is used for quick (1–2 h) effect; Prednisolone Sodium Phosphate Inj. is an alternative. For continuous effect about 8-hourly administration is appropriate. **Oral tablet** strengths, see Table 34.1.

Prednisolone is predominantly anti-inflammatory (glucocorticoid), is biologically active and has little sodium-retaining activity.

Prednisone is a pro-drug i.e. it is biologically inert and converted into prednisolone in the liver. Since there is 20% less on conversion and hepatic failure may impair conversion further, there seems no point in using it.

Methylprednisolone is similar to prednisolone.

Fluorinated corticosteroids. Triamcinolone has virtually no sodium-retaining effect but has the disadvantage that muscle wasting may occasionally be severe and anorexia and mental depression may be more common at high doses. **Dexamethasone and betamethasone** are similar, powerful, predominantly anti-inflammatory steroids.

Table 34.1 Relative potencies of adrenal steroids

Compound (tablet strength, mg)		Approximate relative potency Anti-inflammatory (glucocorticoid) effect	Sodium-retaining (mineralocorticoid) effect	Equivalent★ dosage (for anti-inflammatory effect, mg)
Cortisone	(25)	0.8	1.0	25
Hydrocortisone	(20)	1.0	1.0	20
Prednisolone	(5)	4	0.8	5
Methylprednisolone	(4)	5	minimal	4
Triamcinolone	(4)	5	none	4
Dexamethasone	(0.5)	30	minimal	0.75
Betamethasone	(0.5)	30	negligible	0.75
Deoxycortone	—	negligible	50†	—
Fludrocortisone	(0.1)	15	150	—
Aldosterone	—	none	500‡	—

★[1] Note that these equivalents are in approximate accord with the tablet strengths.
[2] The doses in the final column are in the lower range of those that may cause suppression of the hypothalamic/pituitary/adrenocortical axis when given daily continuously. Much higher doses, e.g. 40 mg prednisolone can be given for 5 days without causing clinically significant suppression.
† Sublingual administration.
‡ Injected.

Fludrocortisone has a very great sodium-retaining effect in relation to its anti-inflammatory action, and only as high doses need the nonelectrolyte effects be considered. It is used to replace aldosterone in Addison's disease.

Deoxycortone (DCA, DOCA) has exclusively mineralocorticoid effects. It is eliminated by hepatic first-pass metabolism and so is ineffective when swallowed. It has been superseded by fludrocortisone.

Aldosterone, the main natural salt-retaining hormone, can be given i.m. (0.5 mg) several times a day in acute adrenal insufficiency or shock. After oral administration it is rapidly inactivated in the first pass through the liver and it has no place in routine therapeutics, as fludrocortisone is as effective and is active orally. *Spironolactone* is a competitive aldosterone antagonist and blocks the mineralocorticoid effect of other steroids (see index).

Beclomethasone and budesonide are used by inhalation for asthma (see p. 604). About 90% of an inhalation dose is swallowed and these steroids are inactivated by hepatic first-pass metabolism; the rest, absorbed from mouth and lungs, gives minimal systemic plasma concentration. The risk of suppression of the hypothalamic/pituitary/adrenal axis is thus minimal (but it can happen).

Pharmacokinetics of corticosteroids taken for systemic effect. Absorption of the synthetic steroids given orally is rapid. The *half-life* of most in plasma is 1–3 h but the maximum biological effect occurs later, 2–8 h. They are usually given two or three times a day. They are metabolised principally in the liver and are excreted by the kidney. The half-life is prolonged in hepatic and renal disease and is shortened by hepatic enzyme induction to an extent that can be clinically important.

Conversion in the liver of cortisone to hydrocortisone is much less efficient than that of prednisone to prednisolone. Liver disease must be severe to prevent the conversion.

In the blood adrenal steroids are carried in the free (biologically active) form (5%) and also bound (95% in the case of hydrocortisone) to *transcortin* (a globulin with high affinity, but low binding capacity) and, when this is saturated, to albumin (80% in the case of hydrocortisone). The concentration of the transcortin is increased by oestrogens (e.g. pregnancy, oral contraception, other oestrogen therapy), so that if plasma hydrocortisone concentration is measured the *total* will be found raised, but the amount of *free* hydrocortisone may be normal (though it can be raised), being controlled by the normal feedback mechanism. Patients may be wrongly suspected of Cushing's syndrome if the fact that they are taking oestrogen is unknown and only the *total* concentration is measured (as is usual).

In patients with very low serum albumin, steroid doses should be lower than usual owing to the reduced binding capacity. In addition, the low albumin concentration may be caused by liver disease, which also potentiates steroids by delaying metabolism (half-life of prednisolone may be doubled).

Various spaced-out dosage schedules as a means of minimizing hypothalamic suppression have been used in the hope of reducing hypothalamic/pituitary/adrenal suppression by allowing the plasma steroid concentration to fall enough between doses to provide time for pituitary recovery, e.g. prednisolone 40 mg on alternate days does not cause appreciable pituitary suppression. But none has been both successful in wholly avoiding suppression at the same time as it was successful in controlling symptoms. Where a single daily dose is practicable it should be given in the early morning. *Alternate day schedules* are worth trying, especially where immunosuppression is the objective (organ transplants) rather than anti-inflammatory effect (rheumatoid arthritis); asthmatics taking a systemic steroid may or may not be manageable on such intermittent dosage. *Short courses* (a few days) may be practicable for some.

Another variant is to give *enormous doses* (grams, not mg), orally or i.v., at intervals of weeks or months ('megadose pulses'). The technique is used particularly in collagen diseases. Definitive evaluation of efficacy and side-effects is awaited.

Choice of adrenal steroid

For oral replacement therapy in adrenocortical insufficiency, *hydrocortisone* should be used to supply mineralocorticoid and some glucocorticoid activity. Prednisolone on its own is not effective replacement therapy. In Addison's disease a small dose of a hormone with only mineralocorticoid effect (fludrocortisone) is normally needed in addition.

For anti-inflammatory and anti-allergic effect, *prednisolone*, triamcinolone or dexamethasone. It is not possible to rank these in firm order of merit. One or other may suit an individual patient best, especially as regards incidence of side-effects such as muscle wasting. By *inhalation*, beclomethasone or budesonide.

For hypothalamic/pituitary/adrenocortical suppression, e.g. in adrenal hyperplasia, prednisolone or dexamethasone.

Adverse effects of adrenal steroid pharmacotherapy

These consist of too intense production of the physiological or pharmacological actions listed under actions of hydrocortisone. Some are confined to systemic use and for this reason local therapy (inhalation, intra-articular injection, etc) is preferred where practicable.

Unwanted effects virtually do not occur with one or two doses though some occur with quite short use, e.g. spread of infection. They follow prolonged administration and are sufficiently frequent and dangerous to warrant serious consideration by the physician whether 'the disease which he is attempting to suppress is more dangerous to the patient than the Cushing's syndrome which he might induce'.* The undesired effects recounted below should never be experienced in replacement therapy, but only when the steroid is used as a 'drug' in above physiological amounts. Naturally, the nature of unwanted effects depends on the choice of steroid. Fludrocortisone in ordinary doses does not cause osteoporosis and prednisolone does not normally cause oedema. With this in mind, the principal evil effects of chronic administration are **iatrogenic Cushing's syndrome**: *moon face, characteristic deposition of fat on the body, oedema, hypertension, striae, bruising, acne, hirsutism, muscle wasting and osteoporosis of the spine* (with fractures of vertebrae, ribs, femora and feet). Addition of a small dose of anabolic steroid in the hope of preventing osteoporosis and muscle wasting has been tried, but is ineffective. When these occur, change to corticortrophin may help, as may calcium supplement to diet and *small* doses of vitamin D to arrest progress of osteoporosis (which is largely irreversible). *Avascular* necrosis of bone (femoral heads) is another serious complication. It appears to be due to restriction of blood flow through bone capillaries. Pain and restriction of movement may occur months in advance of radiographic changes. *Diabetes mellitus* may appear.

Depression and psychosis can occur, sometimes with suicide, especially in those with a history of mental disorder; *insomnia* is common.

Peptic ulceration. Patients taking continuous oral therapy have an incidence of peptic ulcer and haemorrhage approximately twice the normal; the incidence rises from about one to two per cent. It is plainly unreasonable to seek to protect all such patients by routinely giving prophylactic antiulcer therapy, i.e. to treat 98 patients unnecessarily in order to help two. But such therapy (histamine H_2-receptor blocker, sucralfate) may be used when ulcer is particularly likely (e.g. a patient with rheumatoid arthritis taking an NSAID) or when ulcer develops whilst taking the steroid. If it is thought appropriate to stop the corticosteroid when an ulcer develops then it probably should not have been given in the first place. In patients with a history of peptic ulcer disease physicians will exercise their critical judgement.

Ulcer may occur with treatment as brief as 30 days and with total amounts of prednisolone equivalent of less than 1000 mg†.

There has been much controversy on this issue, probably because although the incidence of peptic ulcer is doubled (which sounds a lot), it is still very low, an additional 1%. Such small differences are difficult to measure reliably.

Other effects include posterior subcapsular *lens cataract* (risk if dose exceeds 10 mg prednisolone/day or equivalent for above a year), *glaucoma* (also with prolonged use of eye drops), *raised intracranial pressure and convulsions, blood hypercoagulability, menstrual disorders and fever. Delayed*

* Liddle G W. Clin Pharmacol Ther 1961; 2:615.

† Messer J et al. N Engl J Med 1983; 309:21.

tissue healing following surgery is seldom important, but it can disagreeably complicate deep radiotherapy. Major *skin damage* can result from minor injury of any kind.

Suppression of the inflammatory response to infection and immunosuppression causes some patients to present with atypical symptoms and signs and quickly to deteriorate. The incidence of infection may not be increased, but it can be more severe when it occurs. Previously dormant tuberculosis may become active insidiously. Intra-articular injections demand the strictest asepsis.

The incidence of unwanted effects depends on drug used, dosage and duration of therapy but can be as high as 50% of cases.

Hypothalamic/pituitary/adrenal (HPA) *suppression* is dependent on the steroid used, its dose, duration and the time of administration. A single morning dose of less than 20 mg of prednisolone is usually not followed by suppression, whereas a dose of 5 mg given late in the evening is suppressive of the essential early morning activation of the HPA axis (circadian rhythm). Substantial suppression of the HPA axis can occur within a week, but within this period high-dose treatment of severe asthma (with gradual withdrawal) can be accomplished effectively and safely.

Precautions during chronic adrenal steroid therapy. The most important precaution is to see the patient regularly with an awareness of the possibilities of adverse effects including fluid retention (weight gain), hypertension, glycosuria, hypokalaemia (K supplement may be necessary), and back pain (osteoporosis).

Patients must always carry a card on their persons giving details of therapy and simple instructions and they *must* be instructed on the importance of taking the steroid regularly; also, on what to do if they develop an intercurrent illness or other severe stress — to double their next dose and to tell their doctor. If a patient omits a dose then it should be made up as soon as possible so that the total daily intake is maintained, because every patient should be taking the *minimum* dose necessary to control the disease.

Treatment of intercurrent illness

Treatment of intercurrent illness, particularly infections, is urgent, and the dose of steroid should be doubled during the illness and gradually reduced as the patient improves. Effective chemotherapy of bacterial infections is specially important.

Viral infections contracted during steroid therapy can be overwhelming because the immune response of the body may be largely suppressed; continuous use of equivalent of 20 mg prednisolone/day or more is immunosuppressive.* But a steroid may sometimes be useful in therapy after the disease has begun (thyroiditis, encephalitis) and there has been time for the immune response to occur. It then acts by suppressing unwanted effects of immune responses and excessive inflammatory reaction, but see also under adrenal steroids in severe illness.

In the event of the misfortune of **surgery** being added to that of adrenal steroid therapy the patient should receive hydrocortisone 100–200 mg i.m. with premedication. If there is any sign suggestive that the patient may collapse, e.g. hypotension, during the operation, i.v. hydrocortisone (50–100 mg) should be infused at once. The immediate post-operative period is specially dangerous, and hydrocortisone 100 mg should be given i.m. 6-hourly for 72 h.

An emergency operation should be covered by hydrocortisone 200 mg i.m. before, and 100 mg in an i.v. infusion of saline 500 ml during operation, with similar postoperative care.

Minor operations, e.g. dental extraction, may be covered by hydrocortisone 100 mg orally 2–4 h before operation and the same dose afterwards. An i.v. infusion should be available for immediate use in case that is not enough. These precautions should be used in patients who have received substantial treatment with corticosteroid within the past year, because their hypothalamic/pituitary/adrenal system, though sufficient for ordinary life, may fail to respond adequately to severe stress. If steroid therapy has been prolonged, these precautions should be taken for as long as 2 years after stopping it. This will mean that some unnecessary treatment is given, but collapse due to

* A patient whose immune responses are defective, whether due to drugs or to disease or to radiotherapy is at risk if given a *live* vaccine (polio, smallpox, yellow fever). This should be avoided.

acute adrenal insufficiency can be fatal and the ill-effects of short-lived increased dosage of steroid are less grave, being confined to possible increased incidence and severity of infection.

Adrenal steroids and pregnancy

Although a relationship between steroid therapy and cleft palate and other fetal abnormalities has been suspected, there is no doubt that women taking a steroid throughout have both conceived and borne normal babies. Adrenal insufficiency due to hypothalamic/pituitary suppression in the newborn probably only occurs with high doses. Dosage during pregnancy should be kept as low as practicable. Fluorinated steroids should be especially avoided as they may be teratogenic (e.g. dexa- and betamethasone, triamcinolone and various topical steroids, e.g. fluocinolone). Hypoadrenal patients may require an increase in hydrocortisone replacement therapy by about 10 mg per day to compensate for the increased binding by plasma proteins that occurs in pregnancy. Labour should be managed as described for major surgery (above).

Dosage and routes of administration

Dosage depends very much on the purpose for which the steroid is being used and on individual response. It is impossible to suggest a schedule that will suit every case.

The following commencing doses can be used:

For a *serious disease* such as dermatomyositis, which may be fatal: prednisolone 60–75 mg a day, or its equivalent of another steroid. The dose is then increased if necessary until the disease is controlled or adverse effects occur; as much as prednisolone 300 mg a day can be needed.

For a chronic, *less dangerous disease*, such as rheumatoid arthritis: prednisolone 10–17.5 mg daily, adjusted later according to the response.

In some special cases, including adrenal insufficiency, dosage is mentioned in the account of the treatment of the disease.

For continuous therapy the *minimum* amount to produce the desired effect must be used. Sometimes imperfect control must be accepted by the patient because full control, e.g. of rheumatoid arthritis, though obtainable, involves use of doses that must lead to long-term toxicity, e.g. osteoporosis, if continued for years. The decision to embark on such therapy is a serious matter for the patient.

In general, *serious unwanted effects* are unlikely if the daily dose is below the equivalent of hydrocortisone 50–75 mg or prednisolone 10–15 mg.

Topical applications (creams, intranasal, inhalations, enemas) are used in attempts to obtain local, whilst avoiding systemic, effects whenever possible, and solutions are injected into joints and subconjunctivally. However, all these can, with heavy dose, be sufficiently absorbed to suppress the hypothalamus. Individual preparations are mentioned in the text where appropriate.

The relatively high selectivity of inhaled beclomethasone in asthma is due to a combination of route of administration, high potency and rapid conversion to inactive metabolites by the liver of any drug that is absorbed (see asthma, skin).

Contra-indications to the use of adrenal steroids for suppressing inflammation are all relative, depending on the advantage to be expected. They should only be used for serious reasons in patients with diabetes, a history of mental disorder or peptic ulcer, epilepsy, tuberculosis, hypertension or heart failure. The presence of any infection demands that effective chemotherapy be begun before the steroid, but there are exceptions (some viral infections, see above). Topical corticosteroid applied to an inflamed eye (with the very best of intention) can be disastrous if the inflammation is due to herpesvirus.

Steroids containing fluorine (see above) intensify diabetes more than others and so should be avoided in that disease.

Tissue damage due to deep radiotherapy may be enhanced.

Prolonged use of adrenal steroids in children presents essentially the same problems as in adults except that growth is retarded roughly in proportion to the dose. This is unlikely to be important unless therapy exceeds 6 months; there is a spurt of growth after withdrawal. Intermittent dosage schedules (alternate day) may reduce the risk.

Some other problems loom larger in children than in adults. Common childhood viral infections may be more severe, and if a non-immune child taking an adrenal steroid is exposed to one, it is wise to try to prevent it with immunoglobulin.

Live virus vaccination is unsafe as it may cause the disease but active immunisation with killed vaccines or toxoids will give normal response unless the dose of steroid is high, when the response may be suppressed.

Children may develop raised intracranial pressure more readily than adults.

Fixed-dose combinations of adrenal steroids with other drugs in one tablet are objectionable as it is always important to adjust the steroid dose to the minimum that produces the desired effect so that the dose of the other drug is altered, not on the patient's need for it but on his need for steroid.

Indications for use of adrenal steroids

1. **Replacement of hormone deficiency**
2. **Inflammation suppression.**
3. **Immunosuppression.**
4. **Pituitary suppression (uncommon).**

Nabarro* summarises the place of adrenal steroids in therapeutics, and this account of 1960 remains valid:

'The use of physiological amounts of hydrocortisone has greatly improved the replacement therapy available for patients with Addison's disease or hypopituitarism. Larger or pharmacological amounts of steroids have been used in the treatment of diseases unrelated to the adrenal gland. Adrenocortical steroids inhibit the inflammatory reaction, but in many instances the inflammatory reaction is part of the body's defence mechanism and is to be encouraged rather than inhibited. It has, however, become apparent that there are diseases which are really due to the body's reaction being quite disproportionate to the noxious stimulus. The manifestations of the disease are, in fact, those of an exaggerated or inappropriate inflammatory response, and if steroid therapy can inhibit this inappropriate response the manifestations of the patient's disease will be suppressed. The underlying condition is not cured, though it may ultimately burn itself out.

* Nabarro J D N. Br Med J 1960; 2:553.

'The anti-inflammatory action of steroids is used for this purpose in allergic conditions and diseases like rheumatoid arthritis, rheumatic carditis, disseminated lupus erythematosus, and polyarteritis nodosa. Large doses of steroid will also inhibit antibody production and help in the management of auto-immune conditions like some of the haemolytic anaemias and thrombocytopenic purpuras. Steroid therapy may also be used to suppress the patient's adrenal glands; the doses required, however, are nearer the physiological levels. This may be needed in cases of adrenal dysfunction where abnormal androgenic steroids are being made, or in cases of disseminated breast cancer to inhibit adrenal secretion of oestrogens, the so-called medical adrenalectomy.

'When large doses of steroids are given for their pharmacological action, the result will be to produce an iatrogenic Cushing's syndrome. There is a tendency to forget that Cushing's syndrome is a serious illness with a grave prognosis — so serious, in fact, that one has no hesitation in advising total adrenalectomy for its treatment. Admittedly, treatment with high doses of steroid may in some situations be life-saving, or produce a temporary remission in an incurable disease. There has been a tendency to overlook the dangers of treatment with adrenocortical steroids and to use them in cases where the treatment may prove more dangerous or disabling than the original disease.'

An account of the use of steroids in some individual diseases follows.

Acute adrenal insufficiency (*Addisonian crisis*)

This is an emergency and hydrocortisone sodium succinate 100 mg should be given i.v. immediately it is diagnosed. An i.v. infusion of sodium chloride solution (0.9%) is set up immediately and a second 100 mg of hydrocortisone is added to the first litre, which may be given over 2 h. At the time the infusion is started hydrocortisone 100 mg is given i.m. After the infusion the patient should receive hydrocortisone 50 mg i.m. or orally, 8-hourly for 24 h, then 12-hourly for 24 h and then a total of 50–75 mg a day orally in two or three doses. Other treatment to restore electrolyte balance will depend on the circumstances. Intravascular volume replacement may be needed in addition, to help restore the blood pressure. The cause of the crisis should be sought and treated; it is often an infection. When the dose of hydrocortisone falls below 60 mg a day, supplementary mineralocorticoid (fludrocortisone) may be needed (see below).

Chronic primary adrenocortical insufficiency (Addison's disease)

Hydrocortisone orally is used (20–40 mg total daily) with two-thirds of the total dose in the morning to mimic the natural *diurnal rhythm* of secretion. Some patients do well on hydrocortisone alone, with or without added salt, but most patients require a small amount of mineralocorticoid as well (fludrocortisone, 0.1–0.2 mg once a day, orally). If the dose of fludrocortisone should exceed 0.5 mg a day, an unlikely event, then its hydrocortisone-equivalent must be taken into account (for glucocorticoid effect, fludrocortisone 1 mg is equivalent to hydrocortisone 20 mg). The injectable preparations are obviously valuable for patients liable to vomit. The use of a primarily glucocorticoid agent (prednisolone) with a larger dose of fludrocortisone is practicable but pointless.*

Some patients who find hydrocortisone a gastric irritant will tolerate cortisone.

The dosage of the hormones is determined in the individual by following his general clinical progress and particularly by observing his weight, cardiac size, blood pressure, presence of oedema, serum sodium and potassium concentrations and haematocrit. If any complicating disease arises, such as infection, a need for surgery or other stress, the hydrocortisone dosage should immediately be doubled, see above. If there is vomiting, hormone must be given parenterally without delay.

There are no contraindications to replacement therapy. The risk lies in withholding rather than in giving it.

Some patients (particularly those with hypopituitarism), when first treated, cannot tolerate full doses of hydrocortisone because they become euphoric or otherwise mentally upset. 10 mg a day may be all they can take. The dose can usually soon be increased if it is done slowly. Patients with peptic ulcer may be unable to exceed 20 mg of hydrocortisone a day. If diabetes is present the full dose is used and the diabetes controlled with insulin.

Chronic secondary adrenocortical insufficiency

This occurs in hypopituitarism. In theory the best treatment is corticotrophin, but the disadvantages of frequent injection are such that hydrocortisone is preferred. Usually less hydrocortisone is needed than in primary insufficiency. Special sodium-retaining hormone is seldom required, for the pituitary has little control over aldosterone production, so that this is still secreted by the adrenal cortex. Thyroxine is given in appropriate dosage and sometimes sex hormones. The general conduct of therapy does not differ significantly from that in primary adrenal insufficiency.

Iatrogenic adrenocortical insufficiency

This occurs in patients who have received prolonged high-dose steroid therapy, which inhibits hypothalamic production of the corticotrophin releasing hormone and so results in *secondary* adrenal failure. To avoid an acute crisis on stopping, steroid therapy *must* be withdrawn gradually to allow the hypothalamus, the pituitary and the adrenal to regain normal function. Also, when patients taking steroids have an infection or surgical operation (major stress) they should be treated as for primary insufficiency.

After the use of large doses of hormone to suppress inflammation or allergy, sudden withdrawal may not only lead to an adrenal insufficiency crisis but to relapse of the disease, which has only been suppressed, not cured. Such relapse can be extremely severe, sometimes life-threatening.

Withdrawal of steroid therapy. *The longer the duration of therapy the slower must be the withdrawal.* After short-term use, e.g. 2 weeks, if rapid withdrawal is desired a 50% reduction in

* Adrenalectomised patients (for Cushing's syndrome) may become oedematous on an otherwise optimal dose of hydrocortisone; for these, a proportion of the hydrocortisone may be replaced by a glucocorticoid (prednisolone).

dose may be made each day; but if the patient has been treated for a longer period, reduction in dose is accompanied by the dual risk of a flare up of the disease and of iatrogenic hypoadrenalism; then withdrawal should be done very slowly, e.g. 2.5–5 mg prednisolone or equivalent at intervals of 3–7 days.

An alternative scheme is to try halving the dose weekly until 25 mg prednisolone or equivalent is reached, after which it may be reduced by about 1 mg every third to seventh day. Paediatric tablets (1 mg) can be useful during withdrawal.

But these schemes may be found too fast (occurrence of fatigue, 'dish-rag' syndrome, or relapse of disease) and the rate may need to be even as slow as 1 mg prednisolone or equivalent per month, particularly as the dose approaches the level of physiological requirement (equivalent of 5–7 mg prednisolone daily).

The long tetracosactrin test or measurements of plasma corticotrophin concentration, may be used to assess recovery of adrenal responsiveness, but a positive result should not be taken to indicate full recovery of the patient's ability to respond to stressful situations — the latter is best shown by an adequate response to insulin-induced hypoglycaemia.

Corticotrophin should not be used to hasten recovery of the cortex since its effects cause further suppression of the hypothalamic/pituitary axis, on the recovery of which the patient's future depends. Complete recovery of normal hypothalamic/pituitary/adrenal function sufficient to cope with severe intercurrent illnesses or surgery is generally complete in 2 months but may take as long as 2 years.

There have been many reports of collapse, even coma, occurring within a few hours of omission of steroid therapy, e.g. due to patients' ignorance of the risk to which their physicians are exposing them or failing to have their tablets with them and other trivial causes; but it is not invariable. Patients must be instructed on the hazards of omitting therapy and, during intercurrent disease, i.m. preparations should be freely used. Anaesthesia and surgery in adrenocortical insufficiency is discussed above.

Adrenal steroids in severe illness: shock. There has been considerable dispute on the place of adrenal steroids in severe illness, chiefly infections, where there is no evidence of actual adrenal cortical destruction, or of failure of the hypothalamic/pituitary/ adrenal system to respond adequately to the stress. There is reason to expect that adrenal steroids might both help and harm such patients. Corticosteroids in enormous doses have been shown in animals to protect against bacterial endotoxin shock and especially when given before the noxious agent, a situation that has little clinical relevance.

There are many reasons why corticosteroids *might* benefit **septic vascular** shock (see index), but the question *whether* they do so remains. Current evidence, on balance, suggests they do not benefit even if given early, and may even increase mortality where there is evidence of renal impairment, e.g. raised blood creatinine concentration. In septic shock there is initial vasodilatation (hyperdynamic phase) followed by leakage of intravascular fluid through damaged capillary endothelium (hypovolaemic phase). These phases are mediated by vasoactive substances (kinins, leukotrienes, prostaglandins and other products of arachidonic acid, and by endorphins). The formation of these mediators is influenced by corticosteroids in one way or another. But there are obvious dangers, the suppression of useful inflammation and antibody production so that the infection is exacerbated. The doses of corticosteroid used in shock are far higher than replacement doses (which are useless; e.g. dexamethasone 2–6 mg/kg repeated in 2–6 h) and given for 2–3 days only; it may be that ordinary (glucocorticoid) actions are not relevant.

Corticosteroids are sometimes used in any serious disease in which the consequences of infection seem to be so great as to be likely to kill the patient (e.g. cerebral oedema, obstructive symptoms in meningitis) but controlled trials are lacking and there are obvious dangers of exacerbating active infection.

For use of corticosteroids in terminal illness, see p. 314.

Adrenogenital syndrome and adrenal virilism. An attempt may be made to suppress excess adrenal androgen secretion by inhibiting pituitary corticotrophin production by means of prednisolone or dexamethasone. Suppression of androgen production is effective if there is adrenal hyperplasia, but not if an adrenal tumour is present. Hairiness, which women especially dislike in themselves, is often unaffected even though good suppression is achieved, and menstruation recommences.

Adrenal steroids and inflammation and immunosuppression

Adrenal steroids have been used in virtually every hitherto untreatable or obscure disease, e.g. immune complex diseases, nephrotic syndrome, sarcoidosis, with very variable results. Only a brief survey can be given here.

Drugs with primarily *glucocorticoid effects* (e.g. prednisolone) are chosen, so that dosage is not limited by the mineralocorticoid effects that are inevitable with hydrocortisone. But it remains essential to use only the minimum dose that will achieve the desired effect, and sometimes therapeutic effect must be partly sacrificed to avoid adverse effects, for it has not yet proved possible to separate the glucocorticoid effects from each other; indeed it is not known if it is possible to eliminate catabolic effects and at the same time retain anti-inflammatory action. In any case, in some conditions (e.g. nephrotic syndrome) the clinician cannot specify exactly what action he wants the drug developer to provide.

The following list comprises diseases in which adrenal steroids may be useful. The decision to give a steroid commonly depends on knowledge of the likelihood and amount of benefit (bearing in mind that very prolonged high dose *inevitably* brings a serious complications such as osteoporosis) on the severity of the disease and on whether the patient has failed to respond usefully to other treatment. It often requires expertise that can only be imparted by those with wide experience of the disease concerned.

Adrenal steroids are used in all or nearly all cases of:

Exfoliative dermatitis and pemphigus, if severe.

Systemic lupus erythematosus, if severe.

Status asthmaticus

Acute lymphatic leukaemia (see index).

Acquired haemolytic anaemia.

Severe allergic reactions of all kinds, e.g. serum sickness, angioneurotic oedema; trichiniasis. They will not control acute anaphylactic shock as they do not act quickly enough.

Organ transplant rejection.

Aspiration pneumonitis, adult respiratory distress syndrome and pulmonary oedema from near drowning: give prednisolone i.v., up to 50 mg, 4-hourly for 72 h; given early steroid helps to maintain the integrity of the injured endothelium.

Neonatal respiratory distress syndrome. The steroid increases formation of pulmonary surfactant in the preterm fetus; the corticosteroid is administered to mothers in preterm labour.

Active chronic hepatitis — a corticosteroid improves well being, liver function and histology and patient survival in the short term, but there is considerable uncertainty about the classes of patient that will benefit long term. Prednisone should not be used as the liver may fail to transform it into the active prednisolone.

Giant cell or cranial arteritis, variant of polyarteritis nodosa.

Adrenal steroids are used in some cases of:

The following collagen diseases: rheumatic fever (see index), chronic discoid lupus erythematosus, polyarteritis nodosa, scleroderma, polymyositis, dermatomyositis. If, in the latter disease, vision has been at all affected, steroid administration is urgent.

Rheumatoid arthritis

Ankylosing spondylitis

Ulcerative colitis and proctitis

Regional ileitis.

Bronchial asthma and hay-fever (allergic rhinitis): also some bronchitics with marked airways obstruction.

Sarcoidosis. If there is hypercalcaemia or threat to a major organ, e.g. eye, steroid administration is urgent. Pulmonary fibrosis may be delayed and central nervous system manifestations may improve.

Blood diseases due to circulating antibodies, e.g. haemolytic anaemias; thrombocytopenic purpura (there may also be a decrease in capillary fragility with lessening of purpura even though thrombocytes remain few); agranulocytosis.

Eye diseases. Allergic diseases and non-granulomatous inflammation of the uveal tract. Bacterial and virus infections may be made worse and use of steroids to suppress inflammation of infection is generally undesirable, is best left to ophthalmologists and must be accompanied by effective chemotherapy; this is of the greatest importance in herpesvirus infection. Corneal integrity should be checked before use (by instilling a drop of fluorescein). Prolonged used of corticosteroid eye drops causes glaucoma in 1 in 20 of the population (a genetic trait). Application is generally as hydrocortisone, prednisolone or fluorometholone drops or subconjunctival injection.

Nephrotic syndrome. Patients with 'minimal change' lesions respond well. With 60 mg/day total of prednisolone 90% of those who will lose their proteinuria will have done so within 4–6 weeks. Longer courses only induce adverse effects. Slow withdrawal of the steroid may leave the patient well, but relapses are common (50%) and it is then necessary to find a minimum dose of steroid that will keep the patient well. If a steroid is for any reason undesirable, cyclophosphamide in a dose of 3 mg/kg/day for 8 weeks may be substituted. The prognosis of other forms of glomerulonephritis is not improved by drugs, indeed for some patients the disease may even be made worse.

A variety of skin diseases, such as eczema. Severe cases may be treated by occlusive dressings if a systemic effect is not wanted — though absorption can be substantial (see Ch. 39).

Acute gout resistant to other drugs (see index).

Hypercalcaemia of myelomatosis and other malignant diseases, of sarcoidosis and of vitamin D intoxication responds to prednisolone 30 mg daily (or its equivalent of other steroid) for 10 days. Hyperparathyroid hypercalcaemia does not respond.

Raised intracranial pressure due to cerebral oedema e.g. in cerebral tumour or encephalitis, probably an anti-inflammatory effect, reduces vascular permeability: acts in about 4 h: give dexamethasone 4–10 mg i.m. or i.v. (or equivalent) initially and then oral daily total dose 4–10 mg (or equivalent).

Miscellaneous diseases. In these, other lines of treatment should be tried first where they exist, steatorrhoea, severe nasal allergy (topical application), 'aphthous' ulcers in the mouth (suck a 2.5 mg hydrocortisone tablet [Corlan] four times daily), Bell's palsy, acute polyneuritis, toxic and virus encephalitis, post-irradiation fibrosis, Hunner's ulcer of the bladder, myasthenia gravis, myotonia.

Inhibition of synthesis of adrenal steroids

Metyrapone (Metopirone) was introduced in 1961. It interferes with the enzyme, steroid 11 β-hydroxylase, that coverts 11-deoxy precursors into hydrocortisone, corticosterone and aldosterone. When this happens the fall in plasma hydrocortisone stimulates the hypothalamus to release corticotrophin releasing hormone (corticoliberin, CRH) and so the anterior pituitary to release corticotrophin. Since the block occurs at a late stage of synthesis, there is a build up of biologically active precursors under the influence of corticotrophin (although the final synthetic step remains blocked). This may explain why control of cortical hypersecretion (neoplasm, hyperplasia) is often incomplete. Metyrapone affects synthesis of aldosterone less than that of glucocorticoids. *Trilostane* (Modrenal) blocks the synthetic path earlier (3 β-hydroxysteroid dehydrogenase) and thus also inhibits aldosterone synthesis.

Aminoglutethimide (Orimeten) blocks even earlier, preventing the conversion of cholesterol to pregnenolone. It therefore blocks synthesis of all steroid, hydorcortisone, aldosterone and sex hormones.

These agents have use in diagnosis of adrenal disease and in controlling excessive production of corticosteroids, e.g. by tumours, where the cause cannot be removed. They must be used with special care since they can precipitate acute adrenal insufficiency.

Competitive antagonism of adrenal steroids. Spronolactone (Aldactone; see index) antagonises the sodium-retaining effect of aldosterone and other mineralocorticoids. It is used to treat oedema (see p. 551). There are no competitive antagonists to glucocorticoid effects in clinical use.

GUIDE TO FURTHER READING

1 Hench P S et al. The effect of a hormone of the adrenal cortex (17-hydroxy-11-dehydrocorticosterone: Compound E) and of pituitary adrenocorticotrophic hormone on rheumatoid arthritis. Proceedings of the Staff Meetings of the Mayo Clinic 1949; 24; 181, 277 (acute rheumatism). The classic studies of the first clinical use of an adrenocortical steroid in inflammatory disease. See also p. 298 for an account by E. C. Kendall of the biochemical and pharmaceutical background to the clinical studies. Kendall writes of his collaboration with Hench, 'he can now say "17-hydroxy-11-dehydrocorticosterone" and in turn I can say "the arthritis of lupus erythematosus". In sophisticated circles, however, I prefer to say, "the arthritis of L.E."'.

2 Melby J C. Systemic corticosteroid therapy, pharmacology and endocrinologic considerations. Ann Intern Med 1975; 81:505.

3 Byyny R. Withdrawal from glucocorticoid therapy. N Engl J Med 1976; 295:30.

4 Editorial. Steroid therapy and the adrenals. Lancet 1975; 2:527.

5 Newton R W et al. Adrenocortical suppression in workers manufacturing synthetic glucocorticoids. Br Med J 1978; 1:73.

6 Downie W W et al. Steroid cards: patient compliance. Br Med J 1977; 2:428.

7 Hancock K W et al. Primidone/dexamethasone interaction. Lancet 1978; 2:97.

8 Malone D N S et al. Endocrine response to substitution of corticotrophin for oral prednisolone in asthmatic children. Br Med J 1972; 3:202.

9 Black A K et al. The effect of prednisolone on arachidonic acid and prostaglandin E_2 and F_2 levels in human cutaneous inflammation. Br J Clin Pharmacol 1982; 14:391.

10 Editorial. Emotion, exercise and the adrenal cortex. Br Med J 1958; 2:496.

11 Powell-Tuck J et al. Plasma prednisolone levels after administration of prednisolone-21-phosphate as a retention enema in colitis. Br Med J 1976; 1:193.

12 Malone D N S et al. Hypothalamo-pituitary-adrenal function in asthmatic patients receiving long-term corticosteroid therapy. Lancet 1970; 2:733.

13 Friedman M et al. Effects of long-term corticosteroids and corticotrophin on the growth of children. Lancet 1966; 2:568.

14 Westerhof L et al. Recovery of adrenocortical function during long-term treatment with corticosteroids Br Med J 1972; 2:195.

15 Feiwel M et al. Effect of potent topical steroids on plasma-cortisol levels of infants and children with eczema. Lancet 1969; 1:485.

16 Jenkins J S. Conversion of cortisone to cortisol and prednisone to prednisolone. Br Med J 1967; 2:205.

17 Treatment of polyarteritis nodosa with cortisone: Results after three years. Report to the Medical Research Council by the collagen diseases and hypersensitivity panel. Br Med J 1960; 1:1399.

18 Kocen R S et al. Mumps epididymo-orchitis and its treatment with cortisone. Report of a controlled trial. Br Med J 1961; 2:20.

19 Nixon J E. Early diagnosis and treatment of steroid induced avascular necrosis of bone. Br Med J 1984; 288:741.

20 English J et al. Diurnal variation in prednisolone kinetics. Clin Pharmacol Ther 1983; 33:381.

21 Orth D N. The old and the new in Cushing's syndrome. N Engl J Med 1984; 310:649.

22 Editorial. Prednisolone pulses in collagen disease: grammes or milligrammes. Lancet 1983; 1:280.

23 Budd R. Corticosteroids in bronchitis. Br Med J 1984; 288:1553.

24 Messer J et al. Association of adrenocorticosteroid therapy and peptic-ulcer disease. N Engl J Med 1983; 309:21: also Editorial, Spiro H M, p. 45.

25 Adinoff A D et al. Steroid-induced fractures and bone loss in patients with asthma. N Engl J Med 1983; 309:265: also Editorial, Baylink D J, p. 306.

35

Endocrinology II: Diabetes mellitus: insulin, oral hypoglycaemics

INSULIN

History. Insulin (as pancreatic islet cell extract) was first administered to a 14-year-old insulin-deficient patient on 11 January 1922 in Toronto, Canada. A sufferer from diabetes who developed the disease in 1920 and who because of insulin, lived until 1968, has told* how, 'Many doctors, after they have developed a disease, take up the speciality in it. . . . But that was not so with me. I was studying for surgery when diabetes took me up. I had no symptoms except whilst studying at night I used to fall asleep far too readily, but that is perfectly physiological when you are revising such dull stuff as anatomy. That's not a symptom of diabetes, it's a students' disease, isn't it? The great book of Joslin said that by starving you might live four years with luck.' He went to Italy and, whilst his health was declining there, he received a letter from a biochemist friend which said 'there was something called "insulin" appearing with a good name in Canada, what about going there and getting it. I said "No thank you; I've tried too many quackeries for diabetes; I'll wait and see." Then I got peripheral neuritis. . . . So when [the friend] cabled me and said, "I've got insulin — it works — come back quick"', [I] responded, arrived at King's College Hospital, London, and went to the laboratory 'as soon as it opened. There Dr Harrison went to the fridge, took out a bottle of insulin and we discussed what the dose should be. It was all experimental for I didn't know a thing about it, neither did he . . . So we decided to have 20 units — a nice round figure. I had a nice breakfast. I had bacon and eggs and toast made on the Bunsen. I hadn't eaten bread for months and months . . . by 3 o'clock in the afternoon my urine was quite sugar free. That hadn't happened for many months. So we gave a cheer for Banting and Best'.†

But 'at 4 pm I had a terrible shaky feeling and a terrible sweat and hunger pain. That was my first experience of hypoglycaemia. We remembered that Banting and Best had described an overdose of insulin in dogs. So I had some sugar and a biscuit and soon got quite well, thank you.

'At one time in early 1923 the insulin standardisation was extremely bad. Some batches would be nearly twice as strong as others. Miller and I used to test the batches on ourselves. Thank goodness they soon got a good rabbit test, so we did not have to do it any more.'

Insulin is synthesised and stored in granules in the β-islet cells of the pancreas. Daily secretion amounts to 30–40 units, which is about 25% of total pancreatic insulin content.

Insulin is a polypeptide with two peptide chains (A chain, 21 amino acids and B chain, 30) linked by two disulphide bridges. The basic structure having metabolic activity is common to all species,

* Abbreviated from Lawrence R D King's College Hospital Gazette 1961; 40:220. Transcript from a recorded after-dinner talk to students' Historical Society.

† F G Banting and C H Best, of Toronto, Canada. See also J Lab Clin Med 1922; 7:251.

but there are minor species differences, which result in the development of antibodies in all patients treated with animal insulins as well as to unavoidable impurities in the preparations, minimal though these now are.

Bovine insulin differs from human insulin by three amino acids and is more antigenic to man than is *porcine* insulin, which differs from human by only one amino acid. This difference is seldom clinically important.

Human insulin (1980) is available as two forms, one, *e*nzyme *m*odified *p*orcine (emp), and the other, *c*hain, *r*ecombinant DNA, *b*acterial (crb) insulin, for which the gene for insulin synthesis has been artifically introduced into *Escherichia coli*. Both preparations contain small amounts of contaminants (animal, bacterial), which can cause allergy; and human insulin itself can cause antibody formation. The chief reason for using human insulin is not difference in biological insulin activity, but reduced immunogenicity.

Insulin receptors. Insulin is bound to receptors on the surface of the target cell, and probably also enters the cell along with the receptor. These receptors vary in number inversely with the insulin concentration to which they are exposed, i.e. with *high insulin concentration the number of receptors declines* (*down regulation*) and responsiveness to insulin also declines (insulin resistance); with *low insulin concentration the number of receptors increases* (*up regulation*) and responsiveness to insulin increases. Thus obese maturity-onset diabetics having hypersecretion due to overeating, with insulin resistance, may recover insulin responsiveness as a result of dieting so that the insulin secretion diminishes, cellular receptors increase and insulin sensitivity is restored. Changes in affinity of receptors, as well as in numbers, also contributes to insulin resistance.

Cellular mechanism of action of insulin after combination with the receptor is uncertain; the complex activates the 'second messenger' (uncertain), which in turn causes release of the 'third messenger', Ca^{2+} ions. Insulin also has a membrane effect increasing glucose uptake as well as its utilisation, especially by muscle and adipose tissue. Its effect include:

1. *Reduction in blood sugar* due to increased glucose uptake in the peripheral tissues (which convert it into glycogen or fat), and reduction of hepatic output of glucose (diminished breakdown of glycogen and diminished gluconeogenesis). When the blood-glucose level falls below the renal threshold (10 mmol/l or 180 mg/100 ml) glycosuria ceases in diabetes, as does the osmotic diuresis of water and electrolytes. Polyuria with dehydration and excessive thirst are thus alleviated. If the blood glucose falls much below normal levels appetite is stimulated.

2. *Other metabolic effects*: in addition to enabling glucose to pass across cell membranes, the transit of amino acids and potassium into the cell is enhanced. Insulin regulates carbohydrate utilisation and energy production. It enhances protein synthesis.

3. *An insulin-deficient diabetic* is dehydrated due to osmotic diuresis (see 1 above), and is ketotic because fats break down faster than the ketoacid metabolites can be utilised.

4. There is a *circadian rhythm* in insulin requirement (maximal between 5 a.m. and 9 a.m.).

5. Post-receptor defects also contribute to insulin resistance.

Uses. The main indication is **diabetes mellitus**. Insulin promotes the passage of potassium simultaneously with glucose into cells, and this effect is utilised in *hyperkalaemia* (see index). Its use to stimulate appetite (which it does) is obsolete. Insulin hypoglycaemia can also be used as a test of *anterior pituitary function* (growth hormone and corticotrophin are released) and to test the *completeness of vagotomy* in reducing gastric secretion.

Pharmacokinetics. Insulin must be injected (s.c., i.m. or i.v.) as it is digested if swallowed. It is absorbed into the blood* and is inactivated in the liver and kidney (about 40% in a single passage). About 10% appears in the urine. The plasma $t_{\frac{1}{2}}$ is about 10 min. This is convenient for an accurately controlled continuously functioning biofeedback system, but poses difficulties for routine replacement in insulin deficiency. There-

* Peak-plasma insulin (s.c.) concentration at 60–90 min. Absorption is slower if there is peripheral vascular disease or smoking, and faster if the patient takes a hot bath or uses an ultraviolet light sunbed (which has induced a hypoglycaemic fit) or exercises. The effects are due to changes in peripheral blood flow.

fore *sustained-release preparations* have been developed to provide a nearer approach to natural function compatible with the convenience of daily living. An even closer approach is provided by the development of (at present inevitably expensive) miniaturised pumps.

The engineers have developed two pump systems, which have been dignified with the name 'artificial pancreas'. Both deliver insulin by continuous variable infusion from an electronically controlled pump (s.c. infusion can be managed by the patient) carried in a belt or harness or even implanted s.c. In one a glucose sensor monitors the blood glucose concentration and automatically changes the infused dose accordingly (closed-loop system), and in the other, less complex technically, the infusion is programmed (with varying degrees of manual control) independently of the blood glucose concentration, providing pre- and postprandial doses appropriate to the patient's habits (open-loop system). The kinetics of s.c. infusion differ from those of intermittent injection. Infusion (continuous or pulsed) provides slower absorption that does not allow rapid changes in blood concentration in relation to meals; with changed rate of infusion a steady state is reached in 6–8 h.

Preparations of insulin

There are three major factors:
1. *Strength* (concentration)
2. *Source* (human, porcine, bovine)
3. *Formulation*
a. short-acting solution of insulin for use s.c., i.m., i.v.
b. longer acting (sustained-release) preparations in which the insulin has been modified by combination with other proteins or zinc or by modification of its crystalline form to give a poorly soluble product, which is given s.c. and slowly dissociates to release insulin in its soluble form (given i.m., which is not advised, the time course of release would be different).

Dosage is measured in international units (see below).

Diabetes mellitus may be managed on four insulin preparations having:

1. **Short duration** of action (and rapid onset): the soluble insulins, e.g. Neutral Insulin Inj. (also known as soluble or regular insulin).

2. **Intermediate duration** of action (and slower onset): Insulin Zinc Suspension (Amorphous) Semilente.

3. **Long duration** of action: Insulin Zinc Suspension (Crystalline) Ultralente.

4. **A mixture:** Biphasic Insulin Inj. (25% is in neutral form (1, above) and 75% zinc suspension, crystalline) or other mixtures to suit the individual (see 9 below and Table 35.1). The other insulins (see Table 35.1) will serve. The important thing is for the doctor to get to know well a range that will serve most patients.

General notes

1. *Purity*. Hitherto insulins (beef, pork) have contained substantial impurities both derived from the insulin molecule (proinsulin, the precursor of insulin, and C-peptide which links the A and B chains of proinsulin to form insulin), and some derived from other pancreatic proteins. These impurities cause allergy, but happily advances in technology have now allowed production of a range of *Highly Purified (mixed) Insulins* and *Monocomponent Insulins*, chiefly pork, which are less allergenic than the earlier forms and replace them. They often go under the same names as the conventional insulins, but with identification that they belong to the Highly Purified Group (HP, MC). Human insulins are of high purity and are likely to replace others.

2. There is no need to change a stabilised diabetic to a highly purified insulin if there are no special problems of local or general adverse reactions, or unexplained requirement of above 100 units/day, in which latter case the transfer should be made in hospital as the requirement of highly purified insulin is unpredictable.

3. *Allergy* occurs to both impurities and to insulin itself. It may take the form of local reactions (inflammatory or fat atrophy) or of insulin resistance. Though less common with the highly purified preparations and human insulin it still does occur. Allergy to the preservative (phenol, cresol, methylhydroxybenzoate) may occur.

4. Doses of monocomponent and high purified insulins are about 10% less than that of conven-

tional animal insulins at average doses, but as much as 20% less if the patient has required a high dose of conventional insulin. Human insulin is absorbed slightly more quickly.

5. Patients should continue on the same insulin preparation and should only change between insulins, e.g. to a purified preparation or to insulin from a different species, if there is a clear clinical indication.

6. New cases of diabetes needing insulin should start on a highly purified preparation of animal or human insulin.

7. Pork insulins are slightly quicker and shorter acting than beef insulins, and patients need up to 20% less of them if they have been using beef insulin (due to the greater antigenicity of beef insulin).

8. *Antibodies to insulin*, provided they are moderate in amount, are actually advantageous. They act as a carrier or store, binding insulin after injection and releasing it slowly as the free insulin in the plasma declines. In this way they smooth and prolong insulin action. But too high concentrations cause insulin resistance.

9. *Compatibility*. Neutral Insulin may be mixed in the syringe with Insulin Zinc Suspensions (amorphous, crystalline) and with Isophane and Biphasic Insulin, and used at once: but Protamine Zinc Insulin binds some of the short-acting Neutral Insulin because there is excess protamine.

Preparations of widely differing pH, (see Table 35.1) should not be mixed (except that Acid Insulin Inj, pH3, may, if necessary, be mixed with Isophane Insulin, pH7).

10. *Intravenous insulins: only* Neutral Insulin Inj. or Acid Insulin Inj. should be used.

11. The standard strength of insulin preparations is *100 I.U. per ml* (UK, USA, Australasia). Use of the wide range of strengths previously standard (20, 40, 80, 320 I.U./ml) declines; there is now an increasing consensus that the wide range of formulations of insulin, all in multiple strengths, caused too much confusion and led both doctors and patients into errors of dose.* Use of 100 I.U. per ml insulin in small children requires special care in measurement of the dose.

* *International* agreement on a single concentration has not yet been attained and travelling insulin users must be watchful.

That insulin preparations should be both precise and of uniform strength all over the world is vital to the health and safety of millions of diabetics. Insulin still has to be standardized biologically according to an International Standard (on blood sugar of rabbits). But the day will come when pure insulin is manufactured like other chemicals and then its dose will be by weight.

Neutral Insulin Inj. (soluble, regular insulin) is an aqueous solution of insulin. It is simple to use, being given s.c. two or three times a day, 45 min before meals. There is relatively little risk of hypoglycaemic reaction if it is used sensibly. If it is known that a meal must be delayed, then the insulin injection can be postponed. The dose can easily be adjusted according to the amount of glycosuria. For these reasons it is often used initially to balance diabetics needing insulin, and always for the treatment of diabetic ketosis, when it may have to be given in large amounts both i.v. and i.m. The biggest disadvantages of soluble insulin for long-term use are the need for frequent injections, and the occurrence of heavy glycosuria before breakfast.

There are two principal forms of soluble insulin, Acid Insulin Inj., at pH 3 (which can cause discomfort at the injection site) and Neutral Insulin Inj., at pH 7 (see Table 35.1). The latter is preferred.

Intravenous neutral (soluble) insulin is used in diabetic ketoacidosis. It may be given intermittently but infusion is preferred. If the insulin is *infused* by *drip* in physiological saline (40 units/l) as much as 60–80% can be lost due to binding to the fluid container and tubing. It is necessary to take this into account in dosing. Alternatively a protein, e.g. polygeline (degraded gelatin), or human plasma albumin, or a few ml of the patient's blood, can be added to bind the insulin in competition with the plastic or glass apparatus, so that the full dose enters the patient, where the complex dissociates. Use of a slow-infusion pump with a more concentrated solution (insulin 1 I.U/ml) is preferred.

Insulin loss is much less and control of dosage is more accurate when more concentrated solutions are infused by pump or syringe, and at 1000 units/l (1 unit/ml) such as is convenient for infusion by pump, losses are not of practical importance. For i.v. doses see diabetic ketoaci-

Table 35.1 Some (approximate only) data on some insulins

Preparation (source)	pH	Action (h) given s.c. Onset (h)	Peak	Duration
Short duration				
Acid Insulin Inj. (b)	3	0	2–5	6–8
Neutral Insulin Inj. (h, p, b) (soluble, regular)	7	0	2–5	6–8
Intermediate duration				
Insulin Zinc Susp (IZS) (Amorphous) Semilente (b,p) (prompt)	7	2	5–10	12–16
Isophane Insulin Inj. (h,p,b) (a protamine Zn suspension)	7	2	6–12	20–24
Intermediate duration mixed with short duration				
Biphasic Insulin Inj. (neutral 25%, p: crystalline 75%, b, p)	7	1	3–8	1–22
Mixed: 30/70 (h, p) (Mixtard)	7	0.5	3–8	24
Mixed: 50/50 (h, p) (Initard)	7	0.5	3–8	24
Long duration				
Insulin Zinc Susp (IZS) (Crystalline) Ultralente (h, b)	7	5	10–20	30–36
Insulin Zinc Susp (IZS) (Mixed) Lente (h, p, b) (semilente + ultralente)	7	2	6–14	24–30
Protamine Zinc Insulin Inj. (PZI) (b)	7	4	12–18	24 — 36

Notes: Abbreviations for species: h = human: p = porcine: b = bovine. There is a great complexity of proprietary names for insulins. Though strictly it is imprecise the term 'soluble' insulin is now taken to refer to Neutral Insulin Inj.

dosis, below. Long-acting (sustained-release) preparations *must not* be given i.v.

The *time-course of soluble insulin given i.v.* is shorter than when given s.c. (as in Table 35.1), namely, onset 0.25 h: peak 0.5–1 h: duration 2 h.

Insulin Zinc Suspensions including isophane insulin (see Table 35.1) have been developed following the observation that the pancreatic islet cells store insulin in association with zinc. They are sustained-release formulations in which the rate of release is controlled by modifying particle size. Neutral pH, soluble insulin can be mixed with them without altering the time-course of effect of either (see Table) and these formulations can be a great convenience.

Protamine Zinc Insulin (PZI) contains excess protamine and if soluble insulin is mixed with it some of the soluble insulin is bound and converted to PZI thus altering the otherwise expected time-course of effect.

Duration of action. Patients live by a 24-hour cycle and plainly insulins having a duration of action exceeding 24 hours can cause problems, especially early morning hypoglycaemia.

Choice of insulin

Optimal control is generally best achieved by two doses of soluble insulin/day, 45 min before breakfast and the evening meal.

If this allows too great a fluctuation of blood sugar then smoother control results with Insulin Zinc Susp. (Amorphous) or Isophane Insulin for either one or both doses, with or without added soluble (neutral) insulin (see Table 35.1), and these suit many patients.

Choice of insulin(s) and dose are adjusted to the individual patient. There is no fixed-dose regimen.

If patients cannot (because of age, poor vision), or will not, accept two injections/day, then they may be manageable on a morning dose of Insulin Zinc Susp. (Mixed) with some soluble insulin (neutral) added.

It is preferable to adapt therapy (insulin and diet) to suit the patients' ways of life rather than to coerce them into the physician's favourite routine. Both doctors and patients are faced with a lifetime of collaboration. Compliance is not a one-sided process, and the patients need all the consideration and support they can get.

Human insulins are particularly chosen in patients who have shown allergic or resistance problems with animal insulins.

Dose of insulin

The total daily output of endogenous insulin from pancreatic islet cells is 30–40 units (determined by the needs of completely pancreatectomised patients), and most insulin-deficient diabetics will need 30–50 units/day of human, beef or pork insulin (two-thirds in the morning and one-third in the evening).

Initial treatment for an insulin-deficient diabetic with *soluble (neutral) insulin* may be thus:

blood sugar < 16.5 mmol/l (300 mg/100 ml): 20 units.

blood sugar* 11–16.5 mmol/l (200–300 mg/100 ml): 10 units.

The dose is then adjusted according to the usual monitoring of blood and/or urine glucose. Daily dose increments should be 4 units. When stabilised, two-thirds of the total daily dose is generally given 30 min before breakfast and one-third 30 min before the evening meal.

If it is decided to give the patient only one injection per day, then 10–14 units of an intermediate-duration insulin zinc suspension (mixed or amorphous, see Table 35.1) may be given. Dose increments (4 units) may be given on alternate days.

Soluble insulin (neutral) may be added, or special mixed insulins used, according to the patient's response. Excessive dose of insulin leads to overeating and obesity; it also leads to hypoglycaemia (especially nocturnal), that may be followed by rebound morning hyperglycaemia that is mistakenly treated by increased insulin, thus establishing a vicious cycle (Somogyi effect).

See also *use of insulin* and *ketoacidosis*, below.

Adverse effects of insulin

Adverse effects are mainly those of overdose.† Because the brain relies on glucose as its source of energy, an adequate blood/glucose level is just as essential as an adequate supply of oxygen, and hypoglycaemia may lead to coma, convulsions and even death (in 4% of diabetics under 50 years of age).

It is usually easier to differentiate hypoglycaemia from severe diabetic ketosis than from other causes of coma, which are as likely in a diabetic as in anyone else. If there is doubt as to the aetiology in a comatose patient it is reasonable to give glucose i.v., but only after taking blood for a sugar estimation. If hypoglycaemia of short duration is responsible, then a rapid improvement is usual; in any case a dose of glucose generally (but not always) does no harm. Hypoglycaemia may manifest itself as disturbed sleep and morning headache.

Other adverse reactions to insulin are **lipoatrophy or lipomata** at the injection sites (rare with purified pork and human insulin), after they have been used repeatedly. These are unsightly, but otherwise harmless. The site should not be used further, for absorption can be erratic, but the patient may be tempted to continue if local anaesthesia has developed, as it sometimes does. Generalised **allergic** reactions are very rare, but may occur to any insulin (including human) and to any constituent of the formulation, as more commonly, may, local reactions (itching red lumps and lipoatrophy). Change of brand of insulin, especially to a highly purified or human preparation, may rectify allergic problems. But zinc occurs in all insulins (though very little in soluble insulin) and can be the allergen.

Transient generalised oedema may occur, especially in the early treatment of undernourished patients.

Low pH insulins may cause local discomfort at the injection site.

Treatment of a hypoglycaemic attack

Prevention depends very largely upon patient education. In particular, they should never miss meals and must know the early symptoms of an attack.‡ They should carry glucose sweets or lump sugar about with them and should carry a special card identifying them as diabetics. This card should request that if the bearer is found behaving strangely he should be given sugar (4–5 tablets/lumps [10–20 g]), repeated in 15 min if necessary before the police are called. Treatment is always to give sugar, either by mouth if the patient can still swallow or glucose (dextrose) i.v. (20–50 ml of 50% solution, i.e. 10–25 g). The response is usually dramatic, but if the patient does not respond within 30 min, it may be because of cerebral oedema, which will require treatment with i.v. dexamethasone and perhaps

* The normal (fasting) blood sugar (glucose) range is 3.9–5.8 mmol/l (70–105 mg/100 ml).

† Suicidal overdose (in diabetics) is well recorded. Surgical excision of the skin and subcutaneous tissue at the injection site of an enormous dose of long-acting insulin has been used.

‡ It can be useful to allow a patient to experience hypoglycaemia once by delaying a meal.

mannitol. If the patient has been severely hypoglycaemic for hours or if very large amounts of insulin have been taken, then large amounts of glucose may have to be given by i.v. infusion for several days. Very severe attacks sometimes damage the central nervous system permanently. See also adrenaline and **glucagon** below.

Some advocate (see above) giving i.v. glucose to a comatose diabetic on the basis that it will revive him if he is hypoglacaemic and do no harm if he is hyperglycaemic. The latter assumption is unsound since a minority of comatose insulin-dependent diabetics have hyperkalaemia and the added glucose can cause a brisk and potentially hazardous rise in serum K (mechanism uncertain), in contrast to non-diabetics in whom glucose causes a fall in serum K.

Hypoglycaemia due to other causes, e.g. alcohol, is treated similarly.

Insulin resistance

Insulin resistance may be due to a decline in *number* and/or *affinity* of receptors (see above) or to defects in post-receptor mechanisms.

A diabetic requiring more than 200 units/day is regarded as insulin resistant (some patients have needed as much as 5000 units/day). This is due to *antibodies* binding insulin in a biologically inactive complex (though it can dissociate as with protein binding of drugs, and, in moderation, this is a useful storage mechanism smoothing the insulin action and prolonging it).

As beef insulin is more antigenic than pork, change to a highly purified pork or human insulin may be successful in reducing resistance. Addition of a sulphonylurea to release endogenous insulin (non-antigenic) may also be useful when pancreatic function is not entirely lost (maturity-onset diabetics). Responsiveness to insulin may sometimes be restored by an adrenocortical steroid (prednisolone 20–40 mg/day) over weeks or months, to suppress antibody production. Obviously, if this is successful, insulin dosage will have to be reduced in accordance with the unpredictable reduction in antibodies. Patients need to be carefully monitored to avoid severe hypoglycaemia. Acidosis also reduces the effect of insulin.

HORMONES THAT TEND TO RAISE THE BLOOD SUGAR

Glucagon is a polypeptide hormone (29 amino acids) from the α-islet cells of the pancreas. It is released in response to hypoglycaemia and is a physiological regulator of insulin effect. It releases liver glycogen as glucose. It has been used to treat insulin hypoglycaemia, but in about 45 min from onset of *coma* the hepatic glycogen will be anyway exhausted and glucagon will be useless. Its chief advantage would seem to be that, as it can be given s.c. or i.m. (1 mg; repeated in 10 min) it can be used in severe hypoglycaemic attack by somebody, e.g. a member of the patient's family, who is unable to given an i.v. injection of glucose. If a comatose patient does not recover 15 min after the second injection, i.v. glucose is essential. If recovery does ensue oral glucose will, of course, be needed, or a good meal. Glucagon is ineffective in marked hepatic insufficiency.

Glucagon has a positive cardiac inotropic effect; its use in cardiac disease is experimental. It appears to have value in acute overdose of β-adrenoceptor blockers.

Adrenaline raises the blood sugar by mobilising liver and muscle glycogen; it does not antagonise the peripheral actions of insulin. Adrenaline was once recommended in the treatment of hypoglycaemia, but endogenous adrenaline is secreted reflexly before symptoms occur and glucose provides safer and more effective therapy. Glycosuria and diabetic symptoms may occur in patients with phaeochromocytoma.

Adrenal steroids, either endogenous or exogenous, antagonise the actions of insulin, although this effect is only slight with the primarily mineralocorticoid group; the glucocorticoid hormones *increase* gluconeogenesis and reduce glucose uptake and utilisation by the tissues. Patients with Cushing's syndrome thus develop diabetes very readily and may be resistant to insulin. Patients with Addison's disease and hypopituitarism are abnormally intolerant of insulin.

Oral contraceptives can impair carbohydrate tolerance.

Growth hormone antagonises the actions of insulin in the tissues. Acromegalic patients may develop insulin-resistant diabetes.

Thyroid hormone increases the requirements for insulin.

ORAL HYPOGLYCAEMIC DRUGS

Oral hypoglycaemic drugs are of two kinds, sulphonamide derivatives (sulphonylureas) and guanidine derivatives (biguanides). They are used by 30% of all diabetics. Unlike insulin they are not essential for life.

Following the observation in 1918 that guanidine had a potent hypoglycaemic effect, guanides were tried in diabetes in 1926, but were abandoned a few years later for fear of hepatic toxicity.

In 1930 it was noted that sulphonamides could cause hypoglycaemia, and in 1942 severe hypoglycaemia was found in patients with typhoid fever during a therapeutic trial of a sulphonamide derivative. In the 1950s a similar observation was made during a chemotherapeutic trial in urinary infections. This was followed up and effective drugs soon resulted.

Mode of action: Sulphonylureas act primarily by stimulating the β-islet cells of the pancreas to release stored insulin. They are therefore ineffective in totally insulin-deficient patients and for successful therapy probably require about 30% of normal β-cell function to be present. They cause hypoglycaemia in normal subjects as well as in diabetics.

Biguanides reduce absorption of carbohydrates from the gut and increase the utilization of glucose in peripheral tissues provided insulin is present; and they reduce hepatic gluconeogenesis. They do not (used alone) cause clinical hypoglycaemia in normal subjects nor in diabetics, but they do cause lactic acidosis.

Both groups of drugs are only effective in the presence of insulin. But biguanides, by their effect on gut absorption, modify effects of injected insulin (sulphonylureas do not modify injected insulin though their effects are naturally additive).

Drugs of the two groups may be used together.

Individual Drugs

Absorption from the alimentary tract is good for all the oral agents. If a patient fails to respond to one drug response to another of the same group may yet occur.

The principal oral hypoglycaemic drugs

Drug plasma $t_{\frac{1}{2}}$ h	Total daily dose (tablet size, mg)	Remarks
Sulphonylureas Tolbutamide (Rastinon) ($t_{\frac{1}{2}}$5–8)	0.5–2 g in 2 daily doses (500 mg)	Very safe. Frequent administration. Less effective than chlorpropamide. Dose may be altered daily. Tolerance occurs.
Chlorpropamide (Diabinese) ($t_{\frac{1}{2}}$24–40)	100–500 mg in 1 dose at breakfast (100, 250 mg)	Less safe than tolbutamide: long $t_{\frac{1}{2}}$. May succeed where tolbutamide fails. Taken only once daily and dose increment weekly.
Glibenclamide (Daonil) ($t_{\frac{1}{2}}$10–15)	5–15 mg in 1 dose at breakfast (2.5, 5 mg)	Its $t_{\frac{1}{2}}$ allows once daily dose with less risk of accumulation than with chlorpropamide. Dose increment weekly.
Biguanides Metformin (Glucophage) ($t_{\frac{1}{2}}$, 2)	1.5–3.0 g in 2–3 doses with meals (500, 850 mg)	Capable of controlling some patients when used alone. Chief use in supplementing a sulphonylurea (different mode of action), or insulin.

Sulphonylureas

Tolbutamide is rapidly metabolised by oxidation in the liver ($t_{\frac{1}{2}}$, 6 h; 1–4 doses a day) so that patients with hepatic disease should be treated with caution, as always. Adverse effects are unlikely to occur in more than 3% of patients. They usually consist of mild gastrointestinal upsets, which may be mitigated by taking the drug after food or by antacids, and of rashes. Alcohol intolerance (inhibition of metabolism) occurs occasionally with all sulphonylureas. Other ill-effects are very rare, but include blood disorders. *The question of increased cardiovascular mortality with long-term use continues to be controversial.*

Sulphonamides, as expected, potentiate

sulphonylureas by direct action and by plasma protein displacement.

Tolbutamide (1.0 g i.v.) is sometimes used in **diagnosis of insulinomas**. The blood glucose and, if possible, the plasma insulin, are measured over the succeeding 3 h. In insulinoma (and also severe hepatic insufficiency) the degree of hypoglycaemia is greater and more prolonged than normal.

Chlorpropamide is part metabolised and part excreted unchanged by the kidney and is dangerous in patients with poor renal function because of its long $t_{\frac{1}{2}}$ of 36 h which is even longer in the elderly for whom the drug is unsuitable. Adverse effects are about twice as frequent as with tolbutamide — gastrointestinal upsets, rashes, vertigo, muscle weakness, headache, unpleasant taste, alcohol intolerance, jaundice and blood disorders — but the latter are rare and seldom serious.

Glibenclamide ($t_{\frac{1}{2}}$, 12 h) is shorter-acting than chlorpropamide but is yet suitable for use in single daily dose. It inhibits platelet aggregation.

Other sulphonylureas include acetohexamide, tolazamide, gliclazide, gliquidone, glipizide, glibornuride. **Glymidine** is a related compound (sulphapyrimidine) and may be tried if there is allergy to a sulphonylurea.

Biguanides (diguanides)

Metformin is taken with meals. Minor adverse gut reactions are common, including a metallic taste in the mouth. The plasma $t_{\frac{1}{2}}$ is about 2 h; it is not metabolised and is excreted by the kidney. Heavy prolonged use can cause vitamin B_{12} deficiency due to malabsorption. Its chief *use* is in combination with a sulphonylurea when the latter alone has failed. It is particularly used in obese patients to get their weight down and so to mitigate their (maturity-onset) diabetic state.

With biguanides ketonuria may occur in the presence of normal blood sugar. This is not generally severe and may be treated by reducing the dose; but persistence in overdose may lead to severe lactic acidosis. Indeed the frequency and severity (death) of lactic acidosis with phenformin ($t_{\frac{1}{2}}$ 7–15 h) have caused the drug to be abandoned. Lactic acidosis is treated with large doses of sodium bicarbonate (i.v.).

Adverse effects of oral agents

Hypoglycaemia occurs with sulphonylureas, but is less common than with insulin therapy. However, it can be severe, prolonged for days, and may be fatal, especially in the elderly and in patients with heart failure. Because of its long $t_{\frac{1}{2}}$ chlorpropamide is not suitable for the old.

Renal and hepatic disease. Biguanides should not be used in the patients with either; the risk of lactic acidosis is too great.

Sulphonylureas are potentiated in these diseases and a drug with a short $t_{\frac{1}{2}}$ (*not* chlorpropamide) should be used in low doses.

Age and cardiac disease also add to the hazard of oral agents.

Guar gum, etc.

The addition of fibre or of gel-forming unabsorbable carbohydrate (guar gum, a hydrocolloidal polysaccharide of galactose and mannose from seeds of the 'cluster bean') to the diet of diabetics reduces carbohydrate absorption and flattens the postprandial blood glucose curse. Reduced need for insulin and oral agents has been reported.

THE TREATMENT OF DIABETES MELLITUS

Good control of diabetes always involves diet and some patients need insulin or oral hypoglycaemics in addition.

The *aim* of treatment is to keep the blood sugar level within the normal range* throughout the 24 h, to avoid ketosis and infections, and, it is reasonably hoped, the long-term complications. Each patient must be assessed individually; only an outline of the general principles involved can be given here:

Education. All diabetics should possess a book that contains general information about the treatment of the disease and detailed diets and should *carry* a card stating that they are diabetic and what to do if they are found unconscious. Diabetics should understand that there is a possibility that proper control minimises the risk of serious complication such as blindness.

* Normal fasting range is 3.9–5.8 mmol/l (70–105 mg/100 ml).

They should know how to give their injections and test their urine.

The introduction of simple testing methods has improved control by rendering patients less unwilling to do the tests.

Urine and blood tests for glucose and ketones may be influenced by drugs.*

Some urine tests are enzymic, employing glucose oxidase (Clinistix), and these are specific for glucose; interference by levodopa and small doses of ascorbic acid may cause falsely low results. Other tests employing copper sulphate and sodium hydroxide, e.g. Clinitest, Benedict's or Fehling's solutions, measure reducing substances and give false-positive results with a variety of drugs and metabolites including salicylates and aspirin, nalidixic acid, probenecid, cephalosporins, penicillin (large dose), streptomycin, isoniazid, PAS and chloral.

Ketone test strips may be positive with levodopa and bromsulphalein and Rothera's test also with salicylate.

Users of special test systems should inform themselves of special interfering factors.

Intercurrent infections. It is important to stress that any *infection* or other pyrexial illnss increases insulin need, which means that patients should *increase* their insulin and take enough food or glucose to cover it. In patients taking oral antidiabetics, trivial intercurrent illness does not generally upset control, for this group of patients is not liable to ketosis anyway; but there is great individual variation.

Diet. Patients should be allowed to follow their own preferences as far as is practicable, and drugs should be adjusted to suit the patient rather than the other way round. Some carbohydrate restriction is necessary, but the amount varies from patient to patient according to their total caloric requirements (100–300 g carbohydrate/day generally) and whether weight increase or reduction is desired. The way in which carbohydrate is distributed through the day varies with the type of insulin taken.

In diabetics of normal weight, protein and fat do not need control, and such patients' diets should not be needlessly complicated.

Weight. *Older fat diabetics* (70% of maturity onset type) form a group whose blood often contains much insulin but who are resistant to its action; they seldom develop ketosis. Glycosuria may cease when their weight is reduced. Biguanides particularly help weight reduction (see below). Weight loss is associated with an increase in numbers of insulin receptors and so an increase in responsiveness to insulin.

Young patients with insulin-deficient diabetes (juvenile onset) are often underweight and need insulin to restore normal weight. The blood of these young diabetics contains no insulin (they are sensitive to its action), and they readily become ketotic.

Assessment of drug therapy in diabetes

As in other life-long diseases, e.g. hypertension, drugs are assessed primarily for their capacity to modify favourably easily measurable features of the disease short term. It tends to be assumed that if this is accomplished the desired objective (of controlling the disease until the patient dies of something else) must naturally follow. But this is not necessarily so.

In the case of diabetes mellitus, the initial use of insulin in the young ketotic insulin-deficient (*juvenile-onset*) cases was dramatic and its efficacy for health and indeed for life remains undisputed. There is also a consensus that meticulous control of blood glucose minimises serious complications (sight, kidney).

But in the case of the middle-aged non-ketotic, insulin-resistant (*maturity-onset*) case, the situation is very different. They have a substantial life expectancy and can often be controlled by diet alone.

With the advent of oral hypoglycaemics in the 1950s, the blood sugar of these patients could be controlled without insulin (to which they were

* *Blood glucose estimations* can also be influenced by drugs, and this varies according to the technique used; clinical chemistry laboratories have full information on their method. The following drugs may provide a *falsely high* measure: levodopa, methyldopa, mercaptopurine, hydralazine, propylthiouracil, paracetamol, PAS, ascorbic acid, dextran, iron dextran or sorbitol, isocarboxazid, nalidixic acid, tetracycline.

The following drugs may case *falsely low* measure (in glucose oxidase reactions): ascorbic acid, hydralazine, chlorpropamide, levodopa, nitrazepam, isoniazid, isocarboxazid, tetracycline. Note, some drugs appear on both lists because different drugs affect different methods differently.

often resistant) and the drugs became widely used. There was no evidence of their long-term effects.

A number of studies of long-term use of oral hypoglycaemics have now been done. Unfortunately the results are in disagreement, e.g. whether sulphonylureas do or do not increase cardiovascular mortality. Such studies are hard to do in a way that is not open to serious objection. Evaluation is complicated by the fact that treated and control groups inevitably change in character and diminish in size with the years, and that mortality in all experimental groups must ultimately be 100%. They are also enormously expensive.

The present consensus is that maturity-onset diabetes should be treated by diet. If this is inadequate there is disagreement as to whether an oral agent or insulin should be first chosen. But a short course of an oral agent to abolish glycosuria and relieve symptoms (e.g. polyuria and pruritus vulvae) would seem justified as a temporary expedient until diet is effective.

In one diabetic clinic, 64 patients taking oral hypoglycaemics because they had failed to respond (normoglycaemia) to diet alone were transferred to placebo tablets; 30% did not relapse. Thus the use of oral hypoglycaemics, once started, need not be regarded as permanent.

Selection of therapy for diabetes

Diabetic ketoacidosis — insulin — urgent.

Glycosuria
- Diet — especially if patient overweight,
- or diet + oral hypoglycaemic(s),
- or diet + insulin.

Very approximately, of **diabetics under 30 years**, almost all need insulin; **over 30 years** *one-third* need **insulin**, *one-third* **oral agents** and *one-third* **diet**.

Oral hypoglycaemics should only be used initially when there is no significant ketonuria. Oral drugs are useless if no insulin is present and are most useful in maturity-onset cases. Careful trial is the only sure way of deciding who can be maintained on oral therapy rather than on insulin.

Choice of oral hypoglycaemic agent. When it has been decided to use an oral agent, the choice should fall first on a **sulphonylurea** (except in overweight), for the biguanides, though capable of controlling some patients when used alone, carry too high an incidence of adverse effects, especially on the alimentary tract, and serious lactic acidosis.

The **biguanides** are used: (1) *as a supplement to a sulphonylurea* when this is insufficient to give good control. (2) *in overweight diabetics*, especially those who find diet difficult; patients tend to lose their appetite and therefore to lose weight with a biguanide. (3) *To smooth out the effect of insulin* in 'brittle' (unstable) insulin-dependent diabetics and to reduce insulin requirement in some cases where insulin resistance is not due to antibodies.

Of the principal sulphonylureas, tolbutamide is the safest (short $t_{\frac{1}{2}}$) especially in the elderly, but has to be given up to four times a day. Chlorpropamide is prone to accumulate, but can succeed where tolbutamide fails and need only be given once a day. They thus have their advantages and disadvantages and the choice in any patient is a matter of opinion and of trial. Glibenclamide is popular largely because its kinetics are intermediate (above).

To start a patient on a sulphonylurea, glibenclamide 5 mg is given orally (or 2.5 mg in the aged) with breakfast. The dose is adjusted, according to response, at weekly intervals by increments of 2.5 or 5 mg, to a maximum of 15 mg.

If control is incomplete, metformin may be added.

Failure of oral agents. If the postprandial blood sugar does not fall below 14–16 mmol/l (250–300 mg/100 ml) after four weeks, then other therapy is needed, for not only is this state unsatisfactory but, on the same treatment, control may worsen over succeeding weeks.

Also, unlike insulin, oral agents may fail after months of successful treatment. Disregard of diet is an obvious cause, but there are others, for the mode of action of sulphonylureas is not as simple as has perhaps been implied above. One cause of late failure is progression of the diabetic state, i.e. the insulin-producing capacity falls.

In one study, the relapse rate for patients on tolbutamide was 44%, on chlorpropamide 12% and on chlorpropamide and phenformin 13%. Close supervision is clearly essential.

Withdrawal of oral agents, gradually, may be attempted after the patient has been controlled and stable for 3–6 months. About 30% of patients will be found not to need the drug any longer.

Changeover from insulin to a sulphonylurea. With the shorter-acting tolbutamide and glibenclamide it may be abrupt, but with the longer-acting chlorpropamide it should be made over several days.

If the stopping of insulin leads to ketosis before the sulphonylurea takes effect then the patient is unsuited to oral therapy. In any case insulin should be resumed immediately. Hypoglycaemia may also occur during the changeover. Patients should be watched closely when changing over to oral therapy, with urine tests for sugar and ketones three times a day and blood sugar estimations before and after the drug.

Observation of patients taking these drugs should be at least as close as of those on insulin and probably closer. The patient must be disabused of any notion that substitution of tablets to swallow for the tiresome routine of self-injection carries any implication that his condition is less serious, or that diet can be relaxed.

Use of insulin. If it is decided that insulin is needed as well as diet there is a choice of regimens:

1. *Once-daily insulin* can be used for patients who are not insulin dependent, e.g. maturity-onset cases who have failed on oral agents. A morning dose of intermediate-acting insulin with or without short-acting neutral insulin is used. Plainly this regimen is remote from the physiological profile. A patient needing more than 50 units will be better managed by a twice-daily regimen.

2. *Twice-daily insulin suits most insulin-dependent patients*. A dose of short- plus intermediate-acting insulin (neutral plus isophane) is given before morning and evening meals. The short-acting insulin will not be needed if there is some endogenous insulin production, as in many newly diagnosed patients. Generally two-thirds of the total daily dose is given in the morning, one-third in the evening. The normal circadian peak of insulin need is in the early morning (hyperglycaemia between 5 a.m. and 9 a.m. is known as the 'dawn phenomenon').

3. *Thrice-daily insulin* for those who are not adequately controlled on twice daily (hyperglycaemic in early morning). The three doses may be morning (neutral plus isophane), evening meal (if early; neutral) and a small dose of intermediate acting (isophane) at bedtime.

4. *Intensive insulin regimens*, e.g. short-acting before each of three meals plus intermediate-acting insulin at bedtime; or continuous s.c. infusion with pump plus bolus before each meal.

Diabetic ketosis is an absolute indication for insulin as is any severe illness (e.g. myocardial infarction, surgery) in a diabetic patient; patients taking oral agents should be changed to insulin in acute severe illness.

Other indications for insulin are loss of weight in a thin diabetic or inadequate control with diet plus oral agent.

Generally insulin (intermediate acting) dose may start at 10–20 units each morning, increasing this by 4 units (on alternate days) until glucose concentrations are controlled or mild hypoglycaemia occurs; and then manipulating the class of insulin(s) and their timing according to the results of blood and urine tests.

Muscular activity increases carbohydrate utilisation, so that hypoglycaemia is likely if a well-stabilised patient changes suddenly from an inactive hospital existence to a vigorous life outside. If this is likely to happen the diet may be increased by 250–500 calories* or the dose of insulin reduced by up to one-third and then readjusted according to need. This is less marked in patients on oral agents.

Diabetic complications. A well-controlled diabetic is less liable to ketosis, infections, neuropathy and cataract, but the extent to which good control prevents the serious vascular, eye and renal complications is uncertain, but it seems probable that good control mitigates these.

Peripheral vascular disease and its consequences receive the same treatment as in non-diabetics. Improvement in peripheal neuritis has been dubiously attributed to administration of large amounts of thiamine or hydroxocobalamin.

* 1 calorie ≈ 4.2 joules

Some factors affecting control of diabetes

Intercurrent illnesses can cause fluctuations in the patient's metabolic needs. If these are severe it is prudent to use insulin rather than oral agents. Infections cause an increase in insulin need (about 20%), which may drop briskly on recovery.

Surgery, see later.

Menstruation and oral contraception. Insulin needs may rise slightly.

In pregnancy close control of diabetes is of the first importance to avoid fetal loss. *Insulin* requirements increase steadily after the third month. During *labour* soluble insulin should be given 4-hourly (or by continuous infusion at about 1 unit/h with plenty of glucose orally. Substantially *less* insulin is likely to be needed *immediately* after delivery, when timing and dose of insulin injections should be carefully reconsidered lest hypoglycaemia occur. Insulin need may increase again during lactation. Blood glucose estimations are necessary during the latter part of pregnancy, for glycosuria is not then a reliable guide because the renal threshold for glucose (also of lactose) falls, so that glycosuria and lactosuria may occur in the presence of a normal blood glucose. Some physicians advocate the admission to hospital of all diabetics after the 32nd week of pregnancy for careful control of the diabetes until after delivery.

Maternal hyperglycaemia leads to fetal hyperglycaemia with consequent fetal islet cell hyperplasia and postnatal hypoglycaemia.

Premature labour: use of β_2-adrenoceptor agonists and dexamethasone (to prevent respiratory distress syndrome in the prematurely newborn) causes hyperglycaemia and increased insulin (and K) need.

Oral hypoglycaemic agents and pregnancy. The continued use of these during pregnancy is associated with fetal loss and insulin should be given.

Interactions with other (non-diabetes) drugs

The subject is ill-documented, but whenever a diabetic under treatment takes other drugs it is prudent to be on the watch for disturbance of control, especially with drugs that are known to affect carbohydrate metabolism (adrenal steroids, salicylate).

β-adrenoceptor blocking drugs impair the sympathetic mediated (β_2-receptor) release of glucose from the liver in response to hypoglycaemia and also reduce the symptoms of hypoglycaemia (except sweating). Insulin hypoglycaemia is thus both more profound and less noticeable. A diabetic needing a β-adrenoceptor blocker should be given a β_1-*cardio* selective member, e.g. atenolol. Adrenergic neurone blocking drugs potentiate insulin similarly. Since *thiazides* cause diabetes it is plain the choice of drugs for treating hypertension in diabetics requires care.

The action of sulphonylureas is intensified by heavy *sulphonamide* dosage and some sulphonamides increase free tolbutamide concentrations, probably by competing for plasma protein binding sites.

Monoamine oxidase inhibitors probably potentiate oral agents and perhaps also insulin. They can also reduce appetite and so upset control. Interaction may also occur with alcohol (hypoglycaemia), anticoagulants (competition for liver enzymes), etc. See also *drug-induced diabetes*, below.

Hepatic enzyme inducers may enhance the metabolism of sulphonylureas that are metabolised in the liver (tolbutamide). Displacement from plasma protein may occur due to clofibrate, some NSAIDs and sulphonamides.

Large doses of *aspirin* have their own hypoglycaemic effect.

These examples suffice to show that the possibility of interactions of practical clinical importance is a real one.

Effect of diabetes on pharmacokinetics. Renal complications of diabetes will affect excretion of many drugs. Absorption of i.m. penicillin has shown to be substantially slower in older diabetics than in control subjects. This results in lower peak plasma concentrations; the effect may be due to diabetic micro-angiopathy. It is likely to apply to other drugs, where it may matter more.

Drug-induced diabetes

After the introduction of *thiazide diuretics*, it was soon found that their prolonged use increased hyperglycaemia in diabetics, and, later, that they impaired glucose tolerance in some non-diabetics. With long-term thiazide therapy an increasing proportion of patients develop impaired glucose tolerance. The mechanism of action is uncertain, but it may be associated with inadequate potassium supplement. On stopping therapy, glucose tolerance returns to normal except in some patients who are prediabetic. The risk of diabetes deserves special consideration when hypertensive patients with good life expectancy are treated with a thiazide lest they be made the victim of a second chronic disease. Patients on long-term thiazide therapy should have their urine tested for glucose every few months, and development of polyuria should rouse suspicion of diabetes.

Thiazide-induced diabetes can be controlled by a sulphonylurea.

Research for better antihypertensive thiazides resulted in the discovery of a non-diuretic substance with antihypertensive effect **diazoxide**, but it proved unsatisfactory for long-term use as it often caused diabetes, though it is effective short-term. Diazoxide suppresses insulin release by the pancreatic β-islet cells; it does not affect insulin synthesis. It is useful in treating hypoglycaemia due to islet-cell tumour (insulinoma). The diabetic effect of diazoxide is reversible on withdrawal. Excess effect is amenable to a sulphonylurea.

An antibiotic (*streptozotocin*) is selectively toxic to malignant β-islet cell tumours. It has been used to treat functioning metastases. After a short course remission may occur in 3 weeks and last a year or longer.

Adrenocortical steroids and *oral contraceptives* are also diabetogenic.

Diuretics for diabetics. In general a non-thiazide should be chosen. Frusemide and ethacrynic acid have only rarely precipitated diabetes. Potassium-conserving diuretics are liable to cause hyperkalaemia in patients with nephropathy and should be avoided.

Diabetic ketoacidosis

Severe ketoacidosis. The condition is discussed in detail in medical texts and only the more pharmacological aspects will be dealt with here. The patient urgently needs insulin and i.v. fluid and electrolytes.

Soluble insulin (never a slow-release form) should be given by continuous i.v. infusion, ideally by a pump (which allows independent control of insulin and electrolyte administration more readily than an i.v. drip) in a concentration of 1 unit/ml in isotonic sodium chloride, at a dose of 0.1 unit/kg/h (i.e. 7 units/h in a 70 kg adult). If an i.v. drip is used instead of a pump the concentration used will be lower (40 units/l); stringent precautions against septicaemia are necessary in these patients. It has been shown that continuous infusion i.m. (rather than s.c.) can be equally effective (provided the patient is not in shock, and, presumably, provided there is not an important degree of peripheral vascular disease: see above). If the i.m. route is used, a priming i.v. dose of 15–20 units should be given at the outset and then 5–10 units hourly, then 2-hourly.

Treatment of ketoacidosis by continuous low-dose infusion is highly satisfactory if the dose is tailored to the clinical situation.

But a warning has been sounded* that 'this trend to using lower and lower doses of insulin by continuous infusion must be stopped before it degenerates into a futile, irrational and dangerous race to see who can treat this disorder with the lowest possible dosage'. Some reports have described doses as low as 0.5–2.5 units/h. Common sense must obviously be used with regard to dosage. There is a risk of losing lives through insufficient dosage in the most severe cases and treatment of these should begin with a higher rate of i.v. infusion than that advised above; subsequent dosage being determined by the results of frequent estimations of plasma glucose; when it has fallen to 6 mmol/l (110 mg/100 ml) the rate can be reduced to 1 unit/h.

Milder cases of ketosis can be treated with lower doses (3 units/h) at the outset.

When infusion cannot be adequately supervised, similar total doses given intermittently at hourly intervals can be used.

It has been shown that the rate of fall of blood glucose/hour is proportional to the rate of infusion of insulin over the range of 1–10 units/h. A

* Madison L L. Low-dose insulin: a plea for caution. N Engl J Med 1976; 294:393.

reasonable rate of fall during treatment is 4–5.5 mmol/l (75–100 mg/100 ml) per hour.

Intravenous fluid and electrolytes*. Patients are often more deficient in water than in saline and although initial replacement is by *isotonic (0.9%) sodium chloride* solution, occurrence of hypernatraemia is an indication for half isotonic (0.45%) solution. A dehydrated patient may have a fluid deficit of above 5 l and may be given 500 ml in the first 20 min, followed by 2 litres in 90 min, then 1 litre in 90 min, and 1 litre in 120 min, watching the patient for signs of fluid overload. Fluid replacement causes a fall in blood glucose by dilution.

Dextrose (glucose) should only be given when the blood glucose falls below the renal threshold (8.5–10 mmol/l, i.e. 150–180 mg/100 ml). If it is used at concentrations above the renal threshold it merely increases the diabetic osmotic diuresis causing further dehydration, and potassium and magnesium loss (it is used to treat hyperkalaemia); but see *hypoglycaemia*, above.

Hypokalaemia is usual (though a minority of severe cases show hyperkalaemia) and if the initial serum K is low and renal function is normal, replacement can begin at 20–40 mmol/h. Hypomagnesaemia may also occur rarely.

Bicarbonate† is not useful and may even be harmful (it has been the practice to use it if plasma pH is < 7.0).

Success in treatment of diabetic coma and its complications (hypokalaemia, aspiration of stomach contents, infection, shock) attends on close, constant, informed supervision.

Mild diabetic ketosis. If the patient is fully conscious and there has been no nausea or vomiting for at least 12 h, parenteral therapy is unnecessary. It is reasonable to give small doses of insulin s.c. 3–6 hourly and fluids by mouth.

Hyperosmolar diabetic coma occurs chiefly in non-insulin-dependent diabetics who fail to compensate for their continuing osmotic glucose diuresis. It is characterised by severe dehydration, a very high blood sugar (> 33 mmo/l: 600 mg/100 ml) and lack of ketosis and acidosis. Treatment is with hypotonic fluids (not dextrose) and small doses of insulin. Many patients who recover do not require to continue insulin.

* In this situation dextrose solution does not provide water replacement since the normal capacity to metabolise dextrose (glucose) is fully taken up.

† Hale P J et al. Metabolic effects of bicarbonate in the treatment of diabetic ketoacidosis. Br Med J 1984; 289:1035.

SURGERY IN DIABETIC PATIENTS

Principles:

1. Insulin needs increase with surgery.
2. Avoid ketosis.
3. Avoid hypoglycaemia.
4. High blood glucose level matters little over short periods.

The programme for control should be agreed between anaesthetist and physician *whenever diabetics must undergo general anaesthesia or modify their diets*. There are many different techniques that can give satisfactory results.

For major surgery the patient should be admitted 3 days before operation so that the control of the diabetes can be adjusted according to the results of urine tests and blood sugar analyses. It is specially important to avoid post-anaesthetic vomiting.

There are three main groups of patients:

1. **Diabetics controlled by diet**. To compensate for bed rest, alter the diabetic diet to one containing 250–500 calories less than the patient's usual diet. If glycosuria of over 0.75% persists or the blood sugar is high then treat as in paragraph 2.

Before operation: No glucose by mouth and no insulin.

During operation: No i.v. glucose and no insulin. For operations lasting more than 1 h treat as in paragraph 3.

After operation: Manage as for a normal patient, but test urine for sugar and ketones every 3 h. If there is persistent glycosuria or ketosis give soluble insulin 4–6 hourly to control it.

2. **Diabetics on diet plus oral hypoglycaemic drug**.

Small operations: Omit drug on day of operation (but chlorpropamide will still be acting from the day before)

Big operations: Patient should be transferred to insulin, see 3.

The insulin requirement cannot be accurately predicted, but, as a rough guide, a patient on a short-acting oral agent may be given 12 units soluble insulin 8-hourly; however, much more may be needed and the dose is adjusted according to the urine or blood test results.

If the patient is taking a longer-acting oral preparation (chlorpropamide) less insulin will be needed in the 24 h after stopping it.

3. **Diabetics dependent on insulin and liable to ketosis**. Reduce the diet by 250–500 calories and give only soluble insulin from the night before, or reduce dose of longer-acting insulin by 30%. If the operation is on the following morning set up an i.v. infusion (glucose about 10 g/h) early; 1 h before operation, start insulin diluted in physiological saline (preferably by pump) 1–5 units/h as judged appropriate from known normal requirement and expected metabolic stress. If intermittent administration is unavoidable give glucose 25 g i.v. 1 h before operation plus the above doses of soluble insulin i.m., to the same total every 3 h, and add glucose similarly. If operation is on the following afternoon the patient will need a light breakfast, preceded by about half the usual dose of insulin and then glucose and insulin as above.

After surgery, insulin dose (intermittent or continuous infusion 1–2 units/h) should be decided with knowledge of the blood glucose, and after stabilisation on soluble insulin s.c., a return can be made to the accustomed regimen.

4. **Emergency operations**. When a surgical emergency is complicated by diabetic ketosis, an attempt should be made to control the ketosis before the operation. Management during the operation will be similar to that described in 3 above, except that more insulin may be needed.

In other cases small doses of soluble insulin are given 2–4 hourly, keeping the blood glucose between 8.5 and 10 mmol/l (150 and 300 mg/100 ml).

5. **Minor operations**. For example, simple dental extractions (for multiple extractions or when there is infection the patient should be admitted to hospital). A suitable post-operative diet of appropriate calorie and carbohydrate content must be arranged. Plan the operation for between 12 noon and 5 p.m. Omit the usual dose of long-acting insulin on the morning of the operation and substitute soluble insulin, one-quarter of the usual total daily dose, before a light breakfast 6 h preceding the operation. Take a light evening meal after the operation and soluble insulin, 10–30 units s.c., according to the urine or blood tests. Return to the normal routine the next day.

Patients taking oral agents can continue them normally unless there is likely to be vomiting, when they should be changed to insulin.

GUIDE TO FURTHER READING

1 Lerner P I et al. Abnormalities of absorption of benzylpenicillin G and sulfisoxazole in patients with diabetes mellitus. Am J Med Sci 1964; 248:37.

2 Jankelson O M et al. Effect of coffee on glucose tolerance and circulating insulin in men with maturity onset diabetes. Lancet 1967; 1:527.

3 Viberti G C. Glucose-induced hyperkalaemia: a hazard for diabetics? Lancet 1978; 1:690.

4 Wright A D et al. Beta-adrenoceptor-blocking drugs and blood sugar control in diabetes mellitus. Br Med J 1979; 1:159.

5 Mallory A H et al. Clinitest ingestion. Br Med J 1977; 2:105.

6 Scott J et al. Tolbutamide pharmacogenetics and the University Group Diabetes Program Controversy. JAMA 1979; 242:45.

7 Flier J S et al. Receptors, antireceptor antibodies and mechanisms of insulin resistance. N Engl J Med 1979; 300:413.

8 Editorial. Factitious hypoglycaemia. Lancet 1978; 1:1293.

9 Bergman U et al. Epidemiology of adverse drug reactions to phenformin and metformin. Br Med J 1978; 2:464.

10 Clarke B F et al. Comparison of metformin and chlorpropamide in non-obese, maturity-onset diabetics uncontrolled by diet. Br Med J 1977; 2:1576.

11 Cryer P E et al. Glucose counterregulation, hypoglycemia, and intensive therapy in diabetes mellitus. N Engl J Med 1985; 313:232.

12 Lord J M et al. Effect of metformin on insulin receptor binding and glycaemic control in type II diabetes. Br Med J 1983; 286:830.

13 Stacpoole P W et al. Treatment of lactic acidosis with dichloroacetate. N Engl J Med 1983; 309:390.
14 Dahl-Jørgensen K et al. Rapid tightening of blood glucose control leads to transient deterioration of retinopathy in insulin dependent diabetes mellitus: the Oslo Study. Br Med J 1985; 290:811.
15 Lean M E J et al. Interval between insulin injection and eating in relation to blood glucose control in adult diabetics. Br Med J 1985; 290:105.
16 Critchley J A J H et al. Deaths and paradoxes after intentional insulin overdosage. Br Med J 1984; 289:225.
17 Mecklenburg R S et al. Long-term metabolic control with insulin pump therapy: Report of experience with 127 patients. N Engl J Med 1985; 313:465.
18 Campbell P J et al. Pathogenesis of the dawn phenomenon in patients with insulin-dependent diabetes mellitus. N Engl J Med 1985; 312:1473.
19 Gray R S et al. Influence of insulin antibodies on pharmacokinetics and bioavailability of recombinant human and highly purified beef insulins in insulin dependent diabetics. Br Med J 1985; 290:1687.
20 Marliss E B. Insulin: sixty years of use. N Engl J Med 1982; 306:362.
21 Kinmonth A L et al. Social and emotional complications in a clinical trial among adolescents with diabetes mellitus. Br Med J 1983; 286:952.
22 Watkins P J. Pros and cons of continuous subcutaneous infusion. Br Med J 1985 290:655.
23 Foster D W et al. The metabolic derangements and treatment of diabetic ketoacidosis. N Engl J Med 1983; 309:159.
24 Owens D R et al. Comparative study of subcutaneous, intramuscular, and intravenous administration of human insulin. Lancet 1981; 2:118.
25 Koivisto V A. Sauna-induced acceleration in insulin absorption from subcutaneous injection site. Br Med J 1980; 1:1411.
26 Pickup J. Human insulin. Br Med J 1986; 292:155.

36

Endocrinology III: Thyroid hormones; antithyroid drugs

THYROID HORMONES

L-thyroxine (T_4 or 3,5,3′,5′-tetraiodo-L-thyronine) and **liothyronine** (T_3 or 3,5,3′-triiodo-L-thyronine) are the natural hormones of the thyroid gland. T_4 is a less active precursor of the major peripheral hormone, T_3, which is the major mediator of physiological effect.

For convenience, the term *thyroid hormone* is used to comprise T_4 plus T_3. Both forms are available for oral use as therapy.

Thyroid hormone is stored in the gland as thyroglobulin from which enzymic hydrolysis releases T_4 and a little T_3 into the circulation. About 85% of the released T_4 is deiodinated to biologically active T_3 (30–35%) and biologically inactive *reverse* T_3 (3, 3′, 5′-T_3; 45–50%) in the peripheral tissues; thus most circulating T_3 is derived from T_4. Further deiodination, largely in the liver, leads to loss of activity.

In the blood both T_4 and T_3 are extensively (99.9%) bound to plasma proteins (thyroxine-binding globulin, TBG, and thyroxine-binding prealbumin, TBPA). The concentration of TBG is raised by oestrogens (including doses used in oral contraceptives), clofibrate, and prolonged use of neuroleptics, and in pregnancy. The concentration of TBG is lowered by adrenocortical and androgen (including anabolic steroid) therapy and by urinary protein loss in nephrotic syndrome. Phenytoin and salicylates compete with thyroid hormone for TBG binding sites. Effects such as these obviously can interfere with the assessment of the clinical significance of measurements of plasma protein-bound iodine and *total* thyroid hormone concentration. But measurement of *free* thyroid hormone by ingenious techniques (free thyroxine index) largely avoids these complicating factors.

T_4 (thyroxine). A single dose reaches its maximum effect in about 10 days (its binding to plasma proteins is strong) and passes off in 2–3 weeks ($t_{½}$, 7 days).

T_3 *(liothyronine)* is about five times as biologically potent as T_4; a single dose reaches its maximum effect in about 24 h (its binding to plasma proteins is weak) and passes off in one week ($t_{½}$, 2 days).

Actions. Thyroid hormone passes into the cells of target organs, combines with specific receptors there and induces characteristic metabolic changes: *protein synthesis* during growth; increased *metabolic rate* with raised oxygen consumption; and increased *sensitivity to catecholamines* with proliferation of β-adrenoceptors (particularly important in the cardiovascular system).

Pituitary-thyroid function is assessed by measurement of free plasma concentrations of T_4, T_3 (see above) and of TSH (thyroid stimulating hormone, thyrotrophin) and by the capacity of the pituitary gland to respond to administered TRH (thyrotrophin-releasing hormone).

The above have largely superseded tests involving measurement of *radioiodine uptake*, including the *T_3 suppression (of the pituitary) test*.

Thyroid stimulating hormone (TSH) **thyrotrophin**, a glycoprotein of the anterior pituitary, controls the release of thyroid hormone from the gland, and also the uptake of iodide by the thyroid gland. TSH secretion is inhibited (via the hypothalamus and TRH) by a high level of thyroid hormone in the blood and stimulated by a low level, i.e. there is a feedback mechanism of control.

A stimulation test using TSH is no longer useful now that TSH blood level and free T_4 and T_3 can be measured.

Antithyroid drugs, by reducing thyroid hormone production, cause increased formation of TSH which is the cause of the thyroid enlargement that sometimes occurs during antithyroid drug therapy.

Thyrotrophin-releasing hormone (TRH, protirelin) is a tripeptide formed in the hypothalamus and controlled by free plasma T_4, T_3 concentration. It has been synthesised and can be used in diagnosis to test the capacity of the pituitary to release thyroid-stimulating hormone (TSH), e.g. to determine whether hypothyroidism is due to primary thyroid gland failure or is secondary to pituitary disease or to a hypothalamic lesion.

Eye signs of hyperthyroidism (lid retraction, lid lag, etc.) are doubtfully due to thyroid hormone increasing catecholamine sensitivity. They ordinarily do not require treatment, but if they do, withdrawal of sympathetic drive with an adrenergic-neurone blocking drug (guanethidine eye drops) can help.

Exophthalmos of hyperthyroidism. The cause is unknown. Antithyroid drugs do not help. TSH secretion is not responsible (it is high in primary thyroid gland failure in which exophthalmos does not occur). There may be a special pituitary secretion or immunoglobulin that causes exophthalmos; it has been cleverly named EPS or 'exophthalmos-producing substance'; it is assayed in goldfish.

High systemic doses of an adrenocortical steroid with or without azathioprine may help, but in urgent cases surgery is necessary, i.e. orbital decompression. Artificial tears (hypromellose) are useful when natural tears and blinking are inadequate to maintain corneal lubrication.

The main indication for thyroid hormone is treatment of deficiency (cretinism, hypothyroidism, myxoedema). The adult requirement of hormone is remarkably constant, and dosage does not have to be altered once the optimum is found. Children naturally need more as they grow.

Early treatment of cretinous babies is important if permanent mental defect is to be avoided. It must be life-long.

Hypothyroidism due to panhypopituitarism requires replacement with adrenocortical as well as with thyroid hormones.

Small doses of thyroid in normal subjects merely depress TSH production and consequently reduce the output of thyroid hormone by an equivalent amount.

When thyroid enlargement is associated with excess TSH (puberty goitre, Hashimoto's autoimmune thyroiditis), thyroxine administration can be effective in suppressing TSH secretion with resultant reduction in size of goitre. Thyroxine is also effective, by the same mechanism, in goitre due to inborn thyroid enzyme defect or to iodine deficiency or to other drugs with incidental antithyroid effect.

Thyroxine should not be used to treat simple obesity; if enough is given to 'burn up' the excess fat, then other symptoms of hyperthyroidism are inevitable and appetite is stimulated; also it may lead to dependence on thyroid. But in obese subjects who have been starved there is a reduction in thyroid function, see obesity.

A curious by-way of human nature that can cause diagnostic difficulty is secret thyroxine 'addiction'*. It is associated with overt psychiatric disease and/or emotional immaturity, and aggressive dependence on mothers or mother substitutes. The condition is uncommon, and afflicts women particularly.

Preparations and dosage of thyroid hormones

Thyroid tabs. is a preparation of the dried gland of ox, pig or sheep. Potency varies because irrelevant standardisation procedures have been used and moulds have been known to grow on them. They are deservedly obsolete.

Thyroxine Tabs. (25, 50, 100 μg) contain pure L-thyroxine sodium and should be used **to treat hypothyroidism.**

The intial oral dose may be 50–100 μg daily, but in the old and patients with heart disease or hypertension, this should be achieved gradually, starting with 25 μg daily for the first 2–4 weeks, and then increasing by 25–50 μg every fortnight until symptoms are relieved, usually at 100–200 μg

* Harvey R F. Br Med J 1973; 2:35.

daily. This is usually sufficient to reduce plasma TSH to normal levels. Patients who appear to need more are probably not taking their tablets consistently. The maximum effect of a dose is not reached for about 10 days and passes off over about 2–3 weeks. A cretinous baby should be given 25 μg daily at first and the dose increased by 25 μg fortnightly. The optimum dose is just below that which causes diarrhoea. Absorption is more complete and less variable if thyroxine is taken well apart from food.

Tablets containing supposedly physiological mixtures of *thyroxine* and *liothyronine* are available but offer no advantage.

Hypothyroid patients tend to be intolerant of drugs due to delayed metabolism.

Liothyronine Tabs (20 μg). Liothyronine is the most rapidly effective thyroid hormone, a single dose giving maximum effect within 24 h and passing off over about a week. Its main uses are in *myxoedema coma and psychosis*, both rare conditions. It is not used in routine treatment of hypothyroidism because the fast action can induce heart failure, but in the above conditions, particularly in coma where death is inevitable in the absence of treatment, the risk may be justified.

Myxoedema coma follows prolonged total hormone deficiency and constitutes an emergency. An untreated patient dies of hypothyroidism and a too-vigorously treated patient dies from cardiovascular collapse due to a precipitate rise in metabolism. Thus the physician must steer between the Scylla* of under-treatment and the Charybdis† of overtreatment, both fatal. This may be done by giving thyroxine (T_4) i.v. The biologically weak T_4 is gradually converted into the highly active T_3. A single dose of 500 μg of thyroxine raises the plasma T_4 to about half the normal concentration and suffices for a week, after which routine oral maintenance dose may be used. Oral T_4 is too slow in the emergency. Injectable T_4 is not routinely available.

Alternatively the quick-acting T_3 may be given by stomach tube, 5–10 μg 8–12 hourly (or i.v.). Maximum dose in the first 24 h should probably not exceed 50 μg since 100 μg is the full replacement dose. The dose may be raised after 3 days and the patient transferred to thyroxine after recovery.

Hydrocortisone i.v. is also needed, as prolonged hypothyroidism is associated with hypoadrenalism and hydrocortisone is needed to cope with the increasing metabolism.

Adverse effects of thyroid hormone parallel the increase in metabolic rate. The symptoms and signs are those of hyperthyroidism, minus exophthalmos. Angina pectoris or heart failure are liable to be provoked by too vigorous therapy; should they occur thyroxine must be discontinued for at least a week and begun again at lower dosage. Only slight overdose is needed to precipitate atrial fibrillation in patients over 60 years.

In *pregnancy* a hypothyroid patient should be carefully assessed, and breast feeding is not contraindicated though the baby's thyroid status should be watched.

* *Scylla* was a rival in love to Circe who, using her pharmacological expertise, changed Scylla into a monster having 12 feet, 6 heads and 3 rows of teeth. Terrified by this Scylla threw herself into the sea and was transformed into rocks.

† *Charybdis* stole the oxen of Hercules, was struck by thunder, and became a whirlpool.

Sailors passing between Sicily and Italy were liable to fall victim to one or other of these hazards. The words *Incidit in Scyllam qui vult vitare Charybdim* have become a proverb to show that, in our eagerness to avoid one evil, we often fall into a greater (Lempriere).

ANTITHYROID DRUGS AND RADIOIODINE

Drugs used for the treatment of hyperthyroidism include:

1. **Iodide**, an excess of which reduces the production of thyroid hormone *temporarily* by an unknown mechanism. It is also necessary for the formation of hormone.
2. **Thiourea derivatives**, which block the synthesis of thyroid hormone.
3. **Radioiodine**, which destroys the cells making thyroid hormone.

Iodide

Iodide is well absorbed from the intestine, is distributed like chloride in the body and is rapidly excreted by the kidney. It is selectively taken up and concentrated by the thyroid (× 25 normally), but more in hyperthyroidism and less in myxoedema. A deficiency of iodide reduces the amount of thyroid hormone produced, which stimulates the pituitary to secrete TSH. The result is hyperplasia and increased vascularity of the thyroid, with eventual goitre formation.

Some foods, such as plants of the cabbage family, contain substances that block uptake of iodide by the thyroid or prevent its incorporation into thyroid hormone; these may be a factor in endemic goitre.

Iodide effects are complex and related to dose and to thyroid status of the subject.

In *normal* subjects an excess of iodide has opposite effects to those of TSH on the thyroid.

In *hyperthyroid* subjects a *moderate excess* of iodide may enhance hormone production by providing 'fuel' for hormone synthesis. But a *substantial excess* transiently inhibits hormone release and promotes involution of the gland making it firmer and less vascular so that surgery is easier. The mechanism of this effect is uncertain.

A euthyroid subject with 'hot nodule' (an autonomous adenoma) becomes hyperthyroid if given iodide. Iodide excess also can cause goitre (with or without hyperthyroidism) in subjects with normal thyroids, e.g. use of iodide-containing cough medicines, iodine-containing radiocontrast media, Japanese seaweed eaters. Also iodide added to food with the best of intentions can cause hyperthyroidism in people who are not iodide deficient and may delay the response to antithyroid thiourea derivatives.

Iodide (large dose) is therefore *used* for *thyroid crisis* (*storm*) and *to prepare for thyroidectomy* because it rapidly benefits the patient by reducing hormone release and renders surgery easier and safer (above).

Potassium iodide in doses of 60 mg orally 8-hourly (longer intervals allow some escape from the iodide effect) produces some effect in 1–2 days, maximal after 10–14 days, after which the benefit declines as the thyroid adapts. A traditional alternative is *Iodine Aqueous Solution* (*Lugol's Iodine*) (5% iodine + 10% potassium iodide in water), oral dose 0.5 ml (65 mg total iodine) 12-hourly; the iodine is rapidly converted into iodide in the liver.

Such therapy maximises iodide stores in the thyroid, which delays response to thiourea derivatives.

Prophylactic iodide (1 part in 100 000 parts) should be added to all the salt or bread used where goitre is endemic. In Michigan, USA, the incidence of goitre was inversely proportional to the iodide content of the water supply. In one county 42% of 3645 schoolchildren had goitre in 1924. Four years later, after propaganda for prophylactic iodide, incidence of goitre among children in one town of that county dropped to 9%. Of the 900 children in the town who had used only *iodised* salt, one had a goitre; of 84 using mainly *ordinary* salt, 11 had goitres.*

In underdeveloped communities a method of prophylaxis is to inject 4 ml of iodised oil i.m. every 3 years; given early enough to women, endemic cretinism can be prevented; but long-term safety is unestablished.

A small goitre presumed due to iodine deficiency (a presumption justifiable only in an area of endemic iodine deficiency), which is not producing symptoms, may involute if L-thyroxine in doses similar to those used in hypothyroidism are given (to suppress TSH production) as well as iodide replacement; but nodularity or increase in size of the goitre is an indication for surgery.

As an antiseptic for use on the skin, Weak Iodine Solution (90% alcoholic tincture) is very effective but is painful on broken skin; it is superseded by *povidone-iodine* (a complex of iodine with a sustained-release carrier, providone or polyvinylpyrrolidone) which can be applied repeatedly and used as a surgical scrub, though less concentrated and therefore less effective than the solution.

Bronchial secretion. Iodide is concentrated in bronchial and salivary secretions. It acts as an expectorant (see *cough*), but is unpleasant because it must be given to the limits of tolerance. There is no point in including small amounts in cough mixtures.

Organic compounds containing iodine are widely used as contrast media in radiology. Oily preparations are used, for example, in myelography, retrograde pyelography and bronchography; some solutions liberate iodine so that it is essential to

* Begg T B et al. Q J Med 1963; 32:351.

ask patients specifically whether they are allergic to it before they are used. A few radiogaphic preparations do not contain iodine. For intravenous pyelography water-soluble iodine compounds rapidly excreted by the kidney are used. The biliary system can be outlined by oral or i.v. administration of compounds excreted in the bile. The iodine in these water-soluble compounds is firmly bound, but patients are sometimes allergic to them. An i.v. test dose of 50 μg ought to be given half an hour before the full i.v. dose if there is history of any allergy. If there is any reaction and it is essential to proceed with the investigation, repeated doses every half hour may be given, doubling the dose each time. See also below. Alternatively a substantial dose of a corticosteroid may be given 60 min before the agent (see *drug allergy*).

Adverse reactions. Patients vary enormously in their tolerance of iodine, some are intolerant or allergic to it both orally and when put on the skin. Symptoms of **iodism** include a metallic taste, excessive salivation with painful salivary glands, running eyes and nose, sore mouth and throat, a productive cough, diarrhoea, and various rashes that may mimic chicken-pox. The Weak Iodine Solution (Tincture) used in antisepsis is caustic; it is sometimes drunk by suicidal patients: stomach washouts with solutions of starch are an antidote. Elimination can be enhanced by inducing a saline diuresis.

Goitre can occur (see above) with prolonged use of iodide-containing expectorants by bronchitics and asthmatics. Such therapy should therefore be intermittent, if it is used at all.

Iodide intake above that in a normal diet will depress thyroid *uptake of administered radioiodine*, because the two forms will compete. This may result in normal radioiodine uptake in a hyperthyroid patient who would ordinarily show increased uptake.

Sources of iodide include increased dietary intake (e.g. seaweed bread in South Wales), medication (iodide-containing cough medicines, e.g. Felsol), radiodiagnostic agents, iodoquinoline amoebicides and amiodarone.

In the case of diet, medication and water-soluble radiodiagnostic agents (pyelography, bronchography), interference will cease 2–4 weeks after stopping the source, but with those agents used for cholecystography it may last for 6 months or more (tissue binding).

Naturally, a high uptake remains significant, but a normal or low result may be false. The combination of a low radioiodine uptake with a high level of protein-bound iodine (PBI) in the blood is indicative of unusually high intake of iodine in organic, probably stable, form.

Thiourea derivatives (thioamides)

The *major action* of thiourea derivatives is to *reduce the formation of thyroid hormone* by inhibiting the incorporation of iodine into organic form, iodotyrosines, and by inhibiting the coupling of iodotyrosines to form T_4 and T_3. With heavy dosage the reduction in hormone synthesis may be sufficient to induce the pituitary to produce more TSH, which in turn causes thyroid enlargement (hyperplasia and increase in vascularity). It is possible they may also reduce the formation of thyroid-stimulating immunoglobulins.

History. The association of endemic goitre with hypothyroidism had long been known and there was a supposition that the goitre might represent an attempt by the body to overcome a hormone deficit. It had also been suggested that any agent capable of causing this sort of goitre might be useful in the treatment of hyperthyroidism.

The discovery of the antithyroid activity of thiourea in the 1940s resulted from a variety of further observations. One group of research workers found that the goitrogenic factor in rapeseed was probably allylthiourea. Others, investigating the relation between taste and toxicity in rats, happened to choose the bitter substance phenylthiourea, and found it to be goitrogenic. Yet others noted that workmen manufacturing sulphathiazole, and rats dosed with sulphaguanidine, developed goitres.

Inspired by these observations, two independent groups simultaneously discovered that thiourea was a potent and relatively non-toxic goitrogen. It was, with thiouracil, soon given a clinical trial in hyperthyroidism and found effective. Numerous other drugs have followed it, some being substantially safer.

Thiourea, thus introduced in 1943, was in fact being re-introduced into medicine. Half a century previously it had been used to reduce lupus scars and in arthritis, leprosy and deafness. Its toxicity and therapeutic inefficacy for these purposes led to its abandonment 20 years later, with its ability to prevent thyroxine formation and so to cause goitre still undetected.

Carbimazole ($t_{\frac{1}{2}}$, 6 h), **methimazole** (the chief metabolite of carbimazole) and **propylthiouracil** ($t_{\frac{1}{2}}$, 2 h) are commonly used. Half-lives are shorter in hyperthyroid subjects and lengthen if the patient becomes hypothyroid, but $t_{\frac{1}{2}}$ matters little since the drugs accumulate in the thyroid and act there for 30–40 h; thus a single daily dose suffices.

Propylthiouracil differs from other members of the group in that it also inhibits peripheral conversion of T_4 to T_3 (but this is not quick enough to be clinically useful in a thyroid crisis, see below).

Dose. *Carbimazole* (5 mg), initial, orally, 30–60 mg total/day: maintenance 5–15 mg total/day. *Propylthiouracil* (50 mg) orally, 300–450 mg total/day: maintenance 50–150 mg total/day. Higher doses are sometimes needed (even three times the above).

Use. It is probable that no patient is wholly refractory to these drugs. Failure to respond is likely to be due to the patient not taking the tablets or to wrong diagnosis.

The drugs are used in hyperthyroidism as *principal therapy*, and as *adjuvant to radioiodine* to control the disease until the radiation achieves its effect, and to *prepare patients for surgery*.

Clinical improvement is noticeable in about a week, and the patient should be euthyroid after about 6 weeks. The dose is then reduced and adjusted according to the clinical picture. The best guides to therapy are the patients' feelings, their weight and pulse rate, though measurements of the latter can be misleadingly high in a well-controlled patient if they are only seen in a clinic. Measurement of the ankle reflex time is a useful guide to therapy in both hyper- and hypothyroidism. Simple machines to record this are available.

Symptoms and signs are, of course, less valuable as guides if the patient is also taking a β-adrenoceptor blocker, and reliance is then put on tests, but these drugs also prolong the ankle reflex time.

With optimal treatment the gland decreases in size, but overtreatment leading to low hormone levels in the blood activates the feed-back system, inducing TSH secretion and goitre.

All three drugs give similar results.

Adverse reactions. These drugs are all liable to cause allergic effects including rashes, lymphadenopathy and most serious of all, leucopenia sometimes proceeding to agranulocytosis (~0.3%) or aplastic anaemia. Blood disorders are most common in the first two months of treatment. Repeated leucocyte counts are often advocated but agranulocytosis may be so acute that the counts give no warning; a leucocyte count should be done if the patient develops an infection (patients should be warned to report this), and any suggestion of anaemia should be investigated.

If a *pregnant woman* has hyperthyroidism (2/1000 pregnancies) she should be treated with the *smallest possible* amount of these drugs because they cross the placenta; with overtreatment fetal goitre occurs. Surgery in the second trimester may be preferred to continued drug therapy.

So little of propylthiouracil passes into breast milk that it may safely be used during breast-feeding.

Potassium perchlorate. The thyroid actively, i.e. by an energy-requiring mechanism, takes up iodide from plasma, concentrating it 20–30 times, for the normal plasma iodide concentration is too low for hormone synthesis to be accomplished. Perchlorate ion competes in this active uptake system, reducing iodide uptake, thereby diminishing synthesis of thyroid hormone.

Because aplastic anaemia with perchlorate, though rare, is liable to be fatal, and is commoner than with thioureas, perchlorate is obsolete for the treatment of hyperthyroidism.

Control of antithyroid drug therapy

The aim of drug therapy is to control the hyperthyroidism until a natural remission takes place. Unfortunately, though usual, remission is not invariable and there is no way of predicting which patients will not remit and who should therefore be offered radiation or surgery at the outset

Clinically, it is not possible to decide reliably when remission has occurred, although disappearance of bruit and reduction in gland size suggest it. Treatment should not be stopped whilst a bruit persists.

If there has never been a bruit, treatment may be stopped after the patient has been judged euthyroid for 4–6 months on the minimum dose of the drug. Lid retraction is the only eye sign that improves. But the duration of therapy that minimises the relapse rate is controversial, and 12–18 months total therapy before withdrawal as a routine is commonly advised. Plasma concentrations of T_3 and T_4 (at withdrawal and four weeks later) can be used to determine if remission has occurred, along with clinical monitoring.

Relapse may occur, in a few months or years, in 50–70% of cases and a second course of treatment may be successful. Both successful drug treatment and follow-up requires a compliant patient. For those judged non-compliant surgery may be preferred, though they still need monitoring for late hypothyroidism.

Preparation of hyperthyroid patients for surgery can be satisfactorily achieved by making them euthyroid with one of the above drugs plus a β-adrenoceptor blocker for comfort (see below) and safety*, and *adding* iodide for 7–10 days before operation to reduce the surgically inconvenient vascularity of the gland. This procedure takes about 5 weeks and the gland may be enlarged at the time of operation (probably due to overtreatment, which can be difficult to avoid, leading to increased TSH release).

An alternative is to prepare the patient with a β-adrenoceptor blocker (propranolol, 6-hourly) for 4 days (adjust dose to *eliminate** tachycardia) and to continue thus through the operation and for 7–10 days after.

The important differences with this second technique are that the gland is smaller and less friable, although the patient's *tissues* are still hyperthyroid, and it is essential, in order to avoid a hyperthyroid crisis or storm, that the β-adrenoceptor blocker be continued as above without the omission of even a single 6-hourly dose of propranolol, but erratic plasma concentrations can be a cause of failure.

* No patient should be operated on with a resting pulse of 90/min or above and no dose of β-adrenoceptor blocker, including the important postoperative dose, should be omitted. Toft A D et al. N Engl J Med 1978; 298:643.

Thyroid crisis or storm is rare with modern methods of preparing hyperthyroid patients for surgery. It is probably due to liberation of large amounts of hormone into the circulation. Treatment is urgently required to save life. Propranolol should be given immediately (i.v. *slowly*, 1 mg/min to max of 10 mg, in severe cases preceded by atropine 1–2 mg i.v. to prevent excessive bradycardia); iodide to reduce production of hormone (say 1–2 g/day of potassium iodide orally), and an antithyroid drug and hydrocortisone. Mental disturbance may be treated by chlorpromazine; hyperpyrexia by cooling and aspirin; heart failure in the ordinary way, etc.

Control of hyperthyroid symptoms and signs with drugs that block sympathetic activity. There is evidence that there is increased tissue sensitivity to catecholamines with increased number of β-adrenoceptors in hyperthyroidism and that this is a cause of some of the unpleasant symptoms.

Quick relief can be obtained with a β-adrenoceptor blocking drug (judge dose by heart rate) though these do not block all the metabolic effects of the hormone, e.g. on the myocardium, and the basal metabolic rate is unchanged. For this reason they should not be used as sole therapy; they do not alter the course of the disease, nor tests of thyroid function. Any effect on hormonal action on peripheral tissues is clinically unimportant. Plainly it is desirable to choose a drug that lacks partial agonist effect (intrinsic sympathomimetic activity).

β-adrenoceptor block is specially useful during the long wait for the effect of radioiodine, though it may be used for any patient who feels uncomfortable. Eye signs may respond to eye drops of a β-adrenoceptor blocker (timolol) or of an adrenergic neurone blocker (guanethidine).

A hyperthyroid patient with urgent intercurrent disease, e.g. need for surgery, should at once be treated with a β-adrenoceptor blocker.

In thyrotoxic heart failure patients may need

their sympathetic cardiac drive and may be made worse by β-adrenoceptor block.

Metabolism of drugs is more rapid in hyperthyroidism.

Radioiodine (^{131}I and ^{132}I)

Both isotopes are treated by the body just like the ordinary non-radioactive isotope, so that when swallowed they are concentrated in the thyroid gland. They emit mainly β radiation (90%), which penetrates only 0.5 mm of tissue and thus allows therapeutic effect on the thyroid without damage to the surrounding structures, particularly the parathyroids. However, they also emit some γ rays, which are relatively penetrating and can be detected with a Geiger counter. ^{131}I has a physical (radioactive) $t_{\frac{1}{2}}$ of 8 days.

^{131}I is increasingly used as treatment of choice in hyperthyroidism at all ages, and in combination with surgery in some cases of thyroid carcinoma, especially those in which metastases are sufficiently differentiated to take up iodide selectively.

In hyperthyroidism the beneficial effects of a single dose may be felt in one month but its action is not maximal for 3 months. β-adrenoceptor block and, in severe cases, antithyroid drugs, will be needed to render the patient comfortable whilst waiting. Very rarely the radiation damage to the thyroid causes a release of hormone and a thyroid crisis. Repeated doses are sometimes needed.

In the event of inadvertent overdose, large doses of potassium iodide should be given to compete with the radioiodine for thyroid uptake and to hasten excretion by increasing iodide turnover (increased fluid intake and a diuretic are adjuvants). Radioiodine offers the advantages that treatment is simple and in no way unpleasant (the patient just drinks it) and it carries no immediate mortality. However, it is slow in acting and it is difficult to judge the dose, so that either the patient may remain uncontrolled or permanent hypothyroidism may soon appear (some see no objection to this and would rather stabilise the patient on exogenous hormone than await a slowly developing hypothyroidism (despite the risk of patient non-compliance with therapy that now must be life-long).

In the first year after treatment 6–15% or even more (depending on the dose) of patients will become hypothyroid. After this between 2–3% of patients become hypothyroid *annually* after treatment with radioiodine, perhaps because the capacity of thyroid cells to divide is permanently abolished so that cell renewal ceases. Patients must therefore be followed up indefinitely after radioiodine treatment, for all are likely to need treatment for hypothyroidism sooner or later.

Experience has eliminated the fear that radioiodine causes carcinoma of the thyroid, and it is now used in patients of all ages. But pregnant women should not be treated with radioiodine (^{131}I) because it crosses the placenta.

There is a theoretical risk of germ cell mutagenic effect and patients should not reproduce for a few (say, six) months* after treatment. Larger doses of radioiodine are used for *thyroid carcinoma* than for hyperthyroidism, and there is an increased incidence of late leukaemia in these patients.

Radioiodine uptake can be used to *test thyroid function*, but it has been largely superseded (above).

^{131}I has a physical (radioactive) half-life of 8 days, and even the small amount used for diagnostic purposes is enough to be an appreciable radiation hazard to children so that ^{132}I, which has a half-life of only two hours, or ^{123}I, which gives a lower dose of radiation are preferable for all diagnostic purposes for children, and especially during pregnancy and lactation.

Choice of treatment of hyperthyroidism

There are three possible lines of treatment, each with its special advantages and disadvantages:

1. Antithyroid drug.
2. Radioiodine.
3. Surgery, after preparation as above.

Some pros and cons have already been mentioned, and:

* Even today it can be embarrassing to offer such advice to an excited hyperthyroid unmarried woman or man. Yet to fail to do so could have grave consequences for a child. It is rumoured that some physicians have prescribed an oral contraceptive without telling the patient what it is; a procedure that is understandable if not ethically justifiable.

Antithyroid drugs are generally preferred provided the goitre is small and *diffuse*. A *nodular* goitre is generally large enough to be a source of complaint, relapses when drug therapy is withdrawn (nodules are autonomous), and it is best treated surgically. These drugs do not decrease thyroid size; it may even increase (see above).

Radioiodine is now commonly used for patients for all ages. It affects both diffuse and nodular goitre. The goitre becomes smaller. Hyperthyroidism due to a single hyperfunctioning adenoma ('hot nodule') is particularly suitable for this treatment, and higher doses may be used since the function of the rest of the gland is suppressed by the familiar negative feedback regulatory process.

Surgery is indicated if obstruction of neck veins or trachea exists or is thought to be likely in the future, or if the thyroid is nodular or there are grounds for fearing malignancy.

Drugs that cause unwanted hypothyroidism

In addtion to drugs used for their antithyroid effects, the following substances can cause hypothyroidism: PAS (for tuberculosis), phenylbutazone (antirheumatic), iodide (see above), cobalt salts (for anaemia), sulphonylureas (for diabetes), resorcinol (for leg ulcers), lithium (for mania/depression), amiodarone (cardiac antidysrhythmic): effects are generally reversible on withdrawal.

Goitre may occur as the result of increased TSH secretion elicited by the decreased thyroid hormone synthesis that occurs with antithyroid drugs.

GUIDE TO FURTHER READING

1 Eichelbaum M et al. Influence of thyroid status on plasma half-life of antipyrine in man. N Engl J Med 1974; 290:1040.
2 Yeo P P B et al. Anticonvulsants and thyroid function. Br Med J 1978; 1:1581.
3 Croxson M S et al. Serum digoxin in patients with thyroid disease. Br Med J 1975; 3:556.
4 Toft A D et al. Thyroid function after surgical treatment of thyrotoxicosis: a report of 100 cases treated with propranolol before operation. N Engl J Med 1978; 298:643.
5 Editorial. Beta-adrenergic blocking drugs and thyroid function. Br Med J 1977; 2:1039.
6 Stewart J C et al. Thyrotoxicosis induced by iodine contamination of food — a common unrecognised condition. Br Med J 1976; 1:372.
7 Kimball O P. The efficacy and safety of the prevention of goitre. JAMA 1928; 91:454.
8 Macgregor A G. Why does anybody use Thyroid B.P.? Lancet 1961; 1:329.
9 Sachs B A et al. Bread iodine content and thyroid radioiodine uptake: a tale of two cities. Br Med J 1972; 1:79.
10 Utiger R D. Beta-adrenergic antagonist therapy for hyperthyroid Graves' disease. N Engl J Med 1984; 310:1597.
11 Larsen P R. Thyroid-pituitary interaction: feedback regulation of thyrotropin secretion by thyroid hormones. N Engl J Med 1982; 306:23.
12 Kendall-Taylor P et al. Ablative radioiodine therapy for hyperthyroidism: long-term follow up study. Br Med J 1984; 289:361.
13 Sridma V et al. Long-term follow-up study of compensated low-dose ^{131}I therapy for Grave's disease. N Engl J Med 1984; 311:426.
14 Cavalieri R R, Pitt-Rivers R. The effect of drugs on the distribution and metabolism of thyroid hormones. Pharmacol Rev 1981; 33:55.
15 Frost G J et al. Management of patients with congenital hypothyroidism. Br Med J 1985; 290:1485.
16 Toft A D. Thyroxine replacement treatment: clinical judgement or biochemical control. Br Med J 1985; 291:233.
17 Editorial. Radiation-induced thyroid cancer. Lancet 1985; 2:21.
18 Cooper D S. Antithyroid drugs. N Engl J Med 1984; 311:1353.
19 Abdalla H I et al. Reduced serum free thyroxine concentration in postmenopausal women receiving oestrogen treatment. Br Med J 1984; 288:754.
20 Hamolsky M W. Truth is stranger than factitious. N Engl J Med 1982; 307:436. (The physiology and diagnosis of deliberate self-administration of thyroid hormone).
21 Editorial. Reactor accidents: iodine supplements? Lancet 1983; 1:451.

37

Endocrinology IV: Hypothalamic and pituitary hormones: Sex hormones, contraception, uterus

Once the structure of natural hormones (including hormone-releasing hormones) is defined it becomes possible to synthesise not only the hormones themselves,* but also *analogues* (having a mix of actions of all the main steroid reproductive hormones, oestrogens, progestogens, androgens) and *antagonists*. Thus, increasingly, there become available substances differing in selectivity and duration of action, and active by varying routes of administration.

These substances can be used:

a. to analyse the functional integrity of endocrine control systems,
b. as replacement in hormone deficiency states,
c. to modify malfunction of endocrine systems,
d. to alter normal function where this is inconvenient (e.g. contraception).

The scope of the specialist endocrinologist continues to increase in amount and in complexity and only an outline is appropriate here.

HYPOTHALAMIC/PITUITARY HORMONES

Hypothalamus	Anterior pituitary	Posterior pituitary
Hormone releasing and hormone-release inhibiting hormones	Growth hormone	Vasopressin
	Gonadotrophic hormones	Oxytocin
	Corticotrophin	
	Thyrotrophin	
	Prolactin	

Hypothalamus and anterior pituitary

Some agents have restricted availability. The plasma $t_{\frac{1}{2}}$ of the polypeptide and glycoprotein hormones listed below is 5–30 min; they are digested if swallowed.

Corticotrophin releasing hormone (CRH), or corticoliberin, has diagnostic value, see p. 648.

* Hormones can be synthesised directly in the chemical laboratory or by inserting mammalian genes into microbes (e.g. *Escherichia coli*).

Corticotrophin, adrenocorticotrophic hormone (ACTH; 39 amino acids) is obtained from animal pituitaries or by synthesis (tetracosactrin), see p. 648.

Protirelin, thyrotrophin releasing hormone (TRH) has diagnostic value, see p. 684.

Thyrotrophin, thyroid stimulating hormone (TSH) has diagnostic value, see p. 683.

Somatostatin, or somatotrophin (growth hormone) release inhibitory factor (SRIF), occurs in other parts of the brain as well as in the hypothalamus, and also in some peripheral tissues (e.g. pancreas, stomach). In addition to the action implied by its name, it inhibits secretion of thyrotrophin, insulin, gastrin etc. It is a research tool.

Growth hormone (GH), human growth hormone (HGH), or somatotrophin is available as the biosynthetic **somatrem** (methionyl human growth hormone) (Somatonorm).Growth hormone is secreted by the anterior pituitary. It stimulates cell growth both for number and size. It has complex metabolic effects as it is to be expected. It is used in childhood pituitary insufficiency (the bone epiphyses must be open) to prevent dwarfism and provide normal growth. As supplies and availability increase (by inserting genes into bacteria) the possibilities of abuse have already begun to be discussed (e.g. creation of 'super' sportspeople). Growth hormone is only effective in intact organisms as it acts via an intermediary substance, *somatomedin*.

Gonadorelin is the releasing hormone (RH) for luteinising hormone (LH) and follicle-stimulating hormone (FSH). Its full abbreviation is thus LH/FSHRH, but it is commonly represented as LHRH for brevity, or GnRH. It has use in assessment of pituitary function. Intermittent *pulsatile* administration evokes production of gonadotrophins (LH and FSH) and is used to treat infertility. But *continuous* use evokes tachyphylaxis due to down-regulation of its receptors, i.e. gonadotrophin release is reduced, and this approach is being explored for contraception as well as for prostatic carcinoma, endometriosis and precocious puberty. Frequent nasal administration is required, or use of sustained-release i.m. formulations (using microcapsules), but longer-acting analogues, e.g. *buserelin* and *leuprolide*, have been developed.

Human follicle-stimulating hormone (FSH), menotrophin (Pergonal), urofollitrophin (Metrodin), is prepared from the urine of postmenopausal women (and contains a small amount of LH). It is used in hypopituitary infertility.

Luteinising hormone (LH) is obtained from the urine of postmenopausal women. Generally *human chorionic gonadotrophin* is used when LH action is required.

Human chorionic gonadotrophin (HCG) is secreted by the placenta and is obtained from the urine of pregnant women. Its predominant action is that of luteinising hormone (LH). It is used in hypopituitary and other infertility in both sexes (for LH effect is not confined to females despite its name). It is also used for cryptorchidism in prepubertal boys (about 6 years; if it fails to induce testicular descent, there is time for surgery before puberty to provide maximal possibility of a full functional testis).

Danazol is a synthetic progesterone derivative that inhibits gonadotrophin secretion by the pituitary, see p. 702.

Prolactin is secreted in both women and men, and, despite its name, it influences numerous biological functions (as many as 80), though not all of physiological importance. Prolactin secretion is controlled by an inhibitory dopaminergic path. Thus, dopamine agonists, e.g. bromocriptine and levodopa (converted to dopamine), reduce prolactin secretion and dopamine antagonists increase secretion. This explains the use of bromocriptine for *suppression of lactation* (p. 701) and in *hyperprolactinaemia* from other causes, e.g. pituitary tumours; also the occurrence of hyperprolactinaemia (causing galactorrhoea) during therapy with neuroleptic dopamine antagonist drugs, and with metoclopramide and methyldopa.

Hypopituitarism

In hypopituitarism there is a deficiency of all the hormones secreted by the anterior lobe of the pituitary. The posterior lobe hormones (below) may also be deficient in a few cases (e.g. when a tumour has destroyed the pituitary). Patients suffering from hypopituitarism may present in coma, in which case treatment is as for a severe acute adrenal insufficiency. Maintenance therapy is required, using adrenocortical and thyroid hormones. Sex hormones are not usually required, although androgens will help to establish a positive nitrogen balance in wasted patients.

Infertility: hormone and antihormone use

Hypopituitary female infertility (secondary hypogonadism) can be treated by FSH followed by LH. This sequence mimics natural function and induces maturation of the ovarian follicle followed by ovulation and subsequent development of the corpus luteum so that a pregnancy can be sustained.

Non-hypopituitary anovular infertility may be treated by interfering with the normal negative feedback hormone control system. If hypothalamic oestrogen receptors are blocked, the pituitary responds with a surge of gonadotrophin secretion, which may induce ovulation and result in pregnancy. Antioestrogens are used, e.g. clomiphene, sometimes boosted by a subsequent dose of chorionic gonadotrophin.

Clomiphene is a weak oestrogen with less efficacy than natural oestrogens so that its occupation of hypothalamic receptors results in antagonism, i.e. it is an agonist/antagonist, or partial agonist. Such substances are also referred to as 'impeded oestrogens'. **Cyclofenil** acts similarly though it is less effective. **Tamoxifen** is an alternative (it is also used in oestrogen-dependent breast cancer); it has less agonist action than clomiphene.

Use of these drugs requires great skill. A major adverse effect is multiple pregnancy.

Male infertility due to secondary (hypogonadotrophic) hypogonadism can sometimes be effectively treated by gonadotrophic hormones (HCG), with or without gonadorelin, or by oestrogen antagonist (clomiphene, tamoxifen). Androgen is not generally useful though mesterolone (see *androgens*, below) may improve sperm count and motility.

Posterior pituitary hormones and analogues

Aqueous extracts of posterior pituitary glands (animals) contain both antidiuretic and oxytocic hormones (peptides). Since the different effects are not required simultaneously these extracts have been replaced by separate preparations of the hormones *vasopressin* and *oxytocin*. Synthetic forms are available and are preferred, for biological extracts are always contaminated by some of the other hormone and unwanted protein that causes allergy.

Vasopressin is the antidiuretic hormone (polypeptide). Its official name is unfortunate, for only in high doses does it affect the vascular system and its chief function is to provide renal antidiuresis.

Vasopressin increases permeability and so water reabsorption in the distal tubule. In its absence free water (i.e. water without electrolyte) excretion is increased.

Secretion of the antidiuretic hormone is stimulated by any increase in the osmotic pressure of the blood supplying the hypothalamus and by a variety of drugs, notably nicotine. Secretion is inhibited by a fall in blood osmotic pressure and by alcohol.

In large 'unphysiological' or 'pharmacological' doses vasopressin causes contraction of all smooth muscle, raising the blood pressure and causing intestinal colic. The smooth-muscle-stimulant effect provides an example of tachyphylaxis (frequently repeated doses give progressively less effect). It is not only inefficient when used to raise the blood pressure, but is also dangerous, since it causes constriction of the coronary arteries and sudden death has occurred following its use.

For *replacement therapy of pituitary diabetes insipidus* extracts of pituitary glands were superseded by lypressin (duration of action 3–4 h), which has been superseded by the longer-acting desmopressin.

Desmopressin (DDAVP) has two major advantages, the vasoconstrictor effect has been reduced to near insignificance and the duration of action with nasal instillation is 8–20 h ($t_{\frac{1}{2}}$, 75 min) so that, used two or three times a day, patients are not inconvenienced by frequent recurrence of polyuria during their waking hours and can also expect to spend the night continuously in bed. Duration of action of lypressin is 3–4 h. Desmopressin is available as nasal drops or aerosol and in solution for injection (i.m. or i.v.); it is digested if swallowed. The dose for children is about half that for adults.

Lypressin is synthetic lysine-vasopressin (man secretes arginine-vasopressin); DDAVP is desamino-D-arginine vasopressin.

Nephrogenic diabetes insipidus, as is to be expected, does not respond to antidiuretic hormone.

Bleeding oesophageal varices in hepatic cirrhosis. Use is made of the vasoconstrictor effect of vasopressin (as *terlipressin*, a vasopressin prodrug, 2 mg 4–6 hourly until bleeding is controlled or to a maximum of 72 h) to reduce the pressure in the portal venous system by constricting splanchnic arterioles and reducing blood flow through them so that the amount of blood entering the portal venous system is reduced, despite the concurrently induced rise in systemic arterial pressure due to generalised arteriolar constriction. It is hoped that during the period of reduced portal venous pressure a clot will form at the bleeding point. This is a dangerous treatment for a dangerous disease. It is contraindicated if there is a history of angina pectoris or evidence of myocardial ischaemia. During it, the patient will become pale, arterial pressure will rise and abdominal colic and defaecation may occur. Natural vasopressin (Pitressin) may be used, or lypressin. Some would give nitroprusside i.v. concurrently in the hope of reducing the unwanted general vasoconstriction. A non-selective β-adrenoceptor blocker (propranolol) may be preferred. It reduces cardiac output and enhances splanchnic vasoconstriction by blocking dilator β-adrenoceptors, leaving constrictor α-receptors unopposed. Vasodilators (e.g. isosorbide dinitrate, verapamil) can also reduce portal pressure.

In *haemophilia* desmopressin can enhance blood concentration of factor VIII.

Felypressin is used as a vasoconstrictor with local anaesthetics.

Diabetes insipidus. Desmopressin replacement therapy is the first choice. *Thiazide diuretics* (and chlorthalidone) also have paradoxical antiduretic effect in diabetes insipidus. That this is not due to Na depletion is suggested by the fact that the non-diuretic thiazide, diazoxide (see index) also has this effect. It is probable that changes in the proximal renal tubule result in increased reabsorption and in delivery of less Na and water to the distal tubule, but the mechanism remains incompletely elucidated. Some cases of the *nephrogenic* form, which is not helped by antidiuretic hormone, may be benefited.

Drugs, e.g. lithium and demeclocycline, may cause nephrogenic diabetes insipidus.

Chlorpropamide. A patient with diabetes *insipidus*, wrongly believing himself to suffer from diabetes mellitus, 'at his own discretion' took chlorpropamide.* His physician was surprised at the apparent therapeutic effect and tried the drug on other patients, confirming it.

Chlorpropamide (but not other sulphonylureas) and *carbamazepine* are effective in *partial* pituitary diabetes insipidus (i.e. some natural hormone production remains) because they act on the kidney potentiating the effect of vasopressin. Hypoglycaemia may occur.

Clofibrate probably releases endogenous vasopressin.

Evidently all these drugs may cause difficulty due to their other actions that are not desired, and none are drugs of first choice for this disease.

Syndrome of inappropriate antidiuretic hormone secretion (SIADH). A variety of tumours (e.g. oat cell lung cancer) can make vasopressin, and of course they are not subject to normal homeostatic mechanisms. Dilutional hyponatraemia may occur, and fludrocortisone may be needed along with fluid restriction (soon becomes intolerable) and infusion of hypertonic saline (in acute cases only). Demeclocycline, which inhibits the renal action of vasopressin, can be useful. Chemotherapy to the causative tumour is likely to be the most effective treatment.

Oxytocin, see p. 715.

SEX HORMONES AND ANTAGONISTS

Steroid hormone receptors (for sex steroids and adrenocortical steroids) are complex proteins inside the target cell. The steroid penetrates, is bound and translocates into the cell nucleus, which is the principal site of action and where

* Arduino F et al. J Clin Endocrinol 1966; 26:1325

RNA/protein synthesis occurs. Compounds that occupy the receptor without causing translocation into the nucleus or the replenishment of receptors act as antagonists, e.g. spironolactone to aldosterone, cyproterone to androgens, clomiphene to oestrogens.

Pharmacokinetics. Steroid sex hormones are subject to extensive hepatic metabolic inactivation (some so much that oral administration is ineffective or requires very large doses if a useful amount is to pass through the liver and reach the systemic circulation). There is some enterohepatic recirculation. There are some non-steroid analogues that are slowly metabolised. Sustained-release (depot) preparations are used. The hormones are carried in the blood extensively bound to sex-hormone-binding globulin. In general the plasma $t_{\frac{1}{2}}$ is in relation to the duration of cellular action. Duration of action is implied in the recommended dosage schedules.

Androgens

Testosterone is the natural androgen secreted by the interstitial cells of the testis; it is necessary for normal spermatogenesis, for the development of the male secondary sex characteristics, and for the growth, at puberty, of the sexual apparatus. It is probably converted by hydroxylation to the active dihydrotestosterone.

Protein anabolism is increased by androgens, that is, androgens increase the proportion of protein laid down as tissue, especially muscle. Growth of bone is promoted, but the rate of closure of the epiphyses is also hastened, causing short stature in cases of precocious puberty or of androgen overdose in the course of treating hypogonadal children.

Indications for androgen therapy

Testicular failure may be primary or secondary (due to lack of pituitary gonadotrophins). In either case **replacement** with androgens is often necessary. Unfortunately, sterility is not remedied, although loss of libido and of secondary sex characteristics can be greatly improved. Impotence is helped if it is hypogonadal, but not if it has a psychological cause (which is often the case). If androgens are given to a boy with delayed puberty, a growth spurt and sexual development will occur. Such treatment is not usually indicated until the age of 16 years since up to that age natural delay in pituitary secretion may be responsible and normal development may yet occur. In **hepatic cirrhosis** degradation of oestrogens in the liver may be impaired, leading to raised blood levels of oestrogen with feminisation. Androgens may help such patients and also stop the **itching** of jaundice, though the jaundice may be worsened; methyltestosterone should not be used as it can cause jaundice. Relatively small amounts of androgens can be used to increase the **formation of new tissue**, e.g. in osteoporosis (see below). The **oestrogen-dependent bony metastases** from carcinoma of the breast in premenopausal patients are sometimes made smaller and less painul by large doses of androgen (though an antioestrogen, tamoxifen, is preferred), and the patient may be helped by large doses of an adrenal steroid, especially if there is hypercalcaemia. Androgens may also help in **fibrocystic disease** of the breast and in some cases of **anaemia** due to bone marrow failure.

Preparations and choice of androgens

Testosterone is subject to extensive hepatic first-pass metabolism and therefore orally effective doses must be high. It is therefore best given as sublingual tablets *daily* or as depot injections (of esters) 2–6 *weekly*.

Mesterolone provides alternative oral therapy; its molecular structure is such that it does not inhibit pituitary gonadotrophin secretion, nor does it cause liver injury. *Methyltestosterone* (oral) is likely to cause cholestatic jaundice, as are other 17-α-alkyl derivatives, e.g. *ethyloestrenol* and *stanozolol*, and for that reason should be used briefly, if at all.

Adverse effects are mainly those to be expected of a male sex hormone, increased libido may lead to undesirable sexual activity, especially in mentally unstable patients, and virilisation is obviously undesired by most women. Androgens have a weak *salt and water retaining activity*, which is not often clinically important. Liver injury can occur particularly with methyltestosterone and its allies (see above); it is dose-related and is not an allergy. In patients with malignant disease of bone, e.g. metastases from breast carcinoma, androgen administration may be followed by a rise in blood calcium sufficient to produce symptoms. The cause is uncertain. The less virilising androgens are used to promote anabolism and are discussed below.

Antiandrogens (androgen antagonists). Plainly oestrogens and progestogens are partial physiological antagonists to androgens. But compounds with more selective antiandrogen activity have been made.

Cyproterone is a derivative of progesterone; its combination of structural similarities and differences results in the following:

1. Competition with testosterone for receptors in target *peripheral organs* (but not causing feminisation as do oestrogens); it reduces spermatogenesis even to the level of azoospermia (reverses over about 4 months after the drug is stopped); abnormal sperm occur during treatment.

2. Competition with testosterone in the central nervous system, reducing sexual drive and thoughts, and causing impotence.

3. Some progestogenic agonist activity, which acts on hypothalamic receptors, inhibiting gonadotrophin secretion, which also inhibits testicular androgen production.

Uses. Cyproterone is used for reducing male hypersexuality and severe female hirsutism. A formulation of cyproterone plus ethinyloestradiol (Diane) is offered for this latter purpose as well as for severe acne in women. This preparation acts as an oral contraceptive but should not be used primarily for this purpose. It is also used in prostatic cancer.

Cyproterone causes hepatomas in rats.

Plainly long-term use of the drug poses both medical and ethical problems. It is even advised that for management of male hypersexuality formally witnessed written consent be obtained.

Cyproterone is plainly unsuitable for male contraception (see actions above).

Androgen secretion may be diminished by continued use of luteinising hormone releasing hormone (LHRH), after an initial stimulation. Ketoconazole (antifungal) interferes with androgen synthesis. These agents are used in prostatic carcinoma.

Androgens used as protein anabolic agents

Androgens are effective protein anabolic agents, but their clinical use for this purpose is limited by the amount of virilisation that women* will tolerate. Partially successful attempts have been made to produce compounds with the desired anabolic action but without the other effects. These compounds can be used instead of the ordinary androgens in the treatment of **osteoporosis** in men. They can also prevent the calcium and nitrogen loss in the urine that occurs in patients bedridden for a long time and they have therefore been recommended in the treatment of some severe fractures. **Growth** in hypogonadal children is at first stimulated and the anabolic steroids may be worth using in some cases of dwarfism, but only if bone age is well below chronological age and corresponds with height age. The chief risk of overdose is premature epiphyseal fusion, but this may be avoided by careful intermittent use.

The use of anabolic steroids in conditions of **general wasting** is justifiable in extreme debilitating disease, such as severe ulcerative colitis, after major surgery, and in the later stages of malignant disease they may make the patient feel and look less wretched. Their general use as tonics is scandalous as is their use in sport (see index). They may be tried in *aplastic anaemia*.

The **itching of jaundice** may be relieved and these drugs are perhaps preferable to testosterone for the purpose. There remains, however, a risk of increasing the degree of jaundice. Stanozolol has some *fibrinolytic effect*.

Attempts have been made to use anabolic steroids to counter the unwanted catabolic effects of adrenocortical hormones when the latter are used over long periods, but without notable success.

* In *adult* males androgens can be used as they do not cause hypermasculinisation, though there is risk of prostate hyperplasia in elderly patients; high doses of androgens depress spermatogenesis.

None of these agents is free from virilising properties in high doses; acne and greasy skin may be the early manifestation of virilisation. Salt and water retention may occur; also liver injury (especially with ethyloestrenol, a 17-α-alkyl derivative, see methyltestosterone above), which is usually mild and reversible. If used in carcinoma of the breast with bone metastases there may be hypercalcaemia, as with testosterone.

Oestrogens have only modest anabolic effect.

Administration should generally be intermittent in courses of 3–12 weeks with similar intervals, to reduce the occurrence of unwanted effects, especially liver injury.

There is little to choose between the various available drugs clinically: nandrolone (Durabolin) orally, daily or i.m. once a week; ethyloestrenol (Orabolin); stanozolol (Stromba).

Oestrogens

Oestrone and oestradiol are both natural oestrogens secreted by the ovary. Oestrogens are responsible for the normal development of the female genital tract, of the breast and of the female secondary sex characteristics. The pubertal growth spurt is less marked in females than in males, probably because oestrogens have less protein anabolic action than do androgens, although they are as effective in promoting closure of epiphyses. Blood oestrogen concentrations must be above a critical level for the maintenance of both proliferative and (together with progesterone) secretory phases of the uterine endothelium. If the oestrogen level falls too low then the endothelium can no longer be maintained and uterine bleeding follows. Thus uterine bleeding may be stopped temporarily by giving large doses of oestrogens or may start when they are withdrawn (oestrogen-withdrawal bleeding). Bleeding may occur despite a high blood oestrogen level if large doses are given for a long time, due to infarctions in the greatly hypertrophied endometrium. Oestrogens are necessary for the maintenance of normal pregnancy and for the accompanying breast hyperplasia. The vagina is more sensitive to oestrogens than is the endometrium.

Preparations of oestrogens

Innumerable oestrogen preparations are available, but the following selection should cover all needs. The dose varies greatly according to whether replacement of physiological deficiencies is being carried out (*replacement therapy*) or whether oestrogens are being used as drugs to obtain certain effects by pharmacological force (*pharmacotherapy*). The potency of oestrogens can be measured in women by a method using the occurrence of withdrawal-bleeding as an end point. Natural oestrogens offer no advantage over synthetic oestrogens.

Ethinyloestradiol (10, 50 μg, 1 mg) is a synthetic agent of first choice; it is effective by mouth.

Oestradiol and *oestriol* are orally active natural oestrogens.

Conjugated oestrogens are orally active mixed natural oestrogens obtained from the urine of pregnant mares.

Estropipate (piperazine oestrone sulphate) is an orally active synthetic conjugate.

Quinestrol (4 mg) is orally active, is stored in fat and is released to be metabolised to ethinyloestradiol.

Quinestradol is an alternative.

Stilboestrol is the first synthetic oestrogen: its use is confined to oestrogen-dependent cancers (breast, prostate).

Other oestrogens are used in hormonal (oral) contraception and in cancer (see index).

Choice of oestrogen. Ethinyloestradiol is a satisfactory first choice. However, individual patients may be intolerant of any one agent, when it is worth trying the others. It remains uncertain whether all oestrogens have exactly similar hormonal and non-hormonal effects, including adverse effects.

Indications for oestrogen therapy

Replacement therapy in hypo-ovarian conditions. Ethinyloestradiol (up to 500 μg orally daily for 21 days) followed by a progestagen (norethistrone or medroxyprogesterone 5 mg orally) for 7–10 days per monthly cycle is general acceptable.

Unless the cause of the hypo-ovarian state is primary ovarian failure, treatment should be stopped after every third cycle to see if spontaneous menstruation will occur.

For menopausal symptoms severe enough to demand treatment there are three rules that should be followed:

1. The minimal effective dose should be given.
2. Treatment must be in interrupted courses (cyclical) with a progestogen and not continuous to reduce the risk of endometrial cancer (unless the patient has had a hysterectomy.
3. Treatment should be stopped as soon as possible (usually within 1 year)

The aim is to allow the body gradually to accustom itself to the natural decline of oestrogens. Use of high doses will prevent this.

Cyclical schemes, e.g. oestrogen (11–14 days), oestrogen plus progestogen (7–10 days) and hormone-free period up to 28 days are used in women who have a uterus (to allow a monthly bleed). Special calendar packs of various regimens are available under a range of proprietary names (Menophase, Prempak, etc.). Oestrogens used include ethinyloestradiol, oestradiol and conjugated oestrogens; progestogens include levonorgestrel and norethisterone. Cyclical use is not necessary in hysterectomised women. In resistant cases an androgen may be substituted for the progestogen (Mixogen), but this is liable to cause unwelcome facial hair. Treatment may have to last for a few months to a few years.

Vasomotor symptoms may occasionally be helped by low doses of clonidine (Dixarit).

Postmenopausal hormone replacement therapy (HRT) has been practiced for many years (in the 1970s more than 30% of postmenopausal women were taking prescribed oestrogen) for its benefits on general well being including a hoped for reduction in facial wrinkles, to prevent osteoporosis (accepted) and cardiovascular disease (uncertain)*. Such 'unopposed' oestrogen therapy, if prolonged for years is associated with an increased incidence of endometrial carcinoma. This may obtain whether administration is continuous or cyclical. But it is likely that addition of a progestogen ('opposed' oestrogen therapy) reduces the risk. The evidence is based on case-control studies (see index) and is highly controversial as to amount, i.e. whether any increase is marginal only, or substantial (even 6–15 times that of non-oestrogen users). There is also an increased incidence of gall-bladder disease.

* The evidence on cardiovascular disease is contradictory. In a single issue of the New England Journal of Medicine (October 24, 1985) there was a paper that provided data that 'postmenopausal use of estrogen reduces the risk of severe coronary heart disease' and a paper that provided data that 'mortality from all causes and from cardiovascular disease did not differ for estrogen users and nonusers'. The problem of contradictory research results is discussed in an editorial.

Pharmacotherapy

Contraception (see below). **Menstrual disorders** (see below).

Vaginitis. Senile vaginitis usually responds to daily use of an oestrogen pessary or cream which can also be used in small girls with vaginitis. Absorption can occur sufficiently to cause systemic effects (stillboestrol, dienoestrol, oestriol, etc. are used).

Inhibition of lactation is sometimes necessary e.g. dead child, sick mother, etc. 'One alternative which is not considered often enough is . . . A tight binder, sympathy, and occasional sedatives' which 'will carry many women through the initial discomfort of engorged breasts. Without the stimulus of suckling, the high prolactin concentrations at delivery fall to normal within a week and lactation soon peters out. Fluid restriction is unnecessary;'†

Pituitary secretion of prolactin is normally under inhibitory tone from the hypothalamus via prolactin-inhibiting factor (PIF), which may be dopamine.

Dopamine receptor agonists stimulate the release of hypothalamic prolactin-inhibiting factor, the plasma prolactin concentration falls and lactation stops. **Bromocriptine** (2.5 mg) is used for *prevention* of lactation (oral dose 2.5 mg on day of birth, then 2.5 mg twice a day for 14 days); for *suppression* of lactation (2.5 mg daily for three days, then 2.5 mg twice a day for 14 days); since prolactin

† Editorial. Br Med J 1977; 1:189.

suppresses ovulation during lactation, use of a contraceptive will be appropriate; galactorrhoea from other causes may require higher doses (see *bromocriptine*).

Oestrogens have been used to inhibit lactation since their introduction in the 1930s. They may act by blocking the effect of prolactin on the breast, despite the fact that they increase prolactin secretion by direct hypothalamic–pituitary action. In the doses needed for post-partum prevention they stimulate the endometrium at a time when it should be undergoing involution and they cause thromboembolism. They are less effective for suppressing lactation once it has begun.

Prevention: quinestrol 4 mg orally within 6 hours of delivery. Symptoms of lactation may develop from days 4 to 6. If these persist give a second dose.

Suppression: 4 mg at once when decision is made, repeated in 48 hours if necessary (the patient may experience nausea).

Combinations of oestrogen with a progestogen or androgen are also effective.

Hormone-dependent carcinoma. High doses of oestrogens are used in *prostatic carcinoma*, which is an androgen-dependent neoplasm. Stilboestrol, 5 mg a day, reducing to 1.0 mg a day can be used. If the patient is intolerant other oestrogens can be tried. Feminisation is inevitable and the gynaecomastia is often painful.

Inoperable breast carcinoma in post-menopausal women may also sometimes be favourably influenced temporarily by oestrogens and by an adrenal steroid.

To reduce sexual urge in men whose activities are qualitatively or quantitatively unacceptable to the community and/or to themselves is an occasional indication for oestrogens. 1–2 mg of stilboestrol daily should be enough. See also *antiandrogen* (cyproterone) and *benperidol*.

Epistaxis: as a last resort in recurrent cases, e.g. telangiectasia.

Atrophic rhinitis may benefit, as also may **acne**.

Adverse effects consist largely of overdose causing excess of the physiological actions. Withdrawal uterine bleeding is common but seldom prolonged. In men, reduced libido, impotence and gynaecomastia (which may be painful) occur. In both sexes *oedema* due to salt and water retention, and *thromboembolism* occur.

Oral administration is liable to cause nausea, vomiting and diarrhoea.

Long-term unopposed oestrogen replacement therapy in post-menopausal women is associated with increased incidence of gall bladder disease and endometrial carcinoma.

Stilboestrol has been incriminated as a *transplacental carcinogen*, i.e. administered to the mother in the first 18 weeks of pregnancy (in an attempt to prevent miscarriage) it has caused vaginal adenocarcinoma in the offspring (peak age 18 years).

Oestrogens added to cosmetics (skin and hair creams) can cause precocious puberty in children and postmenopausal bleeding and gynaecomastia in adults. Cosmetics are not subject to the same official controls as are medicines.

Contraindications to oestrogen therapy include women who may have an oestrogen-dependent neoplasm, be pregnant, or have a disposition to thromboembolism. Hypertension, liver disease or gallstones, migraine, diabetes, fibroids or endometriosis may all be made worse by oestrogen.

Antioestrogens. Obviously the virilising effects of androgens and progestogens antagonise physiologically many of the effects of oestrogens. But selective competitive agents blocking the oestrogen receptor are more likely to be clinically useful. There is **clomiphene** (structurally related to stilboestrol), which is a weak oestrogen having less activity than natural oestrogens so that its occupation of receptors results in antagonism, i.e. it is an agnoist/antagonist. Such substances are sometimes referred to as 'impeded oestrogens'. Clomiphene blocks hypothalamic oestrogen receptors so that the negative feedback of natural oestrogens is prevented and the pituitary responds by increased secretion of gonadotrophins, which may induce ovulation. Clomiphene is used to treat anovulatory infertility. Multiple ovulation with multiple pregnancy may occur. **Cyclofenil** acts similarly. **Tamoxifen** competes for oestrogen receptors in target organs; it is used for anovulatory infertility and for treatment of oestrogen-dependent breast cancer.

Osteoporosis

Osteoporosis is an abnormal decrease in amount of bone, but what there is is of normal quality. It has a variety of causes including gonadal hormone deficiency, intestinal malabsorption, hyperthyroidism, corticosteroid excess.

Postmenopausal osteoporosis is due to gonadal deficiency. Oestrogen arrests the process by reducing bone resorption. Progestogen arrests the process by increasing bone formation. A combination of the two may achieve some overall reversal of the osteoporotic process though the bones are unlikely to become fully normal. Unopposed oestrogen has been widely used but carries a risk of endometrial cancer and thromboembolism, which are also diminished by added progestogen.

Oestrogen reduces sensitivity of bone to natural resorbing agents and this results in compensatory stimulation of parathormone secretion. If the oestrogen is suddenly stopped there is a period (as long as 3 years) of enhanced bone loss due to the excess of parathormone. Calcium administration suppresses bone resorbing agents and so does not carry this disadvantage; as a dietary supplement (1.0 g/day of gluconate) is helpful. Where there is concomitant osteomalacia (adult rickets: vitamin D deficiency) oral vitamin D and calcium should be added.

Progesterone and progestogens

Progesterone is produced by the corpus luteum and converts the uterine epithelium from the proliferative to the secretory phase. It is thus necessary for implantation of the ovum, and is essential throughout pregnancy, in the last two-thirds of which it is secreted in large amounts by the placenta.

The production of powerful synthetic progestogens and knowledge of the amounts secreted in the body has led to the realisation that inadequate doses of progesterone have often been used in the past. The decision when to use progestogens as principal therapy is a skilled one, and therapeutic effects are uncertain. A detailed account of what can be attempted is beyond the scope of this book.

The clinical uses of progestational agents are ill-defined, apart from *contraception* (see below) and the menopause (see above). A principal indication is *threatened and habitual abortion*. There is, however, no proof that they are beneficial, although they probably are in cases of *true* progesterone insufficiency.

Vigorous progestogen therapy can seriously virilise female fetuses to the point of sexual ambiguity, and this is least with true derivatives of progesterone (dydrogesterone, hydroxyprogesterone) than with those derived from testosterone.

Other uses include *menstrual disorders* (e.g. menorrhagia), the *premenstrual syndrome, endometriosis*, and *dysmenorrhoea*.

Available *progestogen preparations* include: *oral*: ethisterone, allylestrenol, norethisterone, dydrogesterone, medroxyprogesterone. *suppositories or pessaries*: progesterone. *injectable*: progesterone, hydroxyprogesterone, medroxyprogesterone

An *intra-uterine* contraceptive device that also comprises a slow-release (1 year) progesterone formulation for local endometrial effect has been made.

As progestogen component of *combined oestrogen-progestogen oral contraceptives* (see below).

Antiprogestogens have been made: potential therapeutic applications include abortion, contraception and induction of labour.

Miscellaneous

Danazol (Danol) is a derivative of the progestogen, ethisterone. It is a relatively selective inhibitor of pituitary gonadotrophin secretion (LH, FSH) affecting the surge in the mid-menstrual cycle more than basal secretion. This reduces ovarian function, which leads to atrophic changes in endometrium, both uterine and elsewhere (ectopic), i.e. endometriosis. It lacks oestrogenic and progestogenic agonist activity but blocks these receptors; it has weak androgenic agonist activity, i.e. it is an 'impeded androgen' (see above). It is effective in both sexes. It reduces spermatogenesis.

It is chiefly used for *endometriosis, fibrocystic mastitis, gynaecomastia, precocious puberty, menor-*

rhagia. It increases the concentration of factor VIII in the blood of haemophiliacs.

FERTILITY REGULATION

Induction of ovulation and male infertility, see above.

Drugs and the control of conception

This subject will only be treated here in general terms. Any physician intending to prescribe hormonal contraceptives will need more extensive knowledge.

The requirements of a successful hormonal contraceptive are stringent, for it will be used by millions of healthy people who wish to separate sexual relations from physical reproduction. It must therefore be *extremely safe* as well as *highly effective* and its action must be *quick in onset* and *quickly and completely reversible*, even after years of continuous use. It must not affect libido. The fact that alternative methods are less reliable implies that their use will lead to more unwanted pregnancies with their attendant inconvenience, morbidity and mortality, and this must be taken into account in deciding what risks of hormonal contraception are acceptable.

Possible sites of action include:

1. *Direct inhibition of spermatogenesis* — this presents many problems including the lag in onset of effect due to storage of mature spermatozoa until they are ejaculated or die of old age.

2. *Indirect inhibition of spermatogenesis by suppression of hypothalamic/pituitary activity*, which controls it, e.g. by progestogen–androgen combinations; see gonadorelin.

3. *Immunological techniques* (vaccines), to induce antibodies to pituitary gonadotrophins, sperm, or other components of the reproductive process in either sex, are being developed.

4. *Inhibition of ovulation* presents a different and easier biological problem. There is no need to suppress continuous formation of the gametes, as in the male, but only to prevent their release from the ovary approximately 13 times a year.

Either the pituitary gonadotrophin may be inhibited or the ovary may be made unresponsive to it.

5. *Prevention of fertilisation*: no general progress has been made here, though the female genital tract may be made inhospitable to spermatozoa, e.g. by altering cervical mucus or fallopian tube function.

6. *Antizygotic drugs*: compounds effective in the rat have been developed.,

7. *Inhibition of implantation*: implantation does not occur unless the endometrium is in the right state, and this depends on a delicate balance between oestrogen and progesterone. This balance can readily be disturbed.

Mice fail to become pregnant if, after mating, they are exposed to the smell of alien males (via a chemical communicator or pheromone). This approach does not yet seem to have been explored in man and 'it would be rash indeed to suppose that a contraceptive perfume is on the way'.*

Hormonal and chemical contraception (oral, injectable)

1. Oestrogen and progestogen (combined and phased administration)
2. Progestogen alone

Mode of action of currently used oestrogen–progestogen contraceptives in women. Oral contraceptives have been extensively used since 1956. The principal mechanism is inhibition of ovulation (4, above) by action on the hypothalamus inhibiting the release of hormone-releasing hormones that stimulate the pituitary to release gonadotrophins. In addition the endometrium is altered, so that implantation is less likely (7, above) and cervical mucus may become more viscous and impede the passage of the spermatozoa (5, above).

Oestrogens alone can inhibit ovulation, but they are not completely reliable and cause thromboembolism and endometrial cancer.

Progestogens alone inhibit ovulation in up to 50% of cycles but contraceptive effect is on cervical mucus. There is liable to be break-

* Parkes A S. Practitioner 1965; 194:455.

through bleeding. They are less reliable than a mixture.

An appropriate dose of **oestrogen + progestogen** *gives complete reliability with good menstrual cycle control. The following account applies to these combined preparations.*

The combination is usually started on the 5th day after the start of menstruation and continued for 21 days. Withdrawal bleeding usually begins 1–4 days after discontinuation. After an interval of 7 days,* regardless of menstruation, a new 21-day course is begun, and so on, i.e. daily tablets are taken for 3 weeks out of 4. But packaging of numbered tablets (active and dummy) so that the woman takes a tablet each day without intermission may be best. An alternative method of contraception should be used until the 14th pill has been taken since the first ovulation may not have been suppressed in women who have short menstrual cycles.

An alternative mode is to start the course on the first day of the period. This may lead to some irregular breakthrough bleeding during the first cycle only, but it may be preferred because it does not require use of an alternative method of contraception. The first bleeding cycle will be 23 (not 28) days.

The pill should be taken at the same time every day and preferably not just before intercourse. The monthly bleeds that occur one or two days after the cessation of active hormone administration are hormone withdrawal bleeds not natural menstruation. They are not an essential feature of oral contraception, but women are accustomed to them and they provide monthly reassurance of the absence of pregnancy.

Numerous field trials have shown that progestogen–oestrogen mixtures, if taken as directed, are the most reliable reversible contraceptives known. (The only close competitors are the plastic intrauterine devices.)

Some important aspects of the combined oestrogen–progestogen pill.

Subsequent fertility. So far, the evidence points to a resumption of normal pituitary–ovarian function, with normal fertility, within two cycles of stopping the drug in almost all cases. But amenorrhoea of variable duration may occur. Permanent damage to fertility is rare.

Effect on an existing pregnancy. Although progestogens can masculinise the female fetus, e.g. when used in the hope of preventing habitual abortion, the doses for contraception are lower and the risk of harming an undiagnosed pregnancy is extremely low, probably less than in 1000 (the background incidence of birth defects is 1–2%).

Carcinogenesis. Carcinoma of the breast and cervix may be unaffected or very slightly increased. The risk to life seems to be less than that of moderate smoking (10 cigarettes/day). Carcinoma of the ovary and endometrium are substantially reduced. *Total* incidence of cancer is unaltered.

Effect on menstruation (it is not true menstruation, see above) is generally to regularise it, and often to diminish blood loss, but amenorrhoea can occur. In some women 'breakthrough' intermenstrual bleeding occurs, especially at the outset, but this seldom persists for more than a few cycles. Premenstrual tension and dysmenorrhoea are much reduced.

Libido is not generally directly affected, and removal of fear of pregnancy may permit enthusiasm for the first time. But reduced libido can occur, and there is evidence that the normal increase in female-initiated sexual activity at ovulation time is suppressed.† The effect is limited to current users and is unrelated to duration of use.

Cardiovascular complications. Incidence of venous thromboembolism, hypertension, cerebrovascular accidents (thrombotic and haemorrhagic) and acute myocardial infarction is increased. Increases in specific blood clotting factors have been shown (due to oestrogen).

Increased arterial disease appears to be also associated with the amount of progestogen in the combined pill. The progestogen-only pill does not affect coagulation.

Surgery in patients taking oestrogen–progestogen contraceptives and postmenopausal hormone replacement therapy. Because of the added post-

* A 7-day interval may be too long, i.e. follicles may develop. A safer regimen may be 23 days hormone administration with a 5-day interval.

† Adams D B et al. N Engl J Med 1978; 299:1145.

surgical risk of venous thromboembolism it has been advised that these oral contraceptives should be withdrawn if practicable, four weeks before lower limb operations or major elective surgery (and started again at the first menstruation to occur more than two weeks after surgery).* But increases in clotting factors may persist for many weeks and there is also the risk of pregnancy to be considered. It may be preferable to maintain contraception and to use low-dose heparin (though this may not reverse all the oestrogen effects on coagulation) or other means (mechanical stimulation of venous return) to prevent post-operative thrombosis.

Hepatic function as measured by bromsulphthalein retention may be impaired as may drug-metabolising capacity ($t_{\frac{1}{2}}$ antipyrine, a general indicator of drug-metabolising capacity, may increase by 30%). Gall-bladder disease is more common, and highly vascular hepatocellular adenomas occur (rare).

Cervical erosion occurs. **Crohn's disease** may be promoted.

Decreased glucose tolerance occurs, perhaps due to a peripheral effect reducing the action of insulin.

Plasma lipoproteins may rise.

Plasma proteins: oestrogens cause an increase in proteins, particularly globulins that bind hydrocortisone, thyroxine and iron. As a result, the total plasma concentration of the bound substances is increased, though the concentration of free and active substance remains normal. This can be misleading in diagnostic tests, e.g. of thyroid function. This effect on plasma proteins passes off about 6 weeks after cessation of the oestrogen.

Other adverse effects, often more prominent at the outset and largely due to oestrogen, include, nausea and, rarely, vomiting; breast discomfort; fluid retention; headache (increase in migraine); lethargy; abdominal discomfort; vaginal discharge. A syndrome of lethargy and general 'bitchiness' after about a year has been recognised, though causal attribution of such a phenomenon is naturally difficult. Depression may occur (and some patients have low blood concentration of pyridoxine); it *may* be benefited by pyridoxine (try 25 mg orally/day and stop after 4 weeks if there is no benefit).

* For a detailed review see Guillebaud J. Br Med J 1985; 291:498.

Benefits additional to contraception. Side effects are commonly assumed always to be unpleasant aspects of drug action. But side effects can sometimes also be pleasant.

The oestrogen–progestogen pill is associated with reduced risk of ovarian cysts and cancer, of endometrial cancer, and of benign breast disease; fibroids bleed less; there is perhaps less risk of autoimmune thyroid disease; menses are regular and blood loss is not excessive; menses are accompanied by less premenstrual tension and dysmenorrhoea; and there may even be less ear wax.

Contraindications. Carcinoma of the breast or of the genital tract, past or present, is regarded as an absolute contraindication and so, usually, is a history of thromboembolic disease. In patients with a history of liver disease, they should only be used if liver function tests are normal. Diabetes may become more difficult to control or may be precipitated. Lactation may be reduced by combinations but not by progestogens alone. Migraine may be precipitated. Hypertension will be worsened.

Smoking *greatly* enhances the risks of circulatory disease.

Age. Increasing age above 35 years enhances the risks of circulatory disease.

Duration of use does not enhance risks of itself. The increase in risk with increased duration of use is due to increasing age. The approaching menopause presents an obvious problem. Because cyclic bleeding will continue to occur under the influence of the drugs even after the natural menopause, the only way of deciding whether contraception can be permanently abandoned is by abandoning it (and using another technique) for three months annually to see if natural menstruation is resumed.

Preparations of oestrogen–progestogen combination

The *oestrogen* is usually ethinyloestradiol or mestranol.

The *progestogen* is usually levonorgestrel, norethisterone, ethynodiol, desogestrel or lynoestrenol.

The *most important variable* is the dose of oestrogen, which is usually between 20 and 50 μg.

The incidence of thromboembolism has been found higher with high-dose oestrogen preparations, e.g. 100 μg, but it is not known if there is any difference between doses below 50 μg.

It is now appreciated that the earlier preparations had much more oestrogen than was necessary for efficacy. It seems probable that 20 μg is about the limit below which serious *loss of efficacy* can be expected. Indeed in hepatic enzyme-induced patients (e.g. using antiepileptics, antirheumatics, etc.) it is advisable to use a preparation containing 35 μg oestrogen or more to avoid loss of efficacy due to increased oestrogen metabolism (elimination of breakthrough bleeding is a guide to adequacy of dose).

Inadvertent omission of a dose is less serious on the higher dose preparations, e.g. if one tablet is omitted the woman remains protected for 24 h if she has been taking a 50 μg oestrogen preparation, but for only 12 h if using a 30 μg oestrogen preparation.

If an omitted dose is remembered *within 12 hours* it should be taken at once and the next dose at the usual time, and all should be well.

If *more than 12 hours* has elapsed the same procedure should be followed *but* an alternative barrier method of contraception should be used for 7* days (or abstinence). A missed pill is more serious in the first 7 days of the cycle (because the 7-day pill-free interval is long enough to allow a follicle to develop).

Intercurrent gut upset. Obviously a patient may *vomit* the dose but *diarrhoea* without vomiting can be a cause of failure to absorb or disturb enterohepatic recirculation of hormone. Even a brisk traveller's diarrhoea (rapid transit in small as well as in large intestine) may bring such an unwelcome consequence to a holiday. A prudent user will use a barrier method during and for 14 days after the episode.

Changing of preparation. If a woman is uncomfortable on one preparation she should be changed to another containing a different dose of oestrogen and/or progestogen. The new preparation should start *the day after* she has finished a cycle on the previous preparation. If this is done no extra risk of pregnancy occurs.

Breakthrough bleeding (bleeding on days of active pill taking) can mean a higher dose of oestrogen is required.

Choice of oestrogen–progestogen combination

There is a wide choice of formulations:

1. *low oestrogen* (20–35 μg) plus *low progestogen*, e.g. Ovranette, Trinordiol, Microgynon 30.
2. *low oestrogen* plus *high progestogen*, e.g. Ovran 30, Eugynon 30.
3. *high oestrogen* (50 μg plus *low or high progestogen*, e.g. Ovran, Eugynon 50, Minovlar; Minilyn.

In general users should employ the lowest total hormone dose that suits them (good cycle control and minimal side-effects) and should make a start with a preparation from 1 above.

Postcoital contraception ('morning after pill'). Overall probability of pregnancy following unprotected intercourse is 1:25 to 1:50 (higher in mid cycle, lower at end cycle); it may be prevented by disrupting the normal hormonal arrangements; mode of action is probably by preventing implantation of the fertilized ovum, though there may also be a post-implantation action.

Postcoital contraception may be successfully practised up to 72 hours after the exposure. A usual technique is to take two tablets of an oestrogen–progestogen combined formulation (containing 50 μg of oestrogen) at the earliest opportunity, followed by a further two tablets exactly 12 hours later. Vomiting may occur and must be taken into account as a cause of failure (if tablets are vomited, repeat the dose with an antiemetic). The failure rate is hard to estimate (controlled trials are not practicable, but studies on rape and volunteer cases have been made) and may be about 1:200 (but higher in mid cycle); ectopic pregnancy may perhaps be promoted. It is not known if injury to a pregnancy may occur. If it can, the risk is probably less than 1:1000; some people will consider abortion. The procedure should not be used more than once in a cycle.

Phased-formulation contraceptives employ low doses and variable ratios between oestrogen and

* If these seven unprotected days run beyond the beginning of the routine intended pill-free days the next cycle (packet) should follow without a gap, thus postponing the menses by a month (Family Planning Assoc).

progestogen, in two (*biphasic*) or three (*triphasic*) periods within the menstrual cycle. The dose of progestogen is low at the beginning and higher at the end, the oestrogen remaining either constant or rising slightly in mid cycle. The objective is to achieve effective contraception with minimal distortion of natural hormonal rhythms.

The advantages claimed for these techniques are diminished metabolic changes (e.g. blood lipids) and a particularly reliable monthly bleeding pattern without loss of contraceptive efficacy. But against these (potential) advantages, there is even less latitude of safety if a dose is forgotten. Preparations include BiNovum, TriNovum, Logynon.

Sequential-formulation contraceptives involve using unopposed oestrogen with risk of thromboembolism and are obsolete.

Progestogen-only contraception (mini-pill) oral formulations are taken every day throughout the 28 day cycle (not only for 21 days with a 7-day interval) as when combined with oestrogen (above); a 3-month depot i.m. injection is an alternative. Subcutaneous implants that release hormone for several years are in use; they can be removed surgically if adverse effects develop.

Progestogen-only contraception is less effective but safer (no effect on blood coagulation) than combined formulations. It works by inhibiting ovulation, though much less effectively than the combined pill, and by rendering the cervical mucus inhospitable (thick and scanty) to spermatozoa maximally 6 hours after a daily dose.

Progestogen-only contraception is particularly appropriate to women above 35 years for whom oestrogen carries unacceptable risk, for smokers (who refuse to give it up) and for diabetics; it is used for lactating women as it interferes with the milk less than the combined pill. A missed oral dose allows even less latitude than the combined pill. If a dose is more than 3 hours late it should be taken at once and a barrier method used for two days (though this is controversial and some advocate 14 days) since the chief effect is via cervical mucus.*

An important limitation to the use of the progestogen-only pill is erratic uterine bleeding which many women understandably dislike. There may be no bleeding for months or there may be frequent and irregular bleeding. Ectopic pregnancy may be more frequent due to a fertilized ovum being held up in a functionally depressed fallopian tube.

The progestogens used orally include levonorgestrel (Neogest, Microval), norethisterone (Noriday, Micronor), ethynodiol (Temulen): medroxyprogesterone (Depot-Provera) is a sustained-release i.m. injection given 3-monthly.

The use of i.m. medroxyprogesterone has been much criticised ('ban the jab') on ethical and social grounds (e.g. consent) and there are real ethical issues, especially with mentally retarded women. But it is important that criticism be properly directed (which it has not been) at the *way* the drug is used, not at the safe drug itself. Much has also been made of 'menstrual chaos' by the critics, but the tolerance of this will be a matter of personality and counselling, and some patients will prefer the infrequent (and private) injection according to their own social situation. It is essential that a drug, useful to some, be not banned because some prescribers have used it wrongly or too casually.

Interactions with steroid contraceptives

Particularly now that the lowest effective doses are in use there is little latitude if the absorption, distribution and metabolism are disturbed. Any additional drug taking must be looked at critically lest it reduces efficacy. Also, vomiting and diarrhoea can interfere with absorption and reabsorption of contraceptive steroids (where there is enterohepatic recirculation), i.e. both disease and drugs can cause failure.

The classic example of interference with the combined pill is the increase of breakthrough bleeding and pregnancy in young women being treated with rifampicin for tuberculosis (1971). Rifampicin is a potent inducer of hepatic drug-metabolising enzymes. Enhanced metabolism of the steroids caused failure. Antiepileptics (phenytoin and carbamazepine, but not sodium Valproate) constitute a similar risk.

All drugs that induce metabolising enzymes (see p. 128) constitute a risk to contraceptive efficacy

* Guillebaud J. The Pill. Oxford: Oxford University Press, 1984.

and prescribing should be specifically reviewed for this effect. Self-administered drugs, e.g. alcohol and tobacco smoking, also have this effect. Pregnancies have occurred in women taking a contraceptive who commence an antiepileptic drug.

Subcutaneous implants of progestogen that release hormone for several years are in use. They can be removed easily if adverse effects develop.

Hypothalamic/pituitary hormone approach to contraception, see *gonadorelin*.

Miscellaneous

Intra-uterine devices that are also slow-release formulations of progestogen or copper to enhance their efficacy by local action on the endometrium have been developed.

Vaginal preparations, to immobilise or kill (spermicide) spermatozoa, are used to add safety to various mechanical contraceptives. They are very unreliable and should only be used alone in an emergency. Substances used include nonoxinol-9 (a surfactant that alters the permeability of the sperm lipoprotein membrane), benzethonium, as pessary, gel or pressurised aerosol.

Risks of contraception

Whether a drug should be prescribed involves an assessment of benefit to the patient versus risk to the patient. Even when there is a defined disease the decision can be difficult. It is even more so when the subject is healthy, as is the case with most contraception. Reliable data on nature and incidence of adverse reactions are essential but all too often are not available.

It has been pointed out that a woman having regular sexual intercourse faces a finite chance of death from pregnancy, childbirth or from measures to avoid or interrupt pregnancy. The general problem cannot be discussed here as it goes beyond the use of drugs.

But as well as the risks of unwanted pregnancy, the risk of oral contraceptives should be viewed in the context of the risks of everyday life, which are substantial.

The death rate from oral contraceptives is probably about the same magnitude as deaths from cricket and football (in Britain) and much less than those from swimming (1,000/annum in Britain). A car driver may expect, on average, to be admitted to hospital once in 20 years due to a road accident. A woman would have to use oral contraceptives for 2000 years for a similar chance due to a thrombotic episode. It has been calculated that there is ten times the likelihood of a death in a family that has acquired an outboard motor boat than if an oral contraceptive is being used).*

Any danger oral contraceptives may have for the individual must also be seen in relation to their benefits to the community (fewer self-induced and criminal abortions, fewer unwanted children, slowing down of the speed of increase of world population with less hunger and misery, etc.). Their merits will continue to be debated and new technical advances will continue.

Interpretation of risk estimates

Studies of the effects of drugs ideally involve a *formal experiment* in which subjects are allocated at random to receive or not to receive the treatment. Obviously this is unacceptable with contraception.

Therefore *surveillance studies* (see index) are used, and these are scientifically less satisfactory.

When such a study shows an increased or decreased relative risk of an event, the question arises *whether the association is casual or causal*.

There are *five possible explanations*† *for an association*:

a. *Selection bias*: i.e. women who chose a particular technique may be inherently more or less liable to develop the condition under study.

b. *Information bias*: reporting of events may be influenced by what subjects are motivated to recall, or by their beliefs, e.g. a woman with breast cancer may unconsciously wish to find a 'cause' for her disease; alternatively she may wish to avoid the feeling that her acts may have caused the condition, and these feelings may influence her reporting of her contraceptive history.

c. *Confounding*: i.e. those using or not using a

* Potts D M. Br Med Bull 1970; 26: No 1, 27.

† WHO Scientific Group. Steroid Contraception and the Risk of Neoplasia. Tech. Rep. 619, Geneva: WHO, 1978.

technique may differ in an important respect such as age; if recognised, this can be 'allowed for' by stratification for age, or by calculation of age-standardised risk estimates.

d. *Chance*: see *statistics*

e. *Cause and effect.*

That a large amount of data on oral contraceptives is obtained by surveillance techniques (case-control studies, cohort studies) allows endless vigorous, and sometimes acrimonious, debate on the interpretation of the results, as is also the case with smoking (see index).

But patients need guidance, and an exposition by the doctor of the possible explanations of an observed association is likely to confuse most, though it may give joy to a small minority. These studies, like the science of statistics, provide a *guide to conduct in the face of uncertainty*. They do not eliminate uncertainty. Therefore the results are summarised here, for despite their admitted deficiencies they are a lot better than nothing, and if we wait for certainty before making decisions and giving advice we may sometimes find we have to wait for ever and, perhaps worse, sow alarm and despondency amongst those who are entitled to ask guidance (even if it is only an 'educated guess') of the medical profession in making decisions of great importance to their lives.

Risks and benefits summarised

In order to provide some much-needed general guidance ingeniously useful calculations have been made after putting together data from some major studies of women using different means of contraception*. It is recognised that such assessments provide only crude comparisons and have many limitations, including the fact that oestrogen dosage in some combined preparations has been reduced since some of the figures were collected.

Nevertheless the study probably gives us the most reliable overview that we have (most of the data used have been derived from studies in the UK and cannot certainly be extrapolated in detail to countries with different disease pattern and different risks of childbirth).

* Vessey M P, Doll R. Proc R Soc Lond, Ser B 1976; 195:69. Vessey M P Br Med J 1978; 1:722.

Failure rates†

Oral contraceptives (oestrogen/progestogen)	0.36 pregnancies/100 woman-years
Intra-uterine device	2.0 pregnancies/100 woman-years
Diaphragm (vaginal)	5.0 pregnancies/100 woman-years

If it is assumed that the outcome of unplanned pregnancies is standard throughout the country and that the *increased risk* to oral contraceptive users of gall-bladder disease and cervical erosion is balanced by the *reduced risk* of benign lesions of breast and ovary and of menstrual disorders, *then* **morbidity in 100,000 oral contraceptive users would comprise** (as measured by *excess* of hospital admissions) **per annum**

35 for cerebrovascular accident
70 for venous thromboembolism
10 for acute myocardial infarction
3 for hepatocellular adenoma
360 accidental pregnancies *of which*
200 term births
45 spontaneous abortions
94 terminations, approx

Morbidity in 100,000 intra-uterine device users (as above):

50 for uterine perforation
200 for pelvic inflammatory disease
2000 accidental pregnancies *of which*
495 term births
775 spontaneous abortions
120 ectopic gestations
605 terminations, approx

Morbidity in 100,000 vaginal diaphragm users (as above):

5000 accidental pregnancies *of which*
3045 term births
640 spontaneous abortions
20 ectopic gestations
1295 terminations, approx

† Other *estimates of failure* are expressed as follows: combined pill 0.1–1/100 woman years, progestogen-only pill 0.5–4/100 woman years, intra-uterine device 0.5–4/100 woman years, barrier methods (sheath, cap, diaphragm) about as effective as the intra-uterine device if used meticulously. (Guillebaud J. The Pill Oxford: Oxford University Press, 1984.) For further detail see also Vessey M et al. Lancet 1982; 1:841.

Mortality per 100,000 users per annum

women 20–34 years	
oral contraceptives	2–4 deaths with each method
intra-uterine device	
vaginal diaphragm	
women 35–44 years	
oral contraceptives	20
intra-uterine device	2
vaginal diaphragm	2

Cancer, see p. 704.

Additional risk factors. Age, smoking, hyperlipidaemia, diabetes, hypertension and obesity are all associated with increased risk of cardiovascular complications. It seems likely the associations are causal.

When it is certain that an individual man or woman will not wish to reproduce again then the question arises whether sterilisation is preferable to continuing to use reversible methods of contraception. Vasectomy carries little morbidity and virtually no mortality. Female sterilisation does carry hazard but is safer than continued use of reversible methods. However, further consideration of these matters, which involve many factors in addition to medical safety, is beyond the scope of this book.

Male contraception (systemic)

Suppression of spermatogenesis may be achieved by interfering with:

1. Extra-gonadal endocrine control, i.e. the hypothalamic pituitary gonadal axis,
2. Direct action on gonadal spermatogenesis.
3. Vaccines to produce antibodies to sperm

Approaches include combinations of androgen with danazol, or progestogen, or oestrogen, also gonadorelin. Gossypol, a phenol from the cotton plant*, is being evaluated in China but appears to have unacceptable adverse effects, e.g. hypokalaemia.

Natural regulators of mitosis (chalones) are tissue specific, and their identification should allow synthesis of analogues that might provide the necessary specificity and reversibility to deserve trial as male contraceptives. Whether a risk of genetic damage is inherent in drugs acting on spermatogenesis is unknown. The obvious biological problems of male contraception (need for continuous effect as opposed to elimination of a single regular event) plus the ready availability of female contraception, plus the fact that men do not get pregnant, reduce the incentives to seek and to use contraceptives for men.

Development of new contraceptives (see also Ch. 3)

Extension of the range of contraceptives (chemical or hormonal) to include new mechanisms of action, and especially to include men, has been the subject of social and political demand. This is partly because current contraceptives are imperfect, not only with regard to safety, efficacy and convenience, but also with regard to cultural, socioeconomic and religious aspects. The first combined oestrogen–progestogen pill was developed over 5 years. Development of a new agent that is not just a variant of existing agents is now likely to require 15 to 20 years and the cost will be enormous. The reasons for this are summarised by Diczfalusy†.

Assuming that basic research has discovered *an agent that selectively inhibits sperm motility* and a programme is launched to develop from it a successful contraceptive for men:

1. Variants of the new compound must be synthesised and tested in animals for efficacy, to ensure that the analogue most likely to succeed will go forward (tests in animals are not necessarily reliable predictors for man). This process is likely to take 4–6 years.
2. Once a compound has been selected for development, substantially larger quantities (above those hitherto made in the laboratory) will be needed for toxicological studies in animals, and a pilot manufacturing plant will be required. The plant development and the pharmacokinetic and

* Attention was drawn to gossypol by the high prevalence of male infertility in rural areas where food was cooked in cottonseed oil.

† See Diczfalusy E. In Haspels A A, Rolland R, eds. *Benefits and risks of hormonal contraception,* Lancaster: MTP Press, 1982.

long-duration toxicological studies will occupy another 4–6 years.

3. Application may then be made to an official regulatory body to begin studies in man. The data will be subject to detailed and unhurried scrutiny by regulators concerned for the safety of potential subjects, but also concerned for their own reputations in this particularly sensitive area of drug use in healthy people. Regulatory review will take from months to a year or more.

4. The phase I human studies will then take about one year.

5. At this stage full carcinogenicity studies will be started, and these cannot take less than 2 years in rodents. If studies in longer-lived animals, such as dogs, are required by the regulatory body, these may need about 7 years (in parallel with other development activities).

6. When the phase 2 studies are completed, then large formal phase 3 studies will take place (involving thousands of subjects) for efficacy and safety. There will be detailed studies of all possible adverse biochemical effects. It will be necessary to determine how readily fertility returns after cessation of use and whether there is risk of abnormal offspring. The list of precautions seems almost endless, and most of them will have their advocates.

The formulation must be stable for years in all climates.

The new contraceptive may fail at any stage.

Even if everything also goes well, quite minor side-effects (in a medical sense) will be sufficient to render the agent unacceptable to users.

7. At the end of phase 3 studies there will be major regulatory review that is unlikely to take less than one year.

8. The investment of resources and money in such a programme has to be colossal (10s, even 100s of millions of US dollars) and there is a very real risk that the whole investment will be lost. Whether the research and development is funded by the state (or international consortia or organisations) or by private enterprise, those who are in a position to allocate resources on the scale needed will be few, and they will require a lot of persuading that the techniques currently available are so bad that a fully funded programme for alternatives should be a priority over other social and commerical needs. But, some research is proceeding and it is to be hoped that a happy and serendipitous event may lead to success by a short cut.

Development of new female hormonal contraceptives

Regulatory bodies generally require that the preparation be used in at least 20,000 cycles with a quarter of the data derived from long-term use.

New drugs or methods will be subject to close scrutiny as to whether they truly prevent conception or induce abortion, a distinction that raises moral issues.

MENSTRUAL DISORDERS

Only a note on the simpler uses of hormones in menstrual disorders is appropriate here.

Amenorrhoea, primary or secondary, requires specialist endocrinological diagnosis. Where the cause is failure of hormone production, cyclical replacement therapy is indicated.

Severe menstrual bleeding can be controlled *during bleeding*, generally within 48 hours, by a progestogen (norethisterone 10–15 mg/day but up to 30 mg in very severe cases); it is given for 10 days. To prevent an *anticipated* excessive bleed; give 10 mg/day from 19th to 26th days of the cycle. There will be withdrawal bleeding. This may be followed by cycle control with an oestrogen–progestogen combination (an oral contraceptive will serve). Danazol can also be effective. Other agents that may help resistant cases of excessive menstrual loss include antifibrinolytic agents (aminocaproic acid, tranexamic acid), indomethacin or mefenamic acid (to inhibit prostaglandin synthesis) just before and during menstruation and ethamsylate (to increase capillary resistance), but none of these is treatment of first choice.

Less severe cases, i.e. moderately heavy periods, are likely to respond to prostaglandin synthetase inhibition, e.g. mefenamic acid 500 mg when the blood loss becomes heavy followed by 250 mg × 3/day for 3 days if necessary.

The timing of menstruation

Sometimes there are pressing social reasons for preventing menstruation at the normal time, but obviously this cannot be done at the last moment.

Menstruation can be postponed by giving norethisterone 5 mg ×3/day, from the 20th day of the cycle for up to 20 days; bleeding occurs on withdrawal. If started after the 20th day, then success becomes progressively less likely; but the same dose may be effective if given for 3 days before the expected onset of menstruation. Users of the combined oral contraceptive pill can simply continue with active pills when they would normally stop for 7 days.

The need to bleed monthly is not fundamental to health, and hormone regimens that provide one bleed every 3 months (tricycle regimen) may be used for those who prefer it.

Menstruation can be advanced by giving a progestogen–oestrogen combination such as an oral contraceptive for 14 days, when withdrawal will bring on bleeding. The shorter the time the mixture is given, the less likely becomes success.

Although there is no evidence that harm follows such manoeuvres, it is obviously foolish to practise them frequently in an individual.

Endometriosis. It has been observed that endometriosis is benefited by pregnancy and so a 'pseudopregnancy treatment' has been practised, by giving an oestrogen–progestogen oral contraceptive for about 9 months; marked improvement and even cure may result. But a progestogen (norethisterone) or danazol are now often preferred.

Dysmenorrhoea is due to uterine contractions resulting from excess prostaglandins in the uterus during ovulatory cycles. It can be treated by using inhibitors of prostaglandin synthesis (aspirin, indomethacin, naproxen, etc.) or by inducing anovulatory cycles (oral contraception).

The analgesic prostaglandin synthetase inhibitor (NSAID) may need to be given for several days before menstruation or only at the time of the pain.

Premenstrual tension syndrome may be due to an imbalance of natural oestrogen and progesterone secretion, but knowledge of the syndrome remains imprecise.

There is evidence for and against:

1. Restriction of salt and fluid and a thiazide diuretic in the second half of the menstrual cycle, or

2. Administration of a progestogen in the second half of the cycle, e.g. norethisterone 10–15 mg a day, orally.

3. Use of an oestrogen–progestogen oral contraceptive.

4. Bromocriptine, especially where there is breast pain.

Non-specific treatment includes reassurance, sympathy and, inevitably, a benzodiazepine anxiolytic.

MYOMETRIUM: ERGOT

'He gently prevails on his patient to try
The magic effects of the ergot of rye.'
(attributed to Alfred, Lord Tennyson, 1809–1892)

Ergot is a fungus which preys on grasses, especially rye. For medical production the plant is artificially infected.

The history of ergot is infamous, for consumption of bread made from infected rye has caused epidemics of painful gangrene of the extremities due to its vascular effects. The disease was called St Anthony's Fire because sufferers experienced relief by visiting the saint's shrine in Padova, Italy, because they had left the area where contaminated grain was being used, or by supernatural intervention. Fits and mental disorder were also a feature of these epidemics, but it is not known whether these were partly due to concurrent nutritional deficiencies.

Ergotism is now very rare but an epidemic was reported in England in 1928* and in France in 1951†, although the genuineness of both these has been questioned.

The discovery of the chief alkaloids of ergot, all derivatives of lysergic acid, presents an interesting chapter in the history of both pharmacology and therapeutics. At the beginning of the century pharmacologists investigated ergot and found ergotamine (a principal alkaloid), ergotoxine (later

* Robertson J et al. Br Med J 1928; 1:302.
† Gabbai et al. Br Med J 1951; 2:650 and editorial, ibid., 596.

found to be a mixture of three alkaloids), and histamine, acetylcholine and tyramine, amongst other things. Ergometrine (ergonovine) was found in 1935.

Before 1935 some clinicians maintained that the uterine effect of ergot extracts was not all accounted for by the known constituents, and their view was supported by the fact that the then current Pharmacopoeial method of preparing the extracts effectively removed the known orally active constituents. In 1932, a newly formed Pharmacopoeial Committee decided that it was time that they either stopped the elimination of the active principles or else found out what unknown substance was rendering the extracts active, if indeed they were active. The Committee invited Dr. Chassar Moir* to investigate the subject for them.

The hospital pharmacist prepared an extract according to Pharmocopoeial regulations, i.e. it should, according to current knowledge, have been inert. Moir administered it to parturient patients and recorded the results with a balloon in the uterus attached to a manometer. 'It was with the greatest surprise I found that, far from being inert, this preparation surpassed by great measure the activity of any drug which I had previously used in the same manner.' He also observed that the rate of onset and type of contractions differed from those characteristic of ergotoxine and ergotamine. Moir could only suppose that these effects were due to an entirely new constituent of ergot and that those 'ergot alkaloids hitherto supposed to be all-important play in reality but subsidiary part in the clinical activity of the drug'. Sir Henry Dale, whose early work on the analysis of the constituents of ergot is a pharmacological classic,† commented on Moir's discovery. He wrote that another chapter had been opened 'and probably one of great importance, in the already complicated story of ergot and its active principles . . . Those acquainted with the present position, and its development during a quarter of a century, may be inclined to regard Dr. Moir's observations as a rebuke to the presumption of laboratory pharmacologists. They do, indeed, emphasise the danger of basing therapeutic conclusions on laboratory data, without direct clinical evidence. It is only fair to state, however, that the present position has arisen, not in spite of such evidence as Dr. Moir now supplied, but for lack of it. The need has been recognised and urged by some of us throughout the period in question; but, without such direct experimental guidance from the clinic, we could only search for the principles in ergot producing certain well-defined effects in the laboratory, and hope for the proper clinical trial of the substances so identified . . . I have, indeed, on more than one occasion endeavoured to get a proper experimental comparison made in the clinic. . . . More than one eminent gynaecologist was willing to carry out a test; but only by handing the extracts to a resident officer or ward sister, with an instruction to administer them to alternate patients as a routine and to record impressions of their respective values. It can safely be stated that, so far from affording data for a quantitative comparison, such a method would not even given trustworthy information as to whether either extract was active at all.' X . . . and Y . . . in the case of an extract of ergot 'were content to show that the ward sister could not distinguish its action from that of a "Marmite" solution, when both were given to alternate patients in the puerperium. The inference was that the liquid extract had no action, but Dr. Moir's experimental records show it to contain what may well prove to be the most important substance in ergot from the point of view of practical therapeutics.' This prediction was correct, for the substance was ergometrine.

Fortunately Moir's paper was published in a journal that has a correspondence column so that the subsequent clash of opinion between clinician and pharmacologist could take place in public.*

Aspects of the curiously complex pharmacology of ergot‡

Ergoline is basic to all ergot alkaloids, and it bears structural resemblance to the biogenic amines,

* Moir C. Br Med J 1932; 1:1119, 1189 and 2:75.
† Dale H H. J Physiol 1906; 34:163.

‡ Berde B, Schild H O, eds. (1978) Ergot alkaloids and related compounds. Berlin:Springer, 1978.

noradrenaline, adrenaline, dopamine and serotonin. Therefore it is no surprise that ergot derivatives can act as agonists, antagonists or both simultaneously, at these amine receptors. Indeed, it is combinations of these actions, on the receptors of these amines, that largely account for the multifarious actions of *ergot derivatives*, for example:

Co-dergocrine (Hydergine) is the most active α-adrenoceptor antagonist.

Ergotamine is the most active α-adrenoceptor agonist.

Methysergide is the most active serotonin (5-HT) antagonist.

Bromocriptine and pergolide are the most active dopamine receptor agonists.

Methylergometrine is most active uterine α-adrenoceptor agonist.

(But selectivity alters with changing drug concentrations and specificity may only be attained at carefully adjusted concentrations.)

Lysergide (LSD_{25}) is the most active hallucinogen (mechanism uncertain). But all supply of and research on LSD was stopped by the pharmaceutical firm that invented it following the surge of hallucinogen abuse in the early 1960s.

Bromocriptine provides an example of the exploitation of the extraordinarily wide spectrum of activities of ergot derivatives. Ergotoxine has oxytocic, cardiovascular and prolactin-inhibiting (dopaminergic) effects. Bromocriptine ($t_{\frac{1}{2}}$, 50 h) was the product of a research programme aimed at eliminating the oxytocic and cardiovascular effects whilst retaining the prolactin-inhibiting effect. The result has been a useful dopamine receptor agonist which suppresses lactation, benefits types of hypogonadism associated with hyperprolactinaemia (which affects gonadotrophin secretion), and also has some efficacy in parkinsonism; it increases growth hormone release in healthy people but suppresses it in acromegaly. (see also index.)

In senile cerebral insufficiency there is some evidence that *co-dergocrine* and nicergoline induce a receptor-mediated increase in cyclic-AMP that affects cerebral blood flow and metabolism; three types of receptor seem to be involved, α-adrenoceptors, serotonin receptors and dopamine receptors.

Ergot has been justly termed ‘a treasure chest for pharmacologists’. and it is by no means certain that the treasure chest is yet empty.

Individual alkaloids (see above and also index); they are subject to hepatic metabolism.

Ergotamine, see *migraine*. Ergotamine causes vasoconstriction (arteries and veins), which may be sufficient to cause hypertension, by an α-adrenoceptor agonist action and also by sensitising to endogenously released noradrenaline. The degree of vasoconstriction is determined by the pre-existing vascular tone. The $t_{\frac{1}{2}}$ of ergotamine is about 2 h, but tissue storage allows prolonged action, so that if it is being given several times a day for migraine there is short-term accumulation that can be dangerous, causing peripheral gangrene, for which sodium nitroprusside i.v. may be used. **Dihydroergotamine** constricts veins particularly and has efficacy in prophylaxis of deep vein thrombosis in the legs after surgery (the blood flow faster in the constricted large veins).

Ergometrine (ergonovine) is now the only ergot alkaloid used for stimulating uterine activity, as ergotamine is slow in acting even after i.v. injection, whereas ergometrine acts immediately when injected i.v. Serious circulatory side-effects are also less frequent (see below). The uterus is stimulated at all times, but is much more sensitive in late pregnancy.

Ergometrine and oxytocin differ in their actions on the uterus. In moderate doses oxytocin produces slow generalised contractions with full relaxation in between; ergometrine produces faster contractions superimposed on a tonic contraction. High doses of both substances produce sustained tonic contraction. It will be seen, therefore, that oxytocin is more suited to induction of labour and ergometrine to the prevention and treatment of post-partum haemorrhage, the incidence of which is reduced by its routine prophylactic use (generally i.m.).

Ergometrine (250, 500 μg) may be given:

orally, 0.5–1 mg, when action begins in about 8 min and lasts about 1 hour.

i.v., 100–500 μg; onset of action about 1 min; used as treatment of established post-partum haemorrhage.

i.m., 250–500 μg; action begins in about 2 min; the onset is speeded by mixing hyaluronidase (1500 units) with the injection, and is about as quick as i.v. injection. This combination is appropriate for use by birth attendants who are not allowed to give an i.v. injection. Oxytocin i.m. is an alternative for quick (but brief) action. Plainly speed of onset can be vital if the woman is bleeding profusely. Oxytocin has therefore been mixed with ergometrine (Syntometrine: ergometrine 500 μg plus oxytocin 5 IU) to obtain the advantages of quick onset of action and prolonged effect.

When given during labour the timing of the injection is the subject of disagreement. It is commonly given when the anterior shoulder of the child is delivered, but some give it earlier at the crowning of the head (never before this) or later when the placenta has separated or has been delivered. Ergometrine tablets may be given orally (0.5–1 mg) twice a day in the early puerperium if bleeding occurs, or in incomplete abortion.

The occurrence of **hypertension**, lasting hours or even days after ergometrine has been belatedly recognised. The incidence of this effect may be less with methylergometrine. It seems that in some patients the ergometrine is capable of inducing vascular effects of a magnitude similar to those of ergotamine. It is most likely to occur in toxaemic patients* and in cases where sympathomimetic vasoconstrictors have been used, e.g. with a local anaesthetic. It can be severe and complaints of headache post-partum should be taken seriously. The blood pressure can be reduced by chlorpromazine (10–15 mg) i.v. or i.m. and then larger doses orally, or by any other α-adrenoceptor blocking drug. Ergometrine can also cause hypotension.

Methysergide, see *migraine* and above.

Co-dergocrine (Hydergine) is a mixture of hydrogenated alkaloids, dihydroergocryptine, -cristine, -cornine, see above. Its modest beneficial effects on impaired mental function in the aged are the result of metabolic changes (see above) and not due to changes in blood flow. For this purpose it may be given for up to 8 weeks and abandoned if obvious benefit is not seen.

Adverse effects of ergot derivatives are mostly predictable from the various receptor actions mentioned above.

CNS. Vomiting due to dopaminergic effect on the chemoreceptor trigger zone. Hypotension, especially postural, due to depression of the vasomotor centre, which is enhanced by peripheral α-adrenoceptor block (hydrogenated alkaloids).

Overdose causes, confusion, depression, convulsions and a variety of neurological syndromes, probably vascular in origin.

Peripheral vessels, constriction even to gangrene (ergotamine) occurs and this alkaloid is dangerous in patients with peripheral vascular or ischaemic cardiac disease.

Blood pressure may rise or fall according to the varying central and peripheral receptor effects.

Oxytocin is a hormone of the posterior pituitary gland (see p. 693) it stimulates the contractions of the pregnant uterus, which becomes much more sensitive to it at term. However, patients with diabetes insipidus go into labour normally. The mechanisms governing the initiation and maintenance of labour remain uncertain but oxytocin plays a part.

Oxytocin is reflexly released from the pituitary following suckling (and manual stimulation) and causes contraction of the myoepithelium of the breast; it can be used to enhance milk ejection (nasal spray). The only other clinically important effect is on the blood pressure, which may fall if an overdose is given.

Synthetic oxytocin (Syntocinon) is pure and is not contaminated with vasopressin as is the natural product. It is therefore safer if high doses must be given.

Oxytocin is used in the **induction of labour**, and sometimes for uterine inertia, haemorrhage or during abortion. It produces rhythmic contractions with relaxation between, i.e. it mimics normal uterine activity. The association of oxytocin with neonatal jaundice appears to be due to reduced red cell deformability causing haemolysis.

The decision to use it requires special skill. Oxytocin has a $t_{\frac{1}{2}}$ of 5–10 min and is ordinarily given by i.v. infusion. The buccal route is practicable, but dosage is less controllable due to irregular absorption and uterine rupture can occur.

Oxytocin is structurally close to vasopressin and it is no surprise that it also has antidiuretic activity. Serious water intoxication can occur with prolonged i.v. infusions, especially where accompanied by large volumes of fluid.

* Synthetic oxytocin (Syntocin) is preferable in such patients.

Oxytocin has been supplanted by ergometrine as prime treatment of post-partum haemorrhage except when, as occasionally happens, there is no response to ergometrine. There are advantages in a mixture of oxytocin and ergometrine (Syntometrine, see above).

PROSTAGLANDINS

Prostaglandins (modified fatty acids) were discovered in 1935. They were overhastily named after the prostate gland from which it was supposed that they derived (actually it was the seminal vesicles), but the name has persisted even though it is now known that they occur throughout the body, including the CNS, adrenals, liver, kidney, and gut, where they are both humoural and neurotransmitters.

Prostaglandins are the result of enzymic synthesis from arachidonic acid (Fig. 37.1).

Prostaglandins are principal *mediators of inflammation* and important anti-inflammatory and analgesic drugs (aspirin, indomethacin, etc.) act by inhibiting cyclooxygenase, thus reducing synthesis of prostaglandins; they are prostaglandin synthetase inhibitors; fever may be caused by prostaglandin release.

Prostaglandins induce cellular (including blood platelet) cyclic-AMP production and can stimulate and relax smooth muscle at different sites and affect platelet aggregation.

The arrows in the diagram indicate synthetic paths mediated by enzymes. Selective inhibitors, e.g. of thromboxane synthesis, sparing prostacyclin synthesis, would be of interest as potential therapeutic agents in thrombosis. Aspirin acts at an early stage and so is unselective with regard to the three end products.

An alternative fatty acid precursor to arachidonic acid (occurs in land animal fats), such as eicosapentaenoic acid (occurs in fish oils) promotes prostacyclin synthesis rather than thromboxane synthesis, thus shifting the balance of the system against thrombosis; see also *thrombosis*.

Prostacyclins inhibit platelet aggregation by increasing platelet cyclic AMP, and dipyridamole delays destruction of cyclic AMP (by inhibiting the enzyme phosphodiesterase) and so enhances prostacyclin effect.

All these substances are formed in varying amounts in tissues all over the body, including blood vessels.

Prostaglandins have many actions that differ according to the particular compound used, the activity of enzymic paths and the physiological state of the target organ. According to circumstance they can cause smooth muscle (vascular, uterine, bronchial) to contract or to relax. It is evident that their therapeutic potential involves considerations of great physiological complexity.

There are at least 14 naturally occurring prostaglandins. They are *named* in a complex fashion dictated by their chemical structure. There are six

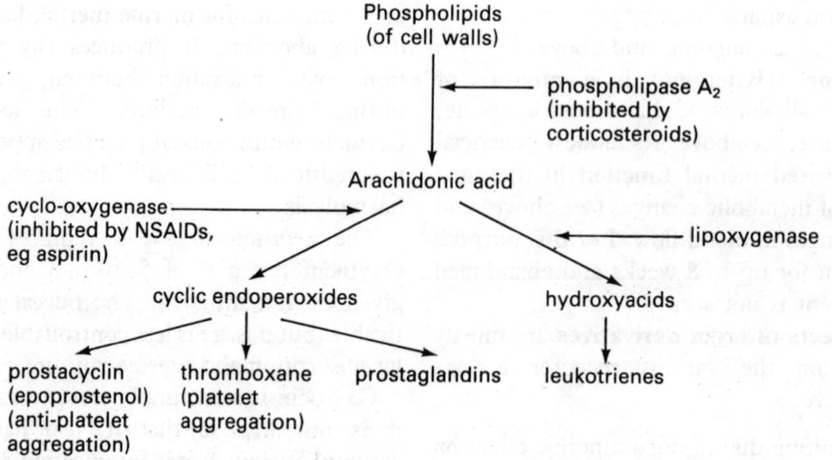

Fig. 37.1 Synthesis of prostaglandins

'primary' natural prostaglandins (PGE_1, PGE_2, PGE_3, $PGF_{1\alpha}$, $PGF_{2\alpha}$, $PGF_{3\alpha}$) and eight other natural prostaglandins derived metabolically from them. Prostaglandins can be synthesised. Their use in a variety of areas of medicine is being explored — asthma, peptic ulcer and vascular disease; but the following have so far found a role:

Dinoprost (prostaglandin $F_{2\alpha}$; $PGF_{2\alpha}$; Prostin F2 alpha) and **dinoprostone** (prostaglandin E_2; PGE_2; Prostin E2) are used to induce abortion, including missed or partial abortion and in the treatment of hydatidiform mole; they are given by intra or extra-amniotic injection, by vaginal tablet, by i.v. infusion or by mouth. Their safe and effective use (including choice of route) requires special skill. Adverse effects include vomiting, diarrhoea, headache, pyrexia, local tissue reaction, etc.

Alprostadil (prostaglandin E_1; PGE_1; Prostin VR) is used to maintain the patency of the ductus arteriosus in neonates with congenital heart abnormalities until corrective surgery can be undertaken. The ductus is normally kept patent by endogenous prostaglandin production and inhibitors of prostaglandin synthetase (NSAIDs) given to the mother can cause its closure (either unintended or intended according to circumstances).

Epoprostenol (prostacyclin; Flolan) is naturally produced by the intima of blood vessels; it is a potent blood platelet aggregation inhibitor (reduces procoagulant activity and the release of heparin neutralising factor) and platelet preserver; it is also a potent vasodilator. It is given by i.v. infusion ($t_{\frac{1}{2}}$, 3 min); the actions cease 30 min after cessation of administration. It is used particularly when it is desired to preserve platelets, e.g. cardiopulmonary bypass, renal dialysis, charcoal haemoperfusion (see index), retinal vein occlusion (first 48 h).

Misoprostol, see peptic ulcer.

Use of drugs and morality. Increasingly, drug use is a cause of moral and social, as well as of technical problems and this is particularly so in the field of reproduction (contraception and abortion).

Some doctors regard such uses as impermissible under any circumstances, as permissible under certain circumstances or as morally indifferent. In any case it is desirable that they should be *technically* informed if they are in any form of practice that may result in their meeting patients who may be taking or seeking such treatment.

Since pharmacological considerations are not fundamental to moral decisions, these contentious issues will not be discussed here.

UTERINE RELAXANTS

β_2-adrenoceptor agonists relax the uterus and are employed by obstetricians to inhibit *premature labour* (e.g. isoxsuprine, orciprenaline, terbutaline ritodrine, salbutamol); their use is complicated by the expected cardiovascular effects.

Alcohol (ethanol) can also inhibit premature labour by inhibiting secretion of oxytocin by the posterior pituitary (just as it causes diuresis by inhibiting vasopressin secretion). Its other effects render it unsuitable in most cases.

GUIDE TO FURTHER READING

1 Hockaday T D R. Assessment of pituitary function. Br Med J 1983; 287:1738.
2 Eaton A C. Cyproterone acetate in treatment of post-orchidectomy hot flushes. Lancet 1983; 2:1336.
3 Reichlin S. Somatostatin. N Engl J Med 1983; 309:1495, 1556.
4 Brook C G D. Management of delayed puberty. Br Med J 1985; 290:657.
5 Dixon A St J. Non-hormonal treatment of osteoporosis. Br Med J 1983; 286:999.
6 Editorial. Diabetes insipidus — turning off the tap. Br Med J 1977; 1:1050.
7 Forrest J N et al. Superiority of demeclocycline over lithium in the treatment of chronic syndrome of inappropriate secretion of antidiuretic hormone. N Engl J Med 1978; 298:173.
8 Yasmuth C et al. Ovarian suppressants in dogs: pilot study of an approach to rabies control. Lancet 1970; 1:1312.
9 Walker S et al. Controlled trial of bromocriptine, quinestrol and placebo in suppression of puerperal lactation. Lancet 1975; 2:542.
10 Horsman A et al. The effect of oestrogen dose on postmenopausal bone loss. N Engl J Med 1983; 309:1405.
11 Underwood L E. Report of the conference on uses and possible abuses of biosynthetic human growth hormone. N Engl J Med 1984; 311:606.
12 Waxman J. Analogies of gonadotrophin releasing hormone. Br Med J 1984; 288:426.
13 Mason P et al. Induction of ovulation with pulsatile luteinising hormone releasing hormone. Br Med J 1984; 288:181.

14 Editorial. Anabolics in meat production. Lancet 1982; 1:721.
15 Goldfarb J M et al. Abnormal vaginal bleeding. N Engl J Med 1980; 302:666.
16 Herbst A L. Diethylstilbestrol exposure — 1984. N Engl J Med 1984; 311:1433.
17 Vaitukaitis J L et al. Premenstrual syndrome. N Engl J Med 1984; 311:1371.
18 Elder M G. Prostaglandins and menstrual disorders. Br Med J 1983; 287:703.
19 Healy D L et al. The antiprogesterones are coming: menses induction, abortion and labour. Br Med J 1985; 290:580.
20 Feeney J G. Water intoxication and oxytocin. Br Med J 1982; 285:243.
21 Editorial. Drug treatment of premature labour Br Med J 1981; 283:395.
22 Abernethy D R et al. Imipramine disposition in users of oral contraceptive steroids. Clin Pharmacol Ther 1984; 35:792.
23 Meffin P J et al. Alterations in prednisolone disposition as a result of oral contraceptive use and dose. Br J Clin Pharmacol 1984; 17:655.
24 Ellinwood E H et al. Effects of oral contraceptives on diazepam-induced psychomotor impairment. Clin Pharmacol Ther 1984; 35:360.
25 Artunes C M F et al. Endometrial cancer and oestrogen use: report of a large case-control study. N Engl J Med 1979; 300:9.
26 Horwitz R I et al. Necropsy diagnosis of endometrial cancer and detection bias in case-control studies. Lancet 1981; 2:66.
27 Petitti D B et al. Uses of oral contraceptives, cigarette smoking and risk of subarachnoid haemorrhage. Lancet 1978; 2:234.
28 Morrison A S et al. Oral contraceptives and hepatitis: a report from the Boston Collaborative Drug Surveillance Program. Lancet 1977; 1:1142.
29 WHO Collaborative Study of Neoplasia and Steroid Contraceptives. Invasive cervical cancer and combined oral contraceptives. Br Med J 1985; 290:961.
30 Royal College of General Practitioners. Breast cancer and oral contraceptives. Br Med J 1981; 282:2089.
31 Wahl P et al. Effect of estrogen/progestin potency on lipid/lipoprotein cholesterol. N Engl J Med 1983; 308:862.
32 Drife J. Which pill? Br Med J 1983; 287:1397.
33 Stalel B V. Oral contraceptives and cardiovascular disease. N Engl J Med 1981; 305:612, 672.
34 Vessey M et al. Efficacy of different contraceptive methods. Lancet 1982; 1:841.
35 Vessey M P et al. Fertility after stopping different methods of contraception. Br Med J 1978; 1:265.
36 Editorial. Drug interaction with oral contraceptive steroids. Br Med J 1980; 2:93.
37 Böttiger L E et al. Oral contraceptives and thromboembolic disease: effects of lowering oestrogen content. Lancet 1980; 1:1097.
38 Fraser H M. New prospects for luteinising hormone releasing hormone as a contraceptive and therapeutic agent. Br Med J 1982; 285:990.
39 Rowlands S. Morning-after pills. Br Med J 1982; 285:322.
40 Drife J O. Drugs and sperm. Br Med J 1982; 284:844.
41 Editorial. Gossypol prospects. Lancet 1984; 1:1108.
42 Royal College of General Practitioners. Reduction in incidence of rheumatoid arthritis associated with oral contraceptives. Lancet 1978; 1:569.
43 Poller L et al. Effects of manufacturing oral contraceptives on blood clotting. Br Med J 1979; 1:1761.
44 Fara G M et al. Epidemic of breast enlargement in an Italian school. Lancet 1979; 2:295.
45 Adams D B et al. Rise in female-initiated sexual activity at ovulation and its suppression by oral contraceptives. N Engl J Med 1978; 299:1145, and comment, 1186.
46 Thomson J et al. Effect of oestrogen on the sleep, mood and anxiety of menopausal women. Br Med J 1977; 2:1317.
47 Weber W W et al. Drug contamination with diethylstilboestrol: outbreak of precocious puberty due to contaminated INH. N Engl J Med 1963; 268:411.
48 Moir J C. The obstetrician bids and the uterus contracts. Br Med J 1964; 2:1025.
49 Embrey M P et al. Use of Syntometrine in prevention of post-partum haemorrhage. Br Med J 1963; 1:1387.
50 Brooke O G et al. Effect of ergotamine and ergometrine on forearm venous compliance in man. Br Med J 1970; 1:139.

38

Malignant disease: Cytotoxic chemotherapy, immunosuppression

Malignant disease is of immense variety. **Prevention**, by drugs, of the genetic change, whether spontaneous or induced by chemicals or viruses, that converts a normal cell to an invasive malignant cell has not yet been attained. However, some cancers can be prevented, wholly or in part, by protecting people or inviting them to protect themselves from exposure to known carcinogens (industrial cancers, bronchial cancer).

Attempts to **cure** cancer employ four principal modes:

1. surgery
2. radiotherapy
3. chemotherapy*
4. endocrine therapy
(5. immunotherapy, experimental)

Details of the exploitation of these techniques, whether alone, sequentially or concurrently is beyond the scope of a book on clinical pharmacology. This account will be substantially confined to drugs.

* Although not in strict accord with the definition of Ch. 11 the word chemotherapy is in general use in this connection and it would be pedantic to avoid it. It arose because some malignant cells can be cultured and the disease transmitted by inoculation as with bacteria. Some prefer to call it anticytotic or cytotoxic therapy.

The possibility of interfering with cancer other than by surgery, e.g. by endocrine alteration, was first tested in 1895 when a Scottish surgeon faced with a woman aged 33 years with advanced breast cancer 'put it to her husband and herself as to whether she should have performed the operation of removal of the tubes and ovaries. Its nature was fully explained to them both, and also that it was a purely experimental one . . . She readily consented . . . as she knew and felt her case was hopeless.'† Eight months after operation 'all vestiges of her previous cancerous disease had disappeared' A second case treated by oophorectomy in a near menopausal woman showed some improvement, and a third in a post-menopausal woman showed none. The surgeon concluded that there may be ovarian influences in breast cancer and added that 'whether (this is) accepted or not, I am sure I shall be acquitted of having acted thoughtlessly or recklessly, and it will be believed that in all I have done I have had some reason for the faith that is in me, and that I have been actuated solely by the motives that guide all of us in the exercise of our profession — primarily the interests of those who place themselves under our care, and secondarily, the progress and advancement of the healing art'.

The treatment had indeed been based on reason. The author, 20 years previously, had agreed to take charge of a Scottish landowner 'whose mind was affected' and went to reside on one of the patient's estates in the rural west of Scotland. His duties 'were at times exciting, but never onerous', and, having the time and the interest to observe the weaning of lambs on a local

† Beatson G T. Lancet 1896; 2: 104, 162.

farm, he began an MD thesis on lactation. He observed a similarity 'up to a point' between the proliferation of epithelial cells of the milk ducts in lactation and in cancer; he learned that some farmers practised oophorectomy to prolong lactation in cows; and he had the idea that cancer of the breast might be due to an abnormal ovarian stimulus and that removal of the ovaries might have therapeutic effect on cancer of the genital tract.

Delayed by an initial unsuccessful operation on advanced uterine cancer, by 'the rise and progress of bacteriology' which gave hope that the true cause of cancer might be found, and by unwillingness 'to do anything of the nature of experiments of my fellow creatures', he eventually, after 20 years, made the first demonstration (above) that some cases of breast cancer are dependent on ovarian function.

In 1941* it was shown that prostatic cancer with metastases was made worse by androgen and made better by oestrogen (stilboestrol). Activity of this cancer was particularly readily observable since the plasma acid phosphatase concentration provides a reliable 'marker'. Indeed the availability of some means of reliably measuring effect is crucial to the use of drugs in cancer (see also later).

Sulphur mustards (oily vesicant liquids) had been developed and used as chemical weapons in World War I (1914–18). Amongst their actions depression of haemopoiesis and of lymphoid tissues were observed.

Preparations for World War II (1939–45) included research to increase the potency and toxicity ('efficacy') of these odious substances. It was found that substitution of a nitrogen atom for the sulphur atom, i.e. making nitrogen mustards, had the desired result. The disappearance of lymphocytes and granulocytes from the blood of rabbits was a useful indicator (marker) of toxicity and gave rise to the idea of possible efficacy in lymphoid cancer. 'The problem was fundamental and simple: could one destroy a tumour with this group of cytotoxic agents before destroying the host?'

* Huggins C et al. Cancer Res 1941; 1:293.

Nitrogen mustards, as anticancer agents, were first tested on experimental lymphoma in mice and the results were sufficiently encouraging to warrant a therapeutic trial in man, 'an X-ray resistant patient in terminal stages of lymphosarcoma was selected as a suitable subject. The tumour masses involved the axilla, mediastinum, face and submental regions, with resulting cyanosis, venous dilatation and oedema of the face and upper part of the chest. Chewing and swallowing had become almost impossible and a tracheotomy set was kept close at hand for immediate use . . . The response of the first patient was as dramatic as that of the first mouse', following 10 days treatment. *But* severe bone marrow depression, delayed for 3–4 weeks, occurred and, disappointingly, as the bone marrow recovered, so did the tumour; in addition, with further courses, it rapidly became resistant. 'Twenty years later (1963) we can appreciate how accurately this first patient reflected the future trials and tribulations of therapy with alkylating agents'.†

The development of other agents, e.g. antimetabolites, soon followed.

Chemotherapy depends on developing drugs that are selective for the malignant cells and leave those of the host unharmed. Development would be greatly assisted if models of the human disease could be set up in the laboratory. Unfortunately this is a great difficulty with cancer; animal tumours and tissue cultures of human tumours are used in screening for effect but their relationship to human cancer is remote and the effectiveness of anticancer agents must finally be determined in humans with cancer.

The comparative success of antimicrobial chemotherapy is due to the fact that the metabolism of the parasite differs qualitatively from that of host cells. But cancer cells are host cells that differ from normal cells quantitatively rather than qualitatively, and to attain adequate selectivity it is necessary to take into account and exploit every possible factor that may improve the therapeutic index, including not only the inherent sensitivity of the malignant cell to drugs but also its endo-

† Gilman A. Am J Surg 1963; 105:574.

crine environment, the number of cells dividing at any one time, the total number of cells (size of the tumour), the kinetics of the drugs and, most important, the rate of recovery of normal tissues from the unavoidable effects of the drugs.

Infection with micro-organisms normally causes an immune response and antibacterial drugs can therefore be cytostatic — the host defence mechanisms of the body eliminating the bacteria whose replication has been arrested. But there is no substantial immune response to cancer (even though attempts are being made to strengthen such response as there is) and cure can only be achieved by killing or removing cancer cells.

Thus in cancer the cells are relatively closely allied to the normal cells and must be killed by treatment. Whereas in bacterial infections the cells are markedly different from the normal host cells and generally a treatment that arrests growth is sufficient.

Drug therapy cannot be conducted rationally without some understanding of the disease as well as of the drugs. Since cancer is not a single disease but many, the following notes must be confined to what is usually true.

CYTOTOXIC CHEMOTHERAPY

Tumour characteristics influencing chemotherapy

A. **Cancers**, despite their variability, share some common characteristics:*

1. Growth that is not subject to normal restrictions for that tissue.
2. Local invasiveness.
3. Tendency to spread to other parts of the body (metastasis).
4. Less differentiated cell morphology.
5. Tendency to retain some characteristics of the tissue of origin.

B. **Survival**. In experimental leukaemia, for example, it has been shown that:

1. survival time is inversely related to the initial number of leukaemia cells, or to the number remaining after treatment.
2. a single leukaemia cell is capable of multiplying and eventually killing the host.

* WHO Tech. Rep. 605 (1977). Chemotherapy of solid tumours. Geneva. A general reference for this chapter.

C. **Cell kinetics**. It used to be thought that cancer cells divided more rapidly than any normal cells, but this is not so, and bone marrow, mucosal surfaces (gut), hair follicles, reticulo-endothelial system, germ cells, are all dividing more rapidly than many cancers and are targets for drugs, as is shown by the occurrence of adverse effects on these tissues during chemotherapy. Most solid tumours in man divide slowly and recovery from cytotoxic agents is slow but normal marrow and gut recover rapidly. This rapid recovery of normal tissues is exploited in devising intermittent courses of chemotherapy.

In cancer, the normal feedback mechanism (perhaps from cell contact phenomena), which restricts cell multiplication when it has reached optimal amount does not function, and cells continue to grow, at first exponentially, i.e. faster and faster as the numbers increase; until later there is a slowing down and the volume-doubling time becomes prolonged due to several factors, most of which conspire to render the *ageing cancer less susceptible to drugs*:

1. increased cell cycle (division) time
2. decrease in the number of cells actively dividing, with more in the resting state.
3. increased cell death within the tumour as it ages
4. overcrowding of cells leading to defective nutrition (poor vascular supply) with defective access of drugs.

All cells engaged in division (cycling) go through a series of phases of synthesis of DNA, RNA, mitosis and rest.

In general *drugs are most active against actively cycling cells, and least active against resting cells.* These latter are particularly sinister in that they retain the capacity to proliferate and may start cycling again after a completed course of chemotherapy. In order to eliminate them it is necessary to develop drugs that are active against the resting phase, to prolong chemotherapy to catch them when they become active, or to induce synchronous activity so that they may all be simultaneously vulnerable to cycle or phase-specific drugs (below).*

Plainly all this has important implications for the practice of chemotherapy.

Principles of chemotherapy

A. Whilst **selectivity** of drugs for the cancer cell is generally low compared with selectivity of drugs against bacteria, in some tumours it can be substantial, as in lymphoma, in which the tumour cell kill with some drugs is 10 000 times as great as that of marrow cells. Techniques for targeting drugs to cancer cells are greatly needed.

B. **Cell destruction by drugs follows first-order kinetics**, i.e. a given dose of drug kills a constant *fraction* of cells (not a constant *number*) regardless of the number of cells present, i.e. a treatment reducing a cell population from 1 000 000 to 10 000 will reduce a cell population of 100 to one. Therefore, where there are many cells (late presentation, macroscopic disease) it is necessary to increase the dose of drug(s) and to repeat administration to the limit of patient (host) tolerance. But where the number of cells is small (microscopic disease), then complete eradication becomes possible at doses that are sub-toxic to the host. But cells remaining after initial doses are likely to be more resistant to drugs since cell sensitivity is not homogeneous at the outset due to random mutations as the tumour grows.

C. **Drug action and resistance**. *Drugs that kill cancer cells may be*:

1. *Cycle non-specific*: kill cells whether resting or actively cycling
2. *Cycle-specific*: kill only cells that are actively cycling
3. *Phase-specific*: kill only cells that are in a particular phase of the active cycle.

These considerations are relevant to the choice of drugs in combination chemotherapy, and to the desirability of attaining synchronisation of cell cycling to achieve maximum cell kill.

However well-chosen the drug, it will be ineffective if it does not reach the malignant cells at a high enough concentration for a long enough time at the right stage of the cell cycle, for the cells are not like receptors, to be acted upon at any time. Considerations of pharmacokinetics in relation to cell kinetics are of the first importance, as drug treatment modifies the activity of both malignant and normal cells.

Cell resistance to single drugs is both frequently present at the outset and develops readily with repeated use. Increased dosage is limited by toxicity, e.g. to bone marrow, which does not become tolerant. Therefore combination therapy is now the routine. Cell resistance may be due to various factors, as with bacteria, including: random mutation, changes in drug uptake by the cell, changes in metabolic activation of the drug, enzyme changes in the cell, development of alternative metabolic paths.

Additional and toxic drugs may then be needed to overcome resistance. Well-designed treatment at the outset lessens this problem. In those tumours where cures can be achieved by chemotherapy (acute lymphoblastic leukaemia in childhood, Hodgkin's lymphoma, choriocarcinoma) *adequate initial chemotherapy is of the first importance*. If inadequate therapy is used, drug-resistant cells emerge and subsequent cure with intensive chemotherapy becomes difficult or even impossible.

D. **Intermittent combination chemotherapy**. *Combinations of drugs are commonly used and repeated* (scheduling) according to the following considerations:

1. having differing biochemical sites of action in the cell
2. attacking cells at differing phases of the growth cycle
3. to synchronise the active cell cycles
4. use of drugs that do not suppress bone marrow in between courses of those that do
5. empirically

The logical basis of 1 and 2 (above) is obvious. But synchronisation (3 above) represents a refinement; for example, cells are killed or are arrested in mitosis by vincristine, which is then withdrawn so that the cells enter a new reproductive cycle more or less synchronously; and when the majority are judged to be in a phase sensitive to

* There are *circadian rhythms* in cell metabolism and proliferation and those of leukaemic cells differ from those of normal leucocytes. There is evidence that maintenance chemotherapy of some leukaemias is more effective if given in the evening. (Rivard G E et al. Lancet 1985; 2:1264.)

a particular phase-specific drug, then that drug is given; an example is vincristine followed by methotrexate or cytarabine.

In spite of the important kinetic considerations previously discussed it remains true that the vast majority of chemotherapy regimens have been devised by using a commonsense empiricism, and do not rely on detailed knowledge of tumour kinetics (which is at best meagre). The *drugs have been chosen,*

a. because they are known to be effective as single agents,
b. because the toxicities do not overlap greatly,
c. because, in trial and error (empirical) use, the margins of safety of the combination have been determined, and
d. because it is reasonably hoped that by mixing differing classes of agents with differing effects in the cell cycle a spectrum of activity against both dividing and non-dividing cells can be achieved, e.g. cycle non-specific agents first to reduce tumour cell mass, and cycle-specific drugs second.

Intermittent chemotherapy. After an attempt to get maximum cell-kill using drugs to the limit of normal host-cell tolerance, an interval must be left for sufficient recovery of the normal cells, including the recovery of immunological mechanisms that have been suppressed. An interval between courses of 2–3 weeks is usually enough.

The aggressive pursuit of cure by total cell kill is conducted with repeated courses of combinations of drugs known by their acronyms, e.g.:

ABVD: doxorubicin (*A*driamycin), *b*leomycin, *v*inblastine, *d*acarbazine

MOPP: *m*ustine, vincristine (*O*ncovin), *p*rocarbazine, *p*rednisolone

MVPP: *m*ustine, *v*inblastine, *p*rocarbazine, *p*rednisolone

But *single drug therapy* is adequate in some cancers (Burkitt's lymphoma, choriocarcinoma).

Adjuvant therapy is therapy given after the initial surgery (or radiation) to eliminate any persisting micrometastases, it is chiefly used for tumours known for their propensity to such spread, e.g. breast cancer. The term includes therapy undertaken after relapses. The objective is to hit tumour cells that may be present but undetectable at the early stage of growth when the cells of a tumour are more rapidly dividing and more sensitive to drugs. Over liberal use of adjuvant therapy carries the risk of treating patients who in fact have been cured by the initial therapy and so exposing them needlessly to the risk of a second, drug-induced, tumour.

E. **Adverse effects** of anticancer drugs acting on dividing normal tissues would be expected to, and indeed do, include:

1. *Bone marrow and lymphoreticular system*: pancytopenia and immunosuppression (depression of both antibody and cell-mediated immunity)
2. *Gut lining* and other *mucosal surfaces*: diarrhoea, mouth ulcers
3. *Hair follicles*: alopecia (recovers 2–6 months after ceasing treatment); loss of hair can be minimised by cooling the scalp, which reduces blood flow and slows down chemical reactions
4. *Delayed wound healing*
5. *Urate nephropathy*: due to rapid destruction of large numbers of cells
6. *Germ cells*: sterility, teratogenesis, mutagenicity
7. *Various tissues*: carcinogenicity.

In general anticancer drugs are unpleasant to take, commonly causing *nausea and vomiting*, which can be extremely severe and cause patients to refuse therapy, see *antiemetics*. Items 1 to 3 are also liable to be troublesome with any vigorously pursued regimen.

Bone marrow suppression is the single most important dose-limiting factor. Repeated blood counts are essential and transfusions of all formed elements of the blood may be needed, e.g. platelet transfusion for thrombocytopenic bleeding or where the platelet count falls below 25 000 per mm^3. Bleomycin and vincristine (but not vinblastine) have relatively low marrow toxicity.

Septicaemia occurs (often opportunistic infection by Gram-negative bacteria from the patient's own flora, e.g. from the gut, which has been injured by the drugs) and vigorous antimicrobial prophylaxis and therapy, often in combination, is used. Granulocyte transfusions are also helpful. Opportunistic infections with virus (herpes zoster), fungus (candida) and protozoa (pneumocystis) are also prominent. *Fever* in a patient under this treatment requires collection of samples for microbiological studies and urgent treatment.

There is evidence that vigorous and prolonged chemotherapy can impair the *immune responsiveness* of patients for as long as 3 years after ceasing therapy.

Effects on *gonadal cells* can lead to reduced sexual drive and to sterility, and the mutagenic effects of anticancer drugs mean that reproduction should be avoided during and for several months after therapy. But both men and women have reproduced successfully (normally) whilst undergoing chemotherapy. It has been recommended that when the long-term outlook for life is good and treatment may cause permanent sterility, e.g. in Hodgkin's lymphoma, men should be offered the facility for storage of sperm before undergoing treatment.

Rapid *destruction of large numbers of malignant cells* results in substantial release of purines and pyrimidines, which are converted to uric acid, which may then crystallise in the urine (*urate nephropathy*). This can be avoided by high fluid intake, alkalinisation of the urine and use of allopurinol during the early stages of chemotherapy. In practice this only occurs when there is a large cell mass and the tumour is very sensitive to drugs (e.g. acute lymphocytic leukaemia and lymphomas).

Carcinogenicity (second tumours). Many cytotoxic drugs are carcinogenic, and a patient may be cured of the primary disease only to succumb to a second, treatment-induced, cancer 5 years later. Alkylating agents are particularly incriminated and also some antimetabolites (mercaptopurine) and antibiotics (doxorubicin). The risk can be as high as 20–30 times that of unexposed people and the cancers include leukaemia, lymphoma and squamous carcinoma. There may be a synergic carcinogenic effect between drugs and radiation.

There is growing concern that over enthusiastic and agressive use of cytotoxic drug therapy has done more harm than good to many patients, destroying the quality of the brief time remaining to them for little or no benefit. This state of affairs is contributed to by our present inability to target the drugs to the cells where they may do good (e.g. monoclonal antibodies used as drug carriers may in the future improve our ability to hit selected targets).

Hazards to staff handling cytotoxic agents. The urine of some nurses and of pharmacists who prepare infusions and injections of anticancer drugs has been found to contain drugs even to the extent of being sometimes mutagenic to bacteria. When they stopped handling the drugs the effect ceased. It cannot be assumed that absorption of these small amounts (compared with therapeutic doses) of drugs is harmless (mutagenesis, carcinogenesis), and it occurs continuously over long periods.

Contamination occurs from spilt drugs, carelessly handled syringes (there should be a swab on the tip of the needle when expelling air), and even open an ampoule can create an aerosol.

Precautions* appropriate to different drugs range from simply avoiding spillage, through gloves, surgical masks, goggles and aprons, to use of laminar flow cabinets. Special training of nominated drug handlers is essential. Pregnant staff should not handle these drugs.

F. **Endocrine therapy**: sex hormones and antihormones. Some cancers are hormone dependent and growth can be inhibited by surgical removal of gonads or by administration of hormones or antihormones, e.g. oestrogens or androgens, or antioestrogens or antiandrogens, or progestogens.

Prostatic cancer is androgen dependent and endocrine treatment may be as follows: (1) *oestrogen*, by stilboestrol, which carries increased risk of thromboembolism; (2) *antiandrogen* (cyproterone); (3) *inhibition of steroid* (*testosterone*) *synthesis* by e.g. aminoglutethimide; (4) *inhibition of gonadotrophin release* from the pituitary by continuous (*not* intermittent) use of gonadorelin (GnRH).

Breast cancers may have receptors for oestrogen, progesterone and androgen, and tumours that have receptors for both oestrogen and progesterone are far more likely to respond to endocrine manipulation than are those that lack them. Receptor analysis of cells from tumours is used in an attempt to choose the most effective therapy. In general, tumours in pre-menopausal women are likely to be oestrogen-dependent and anti-oestrogens, oophorectomy or androgens are used; the

* The Pharmaceutical Society of Great Britain has published useful guidelines. Pharmaceutical Journal Feb 26 (1983) p. 230. See also Williams C J. Handling cytotoxics. Br Med J 1985; 291:1299.

opposite is the case in late post-menopausal women. The anti-oestrogen, *tamoxifen*, has been shown to produce regression in breast cancer. Paradoxically its effect is most marked in post-menopausal women.

Adrenocortical steroids are used for their action on the cancer itself and also to treat some of the complications of cancer (hypercalcaemia, raised intracranial pressure; see index).

Their principal use is in cancer of the lymphoid tissues and blood. In leukaemias they may also reduce the incidence of haematological complications such as haemolytic anaemia and thrombocytopenia. A glucocorticoid is preferred, e.g. prednisolone, as mineralocorticoid actions are not needed and cause fluid retention. High doses, e.g. 200 mg predisolone per day, are used.

Endocrine therapy carries much less serious consequences for normal tissues than do the chemotherapeutic agents.

G. **Immunotherapy** derives from an observation in the 19th century that cancer sometimes regressed after acute bacterial infections, i.e. there may be non-specific immunostimulant effect.

Anticancer drugs are notable as being immunosuppressive and so are likely to diminish what little natural immune resistance to a tumour that there may be.

Exploration of immunotherapy has involved:

1. Non-specific stimulation of immunity with vaccines, e.g. BCG and *Corynebacterium parvum* vaccine. These have efficacy in animals, but results in man are controversial. *C. parvum* vaccine is used in the pleural cavity for malignant effusions but its benefit seems to be due to a local vigorous inflammatory effect rather than to immunostimulation.

2. Non-specific stimulation of immunity with drugs, e.g. *levamisole* (an anthelmintic), which appears to enhance function of phagocytes and T-lymphocytes when this is abnormal. It has also been tried in immune deficiency states and autoimmune disease, e.g. rheumatoid arthritis.

3. use of the natural substance interferon, see p. 265.

4. use of vaccines prepared from the cells of the patient's tumour or from tumours in other people.

5. formation of monoclonal antibodies by tissue culture techniques.

Whilst none of these approaches has found a major role in therapeutics, they may do so in the future.

H. **Assessment of therapy**. Reliable measures of efficacy, and toxicity, of therapy are of particular importance when disease kills and when the treatment often has to be pressed to the point of injuring the patient. The availability of biochemical *markers*, e.g. prostatic carcinoma (acid phosphatase), choriocarcinoma (chorionic gonadotrophin), teratomas (gonadotropin and α-fetoprotein)*, as well as the more routine clinical measures (blood counts, radiology), adds to the precision and safety with which chemotherapy can be conducted. Indeed, intensive chemotherapy should not be used if there is no means of monitoring its effect on the tumour.

I. **Summary of the principles of chemotherapy**

1. Determine that there is no better (more effective and safe) treatment available.
2. Decide whether expected benefit (cure, palliation and the expected quality of life) justifies the risk.
3. Determine the measurable factor (symptom, sign, laboratory measure) that will allow progress to be assessed.
4. With sensitive tumours *treat early* in the course of the disease to increase likelihood of total cell kill.
5. Choose drugs that are cycle non-specific or cycle specific, as appropriate.
6. Use combinations of drugs.
7. Repeated courses of high dose chemotherapy with intervals for recovery of normal tissues is ordinarily more effective than continuous low dose therapy.
8. Contraindications:

very advanced disease
existing bone marrow depression
presence of active infection.

Classes of cytotoxic agents

Drugs used (practical details of administration are of the utmost importance and the manufacturer's Data Sheet should be consulted).

* An onco-fetal protein = protein normally produced by fetus and not by adult, which reappears in adult patients with certain tumours and which provides a 'marker' for cancer.

Alkylating agents (nitrogen mustards and ethyleneimines) act by transferring alkyl groups to DNA in the N-7 position of guanine during cell division. There follows either DNA strand breakage or cross-linking of the two strands so that normal synthesis is prevented.

Examples: busulphan, chlorambucil, cyclophosphamide, ifosfamide, estramustine (a combination of oestrogen and mustine), ethoglucid, mannomustine, melphalan, mitobronitol, mustine, thiotepa, treosulfan, tretamine, uramustine; the nitrosoureas (carmustine, lomustine) have an additional mode of action. Alkylating agents cause nausea and vomiting and bone marrow depression (delayed with the nitrosoureas) and cystitis* (cyclophosphamide, ifosfamide) and pulmonary fibrosis (especially busulphan).

Antimetabolites are analogues of normal metabolites and act by competition, i.e. they 'deceive' or 'defraud' bodily processes.

Folic acid antagonist, methotrexate, competitively inhibits dihydrofolate reductase, preventing the synthesis of tetrahydrofolic acid (the coenzyme important in synthesis of amino and nucleic acids).

A cogent illustration of the need to exploit every possible means of enhancing selectivity is provided by methotrexate. A heavy (potentially fatal) dose of methotrexate is given and is followed about 24 h later by a dose of tetrahydrofolic (folinic) acid (as Ca folinate, Ca leucovorin), to terminate its action. This is called folinic acid or leucovorin 'rescue', since if it is not given the patient will die. The therapeutic justification for this manoeuvre is that high concentrations of methotrexate are obtained and that the bone marrow cells recover better than the tumour cells and some degree of useful selectivity is achieved.

There are also *purine antagonists* (mercaptopurine, azathioprine, thioguanine), and *pyrimidine antagonists* (fluorouracil, cytarabine, floxuridine), which similarly deprive cells of essential metabolites.

Antimetabolites cause gastrointestinal upsets including ulceration and bone marrow depression; renal failure potentiates them, especially methotrexate. Active excretion of methotrexate by the renal tubule is blocked by salicylate, which also displaces it from plasma protein (as do sulphonamides), with increased toxicity.

Natural products

Alkaloids — vincristine, vinblastine and vindesine — cause cell cycle arrest in mitosis, as does demeclocycline. They cause bone marrow depression, peripheral neuropathy (vincristine) and alopecia.

Glucoside — etoposide (derived from epipodophyllotoxin, from a plant) has antimitotic action.

Antibiotics include: actinomycins (dactinomycin, actinomycin D), bleomycin, daunorubicin (rubidomycin), doxorubicin (Adriamycin), and the related mitozantrone and amsacrine, mithramycin, mitomycin, streptozotocin (islet-cell pancreatic tumour); they interfere with DNA/RNA synthesis. They depress the bone marrow, cause gut upsets and stomatitis, alopecia, cardiomyopathy (daunorubicin and doxorubicin) and pulmonary fibrosis and skin rashes (bleomycin). The effects of some are radiomimetic, and use of radiation causes additive toxicity.

Colaspase, asparaginase. It was observed that the serum of guinea-pigs had anticancer activity in experimental animals. This proved to be due to the presence of the enzyme asparaginase, which starved tumour cells dependent on a supply of the amino acid asparagine (except those able to synthesise for themselves or not requiring it). The enzyme is obtained from cultures of *Esch. coli* or *Erwinia carotovora*. Its use is declining.

Miscellaneous: procarbazine, dacarbazine, hydroxyurea, razoxane, urethane and *platinum* derivatives (cisplatin, carboplatin).

Radio-phosphorus (^{32}P, sodium radiophosphate). Phosphorus is concentrated in bone and in cells that are dividing rapidly, so that the erythrocyte precursors in the bone marrow receive most of the β-irradiation when ^{32}P is given. The effects are similar to those of whole-body irradiation, and in **polycythaemia vera** ^{32}P is now a treatment of choice. The maximum effect on the blood count does not occur for 1–2 months after the dose. In polycythaemia, yearly treatments often give good control. Excessive depression of the bone marrow is the main adverse effect. The

* A metabolite, acrolein, of cyclophosphamide and ifosfamide causes haemorrhagic cystits. A high urine volume plus use of *mesna*, which binds acrolein, are used to prevent this serious complication.

disease can also be treated with chlorambucil. Both ^{32}P and chlorambucil increase the incidence of leukaemia (and other cancers) after 5–7 years. Hydroxyurea can also be used.

Radio-gold (^{198}Au) is concentrated in the liver and has been used in various abdominal neoplasms.

Cancer 'Cures'

'So long as conventional medicine cannot cure all patients with cancer some will be willing to try anything that they think might help'.*

Laetrile, a preparation of apricot seeds (pits, pips), contains amygdalin (a β-glucoside). It is claimed to relieve pain, prolong survival and even to induce complete remission of cancer. Benefit is reputed to result from release of cyanide in the body, which is claimed to kill cancer cells but not normal cells.

As has so often been the case in the past, and no doubt will continue to be in the future, the calm evaluation of such claims is obstructed by a mixture of emotionalism and exploitation. Scientific clinical investigation shows no benefit.

Although it is claimed that laetrile has no toxic effects, an 11-month-old girl has died after swallowing tablets (1–5) being used by her father. The toxicity is due to metabolic formation, in the intestine, of hydrocyanic acid. Deaths are also reported from eating material intended for injection.

Interestingly, despite criticism of over-permissive laxity of the drug regulatory authority (FDA) in the USA, the public is unwilling to accept the opinion of the FDA when it advises against the use of laetrile.

There is a long and generally dishonourable history of the promotion of cancer 'cures', but as each new one appears the medical profession must yet again be willing to look dispassionately at the possibility that this time there really may be something in it, whilst avoiding the tragic raising of hopes that will not be realised — a sad and difficult task.

Another currently available substance of this class is H 11, an extract of male urine.

* Editorial. Br Med J 1977; 1:3.

The following tables are included to give a general idea of the scope and range of cancer chemotherapy.

Response to chemotherapy

Group A. Tumours in which *striking response and significant benefit are common, and life expectancy may become normal*

Childhood acute leukaemia (cure)	Choriocarcinoma (cure)
Hodgkin's disease (cure)	Wilm's tumour
Non-Hodgkin lymphoma	Ewing's sarcoma
	Seminoma
	Prostatic carcinoma (oestrogen responsive)
	Small cell bronchial carcinoma
	Burkitt's tumour (cure)

Group B. Tumours in which chemotherapy is *less effective*.

Acute leukaemia in adults	Breast carcinoma
Chronic granulocytic leukaemia	Ovarian carcinoma
Chronic lymphocytic leukaemia	Multiple myeloma
	Cholangiocarcinoma

Group C. Tumours in which chemotherapy is *often ineffective*, or effective only when special techniques of administration are employed.

Cervix uteri carcinoma	Cerebral gliomata
Corpus uteri carcinoma	Oropharyngeal carcinoma
Melanoma	Carcinoma of paranasal sinuses
Osteogenic sarcoma	Squamous bronchial carcinoma
Gastrointestinal carcinomas	Renal carcinoma
Hepatoma	

(Modified from WHO Technical Reports Nos 232 and 605)

Choice of Drugs

Table 38.1 sets out drugs of first and second choice in a number of cancers, but it gives a general indication only. The lists in the table do not indicate desirable combinations, but drugs from amongst which single or combined therapy may be chosen. For interferon see p. 265.

IMMUNOSUPPRESSION

Immunosuppression is a specialised technique; it employs some drugs of use in cancer and so is considered here. The following notes provide a little background.

Table 38.1 Choice of drugs

Disease	1st choice drugs	Alternatives and 2nd choice drugs
Acute leukaemias	prednisolone; mercaptopurine; vincristine; methotrexate; daunorubicin (rubidomycin); doxorubicin (Adriamycin); cytarabine	asparaginase; cyclophosphamide; thioguanine; amsacrine
Chronic granulocytic leukaemia	busulphan	mercaptopurine; hydroxyurea; melphalan; mitobronitol
Chronic lymphocytic leukaemia	chlorambucil; cyclophosphamide; prednisolone	
Hodgkin's lymphoma	cyclophosphamide; vinblastine; procarbazine; prednisolone	other alkylating agents; vincristine; bleomycin; dacarbazine; doxorubicin
Burkitt's lymphoma	cyclophosphamide (used alone)	carmustine; methotrexate
Other lymphomas	prednisolone; cyclophosphamide; vincristine; bleomycin; doxorubicin; cytarabine; methotrexate	vinblastine
Multiple myeloma	melphalan; cyclophosphamide; prednisolone	carmustine; doxorubicin; vincristine
Breast cancer	hormones or anti-hormones depending on endocrine status; cyclophosphamide; methotrexate; fluorouracil; prednisolone	doxorubicin; mitozantrone; vincristine
Prostate cancer	oestrogen (or androgen inhibition)	alkylating agents
Ovary cancer	melphalan; doxorubicin; cyclophosphamide	cisplatin; chlorambucil; fluorouracil; methotrexate
Endometrium cancer	a progestogen	doxorubicin
Cervix cancer	mitomycin; methotrexate; cyclophosphamide	bleomycin
Choriocarcinoma	methotrexate (used alone)	actinomycin D; vinblastine; chlorambucil
Testis cancer (seminoma)	methotrexate; actinomycin D (dactinomycin); chlorambucil; cisplatin	
Small cell carcinoma of bronchus	doxorubicin; cyclophosphamide; vincristine; methotrexate; lomustine	procarbazine; etoposide
Gastrointestinal cancers	fluorouracil; mitomycin	doxorubicin
Bladder cancer	doxorubicin; cisplatin; thiotepa	mitomycin; fluorouracil; ethoglucid
Brain cancers (some)	carmustine; lomustine	procarbazine; vincristine
Wilm's tumour	actinomycin D; vincristine	doxorubicin
Ewing's sarcoma	cyclophosphamide; doxorubicin; vincristine; actinomycin D	
Osteogenic sarcoma	doxorubicin; methotrexate with 'folinic acid rescue'	cisplatin; melphalan

1. Immune responses in man may be antibody (B-cell) mediated or T-cell mediated.

2. Rejection of grafts and delayed allergic (hypersensitivity) reactions are cell-mediated.

3. Suppression of a damaging immune response is employed in allergic and autoimmune diseases and in tissue or organ grafting to prevent rejection.

4. *Effective drugs* act by impairing the reproductive integrity of lymphoid cells during both antibody-mediated and cell-mediated reactions. They include:

a. *adrenal steroids*

b. *cytotoxic agents and antimetabolites* (anticancer drugs)

c. *cyclosporin*
d. *antilymphocytic globulin*

They suppress the development of an immune response after antigenic challenge more readily than they suppress established immunity (which is the usual clinical situation).

The above are all non-specific immunosuppressives so that the general defences of the body against infection are impaired: infections should be treated by bactericidal drugs.

Adrenal steroids destroy lymphocytes, reduce inflammation and impair phagocytosis.

Cytotoxic agents and antimetabolites destroy immunologically competent cells: *azathioprine*, a pro-drug for the purine antagonist mercaptopurine, is used in autoimmune disease. Cyclophosphamide is a second choice. Bone marrow is depressed as is to be expected.

Cyclosporin (ciclosporin, cyclosporine; Sandimmun) (1972) is a polypeptide fungus (soil) metabolite. It is an effective immunosuppressant that spares the bone marrow (unlike azathioprine) and does not depress phagocytosis. It is used to prevent (and to treat) rejection of allogeneic organ transplants including bone marrow. It inhibits cell-mediated immune reactions, inhibiting the multiplication of the immunocompetent T-lymphocyte. It has the hazards inherent in immunosuppression (below) and it can cause kidney and liver injury. It is not teratogenic in animals and may not be so in man. Other adverse effects include gut upsets, hirsutism, tremor, gingival hypertrophy, electrolyte disturbance. It is given orally (or i.v. at first) and then monthly indefinitely. Its use requires careful monitoring (including plasma concentrations where practicable). As with other agents, long-term immunosuppression is associated with increased incidence of lymphoma.

Antilymphocyte immunoglobulin is made by preparing antisera to human lymphocytes in animals (horses): allergic reactions are common.

5. *Hazards of immunosuppression*. Impaired immune responses render the subject more liable to bacterial and viral infections.

Carcinogenicity is also a hazard, generally after 4–7 years of therapy. The cancers most likely to occur are those thought to have viral origin (leukemia, lymphoma). Where cytotoxics are used there is the additional hazard of mutagenicity, which may induce cancer.

Hazards of immunosuppressive drugs include those of long-term corticosteroid therapy, of cytotoxics (bone marrow depression, infertility and teratogenesis).

6. Whilst the hazards are relatively acceptable for treating grave life-endangering disease, they give more cause for concern when immunosuppressive regimens are used in younger patients with less serious disease, e.g. rheumatoid arthritis, ulcerative colitis.

7. Treat all infection early and vigorously (4 above): use human gamma globulin to protect if there is exposure to virus infections, e.g. measles, varicella.

8. *Diseases in which immunosuppression may be useful include*: ulcerative colitis, regional ileitis, rheumatoid arthritis, chronic active hepatitis, systemic lupus erythematosus, glomerulonephritis, nephrotic syndrome, some haemolytic anaemias or thrombocytopenias, tissue transplantations.

9. *Active immunisation during immunosuppressive therapy*. Response to *non-living* antigens (tetanus, typhoid, poliomyelitis) is diminished and 1 or 2 extra doses may be wise. With *living* vaccines (some polio) there is a risk of serious generalised disease; boosters are safer than primary vaccination. If vaccination *must* be performed (an unlikely event) reduce or stop the immunosuppressive therapy and vaccinate lightly. If a severe reaction occurs use an appropriate antiviral agent on a specific immunoglobulin if available.

Immunostimulation: see *Immunotherapy*, p. 725.

GUIDE TO FURTHER READING

1 Green J A. Compliance and cancer chemotherapy. Br Med J 1983; 287:778.
2 Brinkley D. Emotional distress during cancer chemotherapy. Br Med J 1983; 286:663.
3 Emery P W et al. Protein synthesis in muscle measured in vivo in cachectic patients with cancer. Br Med J 1984; 289:584.
4 Editorial. Phase I trials in patients with cancer. Lancet

1983; 1:913.
5 Editorial. Drug targeting in cancer. Lancet 1983; 1:512.
6 Watson J V. What does 'response' in cancer chemotherapy really mean? Br Med J 1981; 283:34.
7 Rosenberg S A. Combined-modality therapy of cancer: what is it and when does it work? N Engl J Med 1985; 312:1512.
8 Mead G M et al. Chemotherapy of solid tumours: trials and tribulations. Br Med J 1984; 288:585.
9 Kinlen L J et al. Collaborative United Kingdom–Australian study of cancer in patients treated with immunosuppressive drugs. Br Med J 1979; 2:1461.
10 Cohn K H. Chemotherapy from an insider's perspective. Lancet 1982; 1:1006.
11 Anonymous. Cancer care: the relative's view. Lancet 1983; 2:1188.
12 Rubens R D et al. Controlled trial of adjuvant chemotherapy with melphalan for breast cancer. Lancet 1983; 1:839.
13 Cavalli F et al. Concurrent or sequential use of cytotoxic chemotherapy and hormone treatment in advanced breast cancer: report of the Swiss Group for Clinical Research. Br Med J 1983; 286:5.
14 Editorial. Cyclosporin and neoplasia. Lancet 1983; 1:1083.
15 Merion R M et al. Cyclosporine: five years' experience in cadaveric renal transplantation. N Engl J Med 1984; 310:148.
16 Salaman J R. Steroids and modern immunosuppression. Br Med J 1983; 286:1373.
17 Moertel G G et al. A clinical trial of amygdalin (laetrile) in the treatment of human cancer. N Engl J Med 1982; 306:201: also Editorial, Relman A S, p. 236.
18 Cassileth B R. After laetrile, what? N Engl J Med 1982; 306:1482.
19 Waxman J. Cancer, chemotherapy, and fertility. Br Med J 1985; 290:1096.
20 Venitt S et al. Monitoring exposure of nursing and pharmacy personnel to cytotoxic drugs: urinary mutation assays and urinary platinum as markers of absorption. Lancet 1984; 1:74.
21 Nolvadex Adjuvant Trial Organisation. Controlled trial of tamoxifen as single adjuvant agent in management of early breast cancer: analysis of six years. Lancet 1985; 1:836.
22 Kirk D. Prostatic carcinoma. Br Med J 1985; 290:875.
23 Tobias J S et al. Doing the best for the cancer patient. Lancet 1985; 1:35.
24 Whitehouse J M A. Risk of leukaemia associated with cancer chemotherapy. Br Med J 1985; 290:261.
25 Mack R M. Lessons from living with cancer. N Engl J Med 1984; 311:1640: a personal account by a 50-year-old surgeon.
26 Mullan F. Seasons of survival: reflections of a (32-year-old) physician with cancer. N Engl J Med 1985; 313:270.
27 Selby P. Acquired resistance to cancer chemotherapy. Br Med J 1984; 288:1252.
28 Manni A. Hormone receptors and breast cancer. N Engl J Med 1983; 309:1383.
29 Baserga R. The cell cycle. N Engl J Med 1981; 304:453.
30 Papadekis J et al. High versus 'low' dose corticosteroids in recipients of cadaveric kidneys: prospective controlled trial. Br Med J 1983; 286:1097.
31 Editorial. Cancer, cancer therapy and hair. Lancet 1983; 2:1177.
32 Anderson M et al. Development and operation of a pharmacy based intravenous cytotoxic reconstitution service. Br Med J 1983; 286:32.
33 Senturia Y D et al. Children fathered by men treated for testicular cancer. Lancet 1985; 2:766.
34 Watson J G et al. Antibiotic prophylaxis for patients in protective isolation. Lancet 1979; 1:1183.
35 Editorial. Relapse in Hodgkin's disease. Lancet 1985; 2:424.
36 Baldwin R W et al. Monoclonal antibodies in cancer treatment. Lancet 1986; 1:603.
37 Rees J K H et al. Principal results of the Medical Research Council's 8th acute myeloid leukaemia trial. Lancet 1986; 2:1236.

39

Drugs and the skin

In this chapter some general aspects of the use of drugs in dermatology will be discussed, but an outline of treatment of a number of afflictions is also provided.

It is well-established that the skin may react to emotion, e.g. in eczema or psoriasis, and sedatives or tranquillisers may be useful adjuvant therapy of skin diseases. To avoid repetition from earlier chapters, the following account is confined to therapy directed primarily at the skin.

It is easy to do more harm than good with potent drugs, and this is particularly true in skin diseases; also, many skin lesions are in fact caused by systemic or local use of drugs. In patients prone to any allergy it is very easy to provoke further reactions during treatment.

Local or *topical* treatment of skin lesions appears to offer a unique opportunity for the trial of different treatments on similar lesions in the same individual at the same time, but substances applied locally are sometimes absorbed and may exert effects on the body as a whole, also, the healing of a lesion at one site, sometimes, for no known reason, may produce improvement in similar lesions elsewhere. Conversely, to provoke a flare-up at one site may make all the other lesions worse as well. Thus a 'control' treatment may at first appear to have caused healing or exacerbation that is in fact due to the effects of a more active substance applied elsewhere.

SOME GENERAL ASPECTS OF DERMAL PHARMACOKINETICS

Substances that are well **absorbed** from intact skin are usually soluble in both water and fats, or combine with skin fatty acids, e.g. heavy metals; those completely insoluble in either are not absorbed. Fats and oils enter the skin partly through the hair follicles and sebaceous glands. From diseased areas most substances are absorbed to some extent so that systemic toxicity is more likely.

There is a greater variety of ways of presenting a drug to the skin than to any other organ. It has been pointed out that 'dermatologic vehicles are drug delivery systems. It does not matter what the preparation looks like in the container. Rather, the environment in which the skin finds itself in the residue left on the skin after application is critical to the rate, intensity and duration of activity'.* Drugs must cross the vehicle-skin interface if they are to affect the skin cells and this involves complex physicochemical issues including those raised in Ch. 8. Most modern dermatological preparations are 'washable hydrophilic oil-in-water systems'.*

* Riegelman S. Clin Pharmacol Ther 1974; 16:873.

The principal barrier to skin permeability (by diffusion) is the keratin layer, and where this is damaged by disease (e.g. eczema, psoriasis) drugs (e.g. corticosteroids) are absorbed more easily. The keratin layer acts as a reservoir for a drug whence it slowly diffuses into the deeper layers of the skin for many hours. When it is absent serious systemic toxicity can occur.

The manner in which drugs are **applied** to the skin is often important and depends upon the nature of the drug and the effect desired, whether it is to be entirely superficial, for instance, to cool, to reduce evaporation or friction, or to protect, or whether penetration of a biologically active substance is required.

In general, acutely inflamed lesions are readily aggravated by drugs and so simple soothing applications (emollients)* should be used.

Intensification of effect can be got by covering the area to which a drug has been applied by a sheet of impermeable plastic (*occlusive dressing*), probably as a result of increased hydration, especially of the keratin layer. Substantial absorption with systemic effects can occur when this is done. Some ointments are mildly occlusive.

Vehicles

Vehicles, listed below, in which drugs or inert substances are formulated for application are important. Whether a drug is offered in a *lotion*, *cream* or *ointment* etc. depends on the drug, the condition and site of the diseased skin, and the objectives of the prescriber, which are rational either on an empirical basis or from knowledge of the pathophysiology of the disease. Those who do not make a special study of dermatology are advised to follow well-trodden paths; they should not dilute formulations or mix one with another without first establishing the pharmaceutical compatibility of the deed.

Lotions or **wet dressings** are generally used to cleanse, cool and relieve pruritus in acutely inflamed lesions, especially where there is much exudation. Water is the most important component. The initial application, and the cooling effect of evaporation of the water, is thought to reduce the inflammatory response by inducing superficial vasoconstriction. Sodium chloride solution 0.9%, or solutions of *astringent*† and weakly antimicrobial substances, e.g. Aluminium Acetate Lotion, are often used. Soaks of approximately 0.05% potassium permanganate are satisfactory if the lesion is on the limbs. Lotions containing more active ingredients (e.g. ichthammol, coal tar) are sometimes used on subacute lesions, but occasionally these irritate the skin further. The use of lotions or wet dressings over very large areas can reduce body temperature dangerously in the old or the very ill.

Shake lotions (e.g. Calamine Lotion) are essentially a convenient way of applying a powder to the skin with additional cooling due to evaporation of the water. They are contra-indicated when there is much exudate because crusts form. They sometimes produce excessive drying of the skin, but this can be reduced if oils are included, as in Oily Calamine Lotion.

Creams are emulsions either of *oil-in-water* (washable; cosmetic vanishing creams) or *water-in-oil*. A cooling effect (cold creams) is obtained with both groups as the water evaporates. *Water-in-oil* creams (e.g. Oily Cream, Zinc Cream) behave like oils in that they do not mix with serous discharges, but their chief advantage over ointment is that the water content makes them easier to spread, and they give a better cosmetic effect. They are specially useful as barrier preparations for protecting the skin, e.g. when it is chapped or dried, or on babies' buttocks, and can be used on hairy parts. They can be used as vehicles, particularly for fat-soluble substances. A dry skin is mainly short of water and oily substances are needed to provide a barrier that reduces evaporation of water; but the presence of oils contributes in some measure to epidermal hydration.

Oil-in-water creams (Aqueous Cream) do mix with serous discharges and are especially useful as vehicles for water-soluble active drugs. They may

* *Emollients* soothe and hydrate the skin, e.g. Aqueous Cream, oils (arachis, castor and cod liver) have a smoothing action on scaly conditions.

† *Astringents* are weak protein precipitants, e.g. tannins, salts of Al and Zn.

contain a wetting (surface tension reducing) agent (cetomacrogol).

Barrier preparations of many different kinds have been devised for use in industry and in medicine to reduce dermatitis. They rely on water-repellent substances, e.g. silicones (Dimethicone Cream), and on soaps as well as on substances that form an impermeable deposit (titanium, zinc, calamine). They are not usually very effective, because it is impossible to maintain a complete barrier that is also easily removed by ordinary washing afterwards. If it is not readily removable, complications due to blockage of sweat glands and follicles and skin irritation follow. Allergic reactions occur.

Barrier creams may make the cleansing of the skin more easy after dirty work, but it is essential that they should be shown to be less harmful than the dirt itself before being used for this.

They are more effective in protecting skin from discharges and secretions (colostomies, napkin rash) than when used under industrial working conditions. Silicone sprays may be effective in preventing and treating pressure sores.

Masking creams for obscuring unpleasant blemishes from view are greatly valued by the victims. They may consist of the inert titanium oxide in an ointment base with colouring appropriate to the site and the patient. Best results are got by consulting a cosmetician.

Ointments are thicker than creams; they are of three kinds:

1. *Non-emulsifying*. These do not mix with water: they adhere to the skin and prevent evaporation (i.e. have some occlusive effect, see above) and heat loss: they can be considered a form of occlusive dressing (with increased systemic absorption of active ingredients): skin maceration occurs: although they are helpful in chronic conditions to soften crusts, and as vehicles, they are not used in acute conditions in which free removal of exudate and cooling are needed: they are difficult to remove except with oil or detergents and are messy and inconvenient, especially on hairy skin: Paraffin Ointment contains beeswax, paraffins and cetostearyl alcohol: Simple Ointment is similar. *Squalane* is a saturated hydrocarbon insoluble in water but soluble in sebum. It therefore penetrates the skin and can deliver active agents, and is water repellent (incontinence, prevention of bed sores). It appears in mixed formulations.

2. *Emulsifying*. These allow evaporation as they mix with water and skin exudate: they are useful as vehicles for active drugs:

Emulsifying Ointment is made from emulsifying wax (cetostearyl alcohol and sodium lauryl sulphate) and paraffins: Aqueous Cream is an oil-in-water emulsion of Emulsifying Ointment.

3. *Water soluble*. These are mixtures of macrogols and polyethylene glycols: the consistency can be varied readily: they are easily removable and are used in burn dressings, as lubricants and as vehicles that readily allow passage of active drugs into the skin (e.g. hydrocortisone).

Gels or **jellies** are semisolid colloidal solutions or suspensions.

Pastes (e.g. Zinc Compound Paste are ointments containing insoluble powders. They are very adhesive and give good protection. Their powder content enables them to absorb a moderate amount of discharge. They are also used as vehicles (e.g. Coal Tar Paste, which is Zinc Compound Paste with 7.5% coal tar).

Dusting powders (e.g. Zinc Starch and Talc* Dusting-powder) may cool by increasing the effective surface area of the skin and they reduce friction between skin surfaces by their lubricating action. Though usefully absorbent, they cause crusting if applied to exudative lesions. They may be used alone as well as a vehicle for, e.g. fungicides.

Some miscellaneous substances and formulations

Caustics are used to destroy unwanted tissue, including warts and corns. Great care is obviously necessary to avoid ulceration. They include trichloracetic acid (10–20%), silver nitrate sticks, salicylic acid (10–50%) and many others. Podophyllin (15%) is also used but may act as an antimitotic

* *Talc* is magnesium silicate. It must not be used for dusting surgical gloves as it causes granulomas if it gets into wounds or body cavities.

rather than as a caustic. They may be localised by application in a nitrated cellulose paint (collodion).

Keratolytics are mild caustics and are used for softening and removing the horny layer of the skin. They are all liable to damage normal skin and should therefore be strictly confined to the lesion. If used too strong or for too long they may cause ulcers. They are used particularly in the chronic scaling conditions, especially psoriasis. Salicylic acid, 2%, is probably the first choice, as in Salicylic Acid Ointment, or Zinc and Salicylic Acid Paste. Tretinoin (Retin-A) is an alternative.

Tars are mildly antiseptic, antipruritic and they modify keratinisation. They are comparatively safe in low concentrations. They are used in chronic conditions associated with parakeratosis, e.g. psoriasis. There are very many preparations, which usually contain other substances, e.g. Calamine and Coal Tar Ointment, or Coal Tar and Salicylic Acid Ointment; it is sometimes useful to add an adrenal steroid. Ichthammol is a sulphurous tarry distillation product of fossilised fish (obtained in the Austrian Tyrol), it is used as a mild antiseptic, Ichthammol Ointment. Tars increase the sensitivity of the skin to sunlight.

Zinc oxide provides mild astringent, barrier and occlusive actions.

Calamine is a basic zinc carbonate that owes its pink colour to added ferric oxide. It has a mild astringent action and is used as a dusting powder and in shake and oily lotions.

Aqueous cream is an emollient (p. 732) and a vehicle for active agents. It consists of emulsifying wax (cetostearyl alcohol and sodium lauryl sulphate, or similar aliphatic alcohols), soft paraffin and liquid paraffin.

Urea is used topically to assist skin hydration, e.g. in ichthyosis.

Insect repellents (against mosquitoes, blackflies, ticks, fleas, etc.), e.g. deet (diethyl toluamide), ethyl hexanediol, dimethyl phthalate. These are applied to the skin and repel insects principally by vapourisation. They must be applied to all exposed skin, and sometimes also to clothes if their objective is to be achieved (some damage plastic fabrics and spectacle frames). Their duration of effect is limited by the rate at which they vaporise (skin and ambient temperature), by washing off (sweat, rain, immersion) and by mechanical factors causing rubbing (physical activity). They can cause allergic and toxic effects. Plainly the vehicle in which they are applied is also important in relation to all the factors, and an acceptable substance achieving persistence of effect beyond a few hours has yet to be developed. But the alternative of spreading insecticide in the environment causing general pollution with indiscriminate insect kill is largely unacceptable. Selective environmental measures against some insects, e.g. mosquitoes are sometimes feasible.

Benzyl benzoate may be used on clothes; it resists one or two washings.

ANTISEPTICS: DISINFECTION OF SKIN WOUNDS

Doctors are seldom actively concerned to exercise personal choice from amongst the huge number of antiseptics and disinfectants. They generally just want to be told which preparation has been found most suitable for each particular task.

There are various techniques: the following will serve:

Surface disinfection of clean objects (glass, stainless steel): hypochlorites with or without a detergent, or 70% solutions of industrial methylated spirit or of isopropyl alcohol are suitable. Cetrimide and povidone–iodine are effective.

Hands: washing with soap *followed* by a chlorhexidine detergent solution (Hibiscrub), used like liquid soap, is usual practice. Single application of alcoholic solution of chlorhexidine rubbed on the hands till dry is also effective.

Skin disinfection prior to surgery or for special needling (blood culture, lumbar puncture). Alcoholic povidone–iodine or alcoholic chlorhexidine are used. Duration of contact is important for special effects, e.g. 60 min for reduction of clostridial spores. Rubbing the antiseptic on the site for 2 min is highly effective; much more so than application by spray. All antiseptic/disinfection applications should be allowed to dry completely before operation or needling. Aqueous chlorhexidine has a narrower antimicrobial spectrum and is used when total evaporation of alcohol cannot be relied on and diathermy is to be used during surgery (face, perineum). Serious burns have occurred due to ignition of alcoholic solutions in the vagina. Chloroxylenol (Dettol), organic Hg, quaternary ammonium compounds (dequalinium, etc.) are less active.

Skin disinfection prior to minor needling (injection, venepuncture): 70% ethyl or isopropyl alcohol is commonly used, though the balance of evidence is that no preparation is necessary, even in diabetics who are more prone to infection than are others. Where the skin is 'socially' clean, the skin burden of bacteria is so low that penetration by a needle will not introduce the minimum number of organisms necessary to start an infection (probably about 10^5 bacteria). But a 5-second skin cleanse with 70% isopropyl alcohol removes 80–90% skin bacteria at injection sites. It is useful to know that an injection may be made safely in the absence of skin preparation, but when it is available it seems likely that the usual ritual will continue to be used for mixed reasons including habit, emotion, the possibility that this patient's skin is exceptionally contaminated,and fear of litigation if anything goes wrong. But bold diabetics have been known habitually to inject themselves through their clothes without harm.

Antiseptics should be allowed to dry before inserting the needle, for maximum efficacy and to avoid pain and contamination of blood taken (haemolysis, interference with coagulation tests) for *laboratory tests.*

Wounds: antiseptics are not generally necessary though irrigation with weak sodium hypochlorite solution (Milton) or calcium hypochlorite (Eusol) is unobjectionable; it should not be left on wound packing as it is inactivated by protein. Chlorhexidine plus cetrimide (Savlon) is an antiseptic–detergent combination that is used on dirty wounds, as also are povidone–iodine or hydrogen peroxide.

Notes on some antiseptics

Alcohol (ethyl, isopropyl) acts by precipitating protein. 70% alcohol is more effective than 100% because 100% alcohol precipitates protein of the outer cell wall, thus reducing penetration of the cell: 70% alcohol reduces surface tension of the microbe and allows better penetration.

Hexachlorophane is a bactericidal chlorinated phenol widely used for prophylaxis of infection in soaps, emulsions and dusting powder. Babies have even been washed or dipped in solutions of various strengths by enthusiasts. But absorption can occur through the skin and it is toxic to the CNS. Therefore recommended strengths and techniques should be adhered to; deaths have occured from thoughtless use.

Iodophors are complexes of *iodine* with a detergent surfactant; the iodine is loosely bound (similarly to drugs bound to plasma protein) and is slowly released, e.g. *povidone–iodine* (Betadine); in presence of blood or exudate, after initial reduction of efficacy, the slow release of iodine allows moderate antibacterial action.

Chloroxylenol (Dettol) is a phenol used as a skin disinfectant; it is inactivated by blood/serum.

Hydrogen peroxide is an unstable weak antimicrobial used for cleansing wounds; it froths (releases O_2) in an encouraging manner, and by mechanical action may help to flush out debris from cavities. It is labelled according to its capacity to produce oxygen from unit volume of solution, e.g. 10 volume, 100 volume.

Chlorhexidine (Hibitane) is a broad-spectrum disinfectant used on the skin for surgery, in obstetrics, for instruments.

Quaternary ammonium compounds: cetrimide (Cetavlon) is a cationic surfactant with antibacterial and detergent properties: *benzalkonium* (Roccal), domiphen and cetylpyridinium are similar.

Nitrofurazone is used for skin infections.

*Hydroxyquinolines. used topically for skin infections include clioquinol** (iodochlorhydroxyquinoline, chinoform, chloriodoquin), *chlorquinaldol* and *hydroxyquinoline.*

Alternatives for various purposes include proflavine, phenols (phenol, cresol, thymol, chloro-

* Clioquinol (Entero-vioform) is no longer used systemically (amoebicide and antidiarrhoeal); between 1956 and 1976 it caused (used in high doses) an epidemic of subacute myelo-optic neuropathy in Japan.

cresol), organic mercury (thiomersal), silver nitrate.

Skin cleansing

Skin cleansing is important because the skin and ulcers often get into a messy state: simple non-irritant and mildly antiseptic (where appropriate) preparations are used as follows:

Scaling disorders: emulsifying ointment (p. 733).

Raw or ulcerated areas: sodium chloride (0.9%): dilute hydrogen peroxide, sodium hypochlorite or potassium permanganate: cetrimide, chlorhexidine, povidone–iodine.

Desloughing agents, e.g. for ulcers: cream or solution containing benzoic, malic and salicylic acids in propylene glycol (Aserbine).

Where some astringent action is desired: potassium permanganate, aluminium acetate.

Acne: soap and water: detergent antiseptic (cetrimide).

SKIN INFECTIONS

Superficial bacterial infections, e.g. impetigo, can best be treated by local application of bactericidal antimicrobials, but severe or *deep infections*, e.g. boils, need systemic administration.

Early use of sulphonamides and then of penicillin on the skin soon showed that allergic reactions to the treatment could be more unpleasant than the disease, and the patient could also be left in a situation where later systemic use for a more serious infection was precluded because of the danger of serious allergic reactions.

To avoid sensitisation, drugs should be applied for as short a time as is reasonable and, to minimise further trouble if sensitisation does occur, the drug should, where practicable, be one that will not be needed for systemic administration in the future.

Topical antibacterial creams/ointments include: gentamicin, neomycin and framycetin (all aminoglycosides that, used to excess on large areas can be absorbed and cause deafness); chloramphenicol; colistin (polymyxin E); polymyxin B; tetracycline; chlortetracycline; fusidic acid; nitrofurazone; mafenide (a sulphonamide); silver sulphadiazine.

Topical antifungals include: amphotericin, benzoic acid, benzoyl peroxide, clotrimazole, econazole, ketoconazole, miconazole, natamycin, nitrophenol, nystatin, salicylic acid, tolnaflate, undecenoates (e.g. zinc).

Topical antivirals: acyclovir: idoxuridine

Topical parasiticides (best as lotions): benzyl benzoate, monosulfiram, malathion, carbaryl.

Minor antiseptics for topical use include: cetrimide, chlorhexidine, proflavine.

General. Antimicrobial creams are generally applied 8-hourly after cleaning the area.

Antimicrobials (bacteria; fungi) are combined with an adrenal steroid in treating infected eczema. The steroid alone will allow the infection to spread by suppressing local inflammatory reaction. The steroid does not prevent an allergic reaction to the antimicrobial.

The following drugs readily induce allergy when used on the skin, penicillin, sulphonamides, streptomycin, chloramphenicol. Neomycin sometimes causes allergy. Tetracyclines do not commonly cause skin allergy, but staphylococci, which are common skin pathogens, are often resistant to them.

Tetracyclines, in combination with adrenal steroids are commonly used for treating, for example, infected eczema in children and stasis eczema in adults.

COUNTER-IRRITANTS: RUBEFACIENTS

Counter-irritants are used to stimulate nerve endings in intact skin to relieve pain in viscera or muscle supplied by the same nerve root. All produce inflammation of the skin which becomes flushed, hence rubefacients. They are often effective, and, though how they act is unknown, there is no lack of theories. The psychological effect is certainly important and other possibilities are:

1. That vasodilatation at the site of the pain, produced by release of prostaglandins may promote relief. This vasodilatation can be blocked by non-steroidal anti-inflammatory drugs (e.g. aspirin, indomethacin).

2. That the arrival in the CNS of numerous afferent impulses from the skin may alter the effect of impulses from other parts supplied by the same nerve root, e.g. via endorphins. The best counter-irritants are physical agents, especially heat. Many drugs have, however, been used for this purpose and suitable liniments (e.g. Turpentine Liniment), ointments (e.g. Methyl Salicylate Ointment), and poultices (e.g. Kaolin Poultice,) and preparations of menthol, camphor and capsicum, are also available to inflame. Histamine and various nicotinates are used in a wide variety of proprietary topical remedies for aches and pains.

ANTIPRURITICS

Impulses responsible for the sensation of itching pass along the same nerve fibres as those of pain, but the sensation experienced differs qualitatively as well as quantitatively from pain. Liberation of histamine and other autacoids in the skin causes itching and may be responsible for much of the itching of urticarial allergic reactions. Many drugs, especially the morphine group, are known to be histamine liberators; bile salts also release histamine and this may explain some, but not all, of the itching of obstructive jaundice. It is likely that other chemical mediators, e.g. serotonin and prostaglandins, are involved.

Treatment of the underlying cause is obviously required (e.g. parasites, renal failure and reticuloses), but there remain those patients in whom the cause either cannot be removed or is not known. Scratching or rubbing seems to give relief by converting the intolerable persistent itch into a more bearable pain, and may even cure the itch at the cost of removing the epidermis. A vicious cycle can be set up in which itching provokes scratching and scratching leads to skin lesions which itch, as in neurodermatitis. Covering the lesion or enclosing it in plaster so as to prevent any further scratching or rubbing may help.

In severe pruritus, sedation is sometimes helpful during the day and a hypnotic is usually required at night.

Antihistamines (H_1-receptor) orally are used in pruritus, but except in urticarial conditions they probably act by their sedative effect; they should not be applied topically due to risk of allergy.

Any cooling application has some antipruritic effect, but a variety of substances, such as *phenol*, menthol or camphor is often added because they have a reputation as antipruritics. Calamine and astringents (aluminium acetate, tannic acid) may help, as may *coal tar*. *Local anaesthetics* do not offer any long-term solution and since they are liable to sensitise the skin they are best avoided; but lignocaine is least troublesome in this respect.

Aspirin (prostaglandin synthesis inhibitor) orally may help some patients with generalised pruritis.

Chlorpromazine or a related drug, e.g. trimeprazine (Vallergan), sometimes helps, probably by altering the patient's attitude to the itching.

Crotamiton, an acaricide, is reputed to have a specific but unexplained antipruritic action, although it may exacerbate an already inflamed skin; convenient proprietary preparations (Eurax) are available. Topical *hydrocortisone* or fluorinated steroid preparations are probably the most effective antipruritics in local inflammatory conditions, e.g. eczema. Obviously they should not be used for generalised pruritus due to systemic disease (see below). Grenz rays are also effective and may be used together with drugs.

The itching of *obstructive jaundice* may be relieved by androgens (e.g. fluoxymesterone orally, up to 5 mg daily; or norethandrolone, 20–30 mg orally daily for women), but jaundice may increase. If obstruction is only partial, cholestyramine can be useful.

ADRENOCORTICAL STEROIDS

'Very few patients are referred to dermatological out-patient departments who have not had one of these preparations applied to their skin.'*

Adrenal steroids topically are effective in suppressing inflammation in the skin (with vasoconstriction), particularly when there is an allergic factor; symptomatic relief can be dramatic. They also reduce epidermal cell division, which is useful

* Milne J A. In: Richardson J, ed. Medical progress 1970–71. London: Butterworths.

in psoriasis. Since the cause of the lesion is not affected it is not surprising that relapse often follows when they are withdrawn. They must not be used in infective inflammation (without effective accompanying chemotherapy) because the infection will exacerbate and spread.

The difficulties and dangers of *systemic* adrenal steroid therapy are sufficient to restrict such use to serious conditions (such as pemphigus and generalised exfoliative dermatitis) not responsive to other forms of therapy.

Local applications of fluorinated steroids can be absorbed from large areas (especially if occlusive dressings, and this includes babies' plastic pants, are used) in amounts sufficient to cause systemic effects, including adrenocortical suppression. Fluorinated steroids are teratogenic in animals and the risk for man is uncertain.

Cortisone and prednisone are ineffective because they are *prodrugs* and must be metabolised to the active forms, hydrocortisone and prednisolone, which should therefore be used instead. The most efficacious and potent steroids for use on the skin are the fluorinated compounds *clobetasol* (Dermovate) and *halcinonide* (Halciderm). Hydrocortisone is now classed as weak.

So potent are these fluorinated steroids that incautious use may be accompanied by enough absorption to cause hypothalamic/pituitary/adrenal suppression and even the classic adverse effects of long-term adrenal steroid use by mouth. It is an excellent thing to have these highly potent substances, but their use carries particular responsibilities.

For this reason, the following useful **guidelines** have been proposed:*

1. Employ the weakest preparation that will control the disorder, especially if long-term use is likely.

2. In cases likely to be resistant, use a high therapeutic potency preparation for three weeks to gain control, after which change to a less potent preparation.

3. Advise the patient to apply the formulation very thinly, just enough to make the skin surface shine slightly.

4. Prescribe in small amounts so that serious overuse is unlikely to occur without the doctor knowing, e.g. weekly quantity by group: high potency 15 g: potent 30 g: others 50 g.

5. Occlusive dressing should only be used briefly. NB. babies plastic pants are an occlusive dressing as well as being a social amenity.

Choice. Corticosteroids are classified according to their therapeutic potency (efficacy). High potency preparations are commonly needed for lichen planus and discoid lupus erythematosus. Potent preparations for psoriasis, and weaker preparations (hydrocortisone 0.5–2.5%) are usually adequate for eczema.

When a skin disorder requiring a corticosteroid is already infected, a preparation containing an antimicrobial is used (neomycin, clotrimazole, nystatin, chlorquinaldol, clioquinol). When the infection is eliminated the corticosteroid may be continued alone.

Examples of preparations of adrenal steroid plus antimicrobial include Canesten (+ clotrimazole), Framycort (+ framycetin) and Hydroderm (+ neomycin). The steroid does not prevent contact dermatitis from the various ingredients.

It is inappropriate to use corticosteroid/antimicrobial preparations in the absence of initial infection.

Adverse effects are more likely with groups 1 and 2 in the table. They include:

Short-term use: spread of infection.

Long-term use: skin atrophy (which may or may not be fully reversible; can occur within 4 weeks); striae (irreversible); local hirsutism; perioral dermatitis (young women), which responds to steroid withdrawal and a course of tetracycline (4–6 weeks); depigmentation (local); acne (local), potent corticosteroids should not be used on the face unless this is unavoidable; systemic absorption can lead to all the adverse effect of systemic corticosteroid use; enough absorption to suppress the hypothalamic/pituitary axis can occur with 20% of the body under an occlusive dressing with the midly potent agents (above), but without occlusion with the very potent agents.

Applications to the eye lids may get into the eye and cause glaucoma.

Rebound exacerbation of the disease can occur after abrupt cessation of therapy. This can lead

* Munro D D. Prescribers Journal 1977; 17:84.

Corticosteroid preparations* may be classified as follows:

1. **Very potent** (% conc.)
   - a. clobetasol (0.05) (Dermovate)
   - b. beclomethasone (0.5) (Propaderm Forte)
   - halcinonide (0.1) (Halciderm)
   - diflucortolone (0.3) (Nerisone Forte)
2. **Potent** (% conc.)
   - beclomethasone (0.025) (Propaderm)
   - betamethasone (0.1) (Betnovate)
   - desonide (0.05) (Tridesilon)
   - diflucortolone (0.1) (Nerisone, Temetex)
   - fluclorolone (0.025) (Topilar)
   - fluocinolone (0.025) (Synalar)
   - fluocinonide (0.05) (Metosyn)
   - fluprednylidene (0.1) (Decoderm)
   - hydrocortisone butyrate (0.1) (Locoid)
   - triamcinolone (0.1) (Adcortyl, Ledercort)
3. **Moderately potent** (% conc.)
   - clobetasone (0.05) (Eumovate)
   - desoxymethasone (0.05) (Stiedex)
   - fluocinolone (0.01) (Synandone)
   - fluocortolone (0.1) (Ultradil)
   - flurandrenolone (0.0125) (Haelan)
   - hydrocortisone (1.0) + urea† (Alphaderm, Calmurid HC)
4. **Mildly potent** (% conc.)
   - hydrocortisone (0.1–2.5) (Cobadex, Cortril, Hydrocortone, etc.), methylprednisolone (0.25) (Medrone)

* Many are available with antimicrobial added under slightly different name.
† The urea increases skin penetration.

the patient to reapply the steroid and so form a vicious cycle.

Occlusive dressings consist of impermeable plastic sheets fixed to the skin at the edges by adhesive tape. By preventing evaporation they allow hydration of the horny layer of the skin so that water-soluble drugs penetrate more readily. They are particularly used with adrenal steroids in highly keratinised lesions, e.g. psoriasis. Dressings are generally kept in place for up to two days or only at night; substantial absorption with systemic effects can occur. Complications include infections (bacterial, monilial) and even heat stroke when large areas are occluded.

Intralesional injections are occasionally used to provide high local concentrations without systemic effects in chronic dermatoses.

SUNBURN AND PHOTOSENSITIVITY

Sunburn is produced by ultraviolet light (UVL) of shorter wavelength than that which produces tanning. However, increased pigment in the skin does protect against sunburn. Ideally, preparations to prevent sunburn should block only the harmful rays and so allow tanning but prevent burn. It is doubtful if this can be achieved, but there are many proprietary preparations that act by screening out a proportion or all the ultraviolet rays. Some skin diseases, e.g. lupus erythematosus, are exacerbated by UVL. Some people like to lie naked in the sun for long periods for psychosocial reasons.

Drug photosensitivity means that an adverse effect occurs as a result of drug plus light; sometimes even the amount of ultraviolet radiation from fluorescent tubes is sufficient. Drugs taken *systemically* that induce photosensitivity include: sulphonamides (including sulphonylurea hypoglycaemics, frusemide, thiazide diuretics), tetracyclines, griseofulvin, phenothiazines, nalidixic acid, oral contraceptives, chlordiazepoxide.

Substances that, applied *locally*, can produce photosensitivity include: various deodorant substances, halogenated salicylanilides (antimicrobials used in soaps, etc.), hexachlorophane, para-aminobenzoic acid and its esters (used as sunscreens), coal tar derivatives, juices of various plants, etc.

There are two forms of **photosensitivity**:

1. **Phototoxicity**: this is, like drug toxicity, a normal effct of too high a dose of the appropriate wavelength. Drugs may lower or raise the threshold for a phototoxic reaction; *the threshold returns to normal when the drug is stopped*.

Protection is needed against the sunburn spectrum (UVB, i.e. 290–320 nm) ultraviolet waveband. These rays inhibit DNA, RNA and protein synthesis and mitosis, and cause release of prostaglandins, i.e. inflammation.

It can be achieved by topical application of substances that absorb or scatter these rays. Effective substances include aminobenzoic acid and dimethyl aminobenzoate (podimate), cinnamates, anthranilates, petroleum jelly and benzophenones (mexenone, Uvistat).* Simple creams are often enough to limit sunburn to a mere erythema. Agents that simply block the sun's rays by their opacity (titanium dioxide, calamine and zinc oxide) are cosmetically unacceptable for social purposes, but titanium is included in some face powders.

If screening blocks the above wavelengths but permits passage of longer waves and visible light, then tanning will occur. Much of the demand for sunscreens is from people who want to be brown, even though they can give no good reason for this; in any case cosmetic acceptability plays a large part in choice. Mexenone (absorbs over range 250–350 nm) is too effective for these people; it prevents tanning, but it is useful against photodermatoses.

Many formulations are available, some are more easily removed by sweating and bathing than others and so need frequent reapplication.

Treatment of mild *sunburn* is usually with a lotion such as Oily Calamine Lotion. Severe cases are helped by Hydrocortisone Lotion (1%) (or a cream). A non-steroidal anti-inflammatory drug can help if given early, by preventing the formation of prostaglandins (e.g. indomethacin).

Spurious suntan. Dihydroxyacetone is used to produce a cosmetic discoloration of the skin resembling suntan. It combines with skin amino acids and the colour develops over hours. Repeated use deepens the 'tan', which, when use ceases, disappears over one to two weeks. It has negligible sunscreen effect. It can cause rashes.

2. **Photoallergy**: is, like drug allergy, an adverse effect that occurs only in some people, and may be severe with a small dose. In relation to drugs it is the result of a photochemical reaction by which the drug combines with tissue protein to form an antigen. *Reactions may persist for years after the drug is withdrawn.*

Photoallergy is caused by longer wavelengths (320–400 nm, i.e. UVA) and so preparations that are adequate against phototoxicity do not suffice. Titanium dioxide, zinc oxide and calamine are effective, but they are cosmetically unattractive. But patients with photoallergy are not concerned with the social oneupmanship of tanning; they simply want protection.

Systemic protection, as opposed to application of drug to exposed areas, should only be considered in the most severe cases of photosensitivity when a patient may be confined indoors. Chloroquine may be effective in polymorphic light eruptions for short periods, but it is contraindicated in porphyria. Claims for vitamin A are not substantiated; it is a cumulative poison.

Psoralens (obtained from citrus and other plants), e.g. methoxsalen, are used to induce photochemical reactions in the skin. After local or systemic administration of the psoralen and subsequent exposure to ultraviolet light there is an erythematous reaction that goes deeper than ordinary sunburn and that may only reach its maximum after 48 h (sunburn maximum 12–24 h). Melanocytes are activated and pigmentation occurs over the following week. This action is used to repigment areas of disfiguring depigmentation. It is also used in some social suntan preparations (as oil of bergamot).

But in the presence of longwave (320–400 nm) ultraviolet irradiation (UVA) the psoralen interacts with DNA and RNA and inhibits DNA synthesis. This action is used in severe psoriasis (a disease characterised by increased epidermal proliferation), mycosis fungoides and some cases of lichen planus.

Severe adverse reactions can occur with psoralens and ultraviolet radiation, perhaps including increased risk of skin cancer (due to mutagenicity inherent in the action) and the treatment is only used by specialists.

DERMAL ADVERSE DRUG REACTIONS

Drugs taken systemically or applied locally often cause rashes. These take many different forms and

* Sunscreen preparations are commonly labelled to indicate their efficacy. A sun protection factor (SPF) number is provided, e.g. SPF10 means the subjects tolerance (duration of exposure without burning) should be increased about ten times.

the same drug will produce different rashes in different people.

Contact dermatitis is commonly eczematous and is often caused by antimicrobials, local anaesthetics and antihistamines. It can also be due to the vehicle in which the active drug is applied.

Reactions to *systemically administered* drugs are commonly erythematous, like those of measles, scarlatina or erythema multiforme. They give no useful clue to the cause.

'Though drugs may change, the clinical problems remain depressingly the same: a patient develops a rash; he is taking many different tablets; which, if any, of these caused his eruption, and what should be done about it? It is no answer simply to stop all drugs, though the fact that this can often be done casts some doubt on the patient's need for them in the first place. All too often potentially valuable drugs are excluded from further use on totally inadequate grounds. Clearly some guidelines are needed but no simple set of rules exist that can cover this complex subject . . .

'We* suggest that the following questions should be asked in every case:

1. Can other skin diseases be excluded?
2. Are the skin changes compatible with a drug cause?
3. Which drug is most likely to be responsible?
4. Are any further tests worth while? and
5. Is any treatment needed? These questions are deceptively simple but the answers are often difficult.'

However, despite great variability, some hints at drug-specific or characteristic rashes, etc. from drugs taken systemically, can be discerned, as follows:*

Toxic erythema commonly occurs at about the 9th day of treatment (or day 2–3 in previously exposed patients); causes include antibiotics, especially ampicillin, sulphonamides and derivatives (sulphonylureas, frusemide and thiazide diuretics), phenylbutazone and PAS.

Erythema multiforme, including Stevens–Johnson syndrome: phenylbutazone, sulphonamides and barbiturates.

* Hardie R A and Savin J A. Br Med J 1979; 1:935, to whom we are grateful for this quotation and the following classification. DRL, PNB.

Erythema nodosum: sulphonamides, oral contraceptives.

Allergic vasculitis: sulphonamides, phenylbutazone, indomethacin, phenytoin.

Purpura: thiazides, sulphonamides, sulphonylures, phenylbutazone, quinine.

Eczema: penicillins, phenothiazines.

Exfoliative dermatitis and erythrodermia: phenylbutazone, PAS, isoniazid, gold, carbamazepine.

Photosensitivity: see above.

Lupus erythematosus: hydralazine, isoniazid, procainamide, phenytoin.

Lichenoid eruption: chloroquine, mepacrine, gold, phenothiazines, PAS, arsenic.

Fixed eruptions are eruptions that recur at the same site, often circumoral, with each administration of the drug: phenolphthalein (laxative self-medication), sulphonamides, quinine, tetracycline, barbiturates.

Toxic epidermal necrolysis: phenytoin, sulphonamides, phenylbutazone, penicillin, barbiturates.

Urticaria, chronic: penicillins, aspirin (salicylates).

Pruritus unassociated with rash: oral contraceptives, phenothiazines, rifampicin (due to biliary stasis).

Hair loss: anticancer drugs, oral contraceptives, heparin, oral anticoagulants, carbimazole, androgenic steroids (women), sodium valproate.

Pigmentation: oral contraceptives, phenothiazines, heavy metals, mepacrine, chloroquine (pigmentations of nails and palate, depigmentation of the hair).

See also *allergy to drugs*, Ch. 9, in relation to the above.

Recovery after withdrawal of the causative drug generally begins in a few days, but lichenoid reactions may not improve until weeks have passed.

Diagnosis: Study of the patient's drug history may give clues. Reactions are commoner during early therapy (days) rather than after the drug has been given for months. Diagnosis by readministration of the drug is safe with fixed eruptions, but not with others.

Patch tests are useful in contact dermatitis, for they reproduce the causative process. Prick and scratch tests introduce all the problems of allergy to drugs, metabolism, combination with protein, etc., see Ch. 9.

Treatment. Remove the cause; use cooling applications and antipruritics; adrenal steroid for severe cases; histamine H_1-receptor blocker systemically for acute urticaria.

SEX HORMONES AND THE SKIN

Androgens stimulate the sebaceous glands. Thus they tend to produce seborrhoea and acne. *Oestrogens* have the opposite effect, but only at doses which have all the other typical effects and so their use for acne in men is seldom justified or acceptable except for a short initial period in severe cases.

Oestrogen-containing creams are advertised as cosmetics to enable women to look younger than they really are, by preventing and removing facial wrinkles. In women before the menopause there is no evidence that oestrogen-containing creams have a greater effect on the skin that the vehicle alone (i.e. hydration) unless sufficient is absorbed for systemic effects to occur. Post-menopausal atrophic changes do sometimes seem to be improved by their topical use, but seldom to the extent claimed by the manufacturers and desired by emotinally immature women obsessed with lost physical youth.

SUMMARY OF THE TREATMENT OF SKIN DISORDERS

The traditional advice, *if it's wet, dry it; if it's dry, wet it*, contains enough truth to be worth repeating. One or two applications a day are all that is usually necessary unless common sense dictates otherwise.

The table below is not intended to give the complete treatment of even the commoner skin conditions but merely to indicate a reasonable approach.

Secondary infections of ordinarily uninfected lesions may require local or systemic antimicrobials in addition. Analgesics, sedatives or tranquillisers may be needed in painful or uncomfortable conditions, or where the disease is intensified by emotion or anxiety.

X-ray therapy is helpful in many chronic skin conditions, but special experience is required and so it is not always included in the table.

Preparations for use on the skin. At the time of writing there are in the UK about 250 preparations for medical prescription (excluding those on direct sale to the public). Many of them are useful and many of them are minor variants. It is not practicable to give other than general guidance on choice. Physicians will select a modest range of products and get to know these well.

Psoriasis

In psoriasis there is increased epidermal cell proliferation with consequent increased numbers of horn cells that contain abnormal keratin. Drugs are used to *dissolve keratin* (keratolysis) and to *inhibit cell division.*

Keratin may be removed by scrubbing followed by a *dithranol* (antimitotic) in Zinc and Salicylic Acid Paste (Lassar's Paste) beginning with 0.1% and increasing to 1%; it stains skin and fabrics. *Tar* preparations are useful alternatives, and are commonly used for psoriasis of the scalp.

Topical *adrenal steroids* reduce epidermal cell division and application, especially under occlusive dressings, can be very effective, but increasing doses (concentrations) become needed and rebound follows withdrawal. They should only be used if dithranol or tar-containing preparations have failed or produced complications. Systemic corticosteroid administration should be avoided if at all possible, for high doses are needed to suppress the disease, which is liable to recur when treatment is withdrawn, as it must be if complications of long-term steroid therapy are to be avoided.

Vitamin A (retinols) play a minor role in epithelial function and the retinoic acid derivative *etretinate* (Tigason, orally) inhibits psoriatic hyperkeratosis. *It is teratogenic*, like other vitamin A derivatives, and can cause serious toxicity (see vitamin A). It must be used with great care.

A *psoralen* followed by ultraviolet light (PUVA) is used in severe cases (see *psoralens* above).

Folic acid antagonists (e.g. methotrexate) also suppress epidermal activity temporarily, but they are too toxic for use unless the psoriasis is life-threatening or severely disabling, and preferably patients should be past their reproductive years.

It is plain from this brief outline that treatment

of psoriasis requires considerable judgement, and it is no surprise that patients have formed a Psoriasis Association.

Acne

The major causative factor is androgen-mediated increased sebum production (in both men and women); the sebaceous glands are colonised by *Propionibacterium acnes*, and there is abnormal keratinization in their ducts.

The following measures are used progressively and selectively as the disease is more severe; they may need to be applied for up to 6 months:

1. Frequent *skin cleansing* and *degreasing*, including weak antiseptics and detergents, e.g. soap and water (merely washing usefully interrupts the logarithmic microbial growth), cetrimide, weak alcoholic solutions.

2. Mild *keratolytic* (exfoliating) formulations to unblock pilosebaceous ducts, e.g. benzoyl peroxide, sulphur, salicylic acid; perhaps with mild abrasive, e.g. aluminium oxide.

3. *Antimicrobial therapy* (tetracycline, erythromycin, co-trimoxazole) are used over months (response begins after 2 months). Bacterial resistance is not a problem; benefit is due to suppression of bacterial lipolysis of sebum, which generates inflammatory fatty acids.

4. A topical *adrenal steroid* reduces inflammation.

5. *Vitamin A derivatives* reduce sebum production and keratinization. Vitamin A is a teratogen.

Tretinoin (Retin-A) is applied topically. It is not known if it is safe in pregnancy.

Isotretinoin (Roaccutane) orally is highly effective (after 4 weeks), but is known to be a serious teratogen; it is used only in the most severe cystic and conglobate cases; its use requires the utmost informed care and supervision. Women of child-bearing potential should use effective contraception throughout treatment and for 2 months after.

6. *Hormone therapy*. The objective is to reduce androgen production or effect by using, (a) oestrogen, to suppress hypothalamic pituitary gonadotrophin production, or (b) an antiandrogen (cyproterone). An oestrogen alone as initial therapy to get the acne under control or, in women, the cyclical use of an oral contraceptive containing 50 μg of oestrogen diminishes sebum secretion by 40%. A combination of ethinyloestradiol and cyproterone (Diane) orally is also effective in women (it has contraceptive effect, which is desirable as the cyproterone may feminise a male fetus).

Drugs and venous ulcer healing. Drugs are not primary treatment for ulcers. But zinc sulphate orally can hasten healing, though its place in routine treatment is still uncertain.

Drugs applied locally are only adjuvants as astringent/protective, e.g. Zinc Gelatin (Unna's Paste), or to remove sloughs, e.g. Aserbine (malic, benzoic, salicylic acids). Allantoin dubiously hastens healing.

Adrenocortical steroids may make ulcers worse, though adjacent eczema may be benefited.

Infections and oedema are treated as usual. A hydrophilic dextran polymer as small beads (Debrisan) absorbs exudate and may reduce local oedema by improving drainage.

Removal of hair

'Unfortunately, our formalised cosmetic standards do not conform with the normal biological range, and this discrepancy brings misery to many individuals'.*

Epilation is removal of the intact hair, one at a time or embedded in wax and pulled out in quantity. This is temporary, and electrolytic destruction of the follicle is the only permanent technique.

Depilation is removal of the hair above the skin surface. Shaving is effective. Women are ashamed to shave their faces, but not their legs. Chemical depilatories are preferred. They act by reducing the disulphide bond between cystine molecules in polypeptide chains. The result is that osmotic pressure within the hair fibre causes swelling and jellification so that it can be wiped off. Many chemicals are effective, including salts of thioglycollic acid and barium sulphide; frequent use can cause dermatitis.

* Editorial. Lancet 1967; 1:488.

Condition	*Treatment*	*Remarks*
Abscess: boils and **carbuncles** (staphylococcal)	Pus should be cultured and antibiotic sensitivities obtained. Carrier sites should be swabbed for culture and sensitivities. Potent local antibiotics (fusidic acid) may be applied to lesions, and nasal carriers are treated with local antibiotic (neomycin). Clorhexidine, hexachlorophane or povidone–iodine in bath water are recommended for a week or so.	Systemic flucloxacillin may be needed in severe cases and may abort an early lesion.
Alopecia: baldness: Alopecia areata	Topical minoxidil is worth trying if the patient is embarrassed by baldness. 'Cosmetically acceptable' results may occur in up to 60%. Further studies are needed to confirm.	Most patients who take minoxidil orally for hypertension experience some increased hair growth. This has led to topical use for baldness. For picture see: Fenton D A et al. Br Med J 1985; 287:1015.
Chilblains	*Prevention*: short-wave diathermy may help. *Cure*: vasodilators and counter-irritants of dubious value. Vitamins are useless.	Use warm clothing even if this impairs elegance.
Dermatitis herpetiformis	Dapsone 25–250 mg daily, effective in 24 h, or sulphapyridine. Adrenal steroid systemically in resistant cases. Prolonged therapy necessary.	Antipruritics locally as required. Not other sulphonamides; beneficial effect *not* due to antimicrobial action. Methaemoglobinaemia may complicate dapsone therapy.
Eczema Allergic states Dermatitis *Acute*: *Subacute*: *Chronic*: *All grades*:	Lotions (Al acetate), wet dressings or soaks (NaCl, tap water). Zinc oxide creams or pastes sometimes with mild keratolytics added, e.g. Zinc Oxide and Salicylic Acid Paste. Zinc Oxide and Coal Tar Paste. Psychiatry can help some. Benefit from adrenal steroid. Treat infection. Moisturising cream if dry skin. Cleansing and emollient agents.	Remove the cause where possible. Often exacerbated by soap and water. Antipruritics (not antihistamines or local anaesthetics) may be added to lotions, creams or pastes.
Erysipelas and other streptococcal infections	Systemic penicillin.	
Exfoliative dermatitis	Chelating agent if due to a heavy metal. Cooling creams and powders locally. Adrenal steroid systemically when severe.	
Herpes simplex	Mild antiseptics for cleansing. Powder for cover. Local antivirus drugs of little or no benefit.	Symptomtic treatment and prevention and treatment of secondary bacterial infection. *No* corticosteroid if cornea involved.
Herpes zoster	Analgesics. Idoxuridine or acyclovir to whole dermatome (not to vesicles alone). Local antibiotics after 48 h until healing occurs.	Prevention of secondary infection reduces scarring. Systemic adrenal steroid in severe cases; may reduce incidence of post-herpetic neuralgia.
Hyperhidrosis	Astringents reduce sweat production, especially aluminium chloride hexahydrate (20%) in ethyl alcohol (95%). Anticholinergics may help and high local concentrations can be obtained with iontophoresis. Surgery, cryotherapy or radiation in extreme cases.	Treatment better in theory than practice; the volume of sweat dilutes the application; the characteristic smell is produced by bacterial action, so cosmetic deodorants contain antibacterials rather than substances that reduce sweat production.

Condition	Treatment	Remarks
Impetigo and sycosis barbae (mainly staphylococcal)	See *skin infections*.	
Intertrigo	Cleansing lotions, powders	To cleanse, lubricate and reduce friction.
Lichen planus	Antipruritics: may be drug caused, e.g. antimalarials, phenothiazines.	Often very resistant to treatment. Adrenal steroid locally but systemically in severe cases.
Lichen simplex (neurodermatitis)	Antipruritics. Sedatives. Grenz rays and adrenal steroid locally of great value	Covering the lesion so as to prevent scratching sometimes breaks the vicious cycle.
Lupus erythematosus affecting the skin	Potent adrenal steroid topically or intralesionally. Chloroquine or hydroxychloroquine, but eye toxicity serious hazard.	A systemic disease
Marginal blepharitis (various organisms)	Ointment containing adrenal steroid and an antimicrobial	Undue persistence can be due to allergy to treatment.
Candida	Nystatin, amphotericin clotrimazole, econazole, miconazole. Gentian violet paint in the mouth.	Suit the formulation to the site of infection: ointment, pessary, paint.
Nappy rash	*Prevention*: rid nappies of soaps, detergents and ammonia by rinsing. Change frequently and use barrier cream to keep skin dry. *Cure*: mild: Zn cream or calamine lotion, plus above measures. Severe: adrenal steroid locally, plus antimicrobial.	Absorption occurs from raw areas, especially under occulsive plastic pants.
Paronychia (candida or bacteria)	Ointment under the nail fold as appropriate to cause; surgery.	Keep fingers dry.
Pediculosis (lice)	Malathion or carbaryl; (anticholinesterases, safety depends on more rapid metabolism in man than in insects, and low absorption)	Ritual of application important. Lindane obsolescent due to resistance in lice.
Pemphigus: pemphigoid	Adrenal steroids systemically: other immunosuppressives, e.g. azathioprine sometimes: gold.	Oral hygiene and general nutrition very important.
Pityriasis rosea	Antipruritics as appropriate	The disease is self-limiting.
Ringworm, tinea (various fungi)	*Acute* lesions need lotions and soaks. *Chronic* lesions on dry skin: Benzoic Acid Cpd. Ointment (Whitfield's ointment). *Nail* and *scalp*: griseofulvin (or ketoconazole) systemically. *Other sites*, topical clotrimazole, econazole, miconazole.	Most preparations are both fungicidal and keratolytic, so the cells containing the fungus are eliminated. Treatment may need to be prolonged. Tolnaftate and undecenoates are now superseded.
Rosacea	1–2% sulphur in emulsion base. Tetracycline, mechanism unknown.	Corticosteroid exacerbates. Flushing makes it worse. Oestrogens for menopausal flushing.
Scabies (*Sarcoptes scabiei*)	Benzyl Benzoate Applic. or monosulfiram to whole body below the neck. Alternative: crotamiton	Correct ritual is essential. Crotamiton is also antipruritic and is useful as a supplementary application, as itching may persist
Scleroderma		No proved therapy

Condition	Treatment	Remarks
Serborrhoeic dermatitis: dandruff (Pityriasis capitis)	*Acute*. Adrenal steroid lotions (Betnovate or Dermovate scalp applications) and frequent use of soapless shampoos (1% cetrimide (Cetavlon) shampoo). *Chronic*. Regular shampooing with detergent shampoo with or without pyrithione zinc helps mild cases. More severe cases need a mild keratolytic (salicylic acid, sulphur) gel or lotion. Occasional corticosteroid application helps where there is much infalmmation	Antimicrobials if badly infected. Sulphur in various forms helps the seborrhoeic state but the reason is not known. Selenium (Selsun) irritates the eyes and is poisonous if swallowed, and offers no advantage.
Urticaria, angioneurotic oedema	As for allergic reactions; histamine H_1-receptor blocker, corticosteroid (or adrenaline in emergency)	
Vitiligo	No safe and reliable treatment. Methoxsalen or other psoralen, topically or systemically, plus daily exposure to UVL (PUVA) is toxic, troublesome and often fails.	Probably an autoimmune disease
Warts	All treatments are *destructive* and should be applied with precision. Cryotherapy (liquid nitrogen, solid CO_2). Salicylic acid 12% in collodion daily. Many other caustic (keratolytic) preparations. Salicyclic and lactic acid lotion (Salactol) topically under occlusion after removing surface layer with coarse emery paper. Surgery	Warts often disappear spontaneously. For plantar warts formalin 3% footsoaks 20 min nightly for 6–8 weeks cures 80% cases. Podophyllin (antimitotic) for plantar or anal warts. Non-surgical remedies may act by disrupting the wart so that virus is absorbed, antibodies develop and the wart is rejected immunologically.
X-ray dermatitis	Andrenal steroid locally.	

GUIDE TO FURTHER READING

1 Hunter J A A et al. Present and future trends in approaches to skin diseases. Br Med J 1974; 1:283.
2 Dineen P. Hand washing and degerming: a comparison of povidone-iodine and chlorhexidine. Clin Pharmacol Ther 1978; 23:63.
3 Editorial. Hexachlorophane — yes or no? Br Med J 1977; 1:337 and subsequent correspondence.
4 Goutières F et al. Accidental percutaneous hexachlorophane intoxication in children. Br Med J 1977; 2:663.
5 Koivisto V A et al. Is skin preparation necessary before insulin injection? Lancet 1978: 1:1072.
6 Lowbury E J L et al. Preoperative disinfection of surgeons' hands: use of alcoholic solutions and effects of gloves on skin flora. Br Med J 1974; 4:369.
7 Khan J S et al. A case of Dettol addiction. Br Med J 1979; 1:791.
8 Editorial. Prophylactic povidone-iodine. Lancet 1976; 1:73.
9 Editorial. Out damned spot (disinfection). Lancet 1978; 2:1349.
10 Speers R et al. Increased dipersal of skin bacteria into the air after shower baths: the effect of hexachlorophane. Lancet 1966: 1:1298.
11 Vollum D I. Skin lesions in drug addicts. Br Med J 1970; 2:647.
12 Ducksbury C F J et al. Contact dermatitis in home helps following use of detergents. Br Med J 1970; 1:537.
13 Editorial. Steroid-antibiotic combinations. Br Med J 1977; 1:1303.
14 Carruthers J A. Observations on the systemic effect of topical clobetasol propionate (Dermovate). Br Med J 1975; 4:203.
15 Editorial. Washing away at acne. Br Med J 1976; 2:834.
16 Editorial. Antibiotics in acne. N Engl J Med 1976; 294:43.
17 Editorial. Iconoclasm in acne. Br Med J 1977; 2:1107.
18 Lane P et al. Treatment of acne with tetracycline HCl: a double-blind trial with 51 patients. Br Med J 1969; 2:76.
19 Fusaro R M et al. Erythropoietic protoporphyria: protection from sunlight. Br Med J 1970; 1:730.
20 Editorial. Artifical tan. Br Med J 1960; 2:285.
21 Editorial. Sensitivity to fluorescent light. Br Med J 1969; 2:185.
22 Editorial. Unhealthy tan. Br Med J 1970; 1:494.
23 Editorial. Sunscreens. Br Med J 1975; 1:237.

24 Stern R S et al. Risk of cutaneous carcinoma in patients treated with oral methoxsalen photochemotherapy for psoriasis. N Engl J Med 1979; 300:809, and subsequent correspondence.
25 Editorial. Risk and benefits of the treatment of psoriasis. N Engl J Med 1979; 300:852; also Editorial. Lancet 1979; 1:1011.
26 Brown D G et al. Psychiatric treatment of eczema: a controlled trial. Br Med J 1971; 2:729.
27 Editorial. Shingles: a belt of roses from Hell.Br Med J 1979; 1:5.
28 Editorial. Epilatories and depilatories. Lancet 1967; 1:488.
29 Shuster S. Over the counter sale of topical corticosteroids: the need for debate. Br Med J 1985; 291:38: and subsequent correspondence.
30 Fenton D A et al, Topical minoxidil in the treatment of alopecia areata. Br Med J 1983; 287:1015.
31 Savin J A. Some guidelines for the use of topical corticosteroids. Br Med J 1985; 290:1607.
32 Ackroyd J F. Fixed drug eruptions. Br Med J 1985; 290:1533.
33 Heddle R J et al, Combined oral and nasal beclomethasone dipropionate in children with atopic eczema: a randomised controlled trial. Br Med J 1984; 290:651.
34 Krame L et al, Mechanism of action of antipruritic drugs. Br Med J 1983; 287:1199.
35 Alexander-Williams J. Pruritus ani. Br Med J 1983; 287:159.
36 Editorial, Preoperative depilation. Lancet 1983; 1:1311.
37 Savin J A. Excessive sweating in the palms and armpits. Br Med J 1983; 286:580.
38 Editorial. Drug induced bullous eruptions. Br Med J 1981; 282:421.
39 Champion R H. Psoriasis and its treatment. Br Med J 1981; 282:343.
40 Marks J M et al, Influence of prophylactic photochemotherapy on incidence of relapse of psoriasis cleared initially with dithranol. Br Med J 1984; 288:95.
41 Henseler T et al, Oral 8-methoxypsoralen photochemotherapy of psoriasis: the European PUVA study: a cooperative study among 18 European centres. Lancet 1981; 1:853.

40

Vitamins, calcium and bone

Vitamins are substances that are essential for normal metabolism and must be chiefly supplied in the diet.

Man cannot synthesise any vitamins in his body except some vitamin D in the skin and nicotinamide from tryptophan. Lack of a particular vitamin may lead to a specific deficiency syndrome. This may be primary (inadequate diet), or secondary, due to failure of absorption (intestinal abnormality or chronic diarrhoea), or to increased metabolic need (growth, pregnancy, lactation, hyperthyroidism, fever).

Vitamin deficiencies are commonly multiple, and complex clinical pictures occur. There are numerous single and multivitamin preparations to provide prophylaxis and therapy.

It has often been suggested, but never proved, that subclinical vitamin deficiences are a cause of much chronic ill-health and liability to infections. This idea has led to enormous consumption of vitamin preparations, which probably have no more than placebo value. Fortunately most of the vitamins are comparatively non-toxic, but prolonged administration of vitamins A and D can have serious ill-effects.

Vitamins fall into two groups:

The water-soluble vitamins: the B group and C.

The fat-soluble vitamins: A, D, K and E.

VITAMIN A

Vitamin A exists in a variety of forms: carotene = provitamin A; retinol = vitamin A_1; 3-dehydroretinol = vitamin A_2.

Functions. Vitamin A is concerned with *sight*; it provides the prosthetic groups for the light-sensitive pigments of the retina; night blindness is an early manifestation of deficiency.

Vitamin A is concerned with the growth and differentiation of *epithelia*; deficiency causes metaplasia and hyperkeratosis of the epithelia throughout the body, which is especially serious in the eye, causing xerophthalmia and keratomalacia, which can lead to blindness; it is this function that has led to use of vitamin A derivatives in hyperkeratotic disorders,e.g. psoriasis and acne. The epithelial metaplasia seen in deficiency is reminiscent of the early stage of transformation of normal tissue to cancer, and vitamin A is being explored for a clinical role in prevention of cancer (inhibition of cancer in animal experimental situations has been shown).

Sources. Carotene is converted into vitamin A in the intestinal wall. Green vegetables and carrots are satisfactory diet sources, and so are milk, cheese, butter, eggs and liver. Margarine has vitamin A added to it.

Fish liver oils are recommended for babies on account of their vitamin D content, but they are also very rich sources of vitamin A.

Daily dietary intake should be 5000 IU for men and 4000 IU for women (who need 6000 IU during pregnancy and lactation). The International Unit is being replaced by the *retinol equivalent* (= 3.33 IU).

A normal Western European diet contains adequate amounts of vitamin A or carotene, but deficiencies are relatively common in Asia (an important cause of blindness). Vitamin A is stored in the liver, which, in normal individuals, contains enough to last for 1–2 years.

Prophylaxis requires the recommended daily intake as one of the numerous available preparations.

Vitamin A is fat-soluble and so is poorly absorbed in steatorrhoea and similar conditions. Once a deficiency has been diagnosed, 30 000 units of vitamin A should be given daily by mouth, and should be continued until the patient recovers. Capsules of the pure vitamin and of fish-liver oil are available, e.g. vitamin A and D Caps (about 4500 IU per capsule). Other uses include *skin diseases* where there is hyperkeratinization, e.g. acne and psoriasis, in which derivatives (tretinol, etretinate and isotretinoin) are used, see index.

Prevention of **cancer** is speculative but smokers have already been advised not to put their hope in vitamin A, but rather to stop smoking.

Toxic effects occur if very large amounts are taken (in children 25 000 to 500 000 IU daily). A diagnostic sign of chronic poisoning is the presence of painful tender swellings over the bones. Anorexia, skin lesions, hepatosplenomegaly and general malaise also occur. Vitamin A is very cumulative and effects take weeks to wear off. Most cases of vitamin A poisoning have been due to mothers administering large amounts of fish-liver oils to their children in the belief that it was good for them, but travellers have been made ill by eating the livers of arctic carnivores.

'Eskimos never eat polar-bear liver, knowing it to be toxic, and husky dogs, with instinctive wisdom, also avoid it . . . Those who pooh-pooh the Eskimos' fears or the husky dogs' instincts and are tempted to enjoy a man's portion of polar-bear liver — appetites get sharp near the North Pole — will consume anything up to 10 000 000 IU of vitamin A. This is too much of a good thing, and the diner will probably soon find himself drowsy, then overcome by headache and vomiting, and finally losing the outer layer of his skin. These are, it is believed, signs of acute poisoning with Vitamin A'.*

Chronic overdose causes an increased liability of biological membranes and of the outer layer of the skin to peel off. An extreme example of this is the case of the Antarctic explorer who in 1913 ate the liver of his husky sledge dogs (see above). His feet felt sore and 'the sight of my feet gave me quite a shock, for the thickened skin of the soles had separated in each case as a complete layer. . . . I did what appeared to be the best thing under the circumstances: smeared the new skin with lanoline . . . and with bandages bound the skin soles back in place.'†

Vitamin A and its derivatives are *teratogenic* at above physiological doses.

THE VITAMIN B COMPLEX

The name 'Vitamin B' was originally given to a dietary factor that was necessary for the growth of rats. It was soon shown not to be a single substance. A number of widely differing substances are now, for convenience, included in the vitamin B complex. *Primary deficiency* occurs with diets in which meat, yeast and whole grains are lacking.

Thiamine (B_1), *riboflavine* (B_2), *pyridoxine* (B_6) and *niacin* (B_7) are discussed here; for *folic acid* and the *cobalamins* (B_{12}) see Chapter 29.

Pantothenic acid, inositol, biotin, and *para-aminobenzoic acid* are not known to be of practical clinical importance as recognisable deficiency states do not occur in man.‡ *Choline* is usually included in the B group of vitamins, although it can be synthesised in the body if sufficient methyl groups are available (e.g. from methionine). Choline deficiency in animals leads to accumulation of fat in the liver, but it has no established

* Editorial. Br Med J 1962; 1:855.

† Shearman J C. Vitamin A and Sir Douglas Mawson, Br Med J 1978; 1:283.

‡ Biotin deficiency may occur with excessive intake of raw egg white.

role in hepatic or in any other disease and a good diet contains enough to prevent deficiency.

B group vitamins are soluble in water and many of them are concerned in essential oxidation–reduction reactions; in addition to dietary sources they are synthesised to a variable extent by bacteria normally present in the colon.

Secondary deficiency may occur as a result of inadequate absorption due to diarrhoea, including that due to antimicrobials that alter colonic flora. It may also be due to increased need (hyperthyroidism, fever) or to defective utilisation (hepatic disease).

Patients maintained by intravenous feeding for more than 2 days need the B vitamins. There is a large number of preparations of the B group vitamins.

Vitamin B Cpd. Tabs: for prophylaxis. Thiamine, 1 mg; riboflavine, 1 mg, nicotinamide, 15 mg. *Dose*: one or two tablets daily.

Vitamin B Cpd Tabs Strong: for treatment of deficiency. Thiamine, 5 mg; riboflavine, 2 mg; nicotinamide, 20 mg; pyridoxine, 2 mg. *Dose*: one or two tablets, thrice daily.

Thiamine (Vitamin B_1)

Gross deficiency of thiamine leads to beri-beri, which is characterised by peripheral neuritis, high-output cardiac failure, oedema and, rarely, demyelination of the central nervous system (Wernicke's encephalopathy).

History. Beri-beri is largely a man-made disease; it became common in the East when steam-driven mills were developed in the mid-19th century and polished rice (i.e. rice without its inner husk) replaced brown rice as the staple diet. Beri-beri occurred in up to 40% of Japanese naval ratings, but was almost abolished by the introduction of a more varied diet. In 1909 an experiment was performed on 300 healthy Javanese labourers building a railway in Malaya. They all preferred polished rice, for its superior taste, and chose it even though it was explained that they might get beri-beri. Half of them, chosen at random, were given polished rice, and the remainder brown rice. After 3 months beri-beri developed only in the group eating polished rice. The groups were switched after 6 months and beri-beri immediately improved when the victims ate the brown rice. Correspondingly, the previously unaffected group began to develop beri-beri now that they were eating polished rice. In all, 20 cases of beri-beri developed on the polished rice diet, as compared with none amongst those eating brown rice. It was soon realised that the anti-beri-beri factor and the 'vitamin B' necessary for growth in rats were similar. Thiamine was synthesised in 1936.

Function. Thiamine is the co-enzyme of carboxylase, and is required for carbohydrate metabolism. In its absence the substrates of carboxylase (pyruvic and other α-keto-acids) cannot be normally metabolised, and so they accumulate. Despite detailed knowledge about its function as a co-enzyme, it is still not known how a deficiency of thiamine leads to the characteristic symptoms of beri-beri.

Sources and requirements. Thiamine is widely distributed in plants and animals. The outer coats of grain kernels are rich in it, but these are removed in the preparation of white flour or polished rice. Requirements of thiamine vary directly with the amount of carbohydrate consumed, but 0.4 mg thiamine for every 1000 calories is about enough, i.e. 1–1.5 mg per day. (with 50% increase in pregnancy and lactation).

For severe beri-beri 50 mg of thiamine should be given × 3/daily, i.m. or i.v. For prophylaxis, 2 mg daily by mouth is adequate.

Indications. Vitamin deficiencies are almost always multiple and although beri-beri is primarily due to a deficiency of thiamine, diets are generally also deficient in riboflavine, nicotinamide, pyridoxine, vitamins A and D and protein. Thus a general improvement in diet is desirable in addition to the specific treatment with thiamine. In Western countries where beri-beri is rare and often atypical, it is due either to a bizarre diet or to malabsorption from the gut, e.g. in chronic diarrhoea. Thiamine is destroyed readily in an alkaline medium and hence deficiency is particularly likely to occur in achlorhydric patients. Thiamine deficiency should always be considered as a possible cause of obscure peripheral neuritis or high-output cardiac failure (which responds to treatment in 12 h). Alcoholic polyneuritis sometimes responds to large doses of vitamin B complex; spirit-drinking alcoholics who take most of their calories in the form of alcohol (which requires thiamine for its metabolism) and do not eat enough thiamine-containing food, may develop beri-beri heart failure.

Adverse effects are rare, but occasionally a patient shows allergy.

Riboflavine (Vitamin B_2)

Deficiency of riboflavine leads to angular stomatitis, ulceration of mucous membranes, 'magenta' tongue, vascularisation of the cornea and seborrhoeic dermatitis, especially of the face. It is very rare in Britain, but occurs in areas where chronic malnutrition is widespread. It usually accompanies other deficiency diseases, such as beri-beri, pellagra and kwashiorkor. Riboflavine deficiency predisposes to snow-blindness.

Riboflavine is an essential component of certain oxidative enzyme systems in intermediary metabolism. It is present in milk, yeast and green vegetables.

Daily requirement is about 1.5 mg. If a deficiency of riboflavine is suspected, a therapeutic test may be performed; improvement of the lesions within a week of giving riboflavine in the absence of other therapy suggests that the lesions were in fact due to its deficiency.

Phototherapy for neonatal jaundice causes transient and probably harmless riboflavine deficiency.

The usual therapeutic dose is 5–10 mg a day orally; parenteral preparations (usually plus vit. C) are available. Toxic effects do not occur.

Nicotinamide (nictonic acid amide, niacinamide), nictoinic acid (niacin)

Deficiency of nictoninamide leads to pellagra, which is a generalised disease affecting especially the whole gastrointestinal tract (diarrhoea, red inflamed tongue, gastritis), the central nervous system (dementia), and the skin, especially where it is exposed to light (dermatitis). It occurs in underfed populations, particularly where maize is a staple food.

Nicotinamide is an essential part of codehydrogenases I and II, and so it is present in every living cell. Tryptophan, which is present in good quality protein, can be converted into nicotinamide, and consequently will substitute for it in the diet. Maize protein is conspicuously lacking in tryptophan. Nicotinamide is also synthesised in the bowel, by bacteria, so that daily needs (about 20 mg) are difficult to measure accurately.

Pellagra is not usually a pure nicotinamide deficiency, so the other B vitamins and ascorbic acid should be given too. The dose is 250–500 mg orally daily in divided doses. Parenteral preparations are available.

Adverse effects do not occur with nicotinamide. Nicotinic acid, which is converted into nicotinamide, causes peripheral vasodilatation accompanied by an unpleasant flushing and itching, and the patient may faint.

Pyridoxine (Vitamin B_6)

Pyridoxine, converted to pyridoxal phosphate, is a coenzyme (including decarboxylases) for transamination and is concerned with many metabolic processes. It is present in liver, yeast and cereals.

Pure pyrodoxine deficiency is very rare. It occurs chiefly in children on peculiar artificial foods (diarrhoea, fits, anaemia); peripheral neuropathy can occur. Familial pyridoxine resistance is also known. The children present with convulsions and dermatitis. Pyridoxine 4 mg/kg orally or parenterally daily should suffice for treatment.

Adults develop an anaemia (hypochromic, microcytic with high serum iron), due to defective haemoglobin synthesis, that may respond to big doses of pyridoxine (0.1–0.3 g a day). That such big doses are needed suggests that it is not a simple pyridoxine deficiency.

Normal adult dietary requirement is 2 mg pyridoxine a day, and the therapeutic dose for suspected deficiency is about 100 mg per day, orally or parenterally.

Isoniazid interferes with pyridoxine (there are structural resemblances) and causes a pyridoxine-deficiency peripheral neuritis that can be prevented by adding pyridoxine without altering the antibacterial effect.

Pyridoxine, even in small doses, can block the therapeutic effect of levodopa in parkinsonism, by enhancing its decarboxylation to dopamine, which does not enter the brain. It does not interfere with the combined levodopa/decarboxylase preparations (e.g. Sinemet) because of the presence of the decarboxylase inhibitor.

It is also advocated in vomiting of pregnancy and radiation sickness, though unequivocal evidence is lacking.

Some cases of homocystinuria (an inborn error of amino acid metabolism with mental defect and thrombosis) respond to pyridoxine. The defect is in an enzyme (cystathionine synthetase) that converts homocystine to cystathionine. This enzyme is activated by pyridoxine, thus lessening the metabolic block.

ASCORBIC ACID, VITAMIN C

Deficiency of ascorbic acid leads to scurvy, which is characterised by petechial haemorrhages, haematomas, bleeding gums (if teeth are present), anaemia and, in children, cessation of ossification in the growing-ends of bone.

History. Scurvy had been a scourge for thousands of years. In the Middle Ages it was treated with a great variety of preparations, among them citrus fruit and fresh vegetables. In 1753, Dr. James Lind performed a simple therapeutic trial on 12 sailors with advanced scurvy. They were all on the same basic diet and were living in the same quarters on board ship at sea. He divided them into pairs and dosed each pair differently. The respective daily treatments were:

1. cyder
2. sulphuric acid
3. vinegar
4. sea-water
5. a concoction of garlic, mustard, balsam and myrrh
6. two oranges and a lemon

The pair receiving the oranges and lemon recovered and were back on duty within a week; of the others, only the pair taking cyder was slightly improved. Lind also recognised the antisorbutic properties of green vegetables and salads. The efficacy of oranges and lemons in the prevention and cure of scurvy was repeatedly confirmed; but 40 years were to pass before any attention was paid and a regular daily allowances of lemon juice provided in the Navy. Unfortunately lime juice* was soon substituted for lemon juice because it could be had cheaply in the West Indian Colonies. Lime juice contains only about a third as much ascorbic acid as lemon juice and failed to prevent scurvy completely. Synthetic ascorbic acid has been available since the 1930s.

Function. Ascorbic acid is a powerful reducing agent and plays a part in intracellular oxidation–reduction systems. In scurvy there is a general breakdown of collagenous connective tissue, which explains the main symptoms. Ascorbic acid is also needed to prevent oxidation of tetrahydrofolic acid, which adds folate deficiency anaemia to the anaemia of bleeding. It is present in high concentration in the adrenal cortex and it may be involved in steroid synthesis. Only man (and other primates), guinea-pigs, the Indian fruit bat and the red-vented bulbul (a bird) get scurvy; other animals are able to synthesise ascorbic acid or themselves.

Detection of deficiency. Ascorbic acid concentration is measured in plasma (or in platelets or leucocytes).

Sources are mainly fresh fruit and vegetables; meat and milk contain a little. Ascorbic acid is rapidly oxidised and destroyed by heating in the presence of air, hence deep-fried potatoes contain more than do boiled. Properly canned fruit and vegetables retain a high proportion of their ascorbic acid. Vitamin C supplements are commonly given to babies (orange juice).

The requirement of ascorbic acid is about 60 mg daily for an adult (with 50% increase during pregnancy and lactation, in smokers and after major surgery). Maintenance of full saturation requires more than 75 mg a day, but there is no certainty that full saturation is necessary. Pregnancy, lactation, active growth or severe disease increase utilisation of the vitamin. Human milk contains 3–4 times as much ascorbic acid as cow's milk, in which the amount is also reduced by heat, including pasteurisation. Hence scurvy

* Hence the term 'limey' for British sailors.

can occur with prolonged bottle-feeding of babies unless a supplement of ascorbic acid is added.

Normal body stores are about 1500 mg, used up at about 3%/day so that scurvy will develop in about 3 months if there is no intake. Scurvy occurs among elderly widowers living alone on bread, bacon, cheese, margarine and tea. Wound healing is delayed in scurvy, hence ascorbic acid supplements may be desirable in surgical patients who are decrepit or who have been eating abnormal diets, and also in patients with pressure sores.

Indications for ascorbic acid are:

The prevention and cure of scurvy. Urinary acidification.

Methaemoglobinaemia, for its properties as a reducing agent (see below).

It is possible that large daily doses (1 g/day) of ascorbic acid may reduce the incidence and severity of coryza. Reliable trials in this disease are difficult and the results are inconclusive. To justify prolonged prophylactic use of such doses in populations, the benefit must be shown to be clinically, as well as statistically, significant. This has not been achieved.

Persistent claims that ascorbic acid is effective treatment in advanced cancer (historical controls were used), receive no support from a double-blind random controlled therapeutic trial (ref at end of chapter).

Dose of Ascorbic Acid Tabs (50, 250, 500 mg) for scurvy is 1 g orally, daily. 75 mg daily is enough to prevent it. Parenteral preparations are available.

Ill-effects do not occur at ordinary doses; it is eliminated in the urine unchanged and metabolised to oxalate. High doses may cause sleep disturbances.

Doses above 4 g/day, which have been taken over long periods to prevent coryza, increase urinary oxalate concentration sufficiently to form oxalate stones. Intravenous ascorbic acid may precipitate a haemolytic attack in subjects with glucose-6-phosphate dehydrogenase deficiency.

Methaemoglobinaemia

A reducing substance is needed to convert the methaemoglobin (ferric iron) back to oxyhaemoglobin (ferrous iron) whenever enough has formed to impair seriously the oxygen carrying capacity of the blood. Ascorbic acid is non-toxic (it acts by direct reduction) but is less effective than methylene blue. Both can be given orally, i.v. or i.m. Excessive doses of methylene blue can *cause* methaemoglobinaemia (it acts by stimulating or ADPH-dependent enzymes).

Methaemoglobinaemia may be drug-induced (phenacetin*, sulphonamides, nitrites, nitrates (may occur in well-water), pamaquin, primaquine, sulfones, phenazopyridine (Pyridium), phenazone, vitamin K analogues, chlorates, aniline and nitrobenzene). In the rare instance of there being urgency, methylene blue 1 mg/kg slowly i.v. benefits within 30 min. (Ascorbic acid competes directly with the chemical cause and is inadequate in severe cases, which are the only ones that need treatment.)

In the congenital form oral methylene blue (3–6 mg/kg/day in divided doses) with or without ascorbic acid (0.5 g/day) gives benefit in days to weeks.

Methylene blue turns the urine blue and high concentrations can irritate the urinary tract, so that fluid intake should be high when big doses are used.

Sulphaemoglobinaemia cannot be treated by drugs. It can be caused by phenacetin, sulphonamides, phenazopyridine, nitrites or nitrates.

VITAMIN D, CALCIUM, PARATHORMONE, CALCITONIN

Deficiency of vitamin D leads to rickets in growing children and to osteomalacia in adults.

Calcium. The skeleton contains about 1200 g of calcium (all the rest of the body contains only about 12 g), and provides a reserve that is drawn upon to maintain the plasma calcium around the normal level of 2.5 mmol/l (10 mg/100 ml); about half of this is normally in the ionised form. Calcium is incompletely (about 30%) absorbed from the proximal small intestine via a carrier process, the amount absorbed being particularly dependent on vitamin D. Calcium is lost from the body in the faeces (faecal calcium is mostly the

* Phenacetin has been withdrawn in the UK and in many other countries.

non-absorbed fraction from the food, but some is excreted into the intestine) and to a lesser extent in the urine. Both absorption and excretion are controlled by vitamin D and parathormone.

A daily intake of 0.5 g of calcium is normally adequate but this should be substantially higher in pregnancy and lactation, and during the treatment of rickets and osteomalacia.

Tetany. A low plasma ionised calcium increases the irritability of the nervous system generally.

Alkalosis (e.g. from vomiting in pyloric stenosis) causes tetany partly by lowering the proportion of ionised calcium in the extracellular fluid. The commonest cause of tetany is probably hysterical overbreathing, leading to respiratory alkalosis; rebreathing from a bag or administration of 10% carbon dioxide in oxygen will help in such a case. Sedation may be necessary to stop the overbreathing. Calcium gluconate is given slowly i.v. in acute hypocalcaemic tetany e.g. following removal of, or damage to, the parathyroid glands or removal of a parathyroid tumour, or associated with very severe rickets or osteomalacia. Dihydrotachysterol is also used to increase Ca absorption. It acts quicker than vitamin D_2 or D_3 (see below). Dietary Ca is increased by giving Ca gluconate (an effervescent tab is available) or lactate, and this and vitamin D (in high dose) may be needed long term for chronic cases.

Aluminium hydroxide binds phosphate in the gut causing hypophosphataemia, which stimulates renal formation of the most active vitamin D metabolite (see below) and so enhances Ca absorption.

Calcium Gluconate Inj. is given i.v. as a 10% solution, 10–20 ml being given at the rate of about 2 ml per min and repeated as necessary (every few hours). It must not be given i.m. as it is painful and causes necrosis.

Adverse effects of intravenous calcium may be very dangerous. An early sign is tingling in the mouth and a feeling of warmth spreading over the body. Serious effects are those on the heart, which mimic and synergise with digitalis; fatal cardiac arrest may occur in digitalised animals and it would seem advisable to avoid i.v. calcium in any patient on digitalis (except in severe symptomatic hypocalcaemia), indeed, reduction of ionised calcium by a chelating agent has been successful in treating digitalis dysrhythmia. The effect of calcium on the heart is antagonised by potassium and similarly the toxic effects of a high serum potassium in acute renal failure may be to some extent counteracted with calcium.

Treatment of acute hypercalcaemia may be needed whether or not the cause can be removed and when severe; generally a plasma concentration of 3.0 mmol/l (12 mg/100 ml) needs urgent treatment if there is also clinical evidence of toxicity (individual tolerance varies greatly). After taking account of the patient's cardiac and renal function, the following measures may be employed selectively.

First, correct *dehydration* (and so enhance renal Ca elimination) and then consider using a high-efficacy *loop diuretic* (frusemide) for rapid renal elimination of Ca; careful attention to fluid balance and plasma electrolytes is essential.

An *adrenocortical steroid* (e.g. prednisolone 20–40 mg/day orally) reduces intestinal absorption of Ca and may inhibit osteolytic cancer, but it is only effective over days and has no effect in hyperparathyroidism. It is most effective in vitamin D intoxication and sarcoid.

Hypercalcaemia due to cancer may be reduced by low doses of *mithramycin* (relatively selective for osteoclasts); a single dose may give benefit for days.

Oral *phosphate* (as Phosphate-Sandoz: equivalent of phosphorus 500 mg, sodium 489 mg, potassium 123 mg) up to two tablets orally 4-hourly is safe and effective (provided the Na load is acceptable and the initial plasma P is not raised), although it causes diarrhoea. Phosphate has a complex reciprocal interrelationship with Ca.

When the hypercalcaemia is at least partly due to mobilisation from bone, *calcitonin* can be used to inhibit bone resorption, and it may enhance urinary excretion of Ca; the effect develops in a few hours, and responsiveness may be lost over a few days (and may sometimes be restored by an adrenal steroid).

Trisodium edetate i.v. can be used; it chelates Ca and is rapidly effective.

Dialysis is quick and effective.

The above measures are temporary only, to give time to tackle the cause.

Sodium cellulose phosphate binds calcium in the intestine and prevents absorption: it is used for renal stone formation (due to hypercalciuria) in patients who overabsorb dietary calcium.

Calcium and phosphorus metabolism are controlled by *parathormone, calcitonin* and *vitamin D*.

Parathormone acts chiefly on bone and kidney; its effects on the gut are indirect due to alteration of renal synthesis of 1α-25-dihydroxycholecalciferol (see vitamin D). It increases the rate of bone remodelling (mineral and collagen) and osteocyte activity, with an overall balance in favour of resorption (osteoclastic activity), so that there is a rise in plasma Ca concentration (and fall in phosphate). It increases the gut absorption of Ca (probably via its effect on vitamin D metabolism).

Impure bovine parathyroid preparations have been used for treatment of acute hypocalcaemic tetany in order to avoid repeated injections of calcium gluconate, but immunological resistance soon occurs and, for this reason also, they do not provide long-term replacement therapy in parathyroid deficiency. (Human parathormone is not generally available.) The D vitamins are both more reliable and more effective in chronic hypoparathyroidism. Owing to the slow action of the vitamin D, acute hypoparathyroidism is better treated by i.v. injections of calcium (see *tetany*) and dihydrotachysterol, or possibly alfacalcidol.

Calcitonin is a peptide hormone produced by the C-cells of the thyroid gland. It decreases the rate of bone turnover and decreases renal tubular reabsorption of Ca and P. It is used in Paget's disease of bone and to control hypercalcaemia. Both natural (porcine) and synthetic (salmon) calcitonin (salcatonin) are available for i.m. and s.c. use. They differ substantially from human calcitonin and antibodies form in a high proportion of cases.

Vitamin D. In the early 1920s there were two theories about rickets, the older that lack of sunlight caused the disease, the other that it was due to a dietary deficiency. Both were correct and were reconciled when it was shown that irradiation of food increased its antirachitic activity. The increased sensitivity to rickets of some dark-skinned races living in temperate climates may be partly due to their skin pigment preventing the comparatively small amount of sunlight that they receive from activating ergosterol in the skin. There is a large number of structurally related compounds with vitamin D-like activity.

Vitamin D

D_2 (calciferol, ergocalciferol), made by ultraviolet irradiation or ergosterol

D_3 (cholecalciferol), made by ultraviolet irradiation of 7-dehydrocholesterol. It is also the form that occurs in natural foods and is formed in the skin.

The above, D_2, D_3, are *25-hydroxylated* into more active forms in the *liver*, which are then 1α-hydroxylated in the *kidney* (under the control of parathormone) into the most active form. Thus the most active natural form of vitamin D is 1α-25-dihydroxycholecalciferol (*calcitriol*). In renal disease this final rate-limited renal α-hydroxylation is inadequate, and administration of the less biologically active precursors is therefore liable to lack efficacy.

But in 1978 there was introduced a 1α-hydoxylated form (1α-hydroxycholecalciferol: *alfacalcidol*: One-Alpha) that only requires *hepatic* 25-hydroxylation to become the highly active 1α-25-dihydroxycholecalciferol (calcitriol). Alfacalcidol is therefore effective in the presence of renal disease since the defective renal hydroxylation stage has been bypassed. Its extraordinary potency and efficacy is indicated by the adult dose, often only 1–2 μg/day.

In addition there is a structural variant of vitamins D_2 and D_3, *dihydrotachysterol* (AT10, Tachyrol), which is also biologically activated by *hepatic* 25-hydroxylation.

The advantages of *alfacalcidol* and *dihydrotachysterol* include a faster onset and shorter duration of *clinical* effect (days) than vitamins D_2 and D_3 (weeks). But these factors are not relevant to the ordinary management of vitamin D deficiency.

Actions are complex. Vitamin D promotes the active transport (absorption) of calcium and therefore of phosphate from the gut, to control, with parathormone, the mineralisation of bone and to promote the renal tubular reabsorption of calcium and phosphate. The plasma calcium concentration rises. After a dose of D_2, D_3 there is a lag of about 21 h before the intestinal effect begins (measured in vitamin D-deficient rats) and this is probably due to the time needed for its metabolic conversion to the more active forms, and also for its action on a protein cellular carrier mechanism for Ca absorption. But after calcitriol the lag is only 2 h.

A large single dose of vitamin D has biological effects for as long as 6 months (because of metabolism and storage, knowledge of the plasma half-life is of no practical importance). Thus the drug is cumulative and overdose by a mother anxious that her child shall have strong bones can cause serious toxicity.

If there is a deficiency of vitamin D, growing metaphysial cartilage and osteoid tissue does not become calcified, and rickets results. An adult, who is not growing, needs much less vitamin D than a child, but a chronic deficiency over many years leads in the adult to skeletal decalcification (*osteomalacia*). Women kept indoors on inadequate diets and who bore many children used to suffer from osteomalacia (the fetus and infant being parasitic upon the mother for both vitamin D and calcium). Nowadays, except in poorly fed populations, osteomalacia usually follows metabolic disorders that appear to produce an increased requirement for vitamin D, for instance steatorrhoea, renal failure, and certain inherited diseases.

Epileptic patients on long-term anticonvulsant therapy may develop osteomalacia (adults) or rickets (children). This may be due to enzyme induction increasing vitamin D metabolism and causing deficiency, or there may be inhibition of one of the hydroxylations that increase biological activity or an effect on calcium metabolism.

Sources and requirements. Milk, liver and egg-yolk are the best sources, but an ordinary diet may not provide enough vitamin D for growing children unless they are exposed to much sunlight. 400 IU (10 μg of calciferol) per day of vitamin D are normally adequate for children; most baby-foods have enough vitamin D added to them by the manufacturers. Fish-liver oil is a usual source for children, some of whom appear not to dislike it. Premature babies require at least 800 IU daily as they are particularly liable to rickets. Adults do not normally need more than 100 IU daily, and this will generally be formed in the skin if it is not present in the diet. Pregnant and lactating women should take about 400 IU daily.

Indications for vitamin D are the prevention and cure of **rickets** of all kinds and **osteomalacia** and the symptomatic treatment of some cases of **hypoparathyroidism**.

In *osteomalacia* secondary to steatorrhoea or renal disease there is defective absorption of calcium from the gut and large amounts of vitamin D are often needed to enhance absorption.

Dosage. The therapeutic dose for primary, diet-deficiency rickets is 3000 to 4000 IU per day, but much more may be needed in malabsorption syndromes (e.g. 40 000 IU) or renal osteodystrophy (200 000 IU), and dosage must then be carefully controlled by measuring plasma calcium concentrations (a rise in total calcium above 2.75 mmol/l (11 mg/100 ml) is dangerous).

The prophylactic dose in diet-deficient people should be about 1000 IU/day for a few months, and then an adequate diet.

The maximum antirachitic effect of vitamin D is delayed for 1–2 months and the plasma calcium concentration reflects the dosage given days or weeks ago. Frequent changes of dose are pointless and confuse the picture.

Preparations are many and the choice is not critical, though the elderly with nutritional osteomalacia due to malabsorption are often best managed by Calciferol Inj. i.m., 6–12 monthly (eliminating problems or patient compliance and gut malabsorption) with biochemical monitoring.

It is important to recognise that, because of the need for very big doses in certain vitamin D-resistant cases, there is an *unusually wide range of dosage in single tablets* available, for example, Calcium with Vitamin D Tabs. each contain 500 IU (12.5 μg calciferol), whereas Calciferol Tabs. High-strength contain 200 times as much. The latter tablets are only for use in exceptional circumstances, e.g. hypoparathyroidism or metabolic rickets; their inadvertent administration to children can lead to disaster.

Alfacalcidol is an alternative to calciferol that may be used to some forms of metabolic rickets; it acts more quickly, i.e. in days rather than in weeks (see above).

Symptoms of overdose are due mainly to excessive rise in plasma calcium. General effects include malaise, drowsiness, nausea, abdominal pain, thirst, constipation and loss of appetite. Other long-term effects include ectopic calcification almost anywhere in the body, renal damage and an increased calcium output in the urine; renal calculi may be formed. It is dangerous to exceed 10 000 IU daily of vitamin D for more than about 12 weeks.

Patients with sarcoidosis are intolerant of vitamin D, possibly even to the tiny amount present in a normal diet, and to that synthesised in their skin by sunlight.

Adrenal steroids antagonise vitamin D by an uncertain mechanism and are used in the treatment of hypercalcaemic sarcoidosis and of severe hypervitaminosis D.

Idiopathic hypercalcaemia of infants, presenting as failure to thrive with vomiting and constipation is related to vitamin D intake. Government action has been taken to limit indiscriminate 'fortifying' with vitamins of children's foods, but much vitamin D toxicity is due to well-meaning, but needless, administration by parents. The US Food and Drug Administration warn that intake of fortified supplements should not exceed 400 IU a day.

PAGET'S DISEASE OF BONE

This disease is characterised by bone resorption and formation (bone turnover) increased as much as 50 times normal. Some therapeutic success has been found with *calcitonin* (which inhibits bone resorption), with *cytotoxic agents* that inhibit osteoclasts (mithramycin, actinomycin D), and with *diphosphonates* (or *bisphosphonates*) (e.g. disodium etidronate), which inhibit crystal formation, growth and dissolution, such as must occur in bone mineralisation and demineralisation (resorption and formation). The overall effects on the disease are modest, but pain, which is the chief indication for treatment, may be alleviated. The therapeutic effects may long outlast the period of administration of therapy.

OSTEOPOROSIS: p. 702

VITAMINE E; THE TOCOPHEROLS

Vitamin E occurs in many foods, especially in vegetable oils. The daily dietary intake should probably be about 15 IU (or 10 mg α-tocopherol equivalent). Its function may be to take up the free radicals generated by normal metabolic process and so to prevent them attacking polyunsaturated fats in cell membranes with resultant cellular injury, including progressive spinocerebellar degeneration.

A deficiency syndrome is not clearly established. Vitamin E has been studied in a variety of diseases with inconclusive results, e.g. spinocerebellar syndromes, peripheral vascular diseases, and, in the premature infant, haemolytic anaemia and retrolental fibroplasia. Vitamin E is particularly subject to therapeutic claims based on poor evidence.

VITAMIN K: see p. 567

GUIDE TO FURTHER READING

1 Editorial. Riboflavine under the lights. Lancet 1978; 1:1191.
2 Editorial. Dusted meat illness. Br Med J 1963; 2:1546.
3 Editorial. Arctic offal. Br Med J 1962; 1:855.
4 Schorah C J et al. Clinical effects of vitamin C in elderly patients with low blood-vitamin C levels. Lancet 1979; 1:403.
5 Editorial. Vitamin C, disease and surgical trauma. Br Med J 1979; 1:437.
6 Davies M et al. The continuing risk of vitamin D intoxication. Lancet 1978; 2:621.
7 Rudman D et al. Megadose vitamins, use and misuse. N Engl J Med 1983; 309:488.
8 Moertel C G et al. High-dose vitamin C versus placebo in the treatment of patients with advanced cancer who have had no prior chemotherapy: a randomized double-blind comparison. N Engl J Med 1985; 312:137: also Editorial, Wittes R E, p. 178.
9 Editorial, Cardiovascular beri-beri. Lancet 1982; 1:1287.
10 Bieri J G et al, Medical uses of vitamin E. N Engl J Med 1983; 308:1063.
11 Avioli L V et al, The vitamin D family revisited. N Engl J Med 1984; 311:47.
12 Raisz L G et al, Regulation of bone formation. N Engl J Med 1983; 309:29, 83.
13 Editorial, Vitamin A and cancer. Lancet 1984; 2:325.
14 Editorial, Diphosphonates: aimed in a chemical sense. Lancet 1981; 2:1326.
15 Austin L A et al. Calcitonin: physiology and pathophysiology. N Engl J Med 1981; 304:269.
16 Wilkinson R. Treatment of hypercalcaemia associated with malignancy. Br Med J 1984; 288:812.

Appendix

Weights and measures: Prescribing: General references

WEIGHTS AND MEASURES

Note: Solid dose form (tablet, capsule) size is given in brackets after drug name throughout the book.

In this book doses are given in the metric system, or occasionally in international units when metric doses are impracticable.

Equivalents: 1 litre (l) = 1.76 pints.
1 kilogram (kg) = 2.2 pounds (lb).

Abbreviations: 1 gram (g).
1 milligram (mg) (1×10^{-3} g).
1 microgram (μg) (1×10^{-6} g).
1 nanogram (ng) (1×10^{-9} g).
1 millilitre (ml) (1×10^{-3} l).
1 micrometre (μm) (1×10^{-6} metres).

Domestic measures. A standard 5 ml spoon is available. Otherwise the following approximations will serve:

1 tablespoonful = 14 ml
1 dessertspoonful = 7 ml
1 teaspoonful = 5 ml

PRESCRIBING

Prescriptions of pure drugs or preparations from the British National Formulary (BNF) are satisfactory for almost all purposes. The composition of many of the preparations in the BNF is laid down in either the British Pharmacopoeia (BP) or British Pharmaceutical Codex (BPC). Hence there is nowadays seldom any need to write a traditional prescription comprising base, adjuvant, corrective, flavouring and vehicle and the skill is virtually lost.

It is both unnecessary and unwise to try to continue the use of traditional forms of prescription writing in Latin, for facility in their use can only be attained by frequent practice. To try to use these old-fashioned terms when they do not come naturally to the mind is to court the embarrassment of issuing an incomprehensible, or worse, an inaccurate, prescription.

It is both easier and safer to state the requirements in English. However, complete consistency is seldom to be achieved in any matter, and there is little doubt that certain convenient Latin abbreviations will survive for lack of English substitutes. These are chiefly used in hospital prescribing where instructions are given to nurses and not to patients for whom such abbreviations would be meaningless. They are listed, without approval, at the end of this appendix. The elementary requirements of a prescription are that is should state *what* is to be given to *whom* and *by whom* prescribed, and give instructions on *how much* should be taken *how often*, by what route and sometimes for *how long*, thus:

1. **Date.**
2. **Address of doctor.**
3. **Name and address of patient.**
4. ℞. This is a traditional esoteric symbol for the word 'Recipe' — 'take thou!', which is addressed to the pharmacist. It is pointless; but since many doctors gain a harmless pleasure from writing ℞ with a flourish before the name of a proprietary preparation of whose exact nature they are ignorant, it is likely to survive as a sentimental link with the past.

5. **The name and dose of the drug or drugs.**

6. **Directions to the pharmacist**, if any, this — 'mix', 'make a solution'. Write the total quantity to be dispensed if this is not stated in 5 above.

7. **Instruction for the patient**, to be written on container by the pharmacist. Here brevity, clarity and accuracy are especially important. It is dangerous to rely on the patient remembering verbal instructions. The BNF provides a list of recommended label wordings representing a balance between 'the unintelligibly short and the inconveniently long'.

8. **Signature of doctor.**

It is now considered exceptional to conceal from patients the nature of their treatment and the name of the preparation should be written on the label unless there is a positive reason for not doing so.

Example of a Prescription for a patient with an annoying unproductive cough.

1, 2, 3, as above.
4. ℞.
5. Codeine Linctus, BNF, 5 ml.
6. Send 60 ml.
7. Label: Codeine Linctus (or NP). Take 5 ml twice a day and on retiring.
8. Signature of doctor.

Legal aspects of prescribing are given in the BNF* which is supplied free to doctors practising in the National Health Service and to medical students.

* For example, Controlled Drugs (CD) (drugs liable to cause dependence or misuse) where prescribers have three main responsibilities: (1) to ensure they do not create dependence, (2) to ensure the patient does not increase the dose and create dependence, and (3) to ensure that they are not used as an unwitting source of supply to addicts.

ABBREVIATIONS (see also *weights and measures*)

ac, ante cibum	before food
bd, bis in die	twice a day (bid is also used)
BNF	British National Formulary
BP	British Pharmacopoeia
BPC	British Pharmaceutical Codex
PC	Pharmaceutical Codex
im, intramuscular	by intramuscular injection
IU	International Unit
iv, intravenous	by intravenous injection
NP, nomen proprium	proper name
od, omni die	every day
om, omni mane	every morning
on, omni nocte	every night
pc, post cibum	after food
po, per os	by mouth
prn, pro re nata	as required. It is best to add the maximum frequency of repetition, e.g. Aspirin and Codeine Tablets, 1 or 2 prn, 4-hourly
qds, quater in die	four times a day (qid is also used)
qq, quaque	every, e.g. qq6h = every 6 h
qs, quantum sufficiat	a sufficiency, enough
rep, repetatur	let it be repeated, as in rep. mist(ura), repeat the mixture
sc, subcutaneous	by subcutaneous injection
sos, si opus sit	if necessary. It is useful to confine sos to prescriptions to be repeated once only and to use prn where many repetitions are intended
stat., statim	immediately
tds, terdie sumendus	three times a day (tid is also used)

GENERAL REFERENCES

The following are sources of further information on any chapter:

Bernard C. *An introduction to the study of experimental medicine*, 1865. Various editions in English. This book should be read by anyone interested in or hoping to practise scientific medicine or research. It is beautifully written and reasoned and it remains the best and most readable short book on the subject.

Goodman and Gilman's, *The pharmacological basis of therapeutics*. New York: Macmillan, current edition. A multiauthor classic, specially valuable to clinicians.

Osol A et al. *The dispensatory of the United States of America*, Philadelphia: Lippincott, an encyclopaedia: current edition.

Martindale: The extra pharmacopoeia, current edition, London: Pharmaceutical Press.An encyclopaedia; invaluable for out-of-the-way information.

AMA drug evaluations: current edition, American Medical Association: Chicago: a clinically oriented encyclopaedia.

Meyler's Side-effects of drugs. Dukes M N G, ed. Amsterdam: Elsevier, current edition.

Side-effects of drugs annual: a worldwide survey of new data and trends, Dukes M N G, Amsterdam: Elsevier.

Drug and Therapeutics Bulletin. Medical Letter on Drugs and therapeutics (USA). Both these are short fortnightly publications that ruthlessly review evidence for and against drugs. The British publication was founded by the American and has since become independent (owned by the Consumers' Association). They are useful sources of up-to-date facts and opinions (a condensation of the views of numerous advisers).

Adverse Drug Reactions Bulletin. Davies D M ed.: 2-monthly: distributed with *Drug and Therapeutics Bulletin*.

Prescribers' Journal. A small bi-monthly review issued by the Departments of Health, Britain, free to all doctors in the National Health Service and medical students.

Clinical Pharmacology and Therapeutics is the monthly publication of the American Therapeutics Society. Original papers and reviews.

European Journal of Clinical Pharmacology: monthly.

Pharmacological Reviews is published quarterly.

British Journal of Clinical Pharmacology: monthly publication of the British Pharmacological Society.

Advances in Pharmacology and Chemotherapy, Garattini S *et al.*, eds. New York: Academic Press. Annual reviews.

Annual Review of Pharmacology, George R *et al.* eds. Annual Reviews Inc., California: Palo Alto, Specialised, largely animal work.

Drugs. Clinical review articles: monthly.

Clinical Pharmacokinetics: monthly.

Trends in Pharmacological Sciences (*TIPS*) monthly: short reviews. Sponsored by the International Union of Pharmacology (IUPHAR).

Index

Proprietary names (an incomplete list, inevitably) are in italic type and are followed by the non-proprietary name. The salts of drugs are generally omitted. Only the first page numbers of accounts are given. Where more than one page number is quoted, the principal account is given in bold print.

ISBN 0-443-03417-6

9 780443 034176